P9-DFZ-716

Histoplasmosis	II
Human immunodeficiency virus infection and acquired immune deficiency syndrome	I
Human papilloma virus diseases	I
Infectious mononucleosis	II
Ludwig's angina	II, III
Lyme disease	II
Mumps	I
Osteomyelitis	I
Syphilis	I, II
Tetanus	I
Toxoplasmosis	I
Tuberculosis	I, II
Varicella-Zoster virus diseases	I

MUSCULOSKELETAL/ CONNECTIVE TISSUE DISEASES

Amyloidosis	I
Cleidocranial dysplasia	II
Dermatomyositis	I
Discoid lupus erythematosus	II
Fibrous dysplasia	II
Gout	I, II
Hereditary hemorrhagic telangiectasia	I
Lichen planus	II
Malignant hyperthermia	III
Marfan's syndrome	I
Muscular dystrophy	I
Osteoarthritis (degenerative joint disease)	I
Osteomyelitis	I
Osteoporosis	I
Polyarteritis nodosa	II
Polymyalgia rheumatica (and associated giant cell arteritis)	I
Polymyositis	I
Psoriasis	II
Raynaud's phenomenon	I
Rheumatoid arthritis	I
Sarcoidosis	I, II
Systemic lupus erythematosus	I
Wegener's granulomatosis	I, II

NEUROLOGIC DISEASES

Alzheimer's disease	I
Cerebral vascular accident	III
Cranial arteritis	II
Delirium tremens	III
Glossopharyngeal neuralgia	II
Headaches: cluster	I, II
Headaches: migraine	I, II
Headaches: tension	I
Ménière's disease	I
Multiple sclerosis	I
Myasthenia gravis	I
Parkinson's disease	I
Postherpetic neuralgia	II
Seizure disorders	I
Seizures	III
Status epilepticus	III
Syncope	III
Transient ischemic attack	III
Trigeminal neuralgia	II

OTHER

Cervical lymphadenitis	II
Medication overdose: epinephrine	III
Medication overdose: local anesthetic	III
Medication overdose: narcotic/analgesic	III
Medication overdose: sedative	III
Neck masses (differential diagnosis)	II
Pregnancy	I
Vitamin deficiencies	II

PHARMACOLOGY

Albuterol	IV
Alendronate	IV
Alprazolam	IV
Amlodipine	IV
Amoxicillin and clavulanic acid	IV
Articaine with epinephrine	V
Atenolol	IV
Atorvastatin	IV
Atropine	V
Bupivacaine with epinephrine	V
Bupropion	IV
Buspirone	IV
Carisoprodol	IV
Cephalexin	IV
Cetirizine	IV
Ciprofloxacin	IV
Citalopram	IV
Clindamycin	IV
Clonazepam	IV
Clopidogrel	IV
Cyclobenzaprine	IV
Desflurane	V
Diazepam	V
Diltiazem	IV
Diphenhydramine	V
Enalapril	IV
Escitalopram	IV
Esomeprazole	IV
Fentanyl	V
Fexofenadine	IV
Fluoxetine	IV
Fluticasone	IV
Furosemide	IV
Gabapentin	IV
Glipizide	IV
Glyburide	IV
Glycopyrrolate	V
Hydrochlorothiazide	IV
Hydrocodone	IV
Isosorbide mononitrate	IV
Ketamine	V
Lansoprazole	IV
Lidocaine	V
Lisinopril	IV
Lorazepam	IV
Lovastatin	IV
Meperidine	V
Mepivacaine	V
Metformin	IV
Methohexital	V
Metoprolol	IV

Midazolam	V
Minocycline	IV
Mirtazapine	IV
Montelukast	IV
Nabumetone	IV
Nifedipine	IV
Nitrous oxide	V
Omeprazole	IV
Oxycodone	IV
Pantoprazole	IV
Paroxetine	IV
Pravastatin	IV
Prednisone	IV
Prilocaine	V
Prilocaine-lidocaine	V
Propofol	V
Propoxyphene	IV
Ramipril	IV
Ranitidine	IV
Sertraline	IV
Sevoflurane	V
Simvastatin	IV
Tizanidine	IV
Tramadol	IV
Trazodone	IV
Triamterene	IV
Triazolam	V
Valsartan	IV
Verapamil	IV
Warfarin	IV
Zolpidem	IV

PSYCHOLOGIC/PSYCHIATRIC DISORDERS

Alcoholism	I
Anorexia nervosa and bulimia nervosa	I
Burning mouth syndrome	II
Child abuse and neglect	I
Delirium tremens	III

RENAL DISEASES

Nephrotic syndrome	I
Reiter's syndrome	I
Renal disease, dialysis, and transplantation	I

RESPIRATORY DISEASES

Airway obstruction	III
Asthma	I
Bronchitis (acute)	I
Bronchospasm	III
Chronic obstructive pulmonary disease	I
Cystic fibrosis	I
Hypertension	I
Hyperventilation	III
Laryngospasm	III
Lung: primary malignancy	II
Malignant hypertension	III
Pneumothorax	III
Sinusitis	II
Sleep apnea	I

Dental
Clinical
Advisor

Dental
Clinical
Advisor

JAMES R. HUPP, DMD, MD, JD, MBA
Dean and Professor, Oral-Maxillofacial Surgery and Pathology
School of Dentistry
University of Mississippi Medical Center
Jackson, Mississippi

THOMAS P. WILLIAMS, DDS
Great River Oral and Maxillofacial Surgery
Dubuque, Iowa
Adjunct Professor
Oral and Maxillofacial Surgery
Oral and Maxillofacial Pathology
University of Iowa
Iowa City, Iowa

F. JOHN FIRRIOLO, DDS, PhD
Associate Professor and Director
Division of Diagnostic Sciences
Department of Diagnostic Sciences, Prosthodontics & Restorative Dentistry
University of Louisville School of Dentistry
Louisville, Kentucky

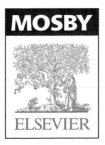

MOSBY

ELSEVIER

MOSBY
ELSEVIER

11830 Westline Industrial Drive
St. Louis, Missouri 63146

DENTAL CLINICAL ADVISOR

ISBN-13: 978-0-323-03425-8
ISBN-10: 0-323-03425-X

Copyright © 2006 by Mosby, Inc.

All rights reserved. No part of this publication may be reproduced or transmitted in any form or by any means, electronic or mechanical, including photocopying, recording, or any information storage and retrieval system, without permission in writing from the publisher.
Permissions may be sought directly from Elsevier's Health Sciences Rights Department in Philadelphia, PA, USA: phone: (+1) 215 239 3804, fax: (+1) 215 239 3805, e-mail: healthpermissions@elsevier.com. You may also complete your request on-line via the Elsevier homepage (http://www.elsevier.com), by selecting 'Customer Support' and then 'Obtaining Permissions'.

Notice

Knowledge and best practice in this field are constantly changing. As new research and experience broaden our knowledge, changes in practice, treatment, and drug therapy may become necessary or appropriate. Readers are advised to check the most current information provided (i) on procedures featured or (ii) by the manufacturer of each product to be administered, to verify the recommended dose or formula, the method and duration of administration, and contraindications. It is the responsibility of the practitioner, relying on their own experience and knowledge of the patient, to make diagnoses, to determine dosages and the best treatment for each individual patient, and to take all appropriate safety precautions. To the fullest extent of the law, neither the Publisher nor the Editors assumes any liability for any injury and/or damage to persons or property arising out or related to any use of the material contained in this book.

The Publisher

ISBN-13: 978-0-323-03425-8
ISBN-10: 0-323-03425-X

Publishing Director: Linda Duncan
Executive Editor: Penny Rudolph
Associate Developmental Editor: Julie Nebel
Publishing Services Manager: Melissa Lastarria
Senior Project Manager: Joy Moore
Design Direction: Mark Oberkrom

Printed in the United States of America

Last digit is the print number: 9 8 7 6 5 4 3 2 1

Working together to grow
libraries in developing countries

www.elsevier.com | www.bookaid.org | www.sabre.org

ELSEVIER   BOOK AID International   Sabre Foundation

Section Editors

F. John Firriolo, DDS, PhD
Associate Professor and Director
Division of Diagnostic Sciences
Department of Diagnostic Sciences, Prosthodontics &
  Restorative Dentistry
University of Louisville School of Dentistry
Louisville, Kentucky

James R. Hupp, DMD, MD, JD, MBA
Dean and Professor, Oral-Maxillofacial Surgery and Pathology
School of Dentistry
University of Mississippi Medical Center
Jackson, Mississippi

Donald P. Lewis, Jr., DDS, CFE
Practice Limited to Oral and Maxillofacial Surgery
Associate Professor of Oral and Maxillofacial Surgery
Case Western Reserve University School of Dentistry
Cleveland, Ohio

Stuart E. Lieblich, DMD
Associate Clinical Professor
Department of Oral and Maxillofacial Surgery
University of Connecticut
Farmington, Connecticut
Senior Attending Staff
Department of Dentistry, Section of Oral-Maxillofacial Surgery
Hartford Hospital
Hartford, Connecticut

Thomas P. Williams, DDS
Great River Oral and Maxillofacial Surgery
Dubuque, Iowa
Adjunct Professor
Oral and Maxillofacial Surgery
Oral and Maxillofacial Pathology
University of Iowa
Iowa City, Iowa

Contributors

Sunday O. Akintoye, BDS, DDS, MS
Assistant Professor
Department of Oral Medicine
University of Pennsylvania
School of Dental Medicine
Philadelphia, Pennsylvania

Daryl E. Bee, DDS, MS
Private Practice, Oral-Maxillofacial Surgery
Dubuque, Iowa

Teresa Biggerstaff, DDS, MD
Resident, Department of Oral-Maxillofacial Surgery
Louisiana State University Health Sciences Center
School of Dentistry
New Orleans, Louisiana

Paul F. Bradley, DDS, MD, MS
Professor and Vice-Chair
Department of Diagnostic Sciences
Nova Southeastern University
College of Dental Medicine
Fort Lauderdale, Florida

Michael T. Brennan, DDS, MHS
Oral Medicine Residency Director
Department of Oral Medicine
Director, Sjögren's Syndrome and Salivary Disorders Center
Carolinas Medical Center
Charlotte, North Carolina

Norbert J. Burzynski, Sr., DDS, MS
Professor of Oral Medicine
Department of Diagnostic Sciences
University of Louisville
School of Dentistry
Louisville, Kentucky

John F. Caccamese, Jr., DMD, MD
Assistant Professor of Surgery
Oral and Maxillofacial Surgery
Baltimore College of Dental Surgery
University of Maryland Medical Center
R. Adams Cowley Shock Trauma Unit
Baltimore, Maryland

James T. Castle, DDS, MS
Chairman and Residency Program Director
Oral and Maxillofacial Department
Naval Postgraduate Dental School
Bethesda, Maryland

Domenick Coletti, DDS, MD
Assistant Professor
Oral and Maxillofacial Surgery
Baltimore College of Dental Surgery
University of Maryland Dental School
Baltimore, Maryland

Michael J. Dalton, DDS
Private Practice, Oral-Maxillofacial Surgery
Dubuque, Iowa

Scott S. DeRossi, DMD
Assistant Dean, Admissions Director, Graduate Dental Education
Director, Oral Medicine Residency
Department of Oral Medicine
University of Pennsylvania
School of Dental Medicine
Philadelphia, Pennsylvania

Andrew M. DeWitt, DDS
Private Practice, Oral-Maxillofacial Surgery
Dubuque, Iowa

Mahnaz Fatahzadeh, DMD
Assistant Professor
Diagnostic Sciences, Division of Oral Medicine
University of Medicine and Dentistry of New Jersey
Newark, New Jersey

Christopher G. Fielding, DDS, MD
Staff Pathologist
Department of Oral and Maxillofacial Pathology
Armed Forces Institute of Pathology
Washington, DC

Michael W. Finkelstein, DDS, MS
Professor
Department of Oral Pathology, Radiology, and Medicine
University of Iowa College of Dentistry
Iowa City, Iowa

F. John Firriolo, DDS, PhD
Associate Professor and Director
Division of Diagnostic Sciences
Department of Diagnostic Sciences, Prosthodontics & Restorative Dentistry
University of Louisville
School of Dentistry
Louisville, Kentucky

Robert D. Foss, DDS, MS
Chairman
Department of Oral and Maxillofacial Pathology
Armed Forces Institute of Pathology
Washington, DC

Darryl T. Hamamoto, DDS, PhD
Assistant Professor
Division of Oral Medicine, Oral Diagnosis, and Oral Radiology
University of Minnesota
School of Dentistry
Minneapolis, Minnesota

John W. Hellstein, DDS, MS
Director of Oral Pathology Laboratory
Clinical Professor
Department of Oral Pathology, Radiology, and Medicine
University of Iowa College of Dentistry
Iowa City, Iowa

Lawrence T. Herman, DMD, MD
Private Practice, Oral and Maxillofacial Surgery Associates
Walpole, Massachusetts
Assistant Clinical Professor, Oral-Maxillofacial Surgery
Boston University
Tufts University
Boston, Massachusetts

Kelly K. Hilgers, DDS, MS
Assistant Professor
Department of Orthodontics and Pediatric Dentistry
University of Louisville
School of Dentistry
Louisville, Kentucky
Diplomate, American Board of Pediatric Dentistry

James R. Hupp, DMD, MD, JD, MBA
Dean and Professor, Oral-Maxillofacial Surgery and Pathology
School of Dentistry
University of Mississippi Medical Center
Jackson, Mississippi

Wendy S. Hupp, DMD
Assistant Professor, Oral Medicine
Department of Diagnostic Sciences
Nova Southeastern University
College of Dental Medicine
Fort Lauderdale, Florida

Cynthia L. Kleinegger, DDS, MS
Associate Professor
Oral Pathology, Radiology, and Medicine
University of Iowa College of Dentistry
Iowa City, Iowa

Robert M. Laughlin, DMD
Senior Resident
Department of Oral-Maxillofacial Surgery
Louisiana State University Health Sciences Center
School of Dentistry
New Orleans, Louisiana

Donald P. Lewis, Jr., DDS, CFE
Practice Limited to Oral and Maxillofacial Surgery
Associate Professor of Oral and Maxillofacial Surgery
Case Western Reserve University School of Dentistry
Cleveland, Ohio

Stuart E. Lieblich, DMD
Associate Clinical Professor
Department of Oral and Maxillofacial Surgery
University of Connecticut
Farmington, Connecticut
Senior Attending Staff
Department of Dentistry, Section of Oral-Maxillofacial Surgery
Hartford Hospital
Hartford, Connecticut

Farideh Madani, DMD
Clinical Associate Professor
Department of Oral Medicine
University of Pennsylvania
School of Dental Medicine
Philadelphia, Pennsylvania

Mansoor Madani, DMD, MD
Associate Professor, Oral and Maxillofacial Surgery
Department of Oral and Maxillofacial Surgery
Temple University
Philadelphia, Pennsylvania
Chair, Department of Oral and Maxillofacial Surgery
Capital Health System
Trenton, New Jersey

Paul Madlock, DMD, MD
Resident
Department of Oral and Maxillofacial Surgery
University of Pennsylvania
School of Dental Medicine
Philadelphia, Pennsylvania

Theresa G. Mayfield, DDS
Clinical Assistant Professor
Department of Diagnostic Sciences
University of Louisville
School of Dentistry
Louisville, Kentucky

Cesar Augusto Migliorati, DDS, MS, PhD
Associate Professor
Department of Diagnostic Sciences/Oral Medicine
Nova Southeastern University
College of Dental Medicine
Fort Lauderdale, Florida

Dale J. Misiek, DMD
Private Practice, Oral-Maxillofacial Surgery
Charlotte, North Carolina

Michael C. Mistretta, DDS, MD
Chief Resident
Department of Oral and Maxillofacial Surgery
Hospital of the University of Pennsylvania
Philadelphia, Pennsylvania

Brian C. Muzyka, DMD, MS, MBA
Associate Professor of Oral Medicine
Department of Oral Medicine
Louisiana State University Health Sciences Center
New Orleans, Louisiana

Ernesta Parisi, DMD
Assistant Professor
Department of Diagnostic Sciences
University of Medicine and Dentistry of New Jersey
Newark, New Jersey
Diplomate, American Board of Oral Medicine

Andres Pinto, DMD
Assistant Professor, Director Medically Complex Patient Care
Department of Oral Medicine
Attending, Oral Medicine
Department of Oral Surgery
University of Pennsylvania
School of Dental Medicine
Philadelphia, Pennsylvania

Nelson L. Rhodus, DMD, MPH
Professor and Director of Oral Medicine, Oral Diagnosis,
  and Oral Radiology
Academy of Distinguished Professors
Department of Diagnostic and Surgical Sciences
University of Minnesota
School of Dentistry
Minneapolis, Minnesota

Sara H. Runnels, DMD, MD
Private Practice, Oral and Maxillofacial Surgery Associates
Walpole, Massachusetts

Douglas Seeger, DMD, MD
Chief Resident
Department of Oral and Maxillofacial Surgery
University of Pennsylvania
School of Dental Medicine
Philadelphia, Pennsylvania

Michael A. Siegel, DDS, MS
Professor and Chair
Department of Diagnostic Sciences
Nova Southeastern University
College of Dental Medicine
Fort Lauderdale, Florida

Sharon Crane Siegel, DDS, MS
Associate Professor and Chair
Department of Prosthodontics
Nova Southeastern University
College of Dental Medicine
Fort Lauderdale, Florida
Clinical Associate Professor
Department of Restorative Dentistry/Graduate School
Baltimore College of Dental Surgery
University of Maryland Dental School
Baltimore, Maryland

Thomas P. Sollecito, DMD
Associate Dean of Academic Affairs
Associate Professor/Clinician Educator
Department of Oral Medicine
University of Pennsylvania
School of Dental Medicine
Attending, Oral Medicine
Hospital of University of Pennsylvania
Philadelphia, Pennsylvania

David C. Stanton, DMD, MD
Assistant Professor, Residency Program Director
Department of Oral and Maxillofacial Surgery
University of Pennsylvania
Attending Surgeon
Oral and Maxillofacial Surgery
Children's Hospital of Philadelphia
Philadelphia, Pennsylvania

Eric T. Stoopler, DMD
Assistant Professor
Department of Oral Medicine
University of Pennsylvania
School of Dental Medicine
Philadelphia, Pennsylvania

Inés Vélez, DDS, MS
Oral and Maxillofacial Pathologist
Associate Professor
Department of Diagnostic Sciences
Nova Southeastern University
College of Dental Medicine
Fort Lauderdale, Florida

Steven D. Vincent, DDS, MS
Professor and Chairman
Department of Oral Pathology, Radiology, and Medicine
University of Iowa College of Dentistry
Iowa City, Iowa

Paul R. Wilson, DMD
Private Practice, Oral and Maxillofacial Surgery Associates
Walpole, Massachusetts

Juan F. Yepes, DDS, MD
Assistant Professor
Division of Oral Diagnosis, Oral Medicine, and Oral Radiology
University of Kentucky
College of Dentistry
Lexington, Kentucky

*To my father, Domenic, and mother, Madeline, for their love, guidance,
unwavering support, and perpetual encouragement.*

—F. John Firriolo

*To my best friend and life-partner, Carmen, and our unbelievable children,
Jamie, Justin, Joelle and Jordan.*

—James R. Hupp

*I would like to thank my family for their many sacrifices on behalf of
my contributions to my specialty.*

—Thomas P. Williams

Preface

Society in general, and health professionals in particular, seem to be moving at an ever-quickening pace, making time a more and more precious commodity. In addition, the steady stream of rapidly changing information challenges the busy clinician's ability to stay abreast of various topics relevant to patient care. Physicians and other providers of medical care have core references readily available to them with large arrays of easy-to-find, succinct presentations of the topics needed to properly provide medical care.

The *Dental Clinical Advisor* seeks to bring these useful features to dental professionals. The book begins with coverage of a large number of medical conditions. Each entry, appearing in alphabetic order, begins with a brief synopsis of the nature of the medical condition. It then goes on to the condition's epidemiology, pathophysiology, usual means of diagnosis, and the typical measures used to manage the condition. The significance of the condition to the dental care of patients is presented to help guide the clinician. In addition, advice is given for how dental care might be modified in the face of the patient's medical situation. Finally, each entry lists recently published, useful references for readers who seek additional information.

The following section covers a sizable number of the most common oral and maxillofacial pathologic entities of importance to dental clinicians. The pathophysiology, histopathology, and relevant laboratory tests and imaging strategies are presented to assist in the differential diagnosis of each topic. Also provided in this section's topics are therapeutic strategies and several comprehensive references.

The next subject area in the book deals with emergencies that may face the dental practitioner in the office setting. Again, the pathophysiology of the emergency is provided and then definitive management techniques follow.

The last two sections of the *Dental Clinical Advisor* focus on the clinical pharmacology of the most commonly used and prescribed drugs currently available in North America. The first of these sections on medications covers drugs used to manage medical and dental conditions, while the second is limited to agents commonly used in dentistry for pain and anxiety control. In both cases the entries provide a very quick overview of the drug so clinicians can obtain the critical information they need on that drug without the need to weed through less relevant data.

Finally, the book offers appendices containing additional information on common medical conditions in tabled and boxed format, and algorithms for the management of various medical conditions and signs or symptoms of disease. This section is for use by those working with other healthcare providers in helping diagnose a particular problem or provide dental support during the investigations leading toward a diagnosis.

A CD-ROM, packaged inside the front cover, will increase opportunities for the busy clinician to use the information contained in this book in everyday practice. All of the topics and materials contained in the text have been placed on this CD. In addition, hundreds of Patient Education Guides provide patients with invaluable drug information and specific instructions, and all are available in both English and Spanish. These sheets are available for printing out and are customizable to include specific practice information. The inclusion of these sheets meets the standards of the 1993 OBRA law mandating patient counseling.

As a total package, the *Dental Clinical Advisor* is designed to be of greatest use to busy general and specialty dentists, dental hygienists, residents in graduate dental programs, and dental and dental hygiene students. It will also be helpful to staff members in the dental office who require diagnosis and treatment codes for insurance and other business forms. The attempt has been made in all sections to limit the information provided to only that of greatest value to dental care providers who have a scarcity of time but require sound, up-to-date information on complex medical and pathologic topics and commonly used medications. Hopefully this will greatly assist in the provision of safe and effective dental care.

ACKNOWLEDGMENTS

I wish to thank my fabulous Executive Assistant Agnes Triplett, and her associate Helen Barnette, as well as our talented and understanding friends at Elsevier, Penny Rudolph and Julie Nebel, for all they did to make this publication come to life.

James R. Hupp

Contents

Section I Medical Diseases and Conditions, **1**

Section II Oral and Maxillofacial Pathology, **225**

Section III Emergencics, **339**

Section IV Drugs, **389**

Section V Anesthesia, **455**

Appendix A Common Helpful Information for Medical Diseases and Conditions, **481**

Appendix B Clinical Algorithms, **489**

Index, **547**

Detailed Contents

SECTION I: MEDICAL DISEASES AND CONDITIONS, 1

Addison's Disease (Adrenocortical Insufficiency), **2**
Alcoholism, **4**
Allergic Reactions (Types I–IV Hypersensitivity), **6**
Alzheimer's Disease, **8**
Amyloidosis, **10**
Anemia: Hemolytic (Congenital and Acquired), **12**
Anemia: Iron Deficiency, **13**
Anemia: Pernicious, **15**
Anemia: Sickle Cell, **17**
Angina Pectoris, **19**
Angioedema, **22**
Anorexia Nervosa and Bulimia Nervosa, **24**
Aplastic Anemia, **27**
Asthma, **29**
Behçet's Syndrome, **32**
Bronchitis (Acute), **33**
Cardiac Dysrhythmias, **35**
Cardiac Septal Defects: Atrial and Ventricular, **41**
Cardiac Valvular Disease, **44**
Cardiomyopathy, **47**
Cat-Scratch Disease, **50**
Child Abuse and Neglect, **51**
Chronic Obstructive Pulmonary Disease, **54**
Coagulopathies (Clotting Factor Defects, Acquired), **58**
Coarctation of the Aorta, **60**
Congestive Heart Failure, **62**
Crohn's Disease, **65**
Cystic Fibrosis, **67**
Deep Venous Thrombosis (Thrombophlebitis), **68**
Dermatomyositis, **70**
Diabetes Insipidus, **71**
Diabetes Mellitus, **72**
Disseminated Intravascular Coagulation, **76**
Down Syndrome, **77**
Endocarditis (Infective), **80**
Epstein-Barr Virus Diseases: Hairy Leukoplakia, **82**
Epstein-Barr Virus Diseases: Infectious Mononucleosis, **83**
Erythema Multiforme (Stevens-Johnson Syndrome), **85**
Gastroesophageal Reflux Disease, **87**
Gout, **89**
Graft-Versus-Host Disease, **90**
Headaches: Cluster, **92**
Headaches: Migraine, **93**
Headaches: Tension, **94**
Hemophilia (Types A, B, C), **95**
Hepatic Cirrhosis, **96**
Hepatitis: General Concepts, **98**
Hepatitis: Alcoholic, **100**
Hepatitis: Viral, **102**
Hereditary Hemorrhagic Telangiectasia, **105**
Herpes Simplex Virus, **106**
Hodgkin's Disease, **108**

Human Immunodeficiency Virus Infection and Acquired Immune Deficiency Syndrome, **110**
Human Papilloma Virus Diseases, **112**
Hyperparathyroidism, **114**
Hypertension, **116**
Hyperthyroidism, **119**
Hypothyroidism, **122**
Idiopathic Thrombocytopenic Purpura, **125**
Inappropriate Secretion of Antidiuretic Hormone, **126**
Langerhans Cell Histiocytosis, **129**
Leukemias (AML, CML, ALL, CLL, Hairy Cell Leukemia), **132**
Marfan's Syndrome, **136**
Ménière's Disease, **138**
Multiple Myeloma, **139**
Multiple Sclerosis, **141**
Mumps, **143**
Muscular Dystrophy, **144**
Myasthenia Gravis, **147**
Myocardial Infarction, **150**
Nephrotic Syndrome, **153**
Non-Hodgkin's Lymphoma, **155**
Osteoarthritis (Degenerative Joint Disease), **157**
Osteomyelitis, **159**
Osteoporosis, **160**
Parkinson's Disease, **162**
Peptic Ulcer Disease, **165**
Peutz-Jeghers Syndrome, **167**
Polymyalgia Rheumatica (and Associated Giant Cell Arteritis), **168**
Polymyositis, **170**
Pregnancy, **172**
Raynaud's Phenomenon, **176**
Reiter's Syndrome, **178**
Renal Disease, Dialysis, and Transplantation, **180**
Rheumatoid Arthritis, **183**
Sarcoidosis, **187**
Seizure Disorders, **189**
Sleep Apnea, **193**
Stroke, **195**
Syphilis, **198**
Systemic Lupus Erythematosus, **200**
Tetanus, **202**
Thrombocytopathies (Congenital and Acquired), **205**
Thrombocytopenia, **208**
Toxoplasmosis, **210**
Tuberculosis, **212**
Ulcerative Colitis, **216**
Varicella-Zoster Virus Diseases, **218**
Von Willebrand's Disease, **220**
Wegener's Granulomatosis, **222**

SECTION II: ORAL AND MAXILLOFACIAL PATHOLOGY, 225

Actinomycosis, **226**
Adenomatoid Odontogenic Tumor, **227**
Amalgam Tattoo, **229**
Ameloblastic Fibroma, **230**
Ameloblastoma, **231**
Aneurysmal Bone Cyst, **233**
Angular Cheilitis, **234**
Aphthous Stomatitis, **235**

Basal Cell Carcinoma, **237**
Benign Lymphoepithelial Cysts, **238**
Burkitt's Lymphoma, **239**
Burning Mouth Syndrome, **241**
Calcifying Epithelial Odontogenic Tumor, **242**
Candidosis, **243**
Central Giant Cell Granuloma, **245**
Cervical Lymphadenitis, **246**
Cherubism, **247**
Chondroma, **248**
Cleidocranial Dysplasia, **249**
Condyloma Acuminatum, **250**
Cranial Arteritis, **251**
Craniopharyngioma, **252**
Dermoid Cyst, **253**
Discoid Lupus Erythematosus, **254**
Fibrous Dysplasia, **255**
Glossitis, **257**
Glossopharyngeal Neuralgia, **258**
Gout, **259**
Hairy Tongue, **260**
Headaches: Cluster, **261**
Headaches: Migraine, **262**
Hemangioma, **263**
Hemangioma (Soft Tissue), **264**
Herpangina, **265**
Herpes Simplex, **266**
Herpes Zoster, **267**
Histoplasmosis, **268**
Hodgkin's Disease, **269**
Hyperparathyroidism, **271**
Infectious Mononucleosis, **272**
Jaw Cysts, **274**
Kaposi's Sarcoma, **275**
Keratoacanthoma, **277**
Keratosis: Actinic, **278**
Laryngeal Carcinoma, **279**
Leukoplakia, **280**
Lichen Planus, **281**
Ludwig's Angina, **282**
Lung: Primary Malignancy, **283**
Lyme Disease, **284**
Malignant Jaw Tumors, **285**
Median Rhomboid Glossitis, **286**
Melanoma, **287**
Mucocele (Mucus Retention Phenomena), **289**
Mucoepidermoid Carcinoma, **290**
Multiple Endocrine Neoplasia Syndromes, **291**
Myeloproliferative Disorders, **292**
Neck Masses (Differential Diagnosis), **294**
Nicotine Stomatitis, **296**
Odontogenic Myxoma, **297**
Odontoma, **298**
Ossifying/Cementifying Fibroma, **299**
Osteoblastoma, **301**
Perioral Dermatitis, **302**
Peripheral Giant Cell Granuloma, **303**
Peripheral Odontogenic Fibroma, **304**
Pleomorphic Adenoma, **305**
Plummer-Vinson Syndrome, **306**
Polyarteritis Nodosa, **307**
Polycythemia Vera, **308**
Polymorphous Low-Grade Adenocarcinoma, **309**

Postherpetic Neuralgia, 310
Psoriasis, 311
Pyogenic Granuloma, 312
Ranula, 313
Reiter's Syndrome, 314
Sarcoidosis, 315
Sialadenitis, 316
Sialolithiasis, 317
Sinusitis, 318
Sjögren's Syndrome, 319
Squamous Cell Carcinoma of the Floor
    of the Mouth, 321
Squamous Cell Carcinoma of the Lip,
    322
Squamous Cell Carcinoma of the
    Tongue, 323
Squamous Odontogenic Tumor, 324
Stevens-Johnson Syndrome (Erythema
    Multiforme), 325
Syphilis, 326
Thyroglossal Duct Cyst, 327
Tori and Exostosis, 328
Traumatic Fibroma, 330
Trigeminal Neuralgia, 331
Tuberculosis, 333
Vitamin Deficiencies, 335
Wegener's Granulomatosis, 337

SECTION III: EMERGENCIES, 339

Acute Adrenal Insufficiency, 340
Airway Obstruction, 341
Anaphylaxis, 342
Angina Pectoris, 344
Angioneurotic Edema, 345
Atrial Tachycardia, 346
Bradycardia, 347
Bronchospasm, 348
Cardiac Arrest, 350
Cerebral Vascular Accident, 351
Delirium Tremens, 352
Diabetic Hypoglycemia, 354
Diabetic Ketoacidosis, 356
Dry Socket, 357
Epistaxis, 358
Hyperventilation, 359
Hypoglycemia, 360
Laryngospasm, 361
Latex Allergy, 362
Ludwig's Angina, 363
Malignant Hypertension, 364
Malignant Hyperthermia, 366
Medication Overdose: Epinephrine, 367
Medication Overdose: Local Anesthetic,
    368
Medication Overdose:
    Narcotic/Analgesic, 369
Medication Overdose: Sedative, 370
Myocardial Infarction, 371
Nausea, 373
Pneumothorax, 375
Postextraction Hemorrhage, 376
Seizures, 377
Status Epilepticus, 379
Syncope, 381
Thyroid Storm, 383
Transient Ischemic Attack, 384
Venous Thrombosis, 386
Ventricular Tachycardia, 388

SECTION IV: DRUGS, 389

Important Reader Information, 390
Albuterol, 391
Alendronate, 392
Alprazolam, 393
Amlodipine, 394
Amoxicillin and Clavulanic Acid, 395
Atenolol, 396
Atorvastatin, 397
Bupropion, 398
Buspirone, 399
Carisoprodol, 400
Cephalexin, 401
Cetirizine, 402
Ciprofloxacin, 403
Citalopram, 404
Clindamycin, 405
Clonazepam, 406
Clopidogrel, 407
Cyclobenzaprine, 408
Diltiazem, 409
Enalapril, 411
Escitalopram, 412
Esomeprazole, 413
Fexofenadine, 414
Fluoxetine, 415
Fluticasone, 416
Furosemide, 417
Gabapentin, 418
Glipizide, 419
Glyburide, 420
Hydrochlorothiazide, 421
Hydrocodone, 422
Isosorbide Mononitrate, 423
Lansoprazole, 424
Lisinopril, 425
Lorazepam, 426
Lovastatin, 427
Metformin, 428
Metoprolol, 429
Minocycline, 430
Mirtazapine, 431
Montelukast, 432
Nabumetone, 433
Nifedipine, 434
Omeprazole, 435
Oxycodone, 436
Pantoprazole, 437
Paroxetine, 438
Pravastatin, 439
Prednisone, 440
Propoxyphene, 441
Ramipril, 442
Ranitidine, 443
Sertraline, 444
Simvastatin, 445
Tizanidine, 446
Tramadol, 447
Trazodone, 448
Triamterene, 449
Valsartan, 450
Verapamil, 451
Warfarin, 452
Zolpidem, 453

SECTION V: ANESTHESIA, 455

Articaine with Epinephrine, 456
Atropine, 457

Bupivacaine with Epinephrine, 458
Desflurane, 459
Diazepam, 460
Diphenhydramine, 462
Fentanyl, 463
Glycopyrrolate, 464
Ketamine, 465
Lidocaine, 466
Meperidine, 468
Mepivacaine, 469
Methohexital, 470
Midazolam, 471
Nitrous Oxide, 472
Prilocaine, 474
Prilocaine-Lidocaine, 475
Propofol, 476
Sevoflurane, 477
Triazolam, 478

**APPENDIX A: COMMON HELPFUL
INFORMATION FOR MEDICAL
DISEASES AND CONDITIONS, 481**

Box A-1 Antibiotic Prophylaxis
    Recommendations by the American
    Heart Association for the Prevention
    of Bacterial Endocarditis (June 11,
    1997), 481
Table A-1 Prophylactic Regimens for
    Dental, Oral, Respiratory Tract, or
    Esophageal Procedures, 482
Box A-2 Presurgical and Postsurgical
    Antibiotic Prophylaxis for Patients at
    Increased Risk for Postoperative
    Infections, 482
Box A-3 Local Anesthetic with
    Vasoconstrictor Dose Restriction
    Guidelines, 482
Box A-4 Dental Management of Patients
    at Risk for Acute Adrenal
    Insufficiency, 483
Box A-5 Dental Management of Patients
    Taking Coumarin Anticoagulants, 484
Box A-6 Drug Use in Hepatic
    Dysfunction, 486
Table A-2 Drug Therapy in Chronic
    Renal Disease, 487

**APPENDIX B: CLINICAL
ALGORITHMS, 489**

Altered Mental Status, 490
Anaphylaxis, 492
Angina: Stable, 494
Angina: Unstable, 495
Arthritis: Monoarticular, 496
Arthritis: Polyarticular, 497
Back Pain, 498
Bite: Human or Animal, 499
Bleeding, 500
Blood Pressure Depression, 501
Blood Pressure Elevation, 502
Bradycardia, 503
Breathing Difficulty: Stridor, 504
Breathing Difficulty: Wheezing, 505
Caustic Ingestion and Exposure, 506
Chest Pain: Ischemic, 507
Chest Pain: Nonspecific, 509
Congestive Heart Failure, 510
Cough, 511

Dizziness, **512**
Dyspepsia, **513**
Dyspnea, **514**
Fever: Unknown Origin, **515**
Foreign Body: Ingestion, **517**
Headache, **518**
Heartburn, **519**
Heart Murmur: Diastolic, **520**
Heart Murmur: Systolic, **521**
Hematuria, **522**
Hepatitis: Exposure, **523**

Hyperlipidemia, **524**
Hypoglycemia, **526**
Lymphadenopathy, **527**
Nausea and Vomiting, **528**
Palpitations, **529**
Pruritus, **530**
Raynaud's Phenomenon, **531**
Rhinitis, **532**
Seizure, **533**
Sjögren's Syndrome, **534**
Smoker, **535**

Status Epilepticus, **536**
Stroke: Acute Ischemic, **538**
Syncope, **539**
Tachycardia. Narrow QRS, **540**
Tachycardia: Wide QRS, **541**
Taste or Smell Disturbance, **542**
Temporomandibular Pain, **543**
Urticaria, **544**
Weight Loss: Involuntary, **545**

INDEX, 547

Medical Diseases and Conditions

SYNONYM(S)

Addison's disease
Primary adrenocortical insufficiency
Corticoadrenal insufficiency

ICD-9CM/CPT CODE(S)

255.4 Corticoadrenal insufficiency—complete

OVERVIEW

- Addison's disease (AD) is a chronic, primary adrenal insufficiency that results from hypofunction of the adrenal cortex.
- It is differentiated from secondary adrenal insufficiency in which adrenocorticotropic hormone (ACTH) levels are abnormally low due to pituitary failure and tertiary adrenal insufficiency due to hypothalamic failure.

EPIDEMIOLOGY & DEMOGRAPHICS

INCIDENCE/PREVALENCE IN USA: Prevalence 4 per 100,000 persons; incidence 0.6 per 100,000 persons.
PREDOMINANT AGE: Occurs at all ages, but most commonly occurs in persons 30 to 50 years old.
PREDOMINANT SEX: Affects females slightly more than males.
GENETICS:
- Autoimmune adrenal insufficiency shows some hereditary disposition.
- Familial glucocorticoid insufficiency may have recessive pattern; approximately 40% of patients have a first- or second-degree relative with one of the associated disorders.

ETIOLOGY & PATHOGENESIS

- Clinical manifestations of adrenocortical insufficiency do not appear until at least 90% of the adrenal cortex has been compromised.
- The etiology of AD includes:
  - Autoimmune adrenalitis (production of antiadrenal antibodies) accounting for approximately 80% of cases of AD
  - Granulomatous infection of the adrenal gland such as tuberculosis (TB), sarcoidosis, or histoplasmosis
  - A component of a hereditary disease of progressive myelin degeneration in the brain (adrenoleukodystrophy) or spinal cord (adrenomyelodystrophy)
  - A complication of acquired immunodeficiency syndrome (AIDS) with involvement of the adrenal glands by opportunistic infection and/or Kaposi's sarcoma
    - Adrenal insufficiency develops in 30% of patients with AIDS.
  - Metastatic cancer infiltration of the adrenal glands
  - Drug-induced (e.g., etomidate, ketoconazole)

CLINICAL PRESENTATION / PHYSICAL FINDINGS

The onset of symptoms of AD are most often insidious and nonspecific:
- Weakness, anorexia, fatigue, nausea, vomiting, fever, dizziness, diarrhea, abdominal pain, weight loss, cold intolerance, hypotension.
- Hyperpigmentation of the skin and mucous membranes:
  - Often precedes all other symptoms by months to years.
  - Is usually generalized but most often prominent on the sun-exposed areas of the skin, extensor surfaces, knuckles, elbows, knees, and scars formed after the onset of disease palmar creases; nail beds, mucous membranes of the oral cavity (especially the dentogingival margins and buccal areas), and the vaginal and perianal mucosa are also frequently affected.
- Other skin findings include vitiligo, which most often is seen in association with hyperpigmentation in idiopathic autoimmune AD and is due to the autoimmune destruction of melanocytes.

DIAGNOSIS

LABORATORY

- Serum chemistry: decreased Na^+, increased K^+, increased BUN, decreased glucose
- Complete blood count: mild normocytic, normochromic anemia, moderate neutropenia, lymphocytosis, eosinophilia (significant dehydration may mask hyponatremia and anemia)
- Deceased plasma cortisol level, high renin level
- Elevated ACTH levels

IMAGING STUDIES

- Chest radiograph may reveal adrenal calcification and decreased heart size.
- Abdominal CT scan: small adrenal glands generally indicate either idiopathic atrophy or long-standing TB, whereas enlarged glands are suggestive of early TB or potentially treatable diseases.

SPECIAL TESTS

- Decreased plasma cortisol and urinary metabolic by-products of cortisol and androgens after challenge with ACTH (Cosyntropin, 0.25 mg)

MEDICAL MANAGEMENT & TREATMENT

PHARMACOLOGIC

- Maintenance cortisol replacement therapy:
  - Hydrocortisone 15 to 20 mg PO every morning and 5 to 10 mg in late afternoon, *plus*
  - Fludrocortisone 0.05 to 0.20 mg PO/day (provides mineralocorticoid replacement necessary for patients with primary adrenocortical insufficiency)
    - Dose is adjusted based on the serum sodium level and the presence of postural hypotension or marked orthostasis.
- Increase corticosteroid dose during exposure to acute neurogenic or systemic stress (including acute illness, surgery, etc.):
  - Typically, this entails doubling the patient's usual steroid dose; once stress has abated, taper gradually to normal maintenance dose over a week or more; monitor vital signs and serum sodium.

COMPLICATIONS

- Addisonian (hypoadrenal) crisis:
  - Acute adrenal insufficiency is characterized by circulatory collapse, dehydration, hypotension, nausea, vomiting, and hypoglycemia.
  - Is usually precipitated by an acute physiologic stressor such as surgery, illness, exacerbation of comorbid process, or acute withdrawal of long-term corticosteroid therapy.

PROGNOSIS

Satisfactory course if adequate daily replacement of cortisone and mineralocorticoids. Doses must be adjusted during periods of physiological stress or adrenal crisis may result.

DENTAL SIGNIFICANCE

- Orofacial manifestations of AD include pale brown to deep-chocolate-colored pigmentation of the oral mucosa, spreading over the buccal mucosa from the commissures and/or developing on the gingiva (typically the dentogingival margins) and lips.
  - In some cases this abnormal oral pigmentation may be the first sign of AD.
- Risk of acute adrenal insufficiency (Addisonian crisis): Acute neurogenic or systemic (physiologic) stress induced by infection, trauma, surgery, general anesthesia, and the like may lead to adrenal crisis in any patient with primary or (less frequently) secondary adrenal insufficiency. The risk of adrenal crisis generally increases with the severity and duration of acute stress.
  - Acute physiologic stress increases the metabolic demand for corticoids. Since this demand cannot be met by the adrenal cortex, the dosage of

exogenous corticoids may need to be increased.

- Increased risk of infection: Dental patients taking corticosteroids are at increased risk of developing severe dental infection, since corticosteroids alter (depress) the host's normal inflammatory response.

DENTAL MANAGEMENT

- Acute orofacial infections may precipitate a hypoadrenal crisis and should be treated aggressively, including appropriate antibiotic therapy.
- The chance of postoperative infection resulting from surgical or other procedures with significant soft tissue manipulation infection can be minimized by employing atraumatic and aseptic techniques and use of adequate perioperative prophylactic antimicrobial therapy (see Appendix A, Box A-2, "Presurgical and Postsurgical Antibiotic Prophylaxis for Patients at Increased Risk for Postoperative Infections").

- Assess the need for perioperative corticosteroid supplementation prior to anticipated dental treatment procedures (see Appendix A, Box A-4, "Dental Management of Patients at Risk for Acute Adrenal Insufficiency").
  - It should be recognized that no uniformly accepted guidelines exist concerning corticosteroid supplementation for patients at risk for adrenal insufficiency.
  - When one is in doubt about the need for supplementation with additional corticosteroids in a patient at risk for adrenal insufficiency, it is best to err on the side of supplementation because patients can tolerate excess levels of corticosteroids for a few (2 to 3) days much better than deficiencies that could result in a hypoadrenal crisis.

- Management of Addisonian (hypoadrenal) crisis: see "Acute Adrenal Insufficiency" in Section III, p 340.

SUGGESTED REFERENCES

Miller CS, Little JW, Falace DA. Supplemental corticosteroids for dental patients with adrenal insufficiency: reconsideration of the problem. *JADA* 2001;132:1570–1579.

Nieman LK. Addison's. Uptodate Online 13.2, updated January 4, 2002, http://www.uptodateonline.com/application/topic.asp?file=adrenal/5492&type=A&selectedTitle=2^94

Salvatori R. Adrenal insufficiency. *JAMA* 2005; 294:2481–2488.

Williams GH, Dluhy RG. Disorders of the adrenal cortex, in Kasper Dl et al. (eds): *Harrison's Principles of Internal Medicine*, ed 16. New York, McGraw-Hill, 2005, pp 2127–2146.

AUTHORS: **JAMES R. HUPP, DMD, MD, JD, MBA; F. JOHN FIRRIOLO, DDS, PHD**

SYNONYM(S)

Ethanol abuse
Alcohol dependence

ICD-9CM/CPT CODE(S)

303.9 Other and unspecified alcohol dependence—incomplete
303.90 Other and unspecified alcohol dependence, unspecified drunkenness—complete
303.91 Other and unspecified alcohol dependence, continuous drunkenness—complete
303.92 Other and unspecified alcohol dependence, episodic drunkenness—complete
303.93 Other and unspecified alcohol dependence, in remission—complete

OVERVIEW

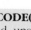

Alcohol dependence is defined (*DSM-IV*, 1994) as three or more of the following symptoms in the past year:

- Tolerance to effects of ethanol
- Withdrawal
- Alcohol use for longer periods than intended
- Desire and/or unsuccessful effort to control alcohol use
- Considerable time spent obtaining, using, or recovering from the effects of alcohol
- Social, work, or recreational activities impacted
- Continued use of alcohol despite knowledge of problems caused by or aggravated by use

Chronic alcohol abuse can have multiple systemic effects including alcoholic liver disease, malnutrition, and toxic effects on bone marrow.

EPIDEMIOLOGY & DEMOGRAPHICS

INCIDENCE/PREVALENCE IN USA: In 2002, 5.9% of U.S. adults reported heavy drinking in past 30 days (heavy drinking defined as > 1 drink/day for women and > 2 drinks/day for men).
PREDOMINANT AGE: Heavy drinking is more predominant in the 18- to 29-year-old age group and decreases with age.
PREDOMINANT SEX: Heavy drinking is more common in men (men 7.1% and women 4.5%). Women who do drink have a higher risk of developing alcoholic liver disease.
GENETICS: Potential genetic factors (genetic polymorphisms) for development of alcoholic liver disease are mutations in tumor necrosis factor promoter, alcohol-metabolizing enzyme systems, and the microsomal ethanol oxidizing system.

ETIOLOGY & PATHOGENESIS

The cause of the systemic effects of alcohol appears to be multifactorial:

- Nutritional impairment
- Metabolism of ethanol to toxic metabolites
- Toxic impact on bone marrow
- Liver damage from toxicity of alcohol and its metabolites

CLINICAL PRESENTATION / PHYSICAL FINDINGS

- Patients with alcohol dependence may deny having a problem and have a maladaptive pattern of alcohol use such as symptoms described by the *DSM-IV* definition of alcohol dependence.
- Nonspecific signs and symptoms of systemic effects of alcohol may include:
  - Nausea
  - Vomiting
  - Abdominal discomfort
  - Diarrhea
- Signs and symptoms associated with alcoholic liver disease, associated portal hypertension, and malnutrition may include:
  - Jaundice
  - Ascites
  - Encephalopathy
  - Dementia
  - Upper gastrointestinal bleeding (gastric erosions or peptic ulcerations)
  - Coagulopathy
  - Infection
  - Renal impairment

DIAGNOSIS

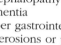

- Screening for alcoholism: "CAGE" questionnaire (≥ 2 suggests alcohol abuse)
  - "C" Have you ever felt the need to <u>c</u>ut down on your drinking?
  - "A" Have you ever felt <u>a</u>nnoyed by criticism of your drinking?
  - "G" Have you ever felt <u>g</u>uilty about your drinking?
  - "E" Have you ever taken a drink (<u>e</u>ye-opener) first thing in the morning?
- Laboratory tests for alcoholic hepatitis
  - Aspartate aminotransferase (AST)
  - Alanine aminotransferase (ALT)
    - Transaminase levels elevated less than 5 to 10 times normal
    - AST level > ALT level
  - Elevated γ-glutamyltransferase
  - Elevated prothrombin/INR
  - Elevated bilirubin
  - Elevated erythrocyte macrocytic volume (MCV)
  - Deficient platelets (thrombocytopenia)
- Liver biopsy offers a definitive diagnosis for alcoholic hepatitis but, due to increased risk from coagulopathy, is typically deferred.

MEDICAL MANAGEMENT & TREATMENT

- Treatment for alcohol dependence:
  - Chemical dependency programs
  - Pharmacotherapy (e.g., naltrexone, disulfiram)
  - Support is vital from family and friends, psychiatry, and support groups (e.g., Alcoholics Anonymous)
  - Medical management of withdrawal symptoms
- For systemic effects of alcoholism:
  - Nutritional support (e.g., vitamin B, protein)
  - Medical management of alcoholic liver disease
    - Pharmacotherapy (e.g., corticosteroids)
    - Standard medical treatment for systemic features such as ascites, esophageal varices, infection, encephalopathy, renal impairment, and coagulopathy
  - Liver transplantation with organ failure and successful alcohol abstinence

COMPLICATIONS

- With marked malnutrition, alcoholic liver disease, and portal hypertension, patient will have increased risks of infection, bleeding from coagulopathies (deficient liver coagulation factors and thrombocytopenia related to portal hypertension/splenomegaly), and bleeding from esophageal varices.
- The risk of oral-pharyngeal esophagus (squamous cell type), prostate, liver, and breast cancer are increased with excessive alcohol.
- Alcohol consumption can exacerbate the hepatitis C virus infection and accelerate disease progression to cirrhosis.

PROGNOSIS

- Despite prolonged alcohol abuse, only 15–20% of patients will develop alcoholic hepatitis and/or cirrhosis.
- Short-term mortality due to acute alcoholic hepatitis is approximately 50%.
- For patients who recover from alcoholic hepatitis, the 7-year survival rate is 50% if they continue drinking alcohol and 80% survival if they abstain.
- For patients who develop liver cirrhosis after alcoholic hepatitis, survival is 60–70% at 1 year and 35–50% at 5 years.

DENTAL SIGNIFICANCE

- Recognition and appropriate referral of patients abusing alcohol can be the first step in helping patient overcome dependency.
- Recognition of oral manifestations
  - Anemia (glossitis)
  - Jaundice appearance of mucosa
  - Submucosal hemorrhages
  - Gingival bleeding
  - Parotid gland enlargement
  - Poor oral hygiene
  - Increased risk of oral cancer
  - Fungal infections
- Alcoholic liver damage can have a major impact on dental treatment.
  - Bleeding from coagulopathies (deficient liver coagulation factors and/or thrombocytopenia)
  - Deficient metabolism of drugs metabolized in the liver

DENTAL MANAGEMENT

- Prior to invasive dental therapy, obtain recent coagulation laboratory values if history of liver disease, signs or symptoms consistent with liver disease, or chronic alcohol abuse.
  - PT/INR
    - May need to consider blood products (e.g., fresh frozen plasma) with INR > 1.5. An INR > 1.5 is a sign of liver disease with a resultant coagulopathy. Note: This is the case when patient is not on concomitant warfarin therapy. With warfarin, the INR will be elevated to therapeutic levels of approximately 2.5–3.5 depending on condition managed by the anticoagulant therapy.
  - Platelets
    - May need platelet transfusion if platelet count < 50,000/mm^3.
  - Limit use of drugs metabolized through liver (see Appendix A, Box A-6, "Drug Use in Hepatic Dysfunction").

SUGGESTED REFERENCES

Centers for Disease Control and Prevention: www.cdc.gov/alcohol/factsheets/general_information.htm

Haber PS et al. Pathogenesis and management of alcoholic hepatitis. *J Gastroenterol Hepatol* 2003;18:1332–1344.

Menon KV et al. Pathogenesis, diagnosis, and treatment of alcoholic liver disease. *Mayo Clin Proc* 2001;76:1021–1029.

Walsh K, Alexander G. Alcoholic liver disease. *Postgrad Med J* 2000;76:280–286.

AUTHOR: **MICHAEL T. BRENNAN, DDS, MHS**

SYNONYM(S)

Type I hypersensitivity reactions
Type II hypersensitivity reactions
Type III hypersensitivity reactions
Type IV hypersensitivity reactions
Allergic reactions

ICD-9CM/CPT CODE(S)

995.3 Allergy, allergic (reaction)

OVERVIEW

In certain individuals, seemingly nonharmful environmental substances (antigens) can trigger an immune system response and future exposure to that substance can lead to an inflammatory reaction. These allergic reactions cause damage to the affected tissue and can lead to sudden death.

These hypersensitivity reactions are classified according to mechanism of reaction:

- Type I reactions (immediate hypersensitivity reactions, anaphylactic hypersensitivity reaction) involve IgE-mediated release of mediators including histamine from mast cells and basophils.
- Type II reactions (cytotoxic hypersensitivity reactions) involve IgG or IgM antibodies binding to cell surface antigen receptors or matrix antigens. The antigens in type II reactions are normally endogenous, although exogenous chemicals agents can also trigger a type II hypersensitivity reaction such as in drug-induced hemolytic anemia. Typical reaction time is a range of minutes to hours.
- Type III reactions (immune–complex reactions) involve circulating antigen–antibody immune complexes that deposit in small blood vessels. These antigens are mostly directed at IgG antibodies. The antigen can be endogenous or exogenous.
- Type IV reactions (delayed hypersensitivity reactions, cell-mediated hypersensitivity reactions) are mediated by T-lymphocytes, not antibodies. An example of type IV hypersensitivity reaction is tuberculosis testing wherein an antigen is injected subcutaneously and localized induration occurs in 48 to 72 hours. Delayed hypersensitivity is

common against intracellular pathogens such as fungi, parasites, and mycobacteria. Type IV reactions also occur in transplant rejection.

See Table I-1 for comparative analysis of hypersensitivity reactions.

EPIDEMIOLOGY & DEMOGRAPHICS

INCIDENCE/PREVALENCE IN USA: Atopic disease has increased steadily in recent years. Approximately 500 people per year die as a result of anaphylaxis. Data on other sensitivity reactions is not readily available.
PREDOMINANT AGE: Atopic diseases tend to wane with increasing age.
PREDOMINANT SEX: No demonstrated gender predilection.
GENETICS: No genetics predilection except as noted for type I reactions.

ETIOLOGY & PATHOGENESIS

- For type I reactions, there is increased vascular permeability and an influx of leukocytes and production interleukins and other proinflammatory agents. The end result is smooth muscle constriction and release of various toxic proteins.
- The severity of the allergic reaction is dependent on the site of mast cell activation. Mast cells are present in epithelial and vascular tissue.
- Inhalation of antigens can result in bronchial constriction (asthma) and mucous secretion (rhinitis).

CLINICAL PRESENTATION / PHYSICAL FINDINGS

- The clinical presentation of type I reactions varies depending on the portal of entry of the allergen and may take the form of localized cutaneous swellings (skin allergy, hives), nasal and conjunctival discharge (allergic rhinitis and conjunctivitis), hay fever, bronchial asthma, or allergic gastroenteritis (food allergy).
- Anaphylaxis is a severe, generalized, systemic, sudden-onset, rapidly progressing, life-threatening manifestation of a type I reaction. Patients experiencing anaphylaxis may demonstrate signs and symptoms including pruritus, flushing, urticaria, angioedema, rhinorrhea, wheezing, weakness,

dizziness, dyspnea, tachycardia, and difficulty swallowing. Nausea, vomiting, abdominal pain, and diarrhea are less common.

- In severe cases, these symptoms may progress over just a few minutes and result in hypotension and hemodynamic collapse (shock), upper airway constriction (due to laryngeal edema), and loss of consciousness.

DIAGNOSIS

- Diagnostic tests for immediate hypersensitivity (type I) include skin testing and enzyme immunoassay (ELISA), which is the measurement of total IgE and specific IgE antibodies against the suspected allergens. Elevated levels of IgE are associated with allergic disease (atopy). Atopy may share an association with presence of human leukocyte antigen HLA-A2.
- Diagnostic tests for type II reactions include study of circulating antibodies and the presence of antibody and complement in the lesional tissue submitted for immunofluorescence studies.
- Diagnosis for type III reactions involves immunofluorescence examination of tissue specimens for immunoglobulin and complement deposits.

MEDICAL MANAGEMENT & TREATMENT

- Treatment of a type I hypersensitivity reaction may include epinephrine, antihistamines, and systemic corticosteroids.
- Antiinflammatory and immunosuppressive agents may be used in the treatment of type II and type III reactions.
- See Medical Management & Treatment in "Anaphylaxis," Section III, p 342.

COMPLICATIONS

- Type I reactions may occur with exposure to exogenous antigens including dust, pollens, foods, drugs, microbiologic agents, environmental agents, and chemicals, and result in potentially fatal disease including bronchial asthma, and anaphylaxis.
  - Possible complications of asthma and anaphylaxis include hypoxemia, cardiac arrest, and death.
- Type II reactions are associated with numerous disease processes including autoimmune hemolytic anemia, autoimmune thrombocytopenic purpura, pemphigus vulgaris, Goodpasture syndrome, acute rheumatic fever, myasthenia gravis, Graves disease, and pernicious anemia.

TABLE I-1	**Types of Allergic Reactions**				
		Antibody	Response Time	Appearance	Examples
Type I (Anaphylactic)		IgE	1–30 minutes	Wheal, flare	Asthma
Type II (Cytotoxic)		IgG, IgM	Minutes to hours	Necrosis	Pemphigus
Type III (Immune Complex)		IgG, IgM	3–8 hours	Erythema, necrosis	Lupus erythematosus
Type IV (Delayed Type)		T-cell-mediated	48–72 hours	Erythema, induration	Tuberculin test

Allergic Reactions (Types I–IV Hypersensitivity)

- Type III reactions are associated with systemic lupus erythematosus; polyarteritis nodosa; poststreptococcal glomerulonephritis; Arthus reaction; serum sickness; acute glomerulonephritis and reactive arthritis (both secondary to bacterial antigens).
- Type IV reactions are associated with multiple sclerosis, type 1 diabetes mellitus, organ transplant rejection, and graft-versus-host disease.

PROGNOSIS

- The prognosis of patients with hypersensitivity reactions varies greatly depending on the specific pathogenesis and severity of the resultant disease.
- Most patients with anaphylaxis respond well to early aggressive management, however outcomes worsen when there is a delay of more than 30 minutes in administration of epinephrine after the onset of symptoms.

DENTAL SIGNIFICANCE

- Adverse hypersensitivity reactions are estimated to occur in 1.4/1000 dental patients. The vast majority of reactions are contact allergic reactions. Allergic contact dermatitis is a type IV hypersensitivity reaction that affects previously sensitized individuals.
- Latex allergy is present in up to 5% of the U.S. population.
- Latex allergy is a delayed (type IV) hypersensitivity reaction that results in a contact dermatitis.
- The primary allergens are by-products of manufacturing and processing of latex; examination gloves or rubber dam material are the most common dental sources.
- Less often, latex allergy may result in a type I hypersensitivity (anaphylaxis) reaction.

DENTAL MANAGEMENT

Avoid exposure of patient to substances known or suspected in causing an allergic reaction (e.g., avoid exposure to latex in latex-sensitive individuals).

SUGGESTED REFERENCES

Johansson SG, Bieber T, Dahl R, Friedmann PS, Lanier BQ, et al. Revised nomenclature for allergy for global use: report of the Nomenclature Review Committee of the World Allergy Organization, October 2003. *Journal of Allergy & Clinical Immunology* 2004;113(5):832–836.

Lygre H. Prosthodontic biomaterials and adverse reactions: a critical review of the clinical and research literature. *Acta Odontologica Scandinavica* 2002;60(1):1–9.

Rajan TV. The Gell-Coombs classification of hypersensitivity reactions: a re-interpretation. *Trends Immunology* 2003;24(7):376–379.

AUTHOR: **BRIAN C. MUZYKA, DMD, MS, MBA**

SYNONYM(S)

Senile dementia

ICD-9CM/CPT CODE(S)
331.0 Alzheimer's disease
290.0 Senile dementia, uncomplicated

OVERVIEW

Dementia is a syndrome characterized by impairment of higher cortical functions, including memory and the capacity to solve the problems of daily living. Dementia leads to a progressive loss of previously acquired cognitive skills including language, insight, and judgment. Alzheimer's disease (AD) is the prototype of cortical degenerative diseases and accounts for the majority (50–75%) of all cases of dementia.

EPIDEMIOLOGY & DEMOGRAPHICS

INCIDENCE/PREVALENCE IN USA: Currently, an estimated 4 million Americans and more than 30 million people worldwide have AD.

PREDOMINANT AGE: AD affects 10–15% of those over age 65 and 20% over age 80. Risk of developing AD doubles every 5 years after the age of 65.

PREDOMINANT SEX: Predominant sex is female (approximately two-thirds of all cases of AD).

GENETICS: The disease affects all races and ethnic groups.

ETIOLOGY & PATHOGENESIS

- The brain of a person with Alzheimer's disease has abnormal areas containing clumps (senile plaques) and bundles (neurofibrillary tangles) of abnormal proteins. These clumps and tangles destroy connections between brain cells.
- Etiology is complex; environmental and genetic factors influence pathogenesis.
- Risk factors include:
  - Age
  - Gender
  - Cerebrovascular disease
  - Myocardial infarction
  - Atherosclerosis
  - Infective agents
  - Immune dysfunction
  - Head trauma
  - Down syndrome
  - Amyloidosis

CLINICAL PRESENTATION / PHYSICAL FINDINGS

- Patients have difficulties learning and retaining new information, handling complex tasks, and have impairments in reasoning, judgment, spatial ability, and orientation.
- A spouse or other family member, not the patient, often notes insidious memory impairment.

- Atypical presentations include early and severe behavioral changes, focal findings on examination, parkinsonism, hallucinations, falls, or onset of symptoms younger than the age of 65.
- As the disease progresses, the following signs or symptoms may be observed:
  - Inability to carry out everyday activities, often called activities of daily living, without help—bathing, dressing, grooming, feeding, using the toilet
  - Inability to think clearly or solve problems
  - Difficulties understanding or learning new information
  - Problems with communication—speaking, reading, writing
  - Increasing disorientation and confusion even in familiar surroundings
  - Greater risk of falls and accidents due to poor judgment and confusion
- Terminal stages of the disease may be indicated by:
  - Complete loss of short- and long-term memory; may be unable to recognize even close relatives and friends
  - Complete dependence on others for activities of daily living
  - Severe disorientation; may walk away from home and get lost
  - Behavior or personality changes; may become anxious, hostile, or aggressive
  - Loss of mobility; may be unable to walk or move from place to place without help
  - Impairment of other movements such as swallowing; increases risk of malnutrition, choking, and aspiration (inhaling foods and beverages, saliva, or mucus into lungs)

DIAGNOSIS

- History and general physical examination.
- Review medications, which may cause mental status changes.
- Patients should be screened for depression.
- On examination, look for signs of metabolic disturbance, presence of psychiatric features, or focal neurologic deficits.
- Mental status testing should be completed. The most commonly used is the Folstein Mini mental status examination (MMSE). A MMSE score < 24 (scores range from 0 to 30) suggests dementia; however, these results must be interpreted with caution since many variables may affect the MMSE score.
- If the MMSE is not available, the following cognitive functions should be assessed:

  - Orientation
  - Attention
  - Verbal recall
  - Language
  - Visual/spatial
  - Patients should be referred for formal neuropsychological testing to confirm screening mental status testing.

LABORATORY TESTS

- CBC
- Serum electrolytes
- Glucose
- BUN/Creatinine
- Liver and thyroid function tests
- Serum vitamin B_{12}
- Syphilis serology, if high clinical suspicion
- Lumbar puncture if there is suspicion of infectious process or when the clinical presentation is unusual
- EEG if there is a history of seizures, episodic confusion, or rapid clinical decline
- Imaging studies (MRI/CT) to rule out brain tumor and/or stroke

MEDICAL MANAGEMENT & TREATMENT

NONPHARMACOLOGIC THERAPY

- Patient safety, including risks associated with impaired driving, wandering behavior, leaving stoves unattended, and accidents, must be addressed with the patient and appropriate measures implemented.
- Family education and support may help reduce need for skilled nursing facility and reduce caregiver stress, depression, and burnout.

PHARMACOLOGICAL THERAPY

- Symptomatic treatment of memory disturbance:
  - Cholinesterase inhibitors: FDA-approved for the treatment of mild to moderate AD. Benefit in severe AD has not been established. These drugs include donepezil, rivastigmine, and galantamine.
- Symptomatic treatment of behavioral disturbances:
  - Agitation, delusions, and hallucinations may be treated with olanzapine and quetiapine.
  - Depression may be treated with citalopram and sertraline.
- Disease-modifying agents include Vitamin E, which has been shown to delay disease progression, and memantine, an NMDA receptor antagonist that improves symptoms and delays progression in patients with moderate to severe AD.

COMPLICATIONS

- Loss of intellectual capacity
- Body wasting

- Seizures
- Inability to walk
- Aggressive behavior
- Infection
- Death

PROGNOSIS

Alzheimer's disease starts slowly but finally results in severe brain damage; it is considered to be a terminal disease. The actual cause of death usually is a physical illness such as pneumonia. On average, a person with Alzheimer's disease will live 8 to 10 years after the disease is diagnosed. Some people live for as long as 20 years with good nursing care.

DENTAL SIGNIFICANCE

- Dental treatment planning, oral care, and behavioral management for persons with AD must be designed with consideration of the severity of the disease and must involve family members.
- Oral dysfunction may limit dental treatment—sucking reflex, involuntary oral movements.
- Changes in oral environment may be disturbing for AD patients.
- Poor gingival health and oral hygiene will increase with the severity of dementia.

DENTAL MANAGEMENT

- Aggressive preventive measures (topical fluoride, chlorhexidine rinses).
- Frequent recall visits.
- Maintain updated medical and medication records.
- Dental appointments or instructions may be forgotten.
- Dentures are frequently broken or lost.
- Progressive neglect of oral health may cause an increase in plaque/calculus.
- Consider IV sedation/general anesthesia for advanced AD patients.
- Avoid complex or time-consuming treatment.

SUGGESTED REFERENCES

Emedicine: www.emedicine.com

Fong TG. Alzheimer's disease, in Ferri FF (ed): *Ferri's Clinical Advisor: Instant Diagnosis and Treatment*. Philadelphia, Elsevier Mosby, 2005, pp 44–45.

Kawas CH. Early Alzheimer's disease. *N Engl J Med* 2003;349:1056.

Kocaelli H, Yaltirik M, Yargic LI, Ozbas H. Alzheimer's disease and dental management. *Oral Surg Oral Med Oral Pathol Oral Radiol Endod* 2002;93:521.

Little JW: Neurological disorders, in Little JW, Falace DA, Miller CS, Rhodus NL (eds): *Dental Management of the Medically Compromised Patient*. St Louis, Mosby, 2002, pp 455–456.

AUTHOR: **ERIC T. STOOPLER, DMD**

SYNONYM(S)

AL amyloidosis
AA amyloidosis

ICD-9CM/CPT CODE(S)

277.3 Amyloidosis

OVERVIEW

Amyloidosis is a disease process in which proteinaceous material is formed and deposited in soft tissues and organs in response to various cell dyscrasias or inflammatory conditions. Amyloid is an amorphous, eosinophilic material that displays birefringence when stained with Congo Red and viewed under polarized light microscopy. There are two major forms of systemic amyloidosis:

- AL (immunoglobulin light chain-related) type affecting the heart, liver, kidneys, skin, intestines, spleen, lungs, and peripheral nervous system.
- AA type is associated with chronic inflammatory diseases such as rheumatoid arthritis. Amyloid is deposited mainly in the liver, kidneys, and spleen.

EPIDEMIOLOGY & DEMOGRAPHICS

INCIDENCE/PREVALENCE IN USA: 1500 to 3500 new cases annually in the U.S. The most common type in the U.S. is AL amyloidosis.
PREDOMINANT AGE: Primarily occurs between the ages of 60 and 70.
PREDOMINANT SEX: Males more likely to be affected.
GENETICS: Only heredofamilial amyloidosis has known genetic transmission.

ETIOLOGY & PATHOGENESIS

In patients with amyloidosis, a soluble circulating protein (serum amyloid P) is deposited in tissues as insoluble β-pleated sheets. Monoclonal plasma cells in the bone marrow are the source of amyloid protein. The amyloidosis can be subdivided into:

- Acquired systemic amyloidosis (immunoglobulin light chain, multiple myeloma, hemodialysis amyloidosis)
- Heredofamilial systemic (familial Mediterranean fever, polyneurpathy)
- Organ-limited (Alzheimer's disease)
- Localized endocrine (medullary thyroid carcinoma, pancreatic islet)

CLINICAL PRESENTATION / PHYSICAL FINDINGS

Findings are variable with organ system involvement.

- Cardiac involvement is common and can lead to predominantly right-sided CHF, JVD, hepatomegaly, and peripheral edema.
- Renal involvement may be indicated by signs and symptoms of nephrotic syndrome.
- Pulmonary involvement may occur and would be evident by fatigue and dyspnea.
- Vascular involvement can result in easy bleeding and periorbital purpura ("raccoon eyes").
- Symmetric polyarthritis, peripheral neuropathy, and carpal tunnel syndrome may be present with joint involvement.
- Diarrhea, macroglossia, malabsorption, hepatomegaly, and weight loss may occur with GI involvement.

DIAGNOSIS

- Should be aimed at demonstration of amyloid deposits in tissues. Biopsy sites to demonstrate amyloid deposition include subcutaneous abdominal fat, rectal mucosa, oral mucosa, renal tissue, or bone marrow.
- Laboratory tests should include CBC, TSH, renal function studies, ALT, AST, alkaline phosphatase, bilirubin, urinalysis, and serum and urine protein immunoelectrophoresis.
- Abnormalities in lab studies may include proteinuria, renal insufficiency, anemia, hypothyroidism, liver function abnormalities, and elevated monoclonal proteins. Monoclonal light chain in the serum or urine (Bence-Jones protein) is diagnostic for immunoglobulin/light-chain diseases, including amyloidosis and multiple myeloma.

IMAGING STUDIES

- Electrocardiogram to reveal cardiac electrical abnormalities
- Echocardiogram to reveal cardiomyopathy
- Chest radiograph to reveal hilar and/or mediastinal adenopathy

MEDICAL MANAGEMENT & TREATMENT

Therapy is variable, depending on the type of amyloidosis.

- Amyloidosis associated with plasma cell disorders may be treated with various chemotherapeutic agents in combination with corticosteroids. The most common combination therapy is melphalan and prednisone. The use of thalidomide has shown promise in the treatment of amyloidosis due to underlying plasma cell disorders; stem cell transplants have also been advocated for treatment of these diseases.
- Long-term treatment may include dialysis and organ transplantation.

COMPLICATIONS

Complications of amyloidosis depend on extent of organ damage. Complications may include:

- Heart failure
- Kidney failure
- Endocrine failure
- Pulmonary failure
- Death

PROGNOSIS

The prognosis is determined primarily by the type of amyloidosis and extent of organ damage.

- Amyloidosis associated with immunocytic processes (AL type) has a very poor prognosis (life expectancy < 1 year).
- Amyloidosis associated with reactive processes (AA type) has a better prognosis. Eradication of the predisposing disease slows and can occasionally reverse the amyloid disease. Survival of 5 to 10 years after diagnosis is not uncommon.
- Median survival in patients with overt CHF is approximately 6 months, or 30 months without CHF.

DENTAL SIGNIFICANCE

- Tongue enlargement/lesions due to amyloid deposition.
- Oral mucosal/gingival lesions due to amyloid deposition.
- Poor oral hygiene depending on extent, severity, and treatment of underlying disease.
- Cardiac involvement may lead to valve dysfunction and/or hypertrophic cardiomyopathy. Use of prophylactic antibiotics to prevent infective endocarditis may be necessary for these patients.
- Blood cell dyscrasias, such as neutropenia, may require use of prophylactic antibiotics to decrease risk of infection.
- Renal/liver dysfunction may affect metabolism of local anesthetic or drugs.
- Liver dysfunction may affect coagulation.

DENTAL MANAGEMENT

- Physician consult recommended prior to dental treatment.
- Review latest CBC with differential, renal function tests, liver function tests, and latest echocardiogram.
- Consider use of antibiotics prior to dental treatment.
- Frequent recall visits if hygiene is poor due to underlying disease.
- Periodic head, neck, and oral evaluations for swellings, nodules, or lesions that may be representative of amyloid deposition.
- Refer to specialist for biopsy, if necessary.

SUGGESTED REFERENCES

Falk RH, Comenzo RL, Skinner M. Medical progress: the systemic amyloidoses. *New Engl J Med* 1997;337: 898.

Ferri FF: Amyloidosis, in Ferri FF (ed): *Ferri's Clinical Advisor: Instant Diagnosis and Treatment.* Philadelphia, Elsevier Mosby, 2005, p 49.

Khan MF, Falk RH. Amyloidosis. *Postgrad Med J* 2001;7:686.

Kyle RA, Gertz MA. Primary systemic amyloidosis: clinical and laboratory features in 474 cases. *Semin Hematol* 1995;32:45.

Stoopler ET, Sollecito TP, Chen SY. Amyloid deposition in the oral cavity: a retrospective study and review of the literature. *Oral Surg Oral Med Oral Pathol Oral Radiol Endod* 2003;95:674.

AUTHOR: ERIC T. STOOPLER, DMD

SYNONYM(S)

Autoimmune hemolytic anemia

ICD-9CM/CPT CODE(S)
283.0 Autoimmune hemolytic anemias
—complete
282.9 Hereditary hemolytic anemia, unspecified
283.9 Acquired hemolytic anemia, unspecified

OVERVIEW

Hemolytic anemia is anemia secondary to premature destruction of red blood cells caused by the binding of autoantibodies and/or complement to red blood cells.

EPIDEMIOLOGY & DEMOGRAPHICS

INCIDENCE/PREVALENCE IN USA: The incidence of autoimmune hemolytic anemia is estimated to be approximately 1 in 100,000 and less than 0.2 in 100,000 in adults and children, respectively.
PREDOMINANT AGE: Occurs at all ages, but with the highest prevalence in midlife.
PREDOMINANT SEX: Autoimmune hemolytic anemia in teenagers and adults is more common in women than in men.
GENETICS: No genetic predilections have been established.

ETIOLOGY & PATHOGENESIS

- Warm antibody-mediated: IgG [often idiopathic (50–70% of cases)] or associated with leukemia, lymphoma, thymoma, myeloma, viral infections, and collagen-vascular disease
- Cold antibody-mediated: IgM and complement in most cases (often idiopathic, at times associated with infections, lymphoma, or cold agglutinin disease)
- Drug-induced: three major mechanisms:
  ○ Antibody directed against Rh complex (e.g., methyldopa).
  ○ Antibody directed against red blood cell (RBC)-drug complex (hapten-induced, such as penicillin).
  ○ Antibody directed against complex formed by drug and plasma proteins; the drug-plasma complex causes destruction of RBCs (innocent bystander, such as quinidine).

CLINICAL PRESENTATION / PHYSICAL FINDINGS

- Chills
- Fatigue
- Dyspnea
- Jaundice
- Dark urine
- Pallor
- Tachycardia
- Hepatomegaly and splenomegaly

DIAGNOSIS

Evaluation consists of laboratory testing to confirm hemolysis and exclude other causes of the anemia.
LABORATORY
There are specific tests that identify the specific types of hemolytic anemia. They are performed after hemolysis has been established.
- Elevated indirect bilirubin levels
- Low serum haptoglobin
- Hemoglobin in the urine
- Hemosiderin in the urine
- Increased urine and fecal urobilinogen
- Elevated absolute reticulocyte count
- Low red blood cell count and hemoglobin
- Elevated serum LDH
Direct measurement of the red cell life span by isotopic tagging techniques shows a decreased life span.
IMAGING STUDIES
- Chest radiograph
- CT scan of chest and abdomen to rule out lymphoma

MEDICAL MANAGEMENT & TREATMENT

NONPHARMACOLOGICAL THERAPY
- Discontinuation of potential offending agents
- Plasmapheresis-exchange transfusion for severe, life-threatening cases only; avoid cold exposure in patients with cold antibody
GENERAL TREATMENT
- Corticosteroids (prednisone 1 to 2 mg/kg/day) are often used in divided doses initially in warm antibody hemolytic anemia. They are usually ineffective with cold antibody disease.
- Splenectomy is common in patients who do not respond favorably to corticosteroid therapy. RBC sequestration studies should indicate splenic sequestration.
- Immunosuppressive drugs and/or immunoglobulins can be used if steroid and splenectomy fail to produce adequate remission.
- Danazol, used in conjunction with corticosteroids, may be useful in warm antibody disease.
- Immunosuppressive drugs such as azathioprine and cyclophosphamide may be useful in warm antibody hemolytic anemia. Their use is indicated only after both corticosteroids and splenectomy have failed to produce adequate remission.

COMPLICATIONS

The complications vary with the specific type of hemolytic anemia. Severe anemia can cause cardiovascular collapse. Severe anemias can aggravate preexisting heart disease, lung disease, or cerebrovascular disease.

PROGNOSIS

Generally good unless anemia is associated with underlying disorder with poor prognosis such as leukemia or lymphoma.

DENTAL SIGNIFICANCE

- Pallor of the oral mucosa (soft palate, tongue, and buccal mucosa)
- Enlargement of extramedullary spaces and more prominent trabeculation on dental radiographs
- Radiolucent areas with prominent lamellar striations
- Jaundice and yellow hue of the oral mucosa

DENTAL MANAGEMENT

- Assess the risk for adrenal suppression and insufficiency in patients being treated with systemic corticosteroids (see Appendix A, Box A-4, "Dental Management of Patients at Risk for Acute Adrenal Insufficiency").
- Patients who are taking cytotoxic or immunosuppressive drugs, including systemic corticosteroids, may have an increased risk of infection and may require perioperative prophylactic antibiotics (see Appendix A, Box A-4, "Dental Management of Patients at Risk for Acute Renal Insufficiency").
- Avoidance of drugs that might induce hemolysis (e.g., dapsone, sulfasalazine, and phenacetin).
- Analgesics and antibiotics can be given safely in therapeutic doses.
- Hemolytic episodes are self-limiting.
- Consider panoramic radiographic studies to evaluate bony changes.

SUGGESTED REFERENCE

Gehrs BC, Friedberg RC. Autoimmune hemolytic anemia. *Am J Hematol (United States)*, 2002; 69(4):258–271.

AUTHOR: SCOTT S. DEROSSI, DMD

SYNONYM(S)

Iron Deficiency Anemia

ICD-9CM/CPT CODE(S)

280 Iron deficiency anemias—incomplete

280.0 Iron deficiency anemia secondary to blood loss (chronic)—complete

280.1 Iron deficiency anemia secondary to inadequate dietary iron intake—complete

280.8 Other specified iron deficiency anemias—complete

280.9 Unspecified iron deficiency anemia—complete

OVERVIEW

Iron deficiency anemia is anemia secondary to inadequate iron supplementation or excessive blood loss.

EPIDEMIOLOGY & DEMOGRAPHICS

INCIDENCE/PREVALENCE IN USA: Most common form of anemia; affects 7–10% of the adult population, 10–20% of infants and toddlers, and 15–45% of pregnant patients.

PREDOMINANT AGE: All ages, but especially toddlers; common in women during their reproductive years as a result of heavy menstruation and during pregnancy.

PREDOMINANT SEX: Female > Male; affects 20% of women, 50% of pregnant women, and 3% of men.

GENETICS: No known genetic pattern.

ETIOLOGY & PATHOGENESIS

Iron deficiency anemia usually develops slowly after the normal stores of iron have been depleted in the body and bone marrow. Women, in general, have smaller stores of iron than men and have increased loss through menstruation, placing them at higher risk than men for anemia.

The etiology of iron deficiency anemia includes:

- Blood loss due to gastrointestinal bleeding associated with ulcers, the use of aspirin or nonsteroidal antiinflammatory medications (NSAIDs); menstrual blood loss (adolescent girls may develop iron deficiency due to heavy menstrual bleeding, as in adult women); certain types of cancer (e.g., esophagus, stomach, colon); or repeated phlebotomy.
- Poor iron intake (in the U.S., dietary deficiency of iron is most often found in infants on a prolonged milk diet or in elderly people with inadequate diets).
- Poor iron absorption due to surgical resection of the proximal intestine, inflammatory bowel disease, and sprue.
- Increased demand for iron as may occur in infancy, adolescence, and pregnancy where fetal needs can outstrip average daily intake.
- Chronic intravascular hemolysis as may be seen in a malfunctioning prosthetic cardiac valve can also result in iron deficiency due to loss of iron in the urine (hemosiderinuria).
- Idiopathic pulmonary hemosiderosis (iron sequestration in pulmonary macrophages).
- Paroxysmal nocturnal hemoglobinuria (intravascular hemolysis).
- Lead poisoning (especially in children).
- Hookworm infestation (rare in the U.S.).

CLINICAL PRESENTATION / PHYSICAL FINDINGS

Patients with mild anemia are usually asymptomatic. Patients with more severe anemia may present with a degree of fatigue that may be disproportionate to the severity of the anemia or any number of additional associated signs and symptoms including:

- Skin pallor and conjunctival pallor
- Irritability
- Weakness
- Shortness of breath
- Brittle, fragile fingernails; spooning of the nails (koilonychia)
- Headache (frontal)
- Decreased appetite (especially in children)
- Pica (unusual food cravings such as for dirt, paint, ice)
- Dysphagia (attributable to an esophageal web, occurs most frequently in elderly women with iron deficiency; this lesion, the Plummer-Vinson or Paterson-Kelly syndrome [see Plummer-Vinson Syndrome in Section II, p 306] may be complicated later by the development of esophageal carcinoma)
- Angular cheilitis, atrophic glossitis

DIAGNOSIS

Evaluation consists of laboratory testing. Most cases of iron deficiency anemia are asymptomatic in early stages. With progressive disease, symptoms and signs become more prominent. A patient's history might suggest GI blood loss (e.g., melena, hematochezia, hemoptysis).

LABORATORY

Laboratory results vary with the stage of deficiency.

- Low serum ferritin (along with absent iron marrow stores; this is the initial abnormality)
- Low hematocrit and hemoglobin (red blood cell indices—hypochromic)
- Small red blood cells (microcytic)
- Low serum iron level
- Elevated RBC distribution width (RDW > 15)
- High iron binding capacity (TIBC) in the blood
- Blood in stool (visible or microscopic)
- Peripheral smear reveals microcytic hypochromic erythrocytes with a wide area of central pallor, anisocytosis, and poikilocytosis when severe

MEDICAL MANAGEMENT & TREATMENT

NONPHARMACOLOGICAL THERAPY

Iron-rich foods include raisins, meats (liver is the highest source), fish, poultry, eggs (yolk), legumes (peas and beans), and whole-grain bread.

GENERAL TREATMENT

- Oral iron supplements are available (ferrous sulfate, 325 mg PO qd for 6 months). The best absorption of iron is on an empty stomach, but many people are unable to tolerate this and may need to take it with food.
- Milk and antacids may interfere with absorption of iron and should not be taken at the same time as iron supplements. Vitamin C can increase absorption and is essential in the production of hemoglobin.
- Supplemental iron is needed during pregnancy and lactation because normal dietary intake rarely supplies the required amount.
- The hematocrit should return to normal after 2 months of iron therapy, but the iron should be continued for another 6 to 12 months to replenish the body's iron stores, which are contained mostly in the bone marrow.
- Intravenous or intramuscular iron is available for patients who cannot tolerate oral forms.
- Transfusions of packed RBCs can be used in patients with severe symptomatic or life-threatening anemia.

COMPLICATIONS

The complications vary with severity of the anemia. Severe anemia can cause angina. Children with this disorder may be more susceptible to infection.

PROGNOSIS

Generally good unless anemia is associated with underlying disorder with poor prognosis such as leukemia or lymphoma.

DENTAL SIGNIFICANCE

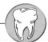

- Oral findings may include angular cheilitis and atrophic glossitis or generalized mucosal atrophy.

The glossitis has been described as a diffuse or patchy atrophy of the dorsal tongue papillae, often accompanied by tenderness or a burning sensation (glossodynia). Such oral changes are rare in the U.S., perhaps because the anemia is usually detected and treated relatively early before the oral mucosal changes have had a chance to develop.

- Esophageal strictures and dysphagia may occur in long-standing cases.

DENTAL MANAGEMENT

- CBC with differential prior to invasive dental treatment
- Physician referral for evaluation and treatment with extremely low hemoglobin levels (< 8 gm/dL)
- Potential for increased clinical bleeding with low hemoglobin (< 8 gm/dL)
- Avoid general anesthesia with low hemoglobin (< 8 gm/dL)

SUGGESTED REFERENCE

Brugnara C. Iron deficiency and erythropoiesis: new diagnostic approaches. *Clin Chem (United States)* 2003;49(10): 1573–1578.

AUTHOR: **SCOTT S. DEROSSI, DMD**

SYNONYM(S)

Megaloblastic anemia

ICD-9CM/CPT CODE(S)

281.0 Pernicious anemia—complete

OVERVIEW

Pernicious anemia (PA) is an autoimmune disease resulting from autoantibodies directed against intrinsic factor (a substance needed to absorb vitamin B_{12} from the gastrointestinal tract) and gastric parietal cells. Vitamin B_{12}, in turn, is necessary for the formation of red blood cells.

EPIDEMIOLOGY & DEMOGRAPHICS

INCIDENCE/PREVALENCE IN USA: In the U.S. the adult form of PA is most prevalent among individuals of either Celtic (i.e., English, Irish, Scottish) or Scandinavian origin. In these groups, 10 to 20 cases per 100,000 people occur per year; the overall prevalence of undiagnosed PA over the age of 60 is 1.9%; prevalence is highest in women (2.7%), particularly in African-American women (4.3%).

PREDOMINANT AGE: Although a juvenile form of the disease can occur in children, PA usually does not appear before the age of 30. The average age at diagnosis is 60 years.

PREDOMINANT SEX: A female predominance has been reported in England, Scandinavia, and among persons of African descent (1.5:1). However, data in the U.S. show an equal sex distribution.

GENETICS: A genetic predisposition is strongly suspected, but no definable genetic pattern of transmission has been discerned.

ETIOLOGY & PATHOGENESIS

- When gastric secretions do not have enough intrinsic factor, vitamin B_{12} is not adequately absorbed, resulting in pernicious anemia and other problems related to low levels of vitamin B_{12}.
- Absence of intrinsic factor itself is the most common cause of vitamin B_{12} deficiency. Intrinsic factor is produced by cells within the stomach. In adults, the inability to make intrinsic factor can be the result of chronic gastritis or the result of surgery to remove the stomach. The onset of the disease is slow and may span decades.
- Antigastric parietal cell antibodies in > 70% of patients.
- Antiintrinsic factor antibodies in > 50% of patients.
- Atrophic gastric mucosa.
- Congenital pernicious anemia is inherited as an autosomal recessive disorder (rare).

- Associated with some autoimmune endocrine diseases such as type I diabetes, hypoparathyroidism, Addison's disease, hypopituitarism, testicular dysfunction, Graves' disease, chronic thyroiditis, myasthenia gravis, secondary amenorrhea, and vitiligo.

CLINICAL PRESENTATION / PHYSICAL FINDINGS

- Shortness of breath
- Fatigue
- Pallor
- Rapid heart rate
- Loss of appetite
- Diarrhea
- Tingling and numbness of hands and feet
- Paresthesias
- Sore or burning mouth
- Unsteady gait, especially in the dark
- Glossodynia
- Impaired sense of smell
- Aphthous ulcers
- Positive Babinski's reflex
- Loss of deep tendon reflexes
- Personality changes, "megaloblastic madness"

DIAGNOSIS

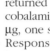

- Evaluation consists primarily of laboratory testing. Initially, patients may be asymptomatic. In advanced stages, memory loss, depression, gait disturbances, paresthesias, and generalized weakness become apparent.
- Endoscopy and biopsy for atrophic gastritis may be performed in selected cases.
- Diagnosis is crucial because of irreversible neurologic deficits.

LABORATORY
- CBC reveals:
  - Macrocytic anemia and leukopenia with hypersegmented neutrophils.
  - MCV is usually significantly elevated in advanced stages.
  - Reticulocyte count is usually normal or low.
  - Since vitamin B_{12} deficiency affects all hematopoietic cell lines, in many cases the white blood cell count and platelet count are reduced (thrombocytopenia), and pancytopenia may be present.
- Low serum vitamin B_{12}.
- Schilling test (measures cyanocobalamin absorption by increasing urine radioactivity after an oral dose of radioactive cyanocobalamin); low absorption in part I (orally administered radioactive cyanocobalamin in water) and corrects (normal) in part II after administration of intrinsic factor.
- Bone marrow examination in some cases.

- Serum LDH is usually markedly increased.
- Methylmalonic acid levels (MMA) may be elevated but do not predict clinical manifestations.

MEDICAL MANAGEMENT & TREATMENT

NONPHARMACOLOGICAL THERAPY
- Avoid folic acid supplementation without proper vitamin B_{12} supplementation.

GENERAL TREATMENT—ACUTE
- Traditional therapy vitamin B_{12} 1000 μg/week injections IM for initial 4 to 6 weeks, followed by 1000 μg/month indefinitely.
- When hematologic parameters have returned to normal, intranasal cyanocobalamin can be used (Nascobal, 500 μg, one spray in one nostril per week).
- Response is monitored and dose increased if serum B_{12} levels decline.

COMPLICATIONS

Neurologic deficits are reversible if they are of relatively short duration (less than 6 months), but they may be permanent if treatment is not initiated promptly.

PROGNOSIS

Generally good prognosis, with anemia resolving with appropriate treatment. Typically, a brisk reticulocytosis occurs in 5 to 7 days, and the hematologic picture normalizes in about 2 months after the initiation of B_{12} therapy.

DENTAL SIGNIFICANCE

Oral findings of pernicious anemia may include:
- Complaints of a burning sensation of the tongue (glossodynia), lips, buccal mucosa, or other mucosal sites
- Focal patchy areas of oral mucosal erythema and atrophy, or the process may be more diffuse, depending on the severity and duration of the anemia
- Erythema and atrophy of the dorsal tongue ("beefy red" and inflamed tongue affects as many as 50–60% of the patients with pernicious anemia but may not show as much involvement as other areas of the oral mucosa in some patients)
- Dysphagia and taste aberrations

DENTAL MANAGEMENT

- Confirm that anemia is controlled prior to dental treatment (review results of recent CBC with differential prior to invasive dental treatment).

- Nitrous oxide oxidizes the cobalt atom in vitamin B_{12}, which renders inactive the vitamin B_{12}-dependent enzyme methionine synthase. Based on nitrous oxide's inactivation of vitamin B_{12}, nitrous oxide sedation should not be used during dental treatment in patients with uncontrolled or poorly controlled pernicious anemia, since it may result in an exacerbation of the disease.

SUGGESTED REFERENCE

Oh R, Brown DL. Vitamin B12 deficiency. *Am Fam Physician (United States)* 2003;67(5): 979–986.

AUTHOR: **SCOTT S. DEROSSI, DMD**

Anemia: Sickle Cell

SYNONYM(S)

Hemoglobin S (HbS) disease
Sickle cell disease
Sickle cell hemoglobinopathies
Homozygous HbS condition

ICD-9CM/CPT CODE(S)
286.60 Sickle cell anemia

OVERVIEW

- Sickle cell anemia [or sickle cell disease (SCD)] is a hemoglobinopathy caused by substitution of the amino acid valine for glutamic acid at position 6 of the beta-globin gene of adult-type hemoglobin (HbA), resulting in a defective, sickle cell hemoglobin (HbS).
  - When exposed to lower oxygen tension, red blood cells (RBCs) with HbS assume a sickle shape resulting in stasis of RBCs in capillaries.
  - Painful crises are caused by ischemic tissue injury resulting from obstruction of blood flow produced by sickling erythrocytes.
- Individuals who are heterozygous for sickle hemoglobin are carriers of the disorder (sickle cell trait) and are typically asymptomatic; individuals who are homozygous for sickle hemoglobin manifest a collection of signs and symptoms that characterize SCD.
  - A patient with SCD will have 80–90% hemoglobin S (HbS), 2–20% hemoglobin F (HbF), and 2–4% hemoglobin A2 (HbA2).
  - A patient with sickle cell trait will have 35–40% HbS and 60–65% hemoglobin A (HbA).

EPIDEMIOLOGY & DEMOGRAPHICS

INCIDENCE/PREVALENCE IN USA: Approximately 1 in 500 African-Americans and 1 in 1000 Hispanics have SCD; 10% of African-Americans have sickle trait.
PREDOMINANT AGE: All ages. Although SCD is inherited and present at birth, symptoms in affected people usually do not occur until after 4 months of age.
PREDOMINANT SEX: Male = female.
GENETICS: Autosomal recessive single-gene defect.

ETIOLOGY & PATHOGENESIS

- Physical findings are variable depending on the degree of anemia and presence of acute vasoocclusive episodes (neurologic, cardiovascular, GU, and musculoskeletal complications).
- SCD may become life-threatening when damaged red blood cells break down (hemolytic crisis); when the spleen enlarges and traps the blood cells (splenic sequestration crisis); or when a certain type of viral infection causes the bone marrow to stop producing red blood cells (aplastic crisis).

- Repeated crises can cause damage to the kidneys, lungs, bones, eyes, and central nervous system.
- Blocked blood vessels and damaged organs can cause acute painful episodes. These painful crises, which occur in almost all patients at some point in their lives, can last hours to days, affecting the bones of the back, the long bones, and the chest.
- Some patients have one episode every few years, while others have many episodes per year. The crises can be severe enough to require admission to the hospital for pain control and intravenous fluids.
- Bones are the most common site of pain. Acute, painful swelling of the hands and feet (dactylitis) is the first manifestation in many infants, along with irritability and refusal to walk.
- In children and adults, vasoocclusive episodes are difficult to distinguish from osteomyelitis, septic arthritis, synovitis, rheumatic fever, or gout.
- Pneumonia develops during the course of 20% of painful events and presents as chest or abdominal pain.
- "Acute chest syndrome" presents as chest pain, wheezing, fever, tachypnea, and cough and is commonly caused by infection, infarction, or fat embolism.
- Leg ulcers are common due to vascular infarcts.
- Endocrine abnormalities include delayed sexual maturation and late physical maturation.
- Seizures and altered mental status are the most common neurologic physical signs.

CLINICAL PRESENTATION / PHYSICAL FINDINGS

The clinical presentation of SCD varies from patient to patient and from region to region, even among those who have apparently similar phenotypes. Signs and symptoms of SCD can include:
- Excessive tiredness and fatigability, dyspnea on exertion, tachycardia, and pallor secondary to anemia
- Cough, dyspnea, chest pain secondary to acute chest syndrome
- Persistent skeletal (bone), joint, chest, and/or abdominal pain associated with sickle cell crisis
- Fever, cough, urinary symptoms (polyuria, hematuria, dysuria) due to infection
- Swollen and painful hands and feet (hand–foot syndrome)
- Leg ulcers, typically forming a shallow depression with a smooth and slightly elevated margin, with a surrounding area of edema
- Priapism (sustained and painful penile erection; this occurs in 10–40% of men with the disease)
- Joint pain and other bone pain

- Notable impairment of growth and development
- Jaundice, mild scleral icterus
- Poor eyesight or blindness due to proliferative retinopathy
- Sudden neurologic deficits and altered consciousness secondary to stroke
Some patients with SCD may remain totally asymptomatic into their late childhood or are only incidentally diagnosed.

DIAGNOSIS

- There is no clinical laboratory finding that is pathognomonic of painful crisis of SCD. The diagnosis is based solely on the physical evaluation.
- Screening of all newborns, regardless of racial background, is recommended and can be performed with a sodium metabisulfite reduction test [Sickle cell (or Sickledex) test]; however, it does not distinguish between sickle cell trait and SCD.

LABORATORY EVALUATION
- Tests commonly performed to diagnose and monitor patients with SCD include:
  - Complete blood count (CBC)
  - Hemoglobin electrophoresis (useful in identifying hemoglobin variants)
  - Sickle cell (or Sickledex) test
- Patients with SCD may have abnormal results on certain tests, as follows:
  - Peripheral smear displaying sickle cells
  - Urinary casts or blood in the urine
  - Decreased hemoglobin
  - Elevated bilirubin
  - High white blood cell count
  - Elevated serum potassium
  - Elevated serum creatinine
  - Blood oxygen saturation may be decreased

IMAGING STUDIES
- Chest radiograph is useful for "chest syndrome" patients.
- CT scan or MRI can display strokes in certain circumstances.
- Bone scans are useful to rule out pain from osteomyelitis.
- Transcranial Doppler is helpful to identify children with SCD at risk for stroke.

MEDICAL MANAGEMENT & TREATMENT

NONPHARMACOLOGICAL THERAPY
Patients should be instructed to avoid conditions that may precipitate a crisis, such as hypoxia, infections, acidosis, and dehydration.
GENERAL TREATMENT—ACUTE
- Aggressive diagnosis and treatment of suspected infections.
- Combination of cephalosporins and erythromycin along with incentive spirometry with acute chest syndrome.

- Provide pain relief during acute vasoocclusive episodes.
  - Meperidine is contraindicated with renal disease.
  - Narcotics should be given on a fixed dose schedule with rescue dosing.
  - Concomitant use of NSAIDs is advisable if not contraindicated.
- Aggressive diagnosis and treatment of complications.
- Transfusions for aplastic crises, severe hemolytic crises, acute chest syndrome, and high stroke risk.
- Hydroxyurea (500 to 700 mg/day) has been shown to increase hemoglobin F levels and reduces incidence of vasoocclusive episodes.
- Replace folic acid (1 mg PO qd).

GENERAL TREATMENT—CHRONIC

- Recommend genetic counseling.
- Avoidance of unnecessary transfusions.
- Allogeneic stem cell transplantation may be curative in some cases.
- Penicillin prophylaxis up to age 5.

COMPLICATIONS

- Recurrent aplastic and hemolytic crises resulting in anemia and gallstones
- Multisystem disease (kidney, liver, lung)
- Narcotic abuse
- Splenic sequestration syndrome
- Acute chest syndrome
- Erectile dysfunction (as a result of priapism)
- Blindness or visual impairment
- Neurologic symptoms and stroke
- Joint destruction
- Gallstones
- Infection, including pneumonia, cholecystitis (gallbladder), osteomyelitis (bone), and urinary tract infection
- Parvovirus B19 infection resulting in aplastic crisis (transient cessation of red cell production often triggered by a viral infection and characterized by pallor, tachypnea, and tachycardia without splenomegaly)
- Tissue death of the kidney
- Loss of function of the spleen
- Leg ulcers

PROGNOSIS

- In the past, death from organ failure often occurred between the ages of 20 and 40 in most SCD patients. More recently, because of better understanding and management of the disease, patients live into their forties and fifties.
- Causes of death include organ failure and infection. Some people with the disease experience minor, brief, and infrequent episodes. Others experience severe, prolonged, and frequent episodes resulting in many complications.

DENTAL SIGNIFICANCE

- Pallor and evidence of jaundice in the oral tissues
- Delayed eruption and hypoplasia of teeth
- Trabeculae between teeth may appear as horizontal rows or as a "stepladder" due to compensatory marrow expansion with increased widening and decreased numbers of trabeculations and generalized osteoporosis
- Dense, more distinct lamina dura
- Areas of opacity and sclerosis of bone
- Prone to develop osteomyelitis
- Trigeminal nerve paresthesias from vascular occlusion of blood supply

DENTAL MANAGEMENT

- Patients with sickle cell trait are not at risk during dental treatment unless severe hypoxia or dehydration occurs.
- Patients with SCD can receive routine dental care during noncrisis periods; however, long and complicated procedures should be avoided.
  - Consultation with the patient's physician is advised prior to any surgical procedure.
    - The dentist needs to establish the patient's current status and if blood transfusion is indicated to correct severe anemia or its complications prior to surgery.
    - Prophylactic antibiotics are recommended for surgical procedures to

prevent wound infection or osteomyelitis.
    - Dehydration must be avoided during surgery and the postoperative period.
  - Treat infections aggressively as soon as possible using local and systemic measures (e.g., incision and drainage, heat, high doses of appropriate antibiotics, pulpectomy, extraction).
    - Intramuscular or intravenous antibiotics should be considered for use in SCD patients who have an acute dental infection.
    - If cellulitis develops, the patient's physician must be consulted and hospitalization considered.
  - The use of a local anesthetic is acceptable; however, inclusion of a vasoconstrictor (e.g., epinephrine) in the local anesthetic is controversial, in that some authors believe it may impair circulation and cause vascular occlusion in patients with SCD.
  - The use of nitrous oxide-oxygen also is controversial; however, if $N_2O\text{-}O_2$ is given with at least 50% oxygen concentration, using a high flow rate and proper ventilation, it appears to have a good margin of safety.
  - General anesthesia or IV sedation must be used with extreme caution in patients with SCD.
  - Routine panoramic radiography can be utilized to assess bony changes.

SUGGESTED REFERENCES

Ballas SK. Sickle cell anaemia: progress in pathogenesis and treatment. *Drugs (New Zealand)* 2002;62(8):1143–1172.

Bunn HF: Pathogenesis and treatment of sickle cell disease. *N Engl J Med* 1997;337(11): 762–769.

Fixler J, Styles L. Sickle cell disease. *Pediatr Clin North Am* 2002;49:1193–1210.

Michaelson J, Bhola M. Oral lesions of sickle cell anemia: case report and review of the literature. *J Mich Dent Assoc (United States)* 2004;86(9):32–35.

Wethers DL. Sickle cell disease in childhood: part I. Laboratory diagnosis, pathophysiology and health maintenance. *Am Fam Physician* 2000;62:1013–1020.

Wethers DL. Sickle cell disease in childhood: part II. Diagnosis and treatment of major complications and recent advances in treatment. *Am Fam Physician* 2000;62:1309–1314.

AUTHOR: SCOTT S. DEROSSI, DMD

SYNONYM(S)

Angina
Myocardial ischemia

ICD-9CM/CPT CODE(S)

411.1 Intermediate coronary syndrome
—complete (*unstable angina*)
413 Angina pectoris—incomplete
413.1 Prinzmetal angina—complete
413.9 Other and unspecified angina
pectoris—complete

OVERVIEW

Angina pectoris (AP) is a syndrome of episodic, paroxysmal, substernal, or precordial chest pain resulting from the inability of diseased coronary vessels to provide adequate blood for myocardial oxygenation.

Three distinct forms of AP have been described.

STABLE ANGINA

- Attacks of chest pain are of limited duration (usually no longer than 15 to 20 minutes) and are predictably induced by exertion (i.e., a temporary increase in demands on the heart).
- The pain usually is relieved by decreasing the cardiac metabolic demand (i.e., rest from exertion) or by administration of nitroglycerin.

UNSTABLE ANGINA (ALSO KNOWN AS PREINFARCTION ANGINA)

- Attacks occur more frequently, are longer, and produce more severe symptoms than those in stable angina; attacks occur with progressively less activity and may occur at rest.
- The term "acute coronary syndrome" (ACS) describes the continuum of myocardial ischemia that ranges from unstable angina at one end of the spectrum to non-ST segment elevation MI at the other end.

VARIANT ANGINA (ALSO KNOWN AS PRINZMETAL'S ANGINA OR VASO-SPASTIC ANGINA)

- Coronary artery spasm appears to be an important mechanism in this disorder.
- Chest pain occurs at rest and is associated with ST segment deviation on electrocardiogram (ECG).
- Patients tend to be younger than patients with chronic stable angina or unstable angina secondary to coronary artery disease (CAD), and many do not exhibit classic coronary risk factors except that they are often heavy cigarette smokers.
- Attacks usually occur in the early morning and most frequently resolve spontaneously, although they may be severe.
- If prolonged, variant angina may result in myocardial infarcts, dysrhythmias, or death.

EPIDEMIOLOGY & DEMOGRAPHICS

INCIDENCE/PREVALENCE IN USA: About half of the 13 million people with coronary artery disease (CAD) experience angina pectoris, and there are 400,000 new cases in the U.S. each year.
PREDOMINANT AGE: Relatively rare in adults under age 35, but prevalence increases after age 35.
PREDOMINANT SEX: Although males tend to present with AP at an earlier age, both genders are affected, typically beginning about age 40 to 50 for men and after menopause for women.
GENETICS: No clearly established genetic pattern has been established for AP; however, there is an increased risk for predisposing factors (e.g., CAD does appear to have strong familial tendencies).

ETIOLOGY & PATHOGENESIS

Common causes of myocardial ischemia leading to AP include:

- Narrowing of coronary artery from atherosclerosis
- Inflammation of coronary artery (e.g., systemic lupus erythematosus, polyarteritis nodosa, rheumatoid arthritis)
- Coronary artery spasm (usually superimposed on atherosclerotic coronary artery disease)
- Aortic stenosis/aortic insufficiency
- Mitral valve prolapse
- Hypertrophic cardiomyopathy
- Hypertensive heart disease
- Primary pulmonary hypertension

CLINICAL PRESENTATION / PHYSICAL FINDINGS

- Substernal chest pain, pressure, or tightness usually precipitated by physical activity. Other precipitating factors include emotional stress, cold exposure, or a large meal. Anginal equivalents include pain in other locations such as the mandible, neck, left shoulder and/or arm, and (rarely) epigastrium and/or back.
  - Discomfort may be described with a clinched fist over the sternum (Levine's sign).
  - Pain is relieved by rest and/or sublingual nitroglycerin.
- Often patient denial, distress.
- Possible transient S3, S4 gallop or heart murmur from left ventricular dysfunction.

FUNCTIONAL CLASSIFICATION

The Canadian Cardiovascular Society (CCS) grading scale (Table I-2) is commonly used to classify the severity of AP, with the most severe symptoms occurring at rest and the least severe only with excessive exercise.

DIAGNOSIS

LABORATORY

- No laboratory abnormalities unless myocardial ischemia progresses to MI. Cardiac enzyme studies may be helpful in determining status of myocardium.

IMAGING/SPECIAL TESTS

- Coronary artery angiography (catheterization) is used to define the location and extent of coronary artery disease.
- Electrocardiogram (ECG) may reveal evidence of old MI and/or myocardial ischemia during the anginal attack.
- Treadmill exercise tolerance (stress) test is useful to identify patients with coronary artery disease who would benefit from cardiac catheterization.
- Echocardiography combined with treadmill exercise (stress echo) or pharmacologic stress with dobutamine can be used to detect regional wall abnormalities that occur during myocardial ischemia associated with CAD.
- Radioisotope imaging (thallium scan/stress test) can used be to detect any disturbance or maldistribution of myocardial blood flow produced by a stenotic coronary artery. It can also differentiate areas of transient myocardial ischemia (such as those resulting from AP) versus persistent ischemia due to infarction.

MEDICAL MANAGEMENT & TREATMENT

NONPHARMACOLOGIC

- Risk reduction and lifestyle modification:
  - Smoking cessation
  - Management of hypertension
  - Control of diabetes
  - Weight loss, regular exercise regimen
  - Dietary changes for weight loss and lipid reduction
  - Limit alcohol ingestion
  - Stress reduction

PHARMACOLOGIC

Acute Management:

- Nitroglycerin, 0.3 to 0.6 mg sublingually or spray is the most effective therapy for acute anginal episodes.
  - Nitroglycerin causes the relaxation of vascular smooth muscle, causing a reduction in systolic, diastolic, and mean arterial blood pressures. Myocardial oxygen consumption or demand is decreased by both the arterial and venous effects of nitroglycerin.

Chronic Management:

- Lipid-lowering therapy (e.g., antihyperlipidemic "statins") has been demonstrated to confer a mortality benefit through reduction of primary and secondary cardiovascular events.
- Aspirin therapy reduces mortality rates. Aspirin should be used in all patients with AP or suspected CAD (unless absolutely contraindicated) since it confers a marked reduction in mortality rates from MI.
  - Other antiplatelet agents such as dipyridamole (Persantine), ticlopidine

(Ticlid), or clopidogrel (Plavix) produce effects equivalent to aspirin and are commonly prescribed for use in a manner similar to aspirin for the treatment of unstable angina and the prevention of MI.

- Beta-blockers (e.g., atenolol, metoprolol) may reduce symptoms in patients with chronic stable angina and improve mortality rates in those who have suffered a prior MI.
- Calcium channel blockers (e.g., nifedipine) decrease myocardial contractile force, which in turn reduces myocardial oxygen requirements and helps relieve angina.
  - Calcium channel blockers also relieve and prevent focal coronary artery vasospasm, the primary mechanism of variant angina. Use of these agents has thus emerged as the most effective treatment for this form of AP.
- Long-acting nitrates (isosorbide mononitrate or transdermal nitrates) have pharmacologic effects similar to nitroglycerin in the treatment of AP.

SURGICAL

- Revascularization surgery is an option for patients with either stable or unstable AP and is more commonly utilized in patients with symptoms that are refractory to pharmacologic therapy. Available procedures for revascularization include:
  - Percutaneous coronary intervention (PCI), typically percutaneous transluminal coronary angioplasty (PTCA)
    - Coronary artery intravascular stents are used in nearly 95% of all percutaneous interventional procedures to help prevent restenosis.
  - Coronary artery bypass grafts (CABG)
    - Particularly beneficial in patients with multivessel disease and reduced left ventricular systolic function, diabetes, or other coronary anatomy not amenable to percutaneous intervention.

COMPLICATIONS

If not treated, AP may result in left ventricular failure, dysrhythmias, and heart failure.

PROGNOSIS

- Typically good prognosis with CABG or PTCA with intravascular stenting.
- Clinical findings suggestive of poor left ventricular function are associated with a worse prognosis.
- May be prodromal to MI; patients with poor exercise capacity and those with evidence of severe ischemia at low exertional capacity are at high risk.

DENTAL SIGNIFICANCE

- The dental care provider must remain aware of the fact that the duration and extent of any dental procedure (including the degree of invasiveness of any surgical intervention) and the resultant physiologic stress to the patient are crucial factors affecting the overall safety of dental treatment in patient with AP.
- Patients with CCS Class IV angina or unstable angina would represent an unacceptable risk for elective dental treatment in most outpatient settings. If dental treatment is indicated for these patients, it is best performed in a hospital dental clinic setting and limited to procedures of short duration (< 30 minutes) and a low degree of surgical invasiveness in conjunction with the precautions outlined in the Dental Management section.

DENTAL MANAGEMENT

The management of the dental patient with a history of AP should start with a comprehensive patient assessment:

- Specific information should be obtained in order to classify the severity of AP (see Table I-2) and to rule out the presence of unstable angina or angina that has become progressively more severe over the past few months.
  - Has the frequency of angina and/or severity increased recently?
  - Have the events precipitating angina become less stressful, or does angina now occur at rest?
- Medications: Determine if there have been any recent changes in medications used to control AP that may indicate a progression (worsening) of the condition (e.g., increase in dosage of and/or increase in the frequency of use of nitroglycerin for angina).
- Determine the presence of continued risk factors for AP including insulin resistance or diabetes, hyperlipidemia or hypercholesterolemia, obesity, sedentary lifestyle, smoking, and so forth.
- Determine the presence of additional high-risk factors secondary to angina, including left ventricular compromise (e.g., clinical evidence of congestive heart failure, radiographic evidence of cardiac enlargement), or ECG abnormalities (e.g., premature ventricular contractions or other dysrhythmias).
  - A medical consultation with the patient's physician is usually indicated to obtain this information.

Specific management considerations for the dental patient with AP would include:

- Appropriate patient monitoring:
  - Record pretreatment vital signs.

TABLE I-2 Canadian Cardiovascular Society (CCS) Functional Classification of Angina Pectoris

Class	Definition	Specific Activity Scale
I	No limitation of ordinary physical activity: Ordinary physical activity, (e.g., walking and climbing stairs) does not cause angina. Angina occurs with strenuous, rapid, or prolonged exertion at work or recreation.	Ability to ski, play basketball, slow jog (5 mph), or shovel snow without angina.
II	Slight limitation of ordinary activity: Walking or climbing stairs rapidly, walking uphill, walking or stair climbing after meals, in cold, in wind, or when under emotional stress, or only during the few hours after awakening. Walking more than two blocks on the level and climbing more than one flight of ordinary stairs at a normal pace and under normal conditions.	Ability to garden, rake, roller-skate, walk at 4 mph on level ground, and have sexual intercourse without stopping.
III	Marked limitation of ordinary physical activity: Angina occurs on walking one to two blocks on level ground or climbing one flight of stairs at a normal pace in normal conditions.	Ability to shower or dress without stopping, walk 2.5 mph, bowl, make a bed, and play golf.
IV	Inability to perform any physical activity without discomfort; anginal symptoms may be present at rest.	Inability to perform activities requiring two or fewer metabolic equivalents (METs) without stopping.

Adapted from Goldman L, Hashimoto B, Cook EF, Loscalzo A. Comparative reproducibility and validity of systems for assessing cardiovascular functional class: advantages of a new specific activity scale. *Circulation* 1981;64:1227–1234.

- Continuous (automated) monitoring of blood pressure, pulse, and blood oxygen saturation during dental treatment is advantageous.
- Stress reduction measures:
  - Keep appointment duration as short as possible. Also, morning appointments are probably preferable for most patients since they may become more fatigued as the day progresses.
  - Consider the use of N_2O-O_2 inhalation sedation and/or premedication with oral antianxiety medications such as benzodiazepines (e.g., triazolam, 0.125 to 0.5 mg the night before appointment and 0.125 to 0.5 mg 1 hour before treatment).
- Ensure adequate oxygenation:
  - Oxygen by nasal cannula at 2 to 4 L/min (if not already using N_2O-O_2 inhalation sedation).
  - A semisupine or upright chair position may be needed for patients with a history of orthopnea.

- Use of pretreatment nitrates:
  - If dental treatment predictably precipitates angina, then consider premedication with nitroglycerin (0.3 mg to 0.6 mg sublingual tablet) prior to initiating dental treatment.
  - Patient should bring own supply of nitroglycerin to appointment for use if necessary. This should be placed within easy reach of the patient in case a dose is necessary during dental treatment.
- Establish profound local anesthesia:
  - For patients with AP who are considered high-risk (i.e., those with CCS Class IV, unstable, or refractory AP), the use of vasoconstrictors in local anesthetics may be contraindicated and should be discussed with the patient's physician.
  - For patients with AP who are considered low- to moderate-risk and where the use of vasoconstrictors in local anesthetics are not contraindicated because of potential drug interactions, it is advisable to limit the total dose of vasoconstrictor (see Appendix A, Box A-3, "Local Anesthetic with Vasoconstrictor Dose Restriction Guidelines").
  - Ensure adequate posttreatment pain control with analgesics as indicated.

SUGGESTED REFERENCES

American College of Cardiology, American Heart Association. ACC/AHA 2002 Guideline update for the management of patients with chronic stable angina. *J Am Coll Cardiol* 2003;41:159–168.

Selwyn AP, Braunwald E. Ischemic heart disease, in Kasper DL et al. (eds): *Harrison's Principles of Internal Medicine*, ed 16. New York, McGraw-Hill, 2005, pp 1434–1444.

Therous P. Angina pectoris, in Goldman L, Ausiello D (eds): *Cecil's Textbook of Medicine*, ed 22. Philadelphia, WB Saunders, 2004, pp 389–400.

AUTHORS: **F. JOHN FIRRIOLO, DDS, PHD; JAMES R. HUPP, DMD, MD, JD, MBA**

SYNONYM(S)
Angioneurotic edema

ICD-9CM/CPT CODE(S)
277.6 Angioedema (hereditary)
995.1 Angioedema (allergic)

OVERVIEW

Angioedema is deep, cutaneous swelling occurring secondary to the release of inflammatory mediators. It can appear as part of an allergic reaction or as an enzyme deficiency syndrome (hereditary type).

EPIDEMIOLOGY & DEMOGRAPHICS

INCIDENCE/PREVALENCE IN USA: Approximately 20%; incidence of hereditary type (HAE) is 1/150,000.
PREDOMINANT AGE: Older than 30 years.
PREDOMINANT SEX: Females affected more than males.
GENETICS: Autosomal dominant (hereditary type).

ETIOLOGY & PATHOGENESIS

- Primary biologic effectors are mast cells, which release histamines, serotonins, and bradykinins, among other potent inflammatory agents. The result of this reaction is vascular leakage, and edema in the deep layers of the dermis and connective tissue.
- Hereditary angioedema (HAE) is caused by a deficiency of the C1 esterase inhibitor. C1 esterase inhibits the action of plasma kallikrein, which cleaves kininogen and is responsible for the production of bradykinins. In the absence of C1 esterase, there will be excess kininogen and circulating kinins.
- Angioedema can appear secondary to infection, connective tissue disorders, physical exertion, or insect bites. Acquired angioedema can result from lumphoproliferative disorders involving B cells.
- IgE-mediated angioedema results from exposure to a specific antigen, resulting in the immediate type reaction. Common antigens include food (milk, eggs, sulfites, chocolate, peanuts) and medications (antibiotics, analgesics [particularly NSAIDs], and sulfonamides). Angioedema can also present as a complement-mediated process, with the development of serum-sickness.

CLINICAL PRESENTATION / PHYSICAL FINDINGS

- Clinical presentation includes absence of pruritus, burning, poorly defined anatomic extension, and slow resolution. Commonly involved areas include the lips, eyelids, tongue, oral mucosa, and extremities. Severe cases can involve the mucosa of the respiratory tract and larynx.
- Urticaria may be part of the clinical presentation.
- Angioedema can be classified as acute or chronic.
  - Acute is defined by the presence of symptoms for less than 6 weeks.
  - Chronic is defined by the presence of symptoms for longer than 6 weeks.

DIAGNOSIS

- Based on a detailed medical history, review of systems, and physical findings.
- Serology is of limited value. However, the following tests are suggested as part of the screening for differential diagnoses:
  - CBC, ESR
  - Stool microbiologic testing
  - Allergy testing in cases of suspected food or medication triggers
  - C4 levels screen for C1 esterase activity; follow up with C1-INH levels if C4 is low
  - Dermatology evaluation in chronic, refractory cases

MEDICAL MANAGEMENT & TREATMENT

- Symptomatic relief in acute attacks of IgE-mediated angioedema is achieved by the use of H1 antihistamines in a majority of patients (greater than 80%). Choices include:
  - Diphenhydramine, 25 to 50 mg q6h
  - Chlorpheniramine, 4 mg q6h
  - Hydroxyzine, 10 to 25 mg q6h
  - Cetirizine, 5 to 10 mg qd
  - Loratadine, 10 mg qd
  - Fexofenadine, 60 mg qd
- H2 antihistamines can be added to H1 antihistamine for resistant cases. Choices include:
  - Ranitidine, 150 mg bid
  - Cimetidine, 400 mg bid
  - Famotidine, 20 mg bid
- Acute, life-threatening, IgE-mediated angioedema involving the larynx is treated with: epinephrine 0.3 mg in a solution of 1:1000 given SC; diphenhydramine 25 to 50 mg IV or IM; cimetidine 300 mg IV or ranitidine 50 mg IV; and methylprednisolone 125 mg IV.
- Long-term combined oral antihistamine and corticosteroid (e.g., prednisone) therapy may reduce the number and severity of attacks in patients with frequent life-threatening episodes of IgE-mediated angioedema.
- Attacks of HAE respond poorly to epinephrine, antihistamines, and corticosteroids. Vapor-heated C1-INH concentrate (recommended dosage 500-2000 U IV) is the first-line therapy for acute attacks of HAE. When vapor-heated C1-INH concentrate is unavailable, fresh frozen plasma (2 U IV) may be used.
  - The regimen indicated for life-threatening IgE-mediated angioedema may be used if vapor-heated C1-INH concentrate or fresh frozen plasma is not available.
- Long-term prophylaxis against HAE is usually indicated in patients experiencing more than 2 attacks per month or for those with severe symptoms. The drugs of choice for prophylaxis are the attenuated androgens (danazol [200 to 600 mg/day], or stanozolol [2 mg/day]), which induce messenger-RNA synthesis in the liver and directly increase C1-INH levels. These drugs should not be given to pregnant women and prepubertal patients.

COMPLICATIONS

- Death from acute IgE-mediated angioedema and respiratory failure
- Esthetic sequelae secondary to facial tissue swelling

PROGNOSIS

- Favorable in mild to moderate cases.
- Trauma-related HAE can pose a significant perioperative and intraoperative challenge.

DENTAL SIGNIFICANCE

- HAE with airway involvement can be triggered by oral or dental procedures.
- Angioedema should be considered in the differential diagnosis of labial or other facial soft tissue swelling.
- NSAIDs and antibiotics used in dental medicine can trigger cases of acquired angioedema.

DENTAL MANAGEMENT

- Obtain a detailed patient history with focus on past episodes, causative (precipitating) factors, and complications of angioedema, especially in relation to dental treatment.
- A detailed diagnosis and classification of angioedema should be sought from patient's physician.
- For patients with IgE-mediated angioedema, avoid exposure to antigens during dental treatment that could precipitate an acute attack.

- For patients with HAE, consultation with patient's physician will guide the practitioner towards an adequate prophylactic drug regimen against HAE administered prior to dental treatment.
  - A combination of fresh frozen plasma (2 U IV), vapor-heated C1-INH concentrate (if available), and androgen therapy is typically the regimen of choice.
- Patients being managed with long-term corticosteroids should be evaluated for possible immunosuppression and/or adrenal suppression prior to receiving invasive dental treatment.

SUGGESTED REFERENCES

Davis AE, III. The pathophysiology of hereditary angioedema. *Clin Immunol* 2005;114:3–9.

Maeda S, Miyawaki T, Nomura S, Yagi T, Shimada M. Management of oral surgery in patients with hereditary or acquired angioedemas: review and case report. *Oral Surg Oral Med Oral Pathol Oral Radiol Endod* 2003;96:540–543.

Turner MD, Oughourli A, Heaney K, Selvaggi T. Use of recombinant plasma kallikrein in hereditary angioedema: a case report and review of the management of the disorder. *J Oral Maxillofac Surg* 2004;62:1553–1556.

Zuraw BL. Current and future therapy for hereditary angioedema. *Clin Immunol* 2005; 114:10–16.

AUTHOR: **ANDRES PINTO, DMD**

SYNONYM(S)

Eating disorder
Wasting
Cachexia

ICD-9CM/CPT CODE(S)

307.1 Anorexia nervosa—complete
307.51 Bulimia nervosa—complete

OVERVIEW

Anorexia nervosa is an eating disorder that is characterized by a disturbed sense of body image, a morbid fear of obesity, and the refusal to maintain a minimally normal weight. In women postmenarche, the disorder includes amenorrhea. The eating disorder is often complicated by bulimia nervosa.

Bulimia nervosa is an eating disorder characterized by recurrent (at least twice per week) episodes of binge eating followed by purging in order to avoid gaining weight. Purging may include self-induced vomiting, laxative or diuretic abuse, and enemas. The disorder is often complicated by anorexia nervosa.

EPIDEMIOLOGY & DEMOGRAPHICS

ANOREXIA NERVOSA

INCIDENCE/PREVALENCE IN USA:
The average rate in young women is 0.3%. The incidence of anorexia nervosa is 8 cases per 100,000 population per year. Approximately 40–50% of anorexic patients are also bulimic.

PREDOMINANT AGE: Approximately 90% of anorexic patients are young (age < 25 years with a peak around age 12 to 13), affluent Caucasian females of at least normal intelligence.

PREDOMINANT SEX: More than 90% of anorexia cases are female.

GENETICS: Often clustered in families, anorexia nervosa may have a genetic component. There is a 50% concordance in monozygotic twins and 7% in dizygotic twins. Furthermore, first-degree relatives of those who are afflicted with anorexia nervosa are predisposed to developing eating disorders when exposed to particular cultural and psychological stresses.

BULIMIA NERVOSA

INCIDENCE/PREVALENCE IN USA:
The incidence of bulimia nervosa is 12 cases per 100,000 population per year. The prevalence rates for bulimia nervosa are 1% and 0.1% for young women and young men, respectively.

PREDOMINANT AGE: Most patients are young (see preceding).

PREDOMINANT SEX: More than 90% of bulimia cases are female.

GENETICS: Often clustered in families and mostly occurring in affluent Caucasian females, bulimia nervosa may have a genetic component. There is a 23% concordance in monozygotic twins

and 9% in dizygotic twins. Similar to anorexia, when exposed to particular environmental stresses, first-degree relatives of those who are afflicted with bulimia nervosa are predisposed to developing an eating disorder.

ETIOLOGY & PATHOGENESIS

- Unknown etiology.
- Often related to other psychiatric disorders such as anxiety, depression, perfectionism, obsessive–compulsive disorder.
- Some evidence suggests a dysfunction of a serotonin-mediated neurotransmission may play an etiological role in the development of eating disorders.
- Possible genetic influence.

CLINICAL PRESENTATION / PHYSICAL FINDINGS

ANOREXIA NERVOSA

The American Psychiatric Association specifies four criteria that must be present for diagnosis:

1. Refusal to maintain body weight at or above a minimally normal weight for age and height:
   - Underweight, generally defined as weight less than 85% of that which is considered normal.
2. Intense fear of gaining weight:
   - Fear is typically not eased by weight loss.
3. Distorted perception of body weight:
   - Many view weight loss as an achievement and weight gain as a lack of self-control.
4. Amenorrhea—absence of at least three consecutive menstrual cycles (postmenarche women):
   - Caused by abnormally low levels of estrogen after pituitary secretion of (follicle-stimulating hormone (FSH) and luteinizing hormone (LH) are diminished.

There are two subtypes of anorexia nervosa distinguished by the presence/absence of regular binge eating and purging:

1. Restrictive/abstaining anorexia nervosa:
   - Weight reduction primarily through caloric restriction, fasting, and excessive exercise.
   - No binge eating or vomiting (a short episode of vomiting may last less than 1 month within this subtype).
2. Bulimic or vomiting or binge/purge anorexia nervosa:
   - Weight reduction primarily through regular purging through self-induced vomiting or through the misuse of laxatives, diuretics, and enemas.

Presenting signs and symptoms of anorexia nervosa include:

- History of weight fluctuation/cachectic appearance
- Dry skin with carotenemia on palms and soles of feet

- Amenorrhea
- Hypothermia/lanugo (fine, soft) hair
- Bradycardia
- Hypotension
- Sleep disturbances
- Mental and motor hyperactivity or report of excessive exercise
- Altered body image
- Paronychia (characterized by inflamed or eroded fingernails due to exposure to acidic vomitus in purging subtype)

BULIMIA NERVOSA

The American Psychiatric Association specifies five criteria that must be present for diagnosis:

1. Recurrent episodes of binge eating (rapid consumption of a large amount of food in a discrete time period).
2. A feeling of lack of control over eating behavior during eating binges.
3. Regularly engaging in either self-induced vomiting, use of laxatives or diuretics, strict dieting or fasting, or vigorous exercise to prevent weight gain.
4. A minimum average of two binge-eating episodes per week for at least 3 months.
5. Persistent overconcern with body shape and weight.

Bulimia is more difficult to detect in patients because they often display no signs of the disorder and may even try to hide the disorder. Presenting signs and symptoms include:

- Preoccupation with weight and food
- History of weight fluctuation
- Dizziness
- Thirst
- Syncope
- Hypokalemia (causing muscle cramps, weakness, paresthesias, and polyuria)
- Postural signs of volume depletion (dehydration)
- Parotitis
- Scars on the dorsum of the hand (characteristic of chronic, self-induced vomiting)

DIAGNOSIS

PHYSICAL EXAMINATION

- History: eating, physical exercise habits, growth patterns, age at menarche, menstruation history, vomiting, use of dieting drugs
- Nutritional status: relative weight (the percent deviation from average weight for a given height), deceleration or cessation of growth
- Clinical exam: phase of puberty, blood pressure, pulse frequency, cardiac auscultation, signs of vasoconstriction and severe malnutrition (edema, skin signs), teeth

LABORATORY TESTS

- Complete blood count (CBC)
- Erythrocyte sedimentation rate
- Serum electrolytes

- Liver function tests
- Blood glucose
- Serum amylase (if vomiting is suspected)
- Thyroid function tests
- Electrocardiogram (ECG)
- Common findings include leukopenia, mild anemia, thrombocytopenia, low serum T4 levels (representing a sick-euthyroid syndrome).
- Less common findings include slightly increased serum creatinine and hepatic enzymes, low albumin concentration.
- Severe conditions may include electrolyte disturbances (hypokalemia or hyponatremia) and ECG abnormalities.
- Laboratory findings can be found to be within a normal range even in severe malnutrition.
- Bone density measurements are indicated for those patients where the disorder has persisted over 12 months, those with a BMI < 15 kg/m^2, or those with a low calcium intake.

PSYCHIATRIC EXAMINATION

- Objectives:
  - To determine if an eating disorder is present
  - To determine if there are other concurrent psychiatric disorders
  - To evaluate if the patient's psychological development is age-appropriate
- Initial patient interview:
  - Symptoms
    - Eating Disorder Examination (EDE)
    - Scoring forms using Eating Disorder Inventory (EDI)
    - Eating habits/food diary
- Patient and family evaluations
- Psychological tests, if necessary
- Family examination

MEDICAL MANAGEMENT & TREATMENT

Management should consist of a combination of psychiatric treatment and nutritional status correction that includes:
- A defined treatment target, which is mutually agreed-upon
- Multidisciplinary eating disorder team approach
- Slow initiation of refeeding in severe malnutrition
- Reverse the most severe weight loss prior to psychotherapy
- Family therapy, particularly in non-chronic adolescents

Pharmacological treatment and other evidence-based treatment studies are limited.
- Indications for inpatient medical/psychiatric treatment:
  - Somatic:
    - Body Mass Index (BMI) < 13 kg/m^2 or < 70% of relative weight corresponding to height or a rapid weight loss (25% in 3 months)
    - Severe disturbances of electrolyte or metabolic homeostasis

- Systolic blood pressure < 70 mm Hg or heart rate < 40/minute or aberrant ECG
  - Psychiatric:
    - Psychotic symptoms
    - Severe self-harm or tendency toward suicide
    - Severe depression
    - Severe problems within family
  - Failure of outpatient treatment
- Indications for outpatient medical or psychiatric treatment:
  - BMI > 13kg/m^2 or > 70% of relative weight
  - High motivation for treatment
  - No severe medical complications
  - Supportive family and social network
  - No previous hospitalizations for anorexia nervosa

COMPLICATIONS

A high level of psychiatric comorbidity is associated with anorexia nervosa and bulimia nervosa. Frequent associated diagnoses include neurotic disorders such as anxiety disorders, phobias, affective disorders, substance abuse disorders, obsessive–compulsive disorder, and unspecified personality disorders.

ANOREXIA NERVOSA

- Cachexia
- Renal damage
- Hepatic damage
- Decreased heart size or cardiac arrhythmias
- Electrolyte imbalances
- Mental impairment
- Amenorrhea due to estrogen deficiency
- Altered metabolism
- Loss of bone density (osteoporosis) and increased risk for fractures
- Seizures
- Hypoglycemic syncope
- Poor wound healing
- Death

BULIMIA NERVOSA

- Electrolyte imbalances
- Diabetes
- Colitis
- Pancreatitis
- Gastric and esophageal rupture
- Superior mesenteric artery syndrome
- Infertility
- Miscarriages
- Seizures
- Arthritis
- Poor wound healing
- Osteoporosis
- Cardiovascular failure
- Renal failure
- Death

PROGNOSIS

ANOREXIA NERVOSA

Approximately 50% of those with anorexia nervosa recover; in 30%,

the symptoms persist; and in 10–20%, the disease is chronic. Unfortunately, death occurs in approximately 6% (often from suicide). This was found to be significantly higher than the mortality rate caused by other psychiatric disorders or of that within populations of the same age range. The prognosis worsens for those whose BMI is dangerously low (< 13 to 15 kg/m^2) and those who have had the disorder for a longer period of time.

BULIMIA NERVOSA

Approximately 50% of those with bulimia eventually no longer demonstrate any symptoms of an eating disorder. However, a long history of the disorder prior to treatment, drug dependence, and vomiting in the final phase of treatment worsen the prognosis for recovery.

DENTAL SIGNIFICANCE

Oral effects result from the presence of stomach acids in the mouth (after chronic and frequent self-induced vomiting), excessive consumption of acidic drinks, and parafunctional habits.

- Dental wear that leads to loss of vertical dimension and anterior guidance and the development of a traumatic group occlusion with premature contacts.
- Dental erosion and perimylolysis:
  - Seen with purging subtype of anorexia nervosa and bulimia nervosa
  - Due to chemical and mechanical effects from regurgitation of gastric contents
  - Lingual, occlusal, and incisal surface enamel erosion with rounded margins
  - Particularly seen on the lingual surfaces of the maxillary anterior teeth
  - Notched incisal edges of anterior teeth
  - Amalgam restorations that appear raised in comparison to tooth structure
  - Loss of contours of unrestored teeth
  - Severity varies with duration and number of incidents of purging per day, oral hygiene, degree of acid dilution (rinsing with neutralizing liquids), and timing of teethcleaning
  - Active erosions are smooth, unstained, and not sensitive to temperature variation
  - Inactive erosions become stained over time
- Dental caries prevalence have conflicting reports.
- Parotid gland hypertrophy:
  - Seen with purging subtype of anorexia nervosa and bulimia nervosa
  - Onset of parotid hypertrophy (swelling) follows purging episode within 2 to 6 days
  - Hypertrophy is bilateral, soft, and painless to palpation

- Ducts of parotids are patent with normal salivary flow and no inflammation
- Magnitude of parotid hypertrophy is proportional to duration and severity of purging
- Xerostomia:
  - Possible causes include psychotropic medications and misuse of diuretics and/or laxatives
- Traumatized oral mucosal membranes and pharynx:
  - Seen with purging subtype
  - Due to rapid ingestion of food, by force of regurgitation, or by use of an object to induce vomiting (resulting in trauma to soft palate)
- Reports of variations in the periodontium are inconsistent.

DENTAL MANAGEMENT

- Recognize the signs and symptoms of eating disorders.
- Remain nonjudgmental and professional, fostering a trusting doctor–patient relationship.
- Ask patient additional questions related to oral manifestations.
- Educate patient regarding diet and oral health.
- Educate the patient regarding perimylolysis when appropriate.

- Recommend sipping water, using artificial saliva preparations, or chewing sugar-free gum for those who have xerostomia due to psychotropic medications.
- Recommend regular professional oral examinations, prophylaxis, and rigorous home care that includes topical fluoride application.
- Refer patients demonstrating signs of eating disorders to the proper specialists (psychologist, psychiatrist, and/or physician experienced in treating eating disorders) but provide palliative treatment when appropriate.
  - Composite bandages, endodontic therapy, and so forth.
  - Defer definitive treatment until control of the eating disorder is established.
- Be aware that anorexic patients are prone to hypoglycemic syncope. Keep simple carbohydrate sources readily available during dental treatment.
- For patients in the initial stage of treatment who may continue to purge, recommend a sodium bicarbonate mouth rinse after purging episodes.
- Definitive restorative treatment depends on the severity of hard tissue destruction and may include composite resins, glass ionomer, porcelain laminate veneers (lingual placement bonded with resin, if necessary), and

for full mouth reconstruction to possibly include endodontic therapy.

SUGGESTED REFERENCES

American Psychiatric Association, *Diagnostic and statistical manual of mental disorders,* ed 4 (text revision). Washington, American Psychiatric Association, 2000, pp 589, 594.

De Moor RJG. Eating disorder-induced dental complications: a case report. *J of Oral Rehabilitation* 2004;31:725–732.

Ebeling H, et al. A practice guideline for treatment of eating disorders in children and adolescents. *Ann Med* 2003;35:488–501.

Gowers S, Bryant-Waugh R. Management of child and adolescent eating disorders: the current evidence base and future directions. *Journal of Child Psychology and Psychiatry* 2004;45(1):63–83.

Little JW. Eating disorders: dental implications. *Oral Surg Oral Med Oral Path* 2002;93(2):138–143.

Seller CA, Ravalia A. Anesthetic implications of anorexia nervosa. *Anaesthesia* 2003;58:437–443.

Steinhausen H. The outcome of anorexia nervosa in the 20th century. *Am J Psychiatry* 2002;159(8):1284–1293.

Studen-Pavlovich D, Elliott MA. Eating disorders in women's oral health. *Dental Clinics of North America* 2001;45(3):491–511.

Waldman HB. Is your next young patient pre-anorexic or pre-bulimic? *ASDC J Dent Child* 1998;Jan-Feb:52–56.

AUTHOR: **KELLY K. HILGERS, DDS, MS**

SYNONYM(S)

Hypoplastic anemia
Progressive hypocythemia
Peripheral pancytopenia
Aregeneratory anemia
Aleukia hemorrhagica
Panmyelophthisis
Bone marrow failure syndrome
Erythroblastphthisis
Panmyelopathy
Progressive hypoerythemia
Refractory anemia
Toxic paralytic anemia

ICD-9CM/CPT CODE(S)

284.9 Aplastic anemia
284.8 Acquired aplastic anemia
284.0 Congenital aplastic anemia

OVERVIEW

Aplastic anemia is a blood disorder caused by bone marrow failure and is characterized by significant reduction or absence of erythroid, granulocytic, and megakaryocytic cells in bone marrow. Affected patients have pancytopenia; however, the erythrocytes are normochromic and normocytic.

EPIDEMIOLOGY & DEMOGRAPHICS

INCIDENCE/PREVALENCE IN USA: It is estimated that about 1000 new cases are diagnosed annually in the U.S.
PREDOMINANT AGE: Aplastic anemia can occur at any age but is most common in young adults (15 to 30 years old) and elderly patients. The peak incidence is observed in people ages 20 to 25, and a subsequent peak in incidence is observed in people older than 60 years.
PREDOMINANT SEX: The male-to-female ratio is approximately equal.
PREDOMINANT RACE: No racial predisposition exists in the U.S.; however, prevalence is increased in Asia.
GENETICS: Twenty percent of cases are believed to be inherited or due to congenital factors. Hereditary aplastic anemia is associated with Fanconi's anemia, dyskeratosis congenital, and Shwachman-Diamond syndrome.

ETIOLOGY & PATHOGENESIS

ACQUIRED (80%)

- Idiopathic (50–65%)
- Drugs: antimetabolites, antimitotic agents, gold, chloramphenicol, phenylbutazone, and sulfonamides
- Infectious causes: viral hepatitis (non-A, non-B, non-C, and non-G), HIV, Epstein-Barr virus, parvovirus B19, and mycobacterial infections
- Toxic exposure to radiation and chemicals such as benzene, solvents, and insecticides
- Transfusional graft vs host disease
- Paroxysmal nocturnal hemoglobinuria

- Pregnancy
- Connective tissue diseases
- Eosinophilic fascitis

CONGENITAL/INHERITED (20%)

- Familial aplastic anemia
- Fanconi's anemia
- Dyskeratosis congenita
- Pearson syndrome
- Shwachman-Diamond syndrome

CLINICAL PRESENTATION / PHYSICAL FINDINGS

- The onset is usually insidious
- The initial symptoms are anemia or bleeding with fever or infections
- Progressive weakness and fatigue
- Cutaneous bleeding or petechial rashes
- Mucosal bleeding (gingival, nasal, vaginal, and gastrointestinal)
- Pallor (cutaneous mucosal and conjunctival)
- Headache
- Palpitations, tachycardia, and heart murmur
- Dyspnea
- Foot swelling
- Neutropenia may manifest as overt infections, recurrent infections, or mouth and pharyngeal ulcerations
- Spontaneous gingival bleeding
- Oral ulcers
- Lymphadenopathy

Review possible exposure to drugs, chemicals, or other potential risk factors.

DIAGNOSIS

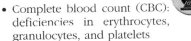

- Complete blood count (CBC): deficiencies in erythrocytes, granulocytes, and platelets
- Bone marrow aspiration and/or biopsy: deficiencies in cellular components (stem cells and progenitors) of bone marrow; replaced with fat cells

MEDICAL MANAGEMENT & TREATMENT

- Withdrawal of the etiologic agent is the most direct approach to the treatment of aplastic anemia. Discontinuation of a suspected drug, thymectomy in patients with thymoma, or delivery or therapeutic abortion in patients with pregnancy-associated aplastic anemia may result in recovery of blood count. Unfortunately, these cases account for a very small proportion of patients.
- Bone marrow transplantation (BMT): 80% response rate with matched, related donor and 50% with matched, unrelated donor; 70% of patients will not have a matched, related donor available.
- Immunosuppressive therapy such as antithymocyte globulin, cyclosporine, cytoxan, cyclophosphamide (alone or in combination).

- Hematopoietic growth factors: erythropoietin, granulocyte colony stimulating factor (G-CSF), granulocyte-macrophage colony stimulating factor (GM-CSF), interleukins1,3 and 6, stem cell factor.
- Peripheral blood stem cell transplant.
- Blood transfusion for acute or symptomatic management of signs or symptoms associated with low blood counts.

COMPLICATIONS

- Up to 87% of patients managed by BMT have chronic graft-vs-host disease (GVHD), with mortality three times higher in BMT patients who develop GVHD.
- Lower survival rates in adults than children due to GVHD.
- Fortyfold increase in late malignancies after bone marrow transplantation (BMT).

PROGNOSIS

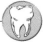

- Depends on cause and severity, as well as the health and age of the patient.
- Cases that are caused by certain medications, pregnancy, low-dose radiation, or infectious mononucleosis often are short-term, and any complications (e.g., anemia, bleeding, increased infections) usually can be treated.
- Women who develop aplastic anemia during pregnancy may have the problem during future pregnancies as well.
- As many as one-fifth of patients may spontaneously recover with supportive care.
- The estimated 5-year survival rate for the typical patient receiving immunosuppression is 75%, and for matched sibling donor, BMT is greater than 90%.
- In cases of immunosuppression, a risk of relapse and late clonal disease exists.
- Patients with severe, chronic aplastic anemia who do not respond to available treatments have an 80% chance of dying within 18 to 24 months.

DENTAL SIGNIFICANCE

In a study of 79 patients with aplastic anemia, the following oral manifestations were found at a baseline visit:

- 27% petechiae
- 15% gingival hyperplasia (associated with cyclosporine use), spontaneous gingival bleeding, herpetic lesions, nonherpetic ulceration
- 10% pallor
- 4% candidiasis
- Herpetic lesions developed in 28% of patients throughout medical therapy

Infection and bleeding are two major problems in patients with aplastic anemia.

- Thrombocytopenia (e.g., platelet count < 50,000/mm^3) increases risk of bleeding episodes.
- Low neutrophils (e.g., absolute neutrophil count < 500/mm^3) increases risk of infection.

DENTAL MANAGEMENT

- No surgical procedures should be performed on a patient suspected of having a bleeding problem based on history and examination findings. Such a patient should be screened with the appropriate clinical laboratory tests and, if indicated, referred to a physician or hematologist for diagnosis and treatment.
- Close coordination with the patient's physician and even hospitalization may be advisable for patients with pancytopenia.
- Have recent CBC available prior to dental treatment. Consider prophylactic antibiotic coverage after invasive dental procedures if absolute neutrophil count < 500/mm^3 (see Appendix A, Box A-2, "Presurgical and Postsurgical Antibiotic Prophylaxis for Patients at Increased Risk for Postoperative Infections).
- Use an antibiotic mouthwash rinse such as chlorhexidine before dental procedures.
- Patients should receive antifibrinolytic drugs such as aminocaproic acid or tranexamic acid to reduce the risk of uncontrolled bleeding. These medications should be given 24 hours prior to oral procedures and must continue for 3 to 4 days afterward.
- To reduce risk of bleeding, local hemostatic measures should be taken as well.
- Patients with aplastic anemia should receive blood transfusion before extraction if the platelet count is less than 50,000/mm^3.
- During dental treatment, avoid intramuscular injections and nerve-block anesthesia because they can lead to uncontrolled bleeding.

SUGGESTED REFERENCES:

Brennan MT, et al. Oral manifestations in patients with aplastic anemia. *Journal of Oral Surgery Oral Medicine Oral Pathology Oral Radiology* 2001;92:503–508, no. 5.

Greenberg MS, Glick M. *Burket's Oral Medicine Diagnosis and Treatment.* Hamilton, Ontario, BC Decker, Inc., 2003, pp 429–453.

Little, JW. Hematologic diseases, in *Dental Management of the Medically Compromised Patient.* St Louis, Mosby, 2002, pp 437–438.

Valdez IH, Paterson LL. Aplastic anemia: current concepts and dental management. *Special Care in Dentistry* 1990;Nov-Dec:185–189.

Young NS: Acquired aplastic anemia. *JAMA* 1999;282(3):271–278.

Websites:

Aplastic anemia:
http://www.emedicine.com/med/topic162.htm

http://my.webmd.com/hw/health_guide_atoz/nord83.asp

Aplastic Anemia and MDS International Foundation:
http://www.aplastic.org/pdfs/ACQUIRED-APLASTIC-ANEMIA-BASIC-EXPLANATIONS.pdf

AUTHORS: **MICHAEL T. BRENNAN, DDS, MHS; FARIDEH MADANI, DMD**

SYNONYM(S)

Bronchial asthma
Extrinsic asthma
Allergic asthma
Intrinsic asthma
Idiosyncratic asthma
Hyperreactive airway disease

ICD-9CM/CPT CODE(S)

493.0 Extrinsic asthma
493.1 Intrinsic asthma
493.9 Asthma unspecified

OVERVIEW

The National Asthma Education and Prevention Program Expert Panel from the U.S. National Institutes of Health define asthma as:

A chronic inflammatory disorder of the airways in which many cells and cellular elements play a role, in particular, mast cells, eosinophils, T-lymphocytes, macrophages, neutrophils, and epithelial cells. In susceptible individuals, this inflammation causes recurrent episodes of wheezing, breathlessness, chest tightness and coughing, particularly at night or in the early morning. These episodes are usually associated with widespread but variable airflow obstruction that is often reversible either spontaneously or with treatment. The inflammation also causes an associated increase in the existing bronchial responsiveness to a variety of stimuli.

EPIDEMIOLOGY & DEMOGRAPHICS

INCIDENCE/PREVALENCE IN USA: Asthma affects 5–10% of the U.S. population (an estimated 17 million persons, including children). It accounts for over 10 million physician visits and 1.9 million emergency room visits annually, with an estimated 500,000 hospitalizations and 5000 deaths annually.

PREDOMINANT AGE: Asthma affects children with an estimated prevalence of 6%. Two-thirds of all asthma cases are diagnosed before age 18, with most being diagnosed before age 5. Approximately 50% of all children diagnosed with asthma have a diminution or disappearance of symptoms by early adulthood.

PREDOMINANT SEX: In childhood asthma, there is a 2:1 male:female gender ratio, while the disease in adults does not have dramatic gender predominance. In fact, asthma prevalence is greater in girls after puberty, and the majority of adult-onset cases occur in women.

GENETICS: Genetic factors are of major importance in determining a predisposition to the development of asthma, including response to asthma medications, but environmental factors are thought to play a greater role in the onset of disease. The ADAM 33 gene is strongly associated with asthma and airway hyperresponsiveness

ETIOLOGY & PATHOGENESIS

- Bronchospasm (see "Bronchospasm" in Section III, p 348), hyperresponsiveness of the airway, and inflammation of the airway are all germane to the disorder. The major inflammatory response in an asthmatic patient involves an interaction between immune cells and immune mediators/cytokines. Mast cells, eosinophils, macrophages, epithelial cells, and activated T-lymphocytes, particularly those which are associated with a Th2 response, are the most important cellular elements in this disorder. These cells either release or are influenced by various mediators/cytokines and adhesion molecules. Together, the cells and mediators act upon the airway and result in significant bronchial changes including subbasement membrane thickening of the airway epithelium as well as airway smooth muscle hypertrophy. Permanent airway changes including airway remodeling, and scarring may ensue.
- Extrinsic asthma (allergic asthma) is brought on by exposure to allergens.
- Intrinsic asthma occurs in patients with no history of allergies but may be triggered by upper respiratory infections.
- Exercise-induced asthma seen frequently in the adolescent age group is triggered by physical activity and diminishes after the activity is completed.

CLINICAL PRESENTATION / PHYSICAL FINDINGS

Signs and symptoms vary with severity of the disease but may include:

- Wheezing
- Tachycardia
- Tachypnea
- Accessory muscle usage with breathing
- Paradoxical abdominal and diaphragmatic movement on inspiration
- Pulsus paradoxus

DIAGNOSIS

LABORATORY TESTS

- Pulmonary function tests
- Methacholine challenge test
- Skin test for atopy
- Arterial blood gas during acute attack can help determine severity of attack

IMAGING TESTS

Chest radiograph; usually normal, may show thoracic hyperinflation

MEDICAL MANAGEMENT & TREATMENT

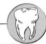

See Tables I-3 and I-4, based on severity

COMPLICATIONS

- Complications of asthma include exhaustion, dehydration, airway infection, cor pulmonale, tussive syncope, and status asthmaticus (small airway obstruction that is refractory to sympathomimetic and antiinflammatory agents and that may progress to respiratory failure without prompt and aggressive intervention).
- Acute hypercapnic and hypoxic respiratory failure occurs in severe disease.

PROGNOSIS

- The long-term outlook for patients with asthma is age-dependent. Whereas 25% or more of childhood asthmatics continue to have symptoms as adults, more than 90% of asthmatics with the onset of symptoms as adults continue to have symptoms throughout their lives.
- Morbidity and mortality rates for asthma have been increasing for more than 15 years. According to the Centers for Disease Control, among persons ages 5 to 24 years, the asthma death rate doubled from 1980 to 1993 (from 4.2 to 8.4 per million population). In 1993, among persons ages 5 to 24 years, African-Americans were four to six times more likely than Caucasians to die from asthma, and males were 1.3 to 1.5 times more likely to die than females.

DENTAL SIGNIFICANCE

- Specific oral conditions have been related to the use of asthma medications, including xerostomia, (from inhaled β-2 agonists), increased caries, and oral pharyngeal candidiasis (presumably from inhaled steroids as well as xerostomia).
- The direct effect of medications may also be manifested by soreness of the oral mucosa. The use of aerosol holding chambers in conjunction with metered dose inhalers, as well as mouth rinsing after medication usage, have been very helpful in preventing oral mucosal disorders.

DENTAL MANAGEMENT

- Optimal asthma control is desirable before dental treatment.
- Some medications used in dentistry may have specific implications when treating the asthmatic patient.
  - Aspirin, as well as other nonsteroidal antiinflammatory medications

TABLE I-3 Classification of Chronic Asthma Based on Severity and Treatment (Step) Protocols (Adults and Children over 5)

Category of Asthma before Treatment	Symptoms	Preferred Treatment
Step 4 Severe Persistent	• Continual symptoms • Limited physical activity • Frequent exacerbations • Frequent nighttime symptoms	Antiinflammatory—high-dose inhaled corticosteroid *and* long-acting bronchodilator *and* systemic corticosteroid (try to reduce and eliminate)
Step 3 Moderate Persistent	• Daily symptoms • Daily use of inhaled short-acting bronchodilator • Exacerbations affect activity • Exacerbations ≥ 2 times/week, which may last weeks • Nocturnal symptoms > 1 time/week	Antiinflammatory—medium-dose inhaled corticosteroid *or* inhaled corticosteroid (low or medium) and a long-acting β-2 agonist bronchodilator [If needed, both inhaled corticosteroid (medium- or high-dose) and a long-acting β-2 agonist]
Step 2 Mild Persistent	• Symptoms > 2 times/week but < 1 time/day • Exacerbations may affect activity • Nighttime symptoms > 2 times/month	Antiinflammatory either low-dose inhaled corticosteroid or cromolyn or nedocromil
Step 1 Mild Intermittent	• Symptoms ≤ 2 times/week • Asymptomatic and normal PEF between exacerbations • Exacerbations brief • Nighttime symptoms ≤ 2 times/month	None needed

- Steps are also based on lung function tests.
- Treatment is individualized and requires a step-up or a step-down based on signs or symptoms.
- Education is extremely important in all Step categories.
- Short-acting bronchodilators (β-2 agonists) are used for quick relief in all categories.
- Use of short-acting β-2 agonist on a daily basis or > 2 times/week in mild intermittent asthma indicates the need for additional long-term control therapy.
- Sustained-release theophylline, long-acting β-2 agonist tablets, and leukotriene modifiers maybe alternatives (see Table I-4).

Source: Reprinted from Sollecito TP, Tino G. Asthma. *Oral Surg Oral Med Oral Pathol Oral Radiol Endod* 2001;92(5):486.

(NSAIDs), should be avoided in aspirin-sensitive asthmatics since they could trigger an acute asthmatic attack. In general, NSAIDs (including aspirin) should be used with caution in all asthmatics since these medications inhibit cyclooxygenase and preferentially generate leukotrienes. Approximately 10–28% of adult asthmatics may be intolerant to aspirin.

○ Opiates, which cause respiratory depression and which can induce histamine release, also should be avoided.

○ Macrolide antibiotics, such as erythromycin, which alter cytochrome P450, may result in elevated serum methylxanthine (theophylline) levels.

○ Patients taking leukotriene modifiers such as Zafirlukast and Zileuton concurrently with Coumadin may have abnormally elevated International Normalized Ratios (INRs) by inhibiting liver metabolism of Coumadin.

○ Sulfite preservatives such as those found in some local anesthetics (i.e., those with vasoconstrictors such as levonordefrin and epinephrine) can precipitate asthmatic attacks. Some practitioners have advocated that the dentist should avoid using a local anesthetic that contains a sulfite preservative. Others have reported that it is safe to use in noncorticosteroid-dependent asthmatics. Further study is required to establish a causal relationship. Of course, patients who report an allergy to sulfites should not be given a sulfite-containing local anesthetic.

• In severe asthmatic patients chronically taking systemic corticosteroids, corticosteroid supplementation prior to stressful or perceived stressful dental procedures may be required (see Appendix A, Box A-4, "Dental Management of Patients at Risk for Acute Adrenal Insufficiency").

• Stress alone, as well as in conjunction with use of various dental materials or chemical irritants, can trigger asthmatic attacks.

• The patient should be advised to bring their short-acting β-2 agonist inhaler medication to the dental appointment. The dentist may need to administer more intensive treatment, including subcutaneous epinephrine administration, to manage an acute asthmatic event.

SUGGESTED REFERENCES

American Dental Association. The dental patient with asthma. An update and oral health considerations. *J Am Dent Assoc* 2001;132(9):1229–1239.

Asthma Management and Prevention: A Practical Guide for Public Health Officials and Health Care Professionals Based on Global Strategy for Asthma Management and Prevention. NHLBI/WHO Workshop Report, publication no. 95–3659A, National Institutes of Health, NHLBI. Bethesda, MD, 1995.

Emedicine: www.emedicine.com (Asthma)

Ferri FF. Asthma, in Ferri FF (ed): *Ferri's Clinical Advisor: Instant Diagnosis and Treatment.* Philadelphia, Elsevier Mosby, 2005, pp 97–99.

Georgitis JW. The 1997 asthma management guidelines and therapeutic issues relating to the treatment of asthma. *National Heart, Lung, and Blood Institute Chest* 1999; 115(1):210–217.

National Institutes of Health. Expert Panel Report 2, *Guidelines for the Diagnosis and Management of Asthma.* NIH publication no. 97–4051. Bethesda, MD, 1997.

Sollecito TP, Tino G. Asthma. *Oral Surg Oral Med Oral Pathol Oral Radiol Endod* 2001;92(5): 485–490.

AUTHOR: THOMAS P. SOLLECITO, DMD

TABLE I-4 Asthma Medications*

Agent	Indication	Mechanism of action	Example
Inhaled β_2-agonist (short-acting)	Acute exacerbation Used in all categories	Bronchodilator • Smooth muscle relaxation after adenylate cyclase activation, resulting in an increase in cyclic AMP • Activation of protein kinase A, which lowers the needed intracellular calcium for smooth muscle contraction	Albuterol Metaproterenol
Inhaled β_2-agonist (long-lasting)	Longer-term prevention usually added to antiinflammatory therapy	Bronchodilator (see above)	Salmeterol
Oral β_2-agonist (long-lasting)	Longer-term prevention usually added to antiinflammatory therapy	Bronchodilator (see above)	Albuterol for sustained relief
Inhaled corticosteroids	Longer-term prevention Daily medication in all persistent forms Low-, medium-, and high-dose formulations depending on asthma severity/control	Antiinflammatory • Inhibits cytokine production and adhesion protein activation • Reverses β_2 downregulation • Suppresses recruitment of airway eosinophils	Beclomethasone Flunisolide Fluticasone Budesonide Triamcinolone
Systemic corticosteroids	Acute exacerbation used in all categories Long-term prevention in severe persistent asthma	Antiinflammatory (see above)	Methylprednisolone Prednisolone Prednisone
Mast cell stabilizers	Longer-term prevention of symptoms Daily medication used in STEP 2 mild persistent asthma	Antiinflammatory • Inhibits sensitized mast cell degranulation and release of mediators from mast cells • Inhibits activation and release of mediators from eosinophils	Cromolyn Nedocromil
Methylxanthines	Longer-term prevention Daily medication used in mild persistent (STEP 2) type asthma or as an adjunct to inhaled corticosteroids in moderate persistent (STEP 3) and severe persistent (STEP 4) categories	Bronchodilator • Smooth muscle relaxation through phosphodiesterase inhibition and increased cAMP • May affect eosinophil infiltration and decrease T cells in epithelium • Increase diaphragm contractility • Increase mucociliary clearance	Theophylline (sustained-release)
Anticholinergics	Acute exacerbation used in patients intolerant to short-acting β_2-agonists	Bronchodilator • Competitive inhibition of muscarinic cholinergic receptors	Ipratropium bromide
Leukotriene modifiers	Long-term control and prevention in STEP 2 mild persistent	Antiinflammatory • Leukotriene receptor antagonist (competitive inhibition) = Zafirlukast/Montelukast • 5-lipoxygenase inhibitor interfering with leukotriene synthesis = Zileuton	Zafirlukast Montelukast Zileuton

AMP, Adenosine monophosphate: *cAMP*, cyclic adenosine monophosphate.
*All medications have side effects with which the dentist should be familiar.
*Medication usage/discontinuance recommendations should be made in light of step-up/step-down protocol (STEP).
*Specific dosage/delivery of medication tailored to patient/severity.
*Children under 5 years old have different regimens.
Source: Reprinted from Sollecito TP, Tino G. Asthma. *Oral Surg Oral Med Oral Pathol Oral Radiol Endod* 2001;92(5):487

SYNONYM(S)

Behçet's disease
Mucocutaneous ocular syndrome

ICD-9CM/CPT CODE(S)

136.1 Behçet's syndrome

OVERVIEW

Behçet's syndrome is a multisystem, inflammatory chronic disorder that may exhibit oral aphthous ulcers, skin lesions, uveitis, and genital ulcers. The clinical course is often characterized by remissions and exacerbations. The syndrome usually begins in the third decade. There have been limited cases involving children. In the U.S., a diagnosis must be considered when patients exhibit oral and genital lesions with uncertain ocular disease.

EPIDEMIOLOGY & DEMOGRAPHICS

INCIDENCE/PREVALENCE IN USA: 0.12 to 0.33 cases per 100,000.
PREDOMINANT AGE: The syndrome generally begins in the third decade.
PREDOMINANT SEX: Males are affected just as often as females.
GENETICS: Areas of prevalence of HLA-B51 are higher in patients with Behçet's syndrome.

ETIOLOGY & PATHOGENESIS

- Etiology is unknown. An immune-related vasculitis is suspected.
- HLA-B51 has been associated with cases in Japan and the Mediterranean area.
- Triggering of the immune response and activation mechanism is not yet known.

CLINICAL PRESENTATION / PHYSICAL FINDINGS

- Painful oral aphthous ulcers are usually less than 1 cm in diameter. The oral lesions are classified as minor, major, and herpetiform ulceration and must occur at least three times in one 12-month period.
- The oral aphthae of Behçet's syndrome are usually continuously present, recur at the same site, may have scarring, usually number more than six, have varying borders and size, and can develop on the soft palate and oropharynx.
- The genital ulcers are similar to the oral ulcers.

- Ocular changes can include uveitis, conjunctivitis, and retinitis.
- Perianal ulcers have been noted, as well as inflammatory bowel disease.
- Other findings include vasculitis, CNS alterations, headaches, infarcts, arthritis in joints, wrists, knees and ankles, polychondritis, and pustules of the skin. Vasculitis (inflammatory or occlusion) can show signs and symptoms of myocardial infarct, intermittent claudication, deep vein thrombosis, hemoptysis, and aneurysm formation.

DIAGNOSIS

- Diagnosis may be based on signs and symptoms listed previously.
- Other signs include epidermal erythema, pustules, uveitis, retinitis, inflammatory bowel disease, arthritis, and polychondritis.
- The diagnosis of Behçet's syndrome is established when recurrent oral ulcerations is accompanied by two of the following:
  ○ Recurrent genital ulcerations
  ○ Eye lesions
  ○ Skin lesions
  ○ Positive pathergy test

DIFFERENTIAL DIAGNOSIS

- Aphthous stomatitis
- Erythema multiform
- Herpes simplex reaction
- Idiosyncratic drug eruption
- Lichen planus
- Recurrent herpes with immunosuppression
- Reiter's syndrome
- Pemphigoid
- Ulcerative colitis
- Crohn's disease
- Sweet syndrome

LABORATORY TESTS

- None are diagnostic.
- Erythrocyte sedimentation rate elevated.
- Hypergammaglobulinemia.
- Histopathology shows no specific diagnosis.

MEDICAL MANAGEMENT & TREATMENT

- Prevent dehydration by increasing fluids.
- Corticosteroids, azathioprine, chlorambucil, pentoxifylline, and cyclosporine have shown beneficial results. Corticosteroids may be of help for oral ulcerations. Topical anesthetics, ointments, and creams have been used.

COMPLICATIONS

- Ocular involvement may result in blindness.
- Involvement of central nervous system after results in serious disability or death.
- Vasculitis may cause aneurysms or thrombosis, which also may involve kidneys.
- A mild, self-limiting, and nondestructive arthritis of knees and other large joints.
- Life-threatening brainstem and spinal cord lesions.
- Crohn's disease.

PROGNOSIS

Behçet's syndrome is generally chronic and manageable. Remission and relapse may extend several decades. Blindness, vena cava obstruction, and paralysis are possible. Occasional fatalities are usually associated with neurologic, vascular, and gastrointestinal tract.

DENTAL SIGNIFICANCE

- Recurrent aphthous ulcerations are painful and impact on patient's overall health.
- Behçet's syndrome demonstrates a triple symptoms complex of recurrent oral ulcerations, ocular inflammation, and recurrent genital ulcerations.

DENTAL MANAGEMENT

- Review differential diagnosis for working diagnosis and treat aphthous ulcers with corticosteroids.
- Refer patient to rheumatologist and/or internal medicine for care. Ophthalmology involvement is mandatory.
- Due to patient's painful oropharyngeal tissues, nutrition input is needed. Oral hygiene must be a part of patient care.
- Oral medicine consultation suggested.

SUGGESTED REFERENCE

Fitzpatrick TB, Johnson RA, Wolff K, Suurmond D (eds): *Color Atlas and Synopsis of Clinical Dermatology. Behçet's Syndrome,* ed 4. New York, McGraw-Hill, 2001, pp 346–348.

AUTHOR: **NORBERT J. BURZYNSKI, SR., DDS, MS**

SYNONYM(S)

Tracheobronchitis
"Chest cold"

ICD-9CM/CPT CODE(S)
466.0 Acute bronchitis—complete

OVERVIEW

Acute inflammatory disease of the trachea and bronchi. Generally self-limited with resolution and return to baseline function. Rarely a cause of hospital admission in children or adults.

EPIDEMIOLOGY & DEMOGRAPHICS
INCIDENCE/PREVALENCE IN USA:
Approximately 5% of the U.S. population per year is afflicted with acute infectious bronchitis.

- Acute bronchitis is a commonly diagnosed condition in general practice during the winter months, approaching a rate of 150 cases per 100,000 population per week. Acute infectious bronchitis shows a consistent January–February peak and an August trough. Illness usually develops following a common cold or other viral infection of the nasopharynx, throat, or tracheobronchial tree. Acute bronchitis is also causally related during epidemics of influenza and measles.

PREDOMINANT AGE: Affects all ages; attack rates are highest in the extremes of life and lowest in the 15 to 44 age group.
PREDOMINANT SEX: Male = female.
GENETICS: None established.

ETIOLOGY & PATHOGENESIS

- In the very young, the most frequently isolated viruses are respiratory syncytial virus (RSV), parainfluenza types 1 to 3, and coronavirus.
- Among those from 1 to 10 years of age, parainfluenza types 1 and 2, enterovirus, RSV, and rhinovirus predominate.
- In those 10 years old and above, influenza A and B, RSV, and adenovirus are found most frequently.
- *Mycoplasma pneumoniae* and *Chlamydia* are reported to cause acute bronchitis in young adults.
- Parainfluenza types 1 and 3 and rhinovirus are found most frequently in the fall; influenza, RSV, and coronavirus cause infections in winter and early spring, while enteroviruses induce infections in summer and early fall.
- In the compromised host and older individuals, herpes simplex virus type 1 as well as gram-negative infections such as klebsiella, serratia, Enterobacter, and pseudomonas may cause acute bronchitis.
- Common bacterial isolates most often include *Haemophilus influenzae, Streptococcus*

pneumoniae, Mycobacterium tuberculosis, Branhamella catarrhalis, Salmonella typhosa, Staphylococcus aureus, and *Bordetella pertussis*.
- There is increasing evidence that yeasts and fungi may produce bronchitis. This is true of *Candida albicans, Candida tropicalis, Cryptococcus neoformans, Histoplasma capsulatum, Coccidioides immitis,* and *Blastomyces dermatitidis*.
- Bronchitis can also occur due to migration of strongyloides and ascaris larvae.
- Acute irritative bronchitis may be caused by mineral and vegetable dusts, fumes from strong acids, ammonia, certain volatile organic solvents, chlorine, hydrogen sulphide, sulphur dioxide, or bromine. Ozone and nitrogen dioxide as well as tobacco or other smokes can be causative.
- Allergen inhalation may trigger acute bronchitis in an atopic individual.

CLINICAL PRESENTATION / PHYSICAL FINDINGS

- Cough
  - Initially dry or nonproductive but later becomes mucoid or mucopurulent (does not abate once the original signs and symptoms of the upper respiratory infection or common cold have ended). The sputum occasionally contains streaks of blood for short periods of time.
- Coryza
- Malaise, headache
- Chilliness, slight fever (101°F to 102°F for 3 to 5 days); persistent fever suggests complicating pneumonia
- Back and muscle pain
- Sternal discomfort or tightness (sometimes described as "burning")
- Sore throat
- Dyspnea (secondary to airway obstruction)
- Scattered high- or low-pitched rhonchi, occasional moist rales at bases (shifts after patient coughs)
- Wheezing
- Acute respiratory failure (in severe cases)

SYSTEMS AFFECTED
- Tracheobronchial tree
  - Hyperemia of the mucous membranes followed by desquamation, edema, leukocytic infiltration of the submucosa, and production of sticky or mucopurulent exudates. Bronchial cilia have disturbed function, and there is spasm of bronchial smooth muscle.

DIAGNOSIS

LABORATORY
- Laboratory evaluation of acute bronchitis is usually not indicated.
- Arterial blood gas: if hypoxia suspected.
- Complete blood count: may reveal mild leukocytosis.

- Sputum culture, Gram's stain (sputum), acid-fast stains.
- Serologic analyses of antibody titers against specific viruses.

IMAGING/SPECIAL TESTS
- Chest radiograph: usually reserved for patients with suspected pneumonia, influenza, or underlying COPD and no improvement with therapy.
  - Bronchoscopy and/or pulmonary function tests may also be indicated under these circumstances.

MEDICAL MANAGEMENT & TREATMENT

GENERAL MEASURES
- Rest until fever subsides
- Oral hydration (3 to 4 L/day)
MEDICATIONS
- Antipyretic analgesics: children 2 to 16 years old should not receive aspirin because Reye's syndrome may occur as a complication in a wide range of viral infections.
- When numerous neutrophils on the Gram's stain (in addition to the historical and physical findings) suggest bacterial etiology, antibiotic therapy should be initiated.
  - If no likely etiologic agent is recovered in culture and there are many neutrophils in the sputum, the possibility of *M. pneumonia* should be considered and treated with either erythromycin 250 to 500 mg qid or tetracycline 250 mg q6h.
  - Trimethoprim/sulfamethoxazole (160 to 800 mg, orally, bid) may be given.
  - In children younger than 8 years old, give amoxicillin 40 mg/kg/day in divided doses tid.
  - If symptoms persist or recur, then the antibiotic is chosen according to the predominant organism and its sensitivity.
  - In general, antibiotics may reduce the possibility of secondary bacterial infections. However, antibiotics are overused in patients with acute bronchitis (70–90% of office visits for acute bronchitis result in treatment with antibiotics); this practice pattern is contributing to increases in resistant organisms.
- Amantadine may also be used prophylactically for the prevention of influenza A in susceptible individuals, such as the elderly and those with coexisting cardiopulmonary disease.
  - Amantadine need only be taken for 2 weeks if an influenza vaccine is given simultaneously.
  - Rimantadine is currently under investigation as an alternative agent and appears to be less prone to produce side effects.

- Bronchodilator therapy is used to help ease cough in patients and is of benefit in those who demonstrate a reduction of FEV1.
- Inhaled corticosteroid therapy and other antiinflammatory agents such as disodium cromolyn may be of benefit in managing this inflammatory condition.

COMPLICATIONS

Can progress to a more serious pulmonary problem such as bronchopneumonia, acute respiratory failure, or bronchiectasis.

PROGNOSIS

Most cases have a benign outcome and ordinarily are not life-threatening. It is unclear whether antibiotics truly make a difference in an uncomplicated acute bronchitis, although the literature suggests that 93% of patients are given antibiotics anyway. The disease may last for up to 6 or 8 weeks. If it persists further, then a careful assessment must be made as to possible pneumonia or a superimposed airway disease.

DENTAL SIGNIFICANCE

Frequent need to cough and to stay upright precludes most dental care.

DENTAL MANAGEMENT

Defer all but emergency dental care until condition subsides.

SUGGESTED REFERENCES

Bartlett J. Acute bronchitis. Uptodate Online 13.2, updated May 12, 2003, http://www.uptodateonline.com/application/topic.asp?file=pulm_inf/4399&type=A&selectedTitle=1^10

Blinkhorn Jr. RJ. Upper respiratory track infections, in Crapo JD et al. (eds): *Baum's Textbook of Pulmonary Disease.* Philadelphia, Lippincott, 2004, pp 413–420.

AUTHOR: **JAMES R. HUPP, DMD, MD, JD, MBA**

SYNONYM(S)

Cardiac arrhythmias
Conduction disorders

ICD-9CM/CPT CODE(S)

426.7	Wolff-Parkinson-White syndrome
427.0	Paroxysmal supraventricular tachycardia
427.1	Paroxysmal ventricular tachycardia
427.2	Paroxysmal tachycardia, unspecified
427.3	Atrial fibrillation and flutter
427.31	Atrial fibrillation
427.32	Atrial flutter
427.4	Ventricular fibrillation and flutter
427.41	Ventricular fibrillation
427.42	Ventricular flutter
427.5	Cardiac arrest
427.6	Premature beats
427.60	Premature beats, unspecified
427.61	Supraventricular premature beats
427.69	Other ventricular premature beats, contractions, or systoles
427.8	Other specified cardiac dysrhythmias
427.81	Sinoatrial node dysfunction (sinus bradycardia, sick sinus syndrome)
427.89	Other rhythm disorder
427.9	Cardiac dysrhythmia, unspecified

OVERVIEW

- Dysrhythmia denotes an alteration of the normal site or rate of electrical impulse generation within the heart, or an alteration of the impulse's orderly spread through the cardiac conducting system resulting in abnormal cardiac rate and/or rhythm.
- Cardiac dysrhythmias may be found in healthy individuals as well as in those with various forms of cardiovascular disease. Some of these dysrhythmias are of little concern to the patient or dentist; however, some can produce symptoms, and some can be life-threatening, including dysrhythmias that occur secondary to anxiety (e.g., those associated with dental care). Therefore, patients with significant dysrhythmias must be identified prior to undergoing dental treatment.

EPIDEMIOLOGY & DEMOGRAPICS

INCIDENCE/PREVALENCE IN USA: An estimated 10% of the population has some form of cardiac dysrhythmia. Specific incidence/prevalence varies with etiology and type of dysrhythmia:

- Atrial fibrillations has an incidence of 20 cases per 1000 persons, and a prevalence of approximately 2% in the general population, affecting approximately 2.2 million persons.

- Paroxysmal supraventricular tachycardia incidence is approximately 1 to 3 cases per 1000 persons; prevalence is 2.25 cases per 1000 persons.

The prevalence of cardiac dysrhythmias in a large population of general dental patients (> 10,000) was reported to be 17.2%, with over 4% of those being serious, life-threatening cardiac dysrhythmias.

PREDOMINANT AGE: Varies by etiology and type of the dysrhythmia. In general, the incidence and prevalence of most dysrhythmias increases with age (e.g., atrial fibrillation is strongly age-dependent, affecting 5% of individuals older than 60 years and almost 10% of persons older than 80 years).

PREDOMINANT SEX: Varies by etiology and type of the dysrhythmia.

GENETICS: Varies by etiology and type of the dysrhythmia, for example supraventricular tachycardia associated with Wolff-Parkinson-White syndrome may be transmitted occasionally in an autosomal-dominant manner; the incidence in first-degree relatives could be as high as 5.5 per 1000 persons.

ETIOLOGY & PATHOGENESIS

OVERVIEW OF THE SPECIAL EXCITATORY AND CONDUCTIVE SYSTEM OF THE HEART

- The primary pacemaker for the heart is the sinoatrial (SA) node, a crescent-shaped structure 9 to 15 mm long located at the junction of the superior vena cava and the right atrium.
  - The SA node regulates the functions of the atria and impulses generated by the SA node result in a normal rhythm of 60 to 100 beats per minute.
  - The impulses from the SA node rapidly travel throughout the atrial myocardium and cause the two atria to contract simultaneously, resulting in the production of the P wave on the electrocardiogram (ECG). At the same time, the impulses are conducted to the atrioventricular (AV) node via the internodal pathways.
- The AV node serves as a gate, preventing too many atrial impulses from entering the ventricle. It also slows the conduction rate of impulses generated in the SA node.
- From the AV node, the impulses rapidly travel through the bundle of His (or the AV bundle). This impulse travels to the right and left bundle branches. These bundle branches extend to the right and left sides of the interventricular septum and the apex of the heart, branching profusely to form the Purkinje fibers that conduct the impulses to the ventricular myocardium.
- The bundle of His, bundle branches and the Purkinje fibers rapidly conduct impulses throughout the ventricular myocardium resulting in depolarization

and contraction of both ventricles simultaneously, which is represented by the QRS complex on the ECG.
- After the ventricular contraction, the myocardial cells repolarize, as reflected in the ECG by the T wave.

ETIOLOGY

- Cardiac dysrhythmias may be found in healthy individuals, in patients taking various medications, and in patients with certain cardiovascular conditions, or with other systemic diseases. The most common causes include:
  - Primary cardiovascular disorders
  - Pulmonary disorders (e.g., embolism or hypoxia)
  - Autonomic disorders
  - Systemic disorders (e.g., thyroid disease)
  - Drug-related side-effects
  - Electrolyte imbalances
- Normal cardiac function depends on cellular automaticity (impulse formation), conductivity, excitability, and contractility.
  - Disorders in automaticity and conductivity form the basis of the vast majority of cardiac dysrhythmias. Under normal conditions the SA node is responsible for impulse formation; however, other cells in the conduction system can generate impulses. Under abnormal conditions, ectopic pacemakers can emerge outside the conduction system. After the generation of a normal impulse and its discharge, the cells of the SA node need time for recovery in what is termed refractoriness. Complete refractoriness results in a block and partial refractoriness in a delay of conductivity.
  - Disorders of conductivity (block or delay) paradoxically can lead to a rapid cardiac rhythm through the mechanisms of reentry. The type of dysrhythmia may suggest the nature of its cause. For example, paroxysmal atrial tachycardia with block suggests digitalis toxicity. However, many cardiac dysrhythmias are not specific for a given cause. In these patients a careful search is made to identify the etiology of the dysrhythmia.

CLASSIFICATION OF DYSRHYTHMIAS

Dysrhythmias are classified on the basis of causing ectopic beats, slowing of the heart rate (bradycardia), speeding of the heart rate (tachycardia), and arresting the heart rate. They encompass a broad spectrum, ranging from incidental dysrhythmias such as premature atrial beats, to lethal ones including ventricular fibrillation.

- **Isolated ectopic beats**
  - **Premature atrial beats:** Premature impulses arising from ectopic foci anywhere in the atrium may result in premature atrial beats.
    - They are common in conditions associated with atria dysfunction such as congestive heart failure.

- **Premature AV beats:** Premature AV beats are less common than premature atrial or premature ventricular ectopic beats.
  - Impulses can spread toward either the atria or the ventricles. When they are present, digitalis toxicity should be suspected.
- **Premature ventricular beats:** The most common form of dysrhythmia, regardless of whether heart disease exists.
  - Common with digitalis toxicity and hypokalemia. Late premature ventricular beats can lead to ventricular tachycardia or fibrillation in the presence of ischemia.
  - More than six late premature ventricular beats per minute may be an indication of cardiac instability.
- **Bradycardias**
  - **Sinus bradycardia:** A sinus rate of less than 60 beats per minute is defined as bradycardia.
    - Bradycardia is a normal finding in young, healthy adults and well-conditioned athletes; also can occur secondary to medication use.
    - Medications with parasympathetic effects (e.g., digoxin, phenothiazine) may slow the heart rate.
    - A sinus bradycardia that persists in the presence of congestive heart failure, pain, or exercise and following atropine administration is considered abnormal.
    - Sinus bradycardia commonly found early in myocardial infarction.
    - It also may occur in infectious diseases, myxedema, obstructive jaundice, and hypothermia.
  - **SA heart block** is relatively uncommon; may occur in stages or degrees:
    - In first-degree SA block, an impulse takes undue time to enter the atrium.
    - In second-degree SA block, one or more impulses fail to emerge from the SA node.
    - In third-degree (complete) SA block, no impulses emerge from SA node.
    - Most cases are caused by rheumatic heart disease, myocardial infarction, acute infection, or drug toxicity (e.g., digitalis, atropine, salicylates, quinidine).
  - **AV heart block** occurs in stages or degrees:
    - First-degree AV block features slow impulses from the atria to the ventricles with increased conduction time.
    - Second-degree heart block is the blockage of some (not all) impulses from atria to ventricles.
    - In third-degree (complete) AV block, none of the atrial electrical activities are transmitted to the ventricles, which contract at an exceedingly slow rate (between 20 and 40 beats per minute); the atria and ventricles exhibit separate, independent rhythms.
    - Rheumatic fever, ischemic heart disease, myocardial infarction, hyperthyroidism, and certain drugs (e.g., digitalis, propranolol, potassium, quinidine) may cause (usually first- or second-degree) AV heart block.
    - Sarcoidosis, Hodgkin's disease, myeloma, and open-heart surgery (e.g., aortic valve replacement or repair, ventricular septal defect repair) may result in complete AV block.
- **Tachycardias**
  - **Sinus tachycardia:** A sinus rate greater than 100 beats per minute is defined as sinus tachycardia.
    - The condition occurs most often as a physiologic response to exercise, anxiety, stress, and emotions.
    - Pharmacologic causes of sinus tachycardia include atropine, epinephrine, nicotine, and caffeine.
    - Pathologic causes include: fever, hypoxia, infection, anemia, and hyperthyroidism.
  - **Atrial tachycardia:** In atrial tachycardia, ectopic impulses may result in atrial rates of 150 to 200 per minute.
    - Atrial tachycardia is seen in some cases of chronic obstructive lung disease, advanced pathology of the atria, acute myocardial infarction, pneumonia, and drug intoxications (e.g., alcohol, catechols).
    - AV block with ectopic atrial tachycardia usually indicates digitalis toxicity or hypokalemia.
  - **Atrial flutter:** A rapid, regular atrial rate of 220 to 360 beats per minute is defined as atrial flutter, which is rare in healthy individuals and most often associated with ischemic heart disease in people over age 40.
    - Atrial flutter also is seen as a complication in patients with mitral stenosis or cor pulmonale and after open-heart surgery.
    - It may result when patients with atrial fibrillation have been treated with quinidine or procainamide.
  - **Atrial fibrillation (AF):** A common dysrhythmia characterized by an extremely rapid atrial rate of 400 to 650 beats per minute with no discrete P waves on the ECG tracing.
    - The ventricular response is irregular since only a portion of the impulses pass through the AV node.
    - The etiologic factors associated with AF are frequently classified into cardiac and noncardiac categories:
      - Cardiac causes of AF include ischemic heart disease, rheumatic heart disease, hypertension, sick sinus syndrome, preexcitation syndrome, cardiomyopathy, mitral valve annular calcifications, mitral valve prolapse, and pericardial disease.
      - Noncardiac causes of AF include acute infections (especially pneumonia), lung carcinoma, pulmonary thromboembolism, and pulmonary conditions that lead to hypoxemia, thyrotoxicosis, and cholinergic drugs.
    - Patients with AF are prone to the development of atrial thrombi.
  - **Ventricular tachycardia:** Three or more ectopic ventricular beats within a minute when the heart rate is 100 or more per minute is defined as ventricular tachycardia.
    - Ventricular tachycardia is almost always associated with underlying structural heart disease, most commonly myocardial infarction.
    - In some instances, drugs such as digitalis, sympathetic amines (e.g., epinephrine), potassium, quinidine, and procainamide may induce ventricular tachycardia.
    - On rare occasions, idiopathic ventricular tachycardia may be found (typically in young, healthy adults) in the absence of structural heart disease.
    - Ventricular tachycardia can be classified according to ECG appearance in to two subgroups: monomorphic and polymorphic.
      - Monomorphic ventricular tachycardia is defined by a repeated QRS wave.
      - Polymorphic ventricular tachycardia is characterized by a QRS complex that varies from beat to beat.
    - Ventricular tachycardia may be unsustained (lasting less than 30 seconds) or sustained, which may be life-threatening and requires activation of advanced cardiac life support.
    - Untreated ventricular tachycardia may degenerate to ventricular fibrillation, resulting in hemodynamic collapse and death.
  - **Wolff-Parkinson-White (preexcitation) syndrome:** Is the most common type of ventricular preexcitation dysrhythmia and is usually found in first, second, or third decade of life. It results from earlier than normal ventricular depolarization following the atrial impulse (called preexcitation) predisposing the affected person to supraventricular tachydysrhythmias.
  - Three events are involved in the Wolff-Parkinson-White syndrome:
    - First, an accessory AV pathway allows the normal conduction systems to be bypassed.

- Second, this accessory pathway allows rapid conduction and short refractoriness, with impulses passed rapidly from atrium to ventricle.
- Third, the parallel conduction system provides a route for reentrant tachydysrhythmias.
  - This pattern constitutes a syndrome when patients display symptoms (e.g., fatigue, dizziness, syncope, angina) from paroxysmal supraventricular tachycardia.
  - Paroxysmal atrial fibrillation and flutter also may occur, leading to ventricular fibrillation and death.
- **Cardiac arrest**
  - **Ventricular fibrillation, agonal rhythm,** and **asystole** are the three types of dysrhythmias associated with cardiac arrest. All are lethal. Patients with these conditions require immediate treatment for survival.
  - **Ventricular fibrillation** is represented as chaotic activity on the ECG, with the ventricles contracting rapidly but ineffectively.
    - It will progress to asystole and is usually lethal unless therapy is administered rapidly.
    - Coronary atherosclerosis is the most common form of heart disease predisposing to ventricular fibrillation.
    - Other causes of this dysrhythmia include rheumatic heart disease, anaphylaxis, blunt cardiac trauma, mitral valve prolapse, digitalis intoxication, cardiac catheterization, and cardiac surgery.
  - **Agonal rhythm** is characterized by wide, bizarre QRS complexes seen on ECG at a slow rate of 10 to 20 beats per minute.
    - It is considered a terminal rhythm and is usually the last rhythm before asystole.
  - In **asystole,** cardiac standstill occurs. There is no cardiac electrical impulse generation (ECG registering a flat line), myocardial contractility, or cardiac output.

CLINICAL PRESENTATION / PHYSICAL FINDINGS

Some dysrhythmias may be asymptomatic while others may produce episodic or chronic symptoms that range from mild (e.g., palpitations, lightheadedness, fatigue, poor exercise capacity) to severe (e.g., angina, dyspnea, syncope).

- The patent may report heart palpitations occurring on a regular or irregular basis. Palpitations, defined as an awareness of the heartbeat, are often disagreeable and may arise as often from increased force of contraction as from rhythm disturbance.
- The impact of an dysrhythmia on the circulation is more important than the

dysrhythmia itself. Dysrhythmias that cause hemodynamic upset are usually sustained bradycardias or tachycardias and may be life-threatening. Light headedness, dizziness, and syncope (usually due to secondary hypotension) are common.

DIAGNOSIS

- Cardiac dysrhythmias may be detected as a change in the rate and/or rhythm of the pulse.
  - A slow pulse may indicate a type of bradycardia, and a fast pulse may indicate a tachydysrhythmia.
- The standard 12-lead electrocardiogram (ECG) remains the principal method for diagnosing dysrhythmias.
  - For paroxysmal or episodic dysrhythmias, 24-hour ambulatory (Holter) ECG monitoring is the most effective method of recording dysrhythmic events, and its value is enhanced by having the patient keep a diary of any associated symptoms.

MEDICAL MANAGEMENT & TREATMENT

- The medical management of cardiac dysrhythmias includes drugs, pacemakers, radiofrequency catheter ablation, cardioversion, and defibrillation.
  - Benign dysrhythmias with no hemodynamic consequence usually require no therapy.
- Antidysrhythmic drug therapy is the mainstay of management for most dysrhythmias.
- Patients who do not respond to antidysrhythmic drug therapy may be candidates for nonpharmacologic intervention (i.e., pacemakers, radiofrequency catheter ablation, or cardioversion). However in some circumstances nonpharmacologic intervention may represent firstline therapy for certain types of dysrhythmia.
  - For example, cardioversion or defibrillation is indicated for any tachydysrhythmias that compromise hemodynamics and/or life; cardiac arrest is also treated by cardioversion.

ANTIDYSRHYTHMIC DRUGS

- The drugs used in the treatment of cardiac dysrhythmias are not easily classified because they often have more than one action. In addition, the drugs within each class vary in their individual magnitude of action or types of effects produced.
  - The Vaughan Williams classification of antidysrhythmic drugs (based on their electrophysiologic effects) has been used for over three decades (see Table I-5).

- There is no universally effective antidysrhythmic drug, and the type of dysrhythmia is a major factor in the selection of an antidysrhythmic drug.
  - Antidysrhythmic drug selection is difficult and often involves trial and error.
  - Various types of dysrhythmias and the degrees of severity will be affected differently with different drugs.
  - All antidysrhythmic drugs have important safety limitations and can worsen or promote dysrhythmias.
- The molecular targets for optimal action of the antidysrhythmic drugs involve channels in the cellular membranes through which ions (Na^+, Ca^{++}, and K^+) are diffused rapidly. With many antidysrhythmic drugs, the toxic/therapeutic ratio is very narrow; therefore, the dosage for a given patient must be individualized. Measurement of the plasma level of the medication is often an important part of therapy.
- Patients with dysrhythmias treated with digitalis are susceptible to digitalis toxicity, especially if they are elderly or have hypothyroidism, renal dysfunction, dehydration, hypokalemia, hypomagnesemia, or hypocalcemia.
- Patients with atrial fibrillation often are prescribed warfarin sodium (Coumadin) to prevent atrial thrombosis.

PACEMAKERS

- Over one million persons in the United States have permanent pacemakers. About 115,000 pacemakers are inserted each year in this country.
- Pacemakers are useful in the management of several conduction system abnormalities including symptomatic sinus bradycardia, symptomatic AV block, and tachydysrhythmias refractory to drug therapy.
- The most common pacing system in use today is the demand ventricular pacemaker with a lithium-powered generator and transvenous leads. Newer units contain pacing circuits that allow for programming, memory, and telemetry.
- Some side-effects can result:
  - Infection at the generator site and thrombosis of the leads or electrodes are uncommon but can occur.
  - Skeletal muscle may be stimulated if insulation is lost around the lead or the generator rotates. In rare cases, myocardial burning can occur.
  - Infective endocarditis secondary to a pacemaker may occur but is rare.
  - Some patients become depressed; suicide attempts have been reported.
- Electromagnetic and RF interference from noncardiac electrical signals may interfere temporarily with the function of a pacemaker. This occurs by a mimicking of the frequency of spontaneous

heartbeats, which causes inappropriate pacemaker inhibition.

- ○ Examples would be transmission from radar antennae, or arc welders.
- ○ Other forms of electrical signals can potentially cause revision of the pacemaker mode to a fixed rate of transmission.
  - ■ These would include microwave ovens, diathermy and electrocautery units, and direct-contact pulse generators in boat or automobile motors.
- Newer design pacemakers have better internal RF shielding and electromagnetic interference-resistant circuitry.

IMPLANTABLE CARDIOVERTER-DEFIBRILLATOR

- Certain patients with ventricular fibrillation or unstable ventricular tachycardias are candidates for an automatic implantable cardioverter-defibrillator (AICD).
- The AICD is a self-contained diagnostic-therapeutic system that monitors the heart, and, when it detects fibrillation or tachycardia of the ventricle, sends a correcting electric shock to restore normal rhythm.
  - ○ By 1996 over 100,000 patients worldwide had had an AICD surgically implanted.
- The AICD is 99% reliable in detecting ventricular fibrillation and 98% reliable in detecting ventricular tachycardias. Its conversion effectiveness is excellent. Usually one 25-joule (J) discharge converts the dysrhythmia.

CARDIOVERSION/DEFIBRILLATION

- Direct-current cardioversion to convert atrial and ventricular dysrhythmias refers to an electrical energy discharge that is synchronized with the large R or S wave of the QRS complex.
  - ○ Synchronization in the early part of the QRS complex avoids energy delivery in the early phase of repolarization when ventricular fibrillation can be easily induced.
- The most common dysrhythmias treated by cardioversion are reentrant dysrhythmias such as atrial flutter, atrial fibrillation, and ventricular tachycardia.
  - ○ Cardioversion of atrial fibrillation or atrial flutter is usually performed on an elective basis, while cardioversion of ventricular tachycardia may be elective or emergent depending on the patient's hemodynamic status.
  - ○ Elective cardioversion is performed under general anesthesia or intravenous sedation.
  - ○ Typical recommended initial energy levels for cardioversion are 50 J for atrial flutter, 100 J for atrial fibrillation and monomorphic ventricular tachycardia, and 200 J for polymorphic ventricular tachycardia.
  - ○ Stepwise increases in energy are used if the initial shock fails to restore normal sinus rhythm.
- Defibrillation refers to an unsynchronized discharge of energy only recommended for ventricular fibrillation. The countershock simultaneously depolarizes the entire myocardium, allowing synchronous repolarization and resumption of normal sinus rhythm.
  - ○ Treatment of ventricular fibrillation always is emergent, and a 200 J shock should be delivered as quickly as possible, followed by one or more 360 J shocks if the initial shock is unsuccessful (i.e., normal sinus rhythm is not established).
  - ○ Cardiopulmonary resuscitation must be used until defibrillation has been successful.

RADIOFREQUENCY CATHETER ABLATION

- Radiofrequency (RF) ablation is a percutaneous catheter technique that can permanently eliminate a variety of dysrhythmias that previously required either chronic pharmacologic treatment for suppression or surgery for cure.
  - ○ It has become the primary modality of therapy for many symptomatic supraventricular dysrhythmias, including atrioventricular nodal reentry tachycardia, reentry tachycardias involving accessory pathways, paroxysmal atrial tachycardia, inappropriate sinus tachycardia, and automatic junctional tachycardia.
- The RF ablation procedure is performed in the cardiac catheterization laboratory as part of diagnostic electrophysiologic testing.
  - ○ Once the diagnosis is made and the abnormal pathway or focus integrally related to the onset and/or maintenance of the dysrhythmia is located precisely, RF energy is delivered through an electrode catheter whose tip is in contact with the target endocardium. This results in resistive heating of the tissue and production of a homogenous hemispheric lesion of coagulative necrosis 3 to 5 mm in radius. If properly placed, such a

TABLE I-5 Vaughan Williams Classification and Action of Antidysrhythmic Drugs

Antiarrhythmic Drug Class	Examples	Primary Antiarrhythmic Action
Ia	Disopyramide Procainamide Quinidine	Medium* sodium channel blockers: • Depress depolarization • Slow conduction velocity • Prolong repolarization
Ib	Lidocaine Mexiletine Phenytoin Tocainide	Fast* sodium channel blockers: • Slow conduction velocity • Shorten repolarization
Ic	Flecainide Moricizine Propafenone	Slow* sodium channel blockers: • Depress repolarization • Slow conduction velocity • Prolong the refractory period
II	Acebutolol Atenolol Metoprolol Propranolol Timolol	β-Adrenergic antagonists: • Decrease atrioventricular node conduction • Decrease automaticity
III	Amiodarone Bretylium Ibutilide Sotalol	Potassium channel blockers: • Prolong repolarization • Decrease automaticity • Decrease conduction • Prolong the refractory period
IV	Bepridil Diltiazem Nifedipine Verapamil	Calcium channel antagonists: • Decrease automaticity • Decrease atrioventricular node conduction • Prolong the refractory period
V (Miscellaneous)	Adenosine Digoxin	*Varies with the specific drug* Adenosine: increases potassium conductance, decreases calcium channel activity, reduces automaticity in the SA node Digoxin: inhibits cardiac sodium-potassium pump and ATPase, decreases automaticity of atrial and junctional pacemakers, prolongs refractory period at the AV node

* The terms *slow*, *medium*, and *fast* refer to the rates of onset of, and recovery from, sodium channel blockade.

lesion may interrupt conduction in an accessory pathway, or eliminate an automatic ectopic focus.

COMPLICATIONS

- Dysrhythmias may be asymptomatic and cause no hemodynamic changes. However, some can affect cardiac output by:
  - Producing insufficient forward flow because of a slow cardiac rate;
  - Reducing forward flow because of insufficient diastolic filling time with a rapid cardiac rate; or
  - Decreasing flow because of poor sequence in AV activation with direct effects on ventricular function.
- The importance of atrial fibrillation as a cause of stroke (due to the formation, and subsequent embolization, of atrial thrombi) is well known. Overall, approximately 15% to 25% of all strokes in the United States (approximately 75,000 per year) can be attributed to atrial fibrillation.

PROGNOSIS

- Primarily dependent on the specific type and severity of the dysrhythmia, as well as any underlying contributory and/or resultant cardiovascular or systemic pathology.
  - Some dysrhythmias cause few or no symptoms but are associated with an adverse prognosis. Others, though symptomatic, are benign.
  - The nature and severity of underlying heart disease is often of greater prognostic significance than is the dysrhythmia itself.
- The effect of a dysrhythmia often is dependent on the physical condition of the patient. For example, a young healthy person with paroxysmal atrial tachycardia may have minimal symptoms, whereas an elderly patient with heart disease with the same dysrhythmia may develop shock, congestive heart failure, or myocardial ischemia. Presence of heart failure can have a dramatic impact on the risk for cardiac arrest.
  - The presence of New York Heart Association (NYHA) grade III or IV congestive heart failure and a low ejection fraction is a predictor of arrhythmic death/cardiac arrest.
  - For every 5% reduction in left ventricular ejection fraction the risk of cardiac arrest/dysrhythmic death increases by 15%.
- Much evidence suggests that prognosis is not necessarily improved treatment/suppression of the dysrhythmia.
  - In some cases, antidysrhythmic drugs appear to contribute to increased mortality.

DENTAL SIGNIFICANCE

- Patients with certain types of cardiac dysrhythmias (i.e., atrial fibrillation) may be more susceptible to ischemic events in the dental office when overly stressed or given excessive amounts of a local anesthetic containing a vasoconstrictor.
- Patients may have their dysrhythmia under control through the use of drugs or a pacemaker but may require special consideration when receiving dental treatment because of the potential increased risks for myocardial infarction, heart failure, and death.
- The severity of a given dysrhythmia may depend on the health of the patient; the patient's age; and the presence of conditions such as severe hypertension, recent myocardial infarction, unstable angina, untreated hyperthyroidism, or congestive heart failure.
- The keys to the dental management of patients susceptible to developing a cardiac dysrhythmia and those with an existing dysrhythmia are in identification and prevention. The identification of patients with an existing dysrhythmia and those susceptible to developing a dysrhythmia is most important.

DENTAL MANAGEMENT

MEDICAL CONSULTATION

- Refer for diagnosis any patient with signs and symptoms suggestive of dysrhythmia:
  - Patients who report experiencing palpitations, dizziness, syncope, angina, or dyspnea should be referred for medical evaluation.
  - Patients who have an irregular cardiac rhythm with or without symptoms should be referred for medical evaluation.
    - Several studies have documented the benefit of the use of a 3-lead ECG unit to screen dental patients for dysrhythmias.
  - Elderly patients with a regular heart rate that varies in intensity with respiration should be referred for an evaluation of possible sinus dysrhythmias and sinus node disease.
- Establish presence and status of any condition that may cause dysrhythmia:
  - Patients with a history of significant heart disease, thyroid disease, or chronic pulmonary disease must be identified and their medical status determined. If their status is uncertain, a medical consultation should be obtained to accurately determine their current status and risk for developing a cardiac dysrhythmia.
  - Patients with underlying cardiac disease must be managed as indicated

by the nature of the underlying cardiac problem (e.g., those susceptible to endocarditis, ischemic heart disease, congestive heart failure, hypertrophic cardiomyopathy).
- Establish the type and severity of the dysrhythmia:
  - Patients with high-risk dysrhythmia (e.g., high-grade atrioventricular block, symptomatic [ventricular] dysrhythmias in the presence of underlying heart disease, supraventricular dysrhythmias with uncontrolled ventricular rate) may not be candidates for elective dental care.
- Establish current status for patient with dysrhythmia
- Determine the method(s) of treatment of the dysrhythmia (e.g., medications, pacemaker or AICD):
  - For patients with pacemakers, determine:
    - Type of dysrhythmia being managed
    - Type of pacemaker being used
    - Degree of shielding provided for the pacemaker
    - Types of electrical equipment that should be avoided
  - Recognize anticoagulant therapy (patients with certain dysrhythmias [e.g., atrial fibrillation] may be receiving anticoagulant therapy with warfarin sodium [Coumadin] to prevent atrial thrombosis):
    - If patient is receiving anticoagulant therapy with warfarin sodium (Coumadin), determine International Normalized Ratio (INR) level if a surgical procedure is planned.
    - Determine whether dosage of warfarin sodium (Coumadin) needs to be adjusted before surgery.
      - Most dental surgeries can be performed if INR is 3.5 or less (see Appendix A, Box A-5, "Dental Management of Patients Taking Coumarin Anticoagulants").

PATIENT MANAGEMENT

- Minimize stressful situations; any increase in sympathetic tone can precipitate a dysrhythmia:
  - Patients with significant dysrhythmias, coronary atherosclerotic heart disease, ischemic heart disease, or congestive heart failure should be managed with short morning appointments; furthermore, the session should be terminated if the patient becomes fatigued, to prevent or minimize acute exacerbation of conditions that might trigger significant dysrhythmias.
  - Complex dental procedures can be performed at several appointments to reduce the stress to the patient.
  - Premedication with a short-acting benzodiazepine (e.g., triazolam 0.25-0.5 mg) the night before the

appointment or 1 hour before the appointment, or both, may be helpful to reduce anxiety.

- Nitrous oxide–oxygen inhalation sedation can also be used during dental treatment.
- An open, honest approach with the patient (i.e., explaining what will happen) is also important in minimizing patient anxiety.

- Periodic or continuous automated monitoring of the patient's pulse rate or rhythm and blood pressure during dental treatment is advantageous.
  - If the patient has a significant change in pulse rate or rhythm during treatment, discontinue treatment and reschedule.

Manage underlying condition(s) that may be contributory to (e.g., ischemic heart disease, hypertension, valvular heart disease), or secondary to (e.g., congestive heart failure), the dysrhythmia:

- Certain cardiac conditions that predispose a person to the development of some dysrhythmias (e.g., atrial fibrillation) may require antibiotic prophylaxis for the prevention of bacterial endocarditis prior to invasive (bacteremia-inducing) dental treatment (see Appendix A, Box A-1, "Antibiotic Prophylaxis Recommendations by the American Heart Association for the Prevention of Bacterial Endocarditis").
  - These conditions include rheumatic heart disease, hypertrophic cardiomyopathy, and mitral valve prolapse and mitral valve annular calcifications when evidence of mitral regurgitation or demonstrated mitral insufficiency is documented.

ANESTHESIA CONSIDERATIONS

- Excessive amounts of epinephrine can trigger a dysrhythmia or other adverse cardiovascular event. At the same time, however, vasoconstrictors in appropriate concentration in the local anesthetic are beneficial. The need to achieve profound local anesthesia and hemostasis far outweighs the very slight risk of using these agents in small amounts (not more than 0.04 mg) of epinephrine (see Appendix A, Box A-3, "Local Anesthetic with Vasoconstrictor Dose Restriction Guidelines").
  - Use local anesthetic without epinephrine in patients with severe dysrhythmias (including high-grade atrioventricular block, symptomatic [ventricular] dysrhythmias in the presence of underlying heart disease, and supraventricular dysrhythmias with uncontrolled ventricular rate), if dental treatment is necessary.
- Caution should be exercised when local anesthetics containing vasoconstrictors are used in patients taking digitalis because of an increased risk of precipitating a dysrhythmia.

- Avoid use of general anesthesia
  - Patients at risk for developing significant cardiac dysrhythmias and those with significant dysrhythmias should not be given general anesthesia in the dental office because of the increased risk of myocardial infarction, congestive heart failure, or death.

PRECAUTIONS FOR PATIENTS WITH PACEMAKERS

- Internal radiofrequency (RF) shielding and electromagnetic interference-resistant circuitry of newer design pacemakers have all but removed the risk that automobile distributors, radar antennae, microwave devices, and airport security detectors once had in suppressing pacemaker function. Some electronic devices may, however, still interfere with pacemaker function.
- Miller et al. demonstrated that the only devices causing significant RF/electromagnetic interference with pacemakers in the dental office were electrosurgery units, ultrasonic bath cleaners, and ultrasonic scaling devices.
  - Amalgamators, electric pulp testers, curing lights, handpieces, electric toothbrushes, microwave ovens, x-ray units, and sonic scalers did not cause any significant electromagnetic interference with pacemakers in the dental office.
- Patients with new, well-shielded generators are at low risk for RF/electromagnetic interference. However, patients with older pacemakers with poor shielding may be at higher risk for complications in pacing because of RF/electromagnetic interference.
  - Studies have identified certain types of equipment that may be safe, but pulp testers, motorized dental chairs, and belt-driven handpieces all may be capable of causing pacemaker malfunction in a patient with poor shielding in the pacemaker generator.
  - Electrosurgery units, ultrasonic bath cleaners, and ultrasonic scaling devices can be of risk to all patients with pacemakers; use in or near these patients is contraindicated.
- The American Heart Association (AHA) does not recommend antibiotic prophylaxis prior to invasive (i.e., bacteremia-inducing) dental procedures for patients with an implanted cardiac pacemaker or an AICD.

PRECAUTIONS FOR PATIENTS TAKING DIGITALIS

- Therapeutic doses of digitalis range from 0.5 to 2.0 ng/mL. Levels greater than 2.5 ng/mL may result in digitalis toxicity.
  - Patients with dysrhythmias treated with digitalis may be susceptible to digitalis toxicity if they are elderly, or have hypothyroidism, renal dysfunc-

tion, dehydration, hypokalemia, hypomagnesemia, or hypocalcemia.
  - Patients with electrolyte imbalances are more susceptible to digitalis toxicity because of the heightened sensitivity of the heart to these changes accompanying certain dysrhythmias.

- Patients should be assessed in light of the signs and symptoms of digitalis toxicity, which are found in three systems: gastrointestinal (e.g., anorexia, excessive salivation, nausea, vomiting, diarrhea), neurologic (e.g., headache, visual disturbances, fatigue, drowsiness), and cardiovascular (e.g., AV block, excessive slowing of the heart, ventricular extrasystoles, other dysrhythmias).
- Dentists should avoid using erythromycin because it can increase the absorption of digitalis by altering the intestinal flora and lead to toxicity.

SUGGESTED REFERENCES

Campbell JH, Huizinga PJ, Das SK, Rodriguez JP, Gobetti JP. Incidence and significance of cardiac arrhythmia in geriatric oral surgery patients. *Oral Surg Oral Med Oral Pathol Oral Radiol Endo* 1996;82(1):42–46.

Defibrillator/monitor/pacemakers. *Health Devices* 2002;31(2):45–64.

Dubernet J, Chamorro G, Gonzalez J, Fajuri A, Jalil J, Casanegra P, et al. A 36 year experience with implantable pacemakers. A historical analysis. *Rev Med Chil* 2002;130(2): 132–142.

Little JW, Falace DA, Miller CS, Rhodus NL. Cardiac Arrhythmias. *Dental Management of the Medically Compromised Patient*, ed 6. St Louis, Mosby, 2002, pp 94–113.

Miller, CS, Leonelli FM, Latham E. Selective interference with pacemaker activity by electrical dental devices. *Oral Surg Oral Med Oral Pathol Oral Radiol Endod* 1998;85:33–36.

Myerberg RJ, Kessler KM, Castellanos A. Recognition, clinical assessment, and management of arrhythmias and conduction disturbances, in Alexander RE, Schlant RC, Fuster V, et al. (eds): *Hurst's The Heart, Arteries, and Veins*, ed 9. New York, McGraw-Hill, 1998, pp 873–942.

Rhodus NL, Little JW. Dental management of the patient with cardiac arrhythmias: an update. *Oral Surg Oral Med Oral Pathol Oral Radiol Endod* 2003;96:659–668.

Stevenson WG, Ellison KE, Sweeney MO, Epstein LM, Maisel WH. Management of arrhythmias in heart failure. *Cardiol Rev* 2002;10(1):8–14.

Wellens HJ. Future of device therapy for arrhythmias. *J Cardiovasc Electrophysiol* 2002;13(1 Suppl):S122–S124.

AUTHORS: **NELSON L. RHODUS, DMD, MPH; F. JOHN FIRRIOLO, DDS, PHD**

SYNONYM(S)

Cardiac septal defects
Septal defect
Atrioventricular septal defects

ICD-9CM/CPT CODE(S)

429.71 Acquired cardiac septal defects
745 Bulbus cordis anomalies and anomalies of cardiac septal closure—incomplete
745.2 Tetralogy of Fallot—complete
745.4 Ventricular septal defect
745.5 Ostium secundum type atrial septal defect—complete
745.9 Unspecified defect of septal closure

OVERVIEW

Defects in the cardiac septa are a broad category of heart diseases, resulting in abnormal communications between opposite chambers of the heart. The most common cardiac septal defects are atrial septal defect (ASD) and ventricular septal defect (VSD).

- An ASD is a deficiency of the atrial septum. It is the most common congenital cardiac lesion presenting in adults.
  - The ostium secundum ASD, accounting for approximately 90% of all ASDs, is a defect located at and resulting from a deficient or fenestrated oval fossa (fossa ovale).
  - Ostium primum anomalies (5% of ASDs) occur adjacent to the atrioventricular (AV) valves and are usually associated with a cleft anterior mitral leaflet. This combination is known as a partial AV septal defect.
  - Sinus venosus defects (5% of ASDs) are located near the entrance of the superior vena cava. They are commonly accompanied by anomalous connections of right pulmonary veins to the superior vena cava or right atrium.
- VSD is a developmental defect of the interventricular septum whereby a communication exists between the cavities of the two ventricles.
- VSDs occur as a primary anomaly with or without additional major associated cardiac defects.
- For anatomic classification of VSDs, the interventricular septum can be divided into four regions.
  - Membranous septum (or infracristal) defects: 75–80% of VSDs; located in a small, translucent area beneath the aortic valve.
  - Canal (or inlet) defects: approximately 8% of VSDs; occur at the crux of the heart between the tricuspid and mitral valves; usually associated with other anomalies of the AV canal.
  - Trabecular or muscular septum defects: 5–20% of VSDs; occur distal to the septal attachment of the tricuspid valve and toward the apex; single or multiple, small or large.
  - Subarterial (or infundibular, or supracristal outlet) defects: 5?% of VSDs; occur in the conal septum above the crista supraventricularis and below the pulmonary valve.
- VSDs may occur as a single component of a wide variety of intracardiac anomalies: tetralogy of Fallot, complete AV canal defects, transposition of great arteries, and corrected transpositions.

EPIDEMIOLOGY & DEMOGRAPHICS

ATRIAL SEPTAL DEFECT

INCIDENCE/PREVALENCE IN USA: ASDs account for about 10–15% of all congenital cardiac anomalies and are the most common congenital cardiac lesion presenting in adults. No racial predilection is known.

PREDOMINANT AGE: ASDs are congenital lesions present at birth. The age at presentation depends on the size of the left-to-right shunt. ASDs in infancy are usually asymptomatic and are detected as a murmur on physical examination.

PREDOMINANT SEX: The female:male ratio is 2:1. No difference in outcome is associated with sex.

GENETICS (FOR ASD AND VSD): Cardiac septal defects occur as a clinical feature of several different syndromes, as autosomal dominant defects, and as sporadically occurring malformations. Consequently, it is clear that there is genetic heterogeneity but, until recently, little else was known about the genes involved in the pathogenesis. Cardiac septal defect is most often found associated with trisomy 21 (Down syndrome), but the responsible gene or genes on chromosome 21 have not been identified. Cardiac septal defect not associated with trisomy 21 usually occurs as a sporadic trait with no indication of the genetic basis. The discovery of cysteine with damage units is the first recognized genetic risk factor for cardiac septal defects, providing new insight into the genetic basis.

VENTRICULAR SEPTAL DEFECTS

INCIDENCE/PREVALENCE IN USA: VSDs occur in approximately 2 to 6 of every 1000 live births and constitutes over 20% of all congenital heart diseases. VSDs are the most common congenital heart defect encountered after bicuspid aortic valve.

PREDOMINANT AGE: VSDs are congenital lesions present at birth. The age at presentation depends on the size of the left-to-right shunt. Ventricular septal defects in infancy are usually asymptomatic and are detected as a murmur on physical examination.

PREDOMINANT SEX: VSDs are slightly more common in females; 44% occur in males, and 56% occur in females. Incidence of ectomesenchymal tissue migration abnormalities (i.e., subarterial type I VSD) is highest in boys.

ETIOLOGY & PATHOGENESIS

ATRIAL SEPTAL DEFECTS

- Abnormality occurs during embryonic development.
- ASDs occur as associated anomalies in many major complex congenital lesions, but sinus venous atrial septal defect usually occurs as an isolated abnormality.
- Other abnormalities may exacerbate ASDs. For example, systemic hypertension in an adult (mitral stenosis, which is either congenital or acquired) may also exacerbate the atrial level left-to-right shunt.

VENTRICULAR SEPTAL DEFECTS

- Maternal factors: maternal diabetes, maternal phenylketonuria, and maternal alcohol consumption and fetal alcohol syndrome
- Genetic syndromes associated with VSD (Table 1-6).

TABLE 1-6 Genetic Syndromes Associated with Congenital Cardiac Malformations

Syndrome	Congenital Cardiac Malformation Type
Del 4q, 21, 32	Ventricular septal defect (VSD), atrial septal defect (ASD)
Del 5p	VSD
Trisomy 13	ASD, VSD, Tetralogy of Fallot (TOF)
Trisomy 18 Edwards	VSD, TOF, double-outlet right ventricle (DORV)
Trisomy 21 Down	VSD, atrioventricular canal (AVC)
Del 22q 11 DiGeorge (single gene etiology, autosomal dominant)	Truncus arteriosus, TOF, VSD

CLINICAL PRESENTATION / PHYSICAL FINDINGS

ATRIAL SEPTAL DEFECTS

ASDs are usually diagnosed upon detection of a murmur in an asymptomatic patient during a routine physical exam. Symptoms are usually associated with the size of the shunt. Dyspnea usually indicates a relatively large shunt.

Physical Exam

- A cardiac murmur secondary to increased pulmonary artery blood flow is heard over the left sternal border.
- The second heart sound is widely split and may be fixed or may vary little with respiration.
- Patients with atrial septal defects may present with a *gracile habitus*. These patients are thin for their height.

VENTRICULAR SEPTAL DEFECTS

Symptoms and physical findings relate to the size of the VSD and the magnitude of the left-to-right shunt. Infants with small defects will present with mild or no symptoms. Feeding or weight gain is usually not affected. In infants with moderate defects, symptoms include tachypnea with increased respiratory effort.

Physical Exam
Physical findings are primarily those of a cardiac examination in a patient with small defects. Infants with small defects will present with normal vital signs and a characteristic murmur. The bigger the defect, the more prominent the signs will be; cyanosis is a sign of a severe defect. Hemoptysis occurs in 33% of patients (never in patients < 24 years of age); it occurs in 100% of patients by age 40 and contributes to cause of death.

DIAGNOSIS

ATRIAL SEPTAL DEFECTS AND VENTRICULAR SEPTAL DEFECTS

Lab Studies
- General laboratory studies are rarely helpful.

Imaging Studies
- Chest radiograph:
  - ASD: cardiomegaly, enlargement of right atrium and ventricle, increased pulmonary vascularity, small aortic knob
  - VSD: cardiomegaly resulting from volume overload directly related to the magnitude of the shunt.
- Two-dimensional echo and color Doppler: usually is sufficient for diagnosis in younger patients and is the noninvasive diagnostic modality of choice to assess the defect and the presence of and degree of shunting.

Other Tests
- Electrocardiogram: right ventricular hypertrophy predominates.
- Cardiac catheterization usually is not required in the preoperative assessment of patients with cardiac septal defects, but it may be considered in special circumstances.

MEDICAL MANAGEMENT & TREATMENT

ATRIAL SEPTAL DEFECTS
Medical Treatment
- Medical care primarily is supportive and is not required for asymptomatic patients.
- Patients presenting in heart failure should be stabilized in anticipation of elective repair.

Surgical Treatment
- Surgical correction is the most important therapy.
  - Asymptomatic children generally undergo repair at ages 3 to 5 years.
  - Sinus venous defects (10% of all ASDs) do not close spontaneously.

VENTRICULAR SEPTAL DEFECTS
Medical Treatment
- Children with small VSDs are asymptomatic and have excellent long-term prognoses. Neither medical therapy nor surgical therapy is indicated.
- In children with moderate or large VSDs, a trial of medical therapy, including furosemide, captopril, and digoxin, is indicated for symptomatic congestive heart failure because many VSDs may get smaller with time.

Surgical Treatment
- Indications for surgical repair:
  - Uncontrolled congestive heart failure, including growth failure and recurrent respiratory infection is an indication for surgical repair
  - Asymptomatic large defects associated with elevated pulmonary artery pressure

COMPLICATIONS

ATRIAL SEPTAL DEFECTS
Common complications of ASDs:
- Sinus node dysfunction
- Pulmonary venous obstruction
- Atrial fibrillation or atrial flutter
- Pulmonary hypertension
- Congestive heart failure
- Pericardial effusion

VENTRICULAR SEPTAL DEFECTS
- Eisenmenger complex is the most severe complication. Fixed and irreversible pulmonary hypertension develops, resulting in reversal of the left-to-right shunt to a right-to-left shunt.
- Secondary aortic insufficiency.
- Right ventricular outflow tract obstruction.
- Infective endocarditis:
  - Infective endocarditis is rare in children younger than 2 years of age.
  - Infection is usually located at the ridge of the VSD itself or the tricuspid leaflet.

PROGNOSIS

ATRIAL SEPTAL DEFECTS
- Treated: Surgical repair in the first two decades of life is associated with a mortality rate near zero. Life expectancy approaches that of the general population if the defect is repaired during this time. Cardiac size rapidly regresses after surgery and the functional result is excellent. In cases of repair during adulthood, the life expectancy is decreased even if the lesion is repaired successfully.
- Untreated: Untreated ASDs are associated with a significantly shortened life expectancy. After age 20, the mortality rate is approximately 5% per decade with 90% of patients dead by age 60. Late problems in untreated patients also include the risk of paradoxical embolus as well as atrial fibrillation, pulmonary hypertension, and right heart failure.

VENTRICULAR SEPTAL DEFECTS
- The current surgical mortality rate is 3% for single VSD repair and 5% for multiple ventricular septal repairs.
- Children with a small VSD are asymptomatic and have excellent long-term prognoses:
  - Many infants improve, showing evidence of a gradual decrease in the magnitude of the left-to-right shunt at ages 6 to 24 months.
  - Most children with VSD remain stable or improve following infancy.
  - A small number of patients who have developed severe pulmonary vascular obstructive disease with predominant right-to-left shunts (Eisenmenger syndrome) at the time of referral require symptomatic therapy.

DENTAL SIGNIFICANCE

- Infective endocarditis (IE) occurs most frequently on or close to a congenital or acquired cardiac septal defect. The defect produces an alteration in the blood flow, resulting in turbulence. IE tends to develop in areas of blood flow turbulence.
- The American Heart Association has identified conditions that pose a risk for development of IE and provides guidelines for antibiotic prophylaxis.
  - IE is rare in patients with an unrepaired ASD; therefore, IE antibiotic prophylaxis is not required for an unrepaired ostium secundum (fossa ovalis) ASD.

SECTION I

- Some cardiac septal defects are classified as moderate risk conditions for IE.
  - The risk of IE in patients with an uncomplicated, unrepaired VSD is between 4% and 10% for the first 30 years of life.
    - All patients with unrepaired VSD require IE antibiotic prophylaxis.
  - Patients with surgically repaired ASD or VSD do not require IE antibiotic prophylaxis if:
    - More than 6 months have passed since the repair; *and*
    - no residual shunting or hemodynamic abnormality exists; *and*
    - no intracardiac prosthetic implant (if used) is exposed in the circulation.

DENTAL MANAGEMENT

As noted previously, patients with some cardiac septal defects without repair or some surgically repaired cardiac septal defects are considered as a moderate-risk condition for IE and require antibiotic prophylaxis prior to bacteremia-inducing dental procedures, according to the AHA recommendations (see Appendix A, Box A-1, "Antibiotic Prophylaxis Recommendations by the American Heart Association for the Prevention of Bacterial Endocarditis").

- If there is any question as to the need for antibiotic prophylaxis in a dental patient with a history of cardiac septal defect (or its subsequent surgical repair), the dentist should consult the patient's physician (preferably their cardiologist).

SUGGESTED REFERENCES

Anderson RH, et al. Normal and abnormal structure of the vetriculo-arterial junctions. *Cardiology Young* 2005; (Feb)(15 Suppl 1):3–16.

Little J, Falace D, Miller C, Rhodus N. Cardiac conditions associated with endocarditis, in *Dental Management of the Medically Compromised Patient*. St Louis, Mosby, 2002, p 56.

Maslen CL. Molecular genetics of atrioventricular septal defects. *Current Opinion Cardiology* 2004;19:205.

Quaegebeur JM, et al. Surgery for atrioventricular septal defects. *Advanced Cardiology* 2004;41:127

Smith P. Primary care in children with congenital heart disease. *Journal Paediatric Nursing* 2001;16:305.

AUTHOR: **JUAN F. YEPES, DDS, MD**

SYNONYM(S)

Aortic stenosis
Aortic insufficiency
Mitral stenosis
Mitral insufficiency

ICD-9CM/CPT CODE(S)

394.0 Mitral stenosis
394.2 Mitral stenosis with insufficiency
395.0 Rheumatic aortic stenosis
396.0 Mitral valve stenosis and aortic valve stenosis
396.1 Mitral valve stenosis and aortic valve insufficiency
424.0 Mitral valve disorders
424.1 Aortic valve disorders
746.3 Congenital stenosis of aortic valve
746.5 Congenital mitral stenosis
758.2 Undiagnosed cardiac murmur

OVERVIEW

Cardiac valvular disease includes different congenital and acquired disorders involving the normal function of the cardiac valves. To control the flow of blood, all valves have thin flaps of muscle tissue that open to let the blood through and close to prevent it from flowing backward. The mitral and the aortic valve are the most common sites of heart valve disease because of their location on the left side of the heart. The left chambers have a greater workload because they pump blood to the entire body; conversely, the right chambers send blood to the lungs with less pressure.

Two major problems may arise in the functioning of the valves: they may fail either to open fully or to close properly. The narrowing of the valve, called stenosis, occurs when the leaflets become rigid, thickened, or fused together, reducing the opening through which the blood passes from one chamber to another. When the valve fails to close properly, a condition referred to as insufficiency and also called incompetence or regurgitation, a portion of the ejected blood flows backward. In some cases, stenosis and insufficiency may occur together. This happens when the leaflets become shrunken and stiff and the valve is fixed in a half-open position.

EPIDEMIOLOGY & DEMOGRAPHICS

INCIDENCE/PREVALENCE IN USA:

- The prevalence of mitral stenosis has decreased because of the decline in the occurrence of rheumatic fever in the U.S. and developed countries. The mitral valve is the most commonly affected valve in patients with rheumatic heart disease.
- Mitral valve prolapse is the most common type of cardiac valvular defect. This condition affects between 5% and 10% of the population in the U.S.
- Aortic insufficiency can be found in up to 10% of elderly persons in the U.S.
- Mitral insufficiency affects approximately 5 in 10,000 people. Mitral valve disease is the second most common valvular lesion, preceded only by aortic stenosis (AS).
- Aortic stenosis is a relatively common congenital cardiac defect. Incidence is 4 in 1000 live births.

PREDOMINANT AGE:

- Mitral valve prolapse tends to be more often seen in adolescents and young adults.
- The onset of symptoms in mitral stenosis usually is between the third and fourth decades of life.
- Significant aortic regurgitation can be found in patients of any age; however, the age at which aortic regurgitation becomes clinically significant varies based on etiology. Patients with Marfan's disease (see "Marfan's Syndrome" in Section I, p 136) and those with bicuspid aortic valve problems tend to present earlier in life and generally are free of disability from left ventricular dysfunction at the time of presentation. If left untreated, significant cardiac symptoms commonly appear in the fifth decade of life and beyond, usually after considerable cardiomegaly and myocardial dysfunction have occurred.
- Mitral insufficiency is associated with advanced age.
- Aortic stenosis usually is not detected until individuals are school-age. Aortic stenosis exists in up to 2% of persons who are younger than 70 years.

PREDOMINANT SEX:

- Mitral valve prolapse is more common in women than in men.
- Mitral stenosis is most common in women. Two-thirds of all patients with this condition are female.
- Aortic insufficiency can be found in men and women equally.
- Mitral insufficiency is independently associated with the female sex.
- Among children, 75% of cases of AS are in males.

ETIOLOGY & PATHOGENESIS

Multiple causes lead to cardiac valvular disease. The most relevant are:

RHEUMATIC FEVER

Although the incidence of rheumatic fever has decreased, it is still an important etiology of cardiac valvular disease, especially in migrant populations. Rheumatic fever is an inflammatory condition that often starts with a streptococcus throat infection. It can affect any tissue in the body, including the joints, brain, and skin, but most important, it can damage the heart, particularly the valves. Damage is caused by an autoim-

mune response. This condition usually affects children ages 5 to 15 years. There is no specific laboratory test for rheumatic fever. The diagnosis is based on signs and symptoms. Usually, rheumatic heart disease affects 60% of the patients who suffered rheumatic fever, and the heart condition develops years later after the rheumatic fever.

INFECTIVE ENDOCARDITIS

Infective endocarditis is a condition that can lead to cardiac valvular disease. It is an infection of the endocardium and occurs when bacteria, fungi, or other microorganisms multiply on the valves' inner lining and form small nodules of cauliflower-like polyps (vegetations). Endocarditis is twice as common in men as in women, and it seldom occurs in people whose valves are completely normal and healthy. Patients with previous rheumatic fever are at high risk to develop infective endocarditis.

MYXOMATOUS DEGENERATION

In the elderly, one of the most common causes of cardiac valvular disease is a process called myxomatous degeneration, which usually affects the mitral valve. This dysfunction is caused by a series of metabolic changes in the course of which the valve's tissue loses its elasticity and becomes weak and flabby. It is not known what triggers myxomatous degeneration.

CALCIFIC DEGENERATION

This is another common cause of valve disease in the elderly. In this condition, calcium deposits build up on the valves. This type of tissue degeneration usually causes aortic stenosis.

CONGENITAL ABNORMALITIES

The most common congenital defect is a defective aortic valve with two leaflets instead of three, and it is referred to as bicuspid. Congenital malformation may also be present in the mitral valve.

CLINICAL PRESENTATION / PHYSICAL FINDINGS

- Aortic stenosis: obstruction to systolic left ventricular outflow across the aortic valve.
  - Classic triad: dyspnea, angina, and syncope. On the physical exam a systolic murmur that usually radiates to the neck is a common finding.
- Aortic insufficiency (regurgitation, incompetence): retrograde blood flow into the left ventricle from the aorta, secondary to incompetent aortic valve.
  - Left ventricular hypertrophy, signs and symptoms of congestive heart failure, and occasionally angina. On the physical exam a diastolic murmur is characteristic.
- Mitral stenosis: a narrowing of the mitral valve orifice.
  - Symptoms of congestive heart failure (typically include dyspnea, orthopnea,

and paroxysmal nocturnal dyspnea) and a diastolic murmur.

- Mitral valve prolapse: a bulging of one or both mitral valve leaflets into the left atrium during systole.
  - Usually asymptomatic; in the physical exam crisp systolic sound or click and a delayed or late systolic mitral regurgitation murmur upon auscultation.
  - Mitral valve prolapse can progress to mitral regurgitation or insufficiency.
- Mitral insufficiency: retrograde blood flow through the left atrium secondary to an incompetent mitral valve.
  - Symptoms of congestive heart failure and a high-pitched murmur present during the entire systole is typical in the physical exam.
  - Eventually there is an increase in left atrial and pulmonary pressures, which may result in right ventricular failure.

DIAGNOSIS

PHYSICAL EXAM

- Auscultation of the heart: when a valve is damaged and fails to open or close completely, blood will create a swirling current as it is squeezed through a narrow opening or regurgitated in the opposite direction, and a murmur is produced. The characteristics of the murmur and the place during the cardiac cycle (diastolic or systolic) will help in the process of differential diagnosis and certainly will give an idea of the type and severity of the disease.
- Chest radiograph may show abnormalities (enlargement) of the cardiac silhouette and other important radiographic signs of cardiac valvular disease (e.g., valvular calcifications, calcification and/or dilation of the ascending aorta).
- Electrocardiogram: may reveal abnormalities suggestive of cardiac (i.e., atrial and/or ventricular) enlargement, as well as any associated dysrhythmias (e.g., atrial fibrillation).
- Echocardiogram and Doppler echocardiogram: this is usually the gold standard in the diagnosis of cardiac valvular disease. It is a noninvasive technique and is painless.
  - Two-dimensional (2-D) echocardiography may indicate abnormal valvular motion and morphology but usually does not indicate the severity of valvular stenosis or regurgitation, except in mitral stenosis.
  - Doppler echocardiography identifies increased velocity of flow across stenotic valves from which the severity of stenosis may be determined. The presence of an abnormal regurgitant jet on Doppler color flow imaging indicates valvular regurgitation and provides semiquantitative information about its severity.

MEDICAL MANAGEMENT & TREATMENT

- Aortic stenosis: valve replacement is usually curative.
- Aortic insufficiency: aortic valve replacement is curative; if not possible, usually medications that reduce the system pressure are used (e.g., vasodilators, diuretics, digitalis, and ACE inhibitors).
- Mitral stenosis: balloon valvuloplasty, diuretics, and anticoagulants.
- Mitral insufficiency: ACE inhibitors, diuretics, vasodilators, and anticoagulants.
- Mitral regurgitation: treatment is not generally necessary unless symptomatic or progressing to mitral insufficiency.

COMPLICATIONS

- The major complication of cardiac valvular disease is congestive heart failure.
- Cardiac valvular disease can also lead to heart muscle disease (cardiomyopathy) and dysrhythmia.
- Systemic thromboembolization secondary to cardiac valvular disease can lead to several complications including stroke, and renal infarction.

PROGNOSIS

The most severe complications, such as congestive heart failure, usually take 20 to 30 years to develop, and by the time that the patient becomes aware of the symptoms, the condition has often progressed to an advanced stage.

DENTAL SIGNIFICANCE

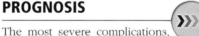

- Medical risk assessment for dental patients with cardiac valvular disease is mainly associated with three situations:
  - Cardiac function (congestive heart failure) and the ability to safely undergo dental treatment (see "Congestive Heart Failure" in Section I, p 62 for additional information).
  - Potential for bleeding problems in patients taking anticoagulant medications [see "Coagulopathies (Clotting Factor Defects, Acquired)" in Section I, p 58 for additional information].
  - Risk for and prevention of infective endocarditis [see "Endocarditis (Infective)" in Section I, p 80 for additional information].
- Cardiac valvular disease can adversely affect cardiac function and place patients at risk for a cardiac emergency (possibly during dental treatment).

- It also important to consider the potential for drug interactions between cardiovascular medications and any medications administered or prescribed in conjunction with dental treatment.

DENTAL MANAGEMENT

- Assessment of the current status and degree of control of the patient's valvular heart disease through a detailed medical history, including signs and symptoms and consultation with the patient's primary physician and/or cardiologist.
- Assessment of hemostasis and risk of prolonged bleeding in patients taking anticoagulant medications [e.g., Coumadin (warfarin)].
- Assessment of the need for antibiotic prophylaxis prior to bacteremia-inducing dental procedures for the prevention of bacterial endocarditis in patients with valvular heart disease.
  - Current American Heart Association guidelines (see Appendix A, Box A-1, "Antibiotic Prophylaxis Recommendations by the American Heart Association for the Prevention of Bacterial Endocarditis") recommend antibiotic prophylaxis (high-risk category) for patients with prosthetic cardiac valves, including bioprosthetic and homograft valves.
  - Current AHA guidelines recommend antibiotic prophylaxis for the following (moderate-risk category) circumstances in patients with valvular heart disease:
    - Most congenital cardiac malformations (e.g., bicuspid aortic valve)
    - Acquired valvar dysfunction (e.g., due to rheumatic heart disease or collagen vascular disease)
    - Mitral valve prolapse (MVP) with valvar regurgitation and/or thickened leaflets:
      - Valve redundancy and thickened leaflets (> 5 mm) as demonstrated by echocardiography.
      - In patients of any age with myxomatous mitral valve degeneration with regurgitation.
      - Men older than 45 years with MVP, without a consistent systolic murmur, may warrant antibiotic prophylaxis even in the absence of resting regurgitation.
      - *Note:* When normal valves prolapse without leaking, as in patients with one or more systolic clicks but no murmurs and no Doppler-demonstrated mitral regurgitation, the risk of endocarditis is not increased above that of the normal population. Antibiotic prophylaxis against bacterial endocarditis is therefore not necessary.

○ If there is any question as to the need for antibiotic prophylaxis for the prevention of bacterial endocarditis in a patient with a history of valvular heart disease, the patient's physician (preferably their cardiologist) should be consulted.

SUGGESTED REFERENCES

Dajani AS, Taubert KA, Wilson W, Bolger AF, Bayer A, Ferrieri P, et al. Prevention of bacterial endocarditis. Recommendations by the American Heart Association. *JAMA*, 1997;277(22):1794–1801.

Little J, Falace D, Miller C, Rhodus N. Cardiac conditions associated with endocarditis, in Little J: *Dental Management of the Medically Compromised Patient*. St Louis, Mosby, 2002, p 56.

Sirois D, et al. Valvular heart disease. *Oral Surg Oral Med Oral Path Oral Radiol Endod* 2001;91:15.

Smith P. Primary care in children with congenital heart disease. *Journal Paediatric Nursing* 2001;16:305.

AUTHOR: **JUAN F. YEPES, DDS, MD**

SYNONYM(S)

Dilated cardiomyopathy:
- Congestive cardiomyopathy

Hypertrophic cardiomyopathy:
- Idiopathic hypertrophic subaortic stenosis (IHSS)
- Hypertrophic obstructive cardiomyopathy (HOCM)

Restrictive cardiomyopathy:
- Obliterative cardiomyopathy

ICD-9CM/CPT CODE(S)

425.1 Hypertrophic obstructive cardiomyopathy—complete
425.4 Other primary cardiomyopathies—complete
425.5 Alcoholic cardiomyopathy—complete
425.7 Nutritional and metabolic cardiomyopathy
425.8 Cardiomyopathy in other diseases classified elsewhere—complete
425.9 Unspecified secondary cardiomyopathy—complete

OVERVIEW

- Cardiomyopathy is a broad term that includes subacute or chronic disorders of the myocardium. It is also used to refer to a group of systemic diseases and processes that are toxic to or alter the myocardium.
- Cardiomyopathies are categorized into three major types:
  - Dilated: Dilated cardiomyopathy (DCM) is the most common form of cardiomyopathy and represents a large subset of congestive heart failure (CHF) cases. DCM is characterized by increased left ventricular or biventricular dimensions with decreased left ventricular ejection fraction in the absence of congenital, coronary, hypertensive, valvular, or pericardial heart disease.
  - Hypertrophic: Hypertrophic cardiomyopathy (HCM) is characterized by marked myocardial hypertrophy not due to other cardiac disease. Thickening of the myocardial walls involves both the atria and the ventricles, although the most characteristic findings involve the left ventricle. The interventricular septum is generally much more massively hypertrophied than the free wall.
  - Restrictive: Restrictive cardiomyopathy (RCM) is the least common of the three major categories of cardiomyopathy and is characterized by restricted filling and diminished diastolic volume of either or both ventricles, with normal or near-normal wall thickness and systolic function.

EPIDEMIOLOGY & DEMOGRAPHICS

INCIDENCE/PREVALENCE IN USA:

- Incidence:
  - DCM: 148 cases per 100,000 persons per year
- Prevalence:
  - DCM: Estimated at 920 cases per 100,000 persons
  - HCM: Estimated at 50 to 200 cases per 100,000 persons
  - RCM: Not established (lower incidence and prevalence than seen in HCM)

PREDOMINANT AGE:

- DCM: Can occur at any age, with half of the patients younger than 65 years.
- HCM: Most commonly presents in the third decade of life, although it may occur throughout the lifespan. Among children, the condition is most likely to present in the second decade.
- RCM: Not established.

PREDOMINANT SEX:

- DCM: Males > females (about 3:1).
- HCM: Slightly more common in males than in females. However, the genetic inheritance pattern is autosomal dominant, without gender predilection.
- RCM: Not established.

GENETICS:

Many cases of cardiomyopathy have a genetic component:
- DCM: Familial inheritance may be responsible for 30–50% of cases of DCM.
- HCM: Up to 90% of cases of HCM are familial, inherited as an autosomal dominant trait with variable penetrance and expressivity.
  - Clinical genetic testing for HCM is becoming available, with significant implications for the physician.
- RCM: Familial inheritance is not characteristic of RCM.

ETIOLOGY & PATHOGENESIS

- The pathogenesis of cardiomyopathy is complex and rests in its categorization. Apoptosis, or programmed cell death, has been reported in clinical and experimental dilated cardiomyopathy, which is characterized by depressed systolic function or systolic pump failure, cardiomegaly, and ventricular dilatation. Reduced left ventricular contractile force leads to decreased cardiac output, resulting in increased residual volumes in end-systole and end-diastole and finally translates in edema. Low cardiac output causes upregulation of the sympathetic nervous system and the renin–angiotensin axis, causing a release of vasopressin and atrial natriuretic peptide. Stimulation of these hormonal tracts results in volume expansion, which induces vasoconstriction and thus further decreases cardiac output.

- Specific etiologies associated with DCM include:
  - Inflammation secondary to infectious disease (e.g., viral, bacterial, fungal, or parasitic infections)
  - Inflammation secondary to noninfectious disease (e.g., collagen vascular disease, transplant rejection)
  - Granulomatous inflammatory disease (e.g., sarcoidosis)
  - Drug or chemical toxicity [e.g., excess alcohol consumption (alcoholic cardiomyopathy)], cocaine, amphetamines, arsenicals, hydrocarbons, chemotherapeutic drugs (e.g., doxorubicin, cyclophosphamide, interferon), heavy metals (e.g., cobalt, lead, mercury)
  - Endocrine disease (e.g., thyroid disease, diabetes, pheochromocytoma, obesity)
  - Metabolic causes [e.g., nutritional deficiencies (thiamine, selenium), electrolyte deficiencies (calcium, phosphate, magnesium)]
  - Genetic disease (e.g., Duchenne's dystrophy, Becker's dystrophy, Friedreich's ataxia, mitochondrial myopathy)
- The specific etiology of HCM remains largely unknown:
  - Up to 90% of cases of HCM are familial and inherited as an autosomal dominant disease and results from any of more than 125 different mutations on at least eight genes, which code for the sarcomeric proteins β-myosin heavy chain, cardiac troponin, T, α-tropomyosin, and myosin-binding C protein genes.
  - A sporadic form of HCM is also recognized and usually occurs in elderly patients.
- RCM may occur idiopathically and is classified as primary or nonobliterative. Obliterative RCM occurs secondary to a number of identifiable etiologies including:
  - Infiltrative disease [e.g., amyloidosis (the most common cause of RCM), sarcoidosis, metastatic carcinoma]
  - Storage disease [e.g., hemochromatosis, mucopolysaccharidosis (Hurler's disease), sphingolipidosis (Fabry's disease, Gaucher's disease), glycogen storage disease (Pompe's disease)]
  - Fibrotic disease (e.g., scleroderma, myocardial fibrosis secondary to radiation)
  - Metabolic disease (e.g., defects in fatty acid metabolism)

CLINICAL PRESENTATION / PHYSICAL FINDINGS

- Table I-7 summarizes some of the significant clinical features of the three major types of cardiomyopathy.

- The severity of the disease, the underlying possible causes, and the type of cardiomyopathy are related to the signs and symptoms. Symptoms are good indicators of the severity of the disease and may include the following:
  - Fatigue
  - Dyspnea on exertion, shortness of breath
  - Orthopnea, paroxismal nocturnal dyspnea
  - Edema
- Medical history, especially the following:
  - Hypertension
  - Angina
  - Coronary artery disease
  - Anemia
  - Thyroid dysfunction
  - Breast cancer
  - Medications
  - Social history (e.g., tobacco, alcohol, illicit drug use)
- On physical examination, signs of heart failure and volume overload are prominent. It is necessary to assess vital signs with specific attention to the following:
  - Tachypnea
  - Tachycardia
  - Hypertension
  - Edema

DIAGNOSIS

A variety of specialized tests are used to diagnose and monitor cardiomyopathy in general. However, depending of the underlying etiology and diagnosis (dilated or restrictive), the exams potentially could be different.

LABORATORY STUDIES
- Cardiac enzymes: help differentiate ischemic heart disease from dilated cardiomyopathy
- Thyroid function tests
- Complete blood count (CBC)
- Urine toxicology screen

DIAGNOSTIC IMAGING
- Chest radiograph
- Echocardiogram: used to help differentiate dilated cardiomyopathy from restrictive and hypertrophic cardiomyopathy

SPECIAL TESTS
- Electrocardiogram: helpful in identifying left ventricular enlargement and estimating the other chamber sizes; it is an important screening tool in differentiating ischemic heart disease from dilated cardiomyopathy.
- Endomyocardial biopsy: may be helpful in diagnosing myocarditis, connective tissue disorders, and amyloidosis.

MEDICAL MANAGEMENT & TREATMENT

Specific therapy according to the underlying disorder must be the final goal of the medical treatment for cardiomyopathies.
  - DCM: The treatment of DCM closely follows that of CHF (see the Medical Management & Treatment section of the Congestive Heart Failure topic for more information).
  - HCM: Beta-blockers (e.g., propranolol) should be the initial drug in symptomatic individuals and is beneficial in resolving dyspnea, angina, and dysrhythmias in about 50% of patients. Calcium channel blockers (e.g., verapamil) have also been effective in the treatment of symptomatic HCM patients. Disopyramide is a useful antidysrhythmic because it is also a negative inotrope. Surgical myotomy-myectomy, or removal of part of the myocardium in the outflow tract, is an option for some patients with symptomatic HCM who are unresponsive to medical therapy.
  - RCM: Treatment of obliterative (secondary) RCM is usually directed at the underlying pathologic process whenever possible (e.g., RCM secondary to sarcoidosis may respond to corticosteroid therapy). There is no effective therapy for idiopathic RCM.

COMPLICATIONS

Complications of cardiomyopathies are directly related with the underlying condition and with the specific type of disease. In a broad overview, the most common complications of cardiomyopathies are:
- Worsening congestive heart failure
- Volume overload: edema
- Pulmonary edema
- Hypoxia
- Cardiogenic shock
- Sudden cardiac death

TABLE I-7 **Characteristics of Symptomatic Primary Cardiomyopathy**

	Dilated (congestive)	Restrictive	Hypertrophic
Ejection fraction (normal > 55%)	< 30%	25–50%	> 60%
Left ventricular diastolic dimension (normal < 55 mm)	60 mm	< 60 mm	Often decreased
Left ventricular wall thickness	Decreased	Normal or increased	Markedly increased
Atrial size	Increased	Increased, may be massive	Increased
Valvular regurgitation	Mitral first during decompensation; tricuspid regurgitation in late stages	Frequent mitral and tricuspid regurgitation	Mitral regurgitation
Common first symptoms*	Exertional intolerance	Exertional intolerance	Exertional intolerance; may have chest pain
Congestive symptoms*	Left side before right side, except right side prominent in young adults	Right side often exceeds left side	Primary exertional dyspnea
Risk for dysrhythmia	- Ventricular tachydysrhythmias	- Ventricular tachydysrhythmias are uncommon except in sarcoidosis	- Ventricular tachydysrhythmias
	- Conduction block in Chagas' disease, giant cell myocarditis, and some families	- Conduction block in sarcoidosis and amyloidosis	
	- Atrial fibrillation	- Atrial fibrillation	- Atrial fibrillation

*Left-sided symptoms of pulmonary congestion: dyspnea on exertion, orthopnea, paroxysmal nocturnal dyspnea. Right-sided symptoms of systemic venous congestion: discomfort on bending, hepatic and abdominal distension, peripheral edema.
(Adapted from Goldman L, Ausiello D (eds): *Cecil Textbook of Medicine*, ed 22. Philadelphia, WB Saunders, 2004, p 442.)

PROGNOSIS

- DCM: Prognosis tends to be related to severity of disease at initial diagnosis. Five-year mortality rate has been estimated at 40–80%. An unfavorable prognosis is more likely in the presence of indicators that include renal dysfunction, anemia, widened QRS, left ventricular ejection fraction < 35%, cardiomegaly seen on chest radiograph, low exercise capacity or poor cardiac reserve during exertion, and so forth.
- HCM: Prognosis is considerably variable and is currently assessed on the basis of family history, symptoms, and the presence of dysrhythmias. Some adults with HCM may experience subtle regression in wall thickness while others (approximately 5–10%) evolve into an end-stage resembling DCM with ventricular enlargement, left ventricular wall thinning, and diastolic dysfunction. Increasing availability and use of clinical genetic testing for HCM should assist prognosis.
- RCM: Fewer than 10% of patients live more than 10 years after initial diagnosis.

DENTAL MANAGEMENT

Patients presenting with any of the three types of cardiomyopathy will potentially be at risk for any combination of three specific cardiovascular complications that must be evaluated and addressed prior to dental treatment, namely:
- Congestive heart failure
- Atrial and/or ventricular dysrhythmias
- Cardiac valvular disease/dysfunction with regurgitation (which places the patient at increased risk of developing bacterial endocarditis secondary to bacteremia-inducing dental treatment)

Please consult the preceding topics elsewhere in this section for additional information.

SUGGESTED REFERENCES

Kushwaha S, et al. Restrictive cardiomyopathy. *New Engl J Med* 2005;336:267.

Murphy RT, et al. Genetics and cardiomyopathy: where are we now? *Cleve Clin J Med* 2005;72:465.

Rhodus N, et al. Dental management of the patient with cardiac dysrhythmias: an update. *Oral Surg Oral Med Oral Path Oral Radiol Endod* 2003;96:659.

AUTHOR: **JUAN F. YEPES, DDS, MD**

SYNONYM(S)

Nonbacterial regional lymphadenitis
Cat-scratch fever
Benign inoculation lymphoreticulosis

ICD-9CM/CPT CODE(S)
078.3 Cat-scratch disease

OVERVIEW

Cat-scratch disease is a condition characterized by progressive regional lymphadenopathy typically following close contact with a feline. It is usually self-limiting, although atypical presentations involve granulomatous inflammation of the eye, spleen, liver, and bone.

EPIDEMIOLOGY & DEMOGRAPHICS

PREDOMINANT AGE: Most common in early and mid-childhood.
PREDOMINANT SEX: No gender-based predisposition.
GENETICS: No genetic predisposition.

ETIOLOGY & PATHOGENESIS

- Transmitted by inoculation through close physical contact with a cat or kitten
- *Bartonella henselae* is the microorganism (bacillus) responsible for the disease
- Two weeks for evidence of lymph node involvement
- Uncommon organ dissemination (liver, bone, spleen)

CLINICAL PRESENTATION / PHYSICAL FINDINGS

- Regional suppurative lymphadenopathy.
- Self-limiting.
- Overlying erythematous skin.
- Fever.
- Malaise and headache in up to one third of patients.
- Common sites include head and neck, axilla, femoral, inguinal, and epitrochlear areas.
- Site of inoculation presents as a pustule or papule.
- Clinical presentation can include osteomyelitis and CNS involvement.

DIAGNOSIS

- Based on detailed medical history and exam; history of progressive lymph node enlargement and recent encounter with a cat.
- Mild leukocytosis and elevated ESR; eosinophilia uncommon; abnormal transaminases secondary to hepatic involvement.
- Diagnostic criteria (at least three positive):
  - History of feline contact with observable inoculation
  - Positive culture of lymphatic aspirate
  - Histology consistent with cat-scratch disease (identification of bacillus)
  - Positive skin test for the disease

MEDICAL MANAGEMENT & TREATMENT

- Antibiotics are recommended for immune-suppressed individuals (aminoglycosides or quinolones).
- Local heat therapy to affected sites.
- NSAIDs and antipyretics.

COMPLICATIONS

Organ or bone involvement and infection in immune compromised individuals

PROGNOSIS

Good prognosis; the disease is self-limited and usually without significant sequelae.

DENTAL SIGNIFICANCE

- Lymphadenopathy may be seen during dental visit.
- May be confused with infection from odontogenic origin.
- Cat-scratch disease can cause acute parotitis.

DENTAL MANAGEMENT

Supportive treatment, adequate hydration, pain control, and antipyretics.
- Parotitis may need antibiotic therapy, especially in immune-compromised patients.
- Referral to physician if multiple nodes or organ involvement.

SUGGESTED REFERENCES:

Batts S, Demers DM. Spectrum and treatment of cat-scratch disease. *Pediatr Infect Dis J* 2004;23:1161–1162.

Brook I. Acute bacterial suppurative parotitis: microbiology and management. *J Craniofac Surg* 2003;14:37–40.

Mandel L, Surattanont F, Miremadi R. Cat-scratch disease: considerations for dentistry. *J Am Dent Assoc* 2001;132:911–914.

AUTHOR: **ANDRES PINTO, DMD**

SYNONYM(S)

Child maltreatment

ICD-9CM/CPT CODE(S)
995.5 Child maltreatment syndrome

OVERVIEW

- *Physical abuse* is the excessive force used upon a child that inflicts an injury. This concept includes "Shaken Baby Syndrome," in which young children present with clinical signs/symptoms of a brain injury, imaging evidence of intracranial trauma (e.g., cerebral edema and subdural blood), retinal hemorrhages, and no history of trauma.
- *Emotional abuse* causes harm to the development of a child's personality through coercive, demeaning acts or words.
- *Child sexual abuse* is any sexual act ranging from indecent exposure, inappropriate touching, improper exposure to sexual acts, prostitution, rape, incest, pornography, and sexual intercourse.
- *Neglect* is the failure to provide for the basic needs of a child such as food, clothing, shelter, and medical/dental care. Dental neglect is not usually separated from the general category of neglect. The American Society of Pediatric Dentists defines dental neglect as dental caries, periodontal diseases, and other oral conditions that, if left untreated, may result in pain, infection, and loss of function.

EPIDEMIOLOGY & DEMOGRAPHICS

INCIDENCE/PREVALENCE IN USA: Over 2 million cases of suspected child maltreatment were reported in 2001 in the U.S. Of these, 903,000 were substantiated, with 59% due to neglect, 19% physical abuse, 10% sexual abuse, and 7% emotional/psychological abuse.
PREDOMINANT AGE: Those most at risk are under 2 years of age, but death from abuse is rare after 1 year. First-order offspring are most affected. More than 80% of all perpetrators are younger than 40 years of age.
PREDOMINANT SEX: Slight male predilection for victims. Approximately two-thirds of perpetrators are female.
GENETICS: No genetic predilection.

ETIOLOGY & PATHOGENESIS

- The leading cause of head injuries to infants and young children is blunt trauma to the head and/or violent shaking.
- The interaction between the perpetrator's personality traits, the child's characteristics, and the environmental condition contributes to the etiology of child abuse, but no specific abusive personality exists. Child maltreatment

(particularly sexual abuse) exists in all social classes, but physical abuse has been more commonly identified in low socioeconomic groups.
- Caregiver risk factors: young parental age, drug and alcohol abuse, mental illness, low self-esteem, poor impulse control, history of prior abuse, inappropriate expectations, marital problems, poor parenting skills, lack of extended family, and unemployment.
- Child risk factors: perinatal complications, complex medical needs, colic, annoying behaviors, rebellious behaviors, and developmental delay.
- Environmental risk factors: low income/poverty, social isolation, external stresses, and prior involvement with social services.
- The strongest predictor for the transmission of violent behavior through generations is childhood exposure of the perpetrator to his/her father abusing his/her mother. Abuse is 20 times more likely to recur if one parent was abused as a child.

CLINICAL PRESENTATION / PHYSICAL FINDINGS

PHYSICAL ABUSE

- Multiple injuries
- Injuries in multiple stages of healing
- Injuries inappropriate for child's stage of development
- Discrepancy in the injury history
- Common head and neck injuries include:
  - Head: skull injuries, traumatic alopecia (bald spots), Battle's sign (bruising behind the ear)
  - Face:
    - Eyes: retinal hemorrhage/detachment, blackened eyes, dislocated lens, traumatic cataract
    - Nose: fracture, displacement
    - Lips: bruises, lacerations, angular abrasions (gag marks)
    - Intraoral: frenum tears (especially in children < 1 year or > 2 years of age), palatal bruises (due to forced fellatio), residual tooth roots
    - Maxilla/mandible: fracture or improperly healed fracture, malocclusion from previous fracture
    - Cheek: bruises to the soft tissue rather than prominences
    - Neck: bruises or cuts
    - Ears: ecchymosis of the pinna
    - Teeth: fractured/mobile/avulsed/discolored teeth without reasonable explanation, untreated rampant caries, untreated obvious infections/bleeding

Specific patterns of abuse include:
- *Gags:* bruising, lichenification, and scarring at the corners of the mouth.
- *Slap marks:* parallel linear bruises on the cheek at finger-width spacing running through more diffuse bruises.

- *Grab marks:* thumb marks on one cheek and two to four finger-mark bruises on the other cheek.
- *Pattern injuries:* "tattoo bruising" from forceful contact with a particular object (e.g., belt buckle, hairbrush), burns with a particular substance/object (e.g., hot/caustic liquids, cigarettes), or burns from submersion in hot fluid.
- *Craniofacial fractures:* (especially children under 3 years of age) 45% affect the nasal bones, 32% the mandible, and 21% the zygomaticomaxillary complex and orbit.
- *Bite marks:* ecchymosis, abrasions, and lacerations in elliptical/ovoid patterns that may have a central area of ecchymosis (contusion). Canine teeth affect the deepest portion. Human bite marks compress flesh rather than tear and rarely avulse tissue. The intercanine distance of a typical child is < 2.5 cm, child/small adult 2.5 to 3.0 cm, and adult > 3.0 cm. If the skin is not broken, the mark usually lasts up to 24 hours, but those that have broken the skin may last several days.

SEXUAL ABUSE

- A child's history is often the most important component since many who have been sexually abused show no physical signs and have normal genital examinations.
- Physical signs include:
  - Oral/perioral gonorrhea/syphilis in a prepubescent child
  - Unexplained petechiae/erythema on the palate
  - Unusual intraoral trauma
  - Very young pregnancy
  - Oral/perioral condyloma acuminata

DENTAL NEGLECT

- Untreated early childhood caries/extensive caries and oral disease.
- Untreated obvious oral infection.

DIAGNOSIS

- Child abuse is not a complete diagnosis and may be a symptom of disordered parenting. There are no specific injuries that are pathognomonic of child physical abuse. Child abuse may be suspected after a thorough history and presentation of clinical signs including:
  - No treatment sought or a delay in seeking medical treatment.
  - Vague story regarding the "accident" that lacks detail, is not compatible with the observed injury, and may vary with each time it is told.
  - Abnormal parental mood that is more preoccupied with his/her own problems rather than with the sake of the child.
  - Erratic parental behavior that may include hostility.

○ Abnormal parent–child interaction in which the child may appear sad, withdrawn, frightened, or excessively submissive.

○ The child may state something that conflicts with the parent's story regarding the injury.

• Bite marks should be swabbed for saliva in order to test for a suspected perpetrator's DNA. Impressions of a suspected perpetrator should also be evaluated by a prosthodontist or forensic odontologist and compared with the bite mark.

• Suspected sexual abuse victims should be evaluated by a sexual assault team at a local hospital:

○ *Neisseria gonorrhoeae* oral cultures should be cultured and should grow and differentiate from *Neisseria meningitides*.

○ Oral semen detection through swabbing the buccal mucosa or tongue is necessary.

○ Dark field examination of syphilis lesions should be performed.

○ Evidence may include unexplained petechiae or erythema of the palate and/or bruising and bite marks around the ears.

○ Oral/perioral wart-like lesions such as condyloma acuminatum should be biopsied for DNA hybridization to rule out sexually transmitted strains of human papilloma virus (HPV). Other causes of intraoral warts should also be considered, such as self-inoculation or verruca vulgaris.

MEDICAL MANAGEMENT & TREATMENT

• Reporting suspected cases of child abuse/neglect to local Child Protective Services (CPS) is required by law of all mandated reporters (e.g., physicians, dentists, nurses, and hospital personnel). A written report should follow.

• Physical abuse injuries should receive proper medical attention.

• Victims should receive psychological counseling.

• Patients in need of dental treatment should receive access to care.

• Suspected cases of abuse that include a facial fracture warrant a full skeletal radiographic series to detect fractures that require less force, such as in long bone.

• Differential diagnoses often include unintentional trauma, uninformed low "dental IQ" with early childhood caries, and condition/radiologic findings that mimic bone fractures. Several of the following conditions may mimic signs of child abuse and could lead to false reporting:

○ Conditions/radiologic findings that mimic bone fractures, including cleidocranial dysostosis, congenital bowing tibia, congenital syphilis, Cornelia de Lange syndrome (infantile muscular dystrophy), eosinophilic granuloma, Gaucher's disease, Hutchinson-Gilford syndrome, hypophosphatasia, infantile cortical hyperostosis, Menkes steely (kinky) hair syndrome, metastatic neuroblastoma, osteogenesis imperfecta, osteoid osteoma, osteomyelitis, osteoporosis, osteoporosis pseudoglioma syndrome, poliomyelitis, rickets, scurvy, septic arthritis, stress fractures, and unicameral bone cysts.

○ Conditions that mimic bruises, burns, bite marks, or scars include contact dermatitis, Ehlers-Danlos syndrome, epidermolysis, erythema multiforme, facial vascular malformation, folk medicine remedy/cupping/coining, fungal infection, seborrheic eczema, hemangiomas, hemophilia, Hereditary Sensory and Autonomic Neuropathies (HSAN), hypersensitivity vasculitis, hypersensitivity reactions, idiopathic thrombocytopenic purpura, leukemia, strawberry nevus, staphylococci infections, scabies, Mongolian spots, purpura, Henoch-Schönlein purpura, vitamin K deficiency, and von Willebrand's disease.

○ Many children begin to crawl and stand at 9 months, with many walking by 12 to 15 months. During this time, bony prominences are typical areas to bruise such as the forehead, elbows, knees, and shins.

COMPLICATIONS

• Shaken baby syndrome is the leading cause of brain injury to infants. Approximately 20–25% of victims die. Nonfatal injuries include blindness, cerebral palsy, and cognitive impairment.

• Approximately 1300 children die per year, with 35% of deaths due to neglect and 26% due to abuse.

• Maltreatment as a child also increases the risk of adverse health effects, violence as an adult, smoking, alcoholism, drug abuse, physical inactivity, severe obesity, depression, suicide, sexual promiscuity, and certain chronic diseases.

• Dental neglect may result in pain, abscess development, fever, Ludwig's angina, and death.

PROGNOSIS

• The prognosis is dependent on the severity of the injury.

• Approximately 20–25% of victims of shaken baby syndrome die.

• Children who are abused are at risk for future problems such as continued abuse as a perpetrator or victim, psychiatric disorders, chronic health conditions, and death.

DENTAL SIGNIFICANCE

• Approximately 50–65% of child abuse cases involve injuries to the craniofacial region, head, face, and neck; many of the signs are evident during a dental examination.

• Physicians often receive minimal training in oral health/dental injuries. Therefore, physicians and dentists should collaborate to improve prevention, detection, and treatment of such conditions.

• Bite marks are signs of physical abuse and require dentists trained in forensic odontology to assist in the evaluation of such cases.

• Dental neglect often occurs even after parents have been informed about the nature and extent of a child's poor oral condition.

• The failure to seek proper dental care may be related to family isolation, finances, ignorance, or the lack of perceived oral health value (even after being alerted by a health care professional about the nature and extent of the child's condition and treatment needed), and access to care.

DENTAL MANAGEMENT

• Interview the patient and parent separately and privately regarding the history of the injury. Ask the child if he/she feels safe at home. Ask the child when and by whom the injury occurred and if it was on purpose.

• Depending on the nature of the injury, consultation with a pediatric dentist, oral and maxillofacial surgeon, or forensic odontologist may be indicated.

• Perform a clinical exam.

• Important considerations regarding injuries:

1. Is it possible that the injury was accidental? How?

2. Is the explanation of the injury compatible with the patient's age and clinical findings? Was it consistent with normal behavior?

3. Was there a delay in seeking treatment for the injury? Why?

4. When asked on different occasions or by different people, does the explanation of the injury vary? Is the caregiver's explanation consistent with the child's?

5. Are there concerns regarding the child's upbringing or lifestyle?

6. Observe the following for abnormalities:
   - Relationship between the caregiver and child
   - Child's reaction to others and to the medical/dental examination
   - Child's general demeanor
- Photograph suspicious injuries (after receiving permission).
- With dental neglect, explain the disease and implications, assist in access to care, and reassure that the appropriate analgesics and anesthesia procedures will be performed for comfort. If the caregiver fails to obtain treatment for the child, he/she should be reported to CPS.
- Bite marks provide both physical and biological evidence. A specialist should evaluate the size, color, and pattern; one may contact a forensic odontologist through the American Board of Forensic Odontology:
  - The mark should be observed and documented with photographs using an identification tag and scale marker (in the photograph, perpendicular to the bite).
  - The suspected perpetrator should also be evaluated (after written consent is obtained).
  - Collect saliva cells from the bite mark (even if dry) with a sterile cotton swab moistened with distilled water, followed by a dry swab. Also collect a control sample from an uninvolved area of the skin. Place the swabs in a sterile tube or envelope and send it to a certified forensic lab.
  - Repeat written observations and photos daily for at least 3 days to document the evolution and age of the bite.
- When appropriate, relay information to the patient and adult caregiver. Simply state that the report is not an accusation and is required by law as a request for assistance, an investigation, and protection for the patient. Reports should be made to the local Child Protective Services agency.
- Prevention of Abuse and Neglect through Dental Awareness (PANDA) is a public–private partnership that educates dental professionals with information and procedures regarding child abuse and neglect through free seminars.
- Dentists who report suspected cases of abuse/neglect in good faith receive immunity from civil/criminal liability from lawsuits that may arise.

SUGGESTED REFERENCES

AAP Committee on Child Abuse and Neglect. AAPD Ad Hoc Work Group on Child Abuse and Neglect. Oral and Dental Aspects of Child Abuse and Neglect. *Pediatrics* 1999;104(2):348–350.

American Board of Forensic Odontology: http://www.abfo.org

Centers for Disease Control: http://www.cdc.gov/ncipc/factsheets/cmfacts.htm

Pretty IA, Hall RC. Forensic dentistry and human bite marks: issues for doctors. *Hospital Medicine* 2002;63(8):476–482.

Senn DR, McDowell JD, Alder ME. Dentistry's role in the recognition and reporting of domestic violence, abuse, and neglect. *Dent Clin N Amer* 2001;45(2):343–363.

Sfikas PM. Reporting abuse and neglect. *JADA* 1999;130(12):1797–1799.

U.S. Department of Health and Human Services Administration for Children and Families: http://www.nccanch.acf.hhs.gov/

Wellbury RR, Murphy JM. The dental practitioner's role in protecting children from abuse 2. The orofacial signs of abuse. *Br Dent J* 1998;184(2):61–65.

Wright FD, Dailey JC. Human bite marks in forensic dentistry. *Dent Clin N Amer* 2001;45(2):365–397.

AUTHOR: **KELLY K. HILGERS, DDS, MS**

SYNONYM(S)

Chronic obstructive lung disease (COLD)
Chronic airflow obstruction
Bronchitis (chronic)
Emphysema

ICD-9CM/CPT CODE(S)

491 Chronic bronchitis—incomplete
491.2 Obstructive chronic bronchitis—incomplete
491.9 Unspecified chronic bronchitis—complete
492.8 Other emphysema—complete
496 Chronic airway obstruction, not elsewhere classified—complete

OVERVIEW

Chronic obstructive pulmonary disease (COPD) is characterized by slowly progressive airway obstruction that is not fully reversible and is not due to another specific cause. COPD encompasses several diffuse pulmonary diseases including chronic bronchitis, cystic fibrosis, bronchiectasis, and emphysema. However, the term usually refers to a mixture of chronic bronchitis and emphysema.

- Chronic bronchitis: excessive secretion of bronchial mucus manifested by productive cough for 3 months or more in at least two consecutive years in the absence of any other disease that might account for this symptom.
- Emphysema: abnormal, permanent enlargement of the respiratory bronchioles and alveoli due to destruction of the interalveolar septa and without obvious fibrosis.

EPIDEMIOLOGY & DEMOGRAPHICS

INCIDENCE/PREVALENCE IN USA:

- Approximately 14.2 million people have COPD (of these, approximately 12.5 million have chronic bronchitis and 1.7 million have emphysema).
- Estimated prevalence of COPD is 8–17% for men and 10–19% for women. The prevalence rates increased in women by 30% in the last decade.

PREDOMINANT AGE: Over 40 years of age.

PREDOMINANT SEX: Male > female (approximately 2:1).

GENETICS: Not established; however:

- Some studies have suggested familial predisposition for development of chronic bronchitis.
- A rare form of emphysema, antiprotease deficiency (due to alpha$_1$-antitrypsin deficiency), is an inherited disorder that is an expression of two autosomal codominant alleles.

ETIOLOGY & PATHOGENESIS

ETIOLOGY

- Tobacco (cigarette) smoking is the most important risk factor for the development of COPD.
  - Cigar or pipe smoking also increases the risk of developing COPD, but to a much lesser extent than cigarette smoking.
  - Since only about 15% of smokers develop COPD, individual host susceptibility to the effect of smoking is believed to be a key factor in the development of COPD.
- Certain chronic occupational exposures, particularly to inorganic dusts (e.g., silica, coal, cement), grain or cotton dusts, or acid fumes (e.g., sulfuric acid).
- The role of exposure to indoor air pollution (e.g., using solid fuels for cooking and heating without adequate ventilation), ambient outdoor air pollution, or a history of recurrent childhood respiratory infections as potential causes of COPD in the absence of smoking is still under investigation.
- Serum alpha$_1$-antitrypsin deficiency causes a rare (< 1% of COPD patients) form of emphysema in young adults or children.

PATHOGENESIS

- Emphysema: pathogenesis remains controversial; probably caused by an imbalance between proteinases and antiproteinases in the lung:
  - Neutrophils are believed to be a major source of proteinases, such as elastase.
  - Respiratory irritants (e.g., tobacco smoke) cause a chronic inflammatory response in the lung characterized by a migration of neutrophils.
  - The neutrophils in the lung release elastase, which overwhelms the local natural antiproteinase activity, resulting in the destruction of lung elastin in the interalveolar septa.
  - Septal destruction has several consequences:
    - Elastic recoil of lung tissue is reduced, restricting air flow to the respiratory portion of the lung and causing airways to collapse during expiration.
    - The alveolar surface area available for gas exchange is reduced.
    - Clinically, this leads to dyspnea and hypoxemia and their resultant consequences:
      - In advanced disease, there is increased pulmonary artery pressure and eventual right-side heart failure (cor pulmonale).
- Emphysema is classified according to its anatomic distribution within the lobule

(i.e., cluster of alveolated terminal respiratory units) into four major types: (1) centriacinar, (2) panacinar, (3) paraseptal, and (4) irregular.

- Chronic bronchitis: pathogenesis is less understood than that of emphysema. Initiation of airway injury by irritant gases (e.g., tobacco smoke), proteinases, and acids results in the characteristic pathologic features of chronic inflammation (predominantly lymphocytes) and hypertrophy of the mucus-secreting glands (and, to a lesser degree, hyperplasia of goblet cells) of the trachea and bronchi.
  - The enlargement in mucous glands can be assessed by the ratio of the thickness of the mucous gland layer to the thickness of the wall between the epithelium and the cartilage ("Reid index").
    - The Reid index (normally 0.4) is increased in chronic bronchitis, usually in proportion to the severity and duration of the disease.

CLINICAL PRESENTATION / PHYSICAL FINDINGS

- COPD has an insidious onset; clinical findings may be completely absent early in the course of the disease.
- COPD characteristically presents in the fifth or sixth decade of life with complaints of excessive cough, sputum production, and shortness of breath.
  - Symptoms have often been present for an average of 10 years.
  - Most patients have smoked at least 20 cigarettes per day for 20 or more years before the onset of symptoms.
- Chronic bronchitis and emphysema often occur together because both are frequent results of the same etiologic factors (i.e., exposure to cigarette smoke). However, symptoms of one disease or the other tend to predominate in any given patient and are historically referred to as *"pink puffers"* and *"blue bloaters."*
  - *"Blue bloaters"* are patients predominately with chronic bronchitis, presenting with:
    - bluish-tinged skin color from peripheral cyanosis secondary to chronic hypoxemia and hypercapnia
    - peripheral edema (secondary to cor pulmonale)
    - tachycardia, tachypnea, and chronic cough with production of large amounts of sputum
  - *"Pink puffers"* are patients predominately with emphysema, presenting with:
    - a cachectic appearance, but pink skin color (indicating adequate oxygen saturation)

- dyspnea manifested by pursed-lip breathing and use of accessory muscles of respiration
- Additional clinical presentation/physical findings in COPD are presented in Table I-8.

DIAGNOSIS

LABORATORY

- Complete blood count (CBC): compensatory polycythemia may develop in severe COPD or in those patients who smoke excessively.
- Arterial blood gases: reveal mild-to-moderate hypoxemia without hypercapnia in the early stages. As the disease progresses, hypoxemia becomes more severe with resultant hypercapnia.
- Sputum examination:
  ○ In stable chronic bronchitis, sputum is mucoid, and macrophages are the predominant cell.
  ○ With an exacerbation, sputum becomes purulent, with excessive neutrophils; most frequently cultured pathogens are *Streptococcus pneumoniae, Haemophilus influenzae,* and *Moraxella catarrhalis.*

IMAGING/SPECIAL TESTS

- Chest radiograph (see Table I-8).

- CT scan: more sensitive than the standard chest radiograph; in emphysema the outlined bullae are not always visible on a radiograph.
- Pulmonary function tests (spirometry):
  ○ Essential for the diagnosis and assessment of the severity of COPD; helpful in following its progress.
    - Forced expiratory volume in one second (FEV_1): volume of air expired during the initial second of forced expiration. This is the most common index of airflow obstruction.
    - Forced vital capacity (FVC): total volume of air exhaled forcefully and rapidly after maximum inhalation.
  ○ Reductions in FEV_1 and in the ratio of forced expiratory volume to forced vital capacity (FEV_1/FVC) occur later in COPD. In severe COPD, the forced vital capacity is markedly reduced.
  ○ Lung volume measurements reveal an increase in the total lung capacity (TLC), a marked increase in the residual volume (RV), and an elevation of the RV/TLC ratio, indicative of air trapping, particularly in emphysema.

CLINICAL CLASSIFICATION

- According to the Global Initiative Chronic Obstructive Lung Disease (GOLD), COPD is now classified (staged) as follows:
  ○ **Stage 0—At Risk:**
    - Spirometry still normal
    - Typically, chronic cough and sputum production
  ○ **Stage I—Mild COPD:**
    - $FEV_1/FVC < 70\%$, but $FEV_1 > 80\%$ of predicted value.
    - Usually, but not always, chronic cough and sputum production.
    - Patient may not be aware that lung function is abnormal.
  ○ **Stage II—Moderate COPD:**
    - $FEV_1/FVC < 70\%$ with FEV_1 between 50% and 80% of predicted value
    - Typically, the stage at which patients first seek medical attention because of dyspnea developing on exertion or an exacerbation of their disease
  ○ **Stage III—Severe COPD:**
    - $FEV_1/FVC < 70\%$ with FEV_1 between 30% and 50% of predicted value
    - Increased shortness of breath and repeated exacerbations, impacting on the quality of life
  ○ **Stage IV—Very Severe COPD:**
    - $FEV_1/FVC < 70\%$ with $FEV_1 < 30\%$ of predicted value, _or_
    - Presence of chronic respiratory failure or clinical signs of right-heart failure due to cor pulmonale
    - Respiratory failure: $pO_2 < 60$ mmHg with or without $pCO_2 > 50$ mmHg while breathing air (21% oxygen) at sea level
    - Patients may have severe COPD even if $FEV_1 > 30\%$ of predicted value when complications of right-heart failure or respiratory failure are present

MEDICAL MANAGEMENT & TREATMENT

GENERAL MEASURES

- The single most important intervention in smokers with COPD is to encourage smoking cessation.
- Aggressive treatment of respiratory infections.
- Chest physiotherapy to mobilize secretions.
- Avoid sedatives and narcotics.
- Maximize nutritional status.
- Moderate exercise program.

PHARMACOLOGIC

- Oxygen (either nocturnal or continuous ambulatory low-flow oxygen):
  ○ Oxygen therapy is primarily used in patients with severe COPD and during exacerbations and should only be administered to patients with documented hypoxemia.

| TABLE I-8 | **Clinical Characteristics of Chronic Bronchitis and Emphysema** |

Feature	Predominant Bronchitis	Predominant Emphysema
Age at presentation	40–45 years	50–75 years
Body habitus	Normal to (frequently) overweight	Typically thin, barrel-chested; recent weight loss common
Respiration	Respiratory rate is usually normal, with no use of the accessory muscles of respiration; intermittent dyspnea late in disease	Dyspnea, tachypnea, use of accessory muscles of respiration, retraction of the lower intercostal spaces with inspiration, and use of pursed lips during expiration are all common
Cough	Chronic productive, with copious mucopurulent sputum	Rare, with scant clear, mucoid sputum
Respiratory infections	Frequent	Occasional
Cyanosis	Common (secondary to cor pulmonale)	Uncommon until disease is very advanced
Peripheral edema	Common (secondary to cor pulmonale)	Uncommon
Chest radiograph findings	Increased bronchovascular (interstitial) markings ("dirty lungs") and cardiomegaly; diaphragms are not flattened.	Abnormal hyperinflation increased A-P dimension, small heart, flat diaphragms and possibly bullous changes
Pulmonary function	Elastic recoil normal; airway obstruction on inspiration and expiration; total lung capacity normal but may be slightly increased	Elastic recoil low; difficulty predominately on expiration as compared to inspiration; total lung capacity increased, some times markedly so
Blood gases	Chronic, moderate to severe hypoxemia with mild to severe hypercapnia	Mild hypoxemia, usually without hypercapnia

- An inspired oxygen fraction of 24–28% is preferred with an oxygen saturation (SaO_2) goal of > 90%.
  - Hypercapnia and further respiratory compromise may occur with high-flow oxygen therapy.
- Antibiotics:
  - Used empirically for respiratory infections.
  - Oral antibiotics of choice are azithromycin, levofloxacin, amoxicillin-clavulanate, and cefuroxime.
- Bronchodilators:
  - May be useful in chronic bronchitis. Obstruction is largely irreversible in emphysema.
    - Anticholinergic:
      - e.g., ipratropium bromide, two puffs qid
    - Sympathomimetics:
      - e.g., albuterol or metaproterenol, one to two puffs from inhaler every 4 to 6 hours
- Methylxanthines:
  - Used in those patients who fail to respond to inhaled bronchodilators or those with sleep-related respiratory disturbances.
    - e.g., theophylline, 400 mg/day orally
- Corticosteroids:
  - Occasional response in bronchitis with eosinophilia.
    - e.g., prednisone, 7.5 to 15 mg/day or qod

SURGICAL

- COPD may be amenable to treatment with bullectomy, lung reduction surgery (reduction pneumoplasty), or lung transplantation in certain cases.

COMPLICATIONS

- Acute or chronic respiratory failure
- Pulmonary hypertension
- Cor pulmonale
- Increased risk for recurrent pulmonary infections

PROGNOSIS

- COPD has a variable prognosis.
- The degree of pulmonary dysfunction (as measured by FEV_1) at the time the patient is first seen is probably the most important predictor of survival.
  - The median survival time of patients with severe COPD ($FEV_1 \leq 1L$ or FEV_1 < 40% predicted) is about 4 years.
- Development of cor pulmonale or hypercapnia and persistent tachycardia are poor prognostic indicators.

DENTAL SIGNIFICANCE

- Patients with COPD already have compromised respiratory function; therefore, efforts must be directed toward the avoidance of anything that could further depress respiration.
- Since patients with COPD often have coexisting heart disease such as congestive heart failure and/or hypertension, these conditions must also be addressed (if present) when considering the dental management of the patient.

DENTAL MANAGEMENT

EVALUATION

- Review patient's medical history pertaining to COPD:
  - Determine time of original diagnosis/duration of disease.
  - Review history for evidence of concurrent heart disease such as hypertension or congestive heart failure (take appropriate precautions if heart disease is present).
  - Determine/record present medication(s) and/or history of surgical treatment for COPD.
- Assess patient's current clinical status (Table I-9) including:
  - Consultation with the patient's physician as needed.
  - Presence and severity of symptoms (e.g., dyspnea, orthopnea).
  - Results of current spirometry (e.g., FEV_1); arterial blood gas (ABG) test results are also useful.
- Determine the presence of factors that may exacerbate COPD (e.g., presence of an acute respiratory infection or continued tobacco smoking).
- Check blood pressure and pulse:
  - Elevated blood pressure, tachycardia, or irregular pulse rhythm may indicate toxic reactions or overdose of a sympathomimetic or anticholinergic bronchodilator, or methylxanthines. Additional symptoms of toxicity or overdose of these drugs include anxiety, tremors, palpitations, dizziness, nausea, and vomiting.
- Consider dental treatment of high-risk patients with COPD (see Table I-9) in a special care facility (e.g., hospital dental clinic).

DENTAL

- Place patients in a semisupine or upright chair position for treatment (as indicated by the presence of orthopnea) in order to avoid orthopnea and the feeling of respiratory discomfort.
- Use of local anesthetic is not contraindicated.
- Patients demonstrating cardiovascular side effects (i.e., elevated blood pressure and/or tachycardia) secondary to their COPD medication may require a dose limitation in the use of local anesthetics containing vasoconstrictors (see Appendix A, Box A-3, "Local Anesthetic with Vasoconstrictor Dose Restriction Guidelines").
- The use of a pulse oximeter during dental treatment is useful in determining the oxygen saturation (SaO_2) of the patient. A drop in SaO_2 to 94% or below indicates impaired oxygen exchange and the need for intervention.
- With severe COPD, the use of a rubber dam may be problematic (unless low-flow oxygen is provided during the dental procedure) because the rubber dam may result in a feeling of compromised air supply.

TABLE I-9	Dental Treatment Risk Assessment of the Patient with COPD	
Risk Category	**Clinical Presentation***	
Low risk	• Dyspnea only on significant exertion • FEV_1 > 65% of predicted • Normal arterial blood gases ($PaCO_2$: 40 mm Hg; PaO_2: 100 mmHg; pH: 7.40)	
Moderate risk	• Dyspnea on exertion • Chronic bronchodilator therapy • Recent use of systemic corticosteroids for treatment of COPD • FEV_1 40–65% of predicted • Hypoxemia (PaO_2 < 85 mmHg), but no CO_2 retention	
High risk	• Previously undiagnosed symptoms of COPD • Acute exacerbation of COPD (e.g., acute respiratory infection) • Chronic respiratory failure, or significant dyspnea at rest, or cor pulmonale who require chronic oxygen therapy • FEV_1 < 40% of predicted • CO_2 retention ($PaCO_2$ > 45 mmHg)	

*When presenting features fall into different categories, the higher category should be selected to classify the patient's risk category.

Chronic Obstructive Pulmonary Disease

○ When needed, low-flow oxygen is generally provided via nasal cannula between 2 and 4 L/min.

- Nitrous oxide-oxygen inhalation sedation is contraindicated or must be used with caution in patients with emphysema and/or severe COPD (patients retaining CO_2):
  ○ Patients with emphysema (or pulmonary cysts) should not have nitrous oxide-oxygen inhalation sedation because nitrous oxide displaces nitrogen from the body. A larger amount dissolves in tissues because it is more soluble than nitrogen. When released, it expands to form a larger volume than was occupied by the nitrogen. It will create pressure if trapped in pockets where it cannot escape quickly.
  ○ Patients with severe COPD (as indicated by the presence of CO_2 retention) are hypoxic drive breathers. They respond to low oxygen levels rather than to the elevated CO_2 levels that drive breathing in disease-free individuals. Therefore, patients with severe COPD may respond with decreased respirations or apnea due

to the high oxygen levels administered with nitrous oxide-oxygen inhalation sedation.

- If sedative medication is required, low-dose oral benzodiazepines (e.g., alprazolam, triazolam) may be used.
- Narcotic analgesics and barbiturates also are to be used with caution (or avoided in patients with more severe COPD) because of their respiratory depressant properties.
- Use of macrolide antibiotics, such as erythromycin, which alter cytochrome P450, may result in elevated serum methylxanthine (theophylline) levels.
- Assess the risk for adrenal suppression and insufficiency in patients being treated with systemic corticosteroids (see Appendix A, Box A-4, "Management of Dental Patients at Risk for Acute Adrenal Insufficiency").
  ○ Patients using inhaled corticosteroids only are usually not considered to be at risk for these complications.

SUGGESTED REFERENCES

Anthonisen, N. Chronic obstructive pulmonary disease, in Goldman L, Ausiello D. Cecil Textbook of Medicine, ed 22. Philadelphia, WB Saunders, 2004, pp 509–515.

Global Strategy for the Diagnosis, Management, and Prevention of Chronic Obstructive Pulmonary Disease. Bethesda, MD, Global Initiative for Chronic Obstructive Lung Disease (GOLD), World Health Organization (WHO), National Heart, Lung and Blood Institute (NHLBI), 2003. http://www.goldcopd.com

Grossman RF. Anaerobic and other infection syndromes, in Crapo JD, et al. (eds): Baum's Textbook of Pulmonary Disease. Philadelphia, Lippincott Williams & Wilkins, 2004, pp 315–317.

Reilly Jr. JJ, Silverman EK, Shapiro SD. Chronic obstructive pulmonary disease, in Kasper Dl, et al. (eds): Harrison's Principles of Internal Medicine, ed 16. New York, McGraw-Hill, 2005, pp 1547–1554.

Stoelting RK, Dierdorf SF. Chronic obstructive pulmonary disease, in Handbook for Anesthesia and Co-Existing Disease, ed 2. New York, Churchill Livingstone, 2002, pp 137–146.

Sutherland ER, Cherniack RM. Management of chronic obstructive pulmonary disease. N Engl J Med 2004;350:2689–2697.

AUTHORS: F. JOHN FIRRIOLO, DDS, PHD; JAMES R. HUPP, DMD, MD, JD, MBA

SYNONYM(S)

Clotting factor deficiency secondary to liver disease or vitamin K deficiency
Hypoprothrombinemia
Anticoagulant therapy

ICD-9CM/CPT CODE(S)

286.7 Acquired coagulation factor deficiency—complete

OVERVIEW

An acquired deficiency of any of the coagulation factors; may be secondary to other disease or to use of medications (e.g., anticoagulants) and therefore may be iatrogenic, as in the treatment of cerebrovascular accident and other conditions.

EPIDEMIOLOGY & DEMOGRAPHICS

INCIDENCE/PREVALENCE IN USA: Varies due to underlying etiology.
PREDOMINANT AGE: Varies due to underlying etiology.
PREDOMINANT SEX: Varies due to underlying etiology.
GENETICS: Not established.

ETIOLOGY & PATHOGENESIS

- With loss of functioning liver parenchymal cells due to liver disease (e.g., hepatitis, cirrhosis, carcinoma), clotting factor deficiencies develop and may become quite severe. Vitamin K-dependent factors, including II, VII, IX, and X, and proteins S and C are affected early. Factor VII, with a half-life of only 4 to 7 hours, is particularly important clinically. As Factor VII levels decrease, there is a progressive increase in prothrombin time (PT). Liver disease (especially cirrhosis) is also associated with both quantitative and qualitative platelet abnormalities.
- Nutritional deficiency of vitamin K or the lack of absorption will interfere with synthesis (e.g., malabsorption syndromes, sprue, obstructive jaundice), resulting in decreased function of the extrinsic coagulation cascade (as seen with liver disease) and a progressive increase in PT.
- Drugs:
  - Coumarin derivative anticoagulants, such as warfarin and dicumarol, act by inhibiting the synthesis of vitamin K-dependent clotting factors, which include Factors II, VII, IX and X, and the anticoagulant proteins C and S. These drugs are only administered orally.
  - Heparin acts at multiple sites in the normal coagulation system. Small amounts of heparin in combination with antithrombin III (heparin cofactor) can inhibit thrombosis by inactivating activated Factor X and inhibiting the conversion of pro-

thrombin to thrombin. Heparin can only be administered intravenously.
- Disseminated intravascular coagulation (DIC, defibrination syndrome, consumption coagulopathy) is characterized by generalized activation of the clotting mechanism with decreases in Factors V and VIII, fibrinogen, and prothrombin, which results in the intravascular formation of fibrin and ultimately thrombotic occlusion of small and midsize vessels along with prolonged bleeding.
- See "Disseminated Intravascular Coagulation" in Section I, p 76 for additional information.

CLINICAL PRESENTATION / PHYSICAL FINDINGS

- A positive history for systemic diseases or conditions leading to the lack of synthesis of clotting factors (e.g., liver disease, biliary obstruction, malabsorption).
- Medications that interfere with the development of a fibrin clot; treatment of atrial fibrillation, prosthetic heart valve, coronary artery disease, cerebrovascular accident, or deep venous thrombosis may involve the use of anticoagulant drugs (e.g., warfarin, dicumarol).
- History of excessive bleeding following previous surgery or tooth extraction; spontaneous bleeding or bruising easily.

DIAGNOSIS

- Table I-10 summarizes the laboratory tests most commonly used for the diagnosis and monitoring of clotting factor defects.
  - Specific coagulation factor assays (e.g., VIII, IX) may be a useful adjunct in the evaluation of some acquired coagulopathies.

MEDICAL MANAGEMENT & TREATMENT

Dependent on the underlying disorder. Most acquired clotting factor deficiencies are iatrogenic; therefore, the patient should be under the care of a physician for the particular condition.

COMPLICATIONS

Bleeding diatheses: gastrointestinal, genitourinary, intracranial bleeding; hematomas.

PROGNOSIS

Prognosis is related to the underlying disease or condition.

DENTAL SIGNIFICANCE

- Excessive bleeding after invasive dental treatment or oral surgery:
  - Anticoagulants present management problems in oral surgery mainly because of prolonged intraoperative and postoperative bleeding. However, about 90% of postextraction hemorrhage is from other causes, including the following:
    - Excessive operative trauma, particularly to oral soft tissues
    - Poor compliance with postoperative instructions
    - Interference with the extraction socket or operation site (e.g., by sucking and tongue pushing; plasminogen activators are present in saliva and oral mucosa and can thus cause fibrinolysis)
    - Inflammation at the extraction or operation site (e.g., due to severe gingivitis), with resultant fibrinolysis

TABLE I-10	**Laboratory Tests for the Diagnosis and Evaluation of Clotting Factor Defects**	
Laboratory Test	**Factors or Functions Measured**	**Normal Values**
Prothrombin Time (PT) International Normalized Ratio (INR)	Evaluation of the extrinsic and common pathway (Factors I, II, V, VII, X)	PT: Normal values vary between laboratories, typically 10–14 seconds INR = 1.0
Partial Thromboplastin Time (PTT)	Evaluation of intrinsic and common pathway (Factors I, II, V, VIII, IX, X, XI, XII)	Normal values vary between laboratories, typically 25–35 seconds or 30–45 seconds
Thrombin Time (TT)	Evaluation of the common pathway (tests the ability to form an initial clot from fibrinogen)	Normal values vary between laboratories, typically 9–13 seconds or 15–20 seconds

- Inappropriate use of analgesia with aspirin or other nonsteroidal antiinflammatory drugs (NSAIDs), which, by interfering with platelet function, induce a bleeding tendency
  - Uncontrolled hypertension
- Aggressive treatment of oral infections and establishment of good oral hygiene is necessary.

DENTAL MANAGEMENT

PATIENTS TAKING COUMARIN ANTICOAGULANTS

- Consultation with physician:
  - Patients on anticoagulants are at risk both from their underlying disorder and their anticoagulation therapy. Both factors must be considered in relation to dental treatment. In most cases routine oral surgery may proceed with an INR ≤ 3.0.
  - Evaluate predental treatment PT/INR results (see Appendix A, Box A-5, "Dental Management of Patients Taking Coumarin Anticoagulants").
- Local hemostatic measures [e.g., absorbable gelatin sponges (Gelfoam®), oxidized cellulose (SURGICEL™), microfibrillar collagen (Avitene®), topical thrombin, tranexamic acid, epsilon-aminocaproic acid (EACA), sutures, surgical splints, and stents].

- Avoid aspirin or nonsteroidal antiinflammatory drugs (NSAIDs).

SUGGESTED REFERENCES

Herman WJ, Konzelman JL, Sutley SH. Current perspectives on dental patients receiving coumarin anticoagulant therapy. *J Am Dent Assoc* 1997;128:327–335.

Schardt-Sacco D. Update on coagulopathies. *Oral Surg Oral Med Oral Pathol Oral Radiol Endod* 2000;90:559–563.

Wahl MJ. Myths of dental surgery in patients receiving anticoagulant therapy. *J Am Dent Assoc* 2000;131:77–81.

AUTHORS: **WENDY S. HUPP, DMD; F. JOHN FIRRIOLO, DDS, PHD**

SYNONYM(S)

Aortic coarctation

ICD-9CM/CPT CODE(S)

747.10 Coarctation of aorta (preductal) (postductal)—complete

OVERVIEW

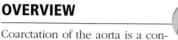

Coarctation of the aorta is a congenital heart disease involving a narrowing of the aorta. This constriction typically consists of a discrete, diaphragm-like ridge extending into the aortic lumen just distal to the left subclavian artery at the site of the aortic ductal attachment. This condition results in hypertension in the arms. Less commonly, the coarctation is immediately proximal to the left subclavian artery, in which case a difference in arterial pressure is noted between the arms. Extensive collateral arterial circulation to the distal body through the internal thoracic, intercostal, subclavian, and scapular arteries frequently develops in patients with this condition.

EPIDEMIOLOGY & DEMOGRAPHICS

INCIDENCE/PREVALENCE IN USA:
Coarctation of the aorta accounts for approximately 5% of all congenital heart disease and is found at necropsy in up to 1:1550 patients, according to recent studies.
PREDOMINANT AGE: Usually diagnosed in infancy; however, the age of presentation is related with the severity rather than the site of obstruction, as a result of cardiac failure or, occasionally, stroke.
PREDOMINANT SEX: Male > female (approximately 3:1)
GENETICS: None established; increased incidence in Turner syndrome.

ETIOLOGY & PATHOGENESIS

- Coarctation of the aorta is manifested when the ductus closes starting at the pulmonary end, with gradual involution of ductal tissue toward the aorta.
- A number of theories exist regarding etiology, including postnatal ductal constriction and a theory that alterations in intrauterine blood flow cause altered flow through the aortic arch and result in the substrate for coarctation.
- Similar to most forms of congenital heart disease (CHD), multifactorial influences appear to affect the occurrence and severity of coarctation, including genetic abnormalities such as Turner syndrome (45,X), in which 15–20% of patients have coarctation of the aorta.
  - Familial patterns of inheritance of coarctation have been reported, as well as other left-heart obstructive lesions.
- An increase in seasonal occurrence is reported in September and November.

CLINICAL PRESENTATION / PHYSICAL FINDINGS

SIGNS/SYMPTOMS

- *Early presentation*: Young patients may present in the first 3 weeks of life with poor feeding, tachypnea, and lethargy and progress to overt congestive heart failure (CHF) and shock. Development of symptoms often is accelerated by the presence of associated major cardiac anomalies, such as ventricular septal defect.
- *Late presentation*: Patients often present after the neonatal period with hypertension or a murmur. These patients often have not developed overt congestive heart failure because of the presence of arterial collateral vessels. Other presenting symptoms may include headaches, chest pain, fatigue, or even life-threatening intracranial hemorrhage. True claudication is rare. Many patients are asymptomatic except for the hypertension that is noted incidentally.

PHYSICAL EXAM

- *Early presentation*: Neonates may present with tachypnea, tachycardia, and increased work of breathing and may even be moribund with shock. Keys to the diagnosis include blood pressure discrepancies between the upper and lower extremities and reduced or absent lower extremity pulses to palpation. The murmur associated with coarctation of the aorta may be nonspecific.
- *Late presentation*: Older infants and children may be referred for evaluation of hypertension or murmur. Most adults with coarctation of the aorta are asymptomatic. Other findings on physical examination may include abnormalities of blood vessels in the retina and a prominent suprasternal notch pulsation. A thrill may be present in the suprasternal notch or on the precordium in the presence of significant aortic valve stenosis. In the rare case of abdominal coarctation, an abdominal bruit may be noted.

DIAGNOSIS

Different exams are used for the diagnosis and monitoring coarctation of the aorta.

SPECIAL TESTS

- Electrocardiogram (ECG): usually shows left ventricular hypertrophy and right atrial enlargement with increasing severity.

IMAGING

- Chest radiography: may reveal cardiomegaly, pulmonary edema, and other signs of CHF. A dilated transverse aorta and the poststenotic dilation of the descending aorta may create a fig-ure-three ("3") sign along the upper left cardiac margin. Rib notching related to intercostal collateral development may become apparent after childhood, usually involving the third to eighth ribs posteriorly.
- Echocardiography: suprasternal notch view allows evaluation of the aortic arch to assess the transverse aortic arch, isthmus, and severity of coarctation.
  - Doppler echocardiography measures the gradient at the area of coarctation and identifies the pattern of diastolic runoff typically seen in patients with severe obstruction.
- MRI: useful in older or postsurgical correction patients to evaluate residual arch obstruction, arch hypoplasia, or formation of aneurysms.

MEDICAL MANAGEMENT & TREATMENT

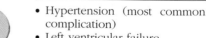

The main treatment of coarctation of the aorta is surgical repair of the defect.

- Surgery should be considered for patients with a high transcoarctation pressure gradient. Although balloon dilatation is a therapeutic alternative, the procedure is associated with a higher incidence of subsequent aortic aneurysm and recurrent coarctation than surgical repair.
- Survival after repair of coarctation of the aorta is also influenced by the age of the patient at the time of surgery.
  - After surgical repair during childhood, 89% of patients are alive 15 years later and 83% are alive 25 years later.
  - When repair of coarctation is performed when the patient is between the ages of 20 and 40 years, the 25-year survival is 75%.
  - When repair is performed in patients more than 40 years old, the 15-year survival is only 50%.

COMPLICATIONS

- Hypertension (most common complication)
- Left ventricular failure
- Aortic dissection
- Premature coronary artery disease
- Infective endocarditis
- Cerebrovascular accidents (due to the rupture of an intracerebral aneurysm)

PROGNOSIS

Two-thirds of patients over the age of 40 who have uncorrected coarctation of the aorta have symptoms of heart failure. Seventy-five percent die by the age of 50 and 90% by the age of 60.

DENTAL SIGNIFICANCE

Patients without surgical treatment have a risk of endarteritis at the site of the narrowing and endocarditis of the aortic and mitral valves.

- Thus, patients with unrepaired coarctation of the aorta require antibiotic prophylaxis. Once the defect is repaired, the risk of endocarditis is minimal and antibiotic prophylaxis is not necessary if more than 6 months have passed after repair (unless a residual valvular disease is present).

DENTAL MANAGEMENT

- A consultation with the patient's cardiologist is recommended if any uncertainty exists regarding the patient's cardiovascular status and risk in relation to contemplated dental treatment procedures.
- Patients without repair are considered a moderate-risk condition for infective endocarditis and require antibiotic prophylaxis according to the American Heart Association recommendations prior to certain dental procedures (see Appendix A, Box A-1, "Antibiotic Prophylaxis Recommendations by the American Heart Association for the Prevention of Bacterial Endocarditis").

SUGGESTED REFERENCES

Brickner ME, et al. Congenital heart disease in adults—first of two parts. *N Engl J Med* 2000;342:256.

Hornung TS, et al. Interventions for aortic coarctation. *Cardiology Review* 2002;10:139.

Little J, Falace D, Miller C, Rhodus N. Cardiac conditions associated with endocarditis, in *Dental Management of the Medically Compromised Patient*. St Louis, Mosby, 2002, p 56.

Moodie DS. Diagnosis and management of congenital heart disease in the adult. *Cardiology Review* 2001;9:279.

Ramnarine I. Role of surgery in the management of the adult patient with coarctation of the aorta. *Postgraduate Medicine Journal* 2005;81:243.

AUTHOR: **JUAN F. YEPES, DDS, MD**

SYNONYM(S)

Coronary failure
Heart failure
Ventricular failure

ICD-9CM/CPT CODE(S)

428.0 Congestive heart failure, unspecified

OVERVIEW

Congestive heart failure (CHF) is a clinical syndrome that happens when the heart is unable to pump sufficient blood for metabolizing tissues or can do so only from an abnormally elevated filling pressure. Different conditions underlie congestive heart failure, and it is important to identify the nature of the cardiac disease and the factors that precipitate acute congestive heart failure. Some of the underlying diseases include states that depress ventricular function (e.g., coronary artery disease, hypertension, dilated cardiomyopathy, valvular heart disease, congenital heart disease) and states that restrict ventricular filling (e.g., mitral stenosis, restrictive cardiomyopathy, pericardial disease).

EPIDEMIOLOGY & DEMOGRAPHICS

INCIDENCE/PREVALENCE IN USA:
Approaching 10 per 1000 population among persons older than 65 years of age; approximately 4.8 million persons have CHF (affecting 1.5% to 2% of the population), with approximately 400,000 to 700,000 new cases each year. CHF is the cause for at least 20% of all hospital admissions among persons older than 65.
PREDOMINANT AGE: Varies by underlying etiology of CHF.
PREDOMINANT SEX: Male > female for ages 40 to 75; male = female for ages 75 and over.
GENETICS: None established.

ETIOLOGY & PATHOGENESIS

The most common causes of congestive heart failure include underlying cardiac diseases—most importantly, coronary artery disease and ischemic or hypertensive heart disease. Some of the possible underlying conditions are:

- Myocardial infarction results in necrosis of myocardial tissue, which is necessary for the heart to function properly.
- Other predisposing cardiac condition, including congenital heart disease and cardiomyopathies.
- Dilated cardiomyopathies are usually idiopathic but may result from toxic effects of alcohol and medications, infectious processes, or collagen-vascular disease. Restrictive cardiomyopathies may result from sarcoidosis, hemochromatosis, or amyloidosis.

- Hypertrophic cardiomyopathies result from different causes, including an autosomal dominant genetic component characterized by massive ventricular hypertrophy.

The most frequent precipitating factors of congestive heart failure include:

- Poor patient compliance with medical therapy
- Poor dietary control, usually an increase in sodium intake
- Acute increase in cardiac metabolic demands such as trauma and sepsis
- Acute dysrhythmias
- Silent myocardial infarction
- Systemic infection
- Pulmonary embolism

CLINICAL PRESENTATION / PHYSICAL FINDINGS

Past medical history may include the following:

- Cardiomyopathy
- Valvular heart disease
- Alcohol use
- Hypertension
- Angina
- Prior myocardial infarction
- Congenital heart disease

CHF may be classified for clinical purposes according to which ventricle is failing.

- Left-sided failure refers to the signs and symptoms caused by failure of the left ventricle or excessive pressure in the left atrium (i.e., clinical features of pulmonary congestion).
  - Clinical manifestations of left-sided failure are the most common because relatively common disorders (e.g., ischemic heart disease, hypertension) cause left ventricular damage.
  - The most common symptoms of left-sided failure are dyspnea, orthopnea, paroxysmal nocturnal dyspnea, cough, and hemoptysis.
    - These features are the result of passive pulmonary congestion, which leads to edema of the alveolar septa and, finally, fluid in the alveolar spaces, or pulmonary edema. With chronic left-sided failure, the

sputum may be rust-colored due to the presence of many hemosiderin-laden alveolar macrophages.
  - The most prominent signs of left-sided failure are pulmonary rales, cardiac enlargement, a S_3 (ventricular filling) gallop, and pulsus alternans.
- Right-sided failure refers to the signs and symptoms caused by failure of the right ventricle or excessive pressure in the right atrium (i.e., clinical features of systemic venous congestion). The leading cause of right-sided heart failure is left-sided heart failure.
  - In most cases, clinical manifestations of right-sided failure are caused by left-sided failure, although cor pulmonale (i.e., right ventricular enlargement due to pulmonary hypertension) is another important cause.
  - The most common signs are related to systemic venous congestion, including jugular venous distention, enlarged and tender liver and spleen, ascites, and peripheral edema.
  - Less significant are symptoms such as fatigue and weakness, anorexia, decreased tissue mass, and cyanosis.
- Biventricular failure (i.e., failure of both ventricles) usually is not simultaneous but develops over time due to the increased stress placed on the remaining ventricle.

FUNCTIONAL CLASSIFICATION OF CHF
The New York Heart Association (NYHA) has devised a functional classification of heart disease that grades the severity of CHF (Table I-11). It is useful in following the course of disease and assessing the effects of therapy.

DIAGNOSIS

A variety of specialized tests are used to diagnose and monitor congestive heart failure, depending on the underlying etiology.
LABORATORY TESTS
- CBC (to rule out anemia, infections), TSH (to rule out hyperthyroidism), BUN, creatinine, liver enzymes.

TABLE I-11 New York Heart Association (NYHA) Classification of Congestive Heart Failure

Class	Clinical Presentation*
I	No limitation of physical activity. No dyspnea, fatigue, or palpitations with ordinary physical activity.
II	Slight limitation of physical activity. These patients have fatigue, palpitations, and dyspnea with ordinary physical activity but are comfortable at rest.
III	Marked limitation of activity. Less than ordinary physical activity results in symptoms, but patients are comfortable at rest.
IV	Symptoms are present at rest, and any physical exertion exacerbates the symptoms.

*Note that, in general, the classification implies the patient's worst level of functioning related to a heart failure symptom (e.g., fatigue, dyspnea, exercise intolerance).

Congestive Heart Failure

- β Natriuretic peptide (BNP): In recent years, BNP has been used to differentiate between dyspnea from asthma and from CHF. In different studies the sensitivity was calculated in 90% and the specificity in 76% for diagnosis of CHF, with a positive predictive value of 79%.

SPECIAL TESTS

- Electrocardiogram (ECG): Nonspecific, but may be useful in diagnosing concomitant cardiac ischemia, prior myocardial infarction, cardiac dysrhythmias, chronic hypertension, and other causes of left ventricular hypertrophy.
- Two-dimensional echocardiography and Doppler: Assesses systolic and diastolic abnormalities involving the right and left sides of the heart and determines the presence of pericardial, endocardial, valvular, and vascular abnormalities.

DIAGNOSTIC IMAGING

- Chest radiograph: Shows cardiomegaly (enlargement of the heart) and pulmonary vascular redistribution.
- Radionuclide ventriculography (RVG): Provides a reliable quantification of right and left ventricular ejection fraction and can characterize wall motion abnormalities in ischemic heart disease.
- Cardiac magnetic resonance imaging (MRI): Can also be used for the evaluation of ventricular function as well as myocardial mass.

ADDITIONAL DIAGNOSTIC DATA

- Ejection fraction: A commonly used index of ventricular function is the ejection fraction (EF). The ejection fraction is defined as the percentage of end-diastolic volume (EDV) ejected during a contraction (systole); therefore:

$$EF = 100 \times systolic \ volume \ (SV) \ / \ EDV$$

A normal ejection fraction is 0.55 (55%) to 0.70 (70%). Patients with ejection fractions of no greater than 0.40 (40%) are considered to have systolic dysfunction.

MEDICAL MANAGEMENT & TREATMENT

The treatment of congestive heart failure is targeted to decrease the symptoms, remove the precipitating factors, and control the underlying cardiac disease.

NONPHARMACOLOGIC THERAPY

- Search, identify, and control underlying correctable conditions responsible for CHF (e.g., anemia, valvular heart disease, hyperthyroidism) when possible.
- Eliminate contributing factors when possible (e.g., smoking cessation, weight loss for the obese patient).
- Supplemental oxygen therapy as needed.

- Fluid and sodium restriction (fluid intake 2 L or less; sodium intake is usually limited to ≤ 3 to 4 g/day). Patient education about this is imperative for long-term control.

PHARMACOLOGIC THERAPY

- Pharmacologic intervention continues to be the mainstay of management of CHF. The pharmacological treatment of CHF has become a combined symptomatic-preventive management strategy. Therapy with angiotensin-converting enzyme (ACE) inhibitors, beta-adrenergic blockers, and diuretics is now standard (see Appendix B, Clinical Algorithms, "Algorithm for the Recommended Pharmacologic Management of Congestive Heart Failure").

SURGICAL MEASURES

- Heart valve surgery may be considered in cases were a defective heart valve is responsible for CHF.
- Ventricular assist devices (VADs) are a variety of mechanical blood pumps employed singly to replace the function of either the right (RVAD) or left (LVAD) ventricle. Two blood pumps can be utilized for biventricular support. The VAD is designed to effectively unload either the right (RVAD) or left (LVAD) ventricle while completely supporting the pulmonary or systemic circulation. The VAD is typically used to support the patient until a suitable donor heart is available for cardiac transplantation.
- Cardiac transplantation may be considered in patients less than 55 to 60 years old with CHF that is unresponsive to other medical therapy and are without other disqualifying medical problems.

COMPLICATIONS

- Acute myocardial infarction
- Cardiogenic shock
- Dysrhythmias (most commonly, atrial fibrillation)
  - Ventricular dysrhythmias, such as ventricular tachycardia, often are seen in patients with significantly depressed left ventricular function
- Electrolyte disturbances
- Mesenteric insufficiency
- Protein enteropathy
- Digitalis intoxication: mental status changes, agitation, lethargy, visual disturbances, anorexia, nausea, vomiting, and diarrhea

PROGNOSIS

- Based on voluminous data collected in the past few years, the total in-hospital mortality rate was 19%, with 30% of deaths occurring from noncardiac causes. Thirty-year data from the Framingham heart study demonstrated a median survival of 3.2

years for male patients and 5.4 years for female patients.
- Long-term prognosis is variable. Mortality rates range from 10% in patients with mild symptoms to 50% in patients with advanced, progressive symptoms.

DENTAL SIGNIFICANCE

- The dentist should have an understanding of the cause of the individual patient's heart failure and current medications and, most importantly, should be aware of any recent changes in signs and symptoms or therapy.
- Patients should avoid excessive fluid intake, excessive sodium in their diets, and smoking.
- An increased gag reflex and an increased tendency for nausea and vomiting may be seen in patients taking digitalis (especially with higher doses); the patient should be instructed to avoid a heavy meal before their dental appointment.
- Some underlying etiologies of CHF (e.g., valvular heart disease) may place the patient at increased risk for bacterial endocarditis and may require antibiotic prophylaxis prior to bacteremia-inducing dental procedures.

DENTAL MANAGEMENT

EVALUATION

- Assessment of the patient's current status including:
  - Identifying the underlying causative factors responsible for the patient's CHF (e.g., coronary artery disease, valvular heart disease, hypertension)
  - Determining the patient's present medications and dosage used to control CHF as well as a history of any recent changes or modifications to CHF medications (that may indicate a worsening or progression of the condition)
  - Determining presence of signs and symptoms of CHF in the patient, including dyspnea, orthopnea, paroxysmal nocturnal dyspnea, cough, hemoptysis, jugular venous distention, ascites, and peripheral edema
  - Determining the severity (see Table I-11) and present status of the patient's CHF
- A medical consultation with the patient's primary physician and/or cardiologist is usually indicated.

MANAGEMENT

- Manage underlying causative factor(s) appropriately.
- For patients with untreated or uncontrolled congestive heart failure, avoid elective dental care.

- For patients with NYHA Class I or II CHF under good medical control, elective dental treatment can usually be accomplished with an acceptable level of risk.
  - It is usually advisable to limit the total dose of local anesthetics containing vasoconstrictors (e.g., epinephrine) with these patients (see Appendix A, Common Helpful Information for Medical Diseases and Conditions).
- For patients with NYHA Class III CHF, consider dental treatment in an outpatient setting or special care facility (e.g., hospital dental clinic).
  - Avoid use of local anesthetics containing vasoconstrictors with these patients.
- For patients with NYHA Class IV CHF, provide dental treatment conservatively (usually emergency or minimally invasive treatment only) in a special care facility.
  - Avoid use of local anesthetics containing vasoconstrictors.
- For patients taking digitalis:
  - Use local anesthetics containing vasoconstrictors (e.g., epinephrine) with caution; avoid gag reflex and also avoid erythromycin that can increase the absorption of digitalis and lead to toxicity.
- Avoid a completely supine position during dental treatment in patients with orthopnea.
- Change chair positions slowly.
- Schedule short, stress-free appointments.
- See Appendix B, Clinical Algorithms, "Algorithm for the Recommended Pharmacologic Management of Congestive Heart Failure."

SUGGESTED REFERENCES

Gomberg-Maitland M, Baran DA, Fuster V. Treatment of congestive heart failure. *Arch Intern Med* 2001;161:342–352.

Jessup M, Brozena S. Heart failure. *New Engl J Med* 2003;348(20): 2007–2018.

Little J, Falace D, Miller C, Rhodus N. Congestive heart failure, in *Dental Management of the Medically Compromised Patient*. St Louis, Mosby, 2002, p 123.

Milore, M. Congestive heart failure. *Oral Surg Oral Med Oral Path Oral Radiol and Endod* 2000;90:9.

Noble J, et al. (eds): *Textbook of Primary Care Medicine*, ed 3. St Louis, Mosby, 2001, p 590, figures 65, 66.

AUTHOR: **JUAN F. YEPES, DDS, MD**

SYNONYM(S)

Regional enteritis
Inflammatory bowel disease

ICD-9CM/CPT CODE(S)
555.0 Crohn's disease, small intestine
555.1 Crohn's disease involving large intestine
555.9 Crohn's disease, unspecified site

OVERVIEW

Chronic inflammation of the gastrointestinal tract, most commonly involving the bowel.

EPIDEMIOLOGY & DEMOGRAPHICS

INCIDENCE/PREVALENCE IN USA: Approximately 7 cases per 100,000 population. Incidence and prevalence of Crohn's has steadily increased in the last 50 years. The condition is more common among Caucasians than African-Americans or Asian-Americans. It is also two to four times more prevalent among the Jewish population in the United States, Europe, and South Africa.
PREDOMINANT AGE: Any age; most common onset occurs between 15 and 30 years of age.
PREDOMINANT SEX: Slight female preponderance.
GENETICS: Twenty to thirty percent of patients with the condition have a family history of inflammatory bowel disease. The relative risk is 10 times higher than that of the general population if a person has a relative with Crohn's and is 30 times greater if the relative is a sibling.

ETIOLOGY & PATHOGENESIS

- Unknown; recent theories have implicated factors such as genetics, microbes, immunologic reactions, environment, diet, and psychosocial factors as potential causes. The condition is thought to occur due to T cell and/or macrophage abnormalities and their interaction. This results in an imbalance between proinflammatory and antiinflammatory mediators.
- Crohn's disease is differentiated from other forms of inflammatory bowel disease by the inflammatory process, which extends through all layers of the bowel and is referred to as "transmural." The inflammation may affect any portion of the gastrointestinal tract; however, the small bowel is most commonly involved, particularly the terminal ileum. It often organizes into noncaseating granulomas, which grow transmurally and into the regional lymph nodes and results in thickening of the bowel wall and narrowing of the lumen.
- "Skip lesions" occur in the bowel since the inflammatory process is frequently discontinuous, resulting in normal bowel separated by portions of diseased bowel. A characteristic feature of Crohn's disease is the tendency for involved bowel loops to be firmly matted together by fibrotic bands or adhesions. This process is often associated with formation of fistulas, which may communicate between loops of bowel. As the disease progresses, abscesses or bowel obstruction may occur.

CLINICAL PRESENTATION / PHYSICAL FINDINGS

SIGNS/SYMPTOMS

- Low-grade fevers, weight loss, fatigue.
- Abdominal pain localized to the right lower quadrant or both lower abdominal quadrants if the colon is involved.
- Intermittent diarrhea.
- Mucus, blood, or pus in the stool.
- Intestinal obstruction can manifest as postprandial bloating, cramping pains.
- Perianal fissures or fistulae, or abscesses, can occur. Patients may also develop fistulae into the mesentery, which may result in intraabdominal or retroperitoneal abscess formation.
- Malnutrition and malabsorption are common at all stages of disease and result in weight loss.
- Extraintestinal manifestations may involve the skin, joints, mouth, eyes, liver, and bile ducts.
- Adolescents commonly experience growth failure and delayed puberty.

DIAGNOSIS

- History and physical findings, along with laboratory, radiologic, endoscopic, and histologic findings.
- Laboratory analysis may detect the presence of inflammatory activity or nutritional deficiencies to support a diagnosis of anemia due to chronic inflammation, iron malabsorption or chronic blood loss, or malabsorption leading to vitamin B_{12} or folate deficiencies. Other laboratory abnormalities include C-reactive protein, which correlates with disease activity, and leukocytosis, which may be due to chronic inflammation, abscess, or steroid treatment.
- Stool samples are usually tested for routine pathogens.
- Specific serologic testing can also give information leading to a diagnosis.
- Positive ASCA (antisaccharomyces cerevisiae antibodies) and negative p-ANCA (antinutrophil cytoplasmic antibody) antigen are highly suggestive of Crohn's disease.
- Imaging studies such as barium contrast studies are helpful in defining the nature, distribution, and severity of disease.
- CT scans can assess complications including fistulas, abscesses, and hepatobiliary complications.
- MRI, ultrasound, and nuclear scans may also be used for disease detection.
- Colonoscopy and upper endoscopy can aid in obtaining biopsies or dilation of strictures.

MEDICAL MANAGEMENT & TREATMENT

Varies depending upon the clinical status of the individual.

- In mild cases, diarrhea and abdominal cramps are effectively treated with diphenoxylate (Lomotil) or loperamide (Imodium), along with codeine for pain. In moderate to severe cases, patients may be admitted to the hospital for evaluation.
- Sulfasalazine is used for colonic disease to delay clinical relapse. Mesalamine (Asacol) is used for small-intestinal Crohn's diseases.
- During acute phases of the condition, steroids may be administered until remission is achieved and slowly tapered. Immunosuppressants such as azathioprine can also be used under careful supervision. If medical therapy fails, surgical resection of the inflamed bowel is indicated.
- Fistulas are rarely treated surgically unless they are complicated by obstruction or abscess formation. Management typically consists of oral metronidazole or ciprofloxacin for at least 1 to 2 months. Total parenteral nutrition (TPN) may promote healing of the fistula during medical therapy.
- Newer medical therapies include antibodies to tumor necrosis factor (TNF-α). Tacrolimus, mycophenolate mofetil (CellCept), and antiinflammatory cytokines such as interleukin-10 have all been proposed as therapeutic agents for treatment of Crohn's disease. Despite promising results, more trials are needed to investigate the effects of these agents.

COMPLICATIONS

- Potential complications include fistulas, abscesses, gastrointestinal blood loss leading to iron deficiency anemia, malabsorption, bowel perforation, and fibrous strictures.
- Patients with colon involvement have an increased risk of colon cancer.

PROGNOSIS

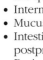

Since Crohn's disease is chronic, patients suffer from recurrent relapses. Medical and surgical therapy help achieve reasonable quality of life.

Medical therapy typically becomes less effective with time, and surgery is required for complications of Crohn's disease in over two-thirds of cases. The mortality rate increases with duration of disease. GI tract cancer is the leading cause of disease-related death.

DENTAL SIGNIFICANCE

- More than 15 specific oral manifestations of Crohn's disease have been described in the literature. The overall prevalence of oral lesions in Crohn's disease is reported to be present in 6–20% of patients. Oral lesions may precede intestinal involvement and are a likely predictor of other extraintestinal involvement.
- The most frequently affected areas are the buccal mucosa, showing a cobblestone pattern; the vestibule, where lesions appear in linear hyperplastic folds with ulceration; and the lips, which have a swollen and indurated appearance. Other orofacial lesions include aphthous ulcers, angular cheilitis, and mucosal tags. The pattern of swelling, inflammation, ulcers, and fissures is similar to that of the lesions occurring in the intestinal tract.

- Nutritional deficiencies may also present with oral manifestations. Burning mouth and atrophic glossitis may be suggestive of B_{12} or folate deficiency. Pallor of the oral mucosa may indicate iron deficiency (see "Vitamin Deficiencies" in Section II, p 335).
- Oral findings warrant a full systemic evaluation for intestinal Crohn's disease. Negative findings on GI evaluations should be repeated in patients with oral symptoms.

DENTAL MANAGEMENT

- Patients presenting with chronic oral lesions should receive a thorough medical history. Oral lesions should be biopsied, and the patient should be referred for a GI evaluation.
- Treatment modalities in oral Crohn's disease include topical corticosteroids, intralesional steroid injections, systemic prednisone therapy, or use of sulfasalazine. Oral lesions typically respond to systemic therapy for intestinal disease.
- Carefully assess treatment medications:
  ○ Assess the risk for adrenal suppression and insufficiency in patients being treated with systemic corticosteroids (see Appendix A, Box A-4, "Management of Dental Patients at Risk for Acute Adrenal Insufficiency").
  ○ Patients taking cytotoxic or immunosuppressive drugs, including systemic corticosteroids, may have an increased risk of infection and may require perioperative prophylactic antibiotics (see Appendix A, Box A-2, "Presurgical and Postsurgical Antibiotic Prophylaxis for Patients at Increased Risk for Postoperative Infections").
- Avoid broad-spectrum antibiotics such as clindamycin in patients taking sulfasalazine; they could reduce the bacterial flora of the colon, leading to diminished cleavage of sulfasalazine.

SUGGESTED REFERENCES

Friedman S. General principles of medical therapy in inflammatory bowel disease. *Gastroenterol Clin North Am* 2004;33(2): 191–208.

Kalmar JR. Crohn's disease: orofacial considerations and disease pathogenesis. *Periodontol 2000* 1994;6:101–115.

Sands BE. Crohn's disease, in Feldman M, Friedman LS, Sleisenger MH (eds): *Sleisinger & Fordtran's Gastrointestinal and Liver Disease*, ed 7. St Louis, WB Saunders, 2002, pp 2005–2038.

AUTHOR: ERNESTA PARISI, DMD

SYNONYM(S)

Mucoviscidosis
Fibrocystic disease of the pancreas

ICD-9CM/CPT CODE(S)

227.0 Cystic fibrosis

OVERVIEW

- Cystic fibrosis (CF) is an autosomal recessive disorder of the exocrine glands primarily affecting the respiratory and gastrointestinal tract.
- Characterized by abnormally thick secretions from mucous glands, pancreatic insufficiency, COPD, and an increase in the concentration of electrolytes in sweat.

EPIDEMIOLOGY & DEMOGRAPHICS

INCIDENCE/PREVALENCE IN USA:
The disorder affects about 1 in 2000 to 3000 Caucasians; 1 in 25 is a carrier. One in 17,000 African-Americans is affected, and incidence is low in Native Americans and Asians. It is the most common fatal hereditary disorder of Caucasians in the U.S.
PREDOMINANT AGE: Infants, children, and young adults.
PREDOMINANT SEX: Male = female.
GENETICS: The gene associated with CF has been localized to 250,000 base pairs of genomic DNA on chromosome 7q. It encodes a membrane-associated protein called the cystic fibrosis transmembrane regulator (CFTR). Over 800 mutations in the gene CFTR have been described, and at least 230 mutations are known to be associated with clinical abnormalities. The mutation known as ΔF508 is associated with about 60% of cases of cystic fibrosis.

ETIOLOGY & PATHOGENESIS

Chromosome mutation (CFTR) results in abnormalities in chloride transport and water flux across the surface of epithelial cells. This affects various organs and causes damage to exocrine tissue. The consequences are recurrent pneumonia, bronchiectasis, atelectasis, diabetes mellitus, biliary cirrhosis, cholelithiasis, internal obstructions, and increased risk for gastrointestinal malignancies.

CLINICAL PRESENTATION / PHYSICAL FINDINGS

Multiple systems are involved.
- The gastrointestinal system of the newborn may have obstruction (meconium ileus). There are pancreatic enzyme insufficiency, frequent bowel movements, stearrhea, creatorrhea, malabsorption, and vitamin deficiency. The patient exhibits failure to grow. The liver shows biliary cirrhosis and fatty infiltration.
- Pulmonary system involvement includes hacking cough, viscous secretions, rapid respiratory rate, frequent pseudomonas/staphylococcus infections with bronchial obstruction, and a high risk for pneumothorax, hemoptysis, and digital clubbing.
- Reproductive system exhibits sterility.
- Salt depletion and heat exhaustion occur frequently in warm climates.

DIAGNOSIS

- Meconium ileus.
- Pancreatic insufficiency.
- Pulmonary manifestations include hacking cough, wheezing, and dyspnea.
- A history of cystic fibrosis in the immediate family.
- Frequent and large bowel movements.
- An increased concentration of Na^+ and Cl^- in the sweat Cl^- test. However, approximately 2% of cystic fibrosis patients have a normal sweat Cl^- level.
- Test for serum concentration of immunoreactive trypsin in newborns with CF.
- 72-hour fecal fat excretion.
- Chest radiographs/imaging.
- Pulmonary function tests.
- Rule out chronic pulmonary disease.

MEDICAL MANAGEMENT & TREATMENT

NONPHARMACOLOGICAL
- Postural drainage and chest percussion
- Exercises/nutrition
- Psychological assistance

GENERAL CARE
Centered on prevention and treatment of various organ dysfunctions and symptoms.
- Antibiotics based on culture.
- Chest physiotherapy; chest percussion and postural drainage to clear purulent secretions.
- Bronchodilator therapy should be considered during exacerbation and in hospitalized patients.
- Proper nutrition and vitamin supplementation.
- Human recombinant deoxyribonuclease cleaving inhalant to increase cough clearance of sputum and decrease the frequency of respiratory exacerbations that require intravenous antibiotics.
- Pancreatic enzyme replacement.
- Glucocorticoids and ibuprofen as anti-inflammatory agents.
- Avoidance of tobacco smoke and other pollutants.

- Adequate immunizations are mandatory; pneumococcal and influenza are a mandatory priority.
- Physical exercise should be encouraged for cardiovascular health and promotion of cough.

COMPLICATIONS

- Pneumothorax incidence increases with age.
- Hemoptysis becomes apparent as bronchiectasis develops.
- Digital clubbing.
- Loss of CFTR function affects upper respiratory epithelium, and chronic rhinitis is common.
- Occurrence of nasal polyps.
- Respiratory failure.

PROGNOSIS

- The course of illness is punctuated with exacerbations.
- Over time, there is a worsening of pulmonary function. The lung disease is progressive. Current median survival is to age 33 years.
- Prognosis has improved because of aggressive treatment before the onset of irreversible pulmonary changes. Long-term survival is improved in patients without pancreatic insufficiency.

DENTAL SIGNIFICANCE

Major and minor salivary glands are involved. Electrolyte, enzyme, and total protein in saliva are altered. Drying of nasal and maxillary sinus mucosa contributes to chronic mouth breathing. Anterior open bite and enamel hypoplasia have been noted. Refer to primary care physician, internal medicine specialist, endocrinologist, and/or pulmonologist for medical care.

DENTAL MANAGEMENT

- General dental and oral care should be pursued emphatically.
- Nutritional consultation should be requested.
- Oral hygiene emphasis.
- Consult with primary physician to understand patient's status, medical care maintenance, and prognosis.

SUGGESTED REFERENCE

Welsh MJ. Cystic fibrosis, in Goldman L, Ansiello D (eds): *Cecil Textbook of Medicine*, ed 22. Philadelphia, WB Saunders, 2004, pp 515–519.

AUTHOR: **NORBERT J. BURZYNSKI, SR., DDS, MS**

SYNONYM(S)
Deep vein thrombosis

ICD-9CM/CPT CODE(S)
453.8 Embolism and thrombosis of other specified veins—complete

OVERVIEW

- Deep venous thrombosis (DVT) is a common condition that develops when a blood clot forms in large veins of the extremities or pelvis. Predisposing factors include venous stasis due to immobilization (e.g., plane flights, bed rest, orthopedic surgery), incompetent ven-ous valves in the lower extremities, hypercoagula-ble states (e.g., malignancy, hormone replacement therapy), obesity, and indwelling venous cath-eters.
- The sequelae of DVT vary from com-plete resolution of the clot without any ill effects to death due to pulmonary embolism. DVT and pulmonary embo-lism (PE) most often complicate the course of sick, hospitalized patients but may also affect healthy ambulatory patients.

EPIDEMIOLOGY & DEMOGRAPHICS

INCIDENCE/PREVALENCE IN USA: DVT occurs in approximately 2 million Americans each year. It is estimated that each year 600,000 patients develop PE and 60,000 die of this complication.
PREDOMINANT AGE: Mean age of 60 years (increasing age is an independent risk factor).
PREDOMINANT SEX: Males slightly greater than females (1.2:1).
GENETICS: Inherited thrombogenic states increase the risk for DVT.

ETIOLOGY & PATHOGENESIS

- Vein thrombi are intravascular deposits composed of fibrin and red cells with variable platelet and leukocyte compo-nents. They usually are formed in the areas of slow or disturbed flow in large venous sinuses and in valve cusp pockets in the deep veins of the calf or in vein segments that have been exposed to trauma.
- The thrombus is the final consequence of an imbalance between the effects of thrombogenic stimuli and different protective mechanisms. Various factors have been implicated in the formation of the thrombus, such as activation of the coagulation cascade in an intact vascular system, vein stasis, and, in some cases, vascular injury.
- Vascular damage directly or indirectly is a major contributor to the develop-ment of venous thrombosis. Blood coagulation can be activated by intravascular stimuli released at a remote site or it can be activated

locally by vessel wall damage. Venous stasis is an important factor that pre-disposes to the development of DVT by impairing the clearance of activated coagulation factors.

CLINICAL PRESENTATION / PHYSICAL FINDINGS

- Classical presentation of DVT is sud-den onset of pain, redness, and swelling of one leg spreading from the calf to the thigh with marked swelling of the dorsum of the foot and tender-ness along the deep venous system.
- The more severe condition can result in marked swelling and femoral arterial compression.
- Marked venous thrombosis produces swelling/hemorrhage in compartments of the lower limbs, resulting in the absence of an arterial pulse.
- DVT can be completely asymptomatic with the first manifestation being a massive pulmonary embolism causing sudden death.
- PE presents with chest pain and sud-den dyspnea. The differential diagnosis of swelling in one leg includes cel-lulites, lymphangitis, gout, and arthritis.

DIAGNOSIS

- Clinical history of DVT should always be confirmed by objec-tive test.
- Some patients with minimal leg symp-toms have extensive venous thrombo-sis, but classical symptoms and signs of pain, tenderness, and swelling of the leg can by produced by nonthrombotic disorders.
- History and physical examination are important.
- Various tests have been used, but only three have been shown to be useful for the diagnosis of DVT in symptomatic patients: venography, impedance plet-hysmography, and venous ultrasound. The Doppler is reliable and is rapidly replacing contrast venography for demonstration of vein thrombosis of the lower limbs up to the femoral region.
- The gold standard is venography, but it is invasive.

MEDICAL MANAGEMENT & TREATMENT

- Main treatment of DVT is unfractionated heparin as soon as diagnosis is made or with high clin-ical suspicion, followed by the oral anticoagulant warfarin. Warfarin is ini-tiated usually in the first 24 to 48 hours after the initial diagnosis.
- Objectives of treating DVT are to pre-vent local extension of the thrombus

and prevent the thrombus from embolizing.
- First episode of DVT should be treated for 6 weeks to 3 months if a reversible risk factor is present and for 3 to 6 months if idiopathic vein thrombosis occurs.
- *Important:* In some patients with more than two documented episodes of DVT, treat with warfarin indefinitely.
- Strict control is required to maintain the INR between 2.0 and 2.5 to prevent excessive bleeding.

COMPLICATIONS

- Patients who develop compli-cations during anticoagulation therapy require management of the actual complications and subsequent management of the thromboembolic event for which the patient is being treated.
- Bleeding is by far the most important complication of anticoagulant therapy. The approach to bleeding depends on the severity of bleeding, anticoagulant and dose used, results of the laboratory test at the time of the bleeding, and severity of the thromboembolic event for which the patient is being treated. Different studies have reported bleed-ing as a complication in 5–10% of all patients under anticoagulation therapy.

PROGNOSIS

Prognosis depends on the num-ber of risk factors present. Severe deep vein thrombosis and throm-boembolic disease are associated with poor prognosis; both result in suffering and death if not recognized and treated effectively. Deep vein thrombosis is the major cause of morbidity and death, together with pulmonary embolism (PE).

DENTAL SIGNIFICANCE

The majority of patients treated with heparin are hospitalized and placed on warfarin once discharged. Dental emergencies in hospitalized patients should be treated as conserva-tively as possible. Invasive procedures are contraindicated. Consultation with the patient's physician is mandatory.

DENTAL MANAGEMENT

Patients taking warfarin:
- Consultation with physician:
  - Patients on anticoagulants are at risk both from their underlying disorder and their anticoagulation therapy. Both factors must be considered dur-ing treatment.

- ○ Evaluate predental treatment PT/INR results (see Appendix A, Box A-5, "Dental Management of Patients Taking Coumarin Anticoagulants").
- Be aware that some medications will affect the action of warfarin.
  - ○ Drugs the dentist may use that potentiate the anticoagulation action of warfarin are acetaminophen, metronidazole, salicylates, nonsteroidal antiinflammatory drugs (NSAIDs), broad-spectrum antibiotics, and erythromycin.
  - ○ Drugs that the dentist may use that will antagonize the action of warfarin are barbiturates, steroids, and nafcillin.
- If infection is present, surgery should be avoided until the infection is under control.
- Several products currently available on the market help with the stabilization of the fibrin.
- See "Venous Thrombosis" in Section III, p 386 for more information on this topic.

SUGGESTED REFERENCES

Hirsh J, Hoak J. Management of deep vein thrombosis and pulmonary embolism: a statement for health care professionals. *Circulation* 1996;93:2212–2245.

Lopez JA, Kearon C, Lee A. Deep vein thrombosis. *Hematology* 2004;52:439–456.

Little J, Miller C, Henry R, McIntosh B. Antithrombotic agents: implications in dentistry. *Oral Surg Oral Med Oral Path Oral Radiol Endod* 2002;93:544–551.

Tovey C, Wyatt S. Diagnosis, investigation, and management of deep vein thrombosis. *Brit Med J* 2003;326:1180–1184.

AUTHOR: **JUAN F. YEPES, DDS, MD**

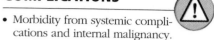

SYNONYM(S)

Idiopathic inflammatory myopathy

ICD-9CM/CPT CODE(S)

710.3 Dermatomyositis

OVERVIEW

- Dermatomyositis (DM) is a chronic idiopathic inflammatory myopathy characterized by a skin rash and proximal muscle weakness.
- DM is a common form of a family of acquired, systemic, connective tissue diseases characterized by the clinical and pathologic effects of chronic muscle inflammation of unknown etiology.
- The idiopathic inflammatory myopathies are diagnosed by a combination of pathologic, clinical, and laboratory data.

EPIDEMIOLOGY & DEMOGRAPHICS

INCIDENCE/PREVALENCE IN USA: The incidence of DM is 1:100,000. It has a prevalence of 1 to 10 cases per million in adults and 1 to 32 cases per million in children.
PREDOMINANT AGE: Average age at diagnosis is 40 years. The average age of onset in children is between 5 and 14 years.
PREDOMINANT SEX: More common in females than males (2:1).
GENETICS: Certain ethnic groups, African-Americans, and Hispanics may be at increased risk for idiopathic inflammatory myopathy with poor outcomes. Dermatomyositis can be associated with mixed connective tissue disease and systemic sclerosis. Described serological abnormalities, known as myositis-specific antibodies, suggest that this disorder is distinct from all other collagen-vascular diseases.

ETIOLOGY & PATHOGENESIS

- Unknown, but appears to be an immune-related phenomenon.
- Evidence implies that immune activation in genetically susceptible individuals, when exposed to environmental triggers, affects the etiology of dermatomyositis.
- Pathology in the muscle and affected tissues is characterized by the presence of mononuclear cells.
- Genetic risk factors: polymorphic genes that regulate the human immune responses in the major histocompatibility complex, HLA genes.
- Immunochemical and other studies implicate different pathogeneses in the various forms of myositis.

CLINICAL PRESENTATION / PHYSICAL FINDINGS

- Subacute onset, over weeks to months.
- Progressive muscle tenderness and weakness affecting proximal limb girdle muscles.
- Occasional involvement of facial, pharyngeal, and esophageal muscles.
- Dysphagia, dyspnea and respiratory failure, and periorbital heliotrope flush.
- Papular dermatitis and scaling on face, scalp, neck, and upper chest.
- Gottron papules over knuckles and interphalangeal joints.
- Calcification in facial tissues noted later in course of juvenile dermatomyositis.
- Photosensitivity is noted.

DIAGNOSIS

DIFFERENTIAL DIAGNOSIS

- Lupus erythematosus
- Mixed connective tissue disease
- Polymyositis
- Muscular dystrophies
- Steroid myopathy
- Amyotrophic lateral sclerosis
- Lambert-Eaton myasthenic syndrome
- Drug-induced myopathies
- Diabetic amyotrophy

The diagnosis of dermatomyositis requires:
- History and physical findings of proximal muscle weakness
- An EMG for noting myopathic process
- Muscle biopsy
- Characteristic skin rash
- Specific blood tests

LABORATORY EXAMINATIONS

- ESR elevation
- Creative phosphokinase elevation
- Elevated creatine urinary excretion
- Autoantibodies
- Electromyography to distinguish a myopathic from a neuropathic process
- MRI for focal lesions
- ECG for myocarditis, irritability, and/or blockage
- Radiograph or imaging of chest for intestinal fibrosis
- Radiograph or imaging of esophagus for state of peristalsis
- Skin and muscle pathology

MEDICAL MANAGEMENT & TREATMENT

NONPHARMACOLOGICAL

- Sun blocking agents for skin; sun avoidance
- Physical, occupational, and speech therapy

ACUTE CARE

- Prednisone. Dosage varies as to patient needs; 1.5 mg/kg/d acceptable. Note possible steroid myopathy. May be combined with an alternative by use of azathioprine, cyclophosphamide, or methotrexate.
- Hydroxychloroquine is used for cutaneous lesions.

CHRONIC CARE

- Prednisone may be needed for years.
- Other drugs of choice are azathioprine, methotrexate, cyclophosphamide, cyclosporine, hydroxychloroquine, and IV immunoglobulins.

COMPLICATIONS

- Morbidity from systemic complications and internal malignancy.
- Cardiomyopathy, cardiac conduction defects, aspiration pneumonia secondary to respiratory muscle weakness, interstitial pneumonitis-fibrosis, vasculopathy, muscle atrophy and calcification, and ocular complications.

PROGNOSIS

- Poor prognostic indicators include delay in diagnosis, older age, recalcitrant dysphagia, pulmonary fibrosis, leukocytosis, fever, and anorexia.
- Most common causes of death are infection, cardiac and pulmonary dysfunction, and malignancy. Early treatment allows for a 5-year 80% and an 8-year 73% survival rate.

DENTAL SIGNIFICANCE

Dysphagia from pharyngeal muscle involvement; fever; anorexia; difficulty in getting up from chair, climbing stairs, brushing teeth and flossing; respiratory compromise; and attitude to oral hygiene and appropriate diet.

DENTAL MANAGEMENT

- Carefully assess risk for adrenal suppression and insufficiency in patients being treated with systemic corticosteroids (see Appendix A, Box A-4, "Dental Management of Patients at Risk for Acute Adrenal Insufficiency").
- Patients who are taking cytotoxic or immunosuppressive drugs, including systemic corticosteroids, may have an increased risk of infection and may require perioperative prophylactic antibiotics (see Appendix A, Box A-2, "Presurgical and Postsurgical Antibiotic Prophylaxis for Patients at Increased Risk for Postoperative Infections").
- Emphasis on personal oral hygiene by assisting, delivering, and monitoring oral hygiene. Any suspected case should be referred to rheumatology.
- Work with medical team for optimal care. Must appreciate patient's loss of muscle strength, systemic disease, and potential of malignancy.

SUGGESTED REFERENCES

Fitzpatrick TB, Johnson RA, Wolff K, Suurmond D. Dermatomyositis, in *Color Atlas and Synopsis of Clinical Dermatology*, ed 4. New York, McGraw-Hill, 2001, pp 349–352.

Koler RA, Montemarano A. Dermatomyositis. *Am Fam Physician* 2001;64:1565–1572.

AUTHOR: NORBERT J. BURZYNSKI, SR., DDS, MS

SECTION 1

SYNONYM(S)

Central diabetes insipidus
Neurogenic diabetes insipidus

ICD-9CM/CPT CODE(S)

253.5 Diabetes insipidus
588.1 Nephrogenic diabetes insipidus

OVERVIEW

Diabetes insipidus (DI) is the production of high volume of very dilute urine due to either deficient secretion of antidiuretic hormone (vasopressin) from the neurohypophysis or inadequate renal response to vasopressin. The specific gravity of the urine is usually less than 1.006.

EPIDEMIOLOGY & DEMOGRAPHICS

INCIDENCE/PREVALENCE IN USA: Uncommon, with a prevalence of about 1 case per 25,000 people.
PREDOMINANT AGE: Vasopressin deficiency may occur at any age, including infancy and childhood. Nephrogenic DI usually presents in infancy.
PREDOMINANT SEX: Central DI: male = female; inherited nephrogenic DI: male > female.
GENETICS:

- Nephrogenic diabetes insipidus can be inherited as X-linked recessive (only males are clinically affected, whereas females are carriers).
- Rare, familial cases of vasopressin deficiency have been reported (commonly autosomal dominant).

ETIOLOGY & PATHOGENESIS

Based on etiology, several types have been identified:

- Primary central DI accounts for one-third of DI cases. It is not associated with any organ damage but may be genetically inherited or associated with autoimmunity to hypothalamic vasopressin-secreting cells.
- Secondary central DI is associated with organ damage to either the hypothalamus or pituitary stalk by infection or primary or metastatic tumor.
- Nephrogenic DI is caused by renal dysfunction affecting water reabsorption. Although the vasopressin level is normal, the kidneys are resistant to cir-

culating vasopressin. The renal dysfunction may be caused by congenitally defective renal vasopressin receptors or a primary renal disorder.
- Adipsic DI occurs in individuals who have lost all ability to self-regulate water metabolism. These individuals have to rely on the medical team to monitor and care for them.
- Loss of the action of vasopressin disrupts the ability of the kidneys to concentrate urine, thereby leading to loss of large volumes of urine.
- The excessive free loss of water leads to cellular and extracellular dehydration.

CLINICAL PRESENTATION / PHYSICAL FINDINGS

- Increase in thirst (polydipsia) and craving for ice-cold water.
- Passage of large volumes of urine (polyuria) that may be up to 20 liters per day depending on water intake.
- Inability to keep up with the increased demand for water intake may lead to cellular dehydration.

DIAGNOSIS

- 24-hour urine collection greater than 2 liters should be followed by other tests for DI.
- Assess the plasma and urine osmolality.
- Dehydration test (also called the water deprivation test or Miller-Moses test).
- Vasopressin challenge test.
- Radioimmunoassay of antidiuretic hormone.
- MRI of pituitary to check for organ damage.

MEDICAL MANAGEMENT & TREATMENT

- Correction of any underlying pathology.
- Neurogenic diabetes insipidus:
  - Desmopressin acetate (synthetic analogue of vasopressin) is the drug of choice for neurogenic diabetes insipidus. Usually administered intranasally at a dose of 100 μg/mL solution every 12 to 24 hours as needed.
- Nephrogenic diabetes insipidus:

  - Assurance of adequate water intake and reduction of polyuria with thiazide diuretics combined with amiloride.

COMPLICATIONS

- Hydronephrosis
- Renal dysfunction leading to confusion, stupor, and coma

PROGNOSIS

The prognosis of DI is dependent on the underlying cause but is generally favorable with proper medical intervention and monitoring, as most cases will require lifelong treatment.

DENTAL SIGNIFICANCE

Fluorosis may result from drinking large volumes of fluoridated water.

DENTAL MANAGEMENT

- Treatment plan for major dental surgery should include replacement of fluid loss with solute-free water.
- The use of high doses of glucocorticoids may increase the renal loss of water and further complicate DI.

SUGGESTED REFERENCES

Aron D, Findling J, Tyrrell B. Hypothalamus and pituitary, in Greenspan F, Strewler G (eds): *Basic and Clinical Endocrinology*, ed 5. New York, McGraw-Hill/Appleton and Lange, 1997, p146–152.
Klein, H. Dental fluorosis associated with hereditary diabetes insipidus. *Oral Surg Oral Med Oral Pathol* 1975;40(6):736–741.
Mizushima T, Kitamura S, Kinouchi K, Taniguchi A, Fukumitsu K. Perioperative management of a child with congenital nephrogenic diabetes insipidus. *Masui* 2001; 50(3):287–289.
Reeves WB, Bichet DG, Andreoli TE. Posterior pituitary and water metabolism, in Wilson JD, Foster DW, Kronenberg HM, Larsen PR (eds): *William's Textbook of Endocrinology*. Philadelphia, WB Saunders, 1998, p 359–372.

AUTHOR: **SUNDAY O. AKINTOYE, BDS, DDS, MS**

SYNONYM(S)

Type 1 diabetes:
- Insulin-dependent diabetes mellitus (IDDM)
- Juvenile-onset diabetes mellitus

Type 2 diabetes:
- Noninsulin-dependent diabetes mellitus (NIDDM)
- Adult-onset diabetes mellitus

ICD-9CM/CPT CODE(S)

250.00 Diabetes mellitus without mention of complication, type II or unspecified type, not stated as uncontrolled—complete

250.01 Diabetes mellitus without mention of complication, type I (juvenile type), not stated as uncontrolled—complete

250.02 Diabetes mellitus without mention of complication, type II or unspecified type, uncontrolled—complete

250.03 Diabetes mellitus without mention of complication, type I (juvenile type), uncontrolled—complete

OVERVIEW

TYPE 1 DIABETES MELLITUS (DM)

- Syndrome with disordered carbohydrate metabolism and inappropriate hyperglycemia due to a deficiency of endogenous insulin secretion, resulting in end-organ complications including accelerated atherosclerosis, neuropathy, nephropathy, and retinopathy.
- Major characteristics of type 1 DM include:
  - Immune-mediated or idiopathic pancreatic beta cell destruction leading to an absolute insulin deficiency
  - Polyuria, polydipsia, and rapid weight loss associated with random plasma glucose > 200 mg/dL
  - Ketonemia, ketonuria, or both

TYPE 2 DIABETES MELLITUS

- Syndrome with disordered carbohydrate metabolism and inappropriate hyperglycemia due to either a deficiency of endogenous insulin secretion and/or a combination of insulin resistance and inadequate insulin secretion to compensate, resulting in end-organ complications including accelerated atherosclerosis, neuropathy, nephropathy, and retinopathy.
- Major characteristics of type 2 DM include:
  - Insulin resistance with relative insulin deficiency to a predominately insulin secretory defect with target cellular insulin resistance.

- Polyuria and polydipsia (ketonuria and weight loss generally are uncommon at time of diagnosis).
- Many patients have few or no symptoms (see following).
- Hypertension, hyperlipidemia, and atherosclerosis are often associated.

GESTATIONAL DIABETES MELLITUS (GDM)

- Disordered carbohydrate metabolism and inappropriate hyperglycemia that occurs during pregnancy, usually resolving after delivery.
- GDM develops in 1–3% of pregnancies and usually in the third trimester.
- Women with GDM will exhibit an elevated risk for perinatal morbidity and mortality. They also are at increased risk (approximately 40–60%) for developing type 2 DM later in life. Control of weight after pregnancy greatly reduces the chance of developing type 2 DM.

SECONDARY DIABETES

Secondary to some other identifiable etiology including:
- Genetic defects of beta cell function
- Genetic defects in insulin action
- Diseases of the exocrine pancreas (pancreatitis, trauma, neoplasia, cystic fibrosis, etc.)
- Endocrinopathies (acromegaly, Cushing's syndrome, hyperthyroidism, pheochromocytoma, etc.)
- Drug- or chemical-induced (glucocorticoids, pentamidine, nicotinic acid, thiazides, phenytoin, etc.)
- Infections (congenital rubella, cytomegalovirus, etc.)
- Other genetic syndromes sometimes associated with diabetes (Down, Klinefelter's, Turner's, or Wolfram syndromes, Friedreich's ataxia, Huntington's chorea, etc.)

EPIDEMIOLOGY & DEMOGRAPHICS

TYPE 1 DIABETES:

INCIDENCE/PREVALENCE IN USA: Incidence of 15 per 100,000 persons per year; prevalence 0.3 to 0.4%. Racial predilection for Caucasians, with African-Americans having the lowest overall incidence.

PREDOMINANT AGE: Mean age of onset at 8 to 12 years, peaking in adolescence; onset about 1.5 years earlier in girls than boys, with a rapid decline in incidence after adolescence.

PREDOMINANT SEX: Male = female.

GENETICS:
- The role of genetics in the etiology of type 1 DM is weak, with data from monozygotic twins showing concordance for development of the disease of 30–50%.
- Two genes linked to type 1 DM have been identified, with one located within the insulin promoter region on

chromosome 11 and another involving the HLA region on the short arm of chromosome 6.
- Specific HLA haplotypes linked to type 1 DM include DR3 and/or DR4 class II HLA molecules.
  - Ninety to ninety-five percent of type 1 DM patients express either HLA DR3 or HLA DR4 II, as compared with an incidence of 50–60% in the general population, and represents a fourfold increase in relative risk of developing type 1 DM.
  - Sixty percent of patients express both alleles, a rate more than 10 times that of the general population, and represents a twelvefold increase in the relative risk of developing type 1 DM.
- HLA B8 and B15 may also be associated with an increased risk of developing type 1 DM.

TYPE 2 DIABETES:

INCIDENCE/PREVALENCE IN USA: Incidence is 300 per 100,000 (males: 230 per 100,000, females: 340 per 100,000). Prevalence is 5000 per 100,000, more common in African-Americans, Hispanic descendants, and in Native Americans, where in some groups (such as Pima Indians) there is a 35% prevalence.

PREDOMINANT AGE: Typically occurs after age 40; may occur at an earlier age, especially in certain populations including Native Americans, Hispanic descendants, and African-Americans, where the appearance of type 2 diabetes may occur as early as adolescence.

PREDOMINANT SEX: Female > male in Caucasian populations.

GENETICS: Strong polygenic familial susceptibility from undefined genetic defect(s) (concordance rates in identical twins are nearly 100%), the expression of which is modified by environmental factors.

ETIOLOGY & PATHOGENESIS

TYPE 1 DIABETES:

- Pancreatic islet beta cells in genetically susceptible individuals are destroyed by an autoimmune response mediated by T-lymphocytes and humoral mediators (TNF, IL-1, NO) that react specifically to one or more beta-cell proteins (autoantigens), resulting in an absolute deficiency of endogenous insulin secretion (insulinopenia) and dependence on exogenous insulin therapy for survival.
- Due to endogenous insulinopenia, patients with type 1 DM are prone to ketosis (and possible ketoacidosis) even under basal conditions.

TYPE 2 DIABETES:

- Impaired beta cell function (defective insulin secretion) and marked resistance or insensitivity to the metabolic actions of endogenous as well as exogenous insulin, in part as the result of decreased tissue insulin receptors (liver, skeletal muscle, adipose). Failure of postreceptor coupling and of intracellular insulin action is a more important cause of insulin resistance.

- Patients with type 2 DM maintain some endogenous insulin secretory capability despite the overt abnormalities of glucose homeostasis, including fasting hyperglycemia and/or carbohydrate intolerance. They are relatively resistant to the development of ketosis under basal conditions because of the retention of endogenous insulin secretory capabilities. However, they are more susceptible to the development of extreme hypertonic dehydration.
- Mild to marked obesity is present in approximately 80% of type 2 DM patients at the time of diagnosis. Obesity is a major risk factor for the development of this type of DM, owing in part to the associated insulin resistance.

CLINICAL PRESENTATION / PHYSICAL FINDINGS

- Almost all initial symptoms of DM are secondary to hyperglycemia (or, if diagnosis and management are not timely, to ketosis and acidosis). Clinical manifestations of hyperglycemia include:
  - Polyuria, polydipsia, polyphagia, and weight loss (with marked glucosuria and an osmotic diuresis, resulting in dehydration)
  - Weakness
  - Fatigue
  - Nausea with abdominal discomfort
  - Blurred vision (due to diffusion of glucose into the lens with subsequent swelling and increased optical density)
  - Candidal infections of the vagina and intertriginous spaces
  - Frequent infections (especially acute urinary tract infections in female patients and wound infections)
- The initial signs and symptoms of type 1 DM are relatively more abrupt and severe than those of type 2 DM, which tends to have a much more slow and insidious onset. In type 2 DM, the initial manifestation of hyperglycemia may be mild or insufficient to produce symptoms, and the disease may become evident only after chronic complications develop.

DIAGNOSIS

- Symptoms of diabetes (polyuria, polydipsia, weight loss) plus a random plasma glucose ≥ 200 mg/dL (11.1 mmol/L)

or

- Fasting plasma glucose ≥ 126 mg/dL (7.0 mmol/L) on two occasions

or

- 2-hour plasma glucose ≥ 200 mg/dL (11.1 mmol/L) during oral glucose tolerance test (OGTT) with 75 g glucose load

Glycosylated hemoglobin (HbA1c) level is not recommended for diagnosis of DM but is extremely useful in monitoring the progress of diabetic patients. HbA1c testing should be performed routinely in all patients with DM, first to document the degree of glycemic control at initial assessment and then approximately every 3 months as part of continuing care.

MEDICAL MANAGEMENT & TREATMENT

DIET

- Weight reduction, gain, or maintenance (as appropriate)
- Carbohydrates: 45–60% (depending on the severity of diabetes and triglyceride levels)
- Restriction of saturated fat (to < 10% of calories)
- Increased monounsaturated fat (depending on the need to limit carbohydrate)
- Decreased cholesterol intake to < 200 mg/day
- Sodium restriction in patients prone to hypertension

EXERCISE

- Limitations are imposed by preexisting coronary or peripheral vascular disease, proliferative retinopathy, peripheral or autonomic neuropathy, and poor glycemic control.
- Aerobic strongly preferred. Avoid heavy lifting, straining, and Valsalva maneuvers that raise blood pressure.
- Intensity: Increase pulse rate to at least 120 to 140 bpm, depending on the age and cardiovascular state of the patient.
- Frequency: 3 to 4 days per week.
- Duration: 20 to 30 minutes preceded and followed by stretching and flexibility exercises for 5 to 10 minutes.

PHARMACOLOGIC THERAPY

(Adapted from Ferri FF. Diabetes mellitus, in *Ferri's Clinical Advisor*. St Louis, Elsevier, 2006.)

- When dietary and exercise measures fail to normalize the serum glucose, oral hypoglycemic agents (e.g., metformin, glitazones, or a sulfonylurea) should be added to the regimen in type 2 DM. The sulfonamides and the biguanide metformin are the oldest and most commonly used classes of hypoglycemic drugs.
- Metformin's primary mechanism is to decrease hepatic glucose output. Because metformin does not produce hypoglycemia when used as a monotherapy, it is preferred for most patients. It is contraindicated in patients with renal insufficiency.

- Sulfonylureas and repaglinide work best when given before meals because they increase the postprandial output of insulin from the pancreas. All sulfonylureas are contraindicated in patients allergic to sulfa.
- Acarbose and miglitol work by competitively inhibiting pancreatic amylase, and small intestinal glucosidases delay gastrointestinal absorption of carbohydrates, thereby reducing alimentary hyperglycemia. The major side effects are flatulence, diarrhea, and abdominal cramps.
- Pioglitazone and rosiglitazone increase insulin sensitivity and are useful in addition to other agents in type 2 diabetics whose hyperglycemia is inadequately controlled. Serum transaminase levels should be obtained before starting therapy and monitored periodically.
- Insulin is indicated for the treatment of all type 1 DM patients and for type 2 DM patients who cannot be adequately controlled with diet and oral agents. The risks of insulin therapy include weight gain, hypoglycemia, and, in rare cases, allergic or cutaneous reactions.
- Combination therapy of various hypoglycemic agents is commonly used when monotherapy results in inadequate glycemic control.
- Continuous subcutaneous insulin infusion (CSII or insulin pump) provides better glycemic control than does conventional therapy and comparable to or slightly better control than multiple daily injections. It should be considered for diabetes presenting in childhood or adolescence and during pregnancy.

COMPLICATIONS

In susceptible individuals, complications secondary to DM begin to appear 10 to 15 years after onset but can be present at time of diagnosis since the disease may go undetected for years.

- Diabetic ketoacidosis (DKA) results from the inability of the body to metabolize ketones (produced by lipolysis from adipose tissue and in hepatic ketogenesis) as rapidly as they are produced and the failure of the body to compensate for the decrease in pH via renal and respiratory mechanisms. The condition primarily affects type 1 DM and is serious, accounting for about 1% of all deaths in diabetic patients (see "Diabetic Ketoacidosis" in Section III, p 356).
- Hyperosmolar, hyperglycemic, nonketotic coma (HHNC) is a diabetic-related coma marked by severe hyperglycemia, resultant extreme hypertonic

dehydration resulting from sustained osmotic diuresis, and absence of significant ketoacidosis. It is predominantly seen in type 2 diabetics. In many patients a precipitating acute illness such as infection, myocardial infarction, or stroke is present in conjunction with the patient not drinking enough water to compensate for urinary losses from chronic hyperglycemia.

- Neuropathies are the most common chronic complications of diabetes and affect:
  - Central nervous system: mono-neuropathies involving cranial nerves III, IV, and VI, intercostal nerves, and femoral nerves
  - Peripheral sensorimotor nerves: symmetric, bilateral paresthesias of extremities (feet more than hands) associated with intense, burning pain, particularly during the night
  - Autonomic nervous system: esophageal motility abnormalities, gastroparesis, diarrhea, neurogenic bladder, impotence, orthostatic hypotension, postural syncope, dizziness, and light-headedness
- Proliferative retinopathy occurs in 15% of diabetic patients after 15 years and increases 1% per year after diagnosis. Up to 20% of patients with type 2 DM have retinopathy at the time of diagnosis.
- Nephropathy and end-stage renal disease (ESRD): Diabetic nephropathy is the leading cause of ESRD, representing 42% of all cases. Patients with type 1 DM have a 30–40% chance of having nephropathy leading to ESRD after 20 years, in contrast to the much lower frequency in type 2 DM patients, in whom only about 15–20% develop ESRD.
- Atherosclerotic cardiovascular and peripheral vascular disease (PVD): DM induces hypercholesterolemia and a markedly increased predisposition to accelerated atherosclerosis, especially in the aorta and large- and medium-sized arteries, and a twofold to sixfold increased risk of heart disease. Other factors being equal, the incidence of myocardial infarction is twice as high in diabetics as in nondiabetics. Patients with DM have a twofold to fourfold increased risk of stroke (primarily due to the accelerated development of cervical carotid artery atheromas) and increased stroke severity.
- Increased risk of infections: Patients with DM exhibit enhanced susceptibility to infections of the skin and to tuberculosis, pneumonia, and pyelonephritis. Such infections are responsible for death in about 5% of patients with DM.
- Gangrene of extremities: The incidence of gangrene of the feet in diabetics is 20 to 100 times the incidence in matched controls. Amputation of the lower extremities is sometimes required, but appropriate prophylactic foot care has greatly reduced its frequency.
- Glaucoma occurs in approximately 6% of persons with diabetes.
- Neuropathic arthropathy (Charcot's joints): Bone or joint deformities from repeated trauma, which occur secondary to peripheral neuropathy.
- Cataracts: Premature cataracts occur in diabetic patients and seem to correlate with both the duration of diabetes and the severity of chronic hyperglycemia.
- Skin ulcerations, including chronic pyogenic infections, eruptive xanthomas (secondary to hypertriglyceridemia), and necrobiosis lipoidica diabeticorum (NLD).

PROGNOSIS

- The Diabetes Control and Complication Trial (1983–1993) proved that intensive treatment decreases the development and progression of complications in patients with type 1 DM. The same was found in patients with type 2 DM in the United Kingdom Prospective Diabetes Study (1977–1991).
- In both types of DM, the diabetic patient's intelligence, motivation, and awareness of the potential complications of the disease contribute significantly to the ultimate outcome.
- In patients with type 1 DM, complications from end-stage renal disease are a major cause of death, whereas patients with type 2 DM are more likely to have vascular diseases leading to myocardial infarction and stroke as the main causes of death.
- Aggressive therapy to lower blood pressure in hypertensive DM patients decreases the rates of complications, death, stroke, heart failure, and microvascular complications.

DENTAL SIGNIFICANCE

- Oral complications of DM include:
  - Salivary gland dysfunction resulting in xerostomia and possible asymptomatic bilateral parotid swelling
  - Increased risk of oral infections: candidiasis (including median rhomboid glossitis, denture stomatitis, and angular cheilitis) and periapical abscesses
  - Increased incidence and severity of gingival inflammation, periodontal abscesses, and chronic periodontal disease
  - Increased incidence and severity of caries
  - Glossodynia and burning mouth syndrome
  - Dysgeusia
- Dentists treating patients with type 2 DM should review their panoramic radiographs carefully for evidence of carotid artery atheroma formation. Patients with atheromatous lesions must be referred to their physicians for further evaluation and treatment because the modification of atherogenic risk factors and the surgical removal of atheromas in certain patients have been shown to reduce the likelihood of stroke.

DENTAL MANAGEMENT

General evaluation to determine:
- Time since diagnosis (age of onset) of DM
- Type of DM
- Type of therapy required:
  - Control of diet
  - Oral hypoglycemic agents (types and dose)
  - Insulin therapy (types and regimen)
- Adequacy of control:
  - Most recent glycosylated hemoglobin (HbA1c) and fasting blood glucose (FBG) test results
  - History and frequency of hypoglycemic episodes
  - History and frequency of ketoacidosis
  - Method and frequency of self-monitoring of blood glucose
  - Frequency of physician visits for evaluation of diabetes status and control
- Presence of chronic complications of diabetes:
  - Cardiovascular, neurologic, renal, retinal, infectious

In general, elective dental treatment on an outpatient basis should be deferred for diabetic patients demonstrating:
- Poor metabolic control of diabetes
- Frequent symptoms of uncontrolled diabetes
- Frequent problems with ketoacidosis and hypoglycemia
- Multiple chronic complications of diabetes
- Fasting blood glucose level greater than 250 mg/dL
- Glycosylated hemoglobin (HbA1c) level greater than 9%

Specific dental management considerations:
- Morning appointments are usually best.
- For patients taking insulin, advise patient to take usual insulin dosage and normal meals on day of dental appointment; confirm when patient comes for appointment. [Some sources recommend having the patient take half their normal insulin dose prior to dental treatment and then taking the

remainder of their insulin dose after dental treatment, provided that normal oral intake of nutrition (food) will not be impaired as a result of dental treatment.]
- Check patient's blood glucose chairside just prior to initiating dental treatment.
  - If patient's blood glucose is less than 70 to 90 mg/dL, have the patient eat (i.e., give carbohydrates) prior to dental treatment to help avoid a hypoglycemic reaction during dental treatment.
  - If patient's blood glucose is greater than 200 mg/dL, then:
    - defer elective dental treatment (and possibly refer patient to physician for evaluation), *or*
    - have patient take a hypoglycemic drug (e.g., insulin), if appropriate.
- Advise patient to inform you or your staff as soon as they become aware of symptoms of hypoglycemia (e.g., hunger, weakness, tachycardia, sweat-

ing, paresthesias) may that occur during dental visit.
- Have approximately 15 grams of a fast-acting oral carbohydrate such as glucose tablets, sugar, candy, soft drinks, or juice available and give to patient if symptoms of hypoglycemia occur.
- If extensive dental surgery is needed:
  - Consult with patient's physician concerning dietary needs during postoperative period.
  - Consider prophylactic (postoperative) antibiotics for a patient with brittle diabetes or one taking high doses of insulin to prevent postoperative infection.
- Additional precautions may be needed for patient with complications of diabetes such as renal disease, heart disease.

SUGGESTED REFERENCES

American Diabetes Association Clinical Practice Recommendations 2003. *Diabetes Care* 2002;26:Supp 1.

Ferri FF. Diabetes mellitus, in *Ferri's Clinical Advisor*. St Louis, Elsevier, 2006, pp 252–253.

Friedlander AH, Garrett NR, Norman DC. The prevalence of calcified carotid artery atheromas on the panoramic radiographs of patients with type 2 diabetes mellitus. *JADA* 2002;133(11):1516–1523.

Guggenheimer J, et al. Insulin-dependent diabetes mellitus and oral soft tissue pathologies I. Prevalence and characteristics of non-candidal lesions. *Oral Surg Oral Med Oral Pathol Oral Radiol Endod* 2000;89:563–569.

Guggenheimer J, et al. Insulin-dependent diabetes mellitus and oral soft tissue pathologies II. Prevalence and characteristics of Candida and candidal lesions. *Oral Surg Oral Med Oral Pathol Oral Radiol Endod* 2000;89:570–576.

Lalla RV, D'Ambrosio JA. Dental management considerations for the patient with diabetes mellitus. *JADA* 2001;132(10):1425–1432.

Maitra A, Abbas AK. The endocrine system, in Kumar V, Abbas AK, Fausto N (eds): *Robbins and Cotran: Pathologic Basis of Disease*. St Louis, Elsevier, 2005, pp 1189–1205.

AUTHOR: **F. JOHN FIRRIOLO, DDS, PHD**

SYNONYM(S)

Defibrination syndrome
Afibrinogenemia
Consumption coagulopathy
Diffuse intravascular coagulation (DIC)
Acquired fibrinolytic hemorrhage
Hemorrhagic fibrinogenolysis
Pathologic fibrinolysis
Fibrinolytic purpura
Purpura fulminans

ICD-9CM/CPT CODE(S)

286.6 Disseminated intravascular coagulation

OVERVIEW

Disseminated intravascular coagulation (DIC) is a pathologic activation of the coagulation system that leads to consumption of clotting factors and results in bleeding. It is invariably the consequence of an underlying disease process such as overwhelming infection, snake bite, or obstetric conditions such as abruptio placentae, amniotic fluid embolism, or preeclampsia.

EPIDEMIOLOGY & DEMOGRAPHICS

INCIDENCE/PREVALENCE IN USA: Unknown; more than 50% of cases are associated with gram-negative sepsis or other septicemic infections.
PREDOMINANT AGE: Not established.
PREDOMINANT SEX: Male = female.
GENETICS: Can be associated with homozygous protein C or protein S deficiency.

ETIOLOGY & PATHOGENESIS

- Initial activation of platelets (by infection, endotoxins, snake bite venom, autoimmune reaction, damage to endothelial cells) leads to intravascular fibrin deposition.
- Mechanical damage to red blood cells as a result of fibrin strands leads to haemolytic anemia and secondary fibrinolysis.
- Organ damage results from fibrin thrombi, especially in the kidneys, gastrointestinal tract, and central nervous system.
- Platelets and coagulation factors are consumed; fibrinolysis degrades the clots and releases natural anticoagulants.

CLINICAL PRESENTATION / PHYSICAL FINDINGS

- Wide spectrum of severity, from mild oozing from venipuncture sites and mucous membranes to serious internal hemorrhage and organ failure.
- A chronic form of DIC can occur in patients with a malignancy or a vascular disorder.

DIAGNOSIS

- Peripheral blood smear shows microangiopathic changes.
- Decreased platelet count.
- Prothrombin time, partial thromboplastin time, and thrombin time are all prolonged.
- Factor V and VIII are consumed, but fibrin degradation products must be demonstrated.

MEDICAL MANAGEMENT & TREATMENT

- Elimination of underlying cause
- Replacement of platelets and coagulation factors (fresh frozen plasma, cryoprecipitate)

COMPLICATIONS

- Spontaneous bleeding, petechiae, ecchymoses

PROGNOSIS

Dependent on the underlying disease or condition

DENTAL SIGNIFICANCE

- Acute DIC: all dental treatment should be deferred until DIC is controlled.
- Chronic DIC: urgent dental care only.

DENTAL MANAGEMENT

- Consultation with patient's physician.
- Replace platelets and coagulation factors as indicated.
- Use good surgical technique.
  - Control bleeding with local hemostatic measures [e.g., absorbable gelatin sponges (Gelfoam®), oxidized cellulose (SURGICEL™), microfibrillar collagen (Avitene®), topical thrombin tranexamic acid, epsilon-aminocaproic acid (EACA), sutures, surgical splints, and stents].
- Monitor patient progress within 24 to 48 hours.
- Avoid aspirin or nonsteroidal antiinflammatory drugs (NSAIDs).

SUGGESTED REFERENCES

Catalono PM. Disorders of the coagulation mechanism, in Rose LF, Kaye D (eds): *Internal Medicine for Dentistry.* St Louis, Mosby, 1990, pp 353–359.

Schardt-Sacco D. Update on coagulopathies. *Oral Surg Oral Med Oral Pathol Oral Radiol Endod* 2000;90:559–563.

AUTHOR: **WENDY S. HUPP, DMD**

SYNONYM(S)

Down's Syndrome

Trisomy 21

Mongoloidism (a term that is no longer considered appropriate because this designation is considered pejorative and stigmatizing)

ICD-9CM/CPT CODE(S)

758.0 Down syndrome—complete

OVERVIEW

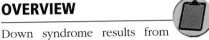

Down syndrome results from nondisjunction causing trisomy of chromosome 21. It is characterized by flattening of the occiput and face, upward slant to eyes with epicanthal folds, and mental retardation.

EPIDEMIOLOGY & DEMOGRAPHICS

INCIDENCE/PREVALENCE IN USA: The most common autosomal chromosome abnormality in humans. Occurs in 1:700 live births, affecting > 250,000 people in the U.S.

PREDOMINANT AGE: Down syndrome is a congenital disorder (present at birth).

PREDOMINANT SEX: No sex predilection.

GENETICS: As described previously. Extra chromosome comes from mother in > 90% of the cases.

ETIOLOGY & PATHOGENESIS

- Ninety-five percent of the genetic abnormalities resulting in Down syndrome are of maternal origin, while only 5% occur during spermatogenesis. Abnormalities include:
  - Free trisomy 21 (95% of cases)
  - Unbalanced translocation between chromosome 21 and other acrocentric chromosomes, especially 14 and 21 (4% of cases)
  - Mosaicism with two cell lines (one normal and one trisomy) (1% of cases)
- The risk for carrying a child with Down syndrome is greatly increased with increasing maternal age.
  - At a maternal age of 30 years, the odds of such occurrence are 1:900.
  - At 35 years, the odds increase to 1:400.
  - At 40 years, the odds increase to 1:100.

CLINICAL PRESENTATION / PHYSICAL FINDINGS

Hall's 10 cardinal signs of Down syndrome during the neonatal period are:

1. Poor Moro reflex
2. Hypotonia
3. Flattening of the occiput and face
4. Upslanting palpebral fissures
5. Simple, small, rounded ears
6. Redundant, loose neck skin
7. Single palmar crease
8. Hyperextensible large joints
9. Abnormal pelvis radiograph
10. Fifth finger hypoplasia

GASTROINTESTINAL (~ 12% PREVALENCE)

- Duodenal atresia, gastroesophageal reflux, annular pancreas, Hirschsprung disease, anorectal anomalies, celiac disease (7–16%).
- Etiology may be anatomical, functional, or due to a nutritional disorder.
- Often results in abnormal growth and development and a small stature.

CENTRAL NERVOUS SYSTEM

- Increased mobility at atlantoaxial joint (cervical vertebrae or ligament abnormalities) occurs in approximately 15% of cases and may result in subluxation and neurological symptoms.
- Approximately 30% of patients develop dementia or early-onset Alzheimer's disease.
- Mental retardation to some degree is universal (mostly ranges from mild to moderate).
- Delayed motor function and expressive speech.
- Approximately 10% of patients develop a seizure disorder.

ENDOCRINE

- Approximately 40% of patients have either a congenital or adult hypothyroid disorder, possibly due to autoantibodies.
  - Unlike congenital hypothyroid seen in otherwise normal patients, the treatment of congenital hypothyroid in patients with Down syndrome does not prevent mental retardation.
- Insulin-dependent diabetes mellitus (possibly a result of lifestyle or autoantibodies).
- Inadequate growth which may require growth hormone for treatment.
  - Special growth charts have been formulated for patients with Down syndrome.
- Infertility.
  - In males, this often results from low testosterone levels.
  - In females, this may result from ovarian dysfunction or hypothalamic–pituitary–ovarian adrenal axis involvement.

BEHAVIOR

- Most Down syndrome patients are gregarious, cooperative, and friendly.

EYES

- Structural abnormalities: Brushfield's spots in the iris, epicanthal folds.
- Functional abnormalities: Congenital glaucoma, cataracts, nystagmus, refractive errors.

SKIN

- Frequent: Increased loose skin on the back of neck, fissured tongue, change in infants' skin color, fungal infections, seborrheic dermatitis, cheilitis.
- Less frequent: Alopecia areata, vitiligo, severe atopic dermatitis.

IMMUNE SYSTEM

- Slow maturation of immune system in children results in repeated upper respiratory infections.
- Deficient immune system:
  - Impaired cell-mediated and humoral immunity.
  - Deficient phagocytic system caused by impaired chemotaxis.
  - Reduced phagocytic ability of polymorphonuclear leukocytes.
  - Results in:
    - Increased risk for chronic hepatitis (seven times higher in Down syndrome patients who are institutionalized than in those who are not institutionalized).

EARS, NOSE, AND THROAT (ENT)

- Increased chronic otitis media and anatomic anomalies of eustachian tube.
- External ear canal stenosis which causes hearing loss (~ 38–78%) by canal collapse or cerumen obstruction.
- Enlarged tonsils and adenoids.

ORTHOPEDIC

- Changes in bones and structure of connective tissue.
- Low muscle tone (hypotonia) is seen in ~ 75%.
- Genu valgus, hip instability, pes planovalgus, scoliosis, frequent joint dislocation.

HEMATOLOGY

- Approximately 10 to 20 times increased incidence of acute lymphocytic leukemia (ALL), particularly in the first 4 years of life, but likely still at increased risk into adulthood:
  - Persistent gingival lesions and gingival hemorrhage may be evident.

RESPIRATORY

- Increased incidence of upper respiratory infection.
- Increased airway obstruction and sleep apnea.
- Increased subglottic stenosis in children.

CARDIAC

- Approximately 40% of patients have a congenital cardiac anomaly.
  - In order of descending frequency: ventricular septal defects, A/V communication, arterial septal defects, and patent ductus arteriosus.
- Mitral valve prolapse (MVP) is common in adults, with ~ 50% requiring bacterial endocarditis prophylaxis prior to invasive dental treatment. Approximately one-third have negative auscultatory findings and require an echocardiogram for diagnosis.
- Increased morbidity and mortality with cardiac surgery compared to the otherwise normal population.

DIAGNOSIS

Clinical assessment and chromosomal analysis.

MEDICAL MANAGEMENT & TREATMENT

- Evaluation by a sleep disorders clinic.
- Predisposition for infection:
  - Hepatitis B vaccine and standard immunization protocol to prevent infection.
  - Strict asepsis for invasive procedures.
  - Remove venous/arterial cannulas and urinary catheters as soon as possible.
- Screening and treatment of celiac disease.
- Screening and treatment of hypothyroid.
- Aggressive approach to prevent ear canal collapse and hearing loss.
- Surgical correction of congenital heart defects.
- Echocardiogram to rule out MVP in undiagnosed adults.
- Careful monitoring during and after general anesthesia to prevent predisposed complications:
  - May require smaller endotracheal tube.
  - Postoperative agitation.
  - Monitor ventilation in recovery.
  - Avoid the use of atropine.
  - Prevent postoperative respiratory tract infection.
  - Prevent postextubation stridor by administering a short period of corticosteroids prior to extubation.
- Radiologic screening for atlantoaxial instability in patients with neurologic/physical signs:
  - Careful manipulation of head.
  - Limited activities in those with signs of instability until properly screened.

COMPLICATIONS

- Common complications after general anesthesia include:
  - Increased airway obstruction and sleep apnea.
  - Inability to maintain airway (hypoventilation) due to hypotonia.
  - Postoperative respiratory tract infection.
  - Postextubation stridor (30–40% vs 2% in the normal population).
- Exaggerated response to atropine.
- Atlantoaxial subluxation:
  - Common when the distance between the odontoid process of the axis and the anterior arch of atlas is > 4.5 mm or if there is atlantooccipital and rotational instability.
  - Injury occurs with hyperextension or radical flexion of the neck or direct pressure on the neck/upper spine.

- May result in irreversible spinal cord damage.
- Neurological signs: abnormal gait, clumsiness, walking fatigue, preference to sit.
- Physical signs: hyperreflexia, clonus quadriparesis, extensor plantars, neurogenic bladder, hemiparesis, ataxia, sensory loss.

PROGNOSIS

- Overall prognosis and longevity may be dependent on the presence congenital heart disease. Most patients die at age 50 to 60 (earlier if there is heart disease).
- Increased morbidity and mortality postcardiac surgery, but most have a good prognosis.
- Alzheimer's disease occurs in 25% of adults with Down syndrome.
- Patients often lose teeth due to periodontal disease.

DENTAL SIGNIFICANCE

OROFACIAL STRUCTURES

- Palate:
  - An underdeveloped midface results in decreased length, height, and depth of palate (not width).
  - Patients may have soft palate insufficiency. "Staired" palates with V-shaped, high vaults are common.
- Lips and oral cavity:
  - Hypotonic orbicularis, zygomatic, masseter, and temporalis muscles may result in altered facial features such that the angle of the mouth appears "pulled down" and the lower lip is everted.
  - The mouth appears open due to a large tongue and small oral cavity.
  - Mouth breathing, drooling, chapped lower lips, angular cheilitis, chronic periodontitis, respiratory tract infections, bifid uvulae, cleft lip/palate, enlarged tonsils and adenoids, and xerostomia are common.
- Tongue:
  - Scalloped due to abnormal pressure.
  - Fissured dorsal surface of anterior two-thirds (probably developmental etiology).
  - Geographic tongue.
  - Hypotonic musculature may result in protrusion and tongue thrusting.
  - Macroglossia relative to small oral cavity.
  - Desiccated (secondary to mouth breathing and/or xerostomia).

DENTAL

- Microdontia:
  - Occurs in 35–55% of patients with Down syndrome, affecting both the primary and secondary dentitions.
  - Short, conical, small clinical crowns.

- Spacing, particularly in the mandibular arch.
- Hypoplasia and hypocalcification:
  - May be congenital generalized/localized in infants.
  - Ranges from intrinsic to overt defects.
  - Related to significant illness, prolonged fever, and antibiotic therapy.
- Hypodontia:
  - Occurs in approximately 50% of patients with Down syndrome, possibly of a genetic etiology.
  - Prevalence of absent teeth is similar to that seen in the normal population:
    - Third molars > second premolars > lateral incisors > mandibular incisors.
  - May result in mandibular spacing (the maxilla is commonly crowded).
- Taurodontism:
  - Occurs in approximately 0.54–5.6% of patients with Down syndrome.
  - Primarily involves mandibular second molars.
- Crown variation:
  - Labial surfaces, incisal edges of anterior teeth, altered cuspal inclines on canines, missing or deficient distolingual cusps of maxillary molars, displaced distal cusps of mandibular molars, tooth agenesis.
    - Approximately tenfold increase in occurrence in patients with Down syndrome as compared to the general population.
    - Male > female.
    - Mandible > maxilla.
    - Left side > right side.
    - Prevalence of teeth affected: mandibular central incisor > maxillary lateral incisor > maxillary second premolar > mandibular second premolar.
- Dental caries:
  - Reported as a decreased incidence but may be due to environmental factors, as many studies performed were on institutionalized patient populations who have well-controlled diets.
- Primary tooth eruption:
  - Delayed timing and sequence, especially for the anterior teeth and first molars.
    - Sequence usually involves the central incisors erupting first and the second molars last, but a varied sequence in between.
    - Eruption of the first tooth often at 12 to 14 months but may occur as late as 24 months.
    - May not complete primary dentition until age 4 to 5 years.
- Secondary tooth eruption:
  - Delayed eruption.
    - Six-year molars and mandibular incisors may erupt at 8 to 9 years of age.

- Overretained primary teeth may be present even after the successor has erupted.
- Normal sequence.

PERIODONTIUM

- Increased periodontal breakdown when compared to similar plaque levels in normal patients.
- Earlier periodontal breakdown (often begins at age 6 to 15 years; most commonly developed by mid-thirties).
- Common findings include marginal gingivitis, acute/subacute necrotizing ulcerative gingivitis, advanced periodontal disease, gingival recession and pockets, horizontal/vertical bone loss with suppuration, bifurcation/trifurcation involvement with molars, mobility, and frequent tooth loss.

OCCLUSION

- Malalignment and malocclusion: crowding, Angle Class III molars, impacted maxillary canines, transposed maxillary first premolars and canines.
- Jaw relationships: approximately 69% of patients have prognathic mandibles (most with maxillary deficiency), 54% have anterior open bite, 97% have posterior cross bite and/or anterior cross bite, and 65% have Class III malocclusion.
- Platybasia: obtuse angle of anterior cranial base to posterior cranial base (Nasion-sella-basion) such that it forms a straight line, indicating a flat cranial base.

DENTAL MANAGEMENT

- Treatment objectives usually do not differ from those for the general population.
- Treatment may often be performed in a normal dental setting but often requires additional time to improve communication and trust.
- Consider potential postoperative anesthetic issues.
- Careful manipulation of the head in patients who have a history of atlantoaxial instability.
- Follow American Heart Association guidelines for antibiotic prophylaxis as indicated for patients with cardiovascular pathology that places them at increased risk for bacterial endocarditis (see Appendix A, Box A-1, "Antibiotic Prophylaxis Recommendations by the American Heart Association for the Prevention of Bacterial Endocarditis").
- Early preventive health program with frequent recalls (every 3 months) beginning at 6 to 18 months:
  - Counsel parents (including growth and development).
  - Consider fluoride sources.
  - Dietary counseling.
  - Oral hygiene instructions with patient and caregiver.
  - Recommend tongue brushing to prevent halitosis with fissured tongues.
    - Delayed motor skills and hypoplastic defects predispose patients to poorer oral hygiene.
  - Watch for signs of leukemia and other disorders that have oral manifestations.
  - Periodontal disease prevention:
    - Frequent cleanings (prophylaxis).
    - Consider 0.12% chlorhexidine gluconate rinses.
- Carefully monitor wound healing.
- Poor candidates for removable prosthodontics (dementia and decreased palatal retention).
- Extract overretained primary teeth.
- Consider splint fabrication (night guards) for those with tooth wear from bruxism.

SUGGESTED REFERENCES

Desai SS. Down syndrome—a review of the literature. *Oral Surg Oral Med Oral Path Oral Radiol Endod* 1997;84:279–285.

Mitchell V, Howard R, Facer E. Clinical review Down's syndrome and anaesthesia. *Paediatric Anaesthesia* 1995;5:379–384.

Roizen NJ, Patterson D. Down syndrome. *Lancet* 2003;361:1281.

Sixth World Congress on Down Syndrome: http://www.altonweb.com/cs/downsyndrome/pilcher.html

AUTHOR: **KELLY K. HILGERS, DDS, MS**

SYNONYM(S)

Infective endocarditis
Bacterial endocarditis

ICD-9CM/CPT CODE(S)
036.42 Meningococcal endocarditis
074.22 Coxsackie endocarditis
098.84 Gonococcal endocarditis
391.1 Acute rheumatic endocarditis
421.0 Acute and subacute bacterial endocarditis
421.9 Acute endocarditis

OVERVIEW

- Infective endocarditis (IE) is defined as an infection of the endocardial surface of the heart, which may include one or more heart valves, the mural endocardium, or a septal defect.
- Although it might result from a bacteremia originating from any source and representing almost any microorganism, it is of interest to dentistry as it relates to oral flora as a potential source for bacteremia and endocarditis.

EPIDEMIOLOGY & DEMOGRAPHICS

INCIDENCE/PREVALENCE IN USA:
Incidence of 1.4 to 4.2 cases per 100,000 people per year.
PREDOMINANT AGE: Although endocarditis can occur at any age, the mean age of patients has gradually risen over the past 50 years. Currently, more than 50% of patients are older than 50 years.
PREDOMINANT SEX: Male > female (approximately 2:1).
GENETICS: Not applicable.

ETIOLOGY & PATHOGENESIS

- Microorganisms (usually bacteria) responsible for IE must gain access to the circulation (resulting in transient bacteremia) in sufficient numbers, for a sufficient interval of time, for endocarditis to result. Transient bacteremias can be the result of many causes, including:
  - Skin infections
  - Pulmonary infections
  - Genitourinary tract manipulation or infections
  - Hemodialysis
  - Intravenous drug abuse
  - Dental treatment and/or odontogenic infections
- IE usually arises following localization and subsequent colonization of micro organisms on sterile thrombotic vegetation (called nonbacterial thrombotic endocarditis or NBTE). NBTE may form as a result of trauma to the endothelial cells or over a subendothelial inflammatory reaction. The sites of involvement suggest an important role for hydrodynamic forces in the etiology of IE as well. IE occurs downstream from where blood flows through a narrow orifice at a high velocity from a high- to low-pressure chamber. In summary, examples of factors that may be responsible for cardiac endothelial trauma predisposing a patient to IE include:
  - High blood flow turbulence (hemodynamic forces) such as congenital cardiac lesions or shunts between arterial and venous channels.
  - Previous heart surgery (e.g., prosthetic heart valves, surgical correction of cardiac lesions).
  - Cardiovascular damage secondary to disease (e.g., previous infective endocarditis, systemic lupus erythematosus, rheumatic heart disease).
- Pathologic effects of IE can include:
  - Local (cardiac) tissue destruction leading to:
    - Valvular incompetence (insufficiency)
    - Congestive heart failure (secondary to aortic valve insufficiency)
    - Myocardial abscess
    - Conduction abnormalities (dysrhythmias)
  - Septic emboli: IE vegetations form in areas of endothelial damage. They are friable and easily detached (becoming septic emboli) and may travel through the bloodstream and cause tissue and organ infarctions including cerebral embolic infarction (stroke) or renal, splenic, or retinal infarctions.
  - Secondary autoimmune effects, such as immune complex glomerulonephritis, arthritis, and vasculitis.
- IE can generally be classified into the following categories:
  - Native valve (acute and subacute) endocarditis:
    - Native valve acute endocarditis usually has an aggressive course. Virulent organisms such as *Staphylococcus aureus* and *group B streptococci* are typically the causative agents of this type of endocarditis. Underlying structural valve disease may not be present.
    - Subacute endocarditis usually has a more indolent course than the acute form. *Alpha-hemolytic streptococci* or *enterococci*, usually in the setting of underlying structural valve disease, typically are the causative agents of this type of endocarditis.
  - Prosthetic valve (early and late) endocarditis:
    - Early prosthetic valve endocarditis occurs within 60 days of valve implantation. *Staphylococci, gram-negative bacilli*, and *Candida* species are the common infecting organisms.
    - Late prosthetic valve endocarditis occurs 60 days or more after valve implantation. *Alpha-hemolytic streptococci, enterococci*, and *staphylococci* are the common causative organisms.
  - Endocarditis related to intravenous drug use:
    - Endocarditis in intravenous drug abusers commonly involves the tricuspid valve. *S. aureus* is the most common causative organism.

CLINICAL PRESENTATION / PHYSICAL FINDINGS

The patient history in IE is highly variable.
- Common symptoms include fever and chills. Anorexia, weight loss, malaise, headaches, myalgias, night sweats, shortness of breath, cough, or joint pain are symptoms that potentially are present in the review of systems.
- In intravenous drug users, dyspnea could be the most important symptom; this is related with right-heart involvement (tricuspid or pulmonary valves).

The the most common findings in the physical exam are:
- Fever, possibly low-grade and intermittent, is present in 90% of patients.
- Heart murmurs are heard in approximately 85% of patients.
- One or more classic signs of IE are found in as many as 50% of patients.
  - Petechiae: Common but nonspecific finding
  - Splinter hemorrhages: Dark red linear lesions in the nailbed
  - Osler nodes: Tender subcutaneous nodules usually found on the distal pads of the digits
  - Janeway lesions: Nontender maculae on the palms and soles
  - Roth spots: Retinal hemorrhages with small, clear centers; rare and observed in only 5% of patients
- Signs of neurologic disease occur in as many as 40% of patients. Embolic stroke with focal neurologic deficits is the most common etiology.

DIAGNOSIS

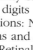

Clinical criteria (commonly referred to as the Duke criteria) for the diagnosis of endocarditis have been proposed.
- Major criteria include:
  1. A positive blood culture for a microorganism that typically causes infective endocarditis from two separate blood cultures.
  2. Evidence of endocardial involvement documented by echocardiography (definite vegetation, myocardial abscess, or new partial dehiscence of a prosthetic valve) or development of a new, regurgitant murmur.
- Minor criteria include:
  1. The presence of a predisposing heart condition or intravenous drug abuse.
  2. Fever of = 100.4°F (38°C).
  3. Embolic disease.
  4. Immunologic phenomena (e.g., glomerulonephritis, Osler nodes, Roth spots, rheumatoid factor).

5. Positive blood cultures but not meeting the major criteria.
6. A positive echocardiogram but not meeting the major criteria.

- A "definite" diagnosis of endocarditis can be made with 80% accuracy if:
  o two major criteria are met *or*
  o one major criterion and three minor criteria are met *or*
  o five minor criteria are met
- If none of these criteria is met and either an alternative explanation for illness is identified or the patient has become afebrile within 4 days, then endocarditis is highly unlikely.

LABORATORY STUDIES

- Complete blood count (CBC), electrolytes, creatinine, BUN, glucose, and coagulation panel.
- Two sets of blood cultures have greater than 90% sensitivity when bacteremia is present.
- Anemia of chronic disease is common in subacute endocarditis.
- Erythrocyte sedimentation rate (ESR), while not specific, is elevated in more than 90% of cases.
- Proteinuria (proteins in the urine) and microscopic hematuria (blood in the urine) are present in approximately 50% of cases.
- Leukocytosis (elevated leukocyte count) is observed in acute endocarditis.

IMAGING STUDIES

- Echocardiography may provide adjunctive information useful for identifying the specific valve or valves that are infected.
- Chest radiograph.
- Ventilation/perfusion (V/Q) scanning.
- CT scanning.

OTHER TESTS

- Electrocardiography: nonspecific changes are common.
- Cardiac catheterization may be indicated to evaluate the degree of valvular damage.

MEDICAL MANAGEMENT & TREATMENT

- In the emergency room, the focus of care is to make the correct diagnosis and stabilize the patient. In most cases, the etiological factor is not known while the patient is in the emergency room. Three sets of blood cultures over a few hours is the standard protocol.
- Empiric antibiotic therapy may be considered according to the patient history and is chosen based on the most likely infecting organisms. Native valve disease usually is treated with penicillin G and gentamicin for synergistic treatment of *streptococci*.
- Patients with a history of IV drug use may be treated with nafcillin and gentamicin to cover for methicillin-sensi-

tive staphylococci. Infection of a prosthetic valve may include methicillin-resistant *Staphylococcus aureus*; thus, vancomycin and gentamicin may be used, despite the risk of renal insufficiency.

COMPLICATIONS

The most common complications of patients with IE are:

- Myocardial infarction, pericarditis, cardiac dysrhythmia
- Cardiac valvular insufficiency
- Congestive heart failure
- Sinus of Valsalva aneurysm
- Aortic root or myocardial abscesses
- Arterial emboli, infarcts, mycotic aneurysms
- Arthritis, myositis
- Glomerulonephritis, acute renal failure
- Stroke syndromes
- Mesenteric or splenic abscess or infarct

PROGNOSIS

- Increased mortality rates are associated with increased age, infection involving the aortic valve, development of congestive heart failure, central nervous system complications, and underlying disease. Mortality rates also vary with the infecting organism.
- Mortality rates in native valve disease range from 16–27%. Mortality rates in patients with prosthetic valve infections are higher. More than 50% of these infections occur within 2 months after surgery.

DENTAL SIGNIFICANCE

- Different epidemiologic studies in different countries have shown that 14–20% of the cases of IE are associated with a possible oral origin. These results should be interpreted with caution because a majority of the studies are retrospective and the prevalence of IE of dental origin is estimated only from the medical/dental records (previous dental manipulations or presence of oral infections, or both), and in many cases the microorganism responsible is not identified.
- The number of patients with cardiovascular conditions that place them at risk for IE has been estimated to be as high as 5–10% of the general population.
- The American Heart Association has established recommendations for the use of antibiotic prophylaxis for the prevention of IE and stratifies cardiac conditions into high- and moderate-risk categories primarily on the basis of potential outcome if endocarditis occurs.
  o High-risk category:

- Prosthetic cardiac valves, including bioprosthetic and homograft valves
- Previous bacterial endocarditis
- Complex cyanotic congenital heart disease (e.g., single ventricle states, transposition of the great arteries, tetralogy of Fallot)
- Surgically constructed systemic pulmonary shunts or conduits
  o Moderate-risk category:
- Most other congenital cardiac malformations
- Acquired valvar dysfunction (e.g., rheumatic heart disease)
- Hypertrophic cardiomyopathy
- Mitral valve prolapse with valvar regurgitation and/or thickened leaflets

- A patient with previous history of IE is at high risk of redeveloping IE, according to the AHA guidelines. Repeat infections of IE are common and found in 2–31% of cases after initial IE. Patients remain permanently at risk for reinfection because of residual damage to the cardiac valves.

DENTAL MANAGEMENT

- The main role of the dentist is identifying patients at risk for IE and following the current AHA guidelines for the use of antibiotic prophylaxis prior to bacteremia-inducing dental procedures (see Appendix A, Box 1, "Antibiotic Prophylaxis Recommendations by the American Heart Association for the Prevention of Bacterial Endocarditis" and Table A-1, "Prophylactic Regimens for Dental, Oral, Respiratory, or Esophageal Procedures").
- If there is any question as to the need for antibiotic prophylaxis for the prevention of IE in a patient with a history a cardiovascular disease, the patient's physician (preferably cardiologist) should be consulted.

SUGGESTED REFERENCES

Carmona IT, et al. An update on the controversies in bacterial endocarditis of oral origin. *Oral Surg Oral Med Oral Path Oral Radiol Endod* 2002;9:660

Dajani AS, Taubert KA, Wilson W, Bolger AF, Bayer A, Ferrieri P, et al. Prevention of bacterial endocarditis. Recommendations by the American Heart Association. *JAMA* 1997;277(22):1794–1801.

Lessard E, et al. The patient with a heart murmur: evaluation, assessment and dental considerations. *JADA* 2005;136:347.

Little J, Falace D, Miller C, Rhodus N. Cardiac conditions associated with endocarditis, in Little J: *Dental Management of the Medically Compromised Patient*. St Louis, Mosby, 2002, p 52.

Seymor RA. Dentistry and the medically compromised patient. *Surgeon* 2003;1:207.

Sirois D, et al. Valvular heart disease. *Oral Surg Oral Med Oral Path Oral Radiol Endod* 2001;91:15.

AUTHOR: **JUAN F. YEPES, DDS, MD**

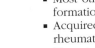

SYNONYM(S)

Oral hairy leukoplakia (OHL)

ICD-9 CM/CPT CODE(S)
529.0 Diseases and other conditions of the tongue—incomplete
528.7 Other disturbances of oral epithelium, including tongue—complete
529.8 Other specified conditions of the tongue—complete

OVERVIEW

- In 1984, an unusual white lesion was first described along the lateral margins of the tongue, predominantly in male homosexuals. Evidence indicates that this white lesion, known as oral hairy leukoplakia (OHL), represents an opportunistic infection related to the presence of Epstein-Barr virus (EBV) and is almost exclusively found in human immune deficiency virus (HIV)-infected individuals.
- Hairy leukoplakia (HL) may be seen in patients with other forms of immunosuppression, such as organ transplantation. A few cases have been reported in patients who are taking corticosteroids and in a few patients who are otherwise healthy.
- There is a positive correlation with depletion of peripheral CD4 cells and the presence of hairy leukoplakia.

EPIDEMIOLOGY & DEMOGRAPHICS

INCIDENCE/PREVALENCE IN USA:
Incidence of OHL in homosexual men and IV drug users who are infected with HIV is approximately 4%. OHL is reported in about 25% of adults with HIV infection but is not as common in HIV-infected children. Its prevalence reaches as high as 80% in patients with acquired immunodeficiency syndrome (AIDS). Some evidence suggests that incidence is decreasing. The decreasing prevalence may be partially due to use of protease inhibitors.
PREDOMINANT AGE: HL is less common in children than adults.
PREDOMINANT SEX: OHL is observed more commonly in homosexual men who are HIV-positive. In general, OHL is more common in men than women.
PREDOMINANT RACE: No racial predilection has been established.

ETIOLOGY & PATHOGENESIS

- Epstein-Barr virus (EBV) is implicated as the causative agent in OHL. Viral particles have been localized within the nuclei and cytoplasm of the oral epithelial cells of hairy leukoplakia.
- OHL has been associated with HIV infection and is a sign of AIDS. More recently, it has been described in patients with other forms of severe immunodeficiency, including those associated with chemotherapy, organ transplant, and leukemia.
- Rarely, it may occur in patients who are immunocompetent.
- OHL has been described in association with Behçet's syndrome and ulcerative colitis.
- Smoking more than a pack of cigarettes a day is correlated positively with development of OHL in men who are HIV-positive.

CLINICAL PRESENTATION / PHYSICAL FINDINGS

- Most commonly involves the lateral border of the tongue but may extend to the dorsal and ventral surface of the tongue.
- White lesion that varies in architecture.
- May appear as flat, plaquelike, or corrugated.
- Unilateral or bilateral.
- May be seen on the buccal mucosa, floor of the mouth, palate, pharynx, or esophagus.
- Usually is asymptomatic.
- Symptoms include mild pain and dysesthesia (alteration of the taste).

DIAGNOSIS

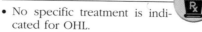

- Diagnosis of OHL can be made by biopsy and histologic examination of the lesion that reveals hyperkeratosis and parakeratosis of superficial epithelial layer, acanthosis of the stratum spinosum with foci or layers of ballooning "koilocyte"-like cells, minimal or absent inflammation in the epithelial and subepithelial tissues, and normal basal epithelial layer. Although these features are highly suggestive of the diagnosis, a definite diagnosis requires demonstration of EBV within the epithelial cells of the lesion that can be achieved by in situ hybridization, PCR, immunohistochemistry, Southern blotting, or electron microscopy.

MEDICAL MANAGEMENT & TREATMENT

- No specific treatment is indicated for OHL.
- The condition usually disappears when antiviral medications such as zidovudine, acyclovir, or ganciclovir are used in the treatment of the HIV infection and its complicating viral infections.
- Responses to topical application of podophyllin resin or tretinoin have been reported, but relapse is often seen with discontinuation of therapy.

COMPLICATIONS

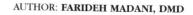

- Use of alcohol and tobacco in patients with OHL contributes to formation of squamous cell carcinomas in these patients.
- Immunosuppression is a risk factor for oral cancer.

PROGNOSIS

- Approximately 10% of individuals with OHL have AIDS at the time of diagnosis, and an additional 20% develop this disease in the following year.
- The probability of developing AIDS in individuals with HIV-associated hairy leukoplakia is approximately 50% within 1.5 years and 80% within 2.5 years.

DENTAL SIGNIFICANCE

- Hairy leukoplakia should be in differential diagnosis of a white lesion on the lateral border of the tongue.
- For patients whose immune status is unknown and in whom biopsy findings indicate hairy leukoplakia, investigation for HIV infection or other causes of immunosuppression should be undertaken.

DENTAL MANAGEMENT

- OHL has been associated with subsequent or concomitant development of the clinical and laboratory features of acquired immunodeficiency syndrome (AIDS) in as many as 80% of cases, and there is a positive correlation between OHL and depletion of peripheral CD4 cells.
- Biopsy must be obtained from the suspected lesions in order to initiate proper referral and medical management as early as possible.

SUGGESTED REFERENCES

Emedicine website: www.emedicine.com
Kabani S, Greenspan D, deSouza Y. Oral hairy leukoplakia with extensive oral mucosal involvement. Report of two cases. *Oral Surg Oral Med Oral Pathol* 1989;67(4):411–415.
Lozada-Nur F, Robinson J, Regezi JA. Oral hairy leukoplakia in nonimmunosuppressed patients. Report of four cases. *Oral Surg Oral Med Oral Pathol* 1994;78(5):599–602.
Red and white lesions of the oral mucosa, in Greenberg MS, Glick M (eds): *Burket's Oral Medicine. Diagnosis and Treatment*, ed 10. Hamilton, Ontario, BC Decker, Inc., 2003, pp 85–125.
White lesions, in Regezi JA, Sciubba JJ, Jordan RCK (eds): *Oral Pathology, Clinical Pathologic Correlations*. St Louis, WB Saunders, 2003, pp 75–109.

AUTHOR: FARIDEH MADANI, DMD

SYNONYM(S)

Acute infectious mononucleosis
Infectious mononucleosis
Mono
EBV
Human herpes virus 4 (HHV-4)
Kissing disease
Glandular fever

ICD-9CM/CPT CODE(S)

075: Infectious mononucleosis—complete

OVERVIEW

- Infectious mononucleosis (IM) or "mono" is a symptomatic disease caused by Epstein-Barr virus (EBV) (named after Tony Epstein and Yvonne Barr, who first isolated and described the virus in 1964).
- EBV is a herpes virus 4 (HHV-4) that only occurs in humans. Infection during childhood usually causes asymptomatic or mild disease and most symptomatic disease arises in young adults. The infection usually occurs by intimate contact; intrafamilial spread is common. Once infected, the individual is a lifelong carrier.
- Children usually become infected through contaminated saliva on fingers, toys, or other objects. Adults usually contract the virus through direct salivary transfer, such as shared straws or kissing, hence the nickname "kissing disease."
- EBV can also spread via blood transfusions and organ transplantation. After exposure to the virus, an incubation period of 2 to 7 weeks follows before the onset of symptoms.

EPIDEMIOLOGY & DEMOGRAPHICS

INCIDENCE/PREVALENCE IN USA: EBV is not a reportable infection, and exact frequency of symptomatic primary infection is not known. More than 95% of adults in the world are seropositive for EBV. In the U.S., by age 5 approximately 50% of children are infected. By age 25, 90–95% of adults between 35 and 40 years of age have been infected with the virus.

PREDOMINANT AGE: EBV infection usually occurs during infancy or childhood and remains latent throughout life. In developed nations, infection may not occur until adolescence or adulthood, and approximately 50% of adolescents who acquire EBV develop the infectious mononucleosis syndrome. Acute infectious mononucleosis has been reported in middle-aged and elderly adults, and usually they are heterophil antibody-negative.

PREDOMINANT SEX: Incidence of infectious mononucleosis is the same in men and women, although the peak incidence occurs 2 years earlier in women.

RACE: No racial predilection exists.

ETIOLOGY & PATHOGENESIS

- EBV is the etiologic agent in approximately 90% of acute infectious mononucleosis cases.
- Cytomegalovirus (CMV) is most commonly associated with EBV-negative infectious mononucleosis syndrome.
- Other viruses associated with a similar acute illness include adenovirus; hepatitis A, hepatitis B, or hepatitis C; herpes simplex 1 and herpes simplex 2; human herpes virus 6; rubella; and primary human immunodeficiency virus in adolescents or young adults.
- Etiology of most EBV-negative infectious mononucleosis cases remains unknown.

CLINICAL PRESENTATION / PHYSICAL FINDINGS

Infectious mononucleosis is considered a triad of fever (as high as 102°F to 104°F, pharyngitis, and lymphadenopathy. Other signs and symptoms include:

- Malaise (constant fatigue and weakness).
- Anorexia.
- Chills.
- Headaches.
- Myalgias.
- Difficulty in swallowing due to pharyngitis and tonsillitis.
- Hepatomegaly and splenomegaly develop in one-quarter to one-half of the patients.
- Nausea.
- Abdominal pain.
- Cervical lymphadenopathy.
- Palatal and gingival petechiae and ecchymosis.
- Cardiac, renal, pulmonary, and nervous system involvement occurs only rarely.
- Autoimmune hemolytic anemia, mild thrombocytopenia, hepatitis, and jaundice may occur as complications of the disease.
- Recovery is in 4 to 6 weeks with general supportive care.

DIAGNOSIS

Usually based on reported symptoms. Diagnosis can be confirmed with specific blood tests and other laboratory tests:

- Classic criteria: The three classic criteria for laboratory confirmation of acute infectious mononucleosis are (1) lymphocytosis, (2) the presence of at least 10% atypical lymphocytes on peripheral smear, and (3) a positive serologic test for EBV.
- Complete blood count:
  - Leukocytosis with total white blood cell (WBC) count usually in the range of 10,000 to 20,000 cells/mm³ occurs in 40–70% of patients with acute infectious mononucleosis.
  - Approximately 80–90% of patients have lymphocytosis, with greater than 50% lymphocytes.
- Liver function tests:
  - Most (i.e., 80–100%) patients with acute infectious mononucleosis have elevated liver function test results.
- EBV serology:
  - Infection with EBV is characterized by development of the specific antibodies to antigenic components of the virus. Viral specific serologic tests which include IgM and IgG antibody titer to viral capsid antigen should be used in children, especially those younger than 4 years of age.
- Heterophile antibody test (Monospot test):
  - Heterophile antibodies are nonspecific IgM antibodies induced by EBV against antigens unrelated to the virus, found on sheep, horses, and cattle red blood cells which can cause agglutination of these cells. Children often do not develop a heterophile antibody response to EBV.

MEDICAL MANAGEMENT & TREATMENT

In most cases, infectious mononucleosis is a self-limited illness that resolves within 4 to 6 weeks.

- Supportive treatment such as bed rest, adequate fluid, and soft diet is usually sufficient.
- Fever should be treated with antipyretics that do not contain aspirin.
- Patient with splenomegaly should avoid contact sports to prevent spleen rupture.
- Penicillin and ampicillin use during the course of the disease has been associated with a higher than normal prevalence of allergic morbilliform skin rashes.
- Corticosteroids should be restricted to life-threatening cases such as airway obstruction, hemolytic anemia, and severe thrombocytopenia.
- Because of low transmissibility of EBV, isolation is not indicated.

COMPLICATIONS

- Hepatitis occurs in more than 90% of patients with infectious mononucleosis but usually is mild and rarely symptomatic.
- Mild thrombocytopenia occurs in approximately 50% of patients with infectious mononucleosis.
- Hemolytic anemia occurs in 0.5–3% of patients with infectious mononucleosis.

- Upper airway obstruction due to hypertrophy of tonsils and other lymph nodes of Waldeyer's ring occurs in 0.1–1% of patients.
- Splenic rupture occurs in 0.1–0.2% of patients with infectious mononucleosis.
- CNS complications such as encephalitis, meningitis, Guillain-Barré syndrome, and Bell's palsy have been reported.

PROGNOSIS

- Immunocompetent individuals with acute infectious mononucleosis have a good prognosis with full recovery expected within several months.
- The common hematologic and hepatic complications resolve in 2 to 3 months.
- Neurologic complications usually resolve quickly in children. Adults are more likely to be left with neurologic deficits.
- All individuals develop latent infection, which usually remains asymptomatic.

DENTAL SIGNIFICANCE

- Anterior and posterior cervical lymphadenopathies that appear as enlarged, symmetric, and tender nodes are common.
- Facial nerve palsy and enlargement of parotid lymphoid tissue rarely has been reported.
- More than 80% of affected young adults have oropharyngeal tonsillar enlargement, sometimes with exudates and secondary tonsillar abscesses.
- 25% of the patients present with petechiae on the hard and soft palate.
- Necrotizing ulcerative gingivitis and periodontitis has been reported.

DENTAL MANAGEMENT

- Dentists should be familiar with the signs and symptoms of the disease, particularly the presence of cervical lymphadenopathy and oral lesions, to be able to refer the suspected patient to their physician for proper diagnosis, management, and monitoring for possible complications.

- EBV can be detected in saliva of many patients with infectious mononucleosis over several months after recovery, and they are able to spread the infection to others. Many healthy individuals can carry the virus in their saliva and are the primary reservoir for person-to-person transmission. Therefore, universal precautions should be followed.

SUGGESTED REFERENCES

Emedicine website: http://www.emedicine.com
CDC website: http://www.cdc.gov
Maddern BR, Werkhaven J, Wessel HB, et al. Infectious mononucleosis with airway obstruction and multiple cranial nerve paresis. *Otolaryngol Head Neck Surg* 1991; 104(4):529–532.
Neville BW, et al. *Oral & Maxillofacial Pathology.* Philadelphia, WB Saunders, 2002, pp 224–226.
Straus SE, Cohen JI, Tosato G, et al. NIH conference. Epstein-Barr virus infections: biology, pathogenesis, and management. *Ann Intern Med* 1993;118(1):45–58.
Topazian R, Goldberg M, Hupp J. Fungal, viral, and protozoal infections of the maxillofacial region, in *Oral and Maxillofacial Infection.* Philadelphia, WB Saunders, 2002, pp 243–278.

AUTHOR: **FARIDEH MADANI, DMD**

SYNONYM(S)

EM

SJS

Major erythema multiforme (Stevens-Johnson syndrome)

Erythema multiforme exudativum (Stevens-Johnson syndrome)

ICD-9CM/CPT CODE(S)

695.1 Erythema multiforme and Stevens-Johnson syndrome

OVERVIEW

EM

An inflammatory disease associated with immune complex formation with diffuse hemorrhagic lesions of the lips, oral mucous membranes, and skin.

SJS

A severe form of EM noted by bulla of the oral mucous membranes, pharynx, anogenital region, and conjunctiva, also considered a hypersensitivity reaction. Signs include target-like lesions and symptoms of fever. See "Stevens-Johnson Syndrome (Erythema Multiforme)" in Section II, p 325 for more information.

EPIDEMIOLOGY & DEMOGRAPHICS

INCIDENCE/PREVALENCE IN USA: Estimates range from 1 in 1000 to 1 in 10,000 persons.

PREDOMINANT AGE: EM is most frequent in the age group of 20 to 40 years. SJS is most frequent in children and young adults.

PREDOMINANT SEX: Male > female (3:2).

ETIOLOGY & PATHOGENESIS

EM

Implied cause is antigen-antibody response with eventual deposition in the cutaneous microvasculature. IgM and C3 have been detected in early antibody response. Frequent EM cases are associated with herpes simplex. Drugs are the most frequent reported etiologic agents for major cases. Etiology unknown in more than 50% of patients.

SJS

An overzealous immune response has been implicated. Drugs, upper respiratory tract infections, herpes simplex virus, and vaccinations are implicated in severe cases.

CLINICAL PRESENTATION / PHYSICAL FINDINGS

EM

Febrile complaints, joint pain and painful skin, oral, and lip ulcers. Target-like skin lesions appear. Common sites on hands, feet and legs, and trunk. Papules vesicles and bullae can appear in oral cavity and skin locations. Some ulcers can attain 2 to 3 cm. Healing of outbreak in 1 to 2 weeks without scarring.

SJS

Nonspecific symptoms of fever, cough, and fatigue occurring before oral and skin lesions. Corneal ulcerations can result in blindness. Ulcerative stomatitis of oral mucous membranes and lips result in hemorrhagic crusting. Dehydration and compromised breathing are observed. Attacks can last 2 to 4 weeks.

DIAGNOSIS

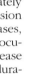

DIFFERENTIAL DIAGNOSIS

- EM
  - ○ Acute drug reaction, lichen planus, contact dermatitis, pityriasis rosea, pemphigus vulgaris, dermatis herpetiformis, granuloma anulare, oral aphthous, or herpetic stomatitis.
  - ○ EM must be differentiated from allergic stomatitis primary herpetic stomatitis and, in older age, from pemphigus. Also, EM skin lesions must be differentiated from urticaria, dermatitis herpetiformis, and possibly Coxsackie virus lesions.
- SJS
  - ○ Acute drug reaction, urticaria, hemorrhagic fevers, serum sickness, Behçet's syndrome, Reiter's syndrome, and pemphigus.

LABORATORY

- EM
  - ○ CBC, cytology for herpetic etiology, serology, toxicology for drug evaluation, ANA, liver panel for hepatitis, glucose for steroid therapy and diabetes.
- SJS
  - ○ CBC differential, cultures for infection, and like tests as listed previously.

IMAGING

- Chest radiograph with suspected lung involvement.

MEDICAL MANAGEMENT & TREATMENT

Rule out any other disease, monitor dehydration and secondary infected lesions.

ACUTE GENERAL CARE

- EM: Treatment of associated diseases as herpes simplex with acyclovir and mycoplasma with erythromycin.
- SJS: Treat associated disease as above. Utilize antihistamines for pruritus, relieve oral symptoms with appropriate rinses, treat secondary infections with antibiotics, maintain liquid and soft diet, use topical and systemic steroid treatment cautiously.

CONTINUED CARE

- EM: Rash developments are 2 weeks, resolving within 3 to 4 weeks without scarring. High-burst glucocorticosteroids IV or oral dosing. Disease course dictates tapering or maintenance on therapy. Steroids contraindicated in presence of infection. Oral and IV fluids for dehydration. Steroid therapy taken into account in diabetes and impact to lower immune response.
- SJS: Severe bullous form can occur. Severity of disease dictates steroid therapy. Death may occur in approximately 10% of patients with extensive signs and symptoms. Scarring and corneal changes may impact in approximately 20% of patients. Hospital admission should be considered in severe cases, especially with skin, urethral, and ocular involvement. In most cases, disease is self-limiting with a 4- to 6-week duration.

COMPLICATIONS

Dehydration, infections, bullous ulcerations, impact on systemic disease such as diabetes mellitus and depressed immune reaction, and possible death.

PROGNOSIS

- Usually self-limited disease lasting 4 to 6 weeks.
- Patient very uncomfortable, especially in mouth, hand, and foot areas.
- Ulceration invites possible infections, eye damage, and urinary tract involvement.
- Mortality possible.

DENTAL SIGNIFICANCE

Initial dental care should be postponed or limited. Pain and discomfort will impact on level of care. Palliative care may be instituted for oral/lip reactive sites. Caution on oral steroid use if infection is present. Advise patient on possible dehydration. Encourage fluid intake. Refer to primary care physician or infectious disease specialist. Consult with oral medicine specialist.

DENTAL MANAGEMENT

Defer oral/dental intervention until symptoms abate. Immediate care, if needed, should be palliative. Medical intervention is a necessity. Reassure patient that this disease is usually self-limiting. General oral/dental care is recommended post patient stability.

SUGGESTED REFERENCES

Duvic M. Urticaria, drug hypersensitivity rashes, nodules and tumors, and atrophic diseases, in Goldman L, Ansiello D (eds): *Cecil Textbook of Medicine*, ed 22. Philadelphia, WB Saunders, 2004, pp 2475–2486.

Korman, NJ. Macular, popular and vesiculobullous and pustular diseases, in Goldman L, Ansiello D (eds): *Cecil Textbook of Medicine*, ed 22. Philadelphia, WB Saunders, 2004, pp 2466–2475.

AUTHOR: **NORBERT J. BURZYNSKI, SR., DDS, MS**

Gastroesophageal Reflux Disease

SYNONYM(S)

GERD

ICD-9CM/CPT CODE(S)

530.81: Esophageal reflux—complete

OVERVIEW

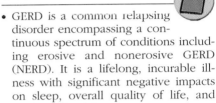

- GERD is a common relapsing disorder encompassing a continuous spectrum of conditions including erosive and nonerosive GERD (NERD). It is a lifelong, incurable illness with significant negative impacts on sleep, overall quality of life, and work productivity.
- Erosive GERD (reflux esophagitis or acid-induced mucosal injury) is the result of chronic abnormal exposure of the lower esophagus to gastric contents.
- More than half of reflux sufferers have NERD or silent reflux.
- NERD patients complain of the same symptoms but have no or minimal mucosal injury or long-term complications. In some cases, silent GERD may be attributed to an increase in esophageal acid reflux or mucosal hypersensitivity to acid. Patients with nonerosive reflux whose symptoms are not related to acid reflux are thought to suffer functional heartburn.

EPIDEMIOLOGY & DEMOGRAPHICS

INCIDENCE/PREVALENCE IN USA: About 10–25% of the U.S. population suffers from GERD.
PREDOMINANT SEX: More prevalent in males.

ETIOLOGY & PATHOGENESIS

- Multifactorial
- Primarily caused by motor dysfunction of the lower esophageal sphincter and retrograde flow of gastric contents through an incompetent gastroesophageal junction.
- Foods such as fat or chocolate, alcohol, smoking, and medications (anticholinergics, nicotine) may transiently decrease the pressure of lower esophageal sphincter or delay gastric emptying and result in esophageal mucosal injury associated with the reflux of acid, bile, pepsin, and pancreatic enzymes.
- Bisphosphonate drugs used to treat osteoporosis are associated with the risk of esophageal ulcers.
- Common in patients with asthma and may be aggravated by the use of β-agonists and theophylline.
- Other etiological factors include obesity, pregnancy, large meals, hiatal hernia, low saliva output, poor esophageal clearance, delayed gastric emptying, and impaired mucosal defensive factors.

CLINICAL PRESENTATION / PHYSICAL FINDINGS

- Recurrent retrosternal burning sensation rising from the stomach or lower chest up toward the neck (heartburn)
- Regurgitation with sour or bitter taste
- Dysphagia
- Odynophagia
- Gastrointestinal bleeding
- Sleep disturbance
- Iron deficiency anemia
- Unintentional weight loss
- Noncardiac chest pain
- Pulmonary symptoms (laryngitis, chronic cough, asthma)
- Otolaryngologic symptoms

DIAGNOSIS

- Primarily a clinical diagnosis (frequent heartburn), often supplemented by response to a therapeutic course of antisecretory agents.
- The following may prove beneficial in selected cases:
  - Air-contrast barium radiography (low sensitivity in diagnosis)
  - Endoscopy (gold standard for detection of mucosal injury)
  - 24-hour esophageal pH monitoring (useful in patients with atypical symptoms)
  - Esophageal manometry (to evaluate esophageal function and to measure sphincter pressure)

MEDICAL MANAGEMENT & TREATMENT

- Medical management is intended to provide symptomatic relief, heal esophageal erosions, and improve quality of life.
- Maintenance therapy is essential to prevent disease relapse.
- Follow-up is important for prevention of complications.
- Management involves:
  - Lifestyle modification:
    - Adjust size and content of meals
    - Avoid foods and drugs precipitating symptoms
    - Smoking cessation and avoidance of alcohol
    - Maintaining normal weight
    - Avoiding lying down within 3 hours after dinner
    - Elevate head of the bed
  - Proton pump inhibitors are mainstay of treatment (first-line therapy).
  - Acid suppressant medications (H2-blockers or proton pump inhibitors).
  - Antacids.
  - Esophageal and gastric prokinetic drugs can be useful when inadequate gastroesophageal motility is present.
  - Open or laparoscopic antireflux surgery in recalcitrant cases.

COMPLICATIONS

- Esophagitis
- Esophageal ulcer
- Esophageal strictures
- Metaplastic changes in esophageal lining (Barrett's esophagus) in 5% of those with erosive GERD
- Esophageal adenocarcinoma (annual risk of 1% in patients with Barrett's esophagus)
- Reflux-induced asthma
- Chronic hoarseness of voice
- Sleep dysfunction

PROGNOSIS

- A chronic, incurable illness with high relapse potential with cessation of medical therapy.
- Risk factors for development of Barrett's esophagus to esophageal adenocarcinoma includes family history, male sex, age over 45, and long-standing GERD.

DENTAL SIGNIFICANCE

- Dental erosion (palatal aspect of maxillary teeth) and dental sensitivity secondary to frequent acid reflux and regurgitation.
- Some acid blockers such as cimetidine may reduce the metabolism of certain dental drugs (diazepam, lidocaine, etc.) and prolong duration of their action.
- Cimetidine may interfere with the absorption of systemic antifungals such as ketoconazole.
- Antacids may significantly impact the absorption of tetracycline, erythromycin, oral iron, and fluoride.
- Frequent regurgitation as well as medical therapy with proton pump inhibitors may cause dysgeusia.
- Some acid blockers (cimetidine, ranitidine) are toxic to bone marrow, leading to anemia (mucosal pallor), agranulocytosis (mucosal ulceration), or thrombocytopenia (petechiae and gingival bleeding).
- Some acid blockers (famotidine) and anticholinergics may cause xerostomia and predispose to dental caries.
- Erythema, mucosal atrophy, fibrosis, or stricture of esophageal mucosa may result from prolonged exposure of tissues to acid.

DENTAL MANAGEMENT

- Periodically update patient's medical status, type and dose of patient's medications.
- Be vigilant about signs and symptoms indicating relapse of the disease.
- Encourage periodic medical evaluations for prevention and early detection of cancer in high-risk patients.

- Avoid prescribing ASA, aspirin-containing compounds, NSAIDs, or exogenous steroids, which cause gastrointestinal distress.
- Avoid or limit prescribing narcotic analgesics, which increase the likelihood of regurgitation.
- Instruct patients to take their prescribed antibiotics or dietary supplements 2 hours before or after the intake of antacids.
- Instruct patient on rinsing mouth after regurgitation to prevent enamel dissolution.
- Recommend baking soda mouth rinses to alleviate reflux-induced altered taste.
- Recommend regular, effective oral hygiene practices and the use of topical fluoride within a custom tray to allow dental mineralization.
- Prescribe artificial saliva or sugarless gum in those with medication-induced xerostomia.
- Encourage patients to avoid stress and other factors aggravating their symptoms.

- Arrange dental care over multiple, short appointments to minimize stress.
- Consider sedation in patients with excessive stress response to dental procedures.
- Treat patients in a semisupine position to reduce reflux-associated symptoms.
- Consider premedication of patients with H2-blockers or antacids prior to dental treatment.
- Consider preoperative workup (CBC with differential) for patients on H2-blockers who are scheduled for invasive oral surgery.

SUGGESTED REFERENCES

Bello IS, et al. Gastroesophageal reflux disease: a review of clinical features, investigations and recent trends in management. *Niger J Med* 2004;13(3):220–226.

Biddle W. Gastroesophageal reflux disease: current treatment approaches. *Gastrenterol Nurs* 2003;26(6):228–236.

Castell DO, et al. Review article: the pathophysiology of gastroesophageal reflux disease-esophageal manifestations. *Aliment Pharmacol Ther* 2004;20(Suppl 9):14–25.

Fass R, et al. Review article: supra-esophageal manifestations of gastro-esophageal reflux disease and the role of night-time gastro-esophageal reflux. *Aliment Pharmacol Ther* 2004;20(Suppl 9):26–38.

Kahilaris PJ. Review article: gastro-esophageal reflux disease as afunctional gastrointestinal disorder. *Aliment Pharmacol Ther* 2004;20 (Suppl 7):50–55.

Little JW, Falace DA, Miller GS, Rhodus NL. Gastrointestinal disease, in Little, et al. (eds): *Dental Management of the Medically Compromised patient*. St Louis, Mosby, 2002, pp 188–202.

Mahoney EK, Kilpatrick NM. Dental erosion: part 1. Aetiology and prevalence of dental erosion. *N Z Dent J* 2003;99(2):33–41.

Savarino V, Dulbecco P. Optimizing symptom relief and preventing complications in adults with gastroesophageal reflux disease. *Digestion* 2004;69(Suppl 1):9–16.

Siegel MA, Jacobson JJ, Braum RJ. Diseases of the gastrointestinal tract, in Greenberg M, Glick M (eds): *Burket's Oral Medicine Diagnosis and Treatment*, Hamilton, Ontario: BC Decker Inc., 2003, pp 389–392.

AUTHOR: **MAHNAZ FATAHZADEH, DMD**

SECTION 1

SYNONYM(S)

None

ICD-9CM/CPT CODE(S)

274.9: Gout, unspecified—complete

OVERVIEW

Common disease characterized by a disturbance of urate metabolism, elevation of serum concentrations of uric acid, accumulation of urate crystals in the joint and soft tissues, and an inflammatory response to crystal deposits. Four phases for development of gout have been described: asymptomatic hyperuricemia, acute gouty arthritis, intercritical gout, and chronic tophaceous gout. While primary gout is an inborn error of purine metabolism, secondary gout is often caused by certain medications or radiotherapy for myeloproliferative disorders affecting uric acid levels in blood. (See "Gout" in Section II, p 259.)

EPIDEMIOLOGY & DEMOGRAPHICS

INCIDENCE/PREVALENCE IN USA: 3 cases/1000 persons.

PREDOMINANT AGE: Predominantly a disease affecting middle-age adults (30–50 years).

PREDOMINANT SEX: 95% of cases affect males; rare in females before menopause.

GENETICS: Primary gout is partially genetically determined.

ETIOLOGY & PATHOGENESIS

- Risk factors:
  ○ Prolonged asymptomatic hyperuricemia (the major risk factor)
  ○ Obesity
  ○ High-purine diet
  ○ Regular intake of alcohol
  ○ Antihypertensive diuretic therapy (reduce renal excretion of uric acid)
  ○ Radiotherapy for myeloproliferative disorders

- Overproduction or underexcretion of uric acid
- Environmental/occupational exposure to lead
- High incidence of hyperlipidemia, hypertension, atherosclerosis, and diabetes mellitus in patients with gout

CLINICAL PRESENTATION / PHYSICAL FINDINGS

- Acute or chronic arthritis
- Recurrent painful episodes affecting multiple joints (most often affects first metatarsal joint of the foot)
- Tophaceous deposits in tissues and organs
- Interstitial renal disease
- Uric acid nephrolithiasis
- Severe functional disability in chronic gout

DIAGNOSIS

Identification of uric acid crystals in joint aspirate, tissues, or body fluids using polarized light microscopy

MEDICAL MANAGEMENT & TREATMENT

- Encourage lifestyle changes to manage asymptomatic hyperuricemia and prevent gout by:
  ○ Weight loss
  ○ Restrict protein and caloric intake in diet
  ○ Limiting alcohol intake
  ○ Avoid environmental/occupational exposure to lead
- Terminating acute attacks using NSAIDs, colchicines, corticosteroids, or adrenocorticotropic hormone
- Prevention of recurrent attacks
- Uricosuric agents and xanthine oxidase inhibitors for long-term management
- Management of complications caused by deposition of urate crystals in tissues

COMPLICATIONS

- Chronic tophaceous gout leads to interstitial renal disease and renal failure.
- Uric acid nephrolithiasis.

PROGNOSIS

- Severe functional disability in those afflicted with chronic gout.
- Fatal renal failure occurs in 25% of patients.

DENTAL SIGNIFICANCE

- Temporomandibular joint (TMJ) gouty arthritis (rare).
- Allopurinol used in the management of gout may cause severe oral ulcerations.

DENTAL MANAGEMENT

- Although rare, consider gouty TMJ arthritis in the differential diagnosis of TMJ pain.
- Avoid prescribing aspirin for analgesia since it interferes with the action of uricosuric patients.
- Be cognizant of the association between hypertension, ischemic heart disease, cerebrovascular disease, diabetes mellitus, renal disease, and gout.

SUGGESTED REFERENCES

Emmerson BT. The management of gout. *N Eng J Med* 1996;334(7):445–451.

Monu JU, Pope TL Jr. Gout: a clinical and radiologic review. *Radiol Clin North Am* 2004;42(1):169–184.

Van Doornum S, Ryan PF. Clinical manifestations of gout and their management. *Med J Aus* 2000;172(10):493–497.

AUTHOR: **MAHNAZ FATAHZADEH, DMD**

SYNONYM(S)

GVHD
Acute GVHD
Chronic GVHD

ICD-9CM/CPT CODE(S)

996.85 Complications of bone marrow transplant—complete

OVERVIEW

- GVHD refers to immunologically competent cells from a donor (the graft) reacting against an immunocompromised host to cause significant medical consequences.
- Occurs primarily after hematopoietic cell transplantation.
- The reaction occurs in both an acute form (within the first 100 days of transplant, usually noted in 10 to 30 days) as well as a chronic form (greater than 100 days posttransplant).

EPIDEMIOLOGY & DEMOGRAPHICS

INCIDENCE/PREVALENCE IN USA:
Directly correlated with the degree of mismatch of the major histocompatibility complex human leukocyte antigen (HLA) between the donor and the recipient.
- Acute GVHD can occur in 7–10% of autologous hematopoietic cell transplantation (HCT) patients, in 19–66% of matched sibling donors based on age, sex matching, and donor parity, and 70–90% of matched unrelated donors and nonidentical related donors.
- Chronic GVHD can occur in 33% of identically HLA-matched siblings, in 64% of HLA-matched unrelated donors, and 80% in those with one HLA mismatch in an unrelated donor.

PREDOMINANT AGE: Risk increases with age: 20% risk for those younger than 20; 80% risk for those older than 50.

PREDOMINANT SEX:
- Incidence for male and nulliparous female is equal.
- Incidence of GVHD increases for sex-mismatched donors with recipients.
- Incidence increases with donor parity.

ETIOLOGY & PATHOGENESIS

- Requires immunologically competent graft cells in which the host appears foreign to the graft and the host is not capable of mounting a response against the graft.
- Involves the recognition of epithelial target tissues as being foreign.
- Subsequent induction of an inflammatory response with apoptotic death of the epithelial tissue.
- Extent of histoincompatibility and number of T cells in the donor result in the major effect in causing GVHD.

CLINICAL PRESENTATION / PHYSICAL FINDINGS

ACUTE GVHD

- Pruritic rash on the palms and soles, cheeks, and upper trunk.
- Erythrodermia and desquamation in hyperacute type.
- Hepatic dysfunction: Elevation of alkaline phosphatase is one of the early signs of liver involvement by GVHD; hyperbilirubinemia can manifest as jaundice and can cause pruritus and lead to excoriations from the patient's scratching.
- GI manifestations of distal small bowel and colon inflammation resulting in secretory diarrhea, abdominal pain and cramping, occasional bleeding and ileus, and occasional dyspepsia.
- Increased risk of infectious and noninfectious pneumonia.
- Hemorrhagic cystitis.
- Anemia and thrombocytopenia.
- Possible hemorrhagic conjunctivitis.

CHRONIC GVHD

- Lichenoid and/or sclerodermatous skin thickening
- Keratoconjunctivitis sicca: Ocular dryness resulting in burning and irritation punctuate keratopathy
- Oral ulceration, atrophy, erythema, and lichenoid-appearing tissues
- Salivary hypofunction/xerostomia
- Obstructive lung disease with wheezing unresponsive to bronchodilator therapy

DIAGNOSIS

BASED ON CLINICOPATHOLOGY

- Diagnosis of acute GVHD is based on staging and grading of the GVHD. Staging of the skin, liver, and gut is based on the severity of the signs and symptoms from each entity. Staging ranges from "+" to "++++." The clinical stage of each entity is combined to form the overall grade of the disease. The grade also includes a functional impairment assessment. The grading ranges from Grade 0 (none) to Grade IV (life-threatening).
- Chronic GVHD is classified as either Limited (localized skin involvement and hepatic dysfunction) or Extensive (generalized skin involvement or local skin involvement with involvement of another target organ such as the liver, eye, or mouth).

LABORATORY

- Liver function tests including bilirubin, alkaline phosphatase, ALT, AST total protein, albumin, and bilirubin.
- A cholestatic liver disease picture is usually seen.
- Alkaline phosphatase is usually elevated early in this disorder.

- Hypoalbuminemia is also seen.

HISTOPATHOLOGY

- Skin or mucosal biopsy help establish the diagnosis.

MEDICAL MANAGEMENT & TREATMENT

- Therapy is based on severity of disease.
- Acute GVHD is treated with corticosteroids, cyclosporin, or tacrolimus. Occasionally other therapies such as antithymocyte globulin, muromonab (a monoclonal antibody directed against CD3 T cells), or mycophenolate mofetil are used.
- Chronic GVHD is treated with corticosteroids, cyclosporin, tacrolimus, antimetabolites (such as azathioprine, mycophenolate mofetil). Thalidomide is also used.
- Psoralen and UV A irradiation (PUVA) is also beneficial in cutaneous lesions.

COMPLICATIONS

- Infections due to impaired barriers of skin and mucosa protection and immunosuppression
- Increased incidence in secondary malignancy with long-term immunosuppression

PROGNOSIS

Based on overall grade of GVHD and response to treatment

DENTAL SIGNIFICANCE

- Patients with GVHD may present to their healthcare practitioner with oral complaints, including oral mucosal disease and dry mouth.
- GVHD clinically resembles lichenoid inflammation/lichen planus. Oral GVHD appears as an area of wispy hyperkeratosis on an erythematous base in various areas of the oral mucosa. In more severe GVHD, the lesions can be eroded and may be associated with chronic mucosal ulceration. These ulcerations may serve as a systemic port of entry for oral pathogens.
- Patients may have oral infection related to their immunosuppression needed to control GVHD, including bacterial, viral, and fungal etiologies.
- Cyclosporin, used to treat GVHD, has been related to gingival overgrowth. Gingival overgrowth should be biopsied since case reports of malignant tumors have been reported to be associated with some of these growths. Impeccable oral hygiene has been

noted to be helpful in preventing gingival overgrowth.

- Salivary gland dysfunction is also a quite common finding in GVHD, from a lymphocytic infiltrate of salivary gland tissue.

DENTAL MANAGEMENT

- Dental treatment planning must take into account the severity of the GVHD. If large, ulcerated lesions are present, elective treatment should be postponed.
- Dental treatment planning must consider the side effects of immunosuppressive medications taken to control the GVHD:

  ○ Assess the risk for adrenal suppression and insufficiency in patients being treated with systemic corticosteroids.

  (See Appendix A, Box A-4, "Dental Management of Patients at Risk for Acute Adrenal Insufficiency.")

  ○ Patients who are taking cytotoxic or immunosuppressive drugs, including systemic corticosteroids, may have an increased risk of infection and may require perioperative prophylactic antibiotics.

  (See Appendix A, Box A-2, "Presurgical and Postsurgical Antibiotic Prophylaxis for Patients at Increased Risk for Postoperative Infections.")

- Other considerations involve medication interactions that immunosuppressive medications have with medications that a dentist may prescribe.

SUGGESTED REFERENCES

Emedicine: www.emedicine.com Graft Versus Host Disease

Peterson DE, Shubert MM, Silverman S, Eversole LR. Blood dyscrasias, in Silverman S, Eversole LR, Truelove EL (eds): *Essentials of Oral Medicine*. Hamilton, Ontario, BC Decker, Inc., 2002.

Schubert MM, Sullivan KM. Recognition, incidence, and management of oral graft-versus-host disease. *NCI Monogr* 1990;9:135–143.

Woo SB, Lee SJ, Schubert MM. Graft-vs.-host disease. *Critical Reviews in Oral Biology & Medicine* 1997;8(2):201–216.

AUTHOR: **THOMAS P. SOLLECITO, DMD**

SYNONYM(S)

All previous terms are obsolete.

ICD-9CM/CPT CODE(S)

Variants of migraine headache
784.0 Cluster headache

OVERVIEW

Severe, unilateral, paroxysmal, and recurring headaches noted around the periorbital and temporal area lasting 15 to 180 minutes. Patients with cluster headaches frequently seek medical care because of the intense pain. These headaches can occur up to 8 times per day and last up to 4 to 12 weeks. Episodes appear to be predictable at times and can occur during sleep. Episodes can remit for months to years. Limited cases have been noted to have pain without remission.

(See "Headaches: Cluster" in Section II, p 261.)

EPIDEMIOLOGY & DEMOGRAPHICS

INCIDENCE/PREVALENCE IN USA: Estimated to occur in 0.051% of the U.S. population.
PREDOMINANT AGE: Peak onset between 25 and 50 years.
PREDOMINANT SEX: Males are affected at least five times more commonly than females.
GENETICS: Usually no family history of headache or migraine; however, increased concordance of these headaches in monozygotic twins has been documented.

ETIOLOGY & PATHOGENESIS

- Unknown, but suspected to be vascular in origin and/or may relate to a disturbance of the serotonergic mechanisms.
- Vascular implication presupposes events that activate the trigeminovascular system to cluster headaches. These observations support the clinical cyclicity of cluster headaches as reported by patients.

CLINICAL PRESENTATION / PHYSICAL FINDINGS

- The intensity of the pain is unique for this type of headache.
- See "Headaches: Cluster" in Section II, p 261 for more information on signs and symptoms.

DIAGNOSIS

- Diagnosis is based on severe, unilateral, periorbital pain episodes occurring for several weeks accompanied by nasal congestion, rhinorrhea, lacrimation, redness of eyes, and/or Horner's syndrome.
- Patient may report etiology agents as alcohol, stress, glare, or ingestion of specific foods.
- Differential diagnosis includes migraine headache, tension headache, giant cell arteritis, intracranial neoplasm, postherpetic neuralgia.
- A variant of the headache is called a chronic cluster headache.
- Diagnosis established by history.
- Imaging studies applied when presentation is questionable.

MEDICAL MANAGEMENT & TREATMENT

- See "Headaches: Cluster" in Section II, p 261 for more information.
- Advise patient to avoid tobacco and ethanol during a cluster headache.
- Physical activity during initial symptoms has been noted to abort the attack.
- Ergotamine tartrate has been used for years, especially if prescribed just before a predictable attack.
- Other medications used for an up to a 50% success rate include verapamil, lithium, methysergide, and topiramate.

COMPLICATIONS

Adverse effects of medications such as nausea, vomiting, cramping, angina, esophageal spasms, hypotension, fatigue, and constipation

PROGNOSIS

See "Headaches: Cluster" in Section II, p 261.

DENTAL SIGNIFICANCE

Depending on frequency of attacks and degree of discomfort, oral/dental care could be compromised. The extent of adverse effects of medications such as xerostomia, fatigue, vomiting, dizziness, esophageal spasms, and dyspepsia all can affect dental/oral care and nutrition. The degree of value of dental/oral care can be compromised by the extent of symptoms.

DENTAL MANAGEMENT

Provider must understand disease process and patient reaction to symptoms and signs. Minimize time and limit degree of treatment when patient is in a state of attack or avoid dental treatment until patient is in state of remission. Emphasize valued dental/oral care and its relation to total body care and maintenance. Refer to primary care physician and/or neurologist.

SUGGESTED REFERENCE

Cutrer FM, Moskowitz MA. Headaches and other head pain, in Goldman L, Ansiello D (eds): *Cecil Textbook of Medicine*, ed 22. Philadelphia, WB Saunders, 2004, pp 2224–2230.

AUTHOR: **NORBERT J. BURZYNSKI, SR., DDS, MS**

SECTION 1

SYNONYM(S)

Hemicrania

ICD-9CM/CPT CODE(S)

346.9 Migraine

OVERVIEW

Recurrent vascular headache disorder with variable intensity and duration and associated with visual disturbances, nausea, and vomiting. There are two categories: common migraine without an aura, which occurs in a large majority of patients, and classic migraine with an aura, which occurs in about 15% of patients. Both types may exhibit prodromal symptoms that precede the attack by 24 to 48 hours.

(See "Headaches: Migraine" in Section II, p 262.)

EPIDEMIOLOGY & DEMOGRAPHICS

INCIDENCE/PREVALENCE IN USA: Incidence in the U.S. is estimated at 18 cases per 1000 females and 6 cases per 1000 males.
PREDOMINANT AGE: Predominant age is greater than 10 years of age, but peak prevalence of 25 to 45 years of age.
PREDOMINANT SEX:
- Male ≥ female in childhood
- Female to male ratio of 3:1 after reaching midadult life

GENETICS: High familial predisposition has been demonstrated. Several novel migraine susceptibility genes have been identified in families by linkage analysis. Autosomal dominate transmission has been postulated.

ETIOLOGY & PATHOGENESIS

- Unknown.
- Primary vascular mechanism has been questioned as the major contributor and has been replaced by primary neuronal events as the major factor.
- The systems affected include the central nervous system (CNS), eyes, and the gastrointestinal tract. Serotonin concentrations show changes during an attack and are implicated in the vasomotor changes.

CLINICAL PRESENTATION / PHYSICAL FINDINGS

- Aura can be any focal neurologic function.
- Symptoms may include hyperactivity, euphoria, lethargy, craving for certain food, and yawning.

- Associated nervous system signs may include visual, paresthesias, aphasia, and hemiparesis.
- Headaches recur as severe headaches on regular or infrequent basis but generally follow a pattern.
- Scalp arteries are more pronounced and note an increased pulsation; scalp may be tender to touch.
- Generally consists of 4 to 72 hours of throbbing head pain, worsened by physical movement and associated with nausea, photophobia, and phonophobia. Symptoms may persist from 1 hour to approximately 1 week.

DIAGNOSIS

- Supported on symptom patterns including unilateral nature, family history, nausea and vomiting, and a positive response to ergot.
- Examination must rule out intracranial pathologic changes.
- Physical examination should be within normal limits.
- Diagnosis must meet criteria for migraine with and without aura.
- Clinical characteristics of common headaches such as tension, cluster, sinusitis, and mass lesion must be addressed.
- Potentially catastrophic illness presenting with nontraumatic headache such as meningitis, encephalitis, temporal arteritis, acute angle glaucoma, and subarachnoid hemorrhage are reviewed in the differential diagnosis.

See "Headaches: Migraine" in Section II, p 262 for other diagnostic information.

MEDICAL MANAGEMENT & TREATMENT

NONPHARMACOLOGIC

- Dietary modifications such as avoidance of caffeine, tobacco, alcohol; fixed patterns of eating, sleeping, and exercising regularly.
- Stress management and relaxation (lying down in a quiet, dark room) recommended.

PHARMACOLOGIC

- Depends on frequency of attacks and presence of comorbidity illness.
- Continued treatment can be classified as prophylactic, abortive, and analgesic.
  - Prophylactic treatment administered if patient has more than one migraine attack per week or if headaches impinge on daily activity of 3 or more

days per month. Choice of medication depends on comorbid illness.
  - Abortive medications for acute treatment; usually sufficient for patients with infrequent and uncomplicated attacks.
  - Analgesic should be used cautiously because of rebound headache, with dose escalation as a hazard of analgesic prescriptions.

COMPLICATIONS

Adverse effects and contraindications of prescribed medications and interactions with comorbidity illness. Also, uncertainty of diagnosis or treatment is not effective.

PROGNOSIS

As patient ages, the frequency and severity of migraine headaches tend to decrease.

DENTAL SIGNIFICANCE

Frequency and severity of illness can compromise general dental/oral care. Greatest impact is in patients under age 30 by reinforcing oral/dental care and nutrition.

DENTAL MANAGEMENT

Dental practitioner should understand the signs, symptoms, and outcomes of migraine headaches. Also, the affected patient should be shown empathy by the dental practitioner. Consult with primary care physician and/or neurologist recommended. Degree of care will depend on the degree of the patient symptoms and status of migraine headaches. Avoid precipitants during dental care.

SUGGESTED REFERENCE

Cutrer FM, Moskowitz MA. Headaches and other head pain, in Goldman L, Ansiello D (eds): *Cecil Textbook of Medicine*, ed 22. Philadelphia, WB Saunders, 2004, pp 2224–2230.

AUTHOR: **NORBERT J. BURZYNSKI, SR., DDS, MS**

SYNONYM(S)

Stress headache
Muscle contraction headache
Ordinary headache
Psychomyogenic headache
Chronic headache

ICD-9CM/CPT CODE(S)

307.81 Tension headache

OVERVIEW

Recurrent headache that lasts 30 minutes to 7 days. It is mild to moderate in severity, bilateral, and not aggravated by exertion. The headaches are intense about the neck or back of the head and are not associated with focal neurology symptoms. The complaint consists of a constricting band around the head. This is experienced more frequently in the early afternoon and evening.

EPIDEMIOLOGY & DEMOGRAPHICS

INCIDENCE/PREVALENCE IN USA: Incidence is undetermined but believed to be the most common type of headache, representing as high as 70% of all headaches presenting to primary care physician. Prevalence rates of tension headaches vary from 29–71%. This variation appears to be the result of differences in research study design.
PREDOMINANT AGE: Greater than 10 years, but occurs at all ages.
PREDOMINANT SEX: Tension headaches are noted to be more frequent in women.

ETIOLOGY & PATHOGENESIS

- Etiology undetermined, as the pathophysiology and probable mechanism remain unclear.
- Current information suggests that tension headaches have a muscular origin. Muscle hardness has been noted to increase in the pericranial muscles.
- Nitric oxide may play a role in tension headaches.

CLINICAL PRESENTATION / PHYSICAL FINDINGS

- Headache presents in episodic and chronic forms.

- Pain radiating in a band-like fashion bilaterally from the forehead to the occiput.
- Pain radiating to the neck muscles.
- Described as tightness, dull ache, and/or pressure.
- Spasms and/or tenderness may be present.
- Patient may exhibit tinnitus, dizziness, and/or blurring of vision.

DIAGNOSIS

DIFFERENTIAL DIAGNOSIS

- Migraine
- Intracranial mass
- Head injury
- Cervical spine disease
- Temporomandibular joint (TMJ) problems
- Rebound headache from overuse of analgesics

LABORATORY

- There are no routine laboratory tests.

IMAGING

- Imaging studies may be initiated if brain lesion is suspect.

MEDICAL MANAGEMENT & TREATMENT

- Nonpharmacologic care to include relaxation techniques, physical therapy, massage, biofeedback, stretching exercises, smoking cessation, and heat, if applicable.
- Identifying and eliminating trigger factors need attention.
- In an acute stage, nonnarcotic analgesics may be tried with limited frequency.
- NSAIDs need monitoring for gastric upset and bleeding.
- Antidepressants may be of prophylactic value.
- Avoid narcotics.

COMPLICATIONS

Possibility of overuse of analgesics and the progression to chronic, daily headache syndrome. Medications should be only enough to support limited usage.

PROGNOSIS

When provoking factors are avoided, the prognosis is encouraging. However, most treatments do not produce a complete response. The degree of patient disability may require a multidimensional approach. Recognition of comorbid illness is essential.

DENTAL SIGNIFICANCE

Head and neck discomfort has the potential to result in patient unconcern for dental/oral care. If sign and/or symptoms of tension headache persevere, it is imperative that the patient be referred to a primary care physician and/or neurologist. A correct working diagnosis is essential for the patient to gain control of symptoms.

DENTAL MANAGEMENT

Patients with active tension headaches should receive medical care initially before complete dental care is instituted. Maintenance and immediate oral/dental care may be initiated for patient poststabilization. If analgesics (NSAIDs) and/or antidepressants [e.g., tricyclics (amitriptyline)] are contemplated initially, a consult should be initiated with medical provider to prevent overmedication. General dental/oral care can be continued once there is stabilization of patients with tension headaches.

SUGGESTED REFERENCES

Cutrer FM, Moskowitz MA. Headaches and other head pain, in Goldman L, Ansiello D (eds): *Cecil Textbook of Medicine*, ed 22. Philadelphia, WB Saunders, 2004, pp 2224–2230.

Millea PJ, Brodie JJ. Tension-type headache. *Am Fam Physician* 2002;66:797.

AUTHOR: **NORBERT J. BURZYNSKI, SR., DDS, MS**

SYNONYM(S)

Type A: Antihemophilic globulin (AHG) deficiency; Factor VIII deficiency; classical, familial, hereditary, X-linked, or sex-linked recessive hemophilia

Type B: Factor IX deficiency; Christmas disease; plasma thromboplastin component (PTC) deficiency

Type C: Factor XI deficiency; Rosenthal's disease; plasma thromboplastin antecedent (PTA) deficiency

ICD-9CM/CPT CODE(S)

286.0 Congenital Factor VIII Disorder—complete

286.1 Congenital Factor IX Disorder—complete

286.2 Congenital Factor XI Deficiency—complete

OVERVIEW

A hereditary deficiency of any of the coagulation factors; lack of a factor interrupts the cascade of the development of a fibrin clot, leading to bleeding after injury.

EPIDEMIOLOGY & DEMOGRAPHICS

INCIDENCE/PREVALENCE IN USA: There are approximately 18,000 patients in the U.S. with hemophilia.

- A: (80% of cases of hemophilia) 1 in 10,000 male births
- B: (13%) 1 to 2 in 100,000 male births
- C: (6%) extremely rare; most frequently in patients of Jewish ancestry

PREDOMINANT AGE: Congenital, noted from birth or early childhood.

PREDOMINANT SEX: Males only.

GENETICS: X-linked recessive pattern of inheritance.

ETIOLOGY & PATHOGENESIS

- Congenital deficiency of the gene that codes the formation of the coagulation factor; X linked, recessive although as high as 30% are spontaneous mutations for hemophilia A.
- Males show disease; females are asymptomatic carriers unless < 40% factor level; daughters of affected men are carriers while half of the children of female carriers will have the gene.
- Disease severity depends on percent of factor present: severe < 2%, moderate 2–5%, mild > 6%; patients with > 25% rarely show bleeding except after extensive surgery.

CLINICAL PRESENTATION / PHYSICAL FINDINGS

- Bleeding typically occurs hours or days after injury and may continue for weeks if left untreated.
- A complaint of pain is followed by swelling in the weight-bearing joints such as the hips, knees, or ankles.
- After repeated episodes of blood in the joint (hemarthroses), osteoarthritis and fibrosis develop along with the destruction of articular cartilage and loss of range of motion.

DIAGNOSIS

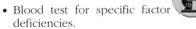

- Blood test for specific factor deficiencies.
- Partial thromboplastin time (PTT) is prolonged while prothrombin time (PT) and platelet count are normal.
- Bleeding time (BT) may be prolonged in 15–25% of hemophilia A patients.

MEDICAL MANAGEMENT & TREATMENT

- Factor replacement transfusions, preferably recombinant forms instead of cryoprecipitate to avoid bloodborne pathogens.
- Epsilon aminocaproic acid (EACA) for inhibition of fibrinolysis.
- Desmopressin (DDAVP) helps for hemophilia A only; increases the amount of Factor VIII for those patients with mild to moderate deficiency (> 5%).

COMPLICATIONS

- Enlargement of joints, pain, and loss of function.
- Soft tissue bleeding can cause peripheral nerve compression from the enlargement of a hematoma; compartment syndrome.
- Other complications include hematuria, intracranial hemorrhage, muscle atrophy, and respiratory obstruction if the tongue is injured.
- Viral hepatitis, chronic liver disease, and HIV/AIDS were potential complications in the treatment of patients with hemophilia prior to the introduction of sterile Factor VIII and IX preparations and screening of blood products for HIV and hepatitis B and C. Up to 70% of hemophiliacs in certain age groups are HIV-seropositive, especially those with severe disease. Patients whose treatment began since the mid- to late 1980s are largely HIV-negative and are not expected to be exposed by modern, sterile replacement products.

PROGNOSIS

The prognosis of patients with hemophilia has been improved by the availability of sterile Factor VIII and IX replacements. The use of recombinant or sterile factor replacement transfusions has reduced the risk of bloodborne diseases. The reduction of fear of becoming infected has led to better management of the disease. With proper treatment using sterile replacement products, a nearly normal life span can be expected even for patients with severe hemophilia, and the crippling sequelae of the disease can be minimized. Genetic counseling has helped to educate patients on the risks to their children.

DENTAL SIGNIFICANCE

- Excessive bleeding after surgery
- Aggressive treatment of oral infections and establishment of good oral hygiene

DENTAL MANAGEMENT

- Consultation with physician.
- Patients with mild to moderate deficiency are usually treated in the dental office.
- For severe deficiency, treatment should be in the hospital.
- For infiltration anesthesia, simple restorative procedures, endodontics, supragingival polishing and calculus removal, there is no factor replacement. Care should be taken when placing bands, wedges, or arch wires.
- Factor replacement may be necessary for those patients with moderate to severe deficiencies, especially for block injections, extractions, and periodontal surgery.
- DDAVP can be given 1 hour before dental procedure by nasal spray (300 mg/kg) or parenterally (0.3 mcg/kg). EACA can be used after extraction (6 g every 6 hours for 3 to 4 days).
  - Local hemostasis with pressure-absorbable gelatin sponges (Gelfoam®), oxidized cellulose (SURGICEL™), microfibrillar collagen (Avitene®), topical thrombin tranexamic acid, epsilon-aminocaproic acid (EACA), sutures, surgical splints, and stents.
- Examine patient 24 hours after procedure for hemostasis or signs of infection.
- Avoid aspirin or NSAIDs.

SUGGESTED REFERENCES

Catalano PM. Disorders of the coagulation mechanism, in Rose LF, Kaye D (eds): *Internal Medicine for Dentistry*. St Louis, Mosby, 1990, pp 353–359

Eastman JR, Nawakoski AR, Triplett MD. DDAVP: a review of indications for its use in treatment of factor VIII deficiency and a report of a case. *Oral Surg* 1983;56:246–250.

Stajcic Z. The combined local/systemic use of antifibrinolytics in hemophiliacs undergoing dental extractions. *Int J of Oral Surg* 1985;18:339.

AUTHOR: **WENDY S. HUPP, DMD**

SYNONYM(S)

Liver cirrhosis
End-stage liver disease

ICD-9CM/CPT CODE(S)
571.5 Cirrhosis of the liver
571.2 Cirrhosis of the liver secondary to alcohol

OVERVIEW

Cirrhosis is defined by the presence of hepatic fibrosis, characterized by nodular changes, portal hypertension, variceal bleeding, and hepatic encephalopathy.

EPIDEMIOLOGY & DEMOGRAPHICS

INCIDENCE/PREVALENCE IN USA: Estimated at 360 per 100,000 population; sixth or seventh leading cause of death for ages 30 to 50; fatality rate of 9 deaths/100,000 persons per year.
PREDOMINANT AGE: Etiology-dependent, but peaks at 40 to 50 years.
PREDOMINANT SEX: Males.
GENETICS: No genetic predilections have been established.

ETIOLOGY & PATHOGENESIS

- The etiology of cirrhosis varies both geographically and socially. In the Western world, the approximate frequency of etiologic categories of cirrhosis is:
  - Alcoholic liver disease: ~ 50%
  - Viral hepatitis: ~ 15%
  - Nonalcoholic steatohepatitis (NASH) related to obesity: ~ 10–15%
  - Biliary diseases including:
    - Primary biliary cirrhosis; primary sclerosing cholangitis; secondary biliary cirrhosis (stones, strictures): ~ 5–10%
  - Primary hemochromatosis: ~ 5%
  - Cryptogenic cirrhosis (cirrhosis of unknown or indeterminate etiology): ~ 15–20%
  - Drug- or toxin-induced liver injury (e.g., acetaminophen, methotrexate, amiodarone): < 5%
  - Other (e.g., Wilson's disease, autoimmune chronic hepatitis, α-1-antitrypsin deficiency, cystic fibrosis, sarcoidosis, galactosemia, glycogen storage disease): < 5%
- The pathogenesis of cirrhosis is characterized by the progressive, irreversible fibrosis and reorganization of the vascular microarchitecture of the liver. The net result is a fibrotic, nodular liver where the delivery of blood to hepatocytes and the ability of hepatocytes to secrete substances into plasma are both severely compromised.

CLINICAL PRESENTATION / PHYSICAL FINDINGS

- Jaundice and palmar erythema, spider angiomas characterize alcoholic signs.
- Jaundice can be seen in the floor of the mouth sometimes before scleral icterus.
- Ecchymosis, caput medusae (dilated periumbilical vein), hemochromatosis, and presence of xanthomas.
- Tremor, choreoathetosis, dysarthria, arthropathy, and peripheral edema.
- Hepatomegaly, splenomegaly, and ascites secondary to portal hypertension and hypoalbuminemia.
- Kayser-Fleischer rings (corneal copper deposition) seen in Wilson's disease, scleral icterus when direct bilirubin levels exceed 0.2 mg/dL.
- Distinct urine and oral odor (musty odor).
- Hemorrhoids, heme-positive stool in the presence of peptic ulcer disease (PUD), variceal bleeding.

DIAGNOSIS

(Adapted from Ferri FF. Cirrhosis, in *Ferri's Clinical Advisor: Instant Diagnosis and Treatment.* St Louis, Mosby, 2005.)

HISTORY

- Alcohol abuse: alcoholic liver disease
- Hepatitis B (chronic active hepatitis, primary hepatic neoplasm, or hepatitis C)
- Inflammatory bowel disease (primary sclerosing cholangitis)
- Pruritus, hyperlipoproteinemia, and xanthomas in middle-aged or elderly women (primary biliary cirrhosis)
- Impotence, diabetes mellitus, hyperpigmentation, arthritis (hemochromatosis)
- Neurologic disturbances (Wilson's disease, hepatolenticular degeneration)
- History of recurrent episodes of right upper quadrant pain (biliary tract disease)
- History of blood transfusions, IV drug abuse (hepatitis C)
- History of hepatotoxic drug exposure
- Coexistence of other diseases with immune or autoimmune features (ITP, myasthenia gravis, thyroiditis, autoimmune hepatitis)
- Family history of "liver disease" [e.g., hemochromatosis (positive family history in 25% of patients), α-1 antitrypsin deficiency]

LABORATORY TESTS

- Decreased Hgb and Hct, elevated MCV, increased BUN and creatinine (the BUN may also be normal or low if the patient has severely diminished liver function), decreased sodium (dilutional hyponatremia), decreased potassium (as a result of secondary aldosteronism or urinary losses).
- Decreased glucose in a patient with liver disease indicating severe liver damage.
- Other laboratory abnormalities include:
  - Alcoholic hepatitis and cirrhosis: there may be mild elevation of ALT and AST, usually < 500 IU; AST > ALT (ratio > 2:3).
  - Extrahepatic obstruction: there may be moderate elevations of ALT and AST to levels < 500 IU.
  - Viral, toxic, or ischemic hepatitis: there are extreme elevations (> 500 IU) of ALT and AST.
  - Alkaline phosphatase elevation can occur with extrahepatic obstruction, primary biliary cirrhosis, and primary sclerosing cholangitis.
  - Serum LDH is significantly elevated in metastatic disease of the liver; lesser elevations are seen with hepatitis, cirrhosis, extrahepatic obstruction, and congestive hepatomegaly.
  - Serum γ-glutamyl transpeptidase (GGTP) is elevated in alcoholic liver disease and may also be elevated with cholestatic disease (primary biliary cirrhosis, primary sclerosing cholangitis).
  - Serum bilirubin may be elevated; urinary bilirubin can be present in hepatitis, hepatocellular jaundice, and biliary obstruction.
  - Serum albumin: significant liver disease results in hypoalbuminemia.
  - Prothrombin time: an elevated PT in patients with liver disease indicates severe liver damage and poor prognosis.
  - Presence of hepatitis B surface antigen implies acute or chronic hepatitis B.
  - Presence of antimitochondrial antibody suggests primary biliary cirrhosis, chronic hepatitis.
  - Elevated serum copper, decreased serum ceruloplasmin, and elevated 24-hour urine may be diagnostic of Wilson's disease.
  - An elevated serum ferritin and increased transferrin saturation are suggestive of hemochromatosis.
  - Elevated blood ammonia suggests hepatocellular dysfunction; serial values are not useful in following patients with hepatic encephalopathy because there is poor correlation between blood ammonia level and degree of hepatic encephalopathy.
  - Serum cholesterol is elevated in cholestatic disorders.
  - Antinuclear antibodies (ANA) may be found in autoimmune hepatitis.
  - Alpha fetoprotein: levels > 1000 pg/ml are highly suggestive of primary liver cell carcinoma.
  - Hepatitis C viral testing identifies patients with chronic hepatitis C infection.
  - Elevated level of serum globulin (especially γ-globulins), positive ANA test may occur with autoimmune hepatitis.

IMAGING STUDIES

- Ultrasonography to detect gallstones and dilation of common bile ducts.
- CT scan to detect mass lesions in liver and pancreas, assess hepatic fat content,

identify idiopathic hemochromatosis, early diagnosis of Budd-Chiari syndrome, dilation of intrahepatic bile ducts, and detect varices and splenomegaly.

- Percutaneous liver biopsy to evaluate hepatic filling defects, diagnose hepatocellular disease or hepatomegaly, evaluate persistently abnormal liver function tests, and diagnose hemochromatosis, primary biliary cirrhosis, Wilson's disease, glycogen storage diseases, chronic hepatitis, autoimmune hepatitis, infiltrative diseases, alcoholic liver disease, drug-induced liver disease, and primary or secondary carcinoma.

MEDICAL MANAGEMENT & TREATMENT

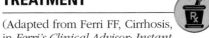

(Adapted from Ferri FF, Cirrhosis, in *Ferri's Clinical Advisor: Instant Diagnosis and Treatment.* St Louis, Mosby, 2005.)

NONPHARMACOLOGIC

Avoid any hepatotoxins (e.g., ethanol, acetaminophen); improve nutritional status.

PHARMACOLOGIC/SURGICAL

- Correct any mechanical obstruction to bile flow (e.g., calculi, strictures).
- Provide therapy for underlying cardiovascular disorders in patients with cardiac cirrhosis.
- Remove excess body iron with phlebotomy and deferoxamine in patients with hemochromatosis.
- Remove copper deposits with D-penicillamine in patients with Wilson's disease.
- Long-term ursodiol therapy slows the progression of primary biliary cirrhosis but is ineffective in treating primary sclerosing cholangitis.
- Glucocorticoids (prednisone 20 to 30 mg/day initially or combination therapy or prednisone and azathioprine) is useful in autoimmune hepatitis.
- Liver transplantation may be indicated in otherwise healthy patients (age < 65 years) with sclerosing cholangitis, chronic hepatitis cirrhosis, or primary biliary cirrhosis with prognostic information suggesting < 20% chance of survival without transplantation.
- Contraindications: AIDS, most metastatic malignancies, active substance abuse, uncontrolled sepsis, and uncontrolled cardiac or pulmonary disease.
- Treatment of complications:
  - Portal hypertension:
    - Ascites [includes dietary sodium restriction, diuretics, large volume paracentesis, transjugular intrahepatic portosystemic shunt (TIPS)].
    - Esophagogastric varices (includes endoscopic band ligation or sclerotherapy, transjugular nonselective β-blockers, TIPS).
  - Hepatic encephalopathy [includes restricting protein intake (40 to 60

g/day) to reduce production of endogenous nitrogenous substances; reducing colonic ammonia production/absorption with lactulose and/or neomycin].
  - Hepatorenal syndrome (includes vasopressin analogues, liver transplantation).

COMPLICATIONS

- Severe hemorrhage in late stages: upper gastrointestinal tract bleeding may occur from varices, portal hypertensive gastropathy, or gastroduodenal ulcer. Hemorrhage may be massive, resulting in fatal exsanguination or portosystemic encephalopathy.
- Cardiovascular organ damage: cardiomyopathy may result from alcohol abuse, impairment of cardiac beta-adrenergic receptors, and altered hemodynamics due to portal hypertension.
- Encephalopathy from failure of the liver to detoxify nitrogenous agents of gut origin because of hepatocellular dysfunction and portosystemic shunting.
- Ascites and edema from portal hypertension (increased hydrostatic pressure); hypoalbuminemia (decreased oncotic pressure) and peripheral vasodilation with resulting increases in renin and angiotensin levels and sodium retention by the kidneys.
- Hepatorenal syndrome: characterized by azotemia, oliguria, hyponatremia, low urinary sodium, and hypotension in a patient with cirrhosis.
- Impaired hemostasis: increased bleeding tendency due to hypoprothrombinemia with prolonged prothrombin time and thrombocytopenia secondary to hypersplenism.
- Hepatocellular carcinoma: cirrhosis is associated with 22.9% increased risk of hepatocellular carcinoma after 3.5 years.

PROGNOSIS

- Varies with etiology of the patient's cirrhosis and whether there is continuing hepatic injury.
- Multiple complications make treatment of cirrhosis challenging. In cases with severe hepatic dysfunction (serum albumin < 3.0 g/dL, bilirubin > 3.0 mg/dL, ascites, encephalopathy, cachexia, and upper gastrointestinal bleeding), only 50% survive 6 months.
- Patients with hepatorenal syndrome have in excess of 80% mortality.
- Liver transplantation has significantly improved the prognosis for patients who are acceptable candidates and are referred for evaluation early.

DENTAL SIGNIFICANCE

- Impaired hemostasis

- Unpredictable/impaired hepatic metabolism of certain drugs
- Increased risk/spread of oral infections
- Delayed healing

DENTAL MANAGEMENT

- A medical consult with the patient's physician is useful in order to help determine the degree of impairment of hepatic function:
  - Establish the underlying etiology of cirrhosis: alcoholism, viral hepatitis.
  - Obtain a list of patient's current medications.
  - Obtains results of most recent lab studies, including:
    - Serum bilirubin, serum albumin
    - AST, ALT, GGTP, alkaline phosphatase
    - Complete blood count (CBC) with differential (including platelet count)
    - PT/INR
  - Determine history or presence of complications of cirrhosis, including:
    - Ascites
    - Encephalopathy
    - Spontaneous bacterial peritonitis
    - Cardiomyopathy
    - Portal hypertension
    - Impaired hemostasis
- Drug use in patients with cirrhosis (see Appendix A, Box A-6, "Drug Use in Hepatic Dysfunction").
- The patient with liver disease and ascites may be uncomfortable in the reclined position because of increased abdominal size and weight, which would place excessive pressure on the abdominal blood vessels. If so, the upright or semi-reclined position is recommended.
- Spontaneous bacterial peritonitis (SBP) is potentially a serious problem in patients with cirrhosis and ascites. The clinician should consider antibiotic prophylaxis with a pre-liver transplant patient who has a history of SBP or with a patient demonstrating liver transplant rejection, as well as with any patient who has ascites or whose medical condition would drastically deteriorate should SBP develop. When antibiotic premedication is indicated to prevent SBP, oral administration of 2 gm of amoxicillin (if nonallergic) in addition to 500 mg of metronidazole 1 hour before the procedure is recommended.

SUGGESTED REFERENCES

Bataller R, Brenner DA. Liver fibrosis. *J Clin Invest.* 2005;115:209–218.

Ferri FF. Cirrhosis, in *Ferri's Clinical Advisor: Instant Diagnosis and Treatment.* St Louis, Mosby, 2005, pp 195–196.

Golla K, Epstein JB, Cabay RJ. Liver disease: current perspectives on medical and dental management. *Oral Surg Oral Med Oral Pathol Oral Radiol Endod.* 2004;98:516–521.

Thomson BJ, Finch RG. Hepatitis C virus infection. *Clin Microbiol Infect.* 2005;11:86–94.

AUTHOR: **ANDRES PINTO, DMD**

SYNONYM(S)

N/A

ICD-9CM/CPT CODE(S)

573.3 Unspecified hepatitis—complete

OVERVIEW

- The liver serves many functions critical to maintenance of life. These functions are both protective and regulatory in nature and include:
  - Glucose homeostasis
  - Plasma protein synthesis
  - Lipoprotein and glycoprotein synthesis
  - Bile acid synthesis and secretion
  - Vitamin storage (B_{12}, A, D, E, and K)
  - Biotransformation of compounds (inactive to active and active to inactive forms)
  - Detoxification drugs, metabolites, and hormones
  - Excretion of wastes (bile, bilirubin, and lipids)
- The liver response to insult and injury is inflammatory in nature; this response is known as hepatitis.
- Hepatitis has a diverse etiology and multiple attributed causes. The end result is hepatic cell inflammation, injury, and cell death. Hepatitis is characterized as being acute (less than 6 months) or, less commonly, chronic (greater than 6 months). Characteristic of hepatic injury is an abnormal elevation of aminotransferases. Aminotransferases (also known as transaminases) are used to assess acute hepatocellular injury and include aspartate aminotransferase (AST) and the alanine aminotransferase (ALT).
  - AST is found in the cells of the liver, cardiac muscle, and skeletal muscle. AST is also found in lesser concentrations in kidneys, brain, pancreas, lung, leukocytes, and erythrocytes.
  - ALT is found mainly in the liver. The aminotransferases are normally present in low concentrations in the serum and are released into the blood in higher concentrations when there is damage to the liver.
- About one-third of people with chronic hepatitis develop it as a result of viral hepatitis. Other causes of chronic hepatitis include Wilson's disease (abnormal copper retention) or autoimmune disease.
- Certain drugs have also been implicated in chronic hepatitis, including acetaminophen, nitrofurantoin, and methyldopa.
- Viral and alcoholic hepatitis will be reviewed more in depth in other topics of this text.

EPIDEMIOLOGY & DEMOGRAPHICS

Dependent upon type of hepatitis

ETIOLOGY & PATHOGENESIS

- Diverse causes include viral, bacterial, protozoal, and fungal infections, immune-mediated disorders, metabolic diseases, hepatic perfusion problems, alcohol and medications, environmental and industrial toxins, and alternative medical therapies.
- Acute hepatitis is usually associated with viral infection. About one-third of people with chronic hepatitis develop it as a result of viral hepatitis.
- Other causes of chronic hepatitis include Wilson's disease (abnormal copper retention) or autoimmune disease.
- Certain drugs have also been implicated in chronic hepatitis including acetaminophen, nitrofurantoin, and methyldopa.
- See "Hepatitis: Alcoholic" and "Hepatitis: Viral" in Section I, pp 100 and 102.

CLINICAL PRESENTATION / PHYSICAL FINDINGS

- The degree of the aminotransferase elevation can be helpful in assessment of hepatitis etiology. In most acute hepatocellular disorders, ALT values are greater or equal to AST values. This relationship differs in alcoholic hepatitis. In alcohol abusers, an AST:ALT ratio > 2:1 is suggestive of alcoholic hepatitis while a ratio > 3:1 is highly suggestive of alcoholic hepatitis.
- Subjective findings may include generalized malaise, poor appetite, and fatigue. Many (but not all) patients with hepatitis will have overt clinical symptoms such as jaundice or icterus. Jaundice is a yellow discoloration of skin due to excessive bilirubin accumulation (> 2.0 mg/dL). Jaundice occurs in three forms:
  - Hemolytic jaundice: resulting from excessive red blood cell (RBC) destruction
  - Hepatocellular jaundice: bilirubin not processed
  - Obstructive jaundice: cholestasis (retention of all constituents of bile)
- Certain clinical signs, when present, may suggest certain etiologies. For example, cutaneous hyperpigmentation and arthralgias are often found with hemochromatosis and acne is found with autoimmune hepatitis. Travel to endemic regions may also suggest certain types of hepatitis (hepatitis A, B, or E).
- It is vital that the clinician note any and all medications and supplements the patient uses. Approximately 30% of patients use supplements and nutraceuticals and, unfortunately, may not share this information with their healthcare providers.
- A summary of the common etiologies and clinical signs associated with hepatitis is seen in Table I-12.

TABLE I-12 **Common Etiologies and Clinical Signs Associated with Hepatitis***

Clinical Sign	Likely Etiology of Hepatitis
Parotid enlargement	Alcohol
Clubbing (of the fingers)	Cirrhosis
Gynecomastia	Alcohol, cirrhosis
Testicular atrophy	Alcohol
Xanthelasmas (benign yellow-white, flat growth of the eyelid consisting of fatty material)	Primary sclerosing cholangitis (PSC), primary biliary sclerosis (PBC)
Skin excoriations	PBC, PSC, drug toxicity
Bronzed skin	Hemochromatosis
Photosensitivity/blisters	Hepatitis C virus (HCV) + iron overload
Blue nails	Wilson's disease
Urticaria	Hepatitis B virus (HBV), drug toxicity
Erythema of the palms	Cirrhosis
Spider angiomas (dilated blood vessel surrounded by smaller dilated capillaries)	Cirrhosis
Kayser-Fleischer rings (a greenish-yellow pigmented ring encircling the cornea just within the corneoscleral margin)	Wilson's disease, PBC
Asterixis (involuntary jerking movements, especially in the hands)	Cirrhosis/portal hypertension
Splenomegaly	Cirrhosis
Ascites	Cirrhosis
Petechiae	HBV, HCV, hemorrhagic fever

*Adapted from Marsano LS. Hepatitis. *Prim Care Clin Office Pract* 2003;30:84.

DIAGNOSIS

- Obtaining a thorough medical history and physical examination is critical in diagnosis of hepatitis.
- The initial evaluation of a suspected hepatitis patient may include various laboratory assays including HBsAg, antibody to HB core, antibodies to HCV or HCV-RNA, antinuclear antibodies (ANA), perinuclear antineutrophil cytoplasmic autoantibodies (pANCA), immunogloblobins IgG, IgA, IgM, iron, transferrin, ferritin, and a host of others. Typically, assays will be ordered to confirm the most probable etiology for the presenting symptoms.
- Although no specific imaging studies are required to make a diagnosis of hepatitis, certain imaging tests may be ordered to assess severity of the disease. These imaging tests include ultrasound and computed tomography, especially if the origin of the hepatitis is thought to be related to gallbladder disease or biliary obstruction.
- In patients with chronic viral hepatic types B or C, a liver biopsy is recommended for initial assessment of disease activity. A small piece of hepatic tissue is analyzed for histological changes associated with chronic hepatitis.
- There are four different methods for obtaining a sample of tissue via a liver biopsy:
  - In percutaneous liver biopsy, local anesthesia is used. A needle is inserted into the liver, and a tissue sample is removed.
  - Percutaneous image-guided liver biopsy involves a similar technique except that the needle is guided to an appropriate location utilizing computed tomography scan (CT scan) or ultrasound images. Percutaneous image-guided liver biopsy is most often used to obtain samples of tissue

from precise locations (i.e., areas of disease activity).
  - Laparoscopic liver biopsy can be done in conjunction with another surgical procedure or as a method to obtain hepatic tissue only. After incisions are made into the abdomen, a laparoscope is inserted and allows for magnified visualization of the external liver surface. Tissue then can be removed.
  - The open surgical liver biopsy technique is rarely done unless it is part of another surgical procedure.

MEDICAL MANAGEMENT & TREATMENT

- Treatment is based on underlying etiology. Therefore, it is important for the clinician to assess the signs and symptoms and ascertain the most likely etiology for hepatitis.
- Additional information may be found in the topics that deal with specific hepatitis etiologies.

COMPLICATIONS

Complications from hepatitis may be self-limiting, or complications may have irreversible effects, including changes in mental status, abnormal collection of fluid in the abdominal cavity (ascites), or fulminant hepatic failure.

PROGNOSIS

- Prognosis is dependent on the etiology of the hepatitis and treatment. Generally, there is good prognosis for acute hepatitis. Chronic hepatitis prognosis is more dependent upon treatment rendered, including hepatic transplantation.

- Further information can be found in the "Hepatitis: Viral" topic, on the next page.

DENTAL SIGNIFICANCE

Patients with hepatitis may have bleeding abnormalities. These abnormalities may be anatomic or specific abnormalities of the coagulation system. In patients with hepatitis, bleeding coagulapathies may be the result of:
- Decreased synthesis of procoagulant and anticoagulant proteins
- Impaired clearance of activated coagulation factors
- Nutritional deficiency (e.g., vitamin K, folate)
- Synthesis of functionally abnormal fibrinogen
- Splenomegaly (sequestration thrombocytopenia)
- Qualitative platelet defects
- Bone marrow suppression of thrombopoiesis

DENTAL MANAGEMENT

- Coagulation status workup for surgical procedures for patients with chronic hepatitis: PT/INR, PTT, platelet count, and bleeding time (or closure time) may be warranted.
- Caution in prescribing drugs metabolized through hepatic mechanisms (see Appendix A, Common Helpful Information for Medical Diseases and Conditions).

SUGGESTED REFERENCE

Marsano LS. Hepatitis. *Prim Care Clin Office Pract* 2003;30:81–107.

AUTHOR: **BRIAN C. MUZYKA, DMD, MS, MBA**

SECTION I

SYNONYM(S)

Alcoholic liver disease (ALD)
Steatosis

ICD-9CM/CPT CODE(S)

571.1 Acute alcoholic hepatitis—complete

OVERVIEW

- Alcoholic hepatitis is part of the continuum of alcoholic liver disease (ALD). Alcoholic liver disease consists of:
  - Fatty liver changes known as steatosis
  - Alcoholic hepatitis
  - Alcoholic cirrhosis

EPIDEMIOLOGY & DEMOGRAPHICS

INCIDENCE/PREVALENCE IN USA:
7.4% of the U.S. population (11% in men and 4% in women) meet the diagnostic criteria for alcohol abuse. (See "Alcoholism" in Section I, p 4.) In the U.S., ALD affects more than 2 million people (i.e., approximately 1% of the population). The true prevalence of ALD, especially of its milder forms, is unknown because patients may be asymptomatic and never seek medical attention.
PREDOMINANT AGE: Can affect any age but is more predominant in 25- to 60-year-old range.
PREDOMINANT SEX: Females are more susceptible to ALD and develop symptoms at lower daily doses of ethanol.
GENETICS: An inherited predisposition to alcoholism has been clearly established, but genetically determined increased susceptibility to liver damage in heavy drinkers is less certain. Increased susceptibility to organ injury may also be associated with certain isoenzymes of alcohol dehydrogenase, the principal metabolizing enzyme of ethanol.

ETIOLOGY & PATHOGENESIS

- Steatosis is usually an incidental, asymptomatic finding that can be reversed.
- Approximately 80% of heavy drinkers, defined as someone who imbibes 80 grams or more of ethanol daily, develop fatty liver. Up to 35% of these heavy drinkers will develop alcoholic hepatitis, while approximately 10% will develop alcoholic cirrhosis.
  - Eighty grams of ethanol equals eight 12-oz beers, a liter of wine, or a half pint of spirits.
- Damage to the liver from alcohol abuse is a result of the metabolism of ethanol and not the presence of ethanol itself.
- Alcohol metabolism involves oxidation into acetaldehyde by the enzyme alcohol dehydrogenase. Acetaldehyde is highly reactive and binds proteins and other compounds forming acetalde-

hyde by-products or adducts. These adducts may stimulate the immune response system (antigenic stimulation) or may attach to cellular proteins and render the proteins nonfunctional. These adducts may initiate harmful cell-mediated and humoral responses. These harmful responses culminate in the expression of proinflammatory cytokines, tumor necrosis factor alpha, transforming growth factor beta, interleukin 1B, and interleukin 6. The end product of these specific cytokines expression is hepatic fibrosis. Reactive oxygen species are also generated through alcohol metabolism and, similarly, contribute hepatic cell damage. Metabolic changes resulting from alcohol metabolism include an increase in triglyceride synthesis and decreased hepatic excretion and lipid oxidation resulting in steatosis.
- Because of differences in alcohol metabolism in women, survival rates are less than those of men. Women who drink 30 grams or more of alcohol daily have a markedly increased chance of being diagnosed with cirrhosis.

CLINICAL PRESENTATION / PHYSICAL FINDINGS

- Steatosis is usually an incidental, asymptomatic finding. In severe cases, right upper quadrant pain, loss of appetite, and nausea may be present.
- Alcoholic hepatitis symptoms may be mild or severe and include:
  - Anorexia
  - Generalized fatigue
  - Weight loss
  - Jaundice
  - Fever
  - Cutaneous signs such as spider nevi
  - Enlarged, tender liver
- Other clinical signs may include:
  - Parotid enlargement
  - Gynecomastia and testicular atrophy in males
- Alcoholic cirrhosis is characterized by a diverse group of findings. These findings include:
  - Bilateral parotid enlargement
  - Dupuytren's contracture: an abnormal thickening of palmar fascia and fingers that can cause the fingers to curl
  - Palmar erythema
  - Multiple spider nevi on the skin
  - Gynecomastia and testicular atrophy in males
  - Hepatomegaly
  - Increased blood pressure in the portal vein (portal hypertension) may also be present as a result of hepatic fibrosis. Portal hypertension is additionally characterized by:
    - Ascites
    - Splenomegaly

  - Distended and engorged umbilical veins (caput medusae)
- Neurological changes also may occur in those with alcoholic liver disease and cirrhosis. These changes include:
  - Altered sleep patterns
  - Behavioral changes
  - Somnolence
  - Confusion
  - Ataxia (total or partial inability to coordinate voluntary bodily movements, especially muscular movements)
  - Asterixis (irregular, flap-like tremor; reflects a brief loss of muscle contraction followed by a rapid recovery)
  - Obtundation

DIAGNOSIS

- In steatosis, abnormal laboratory results such as elevated values of gamma-glutamyl transpeptidase (GGTP), aspartate aminotransferase (AST), and the alanine aminotransferase (ALT) may be seen. Biopsy of the affected tissue is required for a diagnosis of steatosis.
- Alcoholic hepatitis is a potentially life-threatening complication of alcohol abuse resulting in hepatic inflammation and dysfunction. A liver biopsy is also required for the diagnosis of alcoholic hepatitis. Histological findings in alcoholic hepatitis include hyaline deposition, cellular infiltration of PML, and interlobular connective tissue surrounding the hepatocytes. In 90% of those with severe alcoholic hepatitis, cirrhosis is also present.
- In alcoholic abusers an AST:ALT ratio > 2:1 is suggestive of alcoholic hepatitis, while a ratio > 3:1 is highly suggestive of alcoholic hepatitis.
- Biochemical abnormalities noted in those with alcoholic cirrhosis include elevated bilirubin and transaminases (ALT and AST) and decreased serum albumin levels.

MEDICAL MANAGEMENT & TREATMENT

- Treatment for steatosis usually consists of alcohol abstinence and improved dietary intake.
- Treatment for mild to moderate alcoholic hepatitis consists of alcohol abstinence. Alcoholic hepatitis will persist in nonabstainers and will progress into cirrhosis in approximately 40% in an 18-month period. Additional treatment may include thiamine, folate, and multivitamin supplementation and use of corticosteroid agents such as prednisolone. Corticosteroids may improve short-term survival by inhibiting damaging immune responses associated with acetaldehyde product antibody formation.

- Treatment for alcoholic cirrhosis consists of alcohol abstinence. The 5-year survival rate for abstainers reaches 70%. The 5-year survival rate for non-abstainers is approximately 40%.
- Other clinical findings associated with a poorer prognosis include elevated PT/INR values and depressed hemoglobin and albumin values. In addition, the presence of encephalopathy and persistent jaundice is also associated with a poorer prognosis.
- Hepatic transplantation is also a treatment for alcoholic cirrhosis, and survival outcomes are parallel to outcomes of other end-stage hepatic diseases treated with transplantation. Due to the limited availability of organs for transplant and the high economic costs associated with such a procedure, liver transplantation for alcoholic cirrhosis is rare. Approximately 6% of liver transplantation in the U.S. is as a result of alcoholic cirrhosis.

COMPLICATIONS

- The major complication is the development of alcoholic cirrhosis.

PROGNOSIS

- Mild alcoholic hepatitis is a benign disorder with very low short-term mortality. However, when alcoholic hepatitis is of sufficient severity to cause hepatic encephalopathy, jaundice, or coagulopathy, mortality is significantly increased.

- The clinical severity of alcoholic hepatitis can be quantified by using the Maddrey Discriminant Function (DF) index. This index is used to estimate a short-term survival rate.

$$DF = 4.6 \times (\text{Patient's PT} - \text{Control PT}) + \text{serum bilirubin (mg/dL)}$$

or

$$DF = 4.6 \times (\text{Patient's PT} - \text{Control PT}) + (\text{serum bilirubin } [\mu\text{mol/L}] \div 17.1)$$

where PT = prothrombin time (sec)
  - DF scores of greater than 32 are associated with a 30-day survival rate of 50%.
  - DF scores of less than 32 are associated with a 30-day survival rate of 80–100%.
- The long-term prognosis of alcoholic hepatitis depends heavily on whether patients have established cirrhosis and whether they continue to use alcohol. With abstinence, patients with alcoholic hepatitis exhibit progressive improvement in liver function over months to years, and histologic features of active alcoholic hepatitis resolve. If alcohol abuse continues, alcoholic hepatitis invariably persists and progresses to cirrhosis over months to years.

DENTAL SIGNIFICANCE

- Increased risk for oral cancer
- Frequently have poor oral hygiene with increased incidence of caries, gingivitis, and periodontitis

- Xerostomia
- Candidiasis
- Parotid gland enlargement
- Angular and/or labial cheilitis
- Glossitis
- Attrition secondary to bruxism
- Impaired hemostasis
- Unpredictable/impaired hepatic metabolism of certain drugs
- Delayed healing

DENTAL MANAGEMENT

- A medical consult with the patient's physician is usually indicated in order to help determine the degree of impairment of hepatic function and coagulation status, including results of most recent lab studies:
  - Serum bilirubin, serum albumin
  - AST, ALT, GGTP, alkaline phosphatase
  - Complete blood count (CBC) with differential (including platelet count)
  - PT/INR, bleeding time
- Use caution in prescribing drugs metabolized through hepatic mechanisms (see Appendix A, Box A-6, "Drug Use in Hepatic Dysfunction").

SUGGESTED REFERENCES

Mandayam S, Jamal MM, Morgan TR. Epidemiology of alcoholic liver disease. *Seminars in Liver Disease* 2004;24(3):217–232.

Walsh K, Alexander G. Alcoholic liver disease. *Postgraduate Med J* 2000;76(895):280–286.

AUTHOR: **BRIAN C. MUZYKA, DMD, MS, MBA**

SYNONYM(S)

Hepatitis A (HAV)
Hepatitis B (HBV)
Hepatitis C (HCV)
Hepatitis D (HDV)
Hepatitis E (HEV)

ICD-9CM/CPT CODE(S)

070.1   Hepatitis type A
070.21 Hepatitis type B (acute) with delta
070.30 Hepatitis type B (acute)
070.32 Hepatitis type B (chronic)
070.33 Hepatitis type B (chronic) with delta
070.51 Hepatitis type C
070.52 Hepatitis type D (with hepatitis B carrier state)
070.53 Hepatitis type E

OVERVIEW

Viral hepatitis is a major public health issue of global proportions. Viral hepatitis is classified according to causative viral agent. Currently, five different agents are associated with a diagnosis of viral hepatitis. These agents are: hepatitis A virus (HAV), hepatitis B virus, (HBV), hepatitis C virus (HCV), hepatitis D virus (HDV), and hepatitis E virus (HEV).

EPIDEMIOLOGY & DEMOGRAPHICS

INCIDENCE/PREVALENCE IN USA:

- Hepatitis A: approximately 15 cases per 100,000 persons yearly with an estimated 61,000 cases per year in 2003; approximately 33–70% of U.S. population has serologic evidence of prior infection.
- Hepatitis B: estimated 73,000 cases in 2003 and a total of 1 to 1.25 million chronic infections.
- Hepatitis C: estimated 150,000 new cases yearly (37,500 symptomatic; 93,000 later chronic liver disease; 30,700 cirrhosis).
- Hepatitis D: requires coinfection with HBV, approximately 15 million people worldwide have been infected, not established for the U.S.
- Hepatitis E: not established for the U.S.

PREDOMINANT AGE:

- Hepatitis A: in areas of high rates of hepatitis A, virtually all children are infected while younger than 10 years old, but disease is rare; in areas of moderate rates of hepatitis A, disease occurs in late childhood and young adults; in areas of low rates of hepatitis A, most cases occur in young adults.
- Hepatitis B: 30 to 45 years of age, at rates of 5–20%.
- Hepatitis C: highest prevalence in 30- to 49-year-old age group (65%).
- Hepatitis D: more common in adults.
- Hepatitis E: more common in ages 15 to 40 years.

PREDOMINANT SEX:

- Hepatitis A: none.
- Hepatitis B: predominant in males because of increased intravenous drug abuse, homosexuality; fulminant HBV has a male > female (2:1) predominance.
- Hepatitis C: slight male predominance.
- Hepatitis D: none.
- Hepatitis E: none.

GENETICS: No established genetic predisposition for any viral hepatitis diseases.

ETIOLOGY & PATHOGENESIS

- **Hepatitis A**
  - Hepatitis A is picornavirus that causes an acute disease or asymptomatic infection. Hepatitis A virus (HAV) is found in highest concentrations in feces but may also be found in saliva and serum.
  - HAV is transmitted mainly through an oral–fecal route and is often associated with poor sanitation. Person-to-person contact and contaminated food or water or blood have also been associated with HAV transmission. The only host for HAV is humans, and the virus can survive in dried stool up to 4 weeks. Once ingested, the virus replicates in hepatocytes and causes immune-mediated hepatocyte destruction to occur. Those at increased risk are injection drug users, men who have sex with men, international travelers and travelers to endemic regions in the U.S., and consumers of high-risk foods such as shellfish.
  - The normal incubation period for HAV is 15 to 50 days (average 30 days).
- **Hepatitis B**
  - Hepatitis B virus (HBV) is a hepadnavirus that is transmitted both parentally and via sexual contact. Viral concentrations of HBV are high in blood and serum, and moderate in semen and saliva.
  - Those at increased risk are recipients of blood transfusion or blood products, persons undergoing hemodialysis, sharing needles, having sexual contact with an infected person, or having occupational exposure (such as healthcare workers). HBV can also be transmitted perinatally from infected mother to child.
  - The incubation period for HBV infection is approximately 30 to 180 days.
- **Hepatitis C**
  - Hepatitis C virus (HCV) is a hepacivirus that is mainly transmitted via shared needles, blood transfusion or blood products (before screening for this virus in the blood supply), perinatally, and via hemodialysis. HCV can also be transmitted sexually and through saliva, although both are ineffective means of disease transmission. Additionally, healthcare workers are at risk for contraction of HCV.
  - Most infections (up to 70%) are asymptomatic.
  - The incubation time for HCV is 14 to 180 days, and HCV-RNA can be recovered from serum throughout the course of infection.
- **Hepatitis D**
  - Hepatitis D virus (HDV) is a delta virus that requires HBV for propagation. Coinfection of HBV and HDV results in a more severe, acute disease expression but a lower risk of chronic infection of HBV. HDV may also develop as a superinfection (that is, infection at a later point in time) of chronic HBV infection. In this case, there is a higher risk to develop chronic HDV infection and almost an 80% risk of developing severe chronic liver disease.
- **Hepatitis E**
  - Hepatitis E virus (HEV) is an enterically transmitted virus that is clinically similar to HAV infection. HEV is the only member of the herpesvirus genus and is a single stranded RNA virus. There are four genotypes. IgM anti-HEV are used as markers of recent infection and, more recently, IgA anti-HEV in combination with IgM anti-HEV or sole presence of IgA anti-HEV have been reported as markers of HEV infection.
  - HEV is transmitted primarily through the oral-fecal route; waterborne epidemics in developing areas in Africa, Asia, and the Middle East are characteristic. HEV is transmitted less frequently than HAV. To date, there has been only one reported epidemic of HEV in North America. Interestingly, HEV-associated hepatitis occurs among individuals in industrialized countries with no history of travel to endemic areas, and HEV antibodies are routinely found in the blood supply.
  - The incubation period for hepatitis E varies from 15 to 64 days.

CLINICAL PRESENTATION / PHYSICAL FINDINGS

- **Hepatitis A**
  - In 80% of those infected over the age of 5 years, icterus is present. Other symptoms may include generalized malaise, headache, fever, diarrhea, abdominal pains, and muscle aches.
- **Hepatitis B**
  - Initial symptoms may include arthralgias, cutaneous rashes, and arthritic-type pain.
  - Clinical illness later on includes jaundice in 30–50% of persons infected. Other findings may include malaise, anorexia, nausea, vomiting, fever,

muscle pains, and upper right quadrant pain.

- **Hepatitis C**
  - When they occur, symptoms include anorexia, arthralgias, myalgia, and fatigue.
- **Hepatitis D**
  - Signs and symptoms may not develop or be expressed in those who are coinfected or superinfected with HDV. Symptoms when present are similar to those seen in HBV.
- **Hepatitis E**
  - Symptoms are clinically similar to HAV and may include icterus, generalized malaise, headache, fever, diarrhea, abdominal pains, and muscle aches.

DIAGNOSIS

- **Hepatitis A**
  - Diagnosis of HAV is confirmed by presence of IgM antibodies to HAV (IgM anti-HAV) and in the early course of the disease by presence of IgG antibodies. IgG anti-HAV remain for life and are protective (i.e., these antibodies protect against repeat infection to HAV).
- **Hepatitis B**
  - Laboratory diagnostic criteria for HBV include IgM antibody to hepatitis B core antigen (anti-HBc) or hepatitis B surface antigen (HBsAg). In addition, tests that may show elevations include AST, ALT, and bilirubin. In those who recover from the acute episode, HBsAg will no longer be detected in the serum. Immunity is indicated by presence of IgG anti-HBc. Recovery from HBV is indicated by presence of antibodies to hepatitis B surface antigen (anti-HBsAg).
- **Hepatitis C**
  - A diagnostic criterion for HCV is presence of HCV antibodies in addition to one or more of the following: elevation of ALT for 6 months or more, positive anti-HCV for 6 months or longer, and/or liver biopsy consistent with chronic hepatitis. Typically, antibodies are detected using enzyme immunoassay (EIA), the results of which are confirmed with recombinant immunoblot assay (RIBA).
- **Hepatitis D**
  - Diagnosis for HDV coinfection is established with presence of IgM anti-HBc and IgM anti-HD, which will be followed in a few weeks with IgG anti-HD. Diagnosis of a superinfection of HDV is established with anti-HBsAg, anti-HDAg, and IgM anti-HD and IgG anti-HD.

MEDICAL MANAGEMENT & TREATMENT

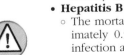

- **Hepatitis A**
  - Treatment for HAV is generally supportive, as the disease is usually self-limiting. Fulminant hepatic failure rarely occurs and is treated with orthotopic hepatic transplantation. HAV is preventable with HAV vaccination, which was approved by the U.S. Food and Drug Administration (FDA) in 1996. HAV vaccination is given in two doses for those ages 2 and older. The second dose is given 6 to 18 months following the first dose. It is generally believed that active immunization against HAV confers immunity for about 20 years.
- **Hepatitis B**
  - In most cases of acute HBV infection, treatment is mainly supportive with > 90% of adults spontaneously clearing the infection.
  - Assessment of viral load is indicated to determine carrier state or a chronic active state of the disease. HBV DNA greater than 10^5 copies/mL is consistent with an active chronic HBV infection, while HBV DNA of less than 10^5 copies/mL is indicative of a carrier state.
  - Interferon-alpha and lamivudine (an antiviral nucleoside analog) are used in the treatment of chronic HBV.
  - In chronic carriers, there is a risk for development of hepatocellular carcinoma, and ultrasound evaluations are recommended every 6 months.
- **Hepatitis C**
  - Current therapy for chronic HCV infection is a 24- or 48-week course of peginterferon-alfa-2a (Pegasys) and ribavirin (Copegus). Pegylated interferon (peginterferon) is the addition of polyethylene glycol molecules to interferon for better absorption and a slower rate of clearance. Ribavirin is a nucleoside analogue and reduces ALT and HCV RNA.
- **Hepatitis D**
  - There is no preventive measure for HDV other than HBV vaccination. Treatment consists of interferon-alpha.
- **Hepatitis E**
  - Prevention is the most effective approach against HEV and there are no current therapies available for treatment.

COMPLICATIONS

- **Hepatitis A**
  - Hepatitis A does not progress to chronic liver disease, though it may persist for up to 1 year, and clinical

and biochemical relapses may occur before full recovery.
  - There is no chronic state of infection associated with HAV.
- **Hepatitis B**
  - Chronic hepatitis B develops in 1–2% of immunocompetent adult patients with acute hepatitis B, but in as many as 90% of infected neonates and infants and a substantial proportion of immunocompromised adults with acute hepatitis B.
  - Such patients are at increased risk for the development of cirrhosis (approximately 40%) and hepatocellular carcinoma (approximately 1–3%).
- **Hepatitis C**
  - Progression to chronic infection is common, 50–84%.
  - 74–86% has persistent viremia; spontaneous clearance of viremia in chronic infection is rare.
  - 15–20% of those with chronic HCV will develop cirrhosis over a period of 20 to 30 years; in most others, chronic infection leads to hepatitis and varying degrees of fibrosis.
  - 0.4–2.5% of patients with chronic infection develop hepatocellular carcinoma.
  - 25% of patients with chronic infection continue to have an asymptomatic course with normal liver function tests and benign histology.
  - Hepatitis C is the main indication for liver transplantation in the U.S. Recurrent infection occurs in almost all patients with progressive fibrosis and cirrhosis; up to 20% progress to cirrhosis within 5 years posttransplant.
- **Hepatitis D**
  - Acute delta infection superimposed on chronic HBV infection may result in severe chronic hepatitis, which may progress rapidly to cirrhosis. Risk for hepatocellular carcinoma for those with HDV is about 40% at 12 years.
- **Hepatitis E**
  - HEV infections are usually self-limiting and hospitalization is generally not required.
  - There is no chronic state of infection associated with HEV.

PROGNOSIS

- **Hepatitis A**
  - The mortality rate is approximately 0.2–0.3%.
- **Hepatitis B**
  - The mortality rate in HBV is approximately 0.5–1% in acute (fulminant) infection and 2–10% in chronic infection.
- **Hepatitis C**
  - The annual mortality rate from chronic hepatitis C is approximately 2%.

- **Hepatitis D**
  - The mortality rate from severe chronic HBV/HDV infection with cirrhosis is approximately 80%.
- **Hepatitis E**
  - The mortality rate for hepatitis E is 0.1–1%, but for unknown reasons it is especially high in pregnant women (10–20%).

DENTAL SIGNIFICANCE

- Since HBV, HCV, and human immunodeficiency virus (HIV) are transmitted in a similar manner, many patients have coinfection. HBV, HCV, and/or HIV coinfection significantly complicates the medical management of the diseases and enhances the probability of the patient's experiencing hepatic dysfunction.
- HBV and HCV are transmissible via infected blood or saliva. Clinicians should comply with the current CDC, OSAP, and ADA infection control recommendations with every patient, regardless of the presence or absence of bloodborne disease.

DENTAL MANAGEMENT

- All patients with histories of viral hepatitis or histories (or clinical findings suggestive thereof) should have laboratory testing to determine the presence of active viral hepatitis or chronic carrier infectivity.
  - Chronic hepatitis B:
    - HBV surface antigen (HBsAg) positive
  - Hepatitis C:
    - Anti-HVC (ELISA, RIBA) positive and qualitative HCV-RNA (PCR) positive
    - A possible indicator of current HCV activity or the patient's response to antiviral therapy is the quantitative HCV-RNA (PCR) test (hepatitis C titer or viral load)
- Patients with active or chronic viral hepatitis need to be evaluated to determine the presence/degree of impairment of hepatic function, including results of most recent laboratory testing:
  - Serum bilirubin, serum albumin AST, ALT, GGTP, and alkaline phosphatase.
- The presence of significant impairment of hepatic function may:
  - Require a dose reduction (or contraindicate the use) of hepatoxic drugs and/or drugs metabolized by the liver (see Appendix A, Box A-6, "Drug Use in Hepatic Dysfunction").
  - Result in clinically significant impaired hemostasis (indicated primarily by an elevated PT/INR due to abnormal synthesis of prothrombin-dependent clotting factors and/or thrombocytopenia secondary to splenomegaly) necessitating a coagulation status work-up prior to surgical procedures.
- Patients being treated for chronic HCV (or recently completing a course of treatment) with peginterferon alfa-2a (Pegasys) and ribavirin (Copegus) should have laboratory testing prior to invasive dental treatment, including a CBC with differential and platelet count to rule out anemia, neutropenia, and thrombocytopenia that may occur as a result of treatment with these drugs.

SUGGESTED REFERENCE

Marsano LS. Hepatitis. *Prim Care Clin Office Pract* 2003;30:81–107.

AUTHOR: **BRIAN C. MUZYKA, DMD, MS, MBA**

Hereditary Hemorrhagic Telangiectasia

SYNONYM(S)

HHT
Osler-Weber-Rendu disease
Osler-Weber-Rendu syndrome
Rendu-Osler-Weber syndrome

ICD-9CM/CPT CODE(S)

448.0 Hereditary hemorrhagic telaniec-
tasia—complete

OVERVIEW

The syndrome encompasses a familial occurrence of multiple capillary and venous dilations of skin and mucous membranes with reoccurring hemorrhage.

EPIDEMIOLOGY & DEMOGRAPHICS

INCIDENCE/PREVALENCE IN USA:
Estimates of frequency have ranged from 1 in 2500 to 1 in 40,000. The syndrome has been noted in all ethnic groups, but more commonly in whites.
PREDOMINANT AGE: Adults; rare in children.
PREDOMINANT SEX: None.
GENETICS: Inheritance is autosomal dominant. Marked intrafamilial and interfamilial variability; penetrance is not complete. At least three genes are capable of causing HHT, and two (HHT1 and HHT2) have been mapped, to 9q33–q34 and to 3p22.

ETIOLOGY & PATHOGENESIS

Hereditary hemorrhagic telangiectasia should be ascertained a generalized pleomorphic angiodysplasia of almost any organ. The telangiectasias are direct arteriovenous connections without an intervening capillary bed. (The telangiectasia ruptures due to the lack of elastic fibers necessary for vasoconstriction.)

CLINICAL PRESENTATION / PHYSICAL FINDINGS

Usually, the patients are pale and show fatigue and weakness due to resultant anemia. Hemorrhage, often nontraumatic, is a concern, especially with advancing age. Hemorrhages are heightened by anemia, resulting in an unwanted vicious cycle. The telangiectasias are red, purple, or violaceous and pinpoint, spider-like, or nodular. Emboli can be formed.

SYSTEMS AFFECTED

- Mucosa: telangiectasias are absorbed in the nasal, upper and lower gastrointestinal tract, conjunctiva, retina, bladder, vagina, uterus, and oral structure.
- Skin: facial, ears, hands, and nail beds.
- Pulmonary: aneurysms and arteriovenous malformations.
- Cerebral: various neurologic symptoms and intracerebral hemorrhage.
- Other: bone, liver, spinal cord, heart.

Seen in CREST syndrome (calcinosis, Raynaud's phenomenon, esophageal dysfunction, sclerodactyly, and telangiectasia).

DIAGNOSIS

HISTORY AND PHYSICAL EXAMINATION

- The most frequent symptom is spontaneous epistaxis. More than half of the patients have epistaxis by age 20 and 90% by age 45.
- Mucosal, skin, gastrointestinal bleeding (endoscopy).
- Telangiectatic lesions on skin, lips, nasal mucosa, fingertips, and toes. Telangiectasia occurs most frequently on the face in two-thirds of patients, on the mouth in half, and on the cheeks, tongue, nose, and lower lip in approximately one-third. In about 40%, the hands and wrists are also involved.
- Pulmonary arteriovenous fistula results in dyspnea, fatigue, cyanosis, or polyerythemia.
- Family history of pulmonary or cerebral arteriovenous malformations.

LABORATORY

- CBC for evidence of iron deficiency anemia

IMAGING

- Angiography for evaluation of arteriovenous malformations

MEDICAL MANAGEMENT & TREATMENT

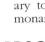

- Laser ablation, surgical resection, or balloon occlusion of the feeding arteries of any sizable malformation to prevent systemic embolization, especially to the brain.
- Transfusions and continuous iron therapy to replace to correct blood loss. In a few patients, epistaxis and gastrointestinal blood loss have been reduced by antifibrinolytic therapy with danazol or aminocaproic acid.

COMPLICATIONS

- Arteriovenous aneurysms, vascular malformations, biliary cirrhosis, encephalic angiomatosis, thrombocytopenia, gastrointestinal tract bleeding, and death.
- Primary morbidity is cerebral secondary to embolic complications of pulmonary arteriovenous malformations.

PROGNOSIS

- Generally, the prognosis is relatively good. Correct diagnosis, appropriate therapy, and patient monitoring improve control of bleeding.
- Death from intestinal bleeding in 12–15% of symptomatic patients.
- Genetic counseling to family cases.

DENTAL SIGNIFICANCE

- The lips and tongue are most frequent sites of telangiectasia. Other oral affected sites are palate, gingiva, buccal mucosa, and mucocutaneous junctions.
- Oral hygiene care must be very careful to avoid traumatized bleeding in affected patients.

DENTAL MANAGEMENT

- Confirm diagnosis.
- Avoid hemorrhaging of oral sites by careful oral hygiene care. Avoid irritation or trauma to potential bleeding sites.
- Advise affected patient of ongoing oral care and avoidance of tissue trauma to prevent bleeding. Inform other office treatment personnel about risks of patient bleeding.
- Consultation and referral to oral medicine, oral-maxillofacial surgeon, and/or primary care physician.

SUGGESTED REFERENCE

Gorlin RJ, Cohen Jr. MM, Hennelsom RCM. *Syndromes of the Head and Neck*, ed 4. New York, Oxford University Press, 2001, pp 576–580.

AUTHOR: NORBERT J. BURZYNSKI, SR., DDS, MS

SYNONYM(S)

HSV
Labial herpes
Genital herpes
Herpes gladiatorum (HSV skin abrasion areas)
Herpes digitalis (herpetic Whitlow)
Eczema herpeticum (diffuse, life-threatening HSV infection associated with chronic ulcerative skin diseases)

ICD-9CM/CPT CODE(S)

054   Herpes simplex—incomplete
054.1   Genital herpes—incomplete
054.9   Herpes simplex without mention of complication
054.10   Unspecified genital herpes—complete

OVERVIEW

Herpes viruses are enveloped DNA viruses. Eight human herpes virus are identified. There are two closely related types of herpes simplex virus. Type 1 (labial/facial, HSV-1) and type 2 (genital, HSV-2); however, each type can infect any location. They demonstrate general similarities and specific differences. Both establish latent infections in humans, their natural host. Following the primary infection, HSV-1 and HSV-2 specifically target nerve tissue in the skin or mucosa immediately adjacent to the lesions and ascend to the dorsal root ganglia where they remain latent until reactivation.

EPIDEMIOLOGY & DEMOGRAPHICS

INCIDENCE AND PREVALENCE IN USA:

- About 90% of adults have serologic evidence of HSV-1 infection, and nearly 25% of adults in the U.S. have been infected with HSV-2.
- HSV infection is more common in lower socioeconomic conditions.
- About 50% of primary HSV infections are subclinical.
- Up to 40% of the population has recurrent labial HSV infections.
- Most cases of ocular or digital herpetic infections are caused by HSV-1.
- Frequency of recurrence of HSV-2 is higher than HSV-1.
- HSV-2 is more virulent than HSV-1.

PREDOMINANT AGE: Primary herpetic gingivostomatitis develops mostly in children and young adults. The higher incidence occurs from 6 months to 5 years of age. Primary genital herpes virus infection usually occurs in young adults (15- to 29-year-old population). Recurrent infections can occur any time during the host's life.

PREDOMINANT SEX: Both sexes are affected equally.

GENETICS: No associated genetic predisposition has been identified. The herpes virus genome contains between 60 and 120 genes. Some of these genes are devoted to the spread of the virus and provide the ability to reply in differentiated cells and adapt to host defense mechanisms.

ETIOLOGY & PATHOGENESIS

- Herpes viruses are extremely successful enveloped DNA viruses. To replicate, they need adaptation to the immune defense of the host. The virus establishes a primary infection during which it replicates to high titers.
- The symptoms are rapidly resolved and the host will present immunity against reinfection. However, the virus is not totally cleared from the host. Some infected cells are able to keep a viral genome without an active infection (latent infection).
- Whenever host immunity is sufficiently suppressed, a usually milder version of the primary infection ensues. Latency does not appear to cause serious problems except in immunosuppressed patients, who may have significant medical problems including disseminated infection in the brain and HSV kerato-conjunctivitis, which can result in blindness.
- During the initial step of infection, the virion membrane fuses with the host's cell membrane. The viral nucleocapsid is transported to the nuclear pores where viral DNA is released into the nucleous of the cell. Interaction of cellular and viral DNA enhances the mechanisms throughout the replication cycle of the viral DNA. The new viral DNA is then packed into mature capsids. These capsids are released from the cellular nucleous, and they can associate with proteins to become mature virions, which are able to spread to uninfected cells.

CLINICAL PRESENTATION / PHYSICAL FINDINGS

- Typically, HSV-1 infection is due to direct contact with active lesions or infected saliva; HSV-2 infection is transmitted predominantly through sexual contact.
- HSV usually enters the body through breaks in the skin, although there is considerable evidence that it can penetrate intact mucous membranes.
- Both HSV-1 and HSV-2 are followed by an incubation period of from 3 to 15 days in which the virus multiplies and spreads into favored tissues. The host responds with expression of interferon and adaptive immunity.
- Clinically evident infections exhibit two patterns:
  1. Primary infection (primary herpetic stomatitis or primary genital infection) is the initial exposure to an individual without antibodies to the HSV. This typically occurs at a young age and sometimes is asymptomatic.
     - Oral primary infection: symptoms include chills, low-grade fever, malaise, headache, myalgias, and irritability, followed by development of grouped, uniform, small vesicles on all mucosal surfaces, which collapse to form small ulcerations covered by yellowish fibrin. Cervical lymphadenopathy may be present. Untreated, the disease usually lasts about 2 weeks.
     - Genital primary infection: may present with similar symptoms but different location, such as genital painful vesicles, ulcers, and inguinal adenopathy. HSV establishes a latent infection by entering a sensory nerve axon near the infection site and migrating to the ganglion. HSV-1 tends to favor the oral mucosa, lips, pharynx, and tonsils for initial infection; hence, the site invaded is the trigeminal ganglion. HSV-2 tends to invade the sciatic nerve ganglia.
  2. Recurrent infection: reactivation of the latent virus is stimulated by sun exposure, cold temperatures, trauma, stress, fever, or immune compromise. Prodromal signs are pain, burning and itching or tingling 1 or 2 days before the development of the lesions.
     - The most common location of recurrent oral HSV is the vermilion and vermilion-skin edge of the lips. However, recurrent intraoral lesions do occur, usually in the keratinized surfaces of the palate and gingiva. In immunosuppressed patients, recurrent herpes is more serious, and the lesions may develop in all mucosal surfaces.
     - The recurrent disease gives rise to a cluster of vesicles identical to those found in primary herpetic gingivostomatitis, but usually involving a smaller area. The labial vesicles rupture in hours, forming a crust. Intraoral lesions seldom form a clinically visible vesicle; instead, they appear as punctuate lesions with red and white basis. The recurrent episode usually lasts 1 to 2 weeks.
     - The recurrent infection of genital HSV presents with unilateral distribution of vesicles and similar symptoms.
- Herpetic Whitlow (herpetic paronychia) is a primary or secondary HSV infection localized to the hands or fingers. It is acquired by direct contact by inoculation of virus via a break in the

epidermal surface or by direct introduction of the virus into the hand through occupational or some other type of exposure. Clinical signs and symptoms of herpetic Whitlow include:

- The abrupt onset of edema, erythema, and localized tenderness of the infected finger.
- Lesions are usually vesicular or pustular and surrounded by a wide zone of erythema.
- Throbbing pain, high fever, and regional lymphadenopathy of the arm or axilla are common.
- Symptoms are often severe enough to incapacitate the patient for 1 or more weeks.
- Healing usually takes 2 to 3 weeks.
- Recurrence is possible and may result in paresthesia and permanent scarring.

Antiviral chemotherapy to limit the severity of the infection and speed healing is usually recommended.

DIAGNOSIS

DIFFERENTIAL DIAGNOSIS

- Oral herpes: herpetic gingivostomatitis may be confused with ulcerative lesions such as necrotizing ulcerative periodontitis, pemphigus vulgaris, erosive lichen planus, and atrophic candidiasis. Recurrent infection may resemble aphthous stomatitis, chickenpox, herpes zoster, herpangina, and Coxsackie virus infection.
- Genital herpes: human papilloma virus infection, molluscum contagiosum, HIV, fungal or bacterial infections, Behcet's syndrome, and cancer of the vulva.

LABORATORY

- The diagnosis of HSV infection is usually made on the basis of the history and clinical features of the lesions. If diagnostic confirmation is necessary, there are several laboratory methods available:
  - Cytologic smear (Tzanck smear of vesicular fluid or cells from an ulcerated lesion).
  - Tissue biopsy (ideally of an intact vesicle).
  - Direct fluorescent monoclonal antibody typing of vesicle scrapings.
  - Virus culture (mean time for results is 2 days, but may take up to 2 weeks for primary infections).
  - Polymerase chain reaction (PCR) for detecting HSV DNA in blood or CSF.

MEDICAL MANAGEMENT & TREATMENT

- The two most effective drugs against HSV are systemic acyclovir (Zovirax) and ganciclovir.
- Primary herpetic gingivostomatitis is self-limiting and should require only supportive care: NSAIDs, hydration, antipyretics, topical anesthetics, and adequate soft, bland nutrition. Local antiseptics may aid resolution of the painful lesions. Antibiotics are needed only if secondary bacterial infection arises.
- Recurrent oral herpes also does not warrant treatment except in cases with multiple debilitating lesions or frequent extensive recurrences: oral acyclovir 200 mg, 5 times/day for 10 days. To prevent frequent, severe outbreaks, maintenance at 400 mg twice daily is recommended. A topical nonprescription medication, docosanol (Abreva), for recurrent orofacial herpes simplex is available. It acts through inhibition of fusion of the cell membrane with the virus membrane and thereby preventing the virus's entry into the cell. Used topically 5 times/day at first sign of cold sore, docosanol produces faster healing and reduces pain and itching (indicated in patients 12 years of age and older).
- Immunocompromised patient may require IV therapy, 30mg/kg per day or ganciclovir 500 mg orally, 3 times/day during the outbreak and prophylactic oral acyclovir, 400 mg/2 times/day (in patients with normal renal function). Foscarnet is either substituted for acyclovir or added to it at a dose of 40 to 60 mg intravenously 3 times/day if acyclovir-resistant strains are found. Any herpes lesions that do not respond to appropriate therapy within 5 to 10 days most likely are the result of resistant strains. Topical acyclovir must be used with caution because of its potential to stimulate resistant viral strains without a strong therapeutic gain.

COMPLICATIONS

- Herpetic encephalitis and herpetic meningitis may occur in rare occasions, especially in immunosuppressed patients.
- Ocular herpes may lead to blindness. HSV is the leading infectious cause of blindness in the United States.
- Newborns may become infected during delivery through a birth canal con-

taminated with HSV, usually HSV-2. Without treatment, there is a greater than 50% mortality rate.

PROGNOSIS

- Good prognosis in immunocompetent patients. However, the risk of recurrence is a lifelong fact.
- Antiviral therapy is effective, particularly if started early in the disease course. Long-term therapy in immunocompromised patients is useful; however, it does not prevent viral shedding in the patient and will not, therefore, prevent transmission of either HSV-1 or HSV-2. Antiviral resistance is becoming a significant problem to immunocompromised persons, especially those with a severe immune defect.
- HSV has been implicated in the development of erythema multiforme, Bell's palsy, and squamous cell carcinoma.
- Congenital herpes may be lethal.

DENTAL SIGNIFICANCE

- HSV is one of the most common oral diseases, and the dentist should be able to diagnose and treat it adequately.
- During the prodrome and the vesicular stage, the patient's saliva and genital secretions are highly contagious. Approximately 33% of persons infected with HSV-1 will occasionally shed infectious viral particles even without the presence of active secondary lesions.

DENTAL MANAGEMENT

- Universal precautions will avoid the contamination of the healthcare providers.
- If the patient has a dental appointment and intact oral/labial vesicles are present, it is preferable to postpone dental treatment (if it is not an emergency) because the intravesicular fluid contains virions and the rupture of the vesicles will allow the release of the virus.

SUGGESTED REFERENCES

Marx S. *Oral and Maxillofacial Pathology*, ed 1. Chicago, Quintessence Publishing Co., 2003, pp 110–114.

Wagner EK, Martinez JH. *Basic Virology*, ed 2. Oxford, UK, Blackwell Publishing Co., 2004, pp 312–333.

AUTHOR: **INÉS VÉLEZ, DDS, MS**

SYNONYM(S)

Hodgkin's lymphoma
Malignant lymphoma
Lymph node cancer

ICD-9CM/CPT CODE(S)

201–201.9 Hodgkin's disease
201.4 Lymphocytic-histiocytic pre-dominance
201.5 Nodular sclerosis
201.6 Mixed cellularity
201.7 Lymphocytic depletion
201.9 Hodgkin's disease, unspeci-fied

OVERVIEW

Hodgkin's lymphoma (HL) is a potentially curable malignancy of lymphoid tissue found in the lymph nodes, spleen, liver, and bone marrow. It has a distinct histology, biologic behavior, and clinical characteristics. Histologically, the picture is unique, with 1–2% of neoplastic cells (Reed-Sternberg cells). HL is of B-cell origin.

EPIDEMIOLOGY & DEMOGRAPHICS

INCIDENCE/PREVALENCE IN USA: It is estimated that 7500 new cases and 1500 deaths are diagnosed annually in the U.S. The age-adjusted incidence rate is 2.9 cases per 100,000 individuals. HL is more common among whites and less common among Asians.
PREDOMINANT AGE: HL can occur in children and adults. It is more common in two age groups: early adulthood (ages 15 to 40, usually around 25 to 30) and late adulthood (after age 55). This type of lymphoma is rare in children under 5. About 10–15% of cases are diagnosed in children 16 years old and younger.
PREDOMINANT SEX: HL is slightly more common in males than in females. This male predominance is particularly evident in children, where 85% of the cases are in males.
GENETICS: Genetic predisposition may play a role in the pathogenesis of HL. Approximately 1% of patients with HL have a family history of the disease. Siblings of an affected individual have a threefold to sevenfold increased risk for developing HL. This risk is higher in monozygotic twins.

ETIOLOGY & PATHOGENESIS

- The etiology of HL remains unknown. It is probably a culmination of diverse pathologic processes such as viral infections, environmental exposures, and genetically determined host response.
- Infectious agents, especially the Epstein-Barr virus (EBV), appear to be a cofactor in HL. It may be more prevalent in people who have contracted infectious mononucleosis.

- In as many as 50% of HL cases, the tumor cells are EBV-positive. Almost 100% of HIV-associated HL cases are EBV-positive.
- Patients with HIV infection have a higher incidence of HL compared to the population without HIV infection. However, HL is not considered an AIDS-defining neoplasm.

CLINICAL PRESENTATION / PHYSICAL FINDINGS

- The most common presentation is a painless enlargement of the lymph nodes without any symptoms.
- Asymptomatic lymphadenopathy above the diaphragm may be present in 80–90% of patients.
- Cervical lymph node enlargements are the initial sites of detection in more than 50% of cases.
- Constitutional symptoms (e.g., unexplained weight loss, fever, night sweats) are present in 40% of patients.
- Chest pain, cough, and/or shortness of breath may be present due to a large mediastinal mass or lung involvement. Back or bone pain occurs rarely.
- Pruritus is a symptom seen most frequently in young women with HL. Intermittent fever is observed in approximately 25% of cases.
- Rarely, the classic Pel-Ebstein fever (a cyclic spiking of high fever) is observed.

DIAGNOSIS

- Diagnosis of HL is made by biopsy. Biopsy specimens are usually from lymph nodes but may occasionally be from other tissues.
- Reed-Sternberg cells must be present for the diagnosis of HL to be established. This cell of lymphocytic origin is characterized by its large size and bilobed nucleus; each lobe contains a large, eosinophilic nucleolus.
- Accurate classification of the disease clinically and histologically is essential because treatment is determined by stage.
- Staging must include lymph node biopsy, chest radiograph, computed tomography scan of the abdomen and pelvis, bone marrow biopsy, and laboratory evaluation of liver, kidney, and bone.
- In selected cases, lymphangiography, exploratory laparotomy, radionuclide scan, and magnetic resonance imaging are indicated.
- HL is classified histologically according to the Rye system:
  - Lymphocyte predominant
  - Nodular sclerosis
  - Mixed cellularity
  - Lymphocyte depleted
- The disease also is staged clinically into four stages according to the criteria

established at the Ann Arbor Conference of 1971 and modified by Cotswold:
  - Stage I : Single lymph node region (I) or one extralymphatic site (IE).
  - Stage II: Two or more lymph node regions, same side of the diaphragm (II) or local extralymphatic extension plus one or more lymph node regions, same side of the diaphragm (IIE).
  - Stage III: Lymph node regions on both sides of the diaphragm (III) that may be accompanied by local extralymphatic extension (IIIE).
  - Stage IV: Diffuse involvement of one or more extralymphatic organs or sites.
  - The presence or absence of significant systemic symptoms such as weight loss, night sweats, and fever is indicated by the suffixes "A" (symptom absent) or "B" (symptoms present). The suffix "E" indicates extralymphatic disease, and "X" indicates the presence of bulky disease (tumor tissue exceeding 10 cm in largest diameter).

MEDICAL MANAGEMENT & TREATMENT

- Radiation therapy: indicated for stage IA or IIA. Radiation commonly consists of 3500 to 4500 cGy.
- Three radiation fields have been developed: mantle field, paraaortic field, and pelvic field.
- The mantle field includes the submandibular region, neck, axillae, and mediastinum.
- Currently, combination chemotherapy of doxorubicin (Adriamycin), bleomycin, vincristine, and dacarbazine (ABVD) is used for most HL patients. Another combination chemotherapy used is MOPP that consists of mechlorethamine, vincristine (Oncovin), procarbazine, and prednisone.
- A combination of radiotherapy and chemotherapy is used for advanced disease. High-dose chemotherapy (HDC) at doses that ablate the bone marrow is feasible with reinfusion of the patient's previously collected hematopoietic stem cells (autologous transplantation) or infusion of stem cells from a donor source (allogeneic transplantation).

COMPLICATIONS

- Cardiac disease: mantle radiotherapy increases the risk of coronary artery disease, chronic pericarditis, pancarditis, valvular heart disease, and defects in the conduction system. ABVD contains Adriamycin, which is also cardiotoxic.

- Pulmonary disease: ABVD contains bleomycin, a drug associated with dose-related pulmonary toxicity, mainly interstitial pneumonitis that may lead to fibrosis. In addition, mantle irradiation enhances lung injury.
- Myelodysplasia/leukemia.
- Infertility.
- Breast cancer, lung cancer.
- Non-Hodgkin's lymphoma.
- Infectious complications.
- Hypothyroidism after neck/mediastinal radiotherapy.
- Immunodeficiency after chemotherapy and/or radiation therapy.

PROGNOSIS

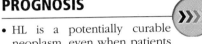

- HL is a potentially curable neoplasm, even when patients present with advanced disease.
- The 5-year, disease-specific survival for patients with stages I and II is 90%; for stage III, 84%; and for stage IV, 65%.
- Prognosis is better among younger individuals as compared to older patients.

DENTAL SIGNIFICANCE

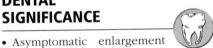

- Asymptomatic enlargement of the cervical lymph node chains is a common early sign of HL; the dentist should play a significant role in early detection by routine examination of the neck.
- Suspicion of lymphoma should increase when lymphadenopathy appears without sings of infection, more than one lymph node chain is involved, or a lymph node of 1 cm or greater in diameter persists for more than 1 month.
- Although primary jaw lesions are uncommon, they have been reported.
- Teeth abnormalities can be a complication of administration of chemotherapy and radiation during tooth development in children. These abnormalities include agenesis, hypoplasia, and blunted or thin roots.

- Patients with HL have a loss of T-lymphocyte function, particularly in advanced stages of the disease. The major clinical infections seen in this group of patients include viral, fungal, and protozoal infection such as histoplasmosis, actinomycosis, and infection with candida albicans, herpes simplex virus, varicella zoster virus, and cytomegalovirus.
- Chemotherapy and radiotherapy may suppress neutrophils and antibody function for years, increasing susceptibility to bacterial infection.

DENTAL MANAGEMENT

- Dentists have an important role in preventing serious, life-threatening infections while patients are neutropenic from cancer chemotherapy. These patients should have a dental evaluation and removal of obvious potential sources of bacteremia, such as teeth with advanced periodontal disease (e.g., pocket depths 5 mm or greater, excessive mobility, purulence on probing), prior to chemotherapy. Additional indicators for extraction of teeth prior to chemotherapy include:
  ○ Periapical inflammation.
  ○ Tooth is broken down, nonrestorable, nonfunctional, or partially erupted, and the patient is noncompliant with oral hygiene measures.
  ○ Tooth is associated with a inflammatory (e.g., pericoronitis), infectious, or malignant osseous disease.
  Extractions should be performed at least 5 days in the maxilla and at least 7 days in the mandible before the initiation of chemotherapy.
- For patients receiving chemotherapy, the dentist should obtain the patient's current WBC and platelet counts before initiating dental care.
  ○ In general, routine dental procedures can be performed if the total WBC count is greater than 2000/mm^3 and the platelet count is greater than 50,000/mm^3. For outpatient care, this is generally about 17 days after chemotherapy.

  ○ If emergency dental care is needed and the platelet count is below 50,000/mm^3, consultation with the patient's oncologist is recommended. Platelet replacement may be indicated if invasive or traumatic dental procedures are to be performed. Topical therapy using pressure, thrombin, microfibrillar collagen, and splints may be required.
  ○ If emergency dental care is needed and the total WBC count is less than 2000/mm^3 or the absolute neutrophil count is less than 500 to 1000/mm^3, consultation with the patient's oncologist is recommended and broad-spectrum antibiotic prophylaxis should be provided to prevent postoperative infection.
- Mucositis is a common side effect of radiation and certain chemotherapy drugs. This can be managed with good oral hygiene, cryotherapy (ice chips), and use of mouthwashes containing sucralfate or sodium bicarbonate. Amifostine (Ethyol) is a drug that protects against the damage of radiation and can reduce dry mouth and prevent mouth sores. Recombinant human keratinocyte growth factor (palifermin) may ultimately reduce mouth soreness and improve function.
- Radiation may cause xerostomia and damage the taste buds. Patients may benefit by using salivary substitutes or pilocarpine (Salagen) to stimulate salivary flow.

SUGGESTED REFERENCES

Cattaneo C. Oral cavity lymphomas in immunocompetent and human immunodeficiency virus infected patients. *Leukemia Lymphoma* 2005;46(1):77–81.

Greenberg MS, Glick M. *Burket's Oral Medicine Diagnosis and Treatment*. Hamilton, Ontario, BC Decker Inc., 2003, pp 429–453.

http://www.emedicine.com/med/topic256.htm

http://www.cancer.org

Little JW, et al. Hematologic diseases, in *Dental Management of the Medically Compromised Patient*. Philadelphia, Elsevier Science, 2002, pp 376–385.

AUTHOR: FARIDEH MADANI, DMD

Human Immunodeficiency Virus Infection and Acquired Immune Deficiency Syndrome

SYNONYM(S)

Human immunodeficiency virus (HIV) infection

HIV disease

Acquired immune deficiency syndrome (AIDS)

ICD-9CM/CPT CODE(S)
042   HIV—complete
042.9 AIDS, unspecified

OVERVIEW

HIV infection is a communicable, retroviral disease. AIDS is composed of a number of diseases resulting from the effect of HIV infection on the immune system. These diseases may be represented by opportunistic infections, malignant tumors, and systemic complications common to the immunocompromised host.

EPIDEMIOLOGY & DEMOGRAPHICS

INCIDENCE/PREVALENCE IN USA: The available statistics on the HIV epidemic demonstrate that it continues to grow. In the U.S., about 980,000 people live with HIV. Approximately 42% of cases are men who have sex with men, 33% are heterosexuals, and 25% are injection drug users. More than half of new infections occur among African-Americans, and the number of new infections in Hispanics is also disproportionate.

PREDOMINANT AGE: Between 25 and 54 years of age.

PREDOMINANT SEX: About 70% of new infections occurs in males.

GENETICS: Not established.

ETIOLOGY & PATHOGENESIS

- Human immunodeficiency virus infection and AIDS are caused by a retrovirus called HIV. This virus may infect several cells in the body, but their main targets are the CD4+ receptor T lymphocytes.
- HIV is transmitted most effectively by sexual intercourse, by exposure to contaminated blood and blood products, perinatally from mother to newborn, and through breastfeeding. After entering the body, HIV fuses with the cell surface receptors of T lymphocytes. The genetic material of HIV enters the cell and integrates into the cell's DNA. When the infected cells divide, new virus material is produced, and the cells release new viruses.
- In addition to CD4+ lymphocytes, monocytes and macrophages also express CD4+ surface receptors and may be infected by HIV. The monocytes transport HIV from lymphoid tissues to the rest of the body. During the progress of HIV disease, HIV-infected cells are destroyed, leading to severe immune dysfunction. As the number of circulating CD4+ lymphocytes declines below 200 cells/mm^3, infected individuals become prone to develop opportunistic infections, autoimmune conditions, and malignant neoplasms.

- The end-stage of HIV disease is the acquired immune deficiency syndrome (AIDS) and is defined by the development of a large number of diseases present in an individual infected with HIV. According to the Centers for Disease Control, an HIV-infected individual with fewer than 200 CD4+ lymphocytes/mm^3 has AIDS. The viral multiplication in the blood (known as the viral load) increases, spreading the infection to virtually all parts of the body. These two markers, the CD4+ cells and the viral load, are used today as predictors of disease progression and prognosis.

CLINICAL PRESENTATION / PHYSICAL FINDINGS

- Classical signs and symptoms of HIV disease may be acute or chronic. Individuals who develop the acute HIV infection may present with severe, flu-like syndrome including fatigue, malaise, fever, lymphadenopathy, night sweats, and sore throat. This syndrome develops when individuals seroconvert after recent exposure to HIV.
- Chronic infection with HIV is characterized by clinical manifestations representing deterioration of the immune system. Patients may present with fever, malaise, unexplained weight loss, lymphadenopathy, night sweats, opportunistic infections, and neoplasms (Kaposi's sarcoma, non-Hodgkin's lymphoma, and squamous cell carcinoma).

DIAGNOSIS

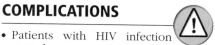

- The diagnosis of HIV infection is initially done by the enzyme-linked immunosorbent assay (ELISA/EIA), which detects general antibody response to HIV infection. Positive test responses are then confirmed by the Western blot test, which identifies specific response to HIV proteins. Approximately 95% of infected individuals will have a positive response within 6 months of exposure.
- The U.S. Food and Drug Administration recently approved a new test for rapid HIV testing. It uses oral fluids collected with the help of a device containing an absorbent pad. The device is positioned on the buccal vestibule against the gingival tissues. The device should gently swab the buccal gingival tissues one time on both the mandible and the maxilla. The collected sample is inserted in a vial containing a solution. A small window on the device will reveal a change in color in about 20 minutes when the sample is positive for antibodies against HIV-1.

MEDICAL MANAGEMENT & TREATMENT

- Therapy with highly active antiretroviral drugs (HAART) is available and may control the natural progression of HIV infection and AIDS.
- The ideal goal of treatment is a complete halt of viral replication, which would prevent future viral resistance by stopping HIV mutation. Regimens that can halt viral growth are more likely to have a more durable effect. Undetectable levels of viral load mean that the plasma viral load is below levels of detection of that particular test, which could be 25 to 400 copies/mL, depending on the test.
- Another goal of the medical therapy is immune reconstitution, which allows for the increase of CD4+ cells and improvement of immune functions. A large number of medications are used, including those that inhibit HIV enzymes including reverse transcriptase, protease, and, more recently, a new medication that inhibits the fusion of HIV with cell surface receptors.
- In addition to antiretroviral medications, patients may be using many other medications for prevention or for treatment of opportunistic infections, anemia, thrombocytopenia, and neoplasms, depending of the stage of HIV disease. Therefore, taking a complete medical history of HIV-infected individuals is of paramount importance.

COMPLICATIONS

- Patients with HIV infection may have several complications during the different stages of the disease. These include wasting syndrome characterized by severe diarrhea, weight loss, loss of appetite, anemia, leukopenia, thrombocytopenia, opportunistic infections, malignant neoplasms, peripheral neuropathy, dementia, and many others.
- Depending on the type of complication present, patients may be at risk for infection and/or bleeding. Several medications used to treat HIV infection may cause oral ulcers, xerostomia, and taste changes or may interact with common medications used in dentistry.

PROGNOSIS

- Depends on several factors; because of the possibility of

early diagnosis, infected individuals are now recognized in very early stages of the disease.

- Initiation of therapy in some cases may delay the progress of the disease for many years. HIV types and individual viral virulence or development of resistance to therapy may accelerate the progress to AIDS.
- It is common today to see infected individuals without any clinical manifestations of the infection. Therefore, many infected people may not even know that they are HIV carriers. Some infected patients may live 10 years or longer without progressing to more advanced stages of the disease.
- HIV disease continues to be universally fatal, leading to death from opportunistic infections, malignant tumors, or multiple organ failure.

DENTAL SIGNIFICANCE

- With the new protocols of antiretroviral therapy available to treat HIV infection, HIV has become a chronic disease. The prolific appearance of oral manifestations found in the early years of HIV and AIDS is no longer observed.
- Highly active antiretroviral therapy (HAART) decreases viral load and improves the immune system. This has led to a change in the prevalence of oral diseases in HIV-infected patients under medical care.
- Several situations make dentistry still very important in the context of HIV disease. The initial clinical manifestation of HIV infection may be in the oral cavity. An undiagnosed patient may develop oral candidal infection, and the dentist may be the first one to suspect a possible HIV infection. In this case, the patient should be immediately referred for medical evaluation.
- A number of oral diseases may be observed in HIV-infected individuals:
  - Oral candidiasis (white or red patches anywhere in the oral mucosa)
  - Hairy leukoplakia (white corrugated patches common on the lateral tongue)
  - Herpes simplex virus (small vesicles or ulcerations on lips or keratinized gingiva)
  - Herpes zoster (intraoral or extraoral ulcerations, unilateral)
  - Cytomegalovirus (deep ulceration, pain, long-lasting)
  - Human papilloma virus (mucosal wart-like growth, pedunculated or sessile)
  - Kaposi's sarcoma (red or purple macule or growth, more common on palate)

- Linear gingival erythema (red line on the marginal gingival, resistant to periodontal therapy)
- Lymphoma (submucosal mass; when around teeth may imitate an abscess)
- Rapidly advancing periodontal disease (severe bone loss and intraosseous pain)
- Oral minor and major ulcerations (aphthous-like lesions of inflammatory origin)
- Xerostomia (secondary to medications, stress, or combination)
- Lymphoepithelial cysts (salivary gland disease with gland enlargement and decreased saliva)

- The diagnosis of oral diseases is made by taking the patient's history, complete clinical examination, and by using one of the available diagnostic techniques. Tumor growths and ulcers may be biopsied under local anesthesia and sent for histopathology. Areas suspected of being infected may be cultured with a swab and sent to the laboratory for identification of the etiological agent.
- After the diagnosis is obtained, oral diseases have to be treated as needed to improve oral health and patient capability of chewing and swallowing. Infections such as candidiasis, herpes, or oral ulcers of different etiologies may cause pain and discomfort, preventing the patient from eating, swallowing, or performing oral hygiene. For specific therapy, the reader will find information in other related topic entries (e.g., candidiasis, Kaposi's sarcoma, lymphoma, ulcers).
- Oral diseases are more common when HIV disease is in its advanced stages and usually result from immune dysfunction. Oral candidiasis, hairy leukoplakia, or Kaposi's sarcoma are commonly observed when CD4+ lymphocyte counts are below 200/mm^3. Nonetheless, oral disease may appear in different stages of HIV disease.
- The development of oral infection, especially candidiasis, in HIV-infected patient who is under treatment by the physician may indicate failure of antiretroviral therapy or lack of adherence to therapy, requiring a referral to the physician for medical evaluation.
- Xerostomia is a common symptom observed in HIV-infected patients. Thus, an immunosuppressed patient with decreased saliva may be at risk for oral mucosal infections, caries, and periodontal disease.
- Good nutrition is an important aspect in the life of an HIV-infected individual. Having a healthy mouth and good teeth will allow for good food intake and improved overall health.

DENTAL MANAGEMENT

- A patient with HIV infection who is medically stable may receive routine dental care like any other patient. Taking the medical history of an HIV-infected patient is very important and allows the dentist to develop an adequate treatment plan.
- Contact the patient's physician before starting any dental treatment for the current status of HIV disease and immune function, laboratory test results, medications, and important medical conditions that may put the patient at risk for complications. Important information for the dentist includes:
  - Stage of disease
  - CD4 count
  - Viral load
  - Tuberculosis status
  - White blood cell counts with differential
  - Platelet count
  - Hemoglobin and hematocrit
  - PT/INR and PTT
  - List of all current medications
- Any required medical adjustments may be discussed with the patient's physician before the treatment is initiated. HIV infection alone is not an indication for antibiotic prophylaxis. Antibiotics should be used based on individual needs, as for any other patient.
- Intravenous drug users may be at risk for bacterial endocarditis and require antibiotic prophylaxis prior to invasive dental treatment. When indicated, the American Heart Association guidelines (see Appendix A) may be used to determine antibiotic coverage.
- Routine dental procedures may be done as needed, including extractions, endodontic and periodontal therapy, as well as restorative or corrective dentistry. There is no evidence of delayed healing in HIV-infected patients after intraoral surgical procedures. Because of possible xerostomia, good oral hygiene practices and frequent recalls are mandatory.

SUGGESTED REFERENCES

Patton LL, Glick M. Clinician's Guide to Treatment of HIV-Infected Patients, ed 3. Seattle, WA, American Academy of Oral Medicine, 2001.

Patton LL. HIV disease. Review. Dent Clin North Am 2003;47(3):467–492.

Revised classification system for HIV infection and expanded surveillance case definition for AIDS. Centers for Disease Control, MMWR 1992;41:1–15.

Silverman Jr. S, Glick M. Human immunodeficiency virus disease, in Silverman Jr. S, Eversole LR, Truelove EL (eds): Essentials of Oral Medicine. Hamilton, Ontario, BC Decker Inc., 2001, pp 128–143.

AUTHOR: CESAR AUGUSTO MIGLIORATI, DDS, MS, PHD

SYNONYM(S)

Verruca vulgaris
Filiform papilloma
Condyloma acuminatum
Squamous papilloma
Focal epithelial hyperplasia

ICD-9CM/CPT CODE(S)
079.4 Human papilloma virus in conditions classified elsewhere and of unspecified site—complete

OVERVIEW

Human papilloma virus (HPV) is a common viral pathogen that can cause a number of different clinical and subclinical infections. Human papilloma virus is a nonenveloped, double-stranded, circular DNA virus. There have been over 90 different types of the virus identified to date. As early as 1933, it was known that HPV lesions may progress to malignancy. A common feature of HPV is an affinity for squamous epithelium and infection of cells of the basal cell layer. The different HPV types have been separated based on their preference for cutaneous or mucosal sites and their risk for malignant transformation, and can be classified as having a low, intermediate, or high risk for malignancy.

The first evidence of papillomavirus in human oral papillomas was published in 1967, and in 1971, investigators demonstrated particles compatible with papillovavirus in oral focal epithelial hyperplasia. To date, 17 HPV DNA types of the more than 90 identified types have been detected in benign, premalignant, and malignant lesions of the oral mucosa. These HPV types of oral lesions are 2, 4, 6, 7, 11, 13, 16, 18, 31, 32, 33, 35, and 57; seven of them (6, 11, 16, 18, 31, 33, and 35) have been isolated from normal oral mucosa. Rarely, HPV types 1, 3, 10, and 52 have been described in the oral cavity.

Oral papillomas are usually benign, localized exophytic lesions that may be solitary or multiple. There are five different presentations of oral papillomas recognized: verruca vulgaris, filiform papilla, condyloma acuminatum, squamous papilloma, and focal epithelial hyperplasia.

Patients receiving immunosuppressive drugs and patients with defects in cell-mediated immunity, including human immunodeficiency virus (HIV), are more susceptible to developing HPV infections.

EPIDEMIOLOGY & DEMOGRAPHICS

INCIDENCE/PREVALENCE IN USA: Oral cavity HPV has been detected in approximately 6% of children and adolescents. The prevalence of HPV in the oral cavity of healthy adults is estimated at 5–80%.

PREDOMINANT AGE: Children and adults.

PREDOMINANT SEX: The overall prevalence of HPV in women is 22–35%. In men, the prevalence is 2–35%, depending on the sexual practices of the population being studied.

GENETICS: Associations between human leukocyte antigens (HLAs) and cervical cancer, cervical cancer precursor lesions, and HPV infections reported.

ETIOLOGY & PATHOGENESIS

- HPV is a member of the papovavirus family and is a nonenveloped double strand of DNA. Replication occurs either through stable replication of the episomal genome in basal cells or vegetative replication in more differentiated cells to generate progeny virus. Virus production only occurs at the epithelial surface where the cells are ultimately sloughed into the environment. All the oral variants of HPV are asymptomatic and are usually an incidental finding.
- HPV infection alone does not cause malignant transformation of infected tissue. Cofactors such as tobacco use, ultraviolet radiation, pregnancy, folate deficiency, and immune suppression are implicated in this process. Patients receiving immunosuppressive drug therapy and patients with cell-mediated immunity defects are more susceptible to developing HPV infections.

CLINICAL PRESENTATION / PHYSICAL FINDINGS

- Verruca vulgaris
  - Verruca vulgaris presents as a white, circumscribed, exophytic, sessile lesion. They are more common on the skin than in the oral cavity. When present intraorally, it is most often a solitary lesion, but it also may be multiple lesions. It is found more frequently on the lips, palate, alveolar mucosa, and the gingiva. The following viral types have been associated with oral verruca vulgaris: HPV-2, HPV-4, and occasionally HPV-1, HPV-3, HPV-27, HPV-29, and HPV-57.
- Filiform papilloma
  - Filiform papillomas are white, exophytic lesions that are usually solitary. These lesions have a more irregular surface morphology than verruca vulgaris and are somewhat pedunculated (attached to the underlying surface by a stalk).
- Condyloma acuminatum (see "Condyloma Acuminatum" in Section II, p 250)
  - These exophytic lesions are also white or flesh-colored, and have an irregular, cauliflower-like surface and are sessile (the attachment of the lesion to the normal mucosa is the greatest diameter of the lesion). Multiple lesions are usually present.

Condyloma acuminate is more commonly found on nonkeratinized surfaces. These lesions may be transmitted via orogenital contact.

- Squamous papilloma
  - Oral squamous papilloma is the most common papillary lesion of the mouth; approximately 3% of all oral lesions are squamous papillomas. Associated HPV subtypes include 2, 6, 11, and 57. These lesions are often found on the hard and soft palate and uvula; they are exophytic and have a cauliflower-like surface appearance.
- Focal epithelial hyperplasia
  - Focal epithelial hyperplasia is also known as Heck's disease and was first identified in 1965. These lesions are typically flat or convex, sessile papules that are generally multiple in number. The color may vary from red to white and is dependent on the degree of keratin present in the affected tissue. The lesions can be found on the buccal and labial mucosa and the tongue.

DIAGNOSIS

- Biopsy of suspected oral lesions is required for a diagnosis of HPV.
- Subtyping of the HPV is recommended.
- Subtypes found in the oral cavity (HPV-16, HPV-18) have been associated with malignant transformation.

MEDICAL MANAGEMENT & TREATMENT

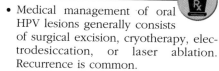

- Medical management of oral HPV lesions generally consists of surgical excision, cryotherapy, electrodesiccation, or laser ablation. Recurrence is common.
- HPV DNA has been found in electrodessication smoke plumes and laser smoke plumes. If either of these treatment modalities is employed, procedures to evacuate the smoke plume must be implemented and equipment to prevent inhalation used.

COMPLICATIONS

- Malignant transformation to squamous cell carcinoma of certain subtypes, especially when cofactors are present. Cofactors include tobacco use, ultraviolet radiation, pregnancy, folate deficiency, and immune suppression.

PROGNOSIS

Recurrence is common.

DENTAL SIGNIFICANCE

May cause esthetic concerns. If large enough, lesions may interfere with mastication.

DENTAL MANAGEMENT

Routine dental care indicated, with no special precautions for immunocompetent individuals.

SUGGESTED REFERENCE

Praetorius F. HPV-associated disease of the oral mucosa. *Clin Derm* 1997;15: 339–413.

AUTHOR: **BRIAN C. MUZYKA, DMD, MS, MBA**

SYNONYM(S)

Primary hyperparathyroidism
Secondary hyperparathyroidism
Tertiary hyperparathyroidism

ICD-9CM/CPT CODE(S)
252.0   Hyperparathyroidism
252.01 Primary hyperparathyroidism
252.02 Secondary hyperparathyroidism, nonrenal
252.08 Other hyperparathyroidism
588.81 Secondary hyperparathroidism (of renal origin)

OVERVIEW

Hyperparathyroidism is excessive secretion of parathyroid hormone resulting in hypercalcemia. Primarily, the parathyroid hormone modulates the extracellular concentration of calcium by controlling intestinal absorption of calcium, mobilization of calcium in bone, and excretion of calcium. A low serum calcium concentration stimulates the secretion of parathyroid hormone. If hypocalcemia is sustained, hyperplasia and hypertrophy of the parathyroid gland occurs in response to the need for sustained secretion of parathyroid hormone. Conversely, high serum calcium concentration decreases parathyroid secretion.

EPIDEMIOLOGY & DEMOGRAPHICS

INCIDENCE/PREVALENCE IN USA: Incidence of 0.1% per year and prevalence of 1%.
PREDOMINANT AGE: Often presents in adults over the age of 50 years.
PREDOMINANT SEX: Three to four times more common in females than males.
GENETICS: Approximately 3–5% of cases of hyperparathyroidism can be linked to an inherited pathology.

ETIOLOGY & PATHOGENESIS

- Eighty percent of primary hyperparathyroidism is caused by a single parathyroid adenoma, while 20% may be caused by parathyroid hyperplasia or carcinoma.
- A presentation of hyperparathyroidism before the age of 30 usually indicates parathyroid gland carcinoma or a multiglandular disease.
- Development of parathyroid adenomas or hyperplasia can be part of the multiple endocrine neoplasia (MEN) type I or type II. Most parathyroid adenomas have chromosome deletion at 11q13 (MEN1 gene). It may also be familial, as in the hyperparathyroid jaw tumor syndrome.
- Secondary hyperparathyroidism may occur in chronic renal failure in response to hyperphosphatemia and low serum calcium that results when activation of 25-hydroxycholecalciferol to 1, 25-dihydroxycholecalciferol is disrupted.
- The compensatory production of parathyroid hormone (secondary hyperparathyroidism) may cause the glands to enlarge and continue to secrete autonomously to precipitate a condition of tertiary hyperparathyroidism.

CLINICAL PRESENTATION / PHYSICAL FINDINGS

- The majority of hyperparathyroidism patients may be symptomatic until the hypercalcemia is discovered in routine blood tests.
- Symptoms develop when serum calcium rises above 12 mg/dL. These cases demonstrate the characteristic manifestation of hyperparathyroidism that has been categorized as "bones-stones-groans-moans and overtones":
  - Excessive parathyroid hormone induces chronic bone resorption that may present as bone pains, arthralgias, pathologic fractures, and cystic bone lesions throughout the skeleton, referred to as osteitis fibrosa cystica or Brown's tumor in the jaw region.
  - In the kidneys, hypercalcuria occurs because of the dominant effect of filtered load over the conserving effect of parathyroid hormone on tubular calcium reabsorption. This induces nephrogenic diabetes insipidus and formation of kidney stones, which may precipitate renal failure. Thus, patients have polydipsia, polyuria, and kidney pains.
  - Urinary Ca^{++} excretion generally is increased, reflecting the dominant effect of filtered load over the conserving effect of PTH on tubular Ca^{++} reabsorption.
  - Other symptoms of hypercalcemia associated with the central nervous system, gastrointestinal, neuromuscular, and cardiovascular systems may include lethargy, fatigue, depression, coma, nausea, vomiting, anorexia, constipation, hypertension, a short QT interval in the electrocardiogram, and cardiac dysrhythmias.

DIAGNOSIS

- The diagnosis of primary hyperparathyroidism is usually confirmed by the presence of hypercalcemia with the serum calcium greater than 10.5 mg/dL or an ionized calcium greater than 5.4 mg/dL (1.4 mmol/L), since ionized calcium is always elevated in primary hyperparathyroidism.
- While the serum phosphate is usually low (less than 2.5 mg/dL) in primary hyperparathyroidism, it is usually high in secondary hyperparathyroidism because of the renal failure.
- In addition to hypercalcemia, an elevated level of parathyroid hormone (usually determined by immunoradiometric assay) will confirm the diagnosis of hyperparathyroidism.
- Alkaline phosphatase level is usually normal unless there is an associated bone disease.
- CT, MRI, and technetium scan are not required but may be useful for preoperative planning.
- Bone radiographs are usually normal but may demonstrate demineralization and subperiosteal bone resorption. Panoramic radiographs may demonstrate loss of lamina dura and presence of the cystic lesions of Brown's tumor.

MEDICAL MANAGEMENT & TREATMENT

- No drugs or agents presently exist that can produce either sustained blockage of parathyroid hormone (PTH) release by parathyroid glands or sustained blockage of hypercalcemia.
- Unless contraindicated, patients should maintain a high intake of fluids (3 to 5 L/day) and sodium chloride (> 400 mEq/day) to increase renal calcium excretion. Calcium intake should be 1000 mg/day.

Subtotal or total parathyroidectomy is the treatment of choice for primary hyperparathyroidism. It is generally indicated in all patients under age 50 with complications from hyperthyroidism, such as nephrolithiasis and osteopenia.

See "Hyperparathyroidism" in Section II, p 271.

COMPLICATIONS

- Bone demineralization and cystic lesions may precipitate pathological fractures.
- Kidney stones may cause urinary tract obstruction and infection.
- Hypercalcemia and generalized dissemination of calcific deposits may cause pancreatitis, chondrocalcinosis, calcific periarthritis, and peptic ulcer.

PROGNOSIS

- Medical treatment of asymptomatic hyperparathyroidism with mild hypercalcemia achieves success.
- In severe cases, surgical removal of parathyroid adenoma achieves complete remission and bone healing.

DENTAL SIGNIFICANCE

- The presence of a clinical or radiographic jaw lesion may indicate Brown's tumor. The clinician should rule out hyperparathyroidism by referring the patient to the medical care provider.

- See "Hyperparathyroidism" in Section II, p 271 for more information on dental implications and management.

SUGGESTED REFERENCES

Current Medical Diagnosis & Treatment 2005. Tierney Jr. LM, McPhee SJ, Papadakis MA (eds), Gonzales R, Zeiger R (online eds): http://www.accessmedicine.com/resourceTOC.aspx?resourceID=1

Harrison's Online: http://www3.accessmedicine.com/home.aspx

Neville BW, Damm DD, Allen CM, Bouquot JE. *Oral and Maxillofacial Pathology.* Philadelphia, WB Saunders, 2002, pp 724–726.

AUTHOR: **SUNDAY O. AKINTOYE, BDS, DDS, MS**

SYNONYM(S)

Primary hypertension
Essential hypertension
Idiopathic hypertension
High blood pressure

ICD-9CM/CPT CODE(S)
401.1 Essential hypertension

OVERVIEW

Hypertension is defined as a persistent elevation in blood pressure that is considered to be higher than normal. More specifically, *The Seventh Report of the Joint National Committee on Detection, Education, and Treatment of High Blood Pressure* (the JNC 7 Report) defines hypertension in adults as a systolic blood pressure greater than or equal to 140 mmHg or a diastolic blood pressure greater than or equal to 90 mmHg as recorded during two or more readings on two or more occasions (office visits) (Table I-13).

EPIDEMIOLOGY & DEMOGRAPHICS

INCIDENCE/PREVALENCE IN USA: Incidence estimated at 50 million in 1988–1991; occurs in 10–15% of white adults and 20–30% of African-American adults.
PREDOMINANT AGE: Primary hypertension usually has an onset between age 25 and 55; it is uncommon before age 20.
PREDOMINANT SEX: Occurs predominantly in males (males tend to run higher blood pressures than females but, more importantly, have a significantly higher risk of cardiovascular disease at any given blood pressure).
GENETICS: No clearly established genetic pattern has been established for primary hypertension; however, blood pressure levels appear to have strong familial tendencies. Children with one (and to a greater degree, two) hypertensive parents tend to have higher blood pressures and are perceived to be at an increased risk to develop hypertension.

ETIOLOGY & PATHOGENESIS

- Primary hypertension accounts for approximately 95% of cases of hypertension and has no single or specific etiology.
- Current evidence suggests the disease is multifactorial, caused by a complex interaction of genetic, environmental, and demographic factors.
- Patients with primary hypertension do not appear to share any one, or a specific combination of, suspected etiologic factors. Some of the potential etiologic factors for primary hypertension include:
  ○ Genetic predisposition
  ○ Defects in the renin-angiotensin system
  ○ Renal retention of excess dietary sodium
  ○ Vascular hypertrophy with increased peripheral resistance
  ○ Sympathic nervous system dysfunction and/or hyperactivity resulting in increased plasma catecholamine levels
  ○ Hyperinsulinemia secondary to insulin resistance
- Additional factors have been implicated as either predisposing or contributing to the development of primary hypertension; these include:
  ○ Cigarette smoking
  ○ Obesity (BMI > 30)
  ○ Dyslipidemia
  ○ Diabetes mellitus
  ○ Microalbuminuria or estimated GFR < 60 mL/min
  ○ Age (> 55 years for men, > 65 years for women)
  ○ Physical inactivity
  ○ Excessive alcohol use
  ○ Chronic nonsteroidal antiinflammatory drug use
- Additional types of hypertension include:
  ○ Secondary hypertension accounts for less than 5% of all cases of systemic hypertension and has an identifiable underlying etiology such as renal vascular or renal parenchymal disease, endocrine disorders, neurological disorders, or induced by drugs or

chemicals. The importance of identifying patients with secondary hypertension is that they can sometimes be cured by surgery or by specific medical treatment.
  ○ Isolated systolic hypertension is a specific form of hypertension most commonly found in elderly individuals (especially in the seventh decade of life). It is defined as a systolic blood pressure of 140 mmHg or more and a diastolic blood pressure of less than 90 mmHg. The most common etiology of isolated systolic hypertension is decreased aortic distensibility (elasticity) secondary to aortic arteriosclerosis.
  ○ Isolated office hypertension, also called white-coat hypertension, is a frequently diagnosed condition characterized by persistently elevated office (clinical) blood pressure (presumably due to patient anxiety/apprehension) combined with normal daytime ambulatory blood pressure. The incidence of this condition is 12–50%, depending on the definition (blood pressure range) of isolated office hypertension and the population studied.
  ○ Malignant hypertension is the syndrome of markedly elevated BP (diastolic BP usually greater than 120 to 140 mmHg) associated with papilledema.

CLINICAL PRESENTATION / PHYSICAL FINDINGS

- Mild to moderate primary hypertension is usually asymptomatic and is often detected only during routine blood pressure screening. A person may be unaware of the consequent progressive cardiovascular damage due to hypertension that remains asymptomatic for as long as 10 to 20 years. Some of the early symptoms of primary hypertension that some patients may eventually experience include:
  ○ Headaches (especially early morning, pulsating, suboccipital headaches)
  ○ Visual disturbances including blurred vision or scotomata
  ○ Tinnitus
  ○ Dizziness
  ○ Coldness or tingling of the extremities
  ○ Fatigue
  ○ Shortness of breath
  ○ Epistaxis
- It should be noted that some of the symptoms often attributed to hypertension, such as headache, fatigue, tinnitus, or dizziness, may be observed just as frequently in normotensive patients.
- Signs and symptoms of severe or later-stage hypertension are usually related to the potential cardiovascular, cerebrovascular, and renal complications of

TABLE I-13	**Blood Pressure Classification for Adults Aged 18 Years or Older***	
Classification[H]	Systolic Blood Pressure (mmHg)	Diastolic Blood Pressure (mmHg)
Normal	< 120	< 80
Prehypertension	120–139	80–89
Stage 1 Hypertension	140–159	90–99
Stage 2 Hypertension	≥ 160	≥ 100

* Based on the mean of two or more seated blood pressure readings taken on each of two or more office visits.
[H] When systolic and diastolic pressures fall into different categories, the higher category should be selected to classify the individual's blood pressure.
(Adapted from Chobanian AV, et al. The seventh report of the joint national committee on prevention, detection, evaluation, and treatment of high blood pressure: the JNC 7 report. *JAMA* 2003;289:2560.)

the disease and may include papilledema, left ventricular hypertrophy, proteinuria, and hematuria.

DIAGNOSIS

Diagnostic examination of a patient with suspected primary hypertension usually includes:

- Blood pressure measurement
- Ocular fundus and retinal examination
- Auscultation of the heart and arteries
- Examination of all major peripheral pulses
- Electrocardiogram
- Laboratory tests including:
  - Complete blood count
  - Complete urinalysis
  - Serum creatinine
  - Serum uric acid
  - Estimated glomerular filtration rate
  - Electrolytes (especially potassium and calcium)
  - Blood urea nitrogen
  - Blood glucose
  - Lipid panel (total cholesterol, VLDL, HDL, LDL cholesterol, and triglycerides)
- Optional or ancillary tests may include:
  - Ambulatory blood pressure monitoring
  - Echocardiography, chest x-ray, CT, or MRI
  - Plasma renin activity
  - Plasma and urinary catecholamines and steroids (vanillylmandelic acid, 17-hydroxy ketosteroids, metanephrine)
  - Renal imaging studies (sonography or angiography)
  - Thyroid panel

MEDICAL MANAGEMENT & TREATMENT

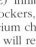

OVERVIEW

- The goal of treatment of hypertension should be to lower patient's blood pressure to normal levels (typically < 140/90 mmHg, or < 130/80 mmHg for patients with diabetes or chronic kidney disease) with minimal adverse effects for the patient.
- It may not be possible to reduce a patient's blood pressure to what would be considered an optimum level; instead, a compromise may be necessary (reducing patient's blood pressure to a level that is as low as can be achieved using an acceptably tolerated therapeutic regimen).
- Treatment of primary hypertension is most frequently accomplished both pharmacologically and nonpharmacologically (adopting a healthy lifestyle).

NONPHARMACOLOGIC THERAPY

- Adoption of a healthy lifestyle is critical for the prevention of high blood pressure in all individuals and is an indispensable part of the management of those with hypertension.
- Lifestyle modification approaches for the management of primary hypertension includes weight reduction, reduced alcohol consumption, a regular exercise program, modification of sodium intake, and cessation of smoking (if applicable).

PHARMACOLOGIC THERAPY

- Thiazide-type diuretics should be used as initial pharmacology therapy, either alone or in combination with one from other classes [angiotensin-converting enzyme (ACE) inhibitors, angiotensin receptor blockers, beta-adrenergic blockers, calcium channel blockers].
- Most patients will require two or more antihypertensive medications to reach blood pressure goals; a second drug should be initiated when use of a single drug in adequate doses fails.
- When initial blood pressure is more than 20/10 mmHg above goal, consider initiating antihypertensive therapy with two drugs (either as separate prescriptions or in fixed-dose combinations).
- When initiating drug therapy with more than one agent, caution is advised for those at risk for orthostatic hypotension, such as patients with diabetic autonomic dysfunction and some older patients.

COMPLICATIONS

The complications of untreated hypertension are numerous. The degree of damage to susceptible target organs is closely related to both the duration and severity of the hypertension. These complications include:

- Cardiovascular disease, including myocardial infarction, congestive heart failure, ventricular dysrhythmias, myocardial ischemia, and sudden cardiac death.
- Cerebrovascular disease; hypertension is the most important risk factor predisposing to stroke (cerebrovascular accident).
- Renal disease including nephrosclerosis and chronic renal failure (end-stage renal disease).
- Peripheral vascular (arterial) disease, including aortic aneurysms.
- Retinopathy, leading to possible blindness.

PROGNOSIS

- If untreated, about 50% of hypertensive patients die of coronary vascular disease or congestive heart failure, about 33% of a cerebrovascular event (stroke), and 10–15% of renal failure.
- Effective medical control of hypertension will prevent or forestall most complications and will prolong life in patients with primary hypertension or isolated systolic hypertension. In contrast, fewer than 5% of patients with malignant hypertension characterized by papilledema survive 1 year without treatment.
- Prolonged elevated systolic blood pressure is generally considered to be a more important predictor of fatal and nonfatal cardiovascular events than is prolonged elevated diastolic blood pressure. Nevertheless, prolonged increases in the usual diastolic pressure of 5 and 10 mmHg are associated, respectively, with at least 34% and 56% increases in stroke risk and with at least 21% and 37% increases in coronary heart disease risk.

DENTAL SIGNIFICANCE

- Patients with hypertension are generally considered to be at increased risk of adverse events during dental treatment approximately in proportion to the severity of hypertension and the presence of end-organ complications.
- Orthostatic hypotension may be a problem for patients taking antihypertensive medications.
- The potential exists for adverse interactions between sympathomimetic vasoconstrictors used in some dental local anesthetic preparations and some antihypertensive agents, including noncardioselective beta-adrenergic blockers, alpha-adrenergic blockers, adrenergic neuronal blockers, and methyldopa.
- Some patients may present with xerostomia of varying severity, secondary to or exacerbated by their antihypertensive medications, particularly diuretics.
- Patients taking ACE inhibitors or beta-adrenergic blockers may complain of taste disturbances and/or present with lichenoid reactions of the oral mucosa; ACE inhibitors are also reported to cause a drug-induced cough.
- Diuretics (especially thiazide-type) and direct-acting vasodilators have been implicated in causing lichenoid or lupus-like oral mucosal changes.
- Patients taking calcium channel blockers may present with drug-induced gingival hyperplasia.

DENTAL MANAGEMENT

The general evaluation of the dental patient with hypertension should include determining the:

- Time of diagnosis of hypertension and type of hypertension.
- Present medications and dosage used to control hypertension as well as a history of any recent changes or

modifications to antihypertensive medications or dosage over the past 6 months.
- Presence of contributing factors to hypertension including:
  - Ischemic heart disease (coronary artery disease, atherosclerotic heart disease)
  - Congestive heart failure in the form of systolic or diastolic ventricular dysfunction
  - Diabetes mellitus
  - Chronic renal disease, defined by either:
    - Reduced excretory function with an estimated glomerular filtration rate of less than 60 mL/min per 1.73 m^2 [corresponding approximately to a creatinine of > 1.5 mg/dL (> 132.6 μmol/L) in men or > 1.3 mg/dL (> 114.9 μmol/L) in women], or
    - The presence of albuminuria (> 300 mg/day or 200 mg albumin per gram of creatinine)
- Presence of any systemic complications secondary to hypertension, including retinopathy, nephropathy, history of cerebrovascular disease, cardiovascular disease, or peripheral vascular disease.

Physical evaluation of the dental patient with hypertension should include:
- Establishing the patient's baseline blood pressure at the first dental appointment.
  - Two to three blood pressure measurements separated by at least 10 to 15 minutes should be taken and the results averaged to determine the patient's baseline blood pressure. The patient's baseline blood pressure will serve as a point of reference from which to make decisions for the emergency management of the patient should a cardiovascular or adverse reaction develop during dental treatment.
- Checking and recording the patient's blood pressure at all subsequent appointments prior to the use of local anesthesia.

Specific management considerations for the dental patient with hypertension would include:
- Reducing stress and anxiety prior to and during dental treatment.
  - Consider the use of N$_2$O-O$_2$ inhalation sedation and/or premedication with oral antianxiety medications such as benzodiazepines (e.g., triazolam, 0.125 to 0.5 mg the night before appointment and 0.125 to 0.5 mg 1 hour before treatment).
- Avoiding the use of local anesthetics with vasoconstrictors in patients with uncontrolled or poorly controlled hypertension. This is defined as any patient with a systolic blood pressure greater than or equal to 180 mmHg and/or a diastolic blood pressure greater than or equal to 110 mmHg.
  - For patients with controlled hypertension where the use of local anesthetics with vasoconstrictors are not contraindicated because of potential drug interactions, it is advisable to limit the total dose of vasoconstrictor (see Appendix A, Box A-3, "Local Anesthetic with Vasoconstrictor Dose Restriction Guidelines").
- Avoiding stimulating the patient's gag reflex during dental treatment.

SUGGESTED REFERENCES

Chobanian AV, et al. The seventh report of the Joint National Committee on Prevention, Detection, Evaluation, and Treatment of High Blood Pressure: the JNC-7 report. *JAMA* 2003;289:2560–2572.

Herman WW, Konzelman JL, Prisant LM. New national guidelines on hypertension: a summary for dentistry. *JADA* 2004;135:576–586.

Kaplan NM. Systemic hypertension: mechanisms and diagnosis, in Braunwal E, Zipes DP, Libby P (eds): *Heart Disease: A Textbook of Cardiovascular Medicine.* Philadelphia, WB Saunders, 2001, pp 941–968.

Little JW. The impact on dentistry of recent advances in the management of hypertension. *Oral Surg Oral Med Oral Pathol Oral Radiol Endod* 2000;90(5):591–599.

Tsai PS. White coat hypertension: understanding the concept and examining the significance. *J Clin Nurs* 2002;11(6):715-722.

AUTHOR: **F. JOHN FIRRIOLO, DDS, PHD**

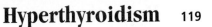

SYNONYM(S)

Thyrotoxicosis

ICD-9CM/CPT CODE(S)

242.9 Hyperthyroidism
242.0 Hyperthyroidism with goiter
242.2 Hyperthyroidism, multinodular
242.3 Hyperthyroidism, uninodular

OVERVIEW

- Hyperthyroidism comprises conditions in which excessive concentrations of free, biologically active thyroid hormone (T4 and T3) are found in the blood and tissues and are derived from an overactive, hyperfunctional thyroid gland (rather than thyroid inflammation or destruction or thyroid hormone administration).
- Thyrotoxicosis applies more broadly and includes all causes of excess thyroid hormone, whether or not they are intrinsic or extrinsic to the thyroid gland.
  - Most clinicians (as well as this text) use the terms hyperthyroidism and thyrotoxicosis interchangeably.

EPIDEMIOLOGY & DEMOGRAPHICS

INCIDENCE/PREVALENCE IN USA:

- Incidence: 100 per 100,000 in women; lower in men.
- Prevalence: Women, 100 per 100,000; men, 33 per 100,000.

PREDOMINANT AGE: Varies with underlying etiology; generally peaks in third and fourth decades.

PREDOMINANT SEX: Varies with underlying etiology; generally female > male (3:1)

GENETICS: Not established for hyperthyroidism in general; Graves' disease has a familial tendency associated with HLA-DRw3 and HLA-B89.

ETIOLOGY & PATHOGENESIS

- Graves' disease:
  - Represents the most common cause of hyperthyroidism (approximately 75% of cases overall and approximately 90% of cases in patients under 40 years old).
  - Much more common in women than in men (8:1).
  - An autoimmune disease that produces IgG-type autoantibodies known as thyroid stimulating immunoglobulins (TSIs).
    - The TSIs bind to the receptors for thyroid stimulating hormone TSH in the thyroid gland and cause the release of triiodothyronine (T3) and thyroxine (T4).
  - Diffuse toxic goiter is the major manifestation of Graves' disease.
- Toxic uninodular goiter (toxic adenoma, Plummer's disease):

- Usually a benign thyroid neoplasm with autonomous hyperfunction. The remaining gland is commonly hypofunctional.
- Toxic multinodular goiter:
  - Usually a benign process that occurs late in life and is generally insidious in nature with a subclinical presentation.
- Hashimoto's thyroiditis (chronic lymphocytic thyroiditis, autoimmune thyroiditis):
  - Autoimmune disease of unknown etiology.
  - More prevalent in women than in men (8:1); incidence increases with age.
  - May cause transient hyperthyroidism during the initial destructive phase.
  - In the final phase of the disease, the thyroid is fibrotic in addition to being atrophic, resulting in usually permanent hypothyroidism.
- Subacute (De Quervain) thyroiditis:
  - Usually idiopathic, but sometimes virally mediated (e.g., Coxsackie, paramyxovirus, adenovirus), inflammation and destruction of the thyroid gland; subsequently, the stored thyroid hormones are released into the circulation, resulting in mild and transient hyperthyroidism.
  - In as many as 50% of patients, hypothyroidism may occur later.
- Thyrotoxicosis factitia (factitious hyperthyroidism):
  - Results from the surreptitious ingestion of synthetic T4 (levothyroxine). Most commonly seen in the mentally handicapped, the elderly, and individuals using thyroid hormone inappropriately as a device for weight control.
  - Jodbasedow disease (iodine-induced hyperthyroidism) may occur in patients with multinodular goiters after intake of large amounts of iodine in the diet or in the form of radiographic contrast materials or drugs, especially amiodarone.
- Rare causes of hyperthyroidism include:
  - Subacute lymphocytic thyroiditis (also called painless thyroiditis or silent thyroiditis): This condition has a suspected autoimmune etiology, is most often seen in middle-aged adults, and is more common in women, especially during the postpartum period (i.e., postpartum thyroiditis). It is characterized by transient hyperthyroidism lasting from 2 to 8 weeks before subsiding.
  - Thyroid stimulating hormone (TSH)-secreting tumors: TSH-secreting pituitary adenoma or pituitary resistance to thyroid hormones.
  - Functioning trophoblastic tumors: These include hydatidiform mole and choriocarcinoma.

- Have extremely high levels of beta human chorionic gonadotropin (bHCG) that can weakly activate the TSH receptor. At very high levels of bHCG, activation of the TSH receptor occurs that is sufficient to cause hyperthyroidism.
  - Struma ovarii: Functioning ectopic thyroid tissue is contained in about 3% of ovarian dermoid tumors and teratomas that can excrete excessive amounts of thyroid hormone.
  - Metastatic functioning thyroid carcinoma.

CLINICAL PRESENTATION / PHYSICAL FINDINGS

Signs and symptoms can include many variations and (in adults) include:
- Enlargement of the thyroid gland (goiter), for example:
  - Diffusely, symmetrically enlarged and slightly firm in most patients with Graves' disease.
  - Asymmetrically irregular, bumpy enlargement to at least two to three times normal size in toxic multinodular goiter.
  - Enlarged, firm, and rubbery thyroid without any tenderness is typically seen in Hashimoto's thyroiditis.
- Nervousness
- Diaphoresis
- Heat intolerance
- Palpitations and tachycardia
- Dyspnea
- Warm and moist skin
- Tremor
- Fatigue and weakness
- Weight loss
- Increased appetite
- Proptosis or exophthalmos
- Emotional lability
- Menstrual dysfunction (oligomenorrhea, amenorrhea)

DIAGNOSIS

LABORATORY

- Thyroid function tests:
  - Serum T4
  - Serum T3 resin uptake
  - Serum T3
  - Free T4
  - Free T3
    - In hyperthyroidism, both total and free thyroid hormone concentrations are elevated, although isolated increases of either T4 or T3 may also occur.
- Thyroid stimulating hormone (TSH):
  - A reliable sensitive TSH assay is the best test for hyperthyroidism; it is below normal except in the very rare cases of pituitary inappropriate secretion of thyrotropin.
- Thyroid autoantibodies:
  - The most specific autoantibody for autoimmune thyroiditis is an enzyme-linked immunosorbent assay (ELISA)

for anti-TPO antibody (thyroperoxidase).
- Other laboratory abnormalities may include hypercalcemia, increased alkaline phosphatase, anemia, and decreased granulocytes.

IMAGING/SPECIAL TESTS
- Thyroid radioactive iodine 123 (I-123) uptake and scan:
  - High radioactive iodine uptake is seen in Graves' disease and toxic nodular goiter but can be seen in other conditions as well.
  - Low radioactive iodine uptake is characteristic of subacute thyroiditis but can also be seen in other conditions.

MEDICAL MANAGEMENT & TREATMENT

GENERAL MEASURES
- Activity should be modified based upon the disease severity.
- Diet should include an adequate number of calories to maintain weight.
- Hospitalization required for life-threatening thyrotoxic crisis (thyroid storm).
- Minimize or avoid exogenous administration of epinephrine.

SPECIFIC TREATMENT
- Antithyroid (thiourea) medications [e.g. methimazole (Tapazole), propylthiouracil (PTU)]:
  - Inhibit the synthesis of thyroid hormones.
  - Have a high rate of recurrent hyperthyroidism (about 50%) after a year or more of therapy.
  - Useful for preparing hyperthyroid patients for surgery and elderly patients for radioactive iodide therapy.
- Radioactive iodine 131 (I-131) therapy (RAIT):
  - Radioactive I-131 is taken up by the thyroid gland and produces destruction of thyroid follicular cells.
  - RAIT is generally avoided in children and is contraindicated during pregnancy and breastfeeding.
  - High incidence of hypothyroidism several years after RAIT, even when small doses are given; permanent, postablative hypothyroidism occurs in about one-third of patients by 8 years after RIAT, requiring lifelong thyroid hormone replacement.
- Subtotal thyroidectomy surgery:
  - Indications include:
    - Patients with large goiters
    - Children who are allergic to antithyroid medications
    - Pregnant women (usually in the second trimester) who are allergic to antithyroid medications
    - Patients who prefer surgery over antithyroid medications or RAIT
  - Complications from subtotal thyroidectomy:

- Hoarseness due to recurrent laryngeal nerve damage and/or hypoparathyroidism occurs in less than 5% of patients.
- Hypothyroidism develops in more than 60% of patients, requiring lifelong thyroid hormone replacement.
- Propranolol (40 to 240 mg/day) is used to treat tachycardia and hypertension associated with hyperthyroid state; it is also used as a first-line drug in treating thyroid storm.

COMPLICATIONS

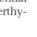

- Exophthalmos:
  - May require surgical decompression to prevent corneal ulceration and loss of vision.
- Cardiac complications:
  - Sinus tachycardia and/or atrial fibrillation are commonly seen in hyperthyroidism and may be the presenting manifestation.
  - Congestive heart failure and dilated cardiomyopathy are also potential complications of untreated hyperthyroidism.
- Thyrotoxic crisis (thyroid storm):
  - This life-threatening complication represents a sudden and severe exacerbation of the signs and symptoms of hyperthyroidism manifested by fever (which is characteristic and may exceed 104°F), restlessness, tachycardia, atrial fibrillation, pulmonary edema, tremor, sweating, stupor, and finally coma and death if treatment is not provided.
  - Most cases occur in patients with Graves' disease (diffuse toxic goiter).
  - Is usually precipitated by physiologic stress, most frequently due to infection, surgery, or trauma in a patient with poorly treated or untreated thyrotoxicosis. Other precipitating factors include emotional stress, cardiovascular disease, systemic illness (including acute oral infection), diabetic ketoacidosis, and vigorous palpation of the thyroid.

PROGNOSIS

- Hyperthyroidism carries a good prognosis with most etiologies when appropriately diagnosed and treated.
- Thyrotoxic crisis (thyroid storm) represents the major complication of the disease, which poses serious morbidity and mortality if untreated. (See "Thyroid Storm" in Section III, p 383 for more information.)

DENTAL SIGNIFICANCE

- Oral findings associated with hyperthyroidism can include:

- Increased susceptibility to caries
- Periodontal disease
- Enlargement of extraglandular thyroid tissue (mainly in the lateral posterior tongue)
- Maxillary or mandibular osteoporosis
- Accelerated dental eruption (in children and adolescents)
- Burning mouth syndrome
- Patients with undiagnosed, untreated, or uncontrolled hyperthyroidism represent a significant risk for dental treatment, primarily due to:
  - The increased risk of thyrotoxic crisis (thyroid storm) precipitated via stress, acute oral infection, or vigorous thyroid gland palpation.
  - Possible concurrent, secondary cardiovascular disease (e.g., atrial dysrhythmia, congestive heart failure, dilated cardiomyopathy).
  - The possible adverse effects of using local anesthetics containing catecholamines (e.g., epinephrine) in patients with nonmedically treated or uncontrolled hyperthyroidism.

DENTAL MANAGEMENT

HISTORY AND PHYSICAL ASSESSMENT
- Establish the specific diagnosis of hyperthyroidism (e.g., Graves' disease, toxic multinodular goiter).
- Determine/record history of past therapy (e.g., surgery, I-131 therapy, antithyroid medication).
- Determine/record present medication(s).
- Perform an assessment of the patient's current clinical status, including:
  - Symptoms of hyperthyroidism (including abnormal blood pressure and pulse).
  - Presence of any concurrent cardiovascular disease (e.g., atrial dysrhythmia, congestive heart failure, cardiomyopathy).
    - If present, make applicable modifications to dental treatment as indicated.
  - Confirm normal physical evaluation and thyroid function tests (e.g., TSH) within the past 6 to 12 months.
- Dental treatment should be deferred if the patient presents with:
  - Symptoms of undiagnosed or uncontrolled hyperthyroidism including tachycardia, irregular pulse, sweating, hypertension, tremor; or
  - An unreliable or vague history of thyroid disease and management; or
  - Neglect to follow physician-initiated control of thyroid disease for more than 6 to 12 months and would require appropriate medical referral.

DENTAL TREATMENT CONSIDERATIONS
- Agranulocytosis is an uncommon but serious complication of thiourea antithyroid drug therapy, being

reported in about 0.1% of patients taking methimazole and about 0.4% of patients taking propylthiouracil; it may be assessed via complete blood count with differential.

- Since emotional stress may precipitate a thyrotoxic crisis, appropriate stress reduction measures should be considered:
  - Keep appointment duration as short as possible. Also, morning appointments are probably preferable for most patients since they may become more fatigued as the day progresses.
  - Consider the use of N_2O-O_2 inhalation sedation and/or premedication with oral antianxiety medications such as benzodiazepines (e.g., triazolam, 0.125 to 0.5 mg the night before appointment and 0.125 to 0.5 mg 1 hour before treatment).
- Establish profound local anesthesia (see following Pharmacologic Considerations).
- Ensure adequate posttreatment pain control with analgesics as indicated.

PHARMACOLOGIC CONSIDERATIONS
- For many years it was believed that thyroid hormone and catecholamines (e.g., epinephrine) interacted synergistically, resulting in tachycardia and other dysrhythmias, a widening of the pulse width, increased cardiac output, and myocardial ischemia. This may be due to the fact that the effects of thyroid hormone on the heart closely resemble those of catecholamines, and many of the signs and symptoms of thyrotoxic crisis are those of adrenergic hyperactivity. However, evidence accumulated over the last three decades shows that in patients with hyperthyroidism:
  - Neither catecholamine sensitivity nor serum catecholamine levels appear to be elevated; and
  - The hemodynamic responses to epinephrine and norepinephrine are not significantly altered.
- Nevertheless, a subset of patients with excessive amounts of thyroid hormone in the circulation will have developed cardiac abnormalities (e.g., atrial dysrhythmia, congestive heart failure, dilated cardiomyopathy) as a result of the chronic overstimulation of myocardial metabolism.
  - Therefore, local anesthetics containing vasoconstrictors should be used with caution in patients with non-medically treated or uncontrolled hyperthyroidism as well as those taking noncardioselective beta blockers (e.g., propranolol).

Management of Thyrotoxic Crisis (Thyroid Storm): see "Thyroid Storm" in Section III, p 383.

SUGGESTED REFERENCES

Dillman WH. The thyroid, in Goldman L, Ausiello D (eds): *Cecil Textbook of Medicine*, ed 22. Philadelphia, WB Saunders, 2004, pp 1391–1402.

Jameson JL, Weetman AP. Disorders of the thyroid gland, in Kasper DI, et al. (eds): *Harrison's Principles of Internal Medicine*, ed 16. New York, McGraw-Hill, 2005, pp 2113–2119.

Pinto A, Glick M. Management of patients with thyroid disease: oral health considerations. *JADA* 2002;133:849–858.

Ross DS. Hyperthyroidism. Uptodate Online 13.2, updated 17 September 2004, http://www.uptodateonline. com/application/topic.asp?file=thyroid/7860

AUTHORS: F. JOHN FIRRIOLO, DDS, PHD; JAMES R. HUPP, DMD, MD, JD, MBA

SYNONYM(S)

Myxedema

ICD-9CM/CPT CODE(S)

243 Congenital hypothyroidism
244.0 Postsurgical hypothyroidism
244.1 Other postablative hypothyroidism, such as following irradiation
244.2 Iodine hypothyroidism
244.3 Other iatrogenic hypothyroidism
244.8 Other specified acquired hypothyroidism; secondary hypothyroidism NEC
244.9 Unspecified hypothyroidism; hypothyroidism, primary or NOS, myxedema, primary or NOS

OVERVIEW

- Hypothyroidism is an endocrine disorder resulting from a deficiency of thyroid hormone production or resistance to thyroid hormone action.
- Myxedema (usually) connotes severe hypothyroidism.

EPIDEMIOLOGY & DEMOGRAPHICS

INCIDENCE/PREVALENCE IN USA:
Hypothyroidism occurs in 0.8–1.0% of the population; in patients over the age of 65, it occurs in as many as 6–10% of women and 2–3% of men.
PREDOMINANT AGE: Over 40 years old.
PREDOMINANT SEX: Female > male (approximately 5–10:1).
GENETICS:

- No genetic pattern established for idiopathic primary hypothyroidism.
- May be associated with type II autoimmune polyglandular syndrome, which is associated with HLA-DR3 and HLA-DR4.
- Secondary hypothyroidism frequently results from treatment for Graves' disease, which may be familial.

ETIOLOGY & PATHOGENESIS

Hypothyroidism is classified as:

- Primary: characterized by failure of the thyroid gland to produce T3 and T4 hormones. This has four basic causes:
1. Autoimmune (atrophic): is a common cause of hypothyroidism in the U.S. and usually represents the late stage of Hashimoto's (chronic lymphocytic) thyroiditis because the majority of the cases have significant elevations of thyroid autoantibody titers.
   - More common in women than men (8:1). Often associated with other autoimmune diseases of the endocrine system, including autoimmune hypoparathyroidism, adrenal failure, hypogonadism,

and type 1 diabetes mellitus. Subacute lymphocytic thyroiditis (also called painless thyroiditis or silent thyroiditis) has a suspected autoimmune etiology and usually evolves through a transient hyperthyroid stage lasting from 2 to 8 weeks before subsiding. A minority of affected individuals eventually progress to hypothyroidism.

2. Postablative (iatrogenic): is quite common and is usually found after radioactive iodine I-31 treatment of hyperthyroidism or subtotal or near-total thyroidectomy surgery for thyroid cancer, Graves' disease, or toxic multinodular goiter. External mantle irradiation for Hodgkin's disease may also lead to thyroid gland failure; this generally evolves over a period of 5 to 10 years.

3. Goitrous: arises because of decreased ability of the thyroid gland to synthesize thyroid hormone, leading to increased thyroid stimulating hormone (TSH) secretion, which results in an increase in the size of the thyroid gland. Causes of goitrous hypothyroidism include:
   - Endemic goiter, which occurs in regions of iodide deficiency such as the mountainous areas of Europe and South America. Children born of parents having an endemic goiter may be born with goitrous hypothyroidism (endemic cretinism).
   - Drugs, including chronic administration of large doses of iodides as in expectorants, lithium, amiodarone, thiourea compounds, alpha-interferon, interleukins, and tumor necrosis factor.
   - Genetic defects: a variety of genetic (congenital) defects affecting thyroid hormone biosynthesis cause goitrous hypothyroidism.

4. Nonautoimmune:
   - Riedel's thyroiditis is of unknown etiology and is the rarest form of thyroiditis; it is found most frequently in middle-aged or elderly women. It is characterized by a dense fibrosis of the thyroid gland and usually results in hypothyroidism and may cause hypoparathyroidism as well.
   - Subacute (De Quervain) thyroiditis:
     - Is usually idiopathic, but sometimes virally mediated, causing inflammation and destruction of the thyroid gland; subsequently, the stored thyroid hormones are released into the circulation, resulting in a mild and transient hyperthyroidism.

     - In as many as 50% of patients, hypothyroidism may occur later, lasting from weeks to months, and may become permanent in 5–10% of patients.
- Secondary: the thyroid gland is normal, and the pituitary fails to secrete adequate TSH due to causes including panhypopituitarism, postoperative panhypopituitarism, infiltrative disease (e.g., sarcoidosis), or isolated TSH deficiency.
- Tertiary: characterized by failure of the hypothalamus to secrete thyrotropin releasing-hormone (TRH) due to causes including congenital defects of the hypothalamus, infiltrative disease (e.g., sarcoidosis), or irradiation of hypothalamus.
   - Congenital: athyreotic cretinism is found in children born with an absence of the thyroid gland.

CLINICAL PRESENTATION / PHYSICAL FINDINGS

The slow and progressive onset of hypothyroidism in most patients can make clinical diagnosis difficult.

- General/Metabolic
   - Weakness; fatigue; lethargy; cold intolerance; decreased basal metabolic rate; decreased T4 and drug turnover; hypercholesterolemia; modest weight gain (~ 10 pounds); low-pitched, hoarse voice; stoic appearance.
- Central Nervous System
   - Decreased (impaired) memory; myxedematous dementia; cerebellar ataxia; slow speech; delayed relaxation of deep tendon reflexes.
- Cardiovascular
   - Decreased cardiac output at rest because of reduction in both stroke volume and bradycardia (reflecting loss of the inotropic and chronotropic effects of thyroid hormones); enlarged heart on chest radiograph (often due to pericardial effusion); reduced systolic blood pressure; increased diastolic blood pressure.
- Respiratory
   - Depressed ventilatory drive (decreased respiratory response to hypercapnia and hypoxia); pleural effusion; dyspnea; sleep apnea.
- Oral/Gastrointestinal
   - Macroglossia; constipation; hypomotility.
- Musculoskeletal
   - Muscle stiffness; cramps; pain; carpal tunnel syndrome.
- Integument
   - Dry, rough skin; hyperkeratosis; yellowish (carotenemic) skin color; decreased sweating; periorbital puffiness and loss of lateral eyebrow; coarse, dry hair that may tend to fall out.
- Endocrine
   - Hyperprolactinemia leading to galactorrhea; heavy menstrual bleeding;

menorrhagia; hypoglycemia; syndrome of inappropriate secretion of antidiuretic hormone (SIADH).

- Hematologic
  - Decreased production of erythropoietin leading to mild normocytic, normochromic anemia; iron deficiency anemia and/or pernicious anemia are less frequent.
- Renal
  - Impaired ability to excrete a free water load leading to edema and dilutional hyponatremia (which can be further exacerbated by SIADH).

DIAGNOSIS

LABORATORY

- Thyroid function tests:
  - Serum T4
  - Serum T3 resin uptake
  - Serum T3
  - Free T4
  - Free T3
    - Clinical, overt hypothyroid patients have reduced free T4 levels; normal and subclinical hypothyroid patients have normal levels.
    - Only one-third of clinical, overt hypothyroid patients have reduced free T3 levels; normal and subclinical hypothyroid patients have normal levels.
- Thyroid stimulating hormone (TSH):
  - The primary test used in the diagnosis (and monitoring the adequacy of and compliance with thyroid hormone therapy) of patients of with hypothyroidism.
  - Serum levels TSH are elevated in more than 99% of the patients with hypothyroidism.
    - TSH levels may be normal or low in suprathyroid (tertiary) hypothyroidism.
- Thyroid autoantibodies: enzyme-linked immunosorbent assay (ELISA) antibody titers for thyroperoxidase and thyroglobulin are elevated in over 90% of patients with autoimmune thyroiditis.
- Other laboratory abnormalities may include:
  - Increased serum cholesterol, liver enzymes, and creatine kinase (CPK).
  - Increased serum prolactin; hyponatremia, hypoglycemia, and anemia (with normal or increased mean corpuscular volume).

MEDICAL MANAGEMENT & TREATMENT

GENERAL MEASURES

- The main goal is to restore and maintain the euthyroid state.
- The diet is modified to avoid constipation mainly by including plenty of high-fiber foods. Also, a low-fat diet may be required for the obese.
- Patient activities are as tolerated.
- Patient education is most important and should stress compliance with medications, adhering to dietary restrictions, and regular follow-up examinations with the primary care physician.

PHARMACOLOGIC

- Levothyroxine (thyroxine, T4) is the treatment of choice:
  - Levothyroxine (Synthroid, Levothroid): 50 to 100 µg/day initially; increase by 25 µg/day every 4 to 6 weeks until TSH levels are in the normal range.
    - In most cases, significant increases in serum T4 levels are seen within 1 to 2 weeks and near maximum levels are seen within 3 to 4 weeks.
    - There is no standardized optimal dose of levothyroxine; so each patient's dose must be based upon careful clinical assessment. Most patients ultimately require 100 to 200 µg daily.
    - It is important to stress to the patient that levothyroxine therapy must be continued for life (in almost all cases) and that regular periodic dosage reassessments will be required.

COMPLICATIONS

- Myxedema (myxedematous) heart disease:
  - In severe, primary hypothyroidism, the heart becomes enlarged due to dilation and pericardial effusion, with consequent electrocardiographic changes.
  - It regresses over several months after initiating thyroid hormone therapy.
- Myxedema (myxedematous) coma:
  - A life-threatening complication of uncontrolled hypothyroidism with a high mortality rate
  - Patients have severe manifestations of hypothyroidism (bradycardia and severe hypotension are invariably present), as well as impaired mentation; hypothermia, hyponatremia, and hypoglycemia are often present.
  - It can be precipitated by exposure to cold (particularly in winter), infection, trauma, surgery, or administration of CNS depressants.

PROGNOSIS

- Hypothyroidism generally carries a good prognosis if treated early. A return to the normal state can usually be expected. However, if compliance is poor or treatment is interrupted, relapse will occur. If left untreated, it may progress to myxedema and coma.

DENTAL SIGNIFICANCE

- Oral findings associated with hypothyroidism can include:
  - Macroglossia (seen in approximately 80% of patients with untreated hypothyroidism)
  - Dysgeusia
  - Delayed eruption of teeth (in children and adolescents)
  - Poor periodontal health
    - Overtreatment of hypothyroidism over long periods can lead to bone demineralization.
  - Delayed wound healing
- Patients with undiagnosed, untreated, or poorly controlled hypothyroidism may represent a significant risk for dental treatment, primarily due to:
  - The increased risk of myxedematous coma as a result of acute oral infections, surgical dental treatment, or administration of CNS depressants (e.g., sedatives, narcotic analgesics)
  - Delayed metabolism of CNS depressants resulting in an exaggerated, prolonged effect

DENTAL MANAGEMENT

HISTORY AND PHYSICAL ASSESSMENT

- Establish the specific diagnosis of hypothyroidism (e.g., postablative).
- Determine/record present medication(s).
- Perform an assessment of the patient's current clinical status, including:
  - Symptoms of persistent hypothyroidism (or iatrogenic hyperthyroidism due to excessive dose of thyroid hormone replacement therapy).
  - Presence of any concurrent cardiovascular disease, since patients with hypothyroidism are at increased risk for cardiovascular disease from arteriosclerosis and elevated LDL, as well as congestive heart failure in the form of myxedematous heart disease.
    - If present, make applicable modifications to dental treatment as indicated.
  - Confirm normal physical evaluation and thyroid function tests (e.g., TSH) within the past 6 to 12 months.
- Dental treatment should be deferred if the patient presents with:
  - An unreliable or vague history of thyroid disease and management; or
  - Neglect to follow physician-initiated control of thyroid disease for more than 6 to 12 months; or
  - Signs and symptoms of undiagnosed or persistent hypothyroidism, which would require appropriate medical referral.

DENTAL TREATMENT CONSIDERATIONS

- Patients with well-controlled hypothyroidism (i.e., asymptomatic with physical and thyroid function tests within normal limits and long-standing, stable dosage of thyroid hormone replacement therapy) require no special precautions for routine or emergent dental treatment in the absence of other concurrent medical problems.
  - During treatment of diagnosed and medicated patients who have hypothyroidism, attention should focus on lethargy, which can indicate an uncontrolled state and become a risk for patients (for example, aspiration of dental materials), and respiratory rate.
- For patients with undiagnosed, untreated, or poorly controlled hypothyroidism:
  - Elective (nonemergent) dental treatment should be deferred until disease is controlled and patient is euthyroid.
  - During treatment, the dentist should remain observant to increasing lethargy in the patient, which can become a risk for complications (e.g., aspiration of dental materials), bradycardia, and decreased respiratory rate.
    - Intraoperative monitoring of vital signs and blood oxygen saturation during dental treatment would be most beneficial.
  - Surgical dental procedures should be avoided since they may precipitate myxedematous coma.
  - Acute orofacial infections may precipitate myxedematous coma and should be treated aggressively, including appropriate antibiotic therapy.
  - No significant immunosuppression per se; total and differential WBC counts and function are usually normal. However, there can be a cardiovascular decrease in blood flow to the tissues and poor glycemic control, which may cause delayed healing and heightened susceptibility to infections.
    - The use of perioperative prophylactic antibiotics (see Appendix A, Box A-2, "Presurgical and Postsurgical Antibiotic Prophylaxis for Patients at Increased Risk for Postoperative Infections") may be indicated if invasive dental procedures are necessary.
  - Establish profound local anesthesia. There are no contraindications to the use of local anesthesia containing vasoconstrictor (in the absence of other concurrent medical problems).
  - Delayed metabolism of CNS depressants (e.g., sedatives, narcotic analgesics) can result in an exaggerated, prolonged effect; therefore, a dose reduction and/or increased dose interval of these medications may be necessary.

SUGGESTED REFERENCES

Dillman WH. The thyroid, in Goldman L, Ausiello D (eds): *Cecil Textbook of Medicine*, ed 22. Philadelphia, WB Saunders, 2004, pp 1402–1405.

Jameson JL, Weetman AP. Disorders of the thyroid gland, in Kasper DI, et al. (eds): *Harrison's Principles of Internal Medicine*, ed 16. New York, McGraw-Hill, 2005, pp 2109–2113.

Pinto A, Glick M. Management of patients with thyroid disease: oral health considerations. *JADA* 2002;133:849–858.

Surks MI. Hypothyroidism. Uptodate Online 13.2, updated 5 January 2005, http://www.uptodateonline.com/application/topic.asp?file=thyroid/18640&type=A&selected Title=1^196

AUTHORS: **F. JOHN FIRRIOLO, DDS, PHD; JAMES R. HUPP, DMD, MD, JD, MBA**

SYNONYM(S)

ITP
Immune thrombocytopenic purpura
Autoimmune thrombocytopenic purpura

ICD-9CM/CPT CODE(S)

287.3 Idiopathic thrombocytopenic purpura

OVERVIEW

Idiopathic thrombocytopenic purpura (ITP) is a hematologic, immune-mediated disease characterized by decreased platelet count and mucocutaneous hemorrhage.

EPIDEMIOLOGY & DEMOGRAPHICS

INCIDENCE/PREVALENCE IN USA: Prevalence of 5 to 10 per 100,000 persons. Incidence of 100 per 1,000,000 persons per year.
PREDOMINANT AGE: Children and persons younger than 40 years of age. More than two-thirds of patients lie within this age range.
PREDOMINANT SEX: Young children have equal female to male distribution. This number increases to more than 70% being female in cases older than 10 years of age.
GENETICS: Some genotypes have been linked to expression of antibodies against the GPIIb/IIIa complex. Interleukin polymorphisms have been linked to severity of ITP.

ETIOLOGY & PATHOGENESIS

ITP is an autoimmune bleeding disorder characterized by the development of autoantibodies to platelet membrane antigens, resulting in the destruction of platelets by phagocytosis in the spleen and, to a lesser extent, in the liver.

CLINICAL PRESENTATION / PHYSICAL FINDINGS

- Physical findings may be absent at time of examination.
- Severe thrombocytopenia presents with mucosal or skin petechiae, purpura, epistaxis, or heme-containing stool.
- Congenital disorders might have ITP as a clinical feature.
- Children often present with sudden appearance of bruising and petechiae.

- Less evident onset of disease in adults; history of prolonged purpura or incidental finding.
- ITP rarely presents with splenic enlargement.

DIAGNOSIS

- CBC with platelet count.
- Peripheral smear.
- Assessment of platelet autoantibodies.
- In the presence of splenomegaly, imaging studies will rule out other causes.

MEDICAL MANAGEMENT & TREATMENT

- Medical follow-up in asymptomatic patients.
- Platelet transfusion in severe hemorrhage.
- High dose corticosteroids (methylprednisolone or prednisone) are given with immunoglobulin in emergency situations. For patients with counts less than 20,000/mm³, tapered dosing of corticosteroid (1 to 2 mg/kg qd) or immunoglobulin (IgG 0.4g/kg/day on 3 to 5 consecutive days) can be used.
- Splenectomy in adults with platelet counts less than 30,000/mm³ if refractory to treatment or after more than 6 weeks therapy with steroids with minimal response. Recommended in pediatrics if child is older than 1 year and significant risk of bleeding.
- Immune monoclonal therapy (i.e., Rituximab) has been used in recalcitrant cases.
- Chemotherapy has been used in chronic cases.

COMPLICATIONS

- Thrombocytopenia will cause severe bleeding.
- Intracranial hemorrhage is the primary cause of death.

PROGNOSIS

- Favorable with close medical follow-up:
  - Children: more than 80% of have a complete remission within a few weeks.

- Adults: the course of the disease is chronic, and only 5% of adults have spontaneous remission.

DENTAL SIGNIFICANCE

- Oral mucosal diathesis can be the presenting symptom.
- Significant hemostatic challenge for oral surgical procedures.

DENTAL MANAGEMENT

- Monitor mucosal hemorrhage.
- Evaluate platelet count prior to dental treatment:
  - Elective dental treatment should be deferred if platelet count is less than 50,000 mm³.
  - Emergency dental treatment will require hospital admission and platelet transfusion and/or immunoglobulin infusion.
  - Consult physician in chronic cases or when platelet count is less than 50,000 mm³.
  - Utilize adjunctive measures to achieve primary hemostasis [e.g., pressure, absorbable gelatin sponges (Gelfoam®), oxidized cellulose (SURGICEL™), microfibrillar collagen (Avitene®), topical thrombin tranexamic acid, epsilon-aminocaproic acid (EACA), sutures, and surgical splints and stents].

SUGGESTED REFERENCES

Cines DB, McMillan R. Management of adult idiopathic thrombocytopenic purpura. *Annu Rev Med* 2005;56:425–442.
Kojouri K, George JN. Recent advances in the treatment of chronic refractory immune thrombocytopenic purpura. *Int J Hematol* 2005;81:119–125.
Vaisman B, Medina AC, Ramirez G. Dental treatment for children with chronic idiopathic thrombocytopaenic purpura: a report of two cases. *Int J Paediatr Dent* 2004;14:355–362.
Wilmott RW. Rituximab for ITP in children. *J Pediatr* 2005;146:A2.

AUTHOR: ANDRES PINTO, DMD

SYNONYM(S)
SIADH

Type 3B euvolemic hyponatremia

ICD-9CM/CPT CODE(S)
276.9 Electrolyte and fluid disorders not elsewhere classified—complete

276.1 Hyposmolality and/or hyponatremia—complete

253.6 Other disorders of neurohypophysis—complete

OVERVIEW

Syndrome of inappropriate antidiuretic hormone secretion (SIADH) is defined as the primary form of euvolemic hyponatremia. It is characterized by continued antidiuretic hormone (ADH) release even though the plasma osmolality is below normal. Vasopressin release continues in the absence of osmotic or nonosmotic stimuli.

EPIDEMIOLOGY & DEMOGRAPHICS

INCIDENCE/PREVALENCE IN USA: Nearly 50% of hyponatremia cases detected in a hospital setting are caused by SIADH.

PREDOMINANT AGE: Not established.*

PREDOMINANT SEX: Not established.*

GENETICS: Not established.*

ETIOLOGY & PATHOGENESIS

- Vasopressin (AVP, antidiuretic hormone) is synthesized in the hypothalamus and secreted by the posterior pituitary in response to the increased osmotic pressure in bodily fluids. Normally, this is regulated by osmoreceptors in the hypothalamus that are very sensitive to changes in serum sodium. The release of vasopressin results in increased water reabsorption in the collecting tubules of the kidney.
- SIADH results from the inappropriate release of vasopressin; this is accompanied by the patient's intake exceeding sensible and insensible losses.
- The ADH release is not osmotically stimulated and results from many associated conditions that are outlined in Box 1–1. Thus, increased intake of free

---

*Some very limited epidemiology can be found in the literature that examines specific associated conditions of SIADH, but the epidemiology research is limited, even when looking at subpopulations within the disease. Specific studies to determine the prevalence and incidence of SIADH could be an area of future research. The authors can only hypothesize that the lack of epidemiology in the literature is due to the extensive number of associated conditions and that SIADH is a diagnosis of exclusion.

water above excreted free water leads to further dilution and extracellular volume expansion. This extracellular expansion stimulates suppression of plasma renin activity and an increase in atrial natriuretic hormone, which increases sodium excretion. This leads to exacerbation of the hyponatremia because the urine is inappropriately high in sodium content. Therefore, the hyponatremia in SIADH is due to an increase in total body water and a decrease in total body sodium.

- In a subtype of SIADH, reset osmostat, ADH (vasopressin) remains responsive to changes in the plasma osmolality, but the set point for release of ADH is abnormally low.

CLINICAL PRESENTATION / PHYSICAL FINDINGS

- Clinical features of SIADH are the same as the features of hyponatremia. The more rapid the onset of hyponatremia, the more dramatic is the presentation of the symptoms.
- The commonly recognized signs and symptoms of hyponatremia include:
  o Mild to moderate: malaise, mild headache, confusion, nausea, vomiting, anorexia, and muscle cramps.
  o Severe (Na$^+$ < 120 mmol/L): confusion, seizures, coma, and death.
- Most often the patient is asymptomatic, and hyponatremia is discovered on a routine serum chemistry panel.
- The volume status of the patient should be euvolemic with no history of CHF, cirrhosis, or nephrosis.
- There should not be signs of cortisol deficiency or hypothyroidism.

DIAGNOSIS

SIADH is a diagnosis of exclusion. Many criteria must be met for a diagnosis of SIADH to be reached.

- Serum sodium below 136 mmol/L.
- Patient has normal renal, thyroid, adrenal, and cardiac function.
- Triglycerides and glucose are normal.
- The urine osmolality must be greater than that of the serum osmolality and must demonstrate excessive sodium excretion (greater than 20 mEq/L in the presence of hyponatremia).
- Plasma levels of ADH can be elevated or inappropriately normal. Unfortunately, due to variability of ADH levels they are of little diagnostic value.
- Patient must be determined to be euvolemic.
- In cases of head trauma or intracranial disease, SIADH must be differentiated from cerebral salt wasting syndrome. The key to differentiating the two entities is volume status. Cerebral salt

wasting syndrome results in a hypovolemic state. Orthostatic blood pressure measurement or central venous pressures can estimate volume status clinically.

MEDICAL MANAGEMENT & TREATMENT

- In patients where an intracranial process or head trauma is the cause of hyponatremia, the first step is to confirm euvolemic volume status. This is especially important because cerebral salt wasting syndrome is frequently confused with SIADH. The treatment of cerebral salt wasting syndrome consists of sodium supplementation and hydration, but treatment for SIADH usually centers on fluid restriction.
- After confirmation of volume status, treatment for SIADH is broken into three groups: mild to moderate, severe, and reset osmostat.
- Mild to moderate cases are treated by restricting fluid intake to less than urine output. A fluid restriction of 1000 to 1500 mL/day will usually correct the hyponatremia. If a 500 mL/day fluid deficit can be reached, then the serum sodium will usually be corrected at a rate of 1–2% per day.
- If fluid restriction fails, then an antibiotic (demeclocycline) is usually the first-line drug used. Demeclocycline acts on the collecting tubule. A dose of 150 to 300 mg is given q6/8h and titrated to effect. The main side effects are phototoxicity and azothemia.
- Lithium also acts on the collecting tubule. It should be considered when the patient exhibits a bipolar diagnosis in addition to SIADH. Renal function should be monitored with both lithium and demeclocycline.
- A third pharmacologic treatment is flurocortisone 0.05 to 0.2 mg q12h. This therapy corrects hyponatremia partially but at the risk of causing edema and congestive heart failure.
- All pharmacologic treatments take 1 to 2 weeks for improvement to show.
- Severe cases are considered to be those cases that have serum sodium less than 120 mmol/L and significant neurological manifestations. These cases are managed in an ICU setting. Intravenous infusion of 3% saline can be considered, but hypertonic saline should be used with caution. Hypertonic saline cannot be infused at a rate of greater than 0.05 mL/kg of body weight/min. Stat sodium levels should be obtained every 2 hours, and once the sodium is corrected to 125 mmol/L, the infusion should be stopped imme-

diately. More rapid correction than the previously mentioned guidelines can result in central pontine myelinolysis. Some practitioners also administer furosemide concurrently with the hypertonic saline infusion.

- In addition to treating the hyponatremia induced by SIADH, the underlying cause should be determined and treated, if possible.
- Reset osmostat is a unique form of SIADH. Attempts at correcting the sodium in these patients are difficult and often futile. With fluid restriction, patients with reset osmostat will be extremely thirsty. Since the hyponatremia is usually mild and the patients are asymptomatic, attempts at water restriction are unnecessary. Treatment should be directed at the underlying cause, if identified.

COMPLICATIONS

- Central pontine myelinolysis occurs when chronic hyponatremia is corrected too rapidly. The complication is potentially fatal and is characterized by abnormal extraocular movements, dysphagia, facial weakness, ataxia, and quadriparesis.
- In cases of increased intracranial pressure, it is imperative to differentiate SIADH from cerebral salt wasting syndrome. Fluid restriction in a patient with cerebral salt wasting syndrome can result in sharp drops in blood pressure resulting in an inadequate cerebral perfusion pressure, which can lead to infarction of brain tissue.
- Rapid hyponatremia can cause intracranial hypertension and brain damage as well as the symptoms of acute hyponatremia.

PROGNOSIS

- Greatly depends on the underlying cause.
- As seen in Box I-1, there are many causes of SIADH but many are self-limiting.
- Most infections can be treated pharmacologically; as a result, the SIADH will be naturally self-limiting.
- When drug reactions cause SIADH, severity of the hyponatremia has to be assessed. Sometimes it is possible to select a different drug to achieve the same disease-modifying outcome. When no alternative therapies are available, then the severity of hyponatremia needs to be considered vs the drug benefit.
- Regardless of the cause, treating SIADH can be challenging. This is due to side effects from pharmacologic

treatment and the difficulty of patient compliance with fluid restriction.

DENTAL SIGNIFICANCE

- SIADH itself has no impact on oral health, but known conditions associated with SIADH can have a direct impact on the oral cavity. Some examples are AIDS, Ewing's sarcoma, and antidepressant drugs.

DENTAL MANAGEMENT

- Dental management and impact of this disease are limited. SIADH should be kept in the differential diagnosis when signs and symptoms of hyponatremia are present. Patient exhibiting mild hyponatremic signs should be referred to an internal medicine physician for

management; a full medical workup should be performed to determine the underlying cause. Patients with signs and symptoms of more severe hyponatremia should be hospitalized.

- A detailed history and sodium trends are helpful to assess for symptoms and establish the time frame for the development of SIADH.
- The seizure threshold is lowered as the sodium levels get farther from normal and with increased rapidity of hyponatremia. The dentist should try to limit or avoid the use of medications that will further reduce the seizure threshold when treating patients with hyponatremia.
- In patients with increased intracranial pressure, neurology or neurosurgery clearance for dental treatment should be obtained. Operative procedures should be delayed until there is no risk

---

BOX I-1 SIADH-Associated Conditions

Neurologic
- Cerebrovascular accident, hemorrhagic or occlusive
- Multiple sclerosis
- Cavernous sinus thrombosis
- Amyotrophic lateral sclerosis
- Hydrocephalus
- Psychosis
- Delirium tremens
- Seizures
- Guillain-Barré syndrome
- Peripheral neuropathies
- Chronic nausea and vomiting
- Head trauma

Lung
- Positive pressure ventilation
- Pneumothorax
- Asthma
- Chronic obstructive pulmonary disease

Infection
- Lung infections/disease
- AIDS
- Brain infections

Cancer
- Lung
- Brain
- Pancreas
- Duodenum
- Urologic
- Ovary
- Ewing's sarcoma
- Carcinoid
- Thymoma

Drugs
- Antidepressive medications
- Nicotine
- Thiazide diuretics
- Narcotics
- Chemotherapeutics

Surgery
- Pituitary
- Major abdominal
- Thoracic

for increasing intracranial pressure to levels that could result in damage of neural tissue.

- SIADH is often associated with a known underlying condition. Consultation with the patient's physician for management of the condition in the dental setting should be obtained. The physician can also provide the dentist with a more detailed history of the present illness than is likely to be obtained from the patient.

- SIADH should always be included in the differential diagnosis of electrolyte disturbances in patients who have incurred facial and head trauma.

SUGGESTED REFERENCES

Albanese A, et al. Management of hyponatremia in patients with acute cerebral insults. *Arch Dis Childhood* 2001;85: 246–251.

Causes of Hyponatremia: Rose, B: www.uptodate.com

Haralampos M, et al. The hyponatremic patient: a systematic approach to laboratory diagnosis. *Canadian Medical Association Journal* 2002;166(8).

Singer G, Brenner R. Fluid and electrolyte disturbances, in Kasper DI, et al. (eds): *Harrison's Principles of Internal Medicine*, ed 16. New York, McGraw-Hill, 2005, pp 252–263.

Singh S, et al. Cerebral salt wasting truths, fallacies, theories, and challenges. *Critical Care Medicine* 2002;30:2575–2579.

Treatment of Hyponatremia: SIADH and Reset Osmostat. Rose, B: www.uptodate.com

Urine Output in the SIADH: Rose, B: www.uptodate.com

AUTHORS: **DAVID C. STANTON, DMD, MD; PAUL MADLOCK, DMD, MD**

SYNONYM(S)

Histiocytosis X
Langerhans cell disease
Idiopathic histiocytosis
Eosinophilic granuloma
Hand-Schüller-Christian syndrome
Letterer-Siwe disease

ICD-9CM/CPT CODE(S)

202.5   Letterer-Siwe disease—incomplete
277.89   Other specified disorders of metabolism

OVERVIEW

Langerhans cell histiocytosis (LCH) is a disorder that is distinguished by a neoplastic proliferation of cells that have the characteristics of the antigen-presenting and -processing Langerhans cell (LC), resulting in a varied clinical presentation ranging from single lesions of bone to multiple skin, bone, and visceral lesions that can be debilitating.

EPIDEMIOLOGY & DEMOGRAPHICS

INCIDENCE/PREVALENCE IN USA: Incidence of LCH can be divided into pediatric and adult populations. LCH in children (newborn to 18 years old) has an incidence of 3 to 5 cases per million. The incidence of LCH in adults is approximately 1 to 2 cases per million.

PREDOMINANT AGE: LCH as a whole is much more common in children, with roughly 75% of all cases presenting in children prior to 10 years old. In pediatric cases, the most common age is between 5 and 10 years old. In adults, the mean age is 32 years old, with the presenting ages ranging from 21 to 69 years old.

PREDOMINANT SEX: Significant male predominance. One large series of 211 patients shows a male:female ratio of 3:1, but this data may be biased as it is from the U.S. armed forces.

GENETICS: Specific associations of LCH and HLA types have been noted. Cw7 and DR4 HLA types are more prevalent in Caucasians with a solitary bone lesion, possibly indicating these patients are at an increased risk for single LCH lesions. There have also been reports of chromosomal instability in multisystem LCH disease. However, to date there are no gene abnormalities that account for these findings.

ETIOLOGY & PATHOGENESIS

- The etiology of LCH is still unknown. The controversy as to the exact etiology is reflected in the various names applied to diseases with the same histopathologic features (see Synonyms).

- The current nomenclature for the disease, Langerhans cell histiocytosis, reflects the consensus on etiology reached by the Histiocyte Society in 1987. The disease is felt to be neoplastic, given that the cells of the disease are of a single, clonal proliferation (all CD1a positive).

- There have been efforts supporting a viral etiology, specifically human herpes virus 6 (HHV-6). However, the studies purporting this link do not consider the significant possibility that the herpes viruses present in LCH are merely a reactivation of a previous herpes infection. This is particularly significant given that an immunologic disease such as LCH could cause this reactivation. As such, the etiological link between HHV-6 and LCH is very rudimentary.

- The LC is an important, efficient antigen-presenting cell in the normally functioning immune system. In LCH, the cell is abnormal and immature and presents antigens poorly.

- The LC also increases significantly in number in LCH. Because they are all of a single clonality, this favors a neoplastic etiology over a polyclonal, reactive etiology.

- The immunologic malfunction due to LCH is thought to be caused by high levels of cytokines. GM-GSF, IL-1, IL-10, and γ-interferon are all produced in high levels by the LC.

- It has been proposed that IL-10 and transforming growth factor (TGF)-β are responsible for the immature LC, as cells have a more mature phenotype when IL-10 production is decreased in their cellular environment.

CLINICAL PRESENTATION / PHYSICAL FINDINGS

- Childhood LCH
  - LCH in children generally presents in one of three forms: single-site, low-risk patient; multisystem disease with high-risk organ involvement; and special sites such as temporal, sphenoid, ethmoid, or orbital bones.
  - LCH with involvement at a single site most commonly presents with lesions of bone, skin, or lymph nodes.
  - Infants can present with dark papules over any portion of the body. This sign is benign and should dissipate with no treatment within the first year.
  - Red, papular rash in the abdomen, chest, back, or groin may appear and ulcerative lesions of the scalp and perineal region are concerning. These lesions may resemble fungal or bacterial infections and, if inappropriately treated, may delay diagnosis of LCH.
  - Intraoral lesions may include ulceration of the buccal mucosa, palate, and lips and tongue.

  - Bone lesions are most commonly lytic skull lesions, although they may appear in any bone of the body (see Figure I-1, A and B).
  - Lymph node lesions usually involve the cervical lymph nodes but can involve mediastinal nodes as well.
  - Multisystem disease generally involves the higher-risk lesions of the liver, spleen, lungs, or some combination thereof. Bone marrow, GI organs, and CNS involvement can occur as well.
  - Liver lesions and enlargement can be accompanied by dysfunction and associated problems such as clotting deficiencies and ascites.
  - Splenomegaly can lead to hypersplenism and cytopenias.
  - Pulmonary involvement is much less common in children than adults, and smoking is a key factor. Widespread fibrosis and destruction of lung tissue can lead to symptoms such as tachypnea, dyspnea, and severe pulmonary disease.

- Adult LCH
  - Presenting symptoms may be skin rash, dyspnea, tachycardia, polydipsia or polyuria, bone pain, lymphadenopathy, or systemic symptoms such as fever or weight loss.
  - Patient may present with isolated diabetes insipidus (15% of patients with isolated DI had LCH).
  - Patients may have skin and oral lesions similar to children's lesions mentioned previously. Pain in the jaw or loosening of teeth can be a presenting symptom.
  - The primary site of bone involvement in adults is the skull or jaw bones.
  - Pulmonary LCH is more common in males and is significantly associated with smoking. Patients usually present with cough or dyspnea. Chest pain could signal a spontaneous pneumothorax.

DIAGNOSIS

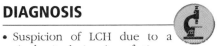

- Suspicion of LCH due to a single-site lesion in soft tissue or bone or in multiorgan disease where the patient presents with pulmonary symptoms or symptoms of liver/spleen dysfunction should have a fairly comprehensive workup to identify other sites of disease.
- Skeletal survey in facial bone/skull plain films, bone scan, and CXR are good frontline imaging exams.
- CBC with differential, liver function tests and erythrocyte sedimentation rate should be evaluated for cytopenias and hepatic abnormalities.
- Bone marrow aspirate and biopsy, stained for CD1a glycoprotein cell membrane antigen, should be performed.

- Urinalysis, serum electrolyte panel, and free water restriction test should be performed if diabetes insipidus is suspected.
- Biopsy of suspicious lesions with staining for CD1a glycoprotein cell membrane antigen (which is specific for LCH) and S100 proteins (which is nonspecific but usually positive) is needed to confirm the diagnosis of LCH.
- Identification of Birbeck granules (characteristic of LC) with electron microscopy is only performed when the diagnosis is in question, as this is time-consuming and costly but is pathognomonic for LCH.

MEDICAL MANAGEMENT & TREATMENT

- Treatment of this disease is still being developed through research and clinical trials.
- Single-site, low-risk lesions may have therapy consisting of prednisone alone, some combination of chemotherapeutic agents (velban) and prednisone, or surgical curettage of lesions in bone.
- Multisystem disease does not respond to prednisone alone, and patients will commonly relapse. These patients typically receive velban and prednisone for extended periods of up to 1 year.

- Multisystem disease with high-risk organ involvement requires extensive chemotherapy with multiple agents over longer periods of time.
- Radiation therapy is no longer used except in cases of lesions of the vertebrae or femoral neck. It can also be used in cases of bone lesions that are surgically inaccessible or those that have recurred despite surgical intervention.
- Some studies suggest that in severe disease bone marrow transplantation can be helpful while the patient is in remission.
- Of most significance is that single drug therapy is ineffective in patients with multiple bone lesions.

COMPLICATIONS

- Pediatric patients with single-site disease generally complete treatment with no complications other than side-effects from chronic steroid use.
- Pediatric patients with diabetes insipidus should be monitored for panhypopituitarism.
- Pulmonary disease can result in decreased pulmonary function chronically, predisposing the patient at risk for infection.

- Hepatic involvement can sometimes cause ascending cholangitis amenable only to the orthotopic liver transplant.
- LCH patients have a higher than average risk of developing a secondary malignancy such as acute myeloid leukemia or lymphoma.

PROGNOSIS

- Prognosis in general is very good because of the slow progression of LCH combined with the usually excellent response to therapy.
- Patients with single-site involvement or even multisite involvement without risk organ involvement generally have greater than 90% survival rates.
- If chemotherapeutics and prednisone are used for 1 year or more, recurrence is less than 20%.
- Pediatric patients with high-risk organ involvement and lack of rapid response (within 6 weeks) to treatment have a mortality rate approaching 70%.
- The majority of life-threatening and refractory cases involve the lungs.
- Developing multisystem disease after initial presentation with a single site is very rare.
- Long-term follow-up is helpful for surveillance of recurrence.

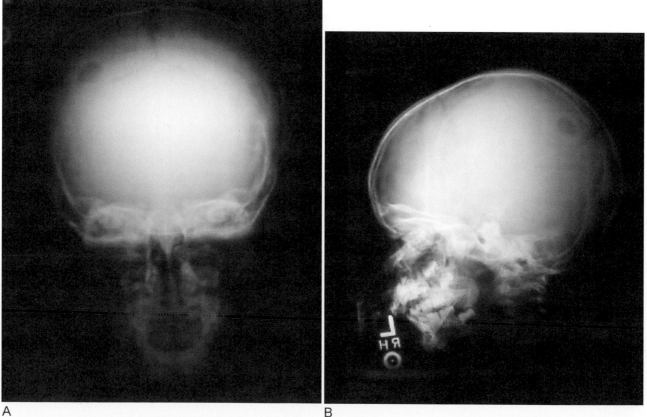

A   B

FIGURE I-1. **A,** PA and **B,** lateral skull films demonstrating a solitary, "punched-out" radiolucency.

DENTAL SIGNIFICANCE

- Single-site LCH can involve the oral cavity in 10–20% of cases, usually with a posterior mandibular lesion.
- May present with mild pain, ulceration of mucosal tissue, periodontal inflammation, mobility of teeth due to alveolar bone loss, or bony expansion.
- Radiographically presents as a radiolucent lesion around or under the tooth roots. The lesion may involve several teeth and appear as a focal area of periodontal disease, where the teeth appear to be floating (Figure I-2).
- This lesion may appear to be an odontogenic cyst, tumor, or osteomyelitis.

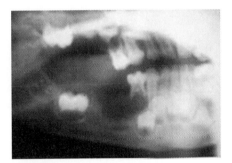

FIGURE I-2. Portion of a Panorex demonstrating the "floating teeth" appearance resultant from jaw radiolucencies from LCH.

- Presentation of a child with loose teeth and alveolar bone loss should alert the practitioner to a differential diagnosis of juvenile periodontitis, LCH, acute lymphocytic leukemia, osteomyelitis, or an odontogenic tumor, as well as malignant disease such as osteosarcoma or fibrosarcoma.

DENTAL MANAGEMENT

- If LCH is being considered as a diagnosis, diagnostic evaluation should be performed in conjunction with a pediatric hematologist.
- Presentation suspicious for LCH requires biopsy, including removal of involved teeth. The pathologist should be alerted that LCH is on the differen-

tial diagnosis; so special stains (CD1a, S100) may be performed.
- For accessible lesions of the facial skeleton, aggressive surgical curettage is the treatment of choice.
- Inaccessible lesions of the skull are treated with low-dose radiotherapy (1400 to 1800 cGy).

SUGGESTED REFERENCES

Hartman KS. Histiocytosis X: a review of 114 cases with oral involvement. *Oral Surg Oral Med Oral Pathol* 1980;49:38.

Henry RJ, Sweeney EA. Langerhans' cell histiocytosis: case reports and literature review. *Pediatr Dent* 1996;18:11.

Histiocytosis Association of America: www.histio.org.

Howarth DM, Gilchrist GS, Mullan BP, et al. Langerhans cell histiocytosis: diagnosis, natural history, management, and outcome. *Cancer* 1999;85:2278.

AUTHORS: **DAVID C. STANTON, DMD, MD; MICHAEL C. MISTRETTA, DDS, MD**

SYNONYM(S)

Acute lymphoblastic leukemia (ALL): lymphoid leukemia

Acute myelogenous leukemia (AML): acute nonlymphoblastic leukemia (ANLL); acute nonlymphocytic leukemia; acute myeloid leukemia (AML)

Chronic myelocytic leukemia (CML): chronic granulocytic leukemia; chronic myeloid leukemia

Chronic lymphocytic leukemia (CLL)

Hairy cell leukemia (HCL): leukemic reticuloendotheliosis

ICD-9CM/CPT CODE(S)

202.4 Hairy cell leukemia
204 Lymphoid leukemia (includes lymphatic, lymphoblastic, lymphocytic, lymphogenous)
204.0 Lymphoid leukemia, acute
204.1 Lymphoid leukemia, chronic
205 Myeloid leukemia (includes granulocytic, myeloblastic, myelocytic, myelogenous, myelosclerotic)
205.0 Myeloid leukemia, acute
205.1 Myeloid leukemia, chronic
206 Monocytic leukemia (includes histiocytic, monoblastic, monocytoid)
206.0 Monocytic leukemia, acute
206.1 Monocytic leukemia, chronic
207 Other specified leukemia
208 Leukemia of unspecified cell type

OVERVIEW

Leukemia is a cancer that begins in blood-forming tissue (such as the bone marrow) and causes large numbers of blood cells to be produced and enter the bloodstream, often infiltrating the spleen, liver, and lymph nodes. Acute leukemia is characterized by proliferation of immature cells called blasts. Chronic leukemia is a proliferation of mature-appearing cells in the marrow, peripheral blood, and various organs.

For decades, leukemia has been broadly categorized by cell of origin and clinical course, as shown in Figure I-3. However, more sophisticated and current classification systems identify leukemias based on morphology, cytochemistry, and immunophenotype as well as cytogenetic and molecular techniques.

More recently, the World Health Organization (WHO) introduced an updated classification of hematologic malignancies including tumors, lymphoid, myeloid, histiocytic, and dendritic cell lineages. The starting point of the disease definition is the cell origin. The classification system takes into account a constellation of morphologic, clinical, and biologic features that make each disease a distinct entity.

EPIDEMIOLOGY & DEMOGRAPHICS

INCIDENCE/PREVALENCE IN USA: It is estimated that over 33,000 new cases of leukemia will be diagnosed in the U.S. this year. Acute leukemias occur more often than chronic leukemias. The most common forms of leukemia in adults are acute myelogenous leukemia (AML), with approximately 11,900 new cases annually, and chronic lymphocytic leukemia (CLL), with an estimated 8,200 new cases per year. Among children, acute lymphocytic leukemia (ALL) is more common.

PREDOMINANT AGE: Most cases of leukemia occur in older adults; more than half of all cases occur after age 67. In 2004, there were 11 times more cases of leukemia in adults than in children ages 0 to 19. Between the years of 1997 and 2001, leukemia comprised 25% of all cancers among children younger than 20 years. The incidence rates by age differ for each type of leukemia. The incident rates of AML, CML, and CLL increase dramatically among people who are over the age of 40. These forms of leukemia are most prevalent in the seventh, eighth, and ninth decades of life.

PREDOMINANT SEX: Overall, leukemia has a higher incidence among males than in females.

GENETICS: High concordance rate among identical twins if acute leukemia develops in the first year of life. Families with an excessive incidence of leukemia have been identified. Acute leukemia has increased frequency in several congenital disorders, including Down, Bloom, Klinefelter, Fanconi, and Aldrich syndromes.

ETIOLOGY & PATHOGENESIS

- Unknown in most patients, but both genetic and environmental factors are important.
- Ionizing radiation: individuals exposed to ionizing radiation, whether it be from the environment, occupational radiation exposure, or those receiving radiation therapy, and survivors of atomic bomb explosions have an increased risk of leukemia.
- Chemical and other exposures: exposure to chemicals such as benzene, alkylating agents, and other chemotherapeutic drugs is also associated with a higher incidence of AML.
- Viruses: RNA retroviruses have been implicated as an etiology for leukemias in animals. However, only adult T cell leukemia is caused by human T cell leukemia virus type I (HTLV-1). Epstein-Barr virus (EBV) has been associated with a form of ALL as well as other types of aggressive lymphomas.
- Other risk factors for leukemia are history of myelodysplastic syndrome and smoking.
- In acute leukemias, there is a clonal proliferation of immature hematopoietic cells. Specifically, there is a malignant transformation of a single hematopoietic progenitor, followed by abnormal cellular replication and clonal expansion. The neoplastic cells of acute leukemia fail to mature beyond the myeloblast or promyelocyte level in AML and the lym-

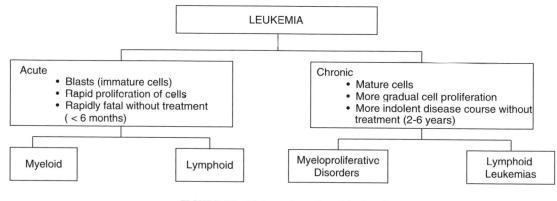

FIGURE I-3. Major categories of leukemia.

phoblast level in ALL. Leukemia cells continue to proliferate and accumulate in the bone marrow, suppressing normal hematopoiesis and ultimately replacing normal elements. This quickly leads to anemia, frequent infections, and bleeding complications that characterize the disease. Leukemic cells then begin to circulate in the blood and may eventually infiltrate tissues such as lymph nodes, liver, spleen, skin, gingiva, or the central nervous system (CNS), causing pain, swelling, and other problems.

- Chronic leukemias also result from clonal proliferation of early progenitor hematopoietic stem cells that may ultimately lead to bone marrow failure states. CML is associated with the Philadelphia chromosome and/or the *bcr/abl* fusion gene. It is characterized by three clinical phases. The first is the chronic phase that may last from 2 to 5 years, during which the disease is often indolent. When there is progression, it is called the accelerated phase, lasting from 6 to 18 months. Ultimately, blast crisis develops, which may behave like aggressive acute leukemia. In CLL there is an accumulation of neoplastic lymphocytes that results from abnormal or absent apoptosis. These neoplastic cells have prolonged survival and cause hypogammaglobulinemia and T cell dysfunction, which puts the patient at high risk for infections.

- Hairy cell leukemia (HCL) is thought to originate from peripheral B cells that display surface cytoplasmic "hairy" projections. These neoplastic B cells release tumor necrosis factor, which may inhibit hematopoiesis and result in cytopenias. About 2% of leukemia cases are of the hairy cell type, and it occurs predominantly in men (M:F = 4:1) between 40 and 60 years of age.

CLINICAL PRESENTATION / PHYSICAL FINDINGS

SIGNS AND SYMPTOMS OF ACUTE LEUKEMIAS

- Most often, patients with acute leukemia present with nonspecific symptoms that begin either gradually or abruptly. Some have symptoms for up to 3 months before receiving a diagnosis.
- Fatigue, weakness, anorexia, weight loss, and unexplained fevers are common complaints.
- Signs of acute leukemia include easy bruising or bleeding, paleness, fatigue, recurrent minor infections, and poor wound healing. Other signs may include lymphadenopathy, headache, or diaphoreses.

PHYSICAL FINDINGS IN ACUTE LEUKEMIAS

- Evidence of infection and hemorrhage are often found at the time of diagnosis

of acute leukemia. In addition, fever, hepatomegaly, splenomegaly, and sternal tenderness may occur. Infiltration of the gingiva, skin, soft tissues, or the meninges with leukemic blasts at diagnosis is characteristic of the monocytic subtypes of acute leukemia.

SIGNS AND SYMPTOMS OF CHRONIC LEUKEMIAS

- The clinical course of chronic leukemia is generally insidious.
- Signs and symptoms may not be present. Often, it may be diagnosed during a periodic medical examination.
- In those who are symptomatic, patients may complain of fatigue, malaise, and weight loss, or have upper left quadrant pain or early satiety resulting from enlargement of the spleen. Less commonly, patients may present with infections, thrombosis, or bleedings.
- Progression of CML is associated with worsening symptoms such as unexplained fever, weight loss, bone and joint pain, bleeding, thrombosis, and infections. Very few newly diagnosed patients with CML present with accelerated disease.

PHYSICAL FINDINGS IN CHRONIC LEUKEMIA

- Splenomegaly is the most common abnormal finding on physical examination. Occasionally, patients may have hepatomegaly. Lymphadenopathy and myeloid sarcoma may be found in later stages of chronic leukemia.

DIAGNOSIS

- When patients present with signs and symptoms of leukemia, physicians will take a detailed medical history.
- Physical examination may reveal hepatomegaly, splenomegaly, and lymphadenopathy.
- CBC with differential is usually abnormal with a very high WBC count. Anemias and other cytopenias are usually present. The acute leukemias may present with pancytopenia without circulating blasts, with a normal leukocyte count, or with marked leukocytosis. Thrombocytopenia is also a common finding in acute leukemia.
- Bone marrow biopsies are performed to help determine the type of leukemia. Both aspirate and solid bone marrow are examined. When leukemia is diagnosed, genetic studies are performed to further classify the disease.
- Other tests such as CT scans, MRI, and plain films may be used to determine the extent of the disease. Lumbar puncture is also performed to detect leukemia in the cerebrospinal fluid.

MEDICAL MANAGEMENT & TREATMENT

- Varies depending on the type.
- The most widely used therapy is chemotherapy, which is classically divided into phases of induction, consolidation, and maintenance. The first phase, induction, is administered with the goal of reducing leukemic cell mass to achieve a complete remission (CR). After remission is achieved, additional chemotherapy may be given to further reduce cell mass and, ideally, eradicate leukemia. This phase is referred to as consolidation. Maintenance is the third phase; it is generally continued over several years and is used to keep the number of leukemic cells low. The doses of chemotherapy during maintenance are lower than in the first two phases. Chemotherapy may be administered by IV, porta-cath (implanted port for central venous access), or intrathecally (into the cerebrospinal fluid).
- In acute leukemias, induction therapy is initiated as quickly as possible. Traditional chemotherapy agents used in AML include cytarabine and anthracyclines. These and other agents are administered based on patient age. Following induction, those who achieve CR undergo some form of consolidation therapy, including sequential courses of high-dose cytarabine, high-dose combination chemotherapy with allogeneic stem cell transplant (SCT), or novel therapies, based on their predicted risk of relapse. Treatment of ALL incorporates a multitude of drugs into regimen-specific sequences of increased dose and time intensity. Almost all patients who achieve remission are given prophylactic chemotherapy to the CNS to prevent leukemic meningitis, since it is the initial site of relapse in up to two-thirds of patients with ALL who do not receive prophylactic therapy. SCT is usually recommended for patients with features of poor prognosis at presentation.
- Chronic leukemia treatment can vary based on the goals of therapy for each individual patient. Goals can range from cure, to improved survival and quality of life, to disease palliation and comfort measures. In CML, the principal goal is to eliminate cellular clones. Hydroxyurea is typically used to manage the chronic phase of the disease. More recently, STI571 (imatinib) and interferon-α have been used for therapy. SCT is also standard therapy for CML with curative potential, although it is associated with significant transplant-related mortality and morbidity.

Individuals with CLL may require no treatment initially. Therapy is indicated when patients develop systemic symptoms, worsening anemia, and/or thrombocytopenia. If treatment is indicated, chemotherapeutic agents such as chlorambucil, cyclophosphamide, vincristine, prednisone, and purine analogues may be used. SCT may also be considered. HCL may be treated with splenectomy and later interferon-α. Recently, pentostatin and cladribine have been found to be effective in achieving long-term remissions.

- Alternative therapy for leukemia may include the use of biological therapeutic agents. In AML and CLL, individuals may receive a monoclonal antibody that targets leukemic cells. Selective drug delivery systems can improve efficacy of the medication and reduce systemic toxicity. Radiation therapy is another treatment used occasionally in some types of leukemia. Radiation can target the brain, bones, or spleen, killing both normal and malignant cells.
- SCT may be used in conjunction with high-dose chemotherapy for treatment of many types of leukemia. High doses of chemotherapy and occasionally total body radiation are followed by transplantation of normal stem cells, rescuing the patient from otherwise lethal myelosuppression. Stem cells may be harvested during remission and used for an autologous SCT, or they may be used from a related or unrelated donor, referred to as allogeneic SCT.

COMPLICATIONS

Complications may be caused either by the disease itself or by the effects of therapy. Common complications related to leukemia are anemia and bleeding associated with thrombocytopenia. In certain types of leukemia, organomegaly (particularly splenomegaly) may increase the risk of infection.

Adverse effects of therapy are:
- Common chemotherapy side-effects, dependent on the type of agent and dosage administered:
  ○ Fatigue/malaise
  ○ Easy bruising
  ○ Hair loss
  ○ Infection
  ○ Nausea/vomiting
  ○ Mucositis
  ○ Infertility
  ○ Dysmenorrhea/amenorrhea
- Common radiation therapy side-effects, localized to the site where radiation is delivered:
  ○ Hair loss
  ○ Dermatitis
  ○ Nausea/vomiting

  ○ Anorexia
  ○ Infertility
- Common effects of stem cell transplant (SCT) are:
  ○ Infection
  ○ Bleeding
  ○ Graft vs host disease (GVHD)

GVHD may occur in patients who receive allogeneic SCT. In this condition, immunologically active donor cells react against the recipient's tissues, most often the liver, skin, and digestive tract. It can occur during the acute stage (within the first 100 days of the transplant) or during the chronic stage (between 3 to 12 months). Medications are administered to the patient to reduce the risk of GVHD

PROGNOSIS

In the past 40 years, the relative 5-year survival rate for patients with leukemia has nearly tripled. In 1960, the relative 5-year survival rate was 14% compared to 1995–2000, when the 5-year survival rate was 46%. Overall, the relative survival rates differ by type of leukemia, stage of patient at diagnosis, age, gender, race, chromosomal findings at diagnosis, and characteristics of leukemic cells. Table I-14 summarizes relative survival rates based on the type of leukemia.

In 2004, approximately 23,300 deaths were due to leukemia. Despite a significant decline in death rate for children below age 14, leukemia is responsible for more deaths than any other cancer among children under the age of 20.

DENTAL SIGNIFICANCE

- Leukemia patients may present with several complications involving the oral cavity. Protective response against oral microbes is lost. These patients are prone to gingival inflammation, periodontal destruction with attachment loss, and mucosal irritations, all of which are worsened by poor oral hygiene.
- Patients with leukemia may develop oral conditions associated with either the malignancy or the therapy. These

include oral ulcerations, mucositis, gingival enlargement, oral infections, and oral GVHD.

- Gingival bleeding may occur spontaneously. The risk is greater when gingival tissue is edematous and if the patient is thrombocytopenic. Even minor trauma such as cheek biting or a tongue bite can cause bleeding.
- Gingival enlargement can be caused by inflammation or infiltration of leukemic cells. A localized mass of leukemic cells is called granulocytic sarcoma or chloroma. Chloromas occur more often in acute leukemia. Generalized gingival enlargement due to inflammation is more common, particularly in patients with poor oral hygiene. It may be controlled with regular plaque control and use of chlorhexidine.
- Mucositis may present 7 to 10 days after the onset of chemotherapy and resolves with the cessation of therapy. Chemotherapy may cause the breakdown of the oral epithelial barrier, leading to oral ulcerations. These sores may become secondarily infected and lead to septicemia and systemic infection. There are protocols in existence for the treatment of mucositis, which include maintenance of oral hygiene, alcohol-free mouth rinses, topical anesthetics and systemic analgesics, and antiseptic antimicrobial rinses such as chlorhexidine. Recently, palifermin (a recombinant human keratinocyte growth factor) has been approved for use in the U.S. to decrease oral mucosal injury induced by cytotoxic therapy and to reduce the duration and severity of mucositis.
- Opportunistic infections are common in leukemic patients because of their immunocompromised state induced by chemotherapy or due to frequent use of broad-spectrum antibiotics. The two most common opportunistic infections are pseudomembranous candidiasis and recurrent herpes (HSV). Individuals with antibodies to HSV are typically given prophylactic antivirals during therapy. Herpetic infections are more chronic, generally taking a longer time to heal. Besides HSV, leukemic patients are also susceptible to varicella-zoster

TABLE I-14 1995–2000 Relative Survival Rates for Leukemia

Type of leukemia	Overall survival rate	Survival rate for children
Acute lymphocytic leukemia (ALL)	64.8%	89.1% (under age 5)
Chronic lymphocytic leukemia (CLL)	72.7%	–
Acute myelogenous leukemia (AML)	19.5%	53%
Chronic myelogenous leukemia (AML)	36.7%	–

virus (VZV) and cytomegalovirus (CMV). They may develop fungal or bacterial infections caused by unusual organisms in the oral cavity. For instance, aspergillosis, mucormycosis, *Pseudomonas*, *Escherichia coli*, or *Enterobacter* can all cause oral infections that may all present as oral ulcerations. In addition, traumatic lesions in the oral cavity may become secondarily infected with these or other organisms.

- It is important to remember that signs and symptoms of infection, even severe, may be masked due to the immunosuppressed state of leukemic patients. Erythema and swelling may be less pronounced in oral infections. Therefore, exudates from oral ulcers should be sent for culture, diagnosis, and antibiotic sensitivity.

- Paresthesia of the face or mandible may also be a complication of leukemic cells infiltrating into peripheral nerves or may be a side effect from chemotherapy, particularly vincristine. Patients with a history of SCT may develop GVHD of the oral cavity. Common presentations of GVHD include mucosal ulcerations, mucositis, xerostomia, salivary gland swelling, or dysphagia. A tissue biopsy may confirm the presence of GVHD.

DENTAL MANAGEMENT

- Oral healthcare providers should be familiar with the signs and symptoms of anemia or white blood cell disorders. Patients presenting with signs or symptoms should be referred immediately to a physician. Surgical procedures in patients with undetected leukemia may lead to serious bleeding problems, poor wound healing, and postsurgical infections.

- When a leukemic patient is identified in the dental office, a consultation with the physician is necessary to establish the patient's current status. With consideration, patients in remission can receive most indicated dental treatment. However, those with signs or symptoms of the disease should only receive conservative emergency care.

- A recent CBC, including platelet count, should be obtained before any surgical procedure is performed.
  - In general, routine dental procedures can be performed if the total WBC count is greater than 2000/mm^3 and the platelet count is greater than 50,000/mm^3. For outpatient care, this is generally about 17 days after chemotherapy.
  - If emergency dental care is needed and the platelet count is below 50,000/mm^3, consultation with the patient's oncologist is recommended. Platelet replacement may be indicated if invasive or traumatic dental procedures are to be performed and topical therapy using pressure, thrombin, microfibrillar collagen, and splints may be required.
  - If emergency dental care is needed and the total WBC count is less than 2000/mm^3 or the absolute neutrophil count is less than 500 to 1000/mm^3, consultation with the patient's oncologist is recommended and broad-spectrum antibiotic prophylaxis should be provided to prevent post-operative infection.

- The oral healthcare provider is an important part of the medical team for patients with newly diagnosed leukemia. Careful planning may help prevent severe oral infections that may become life-threatening. Prior to initiating medical treatment, the focus of dental treatment should be on eliminating the risk of infection by eliminating mucosal or periodontal disease. This may include dental extractions, scaling, or surgical procedures.

- These patients should have a dental evaluation and removal of obvious potential sources of bacteremia, such as teeth with advanced periodontal disease (e.g., pocket depths 5 mm or greater, excessive mobility, purulence on probing), prior to chemotherapy. Additional indicators for extraction of teeth prior to the onset of chemotherapy include:
  - Periapical inflammation
  - Tooth is broken down, nonrestorable, nonfunctional, or partially erupted and the patient is noncompliant with oral hygiene measures
  - Tooth is associated with an inflammatory (e.g., pericoronitis), infectious, or malignant osseous disease

- Extractions should be performed at least 5 days (in the maxilla) to 7 days (in the mandible) before the initiation of chemotherapy. These dental procedures require careful planning with the physician.

- Consideration must be given to risk of infection and bleeding. The patient may require the use of prophylactic antibiotics and/or measures to prevent bleeding, such as platelet transfusion.

SUGGESTED REFERENCES

Appelbaum FR. Acute myeloid leukemia in adults, in Abeloff MD, Armitage JO, et al. (eds): *Clinical Oncology*, ed 3. New York, Elsevier, 2004, pp 2825–2839.

Bruker BJ, Goldman JM. Chronic myeloid leukemia, in Abeloff MD, Armitage JO, et al. (eds): *Clinical Oncology*, ed 3. Elsevier, 2004, pp 2899–2923.

Cheson BD. Chronic lymphoid leukemias, in Abeloff MD, Armitage JO, et al. (eds): *Clinical Oncology*, ed 3. New York, Elsevier, 2004, pp 2921–2958.

http://www.leukemia.org

http://www.cancer.gov/cancer_information/cancer_type/leukemia

Kantarjian HM, Faderl S. Acute lymphoid leukemia in adults, in Abeloff MD, Armitage JO, et al. (eds): *Clinical Oncology*, ed 3. New York, Elsevier, 2004, pp 2793–2822.

Little JW, Falace DA, Miller CS, Rhodus NL (eds): *Dental Management of the Medically Compromised Patient*, ed 6. Philadelphia, Mosby, 2002, pp 369–385.

McKenna SJ. Leukemia. *Oral Surg Oral Med Oral Pathol Oral Radiol Endodon* 2000;89:137–139.

AUTHOR: ERNESTA PARISI, DMD

SYNONYM(S)

Marfan syndrome
Marfan-Achard syndrome

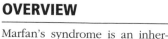

ICD-9CM/CPT CODE(S)
759.82 Marfan's syndrome—complete

OVERVIEW

Marfan's syndrome is an inherited disorder of connective tissue elastic fibers affecting primarily the musculoskeletal system, the cardiovascular system, and the eye.

EPIDEMIOLOGY & DEMOGRAPHICS

INCIDENCE/PREVALENCE IN USA: Prevalence is estimated to be about 1 per 5000 to 10,000.

PREDOMINANT AGE: Congenital (present from birth) but clinical manifestations do not usually become apparent until adolescence or young adulthood.

PREDOMINANT SEX: Both sexes are affected equally.

GENETICS: Approximately 70–85% of cases are familial and transmitted by autosomal dominant inheritance with high penetration. The remainder are sporadic and arise from new mutations.

ETIOLOGY & PATHOGENESIS

Marfan's syndrome results from an inherited defect in an extracellular glycoprotein called fibrillin-1 encoded by the gene *FBN1* mapped to chromosomes 15q21. Fibrillin is the major component of cellular microfibrils found in the extracellular matrix. Although microfibrils are widely distributed in the body, they are particularly abundant in the elastic connective tissues of the aorta, ligaments, and ciliary zonules of the lens, where they support the lens; these tissues are prominently affected in Marfan's syndrome.

CLINICAL PRESENTATION / PHYSICAL FINDINGS

Diagnostic criteria for Marfan's syndrome include:
- Family history of mutation in fibrillin (*FBN1*).
- Skeletal system: tall stature with long, slim limbs and long, tapering fingers and toes (arachnodactyly); minimal subcutaneous fat and muscle hypotonia; joint laxity with scoliosis and kyphosis; chest is classically deformed, presenting either pectus excavatum (deeply depressed sternum) or a pigeon-breast deformity; joint hypermobility (typically the thumb can be hyperextended back to the wrist); head is commonly dolichocephalic (long-headed) with bossing of the frontal eminences and prominent supraorbital ridges; palate typically is highly arched, and the dentition can be crowded and maloccluded.

- Ocular system: ectopia lentis (bilateral subluxation or dislocation, usually outward and upward, of the lens); myopia; retinal detachment.
- Cardiovascular system: mitral valve prolapse occurs in about 80% of cases, and the valve leaflets become progressively thickened (myxomatous on histopathology); the mitral annulus may dilate and calcify; dilation of the ascending aorta owing to cystic medionecrosis beginning in the sinuses of Valsalva and progresses with age at highly variable rates.
- Pulmonary system: apical blebs, spontaneous pneumothorax.
- Skin: striae atrophicae (striae cutis distensae) bands of thin wrinkled skin, initially red but becoming purple and white, which occur commonly on the abdomen, buttocks, and thighs at puberty and/or during and following pregnancy; inguinal or femoral hernia.

DIAGNOSIS

DIFFERENTIAL DIAGNOSIS
Each of the clinical manifestations of the syndrome may meet the specific criteria of that disease and may not be associated with Marfan's syndrome. A Marfan-like habitus may be noted in various disease entities. Some of the diseases include homocystinuria, congenital contractural arachnodactyly, Marfanoid hypermobility syndrome, multiple endocrine adenomatosis type IIb, and Shprintzen-Goldberg syndrome.

DIAGNOSIS

- Diagnosis is made by recognizing the cardiovascular, ocular, and skeletal manifestations, especially with a positive family history.
  ○ Genetic evaluation (*FBN1* gene on chromosome 15)
  ○ Echocardiography evaluation for mitral valve prolapse, mitral regurgitation, tricuspid valve prolapse, aortic regurgitation, dilation of the aortic root
  ○ Transesophageal echocardiography, chest CT scan, chest MRI, or aortography for suspected aortic dissection
  ○ Chest radiograph to evaluate for thoracic cage deformities or distortion, pulmonary apical bullae
  ○ Ophthalmologic examination (slit lamp examination, etc.)

MEDICAL MANAGEMENT & TREATMENT

- All patients should be seen at least annually by a physician who manages the overall care. Most patients require annual ophthalmo-

logic and cardiologic consultation and orthopedic consultation as required by specific problems.
- Restriction of contact sports, weight lifting, and overexertion.
- Genetic counseling and emotional preparation.
- Prophylactic surgical repair of the aortic root has had the greatest beneficial impact.
- Prophylactic use of β-adrenergic blockade from an early age to slow the rate of aortic root dilation and protect from aortic dissection.
- Calcium channel blockers have also been shown to retard aortic growth in children and adolescents.
- Early use of angiotensin-converting enzyme inhibitors in young patients with Marfan syndrome and valvular regurgitation may lessen the need for mitral valve surgery.
- Antibiotic prophylaxis should be prescribed prior to procedures likely to result in bacteremia in patients with echocardiographic evidence of valvular or aortic root abnormalities, or other cardiovascular pathology that represents an increased risk for bacterial endocarditis.
- Physical therapy.

COMPLICATIONS

- Bacterial endocarditis.
- Dissecting aortic aneurysm (cause of death in 30–45% of these individuals).
- Aortic or mitral valve insufficiency.
- Dilated cardiomyopathy.
- Retinal detachment.
- Without diagnosis and proper medical care, sudden death can occur. Excessive physical activities can exacerbate problems.

PROGNOSIS

With appropriate medical intervention, life expectancy in Marfan's syndrome has improved markedly to the point that many patients can expect survival to advanced years. Heterogeneity of disease impacts on the degree of the disease.

DENTAL SIGNIFICANCE

- Cephalometric surveys indicate a 50% prevalence of a high and deep palate.
- Cleft palate or bifid uvula has been reported in several instances.
- The teeth have been noted to be long and narrow and frequently maloccluded, commonly associated with mandibular prognathism.
- Partial anodontia has been reported in association with bilateral aniridia.

- Temporomandibular joint disorders are found more frequently than expected, affecting approximately 50% of patients with Marfan's syndrome.
- A case-control study by De Coster, et al. also found:
  - Enamel defects (mostly local hypoplastic spotting probably related to local trauma or infection) were a significant finding in patients with Marfan's syndrome and may be related to the high caries rate in the deciduous dentition.
  - Root deformity, bilateral abnormal pulp shape, and pulp inclusions, especially when presenting simultaneously, were found to occur significantly more frequently in patients with Marfan's syndrome.
  - Patients with Marfan's syndrome exhibited significantly more severe gingivitis and oral calculus.

DENTAL MANAGEMENT

- Consultation with primary care physician, orthopedic surgeon, and cardiologist.
  - Patients with cardiovascular pathology and/or status postcardiovascular surgery (e.g., prosthetic heart valve) that places them at increased risk for bacterial endocarditis will require antibiotic prophylaxis prior to invasive dental procedures (see Appendix A, Box A-1, "Antibiotic Prophylaxis Recommendations by the American Heart Association for the Prevention of Bacterial Endocarditis").
  - The use of local anesthetics containing vasoconstrictors should be carefully managed in patients with Marfan's syndrome since they may increase cardiac output. Monitoring of blood pressure, systolic time intervals, and aortic pulse wave velocity is strongly recommended during dental treatment. Women have a greater cardiovascular risk if pregnant.
- General dental/oral care followed as needed; oral hygiene should be stressed.

SUGGESTED REFERENCES

Bauss O, et al. Temporomandibular joint dysfunction in Marfan syndrome. *Oral Surg Oral Med Oral Pathol Oral Radiol Endod* 2004;97:592–598.

De Coster P, Martens L, De Paepe A. Oral manifestations of patients with Marfan syndrome: a case-control study. *Oral Surg Oral Med Oral Pathol Oral Radiol Endod* 2002;93:564–572.

Jones KL. *Smith's Recognizable Patterns of Human Malformations*, ed 4. Philadelphia, WB Saunders, 1997, pp 472–475.

Syndromes affecting bone: other skeletal dysplasias, in Gorlin RJ, Cohen Jr MM, Hennelson RCM (eds): *Syndromes of the Head and Neck*, ed 4. New York, Oxford University Press, 2001, pp 327–334.

AUTHORS: **NORBERT J. BURZYNSKI, SR., DDS, MS; F. JOHN FIRRIOLO, DDS, PHD**

SYNONYM(S)

Ménière disease
Ménière's vertigo
Ménière's syndrome
Lermoyez's syndrome
Endolymphatic hydrops

ICD-9CM/CPT CODE(S)

386.00 Unspecified Ménière's disease
—complete
386.01 Active Ménière's disease, cochleovestibular—complete
386.02 Active Ménière's disease, cochlear—complete
386.03 Active Ménière's disease, vestibular—complete
386.04 Inactive Ménière's disease—complete

OVERVIEW

A disorder characterized by tinnitus, hearing loss, vertigo, and a feeling of fullness in the ear. There is an increase in volume and pressure of the innermost fluid of the inner ear. Vertigo may be followed by nausea and vomiting.

EPIDEMIOLOGY & DEMOGRAPHICS

INCIDENCE/PREVALENCE IN USA:
Incidence 15 cases per 100,000 persons; prevalence 100 to 200 cases per 100,000 persons.
PREDOMINANT AGE: The usual age of onset is 20 to 50 years. It is extremely rare in children.
PREDOMINANT SEX: Male = female.
GENETICS: There are no data known to support genetic occurrence.

ETIOLOGY & PATHOGENESIS

The etiology is unknown. Autoimmune, viral, and inner ear response to variety of injuries have been suggested. An association with endolymphatic hydrops has been considered. The pathophysiology data are insufficient.

CLINICAL PRESENTATION / PHYSICAL FINDINGS

- Classic presentation is a quadrad of vertigo, tinnitus, monaural fullness, and hearing loss.
  - Vertigo attacks are of sudden onset, often preceded by low-frequency tinnitus, monaural fullness, or hearing loss. Vertigo is often severe and disabling, with a duration of half an hour to one day and accompanied by nausea, vomiting, and occasionally visual disturbances.
  - Tinnitus is usually perceived as low-frequency prior to an attack and may worsen during a vertigo attack, becoming multifrequency and louder; it then resolves after an attack.
  - Sensation of aural fullness usually affects only one ear and precedes an attack.

- Hearing loss:
  - Sensorineural hearing loss as opposed to conductive loss seen in middle ear disease.
  - Hearing may fluctuate, sensorineural loss being present during a period of attacks and then improving after the disease subsides.
- Clinical manifestation can vary widely, with some patients developing hearing loss after the first attack and others developing no hearing loss after decades of attacks.

DIAGNOSIS

- Evaluation of any hearing loss is recommended.
- Review of any medications or disorders that may alter laboratory results.
- Special tests may be used including otoscopy with air pressure applied to the tympanic membrane; glycerol test and electrocochleography are used by some otolaryngologists; electronystagmography may show peripheral vestibular deficit.
- Imaging studies are needed to rule-out entities such as acoustic neuroma and/or cerebellar or CNS dysfunction.

MEDICAL MANAGEMENT & TREATMENT

- No known medication that influences the disease process. Medications are administered for relief of vertigo and nausea. Activity should be limited during attacks. Bed rest is suggested. Unsteadiness and hearing loss limit patient's activity.
- Streptomycin may be used to intentionally damage the neuroepithelium of the balance centers and reduce their function.
- Surgical intervention varies on the status of hearing; options include:
  - Endolymphatic sac surgery: either decompression or drainage of endolymph into mastoid or subarachnoid space.
  - Severing the vestibular nerve (intracranial procedure).
  - Placement of gentamicin through the tympanic membrane into the middle ear space.
  - Myringotomy with tube placement and use of a Meniett device to apply pressure intermittently to the inner ear several times a day.
- Diet may play a part in nausea. Diuretics, salt restriction, and avoidance of caffeine are traditional recommendations.
- Medications of choice in an acute attack include:
  - Prochlorperazine (Compazine), 5 to 10 mg PO q6h
  - Promethazine (Phenergan), 12.5 to 25 mg PO q4–6h

  - Diazepam (Valium), 5 to 10 mg po q8h
  - Meclizine (Antivert), 25 mg po q6h
- It is advisable that an otolaryngologist administer treatment. Patient education is valuable for quality care.

COMPLICATIONS

- Disease may contribute to loss of hearing.
- Without proper patient workup, failure to diagnose acoustic neuroma may follow.
- Patients may have a limited ability to work and/or may suffer injuries during an attack.

PROGNOSIS

- Prognosis depends on correct diagnosis.
- Attack severity and frequency tends to peak at 2 years, declining thereafter.
- Patients may be vertigo-free after 5 to 8 years; however, hearing loss remains.
- Less than 10% of patients may require some surgical intervention.

DENTAL SIGNIFICANCE

- Vertigo is associated with nausea and or vomiting. These elements would impact on any oral dental care deliverance. Also, oral hygiene might be compromised. Consultation with otolaryngologist is suggested. Modification in oral dental care delivery is a consideration.

DENTAL MANAGEMENT

- Patient education and consultation with an otolaryngologist are recommended for total patient care.
- Recurrent vertigo, tinnitus, hearing loss, and monaural fullness all may impact in oral dental care in varying degrees. Also, stress, noise, and environmental allergies may contribute to the overall background of care.
- Possible nausea and vomiting could contribute to limited and/or guarded care. Possible light-headedness might implicate other entities, such as postural hypotension, anemia, anxiety, hyperventilation, and depression.
- General oral dental care can be provided.

SUGGESTED REFERENCE

Balok RW. Hearing and equilibrium, in Goldman L, Ansiello D (eds): *Cecil Textbook of Medicine*, ed 22. Philadelphia, WB Saunders, 2004, pp 2436–2442.

AUTHOR: NORBERT J. BURZYNSKI, SR., DDS, MS

SYNONYM(S)

Myeloma
Plasma cell myeloma
Myelomatosis
Kahler's disease

ICD-9CM/CPT CODE(S)

203.00 Multiple myeloma—incomplete

OVERVIEW

Multiple myeloma (MM) is a malignant hematologic disorder of plasma cells accounting for nearly 10% of all hematopoietic cancers and 1% of all cancer-related deaths in Western countries. It is an illness characterized by the neoplastic proliferation of a single clone of plasma cells engaged in overproduction of intact monoclonal immunoglobulin IgG or IgA, or free monoclonal κ or λ chains. Multiple myeloma is associated with a constellation of signs and symptoms. Pathological fractures and debilitating bone pain secondary to bone formation/resorption are among the early manifestations of this illness. Anemia, hypercalcemia, and renal insufficiency are other important features.

EPIDEMIOLOGY & DEMOGRAPHICS

INCIDENCE/PREVALENCE IN USA: Annual incidence of 4 cases per 100,000 persons; twice as prevalent in African-Americans as compared to Caucasians.
PREDOMINANT AGE: Incidence is highly age-dependent, with the majority of patients being over 40 years of age. Peak age of onset 65 to 70 years.
PREDOMINANT SEX: Slightly more common in men than in women.
GENETICS: Genetic factors are poorly understood, but occasional familial clusters of disease are noted, indicating recessive heredity.

ETIOLOGY & PATHOGENESIS

- Exact etiology is unknown.
  - Exposure to radiation, organic solvents, chemical resins, herbicides, and insecticides may play a role. Kaposi's sarcoma-associated herpes virus (KSHV) (also known as human herpes virus 8, HHV-8) may possibly play a role in the development of a few cases of MM.
- Neoplastic plasma cells produce IgG in about 55% of MM patients and IgA in about 20%. Of these IgG and IgA MM patients, 40% also have Bence-Jones proteinuria. Light chain MM is found in 15–20% of patients; their plasma cells secrete only free monoclonal light chains (κ or λ Bence-Jones protein), and a homogeneous monoclonal spike (M spike) is usually absent on serum electrophoresis. Patients with the light chain subgroup tend to have a higher incidence of lytic bone lesions, hyper-

calcemia, renal failure, and amyloidosis than do other MM patients.

CLINICAL PRESENTATION / PHYSICAL FINDINGS

- Bone pain (classic symptoms in ~ 80% of patients).
- Skeletal abnormalities, pathologic fractures secondary to lytic bone lesions (~ 70% of cases).
- "Punched out" radiolucent lesions on radiographic examination of the skull, jaws, and long bones.
- Renal insufficiency mainly caused by "myeloma kidney" from light chains or hypercalcemia, rarely from amyloidosis.
- Amyloidosis (heart, liver, CNS, skin, mucosa) develops in ~ 10% of MM patients.
- Neurological complications, including spinal cord or nerve root compression and blurred vision (from hyperviscosity syndrome).
- Weakness or fatigue (often associated with anemia) and weight loss.
- Immunosuppression and recurrent infections (especially respiratory and urinary tract infections caused by gram-positive or gram-negative organisms).
- Hyperviscosity syndrome: mucosal (oronasal) bleeding, vertigo, nausea, visual disturbances, alterations in mental status.
- Anorexia, nausea, vomiting, polyuria, polydipsia, constipation, weakness, confusion, or stupor secondary to hypercalcemia (when present in 15–20% of patients with MM).
- Extramedullary plasma cell tumors (plasmacytomas) occur late in the disease.

DIAGNOSIS

- Bone marrow biopsy: plasma cells usually account for 10% or more of all nucleated cells, but they may range from less than 5% to almost 100%.
- Detection of monoclonal proteins in the serum: tall, homogeneous monoclonal spike (M spike) on protein immunoelectrophoresis in approximately 75% of patients with decreased levels of normal immunoglobulins.
- Detection of free monoclonal κ or λ chain proteins in 24-hour urine specimen (Bence-Jones proteinuria).
- Hypercalcemia, present in 15–20% of patients at diagnosis, due to excess bone resorption.
- Elevated BUN, creatinine, uric acid, and total protein due to renal insufficiency.
- CBC: anemia (normochromic, normocytic with rouleaux formation) leukopenia, thrombocytopenia as a result of bone marrow replacement by plasma cells.
- Serum hyperviscosity (more common with production of IgA).

DIAGNOSTIC IMAGING

- Skeletal images often reveal abnormalities consisting of punched-out lytic lesions, osteoporosis, or fractures in nearly 80% of patients. The skull often shows punched-out lytic lesions with no sclerotic or reactive border. Periosteal reaction is uncommon. Vertebral compression fractures with occasional extraosseous or extradural cord compression are also commonly seen.

MEDICAL MANAGEMENT & TREATMENT

- Goals in the treatment of MM are directed to prevent relapse, prolong remission, manage adverse effects of therapy, provide patient education, and improve quality of life.
- Chemotherapy is the preferred initial treatment for overt, symptomatic MM in patients older than 70 years or in younger patients in whom bone marrow transplantation is not feasible.
  - Oral administration of melphalan and prednisone produces an objective response in 50–60% of patients.
  - Chemotherapy should be continued for 1 year or until the patient is in a plateau state. At that point, α_2-interferon may be given.
  - Almost all patients with MM eventually relapse. Vincristine, doxorubicin (Adriamycin), and dexamethasone (VAD) can be used in patients not responding or relapsing after treatment with melphalan and prednisone.
  - Thalidomide has also been used as frontline therapy in combination with other agents in the initial treatment of MM, as well as in the treatment of relapsed or refractory MM, due to its known antiangiogenic properties.
- Ninety to 95% of patients with MM cannot have allogeneic bone marrow transplantation because of their age, lack of an HLA-matched sibling donor, or inadequate renal, pulmonary, or cardiac function.
- Treatment of complications:
  - Bisphosphonates to delay progression of the skeletal complications.
  - Recombinant erythropoietin to stimulate RBC production.
  - Analgesics for pain control.
  - Dialysis for renal failure secondary to MM.
- Supportive therapy (antibiotics, antifungals, growth factors).

COMPLICATIONS

- Painful lytic bone lesions
- Pathologic bone fractures, spinal cord compression
- Hypercalcemia
- Renal insufficiency
- Anemia and thrombocytopenia

- Immunosuppression and recurrent infections (especially respiratory and urinary tract infections caused by gram-positive or gram-negative organisms)
- Symptomatic hyperviscosity

PROGNOSIS

- MM has a progressive course with no effective curative therapy. The median survival is approximately 3 years; 20–30% of patients survive 5 or more years. Fewer than 5% survive longer than 10 years.
- High rate of relapse after treatment.
- Significant morbidity and mortality associated with available therapies.
- Some chromosomal abnormalities (e.g., partial or complete deletion of chromosome 13) are associated with a particularly poor prognosis.

DENTAL SIGNIFICANCE

- Radiolucent jaw lesions in 3–5% of patients.
- Jaw pain, swelling, paresthesia, and unexplained tooth mobility.
- Extramedullary plasma cell tumors in the oral cavity can occur late in the disease.
- Oral soft tissue deposits of amyloid.
- Hemorrhagic complications after oral surgery due to thrombocytopenia, altered platelet function, hyperviscosity, and inactivation of clotting factors secondary to the disease or chemotherapy.
- Susceptibility to bacterial oral infections (replacement of normal bone marrow by malignant cells and/or effects of chemotherapy).
- Susceptibility to recurrent herpes-zoster in the oral cavity.
- Avascular necrosis and osteomyelitis of the jaw associated with prolonged bisphosphonate therapy.

DENTAL MANAGEMENT

- Prioritize dental treatment in consideration of the poor prognosis of the disease.
- Provide only supportive dental care to patients in terminal stage of MM.
- Oral soft/hard tissue biopsy to establish diagnosis in a patient with signs and symptoms of MM.
- Preoperative workup for surgical procedures (e.g., CBC with differential, platelet count, bleeding time, prothrombin time, partial thromboplastin time).
- Consultation with a hematologist if impaired hemostasis secondary to hyperviscosity is present.
- Consultation with the attending oncologist to determine:
  o Patient's immune status prior to invasive oral surgery and the need for prophylactic antibiotic coverage to prevent postoperative infection (see Appendix A, Box A-2, "Presurgical and Postsurgical Antibiotic Prophylaxis for Patients at Increased Risk for Postoperative Infections").
  o The presence and extent of end-organ complications secondary to MM.
- Aggressive prevention of infection during or after invasive oral surgery for patients on prolonged bisphosphonate therapy.
- Consider hyperbaric oxygen therapy to treat recalcitrant osteomyelitis secondary to chronic bisphosphonate therapy.

SUGGESTED REFERENCES

Barille-Nion S, Barlogie B, et al. Advances in biology and therapy of multiple myeloma. *Hematology* 2003;248–278.

DeRossi SS, Garfunkel A, Greenberg MS. Hematologic diseases, in Greenberg M, Glick M (eds): *Burket's Oral Medicine: Diagnosis and Treatment.* Hamilton, Ontario, BC Decker, Inc., 2003, pp 429–453.

Devenney B, Erickson C. Multiple myeloma: an overview. *Clin J Oncol Nurs* 2004;8(4): 401–405.

Heffner Jr LT, Lonial S. Breakthrough in the management of multiple myeloma. *Drugs* 2003;63:(16):1621–1636.

International Myeloma Working Group. Criteria for the classification of monoclonal gammopathies, multiple myeloma and related disorders: a report of the international Myeloma Working Group. *Br J Haematol* 2003;121:749–757.

Kyle RA, Rajkumar SV. Multiple myeloma. *N Engl J Med* 2004;351:1860–1873.

Little JW, Falace DA, Miller GS, Rhodus NL. Disorders of red and white blood cells, in Little JW, et al. (eds): *Dental Management of the Medically Compromised Patient.* St Louis, Mosby, 2002, pp 365–386.

Lugassy G, Shaham R, et al. Severe osteomyelitis of the jaw in long-term survivors of multiple myeloma: a new clinical entity. *Am J Med* 2004;117:440–441.

Munshi NC. Recent advances in the management of multiple myeloma. *Semin Hematol* 2004;41:2:(Suppl 4):21–26.

AUTHOR: **MAHNAZ FATAHZADEH, DMD**

SYNONYM(S)

MS
Disseminated sclerosis

ICD-9CM/CPT CODE(S)

340 Multiple sclerosis—complete

OVERVIEW

MS is a chronic idiopathic, inflammatory, demyelinating disease of the central nervous system.

EPIDEMIOLOGY & DEMOGRAPHICS

INCIDENCE/PREVALENCE IN USA:

- The most common debilitating and demyelinating illness among young adults.
- 10 to 150 cases per 100,000 persons.
- Approximately 25,000 cases are diagnosed each year.
- More prevalent in the temperate climates/northern latitudes.
- Geographic clustering.
- Incidence is higher for Caucasians.
- Seventy percent of patients present with a relapsing-remitting type of disease pattern that is characterized by acute exacerbations followed by remission vs a chronic progressive type. The chronic progressive type can be primary-progressive, relapsing-progressive (intermediate in severity), and secondary-progressive (which many patients with relapsing-remitting disease progress to over time).

PREDOMINANT AGE:

- MS generally affects those between 20 and 50 years old.
- Rarely seen in those younger than 15 years old.

PREDOMINANT SEX:

- Throughout adulthood the ratio is 2:1 female to male.
- Men have a greater tendency to have a progressive disease at onset.

GENETICS:

- Increased prevalence with HLA DR2, DR 15, and DR4.

ETIOLOGY & PATHOGENESIS

- Unknown.
- Thought to result from an autoimmune process.
  - The autoantigen is most likely a myelin protein.
- Probable genetic predisposition to an environmental agent.
- Pathological hallmark of MS is multicentric, multiphasic CNS inflammation and demyelination.
- Lesions characteristically involve the optic nerve and the periventricular white matter of the cerebellum, brain stem, basal ganglia, and spinal cord.

CLINICAL PRESENTATION / PHYSICAL FINDINGS

SYMPTOMS

- Fatigue
- Diplopia on lateral gaze
- Visual loss
- Hemiparesis
- Aphasia, dysphagia
- Focal weakness
- Sensory loss is a common early complaint
- Ataxia/tremor
- Cognitive impairment
- Depression/psychiatric disease
- Urinary dysfunction
- Trigeminal neuralgia

SIGNS

- Optic neuritis
- Impairment of visual acuity
- Afferent papillary defect in affected eye
- Internuclear ophthalmoplegia
- Paresis of the adducting eye on lateral conjugate gaze with horizontal nystagmus of the abducting eye
- Acute transverse myelitis
- Isolated loss of pain and temperature in dermatomes; dissociated loss of pain and temperature from vibration/position sense
- Spasticity/hyperreflexia reflecting an upper motor neuron dysfunction
- Cerebellar findings such as ataxia, scanning speech, intention tremor, disequilibrium
- Lhermitte's sign: flexion of the neck produces an electric shock-like feeling in the torso and extremities

DIAGNOSIS

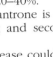

- Clinical diagnosis based on a consistent clinical presentation with evidence of CNS demyelinating lesions disseminated in time and space.
- MRI of the head with gadolinium is the study of choice and can help establish a diagnosis, but a negative MRI cannot rule out the disease.
  - T1 shows active lesions while T2 shows older lesions in the periventricular supratentorial white matter and occasionally in the cerebellum stem. Optic nerve visualization is possible with fat suppression.
- Cerebrospinal fluid analysis from a lumbar puncture is indicated if the diagnosis is uncertain.
  - Positive findings include increase in total protein, mononuclear WBCs.
  - Selective increase in immunoglobulin G (oligoclonal bands and free kappa chains).

- Evoked potential studies demonstrating slow conduction velocities.

MEDICAL MANAGEMENT & TREATMENT

- Acute exacerbations: typically, high-dose IV methylprednisolone (5 days of 1000 mg/day can be used; an alternative dose is 15 mg/kg/day).
- Disease-modifying therapy: includes interferon β-1a (Avonex, Rebif), interferon β-1b (Betaseron), and glatiramer acetate (Copaxone). All four drugs slow progression of relapsing disease and reduce the annual relapse rate by 20–40%.
- Cytotoxic: mitoxantrone is effective in rapidly relapsing and secondary progressive MS.
- Symptoms of disease could be treated by their appropriate pharmacotherapies.

COMPLICATIONS

- Chronic disability is associated with increased mortality.
- Disabilities may include pneumonia, embolism, and skin breakdown/infection.

PROGNOSIS

- The rate of disease progression is highly variable.
- The average interval from initial presentation to death is 35 years.

DENTAL SIGNIFICANCE

- Facial pain symptoms can mimic trigeminal neuralgia.
- V2 and V3 sensory neuropathy.
- Facial paralysis.
- Oral symptoms could include:
  - Dysarthria
  - "Scanning speech"
  - Myokymia

DENTAL MANAGEMENT

- Patients undergoing relapse should have emergency dental treatment only.
- Optimal time for dental treatment is during remission.
- Evaluate level of motor impairment.

SUGGESTED REFERENCES

Calabresi PA. Diagnosis and management of multiple sclerosis. *Am Fam Phys* 2004;70(10): 1935–1944.

Chemaly D, Lefrancois A, Perusse R. Oral and maxillofacial manifestations of multiple sclerosis. *JCDA* 2000;66(11):600–605.

Degenhardt A. Multiple sclerosis, in Ferri FF (ed): *Ferri's Clinical Advisor: Instant Diagnosis and Treatment.* Philadelphia, Elsevier Mosby, 2005, pp 535–536.

Emedicine: www.emedicine.com Multiple Sclerosis

AUTHOR: **THOMAS P. SOLLECITO, DMD**

SYNONYM(S)

Epidemic parotitis

ICD-9CM/CPT CODE(S)

072   Mumps
072.7   Mumps with other specific complications
072.79   Mumps with other specific complications
072.8   Mumps with unspecified complication
072.9   Mumps no complication

OVERVIEW

Mumps is an acute infection of the salivary glands by paramyxovirus. It is contagious and has other systemic manifestations such as meningitis, pancreatitis, and orchitis.

EPIDEMIOLOGY & DEMOGRAPHICS

INCIDENCE/PREVALENCE IN USA: Incidence of mumps has been considerably reduced by widespread use of measles-mumps-rubella (MMR) vaccine, first introduced in the U.S. in 1977. Preimmunization annual cases of mumps were as high as 185,691 in 1968 compared to only 266 cases in 2001.

PREDOMINANT AGE: Prior to widespread use of the MMR vaccine, mumps was predominately a childhood disease, primarily affecting those between the ages of 5 and 14 years. Currently, more than 50% of mumps cases now affect young adults.

PREDOMINANT SEX: Males and females equally affected.

ETIOLOGY & PATHOGENESIS

- Paramyxovirus or mumps virus is a pleomorphic RNA virus. Although there is only one antigenic type, use of PCR technology has shown geographic differences in mumps viruses.
- Mumps is usually spread by saliva droplets and fomites. It is highly contagious with a 90% transmission rate for nonimmune household contacts.
- Incubation period varies from 2 to 3 weeks before clinical symptoms appear. However, infected individuals can still shed viruses during the subclinical period.
- The virus replicates in the upper respiratory tract, leading to viremia and dissemination into glandular tissues and the central nervous system.
- Perivascular and interstitial mononuclear cell infiltrates, edema, and acinar and ductal cell necrosis are prominent in affected glands.

CLINICAL PRESENTATION / PHYSICAL FINDINGS

- Approximately 30% of mumps cases are subclinical and are either asymptomatic or have no specific symptomatology.
- The prodromal symptoms of headache, malaise, anorexia, fever, and myalgia appear first, followed by salivary gland swelling within the next 24 hours.
- Salivary gland swellings are usually bilateral and commonly affect the parotid more than submandibular and sublingual glands.
- Parotid gland swellings may be large enough to mask the postauricular region.
- Mastication is associated with pain; patient may have redness of the orifice of the parotid ducts.
- Up to 20% of postpubertal males with mumps develop orchitis manifesting as painful and considerably enlarged testes, accompanied by fever. While oophoritis may develop in women, it is less common. These women complain of abdominal pain.
- Other manifestations of mumps include meningitis, pancreatitis, myocarditis, mastitis, thyroiditis, nephritis, arthritis, and thrombocytopenic purpura.

DIAGNOSIS

- History of epidemic pattern of bilateral parotitis and recent exposure can easily point to mumps.
- Isolation and culture of mumps virus from saliva of infected individuals.
- Serology for mumps-specific IgM and IgG using highly sensitive ELISA assays.

MEDICAL MANAGEMENT & TREATMENT

- Treatment of mumps is generally symptom-based.
- Patients receive palliative treatment. This is a combination of bed rest, analgesics, and application of warm or cold compress to the parotid glands.

PREVENTIVE MEASURES

- Mumps-attenuated virus vaccine (derived from the Jeryl-Lynn strain of mumps virus) induces antibody in 96% of seronegative recipients and has 97% protective efficacy.
- In the U.S., the recommended immunization schedule for children includes a combination treatment [measles-mumps-rubella (MMR) vaccination] with an initial dose given between 12 and 15 months of age and a second dose recommended between 4 and 6 years of age.

COMPLICATIONS

- Due to the bilateral manifestations of epididymoorchitis, testicular atrophy may lead to sterility in 15% of cases.
- Meningitis occurs in 1–10% of persons with mumps parotitis.

PROGNOSIS

- Mumps is rarely fatal.
- Patients recover very well, and the prognosis is excellent.
- Previously infected people, including those with asymptomatic cases, have long-lasting and possibly lifelong immunity to recurrence.

DENTAL SIGNIFICANCE

- Parotid pain and swelling in one or both glands.
- Inflammatory changes of Stensen's and Wharton's duct orifices but without purulent discharge.

DENTAL MANAGEMENT

- There are no specific dental management protocols in a patient with mumps; however, elective dental treatment is usually postponed until the patient is asymptomatic and noninfectious.
- Usual communicable period is from 48 hours prior to and up to 9 days after parotid swelling.
- Parotid swelling lasts about 3 to 7 days.

SUGGESTED REFERENCES

Greenberg MS, Glick M (eds): *Burket's Oral Medicine: Diagnosis and Treatment*, ed 10. Hamilton, Ontario, BC Decker, Inc., 2003, pp 249–250.

Harrison's Online: http://www3.accessmedicine.com/home.aspx

Neville BW, Damm DD, Allen CM, Bouquot JE. *Oral & Maxillofacial Pathology*. Philadelphia, WB Saunders, 2002, pp 233–234.

AUTHOR: **SUNDAY O. AKINTOYE, BDS, DDS, MS**

SYNONYM(S)
None

ICD-9CM/CPT CODE(S)
359.0 Congenital hereditary muscular dystrophy
359.1 Hereditary progressive muscular dystrophy

OVERVIEW

Muscular dystrophy (MD) is a heterogeneous group of hereditary disorders that are characterized by progressive muscle wasting and weakness associated with skeletal muscle necrosis and regeneration. Muscular dystrophies are classified by mode of inheritance, age of onset, and clinical features (Tables I-15 and I-16). They range in severity from mild to severe and in age of onset from birth to late adult. There are many subtypes within the major types of muscular dystrophy. Most muscular dystrophies are caused by mutations in genes that encode proteins that are important for maintaining the integrity of the muscle fiber during contraction and relaxation.

EPIDEMIOLOGY & DEMOGRAPHICS
INCIDENCE/PREVALENCE IN USA: See Table I-15.
PREDOMINANT AGE: See Table I-16.
PREDOMINANT SEX: Male > female.
GENETICS: See Table I-16.

ETIOLOGY & PATHOGENESIS
- Muscular dystrophies result from mutations in genes that encode for proteins that contribute to the structural integrity of the muscle fiber during contraction and relaxation. See Table I-15 for gene products involved.
- Most congenital muscular dystrophies, some of the limb-girdle muscular dys-

trophies, and Duchenne's and Becker's muscular dystrophies are caused by disruptions of the dystrophin-glycoprotein complex. This transmembrane complex is important for the structure and signaling across the cell membrane of muscle cells.

CLINICAL PRESENTATION / PHYSICAL FINDINGS
- The clinical features of the subtypes of muscular dystrophy are listed in Table I-16. Generally, patients with muscular dystrophy develop weakness in muscle groups that can rapidly or slowly progress depending upon the type of muscular dystrophy.
- Depending upon the muscles affected, patients with muscular dystrophy exhibit symptoms and signs ranging from mild limitations with facial expression and alterations in speech to more severe truncal and limb weakness that confines the patient to a wheelchair.
- Cardiac abnormalities and mental retardation occur in several types of muscular dystrophy.

DIAGNOSIS

- Muscular dystrophies are diagnosed from the clinical presentation of the patient.
- Electromyograms show abnormalities (e.g., fibrillations, positive waves, low-amplitude and polyphasic motor unit potentials) in virtually all cases of muscular dystrophy. Electromyography may help to differentiate muscular from neurologic causes of weakness.
- Serum creatine kinase levels are elevated in many, but not all, of the muscular dystrophies. For example, in Duchenne's and Becker's muscular dystrophies, serum creatine kinase levels are elevated from 25 to 200 times

normal levels. In contrast, serum creatine kinase levels are normal in facioscapulohumeral muscular dystrophy.
- Histopathologic examination of muscle from a biopsy may help to distinguish between various muscle diseases. Analysis of dystrophin protein by immunostaining or immunoblot methods differentiates Duchenne's and Becker's muscular dystrophies from other muscle disorders.
- Duchenne's muscular dystrophy can be recognized during pregnancy by genetic studies of tissue obtained by amniocentesis.
- An electrocardiogram may reveal cardiac abnormalities and various types of arrhythmias.

MEDICAL MANAGEMENT & TREATMENT

- There is no specific treatment for any of the muscular dystrophies.
- Physical therapy and orthopedic procedures may be used to strengthen muscles, treat deformities, and reduce contractures.
- Genetic counseling based on prenatal diagnosis and carrier detection are important for affected families.
- Prednisone appears to retard the tempo of progression of Duchenne's dystrophy for a period of up to 3 years but has significant side-effects.
- Quinine, procainamide, and phenytoin are used to treat myotonia.
- For patients with oculopharyngeal muscular dystrophy who have ptosis that interferes with vision or causes cervical pain due to constant tilting of the head back, surgical resection of the levator palpebral aponeurosis can reduce symptoms. For patients who exhibit marked weight loss, severe chocking, or recurrent pneumonia, cricopharyngeal myotomy will improve symptoms.

COMPLICATIONS

- Depending upon the subtype of muscular dystrophy, complications from MD include cardiomyopathy, cardiac dysrhythmias, varying levels of mental retardation, retinal malformations, and respiratory insufficiency (see Table I-16).

PROGNOSIS

Most patients with muscular dystrophy have a poor prognosis (see Table I-16). In Duchenne's muscular dystrophy, progression is rapid with death occurring usually within 15 years after onset. Similarly, patients with

---

TABLE I-15   Major Types of Muscular Dystrophy

Type of Muscular Dystrophy	Incidence	Mode of Inheritance	Gene Product Affected
Duchenne's	1:3500	X-linked recessive	Dystrophin
Becker's	1:20,000	X-linked recessive	Dystrophin
Emery-Dreifuss	1:100,000	X-linked recessive	Emerin
Limb-girdle	Not reported	Autosomal recessive most common, autosomal dominant	Caveolin 3, Calpain 3, Dysferlin, Sarcoglycan subunits, and other gene products
Congenital	Not reported	Autosomal recessive	Merosin, Fukutin, and other gene products
Facioscapulohumeral	1:20,000	Autosomal dominant	Unknown
Oculopharyngeal	Not reported	Autosomal dominant	Polyadenylation binding protein 2 gene
Myotonic dystrophies	15:100,000	Autosomal dominant	Myotonin protein kinase
Distal	Not reported	Autosomal dominant or autosomal recessive	Dysferlin and other gene products

TABLE I-16 **Clinical Features of Muscular Dystrophy**

Type of Muscular Dystrophy	Age at Onset	Muscles Involved	Signs and Symptoms	Nonmuscular Involvement	Clinical Course
Duchenne's	3–5 yrs	Muscles of the pelvic girdle, extensors of the knees and hips, lumbosacral spine, and shoulders. Facial, sternocleidomastoid, and diaphragm muscle in late stages.	Increasing difficulty in walking, running, and climbing stairs. Lordosis and waddling gait develops. Contractures from limbs remaining in one position.	Mental retardation common, cardiac dysrhythmias.	Relatively rapid, progressive course. Death usually occurs during late adolescence as result of pulmonary infections and respiratory failure.
Becker's	5–15 yrs	Same as Duchenne's MD.	Same as Duchenne's MD.	Cardiac dysrhythmias less frequent than Duchenne's MD.	Relatively benign compared to Duchenne MD. Death usually occurs in the fifth decade, but some patients live to an advanced age.
Emery-Dreifuss	5–30 yrs	Upper arm and pectoral girdle muscles first, then later the pelvic girdle and distal muscles in the lower extremities; occasionally facial muscles.	Early appearance of contractures in the flexors of the elbow, extensors of the neck, and calf muscles.	Severe cardiomyopathy with conduction defects.	Generally benign but sudden death is a frequent occurrence.
Limb-girdle	Late childhood to early adult	Shoulder girdle and pelvic girdle muscles.	Some subtypes resemble a severe form of Duchenne's MD; others are relatively benign with mild weakness and contractures.	Cardiomyopathy, cardiac dysrhythmias.	Ranges from rapidly to slowly progressive.
Congenital	At birth	Difficulty sucking and swallowing.	Contractures of proximal muscles and trunk.	Depending upon the subtype, severe mental retardation, retinal malformations, hydrocephalus, and respiratory insufficiency.	Variable severity and progression.
Facio-scapulohumeral	6–20 yrs	Orbicularis oculi, zygomaticus, orbicularis oris. Masticatory, extraocular, pharyngeal, and respiratory muscles spared.	Often begins with difficulty in raising the arms and winging of the scapulae. Facial weakness including inability to close eyes firmly, purse the lips, and whistle.	Rarely cardiac involvement.	Slowly progressive, may become arrested, but 15% of patients become wheelchair-bound.
Oculopharyngeal	30–50 yrs	Extraocular, facial, masticatory muscles.	Slowly progressive ptosis, dysphagia resulting in cachexia, and change in voice.	None.	Slowly progressive.
Myotonic dystrophies	2nd to 5th decades	Levator palpebrae, facial, masseter, sternocleidomastoid muscles. Forearm, hand, pretibial and diaphragm muscles.	Muscle atrophy and myotonia, facial weakness, ptosis, atrophy of the masseter muscles, malocclusion, weak monotonous, nasal voice. Forward curvature of neck (swan neck) due to weak sternocleidomastoid muscle.	Dystrophic changes in nonmuscular tissues (e.g., lens of the eye, skin, heart). Frontal baldness and wrinkled forehead. Bradycardia and atrioventricular block. Mild to moderate degrees of mental retardation occur.	Slowly progressive. Wheelchair bound within 20 years. Patients may die prematurely due to pulmonary infection, heart block, or heart failure.
Distal	30–80 yrs	Muscles of the hands, forearms, and lower legs.	Depending upon the subtype, weakness begins in the muscles of the wrist and fingers or the ankles and toes.	Occasionally cardiomyopathy and cardiac dysrhythmias.	Slowly progressive.

myotonic dystrophy become wheelchair-bound within 20 years of the diagnosis and die prematurely from pulmonary infection or cardiac abnormalities. Patients with Becker's muscular dystrophy exhibit a milder disease with a slower progression and may have a normal life span. The limb-girdle muscular dystrophies and congenital muscular dystrophies range in severity and rate of progression and can result in severe disability in middle life. The course of Emery-Dreifuss muscular dystrophy is generally benign, but sudden death is a common occurrence.

DENTAL SIGNIFICANCE

- Cardiac abnormalities such as dysrhythmias and cardiomyopathy may increase the risk for a cardiac emergency in a patient with muscular dystrophy.
- In some types of muscular dystrophy, such as myotonic dystrophies or Duchenne's muscular dystrophy, patients may be sensitive to general anesthetics or are at risk for myoglobinuria. Patients with severe anatomic abnormalities may be difficult to intubate endotracheally for general anesthesia. Regurgitation and pulmonary aspiration, may occur following intubation, and pulmonary insufficiency may develop after general anesthesia.
- Patients may have difficulty rising from the dental chair, difficulty walking, and may become wheelchair-bound.

- Recurrent pulmonary infections and respiratory failure may cause dyspnea when the patient is lying back in the dental chair.
- Patients may exhibit mental retardation.
- Upper arm weakness may make it difficult for patients to maintain adequate oral hygiene.
- Two forms of muscular dystrophy affect muscles of the head and neck. In facioscapulohumeral muscular dystrophy, weakness in the perioral muscles may produce deformities of the face and difficulties in mastication and phonation. In oculopharyngeal muscular dystrophy, weakness of the pharyngeal muscles results in dysphagia that may be severe enough to produce cachexia and require a gastrostomy or a nasogastric tube. In both types of muscular dystrophy, weakness in facial muscles causes difficulty with retaining fluids in the mouth during drinking and rinsing.
- In some forms of muscular dystrophy, such as myotonic dystrophy and facioscapulohumeral muscular dystrophy, malocclusions may occur more often.

DENTAL MANAGEMENT

- For all patients with muscular dystrophy, the patient's physician should be consulted to determine the severity of the disease and especially whether cardiac abnormalities are present. Patients should be managed according to the status of their cardiovascular system.

- Patients should be monitored carefully following general anesthesia to reduce the risk for postintubation regurgitation and aspiration.
- Patients with mental retardation may require alterations in the delivery of dental care as indicated by their level of mental function.
- Patients may require assistance in rising from the dental chair and in ambulation or transfer to their wheelchair.
- If the patient exhibits dyspnea, dental treatment may need to be delivered with the patient in a more upright position.
- If the patient has weakness in the perioral muscles, fluids used in dental treatment should be evacuated effectively.
- Patients with upper arm weakness may need assistance with oral hygiene.
- For patients who have facial skeletal abnormalities or dental malocclusion, surgical and orthodontic treatment has been performed.

SUGGESTED REFERENCES

Mathews KD. Muscular dystrophy overview: genetics and diagnosis. *Neurol Clin No Am* 2003;21:795.

Rowland LP. Progressive muscular dystrophies, in Rowland LP (ed): *Merritt's Neurology*, ed 10. Philadelphia, Lippincott Williams & Wilkins, 2000, pp 737–749.

Victor M, Ropper AH. The muscular dystrophies, in *Adams and Victor's Principles of Neurology*, ed 7. New York, McGraw-Hill, 2001, pp 1493–1511.

AUTHOR: **DARRYL T. HAMAMOTO, DDS, PHD**

SYNONYM(S)

None

ICD-9CM/CPT CODE(S)

358.00 Myasthenia gravis

OVERVIEW

Myasthenia gravis is an autoimmune disorder of the neuromuscular junction that is characterized clinically by muscle weakness and fatigability.

EPIDEMIOLOGY & DEMOGRAPHICS

INCIDENCE/PREVALENCE IN USA: Myasthenia gravis is a rare disease, with a prevalence ranging from 40 to 200 cases per million people. Approximately 60,000 people in the U.S. suffer from myasthenia gravis. The reported prevalence of myasthenia gravis has increased over the last 50 years and is now more than four times higher than it was in the 1950s. This increase is likely due to improved recognition of the disease and the use of diagnostic tests with higher sensitivity and specificity. The incidence of myasthenia gravis is higher in older individuals; so as the proportion of elderly in the general population increases, the prevalence of myasthenia gravis will increase.

PREDOMINANT AGE: For males, the incidence of myasthenia gravis is highest in the sixth and seventh decades of life, whereas for females the incidence peaks in the second and third decades.

PREDOMINANT SEX: Myasthenia gravis is twice as prevalent in males than females.

GENETICS:

- Typical adult and juvenile myasthenia gravis do have a familial predisposition (5% of cases) and an increased frequency of HLA-B8 and DR3.
- Neonatal myasthenia gravis is not a genetic disorder. Fifteen percent of infants born to myasthenic mothers have neonatal myasthenia gravis due to the transplacental passage of acetylcholine receptor antibodies. The condition completely resolves in weeks to months.
- Infants with congenital myasthenia gravis syndromes are born to normal mothers. The onset is at birth or in early childhood. Inheritance is typically autosomal recessive. The condition is persistent.

ETIOLOGY & PATHOGENESIS

- Antibody-mediated autoimmune disorder in which at least two different proteins, the acetylcholine receptor and muscle-specific kinase, are the targets of the antibodies.
- Seronegative myasthenia gravis is the term used for patients who do not have detectable levels of antiacetylcholine receptor antibodies. Between 5–30% of patients with myasthenia gravis are seronegative. Up to 70% of seronegative patients actually have antibodies against muscle-specific kinase. The remaining group of seronegative patients likely has antibodies against other proteins involved with neuromuscular transmission.
- Binding of antibodies to the acetylcholine receptor alters receptor function, promotes receptor endocytosis and degradation, and activates complement-mediated destruction of the postsynaptic surface. All of theses processes lead to decreased neurotransmission at the neuromuscular junction and result in impaired muscle function.
- Binding of antibodies to muscle-specific kinase reduces the clustering of acetylcholine receptors at the neuromuscular junction and thereby reduces neuromuscular transmission.
- Autoantibody production in myasthenia gravis is T cell dependent. CD4+ T-helper cells that are specific for the acetylcholine receptor or muscle-specific kinase activate antibody producing B cells.
- The thymus plays an important role in inducing tolerance to self-antigens. In patients with myasthenia gravis, lymphoid follicular hyperplasia and thymomas are often found. These tissues are enriched in acetylcholine receptor-reactive T cells and contain B cells capable of producing antibodies that bind to the acetylcholine receptor.

CLINICAL PRESENTATION / PHYSICAL FINDINGS

- The onset of symptoms and signs are often insidious but can be unmasked by coincidental infection.
- Signs and symptoms may be localized to a few muscle groups (e.g., ocular muscles) or may become generalized.
- Ocular signs and symptoms include ptosis and asymmetrical ocular palsies resulting in diplopia. These are the initial signs in the majority of patients with myasthenia gravis and may remain the only signs in up to 15% of patients.
- Bulbar (i.e., cranial nerve) signs and symptoms include altered speech, facial weakness, and difficulty chewing and swallowing. Weakness in the facial muscles produces a sleepy, expressionless, apathetic appearance.
- Generalized myasthenia gravis refers to patients who have involvement of distal extremity muscles.
- Respiratory difficulties and limb weakness are worsened by sustained muscular activity and are improved by rest.
- Symptoms often fluctuate in intensity both daily and over longer periods with spontaneous remissions and relapses that last for weeks. Generally a slowly progressive disorder that can be fatal due to respiratory complications such as aspiration pneumonia.
- Clinical examination reveals weakness and fatigability of affected muscles.
- Approximately 20% of patients with myasthenia gravis experience myasthenic crisis (see Complications following), usually within the first year of illness.

DIAGNOSIS

- Edrophonium chloride (Tensilon) test: administration of edrophonium chloride enhances neuromuscular transmission by inhibiting the enzyme acetylcholinesterase and delaying degradation of acetylcholine in the neuromuscular junction. Administration of edrophonium chloride to patients suspected to have myasthenia gravis improves strength in the affected muscles (usually resolution of eyelid ptosis). This test is neither absolutely sensitive nor specific for myasthenia gravis but is readily accessible and easy to perform.
- Repetitive nerve stimulation: most commonly used electrophysiological test to evaluate neuromuscular transmission. It is the least sensitive of the diagnostic techniques but is widely available and easy to perform. Repetitive stimulation of a peripheral nerve depletes the store of acetylcholine at the neuromuscular junction of affected muscles and results in a sequential decrease in compound muscle action potentials evoked by the release of acetylcholine. Nerves that innervate muscles in the extremities or face should be tested depending upon the affected muscles.
- Single-fiber electromyography: needle electrodes are used to record the latency from nerve activation to generation of muscle action potentials from individual muscle fibers. Single-fiber electromyography requires special equipment and training. The variation in the latency (i.e., jitter) is small in normal muscles but is increased in muscles with a defect in neuromuscular transmission. Single-fiber electromyography is the most sensitive clinical test for detection of defects in neuromuscular transmission. Virtually all patients with myasthenia gravis exhibit jitter in single-fiber electrophysiology if the appropriate muscles are tested. Other disorders of nerves or muscle may produce jitter and must be excluded by clinical and electrophysiological examination.
- Serological testing: antibodies that bind to the acetylcholine receptor are present in ~ 85% of patients with myasthenia gravis and are thought to be the

most specific diagnostic marker. A large proportion of seronegative patients exhibit antibodies to muscle-specific kinase.

- Computed tomography (CT) or magnetic resonance imaging (MRI) of the chest is important for detecting the presence of a thymoma, which occurs in about 10% of patients with myasthenia gravis.

MEDICAL MANAGEMENT & TREATMENT

- Anticholinesterase inhibitors: as the first line of treatment for myasthenia gravis, these medications (e.g., pyridostigmine) decrease degradation of acetylcholine in the synaptic cleft, resulting in an increase in the amount of acetylcholine available for neuromuscular transmission. Anticholinesterase inhibitors provide symptomatic treatment but may be the only treatment needed. Improvement usually takes a few weeks to several months of treatment.
- Immunomodulating medications: if anticholinesterase inhibitors do not control the weakness, corticosteroids, azathioprine, cyclosporine, or mycophenolate mofetil (MyM) can be added to the treatment regimen. These immunomodulating medications decrease levels of antibodies that bind to the acetylcholine receptor, often through inhibiting proliferation of B- and/or T-lymphocytes. Each medication has significant side effects (e.g., leukopenia, hepatotoxicity, and nephrotoxicity).
- Intravenous immunoglobulin (IVIg): experimental and anecdotal evidence suggests that IVIg is effective in treating myasthenia gravis although its exact mechanism is unknown. IVIg is often used to treat patients with myasthenia gravis who have not responded well to other immunomodulating therapies.
- Plasmapheresis: by removing the plasma proteins from blood, plasmapheresis removes acetylcholine receptor antibodies and is especially useful for patients experiencing myasthenic crisis (see following) because improvement occurs within a few days. However, the effects of plasmapheresis last only a few weeks. Because of the risks of having a chronic indwelling catheter, use of plasmapheresis chronically is unattractive.
- Thymectomy: patients with myasthenia gravis undergoing thymectomy are more likely to achieve remission, become asymptomatic, or show clinical improvement than patients who do not have thymectomies. However, the majority of myasthenia gravis patients having thymectomies still will not have remissions or become asymptomatic,

and the effects of thymectomy may take several years. The presence of a thymoma is an absolute indication for thymectomy.

COMPLICATIONS

- Myasthenic crisis is defined as myasthenic weakness leading to respiratory failure requiring intubation and mechanical ventilation. Myasthenic patients undergoing surgery in whom extubation is delayed for 24 hours or more due to myasthenic weakness are also considered to be in myasthenic crisis.
- Fever, pneumonia, and atelectasis (i.e., absence of gas exchange in the alveoli of the lungs) are the most common complications associated with myasthenic crisis.

PROGNOSIS

Myasthenia gravis is a chronic disorder that can fluctuate in severity from remission to myasthenic crises. Because of improved management approaches, the fatality rate has declined to 6% over the last 40 years. Overall, the prognosis for patients with myasthenia gravis is generally good with a 3-year survival rate of 85% and a 20-year survival rate of 63%. The survival rates for both women and men with myasthenia gravis are slightly lower than for those without the disease. Older age at diagnosis and greater severity of disease were associated with lower survival rates.

DENTAL SIGNIFICANCE

- Weak oropharyngeal muscles may result in collapse of the upper airway and obstruction. Inability to swallow saliva and a weak cough may contribute to obstruction of the airway, hypoxia, and may result in aspiration pneumonia.
- Lipomatous atrophy may result in longitudinal furrowing and flaccidity of the tongue.
- Tongue weakness contributes to difficulty swallowing.
- Lack of strength in the masticatory muscles decreases effective chewing and, along with difficulty swallowing, can lead to malnutrition and dehydration.
- Difficulty elevating the mandible leads some patients to rest their chin on their hand.
- Weakness in the palatal and pharyngeal muscles may result in altered speech and make verbal communication difficult.
- Dropped head syndrome occurs due to weak neck extensor muscles.

- Macrolide antibiotics such as erythromycin and azithromycin may increase myasthenic weakness and trigger a myasthenic crisis.

DENTAL MANAGEMENT

- Consultation with the patient's physician should be obtained for all patients with myasthenia gravis to determine the severity of the disease.
- Chewing and swallowing may be improved by having the patient take their anticholinesterase medication 1 hour before eating. Frequent rest breaks during meals and eating soft foods in small portions can help patients with myasthenia gravis consume more food. Eating the main meal in the morning when muscles are stronger may also be helpful.
- Patients with stable and mild myasthenia gravis can be treated in a private dental office. Patients with significant oropharyngeal, respiratory, or generalized weakness should be treated in a facility with emergency respiratory services, such as a hospital dental clinic.
- Short, morning appointments will take advantage of greater muscle strength associated with the morning and help to reduce muscle fatigue.
- Dental appointments scheduled 1 to 2 hours after the patient takes their anticholinesterase medication will take advantage of the maximum therapeutic effect of their medication and reduce the risk for a myasthenic crisis. Short rest periods during treatment can help reduce muscle fatigue.
- Positioning the patient more upright in the dental chair may prevent respiratory distress.
- Manage oral infections aggressively, since they may precipitate a myasthenic crisis.
- Anticholinesterase medications may result in excess salivation and increase the risk of aspiration in patients with swallowing difficulties associated with myasthenia gravis. High-speed evacuation and/or constant use of a saliva ejector are needed.
- Oral hygiene may be impaired in patients with muscle weakness. Supplemental oral hygiene procedures, such as more frequent recall appointments, use of electric toothbrushes, and use of fluoride mouth rinses may be indicated.
- Patients with myasthenia gravis may have difficulty using complete dentures due to weak oral and facial muscles. Ill-fitting dentures may lead to oral and facial muscle fatigue, impaired speech, and difficulty chewing.
- Patients taking anticholinesterase medications should not be administered ester-type local anesthetics (e.g.,

procaine). Ester-type local anesthetics are metabolized by plasma cholinesterases, and inhibition of these cholinesterases may result in toxic levels of the anesthetic.

- Amide-type local anesthetics (e.g., lidocaine and mepivacaine) should be used with caution due to their potential to produce respiratory depression.
- Avoid the use of medications that potentiate myasthenic weakness (e.g., erythromycin, azithromycin, and clindamycin). Penicillin and its derivatives are relatively safe.

- Narcotic analgesic medications should be used with caution due to their potential for respiratory depression. Cholinesterase inhibitors may potentiate the analgesic effects of narcotics.
- Corticosteroids can exacerbate myasthenia gravis.

SUGGESTED REFERENCES

Meriggioli MN, Sanders DB. Myasthenia gravis: diagnosis. *Sem Neurol* 2004;24:31.

Patton LL, Howard, Jr JF. Myasthenia gravis: dental treatment considerations. *Special Care in Dentistry* 1997;17:25.

Phillips II LH. The epidemiology of myasthenia gravis. *Sem Neurol* 2004;24:17.

Saperstein DS, Barohn RJ. Management of myasthenia gravis. *Sem Neurol* 2004;24:41.

Shaw DH, et al. Dental treatment of patients with myasthenia gravis. *J Oral Med* 1982; 37:188.

AUTHOR: **DARRYL T. HAMAMOTO, DDS, PHD**

SYNONYM(S)

Heart attack
Coronary thrombosis
Coronary occlusion

ICD-9CM/CPT CODE(S)

410.90 Acute myocardial infarction, unspecified site, episode of care unspecified—complete

OVERVIEW

Acute myocardial infarction (MI) refers to irreversible myocardial injury occurring as a result of prolonged ischemia. The result is coagulative necrosis of the myocardial fibers with loss of the normal conductive and contractile properties of the affected myocardial tissue.

EPIDEMIOLOGY & DEMOGRAPHICS

INCIDENCE/PREVALENCE IN USA: 500 to 600 cases exist per 100,000 persons. Each year in the U.S. approximately 1.5 million people sustain a MI, with 460,000 deaths due to coronary artery-related disease.

PREDOMINANT AGE: Incidence of MI rises progressively with increasing age; the majority (55%) of patients who develop an acute MI are older than 65 years. Elderly people also tend to have higher rates of morbidity and mortality from their infarcts.

PREDOMINANT SEX: More prominent in males between age 40 and 70 years; after age 70, there is an equal incidence in both sexes.

GENETICS: No clearly established genetic pattern has been established for MI; however, increased risk for predisposing factors (e.g., atherosclerotic coronary artery disease, hypertension) does appear to have strong familial tendencies.

ETIOLOGY & PATHOGENESIS

- Coronary artery atherosclerosis is the leading cause of MI. The initiating factor in most cases of MI is coronary artery thrombosis resulting from the ruptured margins of an atherosclerotic fibrous plaque resulting in hemorrhage, platelet aggregation, thrombosis, and then occlusion or blocking of a coronary artery.
- Myocardial necrosis begins at approximately 30 minutes after occlusion of a coronary artery. Classic, acute MI with extensive damage occurs when the perfusion of the myocardium is reduced severely below its needs for an extended interval (usually at least 2 to 4 hours), causing profound, prolonged ischemia and resulting in permanent loss of function of large regions of the heart in which myocardial cell death (predominately by coagulation necrosis) has occurred.

- MI most frequently involves the left ventricle due to its greater workload as compared with the other heart chambers. When right ventricular infarction occurs, it almost always represents an extension of severe left ventricular infarction.
- Other less common causes of MI include:
  - Emboli to the coronary arteries (e.g., infective endocarditis, aortic or mitral valve lesions, left atrial or ventricular thrombi, prosthetic heart valves, fat emboli).
  - Coronary artery vasculitis/aneurysms (e.g., Takayasu's disease, Kawasaki's disease, polyarteritis nodosa, systemic lupus erythematosus, scleroderma, rheumatoid arthritis).
  - Coronary artery vasospasm [e.g., idiopathic (vasospastic angina) or drug-induced (nitrate withdrawal, cocaine or amphetamine abuse)].
  - Infiltrative and degenerative coronary vascular disease [e.g., amyloidosis, connective tissue disorders (pseudoxanthoma elasticum), lipid storage disorders and mucopolysaccharidoses, homocystinuria, diabetes mellitus, collagen vascular disease, muscular dystrophies, Friedreich's ataxia].
  - Congenital coronary vascular anomalies (e.g., anomalous origin of left coronary from pulmonary artery, left coronary artery from anterior sinus of Valsalva, coronary arteriovenous fistulas).
  - Myocardial oxygen supply–demand imbalance (e.g., carbon monoxide poisoning, pheochromocytoma, thyrotoxicosis, methemoglobinemia, aortic stenosis/insufficiency, prolonged hypotension).
  - Hematological (in situ) thrombosis due to hypercoagulable states and/or increased blood viscosity (e.g., polycythemia vera, thrombocytosis, thrombotic thrombocytopenic purpura, disseminated intravascular coagulation, antithrombin III deficiency, macroglobulinemia, multiple myeloma, sickle cell anemia).
  - Myocardial trauma [cardiac contusion, radiation (therapy for neoplasia)].

CLINICAL PRESENTATION / PHYSICAL FINDINGS

- Signs and symptoms of acute MI include:
  - Premonitory symptoms: approximately one-third of patients give a history of a change (usually worsening) in the pattern of angina pectoris, recent onset of typical or atypical (unstable) angina, or unusual "indigestion" or pressure or squeezing felt in the chest prior to experiencing an acute MI.

  - Pain of infarction:
    - The most common and best symptom on which to base a consideration of MI is a sudden onset of substernal pain (the location of which may be similar to previous angina pectoris) that is intense, severe, and unremitting for 30 to 60 minutes and may be described as "pressure," "dull," "squeezing," "aching," or "oppressive" and is often associated with apprehension or a sense of impending doom.
    - The discomfort is usually in the center of the chest and may radiate to the left or right arm, neck, jaw, back, shoulders, or abdomen and is not pleuritic in character.
    - Nitroglycerin has little effect in relieving the chest discomfort of MI; even opioids (i.e., morphine) may not relieve the pain.
    - Symptoms of MI usually begin while at rest and only occasionally are brought on by physical exertion that may have previously resulted in anginal episodes.
    - MI most commonly occurs in the morning hours, soon after awakening.
  - Associated symptoms can include profound restlessness, confusion, diaphoresis, weakness, light-headedness, syncope, dyspnea, orthopnea, cough, wheezing, nausea and vomiting, or abdominal bloating which may be present singly or in any combination.
- Additional physical findings associated with MI may include:
  - Mild tachycardia and hypertension (frequently) but bradycardia and hypotension are common in inferior wall MI due to increased vagal tone.
  - Apical systolic murmur caused by mitral regurgitation if papillary muscle ischemia or infarction is present; S_4 is commonly detected, also S_3 if heart failure is present.
  - Bibasilar rales may be present and are indicative of left ventricular heart failure.
  - Jugular vein distension if biventricular heart failure or right ventricular infarction is present.
- In some cases, MI may be clinically silent or associated with only mild discomfort. Studies have indicated that 20–33% of patients diagnosed with MI did not have chest pain upon presentation to the hospital but, rather, presented with less-pronounced symptoms, including generalized weakness, dyspnea, and indigestion. This is particularly true in women, patients with diabetes mellitus, and in patients with a history of prior heart failure or who have undergone cardiac transplantation.

- In contrast to the classic, clinical presentation of acute MI, some women may have less-typical symptoms when experiencing MI. Women are less likely than men to feel severe chest pain and are more likely to report a feeling of severe pyrosis or indigestion in the upper abdomen and/or severe weakness or fatigue.

DIAGNOSIS

Diagnostic tests used in the evaluation of a possible MI include:

- Quantitative determinations of serum troponin I (cTnI), troponin T (cTnT), and CK-MB:
  - Increased serum levels of cTnI and cTnT have been shown to be a specific indicators of myocardial injury. They appear 3 to 6 hours after MI, peak at 16 hours, and decrease for several days after MI (up to 7 days for cTnI and up to 10 to 14 days for cTnT).
  - Elevation of CK-MB in serum is highly suggestive of MI.
- Lactate dehydrogenase (LDH): rises above normal values within 24 to 48 hours of MI, peaks at 3 to 6 days, and returns to baseline within 8 to 12 days.
- Electrocardiography:
  - ST segment elevation in a regional pattern is typical of acute transmural ischemia.
  - ST segment depression with T-wave inversions is typical of subendocardial ischemia.
  - Q waves, representing transmural myocardial necrosis, usually develop over 12 to 36 hours.
- Diagnostic imaging:
  - Chest radiograph: findings dependent on severity of MI; may demonstrate signs of congestive heart failure (CHF).
  - 2-D and M-mode echocardiography: useful in evaluating wall motion abnormalities in MI, overall left ventricular function, postinfarction mitral rupture or regurgitation, or ventricular septal defect.
  - Technetium-99m pyrophosphate scintigraphy: a γ-emitting calcium analog that accumulates in infarcted, necrotic myocardium. When injected at least 18 hours postinfarction, the radiotracer complexes with calcium in necrotic myocardium to provide a radiographic "hot-spot" image of the infarction that can be used to aid in the diagnosis of acute MI.
  - Thallium-201 scintigraphy: a γ-emitting potassium analog that distributes within the myocardium parallel to the blood flow. When injected at rest, thallium 201 accumulates in myocardial cells that are well-supplied with blood and are metabolically active and will demonstrate radiographic "cold spots" in regions of diminished myocardial perfusion (which usually represent infarction) but such abnormalities do not distinguish recent from old infarction.

MEDICAL MANAGEMENT & TREATMENT

- The overall goals in the medical management of acute MI are designed to relieve pain and distress, reverse ischemia, limit infarct size, reduce myocardial oxygen demand, and prevent and treat complications.
- Initial management of acute MI typically includes:
  - Aspirin: administer aspirin 160 to 325 mg PO immediately on suspicion of MI (unless true aspirin allergy is suspected). If the dose is chewed, a therapeutic blood level is achieved more rapidly than if it is swallowed. Clopidogrel may be substituted if a true aspirin allergy is present.
  - Nitrates: nitroglycerin may be used to relieve chest pain associated with MI, alleviate hypertension, and decrease preload in patients with associated CHF. Sublingual nitroglycerin can be administered immediately on suspicion of MI (unless systolic blood pressure is < 90 mmHg or heart rate is < 50 bpm or > 100 bpm). It may be started at sublingual doses of 0.4 mg given every 5 minutes for three doses to relieve chest pain, followed by an intravenous nitroglycerin infusion if necessary as long as hypotension is not present.
  - Oxygen: via nasal cannula at 2 to 4 L/min.
  - Morphine sulfate: 2 to 5 mg IV, repeated every 5 to 30 minutes as necessary for severe pain unrelieved by nitroglycerin.
  - β-Adrenergic blocker (e.g., metoprolol, 5 mg IV every 2 to 5 minutes for three doses) has been shown to decrease the likelihood of ventricular dysrhythmias and recurrent ischemia in acute MI in the absence of contraindications such as bradycardia or CHF.
  - Angiotensin-converting enzyme (ACE) inhibitor: (e.g., captopril 6.25 to 50 mg PO, tid) reduce left ventricular dysfunction and dilation and slow the progression of CHF.
  - Thrombolytic therapy: if the duration of pain has been less than 6 hours and primary angioplasty is not readily available, recanalization of the occluded arteries should be attempted with thrombolytic agents such as tissue plasminogen activator (tPA), reteplase (rPA), or streptokinase, possibly in combination with glycoprotein IIb/IIIa inhibition (e.g., abciximab). Because the effectiveness of thrombolytics is time-dependent, ideally these agents should be administered either in the field or within 30 minutes of the patient's arrival in the hospital. When thrombolytics are used, IV heparin is given to increase the likelihood of patency in the infarct-related artery.
  - Percutaneous coronary intervention (PCI): if readily available without delay, PCI with adjunctive glycoprotein IIb/IIIa inhibition is preferred over thrombolytic therapy. It is effective and generally results in more favorable outcomes than thrombolytic therapy. When PCI is performed, use of IV heparin is recommended. Coronary stents are useful to decrease ischemia, improve long-term patency, and lower the rate of restenosis of the infarct-related artery.

COMPLICATIONS

Possible complications secondary to MI include:

- Dysrhythmias: ventricular dysrhythmias, such as ventricular fibrillation, are the most common cause of sudden cardiac death in the first hour post-MI.
- Heart failure/cardiogenic shock: heart failure develops when the infarct involves 20–25% of the left ventricle. Scar tissue over the infarcted area results in decreased contractility and abnormal ventricular wall motion, with subsequent reduction of cardiac output usually resulting in CHF. Infarction involving 40% or more of the left ventricle leads to cardiogenic shock, which is the most common cause of death among in-hospital patients with acute MI.
- Myocardial rupture: rupture of the myocardium at the site of infarction can occur at any time within about 3 weeks after onset of the infarct, but it tends to occur most frequently between 2 and 10 days postinfarction, when the infarcted zone has minimal structural strength. After cardiogenic shock and dysrhythmias, cardiac rupture is the most common cause of post-MI death, being responsible for up to 20% of all fatal infarcts.
- Thromboembolism: mural thrombi can form on the disrupted endocardial surface over areas of infarcted/necrotic myocardium. Because these thrombi are quite friable prior to fibrous organization, portions of a thrombus may break off and enter the peripheral circulation as emboli. These emboli most frequently occlude arterial vessels that supply the brain, kidneys, spleen, intestine, and extremities and may result in infarction.
- Aneurysm: ventricular aneurysm is a late complication that occurs in 12–20% of patients. It develops when the fibrous scar that forms after infarction

has insufficient structural strength to withstand the intraventricular chamber pressure. The scar stretches, resulting in extreme thinning of the ventricular wall with progressive convex deformity of the external cardiac surface. Stasis of blood within the aneurysm results in mural thrombi in 50% of cases because the affected segment of myocardium cannot contract in phase with the remaining normal ventricle.

- Pericarditis: fibrinous pericarditis can develop soon after infarction in the region overlying the myocardial necrosis, or it may become generalized. It is clinically evident in 7–15% of cases, characterized by a pericardial friction rub heard on auscultation. Complete resolution or conversion to inconsequential fibrous adhesions may occur.
  - Dressler's syndrome: characterized by pericarditis, pericardial effusion, and fever; may develop within 2 weeks to several months postinfarction. It develops in less than 5% of post-MI patients and is thought to be of autoimmune origin.

PROGNOSIS

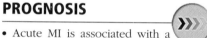

- Acute MI is associated with a 30% mortality rate; half of the deaths occur prior to arrival at the hospital.
- An additional 5–10% of survivors die within the first year after their MI.
- Approximately half of all patients are rehospitalized within 1 year of their MI (index event).
- Overall, prognosis is highly variable and depends on multiple factors, including:
  - The timing and nature of medical intervention and success of the intervention
  - Size (extent) and location (site) of the infarct
  - Ejection fraction after MI (amount of the residual left ventricular function)
  - Presence of dysrhythmias
  - Presence of post-MI angina
  - Use of post-MI β-adrenergic blocker therapy
  - Use of lipid-lowering agents in patients with hyperlipidemia
  - Presence of comorbid conditions (e.g., diabetes, hypertension)

DENTAL SIGNIFICANCE

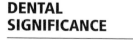

The dental provider must remain aware of the fact that

the duration and extent of any dental procedure (including the degree of invasiveness of any surgical intervention) and the resultant physiologic stress to the patient are crucial factors affecting the overall safety of dental treatment in the post-MI patient.

DENTAL MANAGEMENT

The management of the dental patient with a history of MI should start with a comprehensive patient assessment that would include:

- Determining the time interval from MI as a predictor of dental treatment risk:
  - Recent (> 7 days but ≤ 30 days) MI with evidence of important ischemic risk by clinical symptoms or noninvasive study: high risk
  - Prior MI (> 30 days) by history or pathological Q waves and cardiovascular status stable: moderate to low risk
- Presence of other significant cardiovascular pathology and/or increased surgical risk, including:
  - Congestive heart failure (especially uncontrolled/decompensated)
  - Dysrhythmias (especially high-grade atrioventricular block, symptomatic ventricular dysrhythmias, supraventricular dysrhythmias with uncontrolled ventricular rate)
  - Angina pectoris (especially if severe or unstable)
  - Valvular heart disease
- Presence of continued risk factors for MI including hypertension, hyperlipidemia or hypercholesterolemia, diabetes mellitus, and smoking.
- An individual assessment of the patient's post-MI current status and stability (this will usually require a medical consultation with the patient's physician).
  - If the post-MI dental patient has been established by medical consultation/evaluation as not being at risk for continued ischemia, dental treatment can be considered as early as 6 weeks post-MI.

Specific management considerations for the post-MI dental patient would include:

- Appropriate patient monitoring:
  - Record pretreatment vital signs.
  - Continuous (automated) monitoring of blood pressure, pulse, and blood oxygen saturation during dental treatment is advantageous.

- Stress reduction measures:
  - Keep appointment duration as short as possible. Also, morning appointments are probably preferable for most patients as they may become more fatigued as the day progresses.
  - Consider the use of N_2O-O_2 inhalation sedation and/or premedication with oral antianxiety medications such as benzodiazepines (e.g., triazolam, 0.125 to 0.5 mg the night before appointment and 0.125 to 0.5 mg 1 hour before treatment).
- Ensure adequate oxygenation:
  - Oxygen by nasal cannula at 2 to 4 L/min (if not already using N_2O-O_2 inhalation sedation).
  - A semisupine or upright chair position may be needed for patients with a history of orthopnea.
- Use of pretreatment nitrates:
  - If dental treatment predictably precipitates angina, then consider premedication with nitroglycerin (0.3 mg to 0.6 mg sublingual tablet) prior to initiating dental treatment.
  - Patient should bring own supply of nitroglycerin to appointment for use if necessary. This should be placed in easy reach of the patient in case a dose is necessary during dental treatment.
- Establish profound local anesthesia:
  - For high-risk, post-MI patients, the use of vasoconstrictors in local anesthetics may be contraindicated and should be discussed with the patient's physician.
    - For post-MI patients that are not considered high-risk and where vasoconstrictors are not contraindicated because of potential drug interactions, it is advisable to limit the total dose of vasoconstrictor (see Appendix A, Box A-3, "Local Anesthetic with Vasoconstrictor Dose Restriction Guidelines").
- Ensure adequate posttreatment pain control with analgesics as indicated.

SUGGESTED REFERENCES

Niwa H, et al. Safety of dental treatment in patients with previously diagnosed acute myocardial infarction or unstable angina pectoris. *Oral Surg Oral Med Oral Pathol Oral Radiol Endod* 2000;89:35–41.

Roberts HW, Mitnitsky EF. Cardiac risk stratification for postmyocardial infarction dental patients. *Oral Surg Oral Med Oral Pathol Oral Radiol Endod* 2001;91:676–681.

AUTHOR: F. JOHN FIRRIOLO, DDS, PHD

SYNONYM(S)

Nephrosis

ICD-9CM/CPT CODE(S)

581   Nephrotic syndrome—incomplete

581.0   Nephrotic syndrome with lesion of proliferative glomerulonephritis—complete

581.1   Nephrotic syndrome with lesion of membranous glomerulonephritis—complete

581.2   Nephrotic syndrome with lesion of membranoproliferative glomerulonephritis—complete

581.3   Nephrotic syndrome with lesion of minimal change glomerulonephritis—complete

581.8   Nephrotic syndrome with other specified pathological lesion in kidney—incomplete

581.81   Nephrotic syndrome with other specified pathological lesion in kidney in diseases classified elsewhere—complete

581.89   Other nephrotic syndrome with specified pathological lesion in kidney—complete

581.9   Nephrotic syndrome with unspecified pathological lesion in kidney—complete

OVERVIEW

Nephrotic syndrome consists of clinical and laboratory abnormalities common to a variety of primary and secondary kidney diseases, each characterized by increased permeability of the glomerular capillary wall to circulating plasma proteins, particularly albumin. Nephrotic syndrome results in a constellation of signs and symptoms including protein in the urine (exceeding 3.5 g per 1.73 m² body-surface area per 24 hours), hypoalbuminemia, with plasma albumin levels less than 3 g/dL, generalized edema, and hyperlipidemia. The urine often contains fat (lipiduria) that is visible under the microscope.

EPIDEMIOLOGY & DEMOGRAPHICS

INCIDENCE/PREVALENCE IN USA: In children, 2 new cases per 100,000 per year; in adults, 3 new cases per 100,000 per year.

PREDOMINANT AGE: Occurs predominantly in children 2 to 6 years of age and in adults of all ages.

PREDOMINANT SEX: Males are slightly more likely to be affected than females.

GENETICS: None established.

ETIOLOGY & PATHOGENESIS

- Idiopathic or primary causes of nephrotic syndrome:
  - Minimal change disease (also known as nil disease or lipoid nephrosis) (incidence 5–10%)
  - Focal segmental glomerulosclerosis (incidence 20–25%)
  - Membranous nephropathy (incidence 25–30%)
  - Membranoproliferative glomerulonephritis (incidence 5%)
  - Other proliferative and sclerosing glomerulonephritides (incidence 15–30%)
- Nephrotic syndrome associated with specific causes ("secondary" nephrotic syndrome):
  - Systemic diseases:
    - Diabetes mellitus
    - Systemic lupus erythematosus and other collagen diseases
    - Amyloidosis (amyloid AL or AA associated)
    - Vasculitic-immunologic disease (mixed cryoglobulinemia, Wegener's granulomatosis, rapidly progressive glomerulonephritis, polyarteritis, Henoch-Schönlein purpura, sarcoidosis, Goodpasture's syndrome)
  - Infections:
    - Bacterial (poststreptococcal, congenital and secondary syphilis, subacute bacterial endocarditis, shunt nephritis)
    - Viral (hepatitis B, hepatitis C, HIV infection, infectious mononucleosis, cytomegalovirus infection)
    - Parasitic (malaria, toxoplasmosis, schistosomiasis, filariasis)
  - Medication-related:
    - Gold, mercury, and the heavy metals
    - Penicillamine
    - Nonsteroidal antiinflammatory drugs
    - Lithium
    - Paramethadione, trimethadione
    - Captopril
    - Narcotic analgesic abuse (e.g., "street" heroin)
    - Others: probenecid, chlorpropamide, rifampin, tolbutamide, phenindione
  - Allergens, venoms, and immunizations
  - Associated with neoplasms:
    - Hodgkin's lymphoma and leukemia lymphomas (with minimal change lesion)
    - Solid tumors (with membranous nephropathy)
  - Hereditary and metabolic disease:
    - Alport's syndrome
    - Fabry's disease
    - Sickle cell disease
    - Congenital (Finnish type) nephrotic syndrome
    - Familial nephrotic syndrome
    - Nail-patella syndrome
    - Partial lipodystrophy
  - Other causes of secondary nephrotic syndrome:
    - Pregnancy related (includes preeclampsia)
    - Transplant rejection
    - Serum sickness
    - Accelerated hypertensive nephrosclerosis
    - Unilateral renal artery stenosis
    - Sleep apnea associated with massive obesity
    - Reflux nephropathy

(Adapted from Goldman L, Ausiello D (eds). *Cecil's Textbook of Medicine*, ed 22. Philadelphia, WB Saunders, 2004, p 727.)

CLINICAL PRESENTATION / PHYSICAL FINDINGS

- Edema:
  - Peripheral, especially in the feet and ankles
  - Abdominal (ascites)
  - Periorbital
- Significant weight gain (unintentional) from fluid retention
- Foamy appearance of the urine
- Poor appetite
- Pleural effusion
- Hypertension
- Exertional dyspnea

DIAGNOSIS

Diagnostic workup consists of family and drug history, exposure to toxins, and laboratory evaluation.

LABORATORY

- Urinalysis reveals proteinuria. The presence of hematuria, cellular casts, and pyuria is suggestive of nephritic syndrome. Oval fat bodies are often present in the urine (lipiduria).
- 24-hour urine protein excretion is > 3.5 g per 1.73 m² body-surface area.
- Hypoalbuminemia (< 3 g/dL), hyperlipidemia, hypercholesterolemia, and azotemia may also be present.

Evaluation of the nephrotic patient also includes laboratory tests to define whether the patient has primary, idiopathic nephrotic syndrome or a secondary cause related to a systemic disease. Common screening tests include:

- Fasting blood sugar and glycosylated hemoglobin tests (for diabetes)
- Antinuclear antibody test (for collagen vascular disease)
- Serum complement levels (screens for many immune complex-mediated diseases)
- Antineutrophil cytoplasmic antibodies (ANCAs)
- Anti-GBM antibodies
- Rheumatoid factor
- Cryoglobulins
- Hepatitis B and C serology
- VDRL serology
- Serum protein electrophoresis

Renal biopsy is generally performed in individuals with persistent proteinuria in whom the etiology of the proteinuria is unclear.

IMAGING STUDIES
- Renal ultrasound
- Chest radiograph

MEDICAL MANAGEMENT & TREATMENT

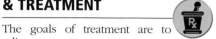

The goals of treatment are to relieve symptoms, prevent complications, and delay progressive kidney damage. Treatment of the causative disorder is necessary to control nephrotic syndrome. Treatment may be required for life.

NONPHARMACOLOGIC
- Bed rest as tolerated, avoidance of nephrotoxic drugs, low-fat diet, and fluid restriction.
- Normal protein diet (usually) unless malnutrition risk.
- Low-fat soy has shown some improvement in urinary protein excretion and serum lipid changes.
- Close evaluation for development of peripheral venous thrombosis.

GENERAL TREATMENT
The goal of treatment is directed toward the underlying disorder:
- Minimal change disease: usually responds to prednisone 1 mg/kg/day. Chlorambucil and cyclophosphamide may also be helpful.
- Focal and segmental glomerulosclerosis: steroid therapy is also indicated. Response rate is 35–40%, and most patients progress to end-stage renal disease within 3 years.
- Membranous glomerulonephritis: prednisone 2 mg/kg/day with adjuvant cytotoxic agents if poor response to steroid.
- Membranoproliferative glomerulonephritis: steroid and antiplatelet therapy. Most patients will progress to end-stage renal failure within 5 years.

GENERAL TREATMENT—ACUTE
- Furosemide is useful for edema.

- ACE inhibitors to reduce proteinuria even in normotensive patients.
- Anticoagulant therapy with proteinuria, albumin levels > 20 g/L.

GENERAL TREATMENT—CHRONIC
- Patients should be monitored for azotemia and aggressively treated for hypertension and hyperlipidemia.
  - If hypertension occurs, it must be treated vigorously. Treatment of high blood cholesterol and triglyceride levels is also recommended to reduce the risk of atherosclerosis. Dietary limitation of cholesterol and saturated fats may be of little benefit since as the high levels that accompany this condition seem to be the result of overproduction by the liver rather than from excessive fat intake. Medications to reduce cholesterol and triglycerides may be recommended.
- Oral vitamin D is useful in the treatment of hypocalcemia due to vitamin D loss.

COMPLICATIONS

- Atherosclerosis and related heart diseases
- Renal vein thrombosis
- Acute renal failure
- Chronic renal failure
- Infections, including pneumococcal pneumonia
- Malnutrition
- Fluid overload, congestive heart failure, pulmonary edema

PROGNOSIS

The outcome varies; the syndrome may be acute and short-term or chronic and unresponsive to therapy. The cause and development of complications also affects the outcome.

DENTAL SIGNIFICANCE

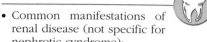

- Common manifestations of renal disease (not specific for nephrotic syndrome):
  - Pallor, hyperpigmentation, ecchymosis of the oral mucosa
  - Renal osteodystrophy of the mandible and maxilla
    - Loss of trabeculation
    - Ground-glass appearance
    - Giant cell lesions
    - Loss of lamina dura
    - Pulp narrowing and calcifications
  - Xerostomia and candidiasis
  - Ammoniacal breath
  - Low caries rate
  - Low-grade gingival inflammation
  - Prolonged bleeding
  - Enamel hypoplasia

DENTAL MANAGEMENT

- Determine extent and chronicity of renal failure and treat as appropriate (see "Renal Disease, Dialysis, and Transplantation" in Section I, p 180 for additional information).
- CBC and serum chemistry prior to invasive dental treatment.
- Assess vital signs each visit.
- Consider antibiotic prophylaxis to prevent postoperative infections for patients taking cytotoxic medications.

SUGGESTED REFERENCE
Robinson RF, Nahata MC, Mahan JD, et al. Management of nephrotic syndrome in children. *Pharmacotherapy (United States)* 2003;23(8):1021–1036.

AUTHOR: SCOTT S. DEROSSI, DMD

SYNONYM(S)

NHL

ICD-9CM/CPT CODE(S)

202.80–202.88 Other malignant neoplasms of lymphoid and histiocytic tissue, other lymphomas

OVERVIEW

- Non-Hodgkin's lymphomas (NHLs) are a heterogeneous group of lymphoproliferative malignancies with differing patterns of behavior and responses to treatment. NHL can be of B-cell (accounting for 85–90% of all NHLs) or T-cell (10–15% of NHLs) origin. Like Hodgkin's lymphoma, NHL usually originates in lymphoid tissues and can spread to other organs. However, NHL is much less predictable than Hodgkin's lymphoma and has a far greater predilection to disseminate to extranodal sites.
- Classification of NHLs is based on pattern of distribution (diffuse or nodular); cell type (lymphocytic, histiocytic, mixed); and degree of differentiation of the cell (well, moderate, poor).
- There are more than 30 types of NHL. The most common types of NHL are:
  - Diffuse large B-cell lymphoma (DLBCL): accounts for 31% of all NHLs. Clinically, DLBCL is an aggressive lymphoma.
  - Follicular lymphoma (FL): accounts for 22% of all NHLs. Clinically, FL (a B-cell lymphoma) is an indolent lymphoma, but it may behave more aggressively or transform into DLBCL.
  - Mucosa-associated lymphoid tissue (MALT) lymphoma: accounts for 8% of all NHLs. Clinically, MALT lymphoma is an indolent tumor but may behave more aggressively or transform into DLBCL.
  - Burkitt's lymphoma: an important, less common form of NHL. Clinically, Burkitt's lymphoma is a highly aggressive tumor and is the most common form of NHL seen in immunocompromised patients (following bone marrow/solid organ transplantation or in HIV infection). Epstein-Barr virus (EBV) infection is also implicated in Burkitt's lymphoma, particularly in Africa (see "Epstein-Barr Virus Diseases: Hairy Leukoplakia" in Section I, p 82; "Epstein-Barr Virus Diseases: Infectious Mononucleosis" in Section I, p 83; and "Burkitt's Lymphoma" in Section II, p 239).

EPIDEMIOLOGY & DEMOGRAPHICS

INCIDENCE/PREVALENCE IN USA: Non-Hodgkin's tumors occur more frequently than Hodgkin's lymphoma. The incidence is 3 in 10,000 people. More than 56,000 cases of non-Hodgkin's lymphoma are diagnosed annually in the U.S. Each year the disease accounts for nearly 25,000 deaths in the U.S.

PREDOMINANT AGE: NHLs can affect people of all ages, although the incidence of NHL increases with age. NHL is more common in patients older than 40 years. About half of all cases are in people aged 60 and older.

PREDOMINANT SEX: Young males are diagnosed more frequently with NHL than are young females, but this difference decreases with increasing age.

GENETICS: Cytogenic and molecular genetic abnormalities with specific mutation and translocation have been well-documented in a number of NHLs.

ETIOLOGY & PATHOGENESIS

- A variety of factors including congenital and acquired immunodeficiency states, as well as infectious, physical, and chemical agents have been associated with an increased risk of developing NHL.
- Infectious agents such as viral infections (EBV, HIV, and the human T-cell leukemia virus) and bacterial infections (such as Helicobacter pylori) have been associated with the development of NHL.

CLINICAL PRESENTATION / PHYSICAL FINDINGS

- More than two-thirds of patients with NHL present with persistent, painless, peripheral lymphadenopathy.
- NHL in the digestive tract can cause nausea, vomiting, or abdominal pain.
- In the chest, shortness of breath or cough may develop.
- If the brain is involved, patients may have headaches, vision changes, or seizures.
- If the bone marrow is affected, lymphoma cells may crowd out red blood cell precursors, causing anemia.
- Other clinical presentations include fever, weight loss, night sweats, and widespread itching.

DIAGNOSIS

- Lymph node biopsy.
- Bone marrow biopsy.
- Peripheral blood smear and CBC with differential.
- Clinical staging of NHL (Box I-2) requires the following: physical examination; CT scan of the abdomen; lymphangiogram; exploratory laparotomy and liver biopsy; chest radiograph; and blood chemistry evaluation (including lactate dehydrogenase and β_2-microglobulin). MRI and other diagnostic imaging studies might also be required.

MEDICAL MANAGEMENT & TREATMENT

- Radiation and chemotherapy are the most successful modes of treatment.
- The National Cancer Institute characterizes NHL according to biologic behavior.
- Low-grade NHL responds to radiotherapy alone and is localized in 10–25% of cases.
- Localized NHL is highly radiosensitive and is treated with 3000 to 5000 cGy to the involved area.
- Intensive combination of chemotherapy is the treatment choice for intermediate and high-grade NHL.
- Commonly used drug protocols include cyclophosphamide, vincristine, and prednisone (CVP), or cyclophosphamide, doxorubicin, vincristine, and prednisone (CHOP).
- More advanced-stage disease requires a combination of radiotherapy and chemotherapy.
- Bone marrow transplant and monoclonal antibody directed against the B-cell surface antigen (e.g., Rituxan) combined with chemotherapy has been shown to be effective for patients who respond poorly to traditional therapies.

COMPLICATIONS

- Complications of NHL include infections as a result of immune suppression from chemotherapy, radiation therapy, or low γ globulin secondary to the disease itself.

PROGNOSIS

- The prognosis depends on the histologic type, stage, and treatment. The NHL can be divided into two prognostic groups: the indolent lymphomas and the aggressive lymphomas.
  - Indolent NHL types have a relatively good prognosis, with median survival as long as 10 years, but they usually are not curable in advanced clinical stages. Early-stage (I and II) indolent NHL can be effectively treated with radiation therapy alone. Most of the indolent types are nodular or follicular in morphology.
  - The aggressive type of NHL has a shorter natural history, but a significant number of these patients can be cured with intensive combination chemotherapy regimens. In general, with modern treatment of patients with NHL, overall survival at 5 years is approximately 50–60%. Thirty to 60% of patients with aggressive NHL can be cured. The vast majority of relapses occur in the first 2 years after therapy. Extranodal lymphoma

in the oral-pharyngeal region has a poor prognosis.

DENTAL SIGNIFICANCE

- Patients with NHL might present with painless cervical lymphadenopathy.
- In the oral cavity, Waldeyer's ring is the most common place to find NHL.
- Intraoral tumors might appear as a swelling of the palate, gingiva, buccal sulcus, or floor of the mouth. This enlargement can be painful or painless.
- Although rarely affecting the primary jawbone, NHL might present as swelling, pain, alveolar bone loss, tooth mobility, and neurologic disturbances, and in severe cases can lead to pathologic fracture of the mandible.
- Primary NHL of the soft tissue might present as an asymptomatic ulceration.
- Presence of any of these orofacial abnormalities requires prompt evaluation followed by biopsy.

DENTAL MANAGEMENT

- Dentists have an important role in preventing serious, life-threatening infections while patients are neutropenic from cancer chemotherapy. These patients should have a dental evaluation and removal of obvious potential sources of bacteremia, such as teeth with advanced periodontal disease (e.g., pocket depths 5 mm or greater, excessive mobility, purulence on probing), prior to chemotherapy. Additional indicators for extraction of teeth prior to chemotherapy include:
  - Periapical inflammation
  - Tooth is broken down, nonrestorable, nonfunctional, or partially erupted, and the patient is noncompliant with oral hygiene measures.
  - Tooth is associated with a inflammatory (e.g., pericoronitis), infectious, or malignant osseous disease.
- Extractions should be performed at least 5 days (in the maxilla) to 7 days (in the mandible) before the initiation of chemotherapy or at least 2 weeks (ideally, 3 weeks) before initiation of radiation therapy that involves the extraction site(s).
- For patients receiving chemotherapy, the dentist should obtain the patient's current WBC and platelet counts before initiating dental care (see "Leukemias (AML, CML, ALL, CLL, Hairy Cell Leukemia)" in Section I, p 132 for information on WBC and platelet counts necessary for routine and emergency dental care).
- Mucositis is a common side effect of radiation and certain chemotherapy drugs. Its management consists of good oral hygiene, cryotherapy (ice chip), and use of mouth washes containing sucralfate or sodium bicarbonate. Amifostine (Ethyol) is a drug that protects against the damage of radiation and can reduce dry mouth and prevent mouth sores. Recombinant human keratinocyte growth factor (palifermin) may ultimately reduce mouth soreness and improve function.
- Radiation may cause xerostomia and damage the taste buds. Patients may benefit by using salivary substitutes or pilocarpine (Salagen) to stimulate salivary flow.

SUGGESTED REFERENCES

Greenberg MS, Glick M (eds): *Burket's Oral Medicine. Diagnosis and Treatment*, ed 10. Hamilton, Ontario, BC Decker, Inc., 2003, pp 385–450.

Little JW. Hematologic diseases, in *Dental Management of the Medically Compromised Patient*. St Louis, Mosby, 2002, p 377.

Long F, De Maria G, Esposito P, Califona L. Primary non-Hodgkin's lymphoma of the mandible: report of a case. *Int J Oral Maxillofac Surg* 2004;33:801–803.

www.cancer.gov/cancerinfo/types/non-hodgkins-lymphoma

www.fda.gov/fdac/features/096_nhl.html

www.patientcenters.com/lymphoma

AUTHOR: **FARIDEH MADANI, DMD**

BOX I-2   Non-Hodgkin's Lymphoma Staging*

Stage I: Involvement of a single lymph node region (I) or a single extralymphatic organ or site (I_E).

Stage II: Involvement of two or more lymph node regions on the same side of the diaphragm (II) or localized involvement of extralymphatic organ or site and one or more lymph node regions on the same side of the diaphragm (II_E).

Stage III: Involvement of lymph node regions on both sides of the diaphragm (III), which may also be accompanied by localized involvement of extralymphatic organ or site (III_E) or by involvement of spleen (III_S), or both (III_{SE}).

Stage IV: Diffuse or disseminated involvement of one or more extralymphatic organs or tissues with or without associated lymph node enlargement.

*Adapted from Carbone PP, Kaplan HS, Musshoff K, et al. Report of the Committee on Hodgkin's Disease Staging Classification. *Cancer Res* 1971;31:1860–1861.

SYNONYM(S)

Degenerative joint disease (DJD)
Osteoarthrosis (when secondary inflammation minimal)
"Wear and tear" arthritis

ICD-9CM/CPT CODE(S)

715.0 Generalized osteoarthritis
715.1 Osteoarthritis, primary localized
715.2 Osteoarthritis, secondary localized

OVERVIEW

Osteoarthritis (OA) is degenerative condition of a joint characterized by deterioration and abrasion of articular tissue and concomitant remodeling of the underlying subchondral bone.

EPIDEMIOLOGY & DEMOGRAPHICS

INCIDENCE/PREVALENCE IN USA: Two to 6% of general population; approximately 60 million patients at any one time are affected with OA.
PREDOMINANT AGE: Common over the age of 50; by seventh decade, 75% of individuals may be affected.
PREDOMINANT SEX: Male = female.
GENETICS: Genetic transmission is unknown.

ETIOLOGY & PATHOGENESIS

- Primary osteoarthritis is idiopathic, although often considered as part of the aging process; there may be genetic and racial factors.
- Biomechanical, biochemical, inflammatory, and immunological factors are all implicated to some degree in the pathogenesis of osteoarthritis. Risk factors include:
  - Age over 50
  - Obesity (resulting increased stress on weight-bearing joints)
  - Prolonged occupational or sports stress to joints
  - Injury to a joint
- Pathologically, the articular cartilage is first roughened and finally worn away, and bone spur formation and lipping occur at the edge of the joint surface. The synovial membrane becomes thickened, with hypertrophy of the villous processes; the joint cavity, however, never becomes totally obliterated, and the synovial membrane does not form adhesions. Inflammation is prominent only in occasional patients with acute interphalangeal joint involvement.
- Secondary osteoarthritis may follow trauma, infection, or systemic inflammatory arthritides such as rheumatoid arthritis.
- Osteoarthrosis occurs once adaptive changes have occurred after osteoarthritis and the joint structures have stabilized with minimization of secondary inflammation and reduction of symptoms.

- In the temporomandibular joint (TMJ), osteoarthritis may follow unrelieved anterior dislocation of the disk with wearing through of the posterior attachment and bone-to-bone contact.

CLINICAL PRESENTATION / PHYSICAL FINDINGS

SYMPTOMS

- Pain and limitation in a joint (commonly hips, knees, feet, spine, and not infrequently the TMJ) in an older age group person is often associated with a sensation of grinding or grating on movement (TMJ "sounds like sandpaper").
- The pain associated with osteoarthritis of the TMJ may be subdivided into retrodiscal pain, capsular pain, and arthritic pain depending on the site of origin. The painful phase in the TMJ often spontaneously regresses after about 8 months, but in weight-bearing joints there may be progressive symptoms.

SIGNS

- Crepitus in all phases of joint excursion. Pain on movement. Limitation of movement; but in the TMJ, this may not be marked. In the TMJ, myogenous involvement, (as in the form of trigger points) is less common than in the myofascial pain dysfunction syndrome (MPD) seen commonly in younger, predominantly female patients.
- There is a rare variant of osteoarthritis of the TMJ called condylosis, often presenting in a younger age group of females, associated with inability to occlude the front teeth due to reduction in the vertical dimension of the vertical ramus of the jaw.

DIAGNOSIS

- No specific laboratory test
  - Synovial fluid may have a slightly increased (predominantly mononuclear) white blood cell count.
  - The erythrocyte sedimentation test (ESR) is usually normal as is the rheumatoid factor (RF). Occasionally the ESR may be mildly raised in generalized primary cases.

IMAGING

- Radiographs usually normal early in OA; later they often demonstrate narrowed joint space, osteophyte formation, subchondral bony sclerosis, and cyst formation. When OA is associated with inflammation, erosions may occur on the surface of distal interphalangeal (DIP) and proximal interphalangeal (PIP) joints.
- Radiographic changes as in the TMJ may be seen including:
  - Erosion
  - Subchondral sclerosis
  - Osteophyte formation
  - Occasionally microcyst formation

MEDICAL MANAGEMENT & TREATMENT

- Heat (local heating pads).
- Topical ointments such as methyl salicylate.
- Energy medicine such as ultrasound, microelectrical stimulation, low-intensity laser therapy.
- Acetaminophen.
- Nonsteroidal antiinflammatory drugs (NSAIDs) if inflammation is present.
- Intraarticular corticosteroid injections may be used if slow to respond to other treatment.
- Physical therapy.
- Weight reduction where weight-bearing joints are involved.
- Surgery may be indicated in advanced disease (e.g., osteotomy, prosthetic joint replacement).

COMPLICATIONS

- In the weight-bearing joints such as the hip, OA may sometimes lead to crippling incapacity or ankylosis requiring joint replacement.

PROGNOSIS

- The prognosis of OA is variable depending on the site and extent of the disease. OA tends to be progressive; however, progression is not always inevitable.
- In the TMJ, the prognosis is usually good since the painful phase will often burn itself out after about 8 months, leaving residual crepitus and only occasional episodes of discomfort.

DENTAL SIGNIFICANCE

The symptomatology is often seen in full-denture wearers where there has been progressive loss of vertical dimension with joint strain.

DENTAL MANAGEMENT

- Attention to a comfortable position in the dental chair, particularly if hips and spine involved; brief appointments.
- Determine the functional ability of the patient, especially regarding any impairment of their ability to perform oral hygiene tasks; address as needed.
- Patients with prosthetic joints may require antibiotic prophylaxis prior to invasive, high-bacteremic incidence dental treatment procedures for the prevention of late prosthetic joint infection (Box I-3 and Table I-17).
- Mild prolongation of bleeding time due to NSAIDs. May require local hemostatic measures after oral surgery.

- Prophylaxis of TMJ pain in elderly full-denture wearers by preventing over-closure with timely denture relining or replacement.
- Historically, patients with intractable pain from TMJ involvement were considered for high condylar shave (Henny procedure), but this does not normally arise with effective, conservative management.

BOX I-3 Patients at Potential Increased Risk of Hematogenous Prosthetic Joint Infection

---

All patients during first 2 years following joint replacement:
- Immunocompromised/immunosuppressed patients:
  ○ Inflammatory arthropathies such as rheumatoid arthritis, systemic lupus erythematosus
  ○ Disease-, drug-, or radiation-induced immunosuppression
- Other patients:
  ○ Insulin-dependent (Type 1) diabetes
  ○ Previous history of prosthetic joint infections
  ○ Malnourishment
  ○ Hemophilia

SUGGESTED REFERENCES

Advisory statement by the American Dental Association (ADA) and the American Academy of Orthopedic Surgeons (AAOS) for antibiotic prophylaxis for dental patients with total joint replacements. *JADA* 2003;(134):895–899.

Greene CS. Temporomandibular disorders in the geriatric population. *J Prosthet Dent* 1994;72:507–509.

Luder HU. Articular degeneration and remodeling in human temporomandibular joints with normal and abnormal disc positions. *J Orofacial Pain* 1993;7:391–402.

Okeson J. Types of TMJ pains, in *Orofacial Pains the Clinical Management of Orofacial Pain*. Chicago, Quintessence Publishing Co., 2005, pp 347–363.

AUTHOR: **PAUL F. BRADLEY, DDS, MD, MS**

TABLE I-17 Suggested Antibiotic Prophylaxis Regimens for Prevention of Late Prosthetic Joint Infection

Patient Type	Suggested Drug	Regimen
Patients not allergic to penicillin	Cephalexin, cephradine, or amoxicillin	2 g orally 1 hour prior to dental procedure
Patients not allergic to penicillin and unable to take oral medications	Cefazolin or ampicillin	Cefazolin 1 g or ampicillin 2 g intramuscularly or intravenously 1 hour prior to the dental procedure
Patients allergic to penicillin	Clindamycin	600 mg orally 1 hour prior to the dental procedure
Patients allergic to penicillin and unable to take oral medications	Clindamycin	600 mg intravenously 1 hour prior to the dental procedure

SYNONYM(S)

Acute osteomyelitis
Chronic osteomyelitis

ICD-9CM/CPT CODE(S)

526.4   Osteomyelitis of jaw
376.03 Orbital osteomyelitis
730.00 Acute osteomyelitis—site un-
        specified, without mention of
        periostitis
730.10 Chronic   osteomyelitis—site
        unspecified
730.18 Chronic osteomyelitis—other
        specified sites
730.19 Chronic osteomyelitis—multi-
        ple sites
730.20 Unspecified   osteomyelitis—
        site unspecified
730.28 Unspecified   osteomyelitis—
        other specified sites
730.29 Unspecified   osteomyelitis—
        multiple sites

OVERVIEW

Osteomyelitis is bacterial infection of trabecular and cortical
bone spreading gradually from the initial
site of involvement. It can present as
acute osteomyelitis in which the individual's immune defense mechanism does
not react quickly to control the infection.
Chronic osteomyelitis, however, results
from the actions of the immune defense
mechanisms; the infection and offending
microbes are isolated into a mass of
granulation tissue surrounded by fibrous
connective tissue within the bony cavity.

EPIDEMIOLOGY & DEMOGRAPHICS

INCIDENCE/PREVALENCE IN USA:
Osteomyelitis is now uncommon in the
U.S. compared to developing counties
with inadequate health care facilities.
PREDOMINANT AGE: Osteomyelitis
can affect any age; however, children,
elderly, and immunocompromised indi
viduals are the most susceptible.
PREDOMINANT SEX: Osteomyelitis predominantly affects males (75% of cases).

ETIOLOGY & PATHOGENESIS

- While it is rare for patients to present
  with classic osteomyelitis in developed
  countries, infection of the jaw can easily
  progress to osteomyelitis when a patient
  does not receive prompt treatment.

- The predisposing factors to osteomyelitis are conditions that diminish
  bone vascularity such as chronic systemic diseases and immunocompromised conditions. Trauma and impaction
  of foreign objects can also predispose to
  osteomyelitis.

- Osteomyelitis is more common in
  the mandible than the maxilla. The microbes invade the bone either through
  a local infection or spread through the
  bloodstream. The infection starts in the
  trabecular bone; if uncontrolled by the
  body immune defense mechanisms, it
  progressively spreads to the cortical
  bone. If it is still unresolved, chronic
  osteomyelitis results.

- Enzymatic activity of macrophages
  causes bone breakdown and pus accumulation. The increased pressure
  within the enclosed bony environment
  further diminishes vascular perfusion.
  The encased bone becomes necrotic
  and detaches to form a sequestrum.
  However, if pus is able to escape and
  track subperiosteally, a subperiosteal
  abscess is formed and new subperiosteal bone formation or involucrum
  is initiated.

CLINICAL PRESENTATION / PHYSICAL FINDINGS

- Pain.
- Fever.
- Swelling.
- Lymphadenopathy.
- Sequestrum.
- Sinus formation.
- Purulent discharge.
- Acute osteomyelitis may progress to
  chronic osteomyelitis if untreated.

DIAGNOSIS

- Biopsy tissue of acute osteomyelitis consists of necrotic
  bone with empty lacunae, microorganisms, and neutrophils. Chronic osteomyelitis contains more of mononuclear
  cells, granulation, and fibrous tissues
  filling the intratrabecular spaces.
- Histopathology and microbial culture
  and sensitivity tests are useful.
- Imaging: radiographs, MRI, or scintigraphy with technetium (^{99m}Tc)-labeled
  phosphorus compounds may be
  required to evaluate extent and spread
  of the infection.

MEDICAL MANAGEMENT & TREATMENT

See Dental Management section
following for information on
treating this condition.

COMPLICATIONS

- Pathological fracture
- Bone loss
- Paresthesia

PROGNOSIS

Usually good if diagnosed early.

DENTAL SIGNIFICANCE

- Preventive measures such as
  meticulous oral hygiene are
  indicated in immunocompromised
  individuals undergoing dental surgery.

DENTAL MANAGEMENT

- The administration of antimicrobial
  agents and drainage of the infection
  site is usually indicated. Antibiotics of
  choice are usually penicillin, clindamycin, gentamicin, tobramycin, and
  cephalexin.
- Surgical removal of necrotic bone is
  necessary in chronic osteomyelitis
  because the microbes associated with
  the dead bone are usually walled off
  by fibrous connective tissue.
- Hyperbaric oxygen therapy to promote
  healing may be indicated in patients
  who do not respond to standard therapy.

SUGGESTED REFERENCES

Lew DP, Waldvogel FA. Osteomyelitis. *N Engl
    J Med* 1997;336(14):999–1007.
Harrison's Online: http://www3.accessmedi
    cine.com/home.aspx
Mader JT, Shirtliff ME, Bergquist SC, Calhoun
    J. Antimicrobial treatment of chronic
    osteomyelitis. *Clin Orthop* 1999;360:47–65.
Neville BW, Damm DD, Allen CM, Bouquot
    JE. *Oral and Maxillofacial Pathology.*
    Philadelphia, WB Saunders, 2002, pp
    126–131.

**AUTHOR: SUNDAY O. AKINTOYE, BDS,
DDS, MS**

SYNONYM(S)

Brittle bone disease
Osteopenia (low bone mass)

ICD-9CM/CPT CODE(S)

268.2 Osteoporosis-osteomalacia syndrome
733.0 Osteoporosis (unspecified)
733.01 Postmenopausal osteoporosis
733.01 Senile osteoporosis
733.02 Idiopathic osteoporosis
733.03 Disuse osteoporosis
733.09 Drug-induced osteoporosis

OVERVIEW

Osteoporosis is a disease of the skeletal system characterized by a compromise in bone strength (bone density and bone quality) predisposing to increased fracture risk of the wrist, hip, and spine. Bones become porous, less dense, brittle, and subject to fracture due to the loss of calcium and other minerals. The World Health Organization further defines osteoporosis as a bone mineral density (BMD) value more than 2.5 standard deviations below the mean for healthy, young, white women. It is common in older persons, postmenopausal women, and those having long-term steroid therapy and other endocrine disorders.

EPIDEMIOLOGY & DEMOGRAPHICS

INCIDENCE/PREVALENCE IN USA:
The prevalence of osteoporosis varies by gender and increases with age. The overall prevalence of osteoporosis in women in the U.S. is 17%. Ninety percent of women over age 75 have osteoporosis. The incidence of fracture varies by race and ethnicity. White postmenopausal women have the highest incidence of all age-related fractures and about 75% of hip fractures. Ten million over age 50 have osteoporosis; 33.6 million over age 50 have osteopenia (low bone mass); 1.5 million suffer fractures annually. Four out of 10 white women will have a fracture caused by osteoporosis. By 2020, 1 in 2 Americans will have osteoporosis or be at risk for osteoporosis.
PREDOMINANT SEX: Eighty percent of those with osteoporosis are women.
PREDOMINANT AGE: The predominant age is over 50 years; incidence increases with age.
GENETICS: Genetics plays a key role in risk for osteoporosis.

- Seventy percent of variance in bone mineral density is genetically determined, with several genes involved (collagen type 1 alpha gene, vitamin D receptor gene, and chromosome 20-BMP 2 gene).
- There is increased risk for Caucasian, Asian, and Hispanic women.

- There is increased risk for those of slender body build.

RISK FACTORS:
- Family history of fractures
- Low body weight
- History of "yo-yo" dieting or anorexia nervosa
- Premature menopause
- Smoking
- Heavy alcohol consumption
- Sedentary lifestyle
- Calcium or vitamin D deficiency
- Lactose intolerance
- Corticosteroid use
- Athletes with amenorrhea due to heavy exercise and disordered eating have increased risk of osteoporosis (the female athlete triad)

ETIOLOGY & PATHOGENESIS

- Osteoporosis occurs as bone resorption outpaces bone formation. Mechanisms for this are complex and diverse.
- During the first 25 years of life, our bodies are programmed to build bone with the amount dependent on calcium, phosphorus, and magnesium ingestion; exercise; and sex hormones available. In the mid-thirties, the balance changes with bone resorption occurring faster than deposition, due to lessened ability to absorb calcium. At menopause, women's bones begin a resorptive process, losing 1–5% of bone mass annually for the first 5 years, which slows to 1–2% per year until the age of 70. By age 85, a woman may have lost one-half the bone she had at her peak.
- Estrogen loss exacerbates osteoporosis in that estrogen is critical for stimulating osteoblastic activity, suppressing osteoclastic activity, and absorbing calcium.
- Osteoporotic bone microarchitecture exhibits trabecular plates that are disrupted, thin, porous, weak, and not well-connected, contributing to bone weakness and risk fracture.
- Bone loss commonly occurs as men and women age, but those who do not reach optimal peak bone mass during childhood may develop osteoporosis without the occurrence of accelerated bone loss.
- Osteoporosis can be primary or secondary.
- Primary osteoporosis is the most common loss of bone not caused by another disorder.
  - Idiopathic osteoporosis:
    - Rarely affects children and adolescents
    - Usually goes into remission at puberty
  - Age-related osteoporosis (most common):
    - Women experience a rapid loss of bone for 4 to 7 years at menopause

and then a slow, continuous loss of bone with aging.
- Most common type for women and men.
- Largely caused by estrogen deficiency.
- Secondary osteoporosis is bone loss caused by specific diseases or medication use:
  - Genetic diseases
  - Endocrine disorders (e.g., diabetes mellitus type 1, Cushing's syndrome, hyperparathyroidism)
  - Hypogonadal states
  - Gastrointestinal diseases (e.g., celiac disease, malabsorption)
  - Hematological disorders
  - Autoimmune/allergic disorders (e.g., rheumatoid arthritis, lupus erythematosus)
  - Neurologic disorders (e.g., anorexia nervosa, epilepsy, major depression)
  - Medications use (e.g., glucocorticoids, anticonvulsants, anticoagulants)

CLINICAL PRESENTATION / PHYSICAL FINDINGS

- This silent disease has no early signs until the patient experiences a fracture.
- Fractures of the hip, wrist, or spine with minimal trauma; but any bone can be affected.
- Thoracic kyphosis (i.e., "Dowager's hump" or stooped posture) caused by wedge spinal fractures.
- Loss of height.
- Back pain, especially in the middle or upper middle back.
- Abdominal distention caused by kyphosis and downward pressure of ribs on viscera.
- Bone Mineral Density (BMD) Score
  - T-score < 2.5, bone mass is lower by more than 2.5 standard deviations (SD) for healthy, young adult women.
  - Z-score < 2.5, bone mass is lower by more than 2.5 SD than average for women the same age.

DIAGNOSIS

- Current choice diagnostic test is dual energy x-ray absorptiometry (DEXA or DXA) of the hip and lumbar spine
- Ultrasound densitometry
- Single x-ray absorptiometry
- Radiographic absorptiometry
- Computerized axial tomography (CT or CAT scan)
- Blood or urine test to determine why and how quickly bone is being lost:
  - Bone turnover test
  - Estradiol test
  - Follicle-stimulating hormone test
  - Thyroid test
  - Parathyroid test
  - Blood calcium levels test

MEDICAL MANAGEMENT & TREATMENT

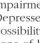

- Adequate calcium intake in diet [dietary reference intake (DRI) in mg/day] or consider supplementation.
  - 9 to 18 years = 1300 mg
  - 19 to 50 years = 1000 mg
  - 51 years and older = 1200 mg
- Adequate vitamin D in diet [DRI in International Units (IU) or µg].
  - 51 to 70 years = 400 IU or 10 µg
  - 71 years and older = 600 IU or 15 µg
- Exercise regimen as part of daily life to maximize peak bone mass during youth and maintain bone mass and prevent resorption during aging.
  - Weight-bearing aerobic activity most days of the week (30 to 60 min/day)
    - Walking, running, stair climbing, etc.
  - Resistance/strength training twice weekly (weight lifting)
  - Balance training to reduce falls
- Medications:
  - Bisphosphonates:
    - Alendronate (Fosamax), 70-mg tablet once weekly or 10-mg tablet once daily.
    - Risedronate (Actonel), 35-mg tablet orally once weekly or 5-mg tablet once daily.
    - Ibandronate sodium (Boniva, approved by FDA March 24, 2005 for treatment and prevention of postmenopausal osteoporosis), 2.5-mg tablet once daily.
  - Parathyroid Hormone (PTH):
    - Teriparatide (Forteo), 20 µg once a day subcutaneous injection into the thigh or abdominal wall.
  - Selective estrogen receptor modulators (SERMs):
    - Raloxifene (Evista), 60-mg tablet once daily.
  - Calcitonin:
    - Calcimar/Cibacalcin, injectable.
    - Miacalcin, nasal spray.
  - Estrogen and hormone therapy:
    - This was once considered the best prevention of osteoporosis but the 2004 Women's Health Initiative showed increased risk of heart disease/ stroke.
    - Short-term use of estrogen is considered effective and is still prescribed for managing age-related bone loss associated with menopause.

COMPLICATIONS

- Reduced quality of life
- Physical debilitation/functional impairment
- Depressed mental health
- Possibility of death due to complications of hip fracture

PROGNOSIS

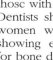

The prognosis is dependent on when the disease is diagnosed, with a more favorable or good prognosis if the diagnosis made when the patient has osteopenia, can make lifestyle changes, and/or take medication that can minimize bone loss or that can build bone. Mortality approaches 20% within 1 year with hip fracture.

The prognosis is becoming more favorable for newer generations with:

- Implementation of preventive measures (eating a diet rich in calcium and vitamin D and exercising regularly for 30 to 60 minutes/day) early in life to maximize peak bone mass
- Current availability of information on bone health as a result of the 2004 Surgeon General's Report
- Implementation of new bone-preserving and -building medications

DENTAL SIGNIFICANCE

- Oral bone loss and tooth loss are associated with estrogen deficiency and osteoporosis.
- Increased severity of alveolar ridge bone loss has been shown in edentulous patients with osteoporosis.
- Increased severity of periodontal disease and tooth loss is seen in patients with osteoporosis.
- There are conflicting studies on the success of implants in osteoporotic postmenopausal women, with the consensus that implant site bone quality is more diagnostic than a DEXA test.
- Dental panoramic radiographs of postmenopausal women are diagnostically accurate to screen for spinal osteoporosis.
- Women taking bisphosphonates for osteoporosis are at an increased risk for developing drug-induced avascular bone necrosis in the jaws.

DENTAL MANAGEMENT

- Recommendations to take the DRI of calcium and vitamin D for patients presenting with osteoporosis, especially those with periodontal disease.
- Dentists should refer postmenopausal women with panoramic radiographs showing eroded mandibular cortices for bone densitometry testing.
- Patients with risk factors for osteoporosis and having periodontal disease and tooth loss should be referred to their physician for bone densitometry testing to assess for osteoporosis.
- Dentists should be aware of the implications of, and preventing, drug-induced avascular osteonecrosis when treating patients taking bisphosphonates for osteoporosis.
- While implants are not contraindicated in patients with osteoporosis, the dentist should inform the patient of the possibility of a compromised prognosis for the implant.

SUGGESTED REFERENCES

Jeffcoat MK, Lewis CE, Reddy MS, Wang CY, Redford M. Post-menopausal bone loss and its relationship to oral bone loss. *Periodontol* 2000;23:94–102.

Migliorati C. Bisphosphonates and oral cavity avascular bone necrosis. *J Clin Oncol* 2003;21(22):4253–4254.

Mulligan R, Sobel S. Osteoporosis: diagnostic testing, interpretation and correlations with oral health-implications for dentistry. *Dent Clin North Am* 2005;49(2):464–484.

National Osteoporosis Foundation: www.nof.org

Nelson ME, Wernick S. *Strong Women, Strong Bones: Everything You Need to Know to Prevent, Treat and Beat Osteoporosis.* New York, The Berkley Publishing Group, 2000, pp 72–77, 101, 107.

U.S. Department of Health and Human Services. *Bone Health and Osteoporosis: A Report of the Surgeon General.* Rockville, MD, U.S. Department of Health and Human Services, Office of the Surgeon General, 2004, p 30.

WHO Scientific Group on the Burden of Musculoskeletal Conditions at the Start of the New Millennium. The burden of musculoskeletal conditions at the start of the new millennium: report of a scientific group. Geneva, Switzerland, *World Health Organization technical report series,* 2003;919:57.

AUTHOR: **SHARON CRANE SIEGEL, DDS, MS**

Parkinson disease
Paralysis agitans
Shaking palsy
Hypokinetic syndrome

ICD-9CM/CPT CODE(S)

332.0 Idiopathic Parkinson's disease, primary
332.1 Parkinson's disease, secondary

OVERVIEW

Parkinson's disease (PD) is a progressive, debilitating movement disorder characterized by tremor, bradykinesia, rigidity, postural changes, and often mental changes. Affliction is a slowly progressive, neurologic, degenerative disorder of the basal ganglia associated with a localized deficiency of the neurotransmitter dopamine.

EPIDEMIOLOGY & DEMOGRAPHICS
INCIDENCE/PREVALENCE IN USA:

- Incidence: 4.5 to 21 cases per 100,000 population per year.
- Prevalence: Affects 0.3% of the general population and 3% of the population over age 65.

PREDOMINANT AGE: Predominately seen in persons between 50 and 65 years of age, with an average age of onset at 55 years.

PREDOMINANT SEX: Males > females (approximately 3:2).

GENETICS: PD is generally considered to be a sporadic disease; however, autosomal dominant and autosomal recessive inheritance have been documented. Familial parkinsonism is estimated to be responsible for approximately 5–10% of PD cases.

ETIOLOGY & PATHOGENESIS
ETIOLOGY

- Primary (idiopathic) PD accounts for approximately 75% of cases:
  - The specific etiology of primary PD is unknown and is believed to be due to a combination of genetic and environmental factors.
- Secondary (acquired) PD accounts for approximately 25% of cases:
  - Familial:
    - Autosomal dominant or autosomal recessive inheritance (accounts for approximately 5–10% of PD cases):
      - Two mutations have been identified in the gene coding for α-synuclein (*PARK1*) on chromosome 4q in families with autosomal dominant PD.
      - Two gene loci on chromosome 1 have been found to be associated with autosomal recessive, early-onset parkinsonism: 1p35–36 (*PARK6*) and 1p36 (*PARK7*).

- Infectious:
  - Including postencephalitic, subacute sclerosing panencephalitis (SSPE), AIDS, Creutzfeldt-Jakob disease, and prion diseases
- Drug-induced:
  - Including neuroleptics (e.g., phenothiazines and butyrophenones), antiemetics (e.g., prochlorperazine, trimethobenzamide), dopamine-depleting agents (e.g., reserpine), tetrabenazine, methyldopa, lithium, flunarizine, cinnarizine, metoclopramide, and valproic acid
- Toxins:
  - Including manganese, cyanide, methanol, carbon monoxide, MPTP (1-methyl-4-phenyl-1,2,3,6-tetrahydropyridine), pesticides, and herbicides
- Vascular:
  - Including multiinfarct cerebrovascular disease, and Binswanger's disease
- Traumatic:
  - Including head trauma and pugilistic encephalopathy

PATHOGENESIS

- PD is characterized by loss of dopaminergic neurons in the substantia nigra, ventricular enlargement, and cortical atrophy. The histologic presentation is one of neuronal loss with depigmentation of the substantia nigra and the presence of Lewy bodies (eosinophilic cytoplasmic inclusions in neurons consisting of aggregates of normal and abnormal proteins).
- At least a 60% loss of dopaminergic neurons in the substantia nigra must appear before the clinical symptoms of PD become evident.

CLINICAL PRESENTATION / PHYSICAL FINDINGS

- Resting tremor and bradykinesia (slowness of movement) are the most typical signs of PD and are virtually synonymous with the diagnosis.
  - Resting tremor:
    - Typically presents with a frequency of 4 to 7 Hz that is often first noted in the hand as a "pill rolling" tremor (thumb and forefinger); can also involve the leg and lip.
    - Tremor improves with purposeful movement.
    - Usually starts asymmetrically but can eventually involve the other hemibody.
  - Bradykinesia accounts for most of the associated PD symptoms and signs:
    - General slowing of movements and activities of daily living
    - Lack of facial expression (hypomimia or masked facies)
    - Staring expression resulting from a decreased frequency of blinking
    - Impaired swallowing causing drooling (sialorrhea)

- Hypokinetic and hypophonic dysarthria, monotonous speech
- Small handwriting (micrographia)
- Difficulties with repetitive and simultaneous movements
- Difficulty in rising from a chair and turning over in bed
- Shuffling gait with short steps
- Decreased arm swing and other automatic movements
- Difficulty in initiating movements and freezing of motion
- Autonomic dysfunction:
  - Orthostatic hypotension
  - Respiratory dysregulation
  - Flushing, excessive sweating ("drenching sweats")
  - Constipation, sphincter and sexual dysfunction
- Sensory dysfunction:
  - Paresthesias, pains, and akathisia
  - Visual, olfactory, and vestibular dysfunction
- Personality changes:
  - Apathy, lack of confidence, fearfulness, anxiety, emotional lability and inflexibility, social withdrawal, and dependency
- Dementia:
  - About 10–20% of patients with PD develop dementia, with increasing incidence with advancing age; it is more common in patients whose disease onset was bilateral.

CLINICAL CLASSIFICATION

- Hoehn and Yahr scale of disability in PD:
  - Stage 0: No visible disease.
  - Stage 1: Mild disease; one side of the body is affected. Symptoms are mild, not disabling.
  - Stage 2: Mild to moderate disease; both sides of the body are affected, and the patient may have difficulty walking. Posture is affected, and the disability may become more apparent.
  - Stage 3: Moderate disease; patient has difficulty with balance and walking, and movement is slow. Moderate to severe generalized dysfunction is present.
  - Stage 4: Moderate to severe disease; patient has great difficulty with balance or walking and is functionally disabled. Symptoms are severe, and the person may not be able to live alone any longer.
  - Stage 5: Severe disease; patient is completely immobile and confined to a bed or wheelchair. He or she loses weight and may require constant nursing care.

DIAGNOSIS

- There are no specific diagnostic tests for PD.
- A presumptive clinical diagnosis can be made based on a comprehensive history and physical examination.

- Use of laboratory tests or imaging studies (e.g., CT, MRI) in the evaluation of suspected PD is necessary only for the purpose of excluding other diagnoses.

MEDICAL MANAGEMENT & TREATMENT

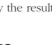

OVERVIEW

- A long-term perspective for treatment is necessary since the PD will be present for the rest of the patient's life.
- Treatment of PD is palliative in an attempt to control tremor and rigidity; currently there is no convincing evidence that any medication or combination of medications slows or stops the progression of this disease.

GENERAL MEASURES

- Physical therapy, patient education and reassurance, treatment of associated conditions (e.g., depression).
- Avoidance of drugs that can induce or worsen parkinsonism.

PHARMACOLOGIC

- Most PD experts agree that drug treatment should not be started until a patient is experiencing some functional impairment.
- Drug therapy with combinations of levodopa, selegiline, dopamine agonists, anticholinergics or amantadine, and catechol-O-methyltransferase (COMT) inhibitors is common.
- The choice of medication is based on patient-specific symptoms and stage of disease.
  - Dopamine precursors [levodopa carbidopa (Sinemet)]:
    - May be the initial drug of choice in older patients with more severe PD symptoms.
    - Neurovegetative symptoms such as speech disorders and postural instability are resistant to levodopa.
    - Side effects include nausea, hypotension, confusion, hallucinations, dyskinesia, and xerostomia.
  - Dopamine agonists (e.g., bromocriptine, pergolide, pramipexole, ropinirole):
    - Often initial drug of choice in younger patients with milder symptoms.
    - Early monotherapy may reduce levodopa use and its long-term effects.
    - Low potency; long half-life; reduces wearing-off effects of levodopa.
    - Side effects include somnolence, confusion, hallucinations, and hypotension.
  - Monamine oxidase (MAO) B inhibitor (e.g., deprenyl):
    - Blocks the metabolism of dopamine.
    - Used as an adjunct to levodopa to diminish motor fluctuations.

- Side effects include xerostomia, sleep disturbance, lightheadedness, and hallucinations.
  - Anticholinergics (e.g., trihexyphenidyl, biperiden):
    - Used for tremor and rigidity in early stages or as an adjunct; results in 30% improvement in 50% of patients.
    - Side effects include confusion, sleepiness, blurred vision, constipation, and xerostomia.
  - Indirect dopamine agonist (amantadine):
    - Used similarly to anticholinergics in the treatment of PD; improves bradykinesia and rigidity.
    - Side effects include hallucinations, xerostomia, livedo reticularis, ankle swelling, and myoclonic encephalopathy in setting of renal failure.
  - Catechol-O-methyltransferase (COMT) inhibitors (e.g., tolcapone, entacapone):
    - Reduces peripheral metabolism of levodopa, permitting increased brain concentration.
    - Used as adjunct to levodopa (similarly to dopamine agonists).
    - May decrease motor fluctuation in late-stage disease and reduce early wearing off of levodopa; requires fewer daily doses of levodopa.
    - Side effects are orthostatic hypotension, somnolence, nausea, diarrhea, dyskinesia, dystonia, and muscle cramps.
  - Neuroleptics; used for psychosis and unusual tremor:
    - Clozapine
    - Side effects include fatal neutropenia, somnolence, and xerostomia.
    - Quetiapine
    - Side effects include somnolence and potential aggravated parkinsonism.
  - Tricyclic antidepressant (amitriptyline):
    - Used to treat sleep fragmentation.
    - Side effects include xerostomia, forgetfulness, blurred vision, and constipation.
  - GABA derivative skeletal muscle relaxant/antispastic (baclofen):
    - Used to treat dystonic cramps.
    - Side effects include sleepiness and dizziness.

SURGICAL

- Adrenal brain transplants and thalamotomy are being investigated as possible therapies for PD.

COMPLICATIONS

- Postural instability often occurs in the more advanced stages of PD and will increase the risk of traumatic injury from falls.

- Patients with PD complain of painful spasms and dystonic posturing of the extremities, usually the lower extremities.
- Neuropsychiatric problems in PD are universal and include dementia and depression.
  - Dementia occurs in approximately 20% of patients with advanced PD.
  - Psychosis and hallucinations occur but are usually the result of dopaminergic therapy.

PROGNOSIS

PD usually follows a slowly progressive degenerative course with increased muscle tremor and rigidity and increased mental changes leading to eventual disability over the course of years.

DENTAL SIGNIFICANCE

- Address the adverse effects of muscle tremor and rigidity on the patient's ability to perform home oral hygiene as well as its effect during delivery of dental treatment.
- Avoid interactions with drugs used to treat PD.
- Oral manifestations and complications:
  - Excess salivation and drooling with decreased swallowing frequency may be associated with PD; conversely, xerostomia may occur due to some drugs (e.g., anticholinergics, amantadine, dopaminergics, levodopa) used to treat PD.
  - Levodopa and dopamine agonists may cause tardive dyskinesia; manifestations include uncontrolled, purposeless chewing movements and bruxism.

DENTAL MANAGEMENT

- Family cooperation is critical for history taking, follow-up for dental treatment, and home oral hygiene for patients with PD.
- Patients with PD should ideally receive dental treatment at the time of day when their anti-Parkinson's medications are at their maximal effect, typically 2 to 3 hours after administration.
  - Blankness of expression should not be interpreted as apathy. Empathetic responses are important.
- Dental treatment for patients with PD may be facilitated by use of benzodiazepines, nitrous oxide-oxygen, or IV conscious sedation and may help reduce tremors or choreiform movements.
- Frequent dental recall visits as needed based on patient's needs.

- An assessment of the patient's ability to perform home oral hygiene tasks (e.g., tooth brushing) should be done at each recall appointment, as well as the need for oral hygiene aids (e.g., mechanical toothbrush, oral hygiene assisted by a caregiver).
- Topical fluoride application is beneficial for patients with xerostomia and/or are unable to maintain good oral hygiene.
- Salivary substitutes are beneficial for easing symptoms of xerostomia.
- Orthostatic hypotension and muscular rigidity are common in patients with PD; patient should be assisted to and from the dental chair.

- Drug interaction concerns:
  - COMT inhibitors (e.g., tolcapone, entacapone) may decrease the metabolism and increase the side effects of vasoconstrictors (e.g., epinephrine) used in some local anesthetic preparations. Concurrent use of these drugs should be approached with caution.
  - Many anti-Parkinson drugs have CNS sedative effects that may be additive with effects with any CNS-depressive drugs (e.g., benzodiazepines, narcotic analgesics, other sedative-hypnotics) administered or prescribed by the dentist.

SUGGESTED REFERENCES

DeLong MR, Juncos JL. Parkinson's disease and other movement disorders, in Kasper DI, et al. (eds): *Harrison's Principles of Internal Medicine*, ed 16. New York, McGraw-Hill: 2005, pp 2406–2415.

Jankovic J. Parkinsonism, in Goldman L, Ausiello D (eds): *Cecil Textbook of Medicine*, ed 22. Philadelphia, WB Saunders, 2004, pp 2307–2310.

Jankovic J. Parkinson's disease. Uptodate Online 13.2, updated 4/19/05, http://www.uptodate online.com/application/topic.asp?file=ped_ne ur/8599&type=A&selectedTitle=4^25

AUTHORS: **F. JOHN FIRRIOLO, DDS, PHD; JAMES R. HUPP, DMD, MD, JD, MBA**

SYNONYM(S)

PUD

ICD-9CM/CPT CODE(S)

533 Peptic ulcer, site unspecified—incomplete

OVERVIEW

- Peptic ulcer disease (PUD) is a common, benign ulcerative disorder of gastric or duodenal lining mucosa involving a complex, multifactorial imbalance between mucosal protective factors and various mucosal damaging mechanisms most commonly resulting from infection with *Helicobacter pylori* (*H. pylori*) and use of nonsteroidal antiinflammatory drugs (NSAIDs).
  - Duodenal ulcer (DU) is commonly located in the duodenal bulb.
  - Gastric ulcer (GU) is commonly located along the lesser curvature of the antrum near the incisura and in the prepyloric area.
  - The incidence ratio of duodenal to gastric ulcers is 4:1.

EPIDEMIOLOGY & DEMOGRAPHICS

INCIDENCE/PREVALENCE IN USA: DU: lifetime prevalence = 10% for men; 5% for women (gender disparity is decreasing) with 200,000 to 400,000 new DU cases annually; GU: 87,500 new cases annually. Incidence of new GU is 50 per 100,000 adults.
PREDOMINANT AGE: DU: twenty-five to 75 years (rare before age 15); GU: peak incidence age 55 to 65; rare < age 40.
PREDOMINANT SEX: DU: male > female (slightly); GU: male = female (however, there is a female predominance among NSAID users).
GENETICS: Higher incidence with HLA-B12, B5, Bw35 phenotypes, and identical twins.

ETIOLOGY & PATHOGENESIS

- The etiology of PUD involves a multifactorial imbalance between mucosal protective factors and various mucosal damaging mechanisms including:
  - *H. pylori*: infection occurs during childhood and persists for life; 20% of infected persons develop PUD.
  - Medications: NSAIDs, corticosteroids, histamine, nitrogen-containing bisphosphonates (used for management of osteoporosis), immunosuppressive agents (e.g., mycophenolate mofetil).
  - Gastric acid hypersecretion and hypersecretory syndromes (e.g., Zollinger-Ellison syndrome or hyperparathyroidism causing elevated gastrin levels and excess acid production).

- Renal dialysis (insufficient removal of circulating gastrin).
- Heavy alcohol consumption.
- Cigarette smoking.
- Caffeine.
- Crack cocaine, amphetamine drug use.
- Psychological stress.
- Family history.

CLINICAL PRESENTATION / PHYSICAL FINDINGS

- Gastric ulcer:
  - Epigastric pain exacerbated by food ingestion
- Duodenal ulcer:
  - Periodic, epigastric pain, nausea, and vomiting starting 1 to 2 hours after ingestion or during sleep
  - Rapid relief of pain with ingestion of food or drinks
  - Frequent recurrence of symptoms, especially with seasonal changes
- Bloody vomit, melena, signs and symptoms of anemia (e.g., gastrointestinal bleeding)
- Aggravation of pain and lack of therapeutic relief (e.g., gastrointestinal perforation)
- Protracted vomiting (e.g., gastrointestinal obstruction)

DIAGNOSIS

- Upper GI barium swallow and radiological examination (to detect the ulcer)
- Endoscopy (to visualize and biopsy superficial ulcers and rule out malignancy)
- Detection of *H. pylori* by:
  - Serologic tests
  - Stool antigen detection
  - Urea breath test
  - Staining and microscopic analysis of biopsy specimen
  - Urease activity test on the biopsy specimen
  - Polymerase chain reaction

MEDICAL MANAGEMENT & TREATMENT

GENERAL MEASURES

- Avoid use of NSAIDs.
- Avoid or eliminate cigarette smoking and alcohol consumption.
- Reduce psychological stress.

PHARMACOLOGIC

Several agents that enhance the healing of peptic ulcers. They may be divided into three categories:

1. Acid-antisecretory agents (acid suppression):
   - H2 blockers [e.g., ranitidine or nizatidine 150 bid or 300 mg hs; cimetidine 400 mg bid or 800 mg hs; famotidine (Pepcid) 20 mg bid or 40 mg hs for 8 to 12 weeks]

  - Proton pump inhibitors (e.g., omeprazole 20 mg, lansoprazole 15 mg qd, rabeprazole 20 mg, esomeprazole 40 mg, or pantoprazole 40 mg daily for 4 weeks)
2. Mucosal protective agents:
   - Sucralfate, 1 g four times daily for the treatment of duodenal ulcers (its efficacy in gastric ulcers is less well-established).
   - Bismuth subsalicylate (Pepto-Bismol), 600 mg qid.
   - Antacids: low-dose aluminum- and magnesium-containing antacid regimens promote ulcer healing through stimulation of gastric mucosal defenses, not by neutralization of gastric acidity.
3. Eradication of *H. pylori* with combination therapy using antibiotics (e.g., metronidazole, tetracycline, amoxicillin, clarithromycin) concurrently with acid-antisecretory agents and/or mucosal protective agents:
   - A frequently used triple-therapy regimen consists of omeprazole 20 mg bid or lansoprazole 30 mg bid plus clarithromycin 500 mg bid and amoxicillin 1000 mg bid for 7 to 10 days.
   - A one-day, quadruple-therapy regimen consists of two tablets of 262 mg bismuth subsalicylate qid, one 500-mg metronidazole tablet qid, 2 g of amoxicillin suspension qid, and two capsules of 30 mg of lansoprazole.

- Surgical treatment approach for complicated ulcers, recalcitrant symptoms, and for removal of affected endocrine glands (e.g., parathyroid adenoma).
- Prevention of NSAID-induced PUD:
  - Misoprostol (Cytotec), 100 μg qid with food, increased to 200 μg qid if well-tolerated, should be considered for the prevention of NSAID-induced gastric ulcers in all patients on long-term NSAID therapy. Note: FDA pregnancy category "X."
  - Proton pump inhibitors are also effective, helping to prevent PUD when used concurrently in patients on long-term NSAIDs.

COMPLICATIONS

- Massive gastrointestinal hemorrhage
- Gastrointestinal perforation
- Gastrointestinal obstruction caused by fibrosis and scarring
- Potential for malignant transformation of some gastric ulcers
- Atrophic gastritis caused by chronic use of proton pump inhibitors (higher risk of gastric cancer)
- Potential for gastric lymphoma in patients with *H. pylori* infection

PROGNOSIS

- Early detection and medical management improves prognosis.
- Late diagnosis and presence of complications will negatively impact the prognosis.

DENTAL SIGNIFICANCE

- Dental erosion (palatal aspect of maxillary teeth) and dental sensitivity secondary to frequent gastric acid regurgitation secondary to gastrointestinal obstruction.
- Dental plaque may be a reservoir for *H. pylori* and the source of persistent (re)infection with this organism.
- The use of systemic antibiotics for *H. pylori* eradication therapy can result in fungal overgrowth (candidiasis) in the oral cavity. The dentist should be alert to identify oral fungal infections, including median rhomboid glossitis, in this patient population. A course of antifungal agents is prescribed to resolve the fungal infection.
- Mucosal pallor, weakness, shortness of breath secondary to anemia caused by gastrointestinal blood loss.
- The presence of vascular malformations of the lip that range from a very small macule ("microcherry") to a large, venous pool has been noted to occur in older men with PUD.
- Some H2 blockers such as cimetidine may reduce the metabolism of certain dental drugs (e.g., diazepam, lidocaine) and prolong duration of their action.
- Cimetidine may interfere with the absorption of systemic antifungals such as ketoconazole.
- Antacids may significantly impact the absorption of tetracycline, erythromycin, oral iron, and fluoride.
- Frequent regurgitation as well as medical therapy with proton pump inhibitors may cause dysgeusia.

- Some acid blockers (e.g., cimetidine, ranitidine) are toxic to bone marrow, leading to anemia (i.e., mucosal pallor), agranulocytosis (i.e., mucosal ulceration), or thrombocytopenia (i.e., petechiae and gingival bleeding).
- Some acid blockers (famotidine) or anticholinergic agents may cause xerostomia and predispose to dental caries.
- Erythema, mucosal atrophy, fibrosis, or stricture of esophageal mucosa may result from prolonged exposure of tissues to acid.

DENTAL MANAGEMENT

- Periodically update patient's medical status and type and dose of patient's medications:
  - Be vigilant about signs and symptoms indicating relapse of the disease.
  - Encourage periodic medical evaluations for prevention and early detection of gastric cancer in high-risk patients.
- Recommend baking soda mouth rinses after acid regurgitation to prevent enamel dissolution and alleviate acid reflux-induced altered taste.
- Recommend regular, effective oral hygiene practices and the use of topical fluoride via custom tray application to promote dental remineralization.
- Avoid prescribing ASA, aspirin-containing compounds, NSAIDs, or corticosteroids that cause gastrointestinal bleeding and/or promote PUD recurrence.
  - If use of NSAIDs is necessary, consider concurrent use of H2 blocker, proton pump inhibitor, or misoprostol during duration of NSAID therapy.
- Recommend regular and effective oral hygiene practices and minimize the potential for *H. pylori* colonization in dental plaque.
- Arrange dental care over multiple, short appointments to minimize stress.

- Consider sedation in patients with excessive stress response to dental procedures.
- Consider premedication of patients with H2 blockers or antacids prior to dental treatment.
- Consider preoperative workup (order CBC with differential) in patients with history of gastric bleeding, anemia, or those treated with H2 blockers scheduled for invasive oral surgery.
  - Anticipate potential poor healing and increased risk of infection with anemia secondary to GI bleeding, as well as potential respiratory depression with narcotic analgesics.
- Select antibiotics to treat odontogenic infections in patients who have recently been treated with antibiotics for the eradication of *H. pylori* with consideration of possible microbial resistance issues.

SUGGESTED REFERENCES

Hansson L. Risk of stomach cancer in patients with peptic ulcer disease. *World I Surg* 2000;24:315–320.

Little JW, Falace DA, Miller GS, Rhodus NL. Gastrointestinal disease, in Little JW, et al. (eds): *Dental Management of the Medically Compromised Patient.* St Louis, Mosby, 2002, pp 188–202.

Nguyen A-M, El-Zaatari F, Graham D. Helicobacter pylori in the oral cavity: a critical review of the literature. *Oral Surg Oral Med Oral Pathol Pral Radiol Endod* 1995;76:705–709.

Quan C, Talley N. Management of peptic ulcer disease not related to *Helicobacter pylori* or NSAIDS. *Am J Gastroent* 2002;97:2950–2961.

Siegel MA, Jacobson JJ, Braum RJ. Diseases of the gastrointestinal tract, in Greenberg M, Glick M (eds): *Burket's Oral Medicine: Diagnosis and Treatment.* Hamilton, Ontario, BC Decker, Inc., 2003, pp 389–392.

AUTHOR: **MAHNAZ FATAHZADEH, DMD**

SYNONYM(S)

Hereditary intestinal polyposis syndrome

ICD-9CM/CPT CODE(S)

759.6 Other congenital hamartoses, not elsewhere classified—complete

OVERVIEW

A hereditary multiple hamartomatous polyposis of the small intestine with multiple pigmented (melanin) macules of the skin and oral mucosa.

EPIDEMIOLOGY & DEMOGRAPHICS

INCIDENCE/PREVALENCE IN USA: Approximately 1 case per 60,000 to 300,000.

PREDOMINANT AGE: Average age of diagnosis is in the mid-twenties.

PREDOMINANT SEX: Male = female.

GENETICS: Autosomal dominant inheritance with variable and incomplete penetrance. Approximately 50% of the reported cases have a family history. The remaining cases are attributed to sporadic mutations.

ETIOLOGY & PATHOGENESIS

Peutz-Jeghers syndrome (PJS) appears to be inherited as a single pleiotropic, autosomal dominant gene with variable and incomplete penetrance causing varied phenotypic manifestations among patients with PJS (e.g., inconsistent number of polyps, differing presentation of the macules) and allowing for a variable presentation of cancer (see Complications section following). The gene responsible for the syndrome appears to be the serine-threonine kinase *STK11 (LKB1)* gene located on chromosome 19p.

CLINICAL PRESENTATION / PHYSICAL FINDINGS

- Oral mucosa and skin presents with pigmentation that occurs as brown to greenish-black melanotic spots (1- to 5-mm macules) on lips, buccal mucosa, gingiva, facial skin, extremities, and perianal area. More than 95% of patients have characteristic patterns of this pigmentation.
- Hamartomatous polyps located predominantly in the small intestine (64–96%), stomach (24–49%), and colon (60%). Histologically, these polyps are benign and unique in that a layer of muscle that extends into the submucosa or muscularis propria may surround the glandular tissue. However, hemorrhage, obstruction,

infarction, and intussusception are noted. Polyps have also been found in the nose and lung.
  - Gastrointestinal bleeding may occur and may lead to iron deficiency anemia.
- Extraintestinal manifestations include ovarian sex cord stromal tumors and polyps of the gallbladder, ureter, and nasal passages.

DIAGNOSIS

PHYSICAL EXAM

- Oral mucosa and skin present with multiple, melanotic-like macules. The gingiva, hard palate, and tongue also contribute to the clinical findings. The facial skin, forearms, hands, and soles have similar findings. Clubbing of fingers is noted in some cases. Frequently, patients can be diagnosed on the basis of the typical cutaneous pigmentation.

LABORATORY

- A CBC count should be obtained because the polyps may be a source of blood loss and anemia.

IMAGING

- Esophagogastroduodenoscopy/colonoscopy: polyps may be found in the stomach, small intestine, or colon; biopsy of polyps is advised.

MEDICAL MANAGEMENT & TREATMENT

- Treatment is focused on management of complications such as hamartomatous polyps in the stomach, small bowel, and colon, with removal of hemorrhagic or large polyps (> 5 mm) by endoscopic polypectomy.
- Surveillance for cancer, including periodic small intestine with small bowel radiography, esophagogastroduodenoscopy, and colonoscopy.
- Prevention and control of this disorder is through genetic counseling of the individual and family.

COMPLICATIONS

- PJS confers an increased risk of developing carcinomas of the pancreas, stomach, breast, lung, ovary, testes, and uterus. The mean age at diagnosis of cancer is approximately 40 to 50 years, with a 93% overall cumulative risk of developing cancer between ages 15 and 64 years. The cumulative risk of colon cancer is

39%, with similar rates for gastric and pancreatic cancer.
- Additional complications of PJS include small intestinal obstruction and intussusception (43%), abdominal pain (23%), hematochezia (14%), and prolapse of a colonic polyp (7%); these typically occur in the second and third decades of life.

PROGNOSIS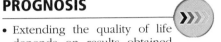

- Extending the quality of life depends on results obtained from colonoscopies with polypectomies, and screening for breast cancer, testicular cancer, and possible ovarian cancer.
  - Almost 50% of patients with Peutz-Jeghers syndrome develop and die from cancer by age 57 years.
- Skin and facial pigmentations tend to fade at puberty. However, oral (buccal) mucosal pigmentation appears to persist.

DENTAL SIGNIFICANCE

Must rule out appropriate disease in a differential diagnosis. These would include Addison's disease, hereditary pigmentation, medication, and/or hematochromatosis. Syndromes in contention include juvenile polyposis, Cowden disease, and Cronkhite-Canada syndrome. Treatment modification is based on functional diagnosis.

DENTAL MANAGEMENT

Postdiagnosis of patient's status and degree of medical intervention would determine level of dental/oral therapy. However, dental/oral care must include maintaining functional oral hygiene, nutrition, and correcting any oral/dental deviation from an acceptable healthy oral cavity. Limited care initially may be the required modality.

SUGGESTED REFERENCE

Hamartoneoplastic syndromes, Peutz-Jeghers syndrome, in Gorlin RJ, Cohen Jr MM, Hennekam RCM (eds): *Syndromes of the Head and Neck*, ed 4. New York, Oxford University Press, 2001, pp 476–480.

AUTHOR: **NORBERT J. BURZYNSKI, SR., DDS, MS**

SYNONYM(S)

Polymyalgia rheumatica: antarthritic rheumatoid syndrome

Giant cell arteritis (GCA): temporal arteritis

ICD-9CM/CPT CODE(S)

725.0 Polymyalgia rheumatica—complete

446.5 Giant cell arteritis—complete

OVERVIEW

Polymyalgia rheumatica (PMR) and temporal arteritis (TA) are considered to be companion systemic inflammatory disorders formed by antigen-driven, cell-mediated mechanisms associated with genetic markers that represent a continuum from severe proximal aches and pains and constitutional symptoms to an occlusive granulomatous vasculitis of medium and large vessels that can lead to permanent blindness or other organ and tissue damage. Similar signs and symptoms for PMR and TA suggest a possible spectrum of a coexisting single disease, but with some limited variations at different stages of the disease.

EPIDEMIOLOGY & DEMOGRAPHICS

INCIDENCE/PREVALENCE IN USA: Average annual incidence of PMR is 52.5 per 100,000 patients age 50 years and older and increases with age. The prevalence is about 0.5–0.7%.

PREDOMINANT AGE: These disorders occur in patients older than 50 years of age; the average age at onset is 70 years.

PREDOMINANT SEX: Observed to be more frequent in women than men (2:1).

GENETICS: A genetic predisposition is suspected. Both entities show familial aggregation and have a genetic association with HLA-DR4 and a demonstrated sequence polymorphism encoded within the hypervariable region of the HLA-DRβ1 *04 gene.

ETIOLOGY & PATHOGENESIS

- The etiology for PMR and associated GCA is unknown.
- GCA has a predilection for arteries containing elastic tissue. The histologic findings in GCA include nodular thickenings with reduction of the lumen and may become thrombosed; granulomatous inflammation of the inner half of the media centered on the internal elastic membrane marked by a mononuclear infiltrate, multinucleate giant cells of both foreign body and Langhans type; and fragmentation of the internal elastic lamina. Fibrinoid necrosis is not observed in GCA.
- Cytokine profiles in PMR and GCA differ.

CLINICAL PRESENTATION / PHYSICAL FINDINGS

- Shared features of the two disorders include fever, fatigue, weight loss, an elevated erythrocyte sedimentation rate, anemia, and thrombocytosis.
- PMR exhibits musculoskeletal proximal, severe, symmetrical persistent stiffness, soreness, and pain in the shoulder, neck, and pelvic girdle. Carpal tunnel syndrome and hand and knee synovitis are also noted. There is no muscle inflammation.
- GCA affects certain blood vessels. Headache and scalp pain are very frequent. Headache is very severe and does not respond to routine medication. Temporal and occipital pain can occur. Mandibular pain due to masseter muscle ischemia on chewing is noted in at least 50% of affected individuals. There can be sudden visual loss.

DIAGNOSIS

- Diagnosis of PMR and GCA are based on clinical findings. Laboratory and biopsy are considered supportive tests.
- Differential diagnosis includes ruling out rheumatoid arthritis, polymyositis, fibromyalgia, systemic lupus erythematosus, polyarteritis nodosa, and viral myalgia.
- PMR signs and symptoms include myalgia, especially in the morning and during inactivity. Fatigue, weight loss, weakness, and a low-grade fever are elicited.
- GCA is a vascular symptom-related disease that might present with headache, scalp tenderness, fatigue, masseter muscle pain on chewing, and tongue and pharyngeal pain on swallowing. The clinical appearance of the tongue exhibits a bluish color. This implicates possible infarction.
- Laboratory tests should include CBC, ESR, and rheumatoid factor.
  - PMR exhibits morning stiffness, pain with active joint movement, anemia, and elevated ESR.
  - GCA is associated with headache, scalp pain, anemia, and elevated ESR.
  These diagnostic variations and likenesses demonstrate the relationships of these two diseases.
- Biopsy of a superficial artery assists in diagnosis of GCA.

MEDICAL MANAGEMENT & TREATMENT

- Both diseases are highly responsive to corticosteroids, which are the treatment of choice:
  - Prednisone 10 to 20 mg/day is given. The positive response is within 24 to 48 hours. This dosage should be reduced by 2.5 mg/day every week to 10 mg/day, then by 1 mg/day every month. The steroids should be tapered over the ensuing weeks.
  - This response is so characteristic that an immediate and dramatic improvement in PMR and GCA symptoms within 1 to 3 days after steroid institution supports the diagnosis. Conversely, a lack of rapid and significant improvement in signs, symptoms, and function within 5 to 7 days should lead to the consideration of an alternative diagnosis (e.g., tumor or infection).
- Alternative immunosuppressive agents including methotrexate and azathioprine have been tested in both PMR and GCA patients in an attempt to "spare steroids" and control the inflammatory state. Results have been inconclusive.
- Tumor necrosis factor is used on an investigational basis for the treatment of GCA.

COMPLICATIONS

- Complications may result from long-term treatment with corticosteroids.
- Musculoskeletal, hematologic, and lines involvement must be addressed as early as possible.
- The cardiovascular form of GCA may lead to occlusion, and visual involvement can lead to blindness.

PROGNOSIS

- PMR is considered to be a self-limiting illness. Prognosis depends on early, correct diagnosis. Delay in treatment can result in severe disability.
- With GCA there is an increased risk of mortality. GCA can contribute to blindness, myocardial infarction, cerebrovascular accident, claudication of extremities, and ischemic manifestations.

DENTAL SIGNIFICANCE

- Medical intervention is necessary for stabilization before oral/dental problems are addressed.
- Patient's complaint of fatigue or pain in masticating muscles when chewing food and pain in tongue and throat while eating or swallowing should alert practitioners to a more extensive rather than localized illness. Blanching of the tongue should cause suspicion.

- If visual involvement is noted, it is imperative that the patient is referred to their primary care physician and/or rheumatologist.

DENTAL MANAGEMENT

- If a dental/oral problem is encountered by a patient with PMR or associated GCA, immediate care may be rendered. This is a judgment call by the dental practitioner. Nevertheless, the patient should be referred to their primary care or rheumatologist before any exclusive care is rendered by the dental practitioner.

Assess the risk for adrenal suppression and insufficiency in patients being treated with systemic corticosteroids (see Appendix A, Box A-4, "Dental Management of Patients at Risk for Acute Adrenal Insufficiency").

SUGGESTED REFERENCE

Paget SA. Polymyalgia rheumatica and temporal arteritis, in Goldman L, Ansiello D (eds.): *Cecil Textbook of Medicine*, ed 22. Philadelphia, WB Saunders, 2004, pp 1693–1696.

AUTHOR: **NORBERT J. BURZYNSKI, SR., DDS, MS**

SYNONYM(S)
Primary idiopathic polymyositis

SYNONYM(S)
Primary idiopathic polymyositis

ICD-9CM/CPT CODE(S)
710.4 Polymyositis—complete

OVERVIEW

Polymyositis is characterized by inflammation in skeletal muscle and moderate to severe muscle weakness affecting mainly the proximal limb and trunk muscles.

EPIDEMIOLOGY & DEMOGRAPHICS

INCIDENCE/PREVALENCE IN USA: The incidence and prevalence of polymyositis is uncertain because previous estimates did not differentiate between polymyositis and related inflammatory myopathies such as dermatomyositis and inclusion-body myositis. However, the annual incidence rate of polymyositis is estimated to be 6 to 10 cases per million people.
PREDOMINANT AGE: Although polymyositis may develop at any age, it is usually seen after the age of 20; most patients are between 30 and 60 years old.
PREDOMINANT SEX: Female > male (2:1).
GENETICS: Mild association with HLA-DR3, HLA-DRw52.

ETIOLOGY & PATHOGENESIS

- Muscle fiber destruction associated with infiltration of T-lymphocytes and lesser numbers of leukocytes and plasma cells
- Increased expression of cytokines (e.g., interleukins 1, 2, 6, and 10; tumor necrosis factor α; interferon γ; and transforming growth factor β), chemokines, and metalloproteinases
- Necrosis and phagocytosis of muscle fibers
- Signs of muscle fiber regeneration
- Autoimmune etiology supported by:
  - The association of polymyositis with other autoimmune disorders such as rheumatoid arthritis and systemic lupus erythematosus
  - The expression of MHC Class I antigen on muscle fibers, which do not normally express MHC Class I or II antigens
  - The presence of autoantibodies against ribonucleoproteins involved in protein synthesis, such as histidyl tRNA synthetase, in 20% of patients with polymyositis

CLINICAL PRESENTATION / PHYSICAL FINDINGS

- The typical onset of polymyositis is usually insidious, beginning with painless weakness of the proximal limb muscles. The hips and thighs are most commonly affected, resulting in increasing difficulty in rising from a deep chair or climbing or descending stairs.
- The disease progresses over a period of weeks to months involving the muscles of the trunk, shoulders, and upper arms and resulting in difficulty putting objects on a high shelf or combing one's hair.
- Involvement of the posterior and anterior neck muscles results in difficulty keeping the head upright (i.e., head loll).
- Weakness in the pharyngeal, esophageal, and laryngeal muscles result in dysphagia and dysphonia.
- Ocular, facial, tongue, and masticatory muscles are rarely affected.
- Affected muscles may atrophy over time.
- Pain in muscles is experienced in only 15% of patients.
- Cardiac abnormalities including dysrhythmias and myocarditis can occur.
- Involvement of thoracic muscles may result in pulmonary symptoms.
- A slightly increased frequency of malignancy has been reported in patients with polymyositis. Ovarian, gastrointestinal, lung, and breast cancer and non-Hodgkin's lymphoma are the most commonly reported.
- Autoimmune and connective tissue disorders such as rheumatoid arthritis and systemic lupus erythematosus are seen in association with polymyositis.

DIAGNOSIS

- The diagnosis of polymyositis is based upon the presence of progressive weakness of proximal muscles of the limbs, elevated muscle enzymes in the serum, myopathic electromyographic findings, and characteristic histological findings upon muscle biopsy. Only 25–30% of patients with polymyositis exhibit all three laboratory findings.
- Creatine kinase is the most sensitive muscle enzyme assay in polymyositis, with increases up to 50 times normal levels found during active disease.
- Aspartate and alanine aminotransferases, lactate dehydrogenase, and aldolase levels are also increased in the serum.
- Needle electromyography reveals increased spontaneous activity with fibrillations, complex repetitive discharges, and positive sharp waves in affected muscles.
- Histopathologic examination of tissue from affected muscles demonstrates widespread destruction of segments of muscle fibers, with multifocal lymphocytic infiltrates surrounding and invading nearby healthy muscle fibers.

MEDICAL MANAGEMENT & TREATMENT

- There have been very few randomized, controlled clinical trials, so optimal therapeutic regimens have not been determined.
- Goals of therapy are to improve muscle strength and decrease extramuscular manifestations, such as cardiac abnormalities.
- Corticosteroids are the main therapeutic agents. Prednisone, 1 mg/kg, divided into 3 to 4 equal doses per day, usually provides some relief in most patients with polymyositis. Response is determined by evaluating muscle strength and monitoring creatine kinase levels. Once recovery has begun, the dose of prednisone is tapered, but the patient may require a low dose of steroids for years.
- In cases where corticosteroids are not sufficiently effective, immunosuppressive drugs such as azathioprine (150 to 300 mg/day) or methotrexate (5 to 20 mg/week) may be added to the treatment regimen. Other immunosuppressive drugs used include cyclosporin, mycophenolate mofetil, and cyclophosphamide, alone or in combinations.
- Intravenous infusion of immunoglobulin has been reported effective for treating polymyositis.

COMPLICATIONS

- Hypertension-induced heart failure associated with long-term corticosteroid use.
- Increased risk of infection due to immunosuppressive drugs.
- Slightly increased incidence (~ 9%) of malignancy, although the cause of this increase is not known.

PROGNOSIS

The prognosis for patients with polymyositis is generally favorable. The active period of polymyositis usually lasts for 2 years, and most patients improve with corticosteroid therapy. A small percentage of patients with polymyositis die from pulmonary or cardiac complications. Approximately 20% of patients recover completely and another 20% achieve long-term remission. Older age and development of polymyositis associated malignancy contribute to a poor prognosis.

DENTAL SIGNIFICANCE

- Increased risk and severity of oral infections due to treatment with immunosuppressive drugs.

- Dysphagia may make it difficult for patients with polymyositis to maintain an adequate diet.
- Dysphonia may hinder effective communication.
- Weakness of the neck muscles may make it difficult for patients to hold their head still during dental treatment.
- Weakness in the hips and thighs may make standing up from a seated position in the dental chair difficult.
- Weakness in the shoulders and upper arms may make it difficult for the patient to raise their arms to brush and floss their teeth.

DENTAL MANAGEMENT

- The patient's physician should be consulted as to the status of any cardiac abnormalities (e.g., dysrhythmias, myocarditis) and their implications regarding dental treatment, including the use of local anesthetics containing vasoconstrictors.
- Medications used for treatment of polymyositis should be carefully assessed:
  - Assess the risk for adrenal suppression and insufficiency in patients being treated with systemic corticosteroids (see Appendix A, Box A-4, "Dental Management of Patients at Risk for Acute Adrenal Insufficiency").
  - Patients who are taking cytotoxic or immunosuppressive drugs (e.g., systemic corticosteroids, azathioprine, methotrexate) may have an increased risk of infection and may require perioperative prophylactic antibiotics (see Appendix A, Box A-2, "Presurgical and Postsurgical Antibiotic Prophylaxis for Patients at Increased Risk for Postoperative Infections").
- Supporting the neck with pillows or towels will help the patient keep their head still during dental treatment.
- Patients should be assisted when sitting down or rising from the dental chair. The dental chair should be raised so that the patient can more easily get to a standing position.
- Patients having difficulty raising their arms may need help from a caregiver to maintain adequate oral hygiene.

SUGGESTED REFERENCES

Dalakas MC, Hohlfeld R. Polymyositis and dermatomyositis. *Lancet* 2003;362:971.

Victor M, Ropper AH. The inflammatory myopathies, in *Adams and Victor's Principles of Neurology*, ed 7. New York, McGraw-Hill, 2001, pp 1480–1492.

AUTHOR: **DARRYL T. HAMAMOTO, DDS, PHD**

SYNONYM(S)

Gravidism
Gestation
Fetation

ICD-9CM/CPT CODE(S)

633.0 Abdominal pregnancy—incomplete

OVERVIEW

The period from conception to birth when a woman carries a developing fetus in her uterus.

EPIDEMIOLOGY & DEMOGRAPHICS

INCIDENCE/PREVALENCE IN USA: Approximately 10,000 births take place per day.

PREDOMINANT AGE: Varies, occurs after puberty and prior to menopause.

PREDOMINANT SEX: Pregnancy is exclusive to females.

ETIOLOGY & PATHOGENESIS

- Conception (fertilization) occurs approximately 14 days before a menstrual period, just after ovulation. A sperm and ovum unite to form a zygote in the uterine tube.
- After some cellular division, within 3 to 5 days the ovum moves to the site of implantation, where it continues to divide, developing into an embryo approximately 10 days after fertilization.

CLINICAL PRESENTATION / PHYSICAL FINDINGS

- Absence of menstrual cycle
- Nausea and vomiting
- Weight gain

DIAGNOSIS

- Pregnancy test to detect human chorionic gonadotropin (hCG) level

MEDICAL MANAGEMENT & TREATMENT

MATERNAL CHANGES

- Cardiovascular
  - Increased total blood volume without a compensatory increase in red blood cell mass may result in a "dilutional anemia."
  - Cardiac output increases 30–50% during 16 to 28 weeks, often resulting in functional systolic or "physiologic" murmurs. These murmurs often do not require subacute bacterial endocarditis (SBE) prophylaxis. A consult with the patient's physician is recommended.
- Respiratory
  - Larger abdominal content displaces the diaphragm upward 3 to 4 cm, causing the ribs to flare out and the chest circumference to increase around 5 to 7 cm.
  - Abdominal contents may press on the diaphragm causing breathing difficulties; therefore, patients should not be placed completely supine.
  - Decreased functional residual capacity of approximately 15–20% and modest hypoxemia occurs in about 25% of pregnant females while supine.
- Endocrine
  - Nausea and vomiting/"morning sickness":
    - Incidence: approximately 50–90% of all pregnancies.
    - Associated with young age and low socioeconomic status.
    - Etiology: likely multifactorial but has been mainly been attributed to an increase in human chorionic gonadotropin (hCG) and estrogen.
    - Treatment: no drug is currently approved for morning sickness. Physicians sometimes prescribe antiemetics, sedatives, or vitamins. Patients with extreme nausea and vomiting (hyperemesis gravidarum) should be referred to an obstetrician. After vomiting, patients should rinse with baking soda and water solution to neutralize acidity of the saliva and prevent enamel erosion.

COMPLICATIONS

- Supine hypotensive syndrome: occurs when the gravid uterus partially obstructs the inferior vena cava, decreasing cardiac return to the right side of the heart, which causes hypotension, syncope, decreased placental perfusion, and fetal hypoxia.
  - Approximately 10% of pregnant females near term show signs of hypotension, pallor, and tachycardia when in a supine position. This should be prevented by placing the patient on her left side with her right hip elevated 10 to 12 cm using a folded towel, avoiding a completely supine position.
- Gestational diabetes:
  - Occurs in 13% of all pregnancies.
  - Increased incidence in adolescents.
  - Etiology: usually due to increased insulin requirements from the additional strain on carbohydrate metabolism.
  - Disease management may include diet modifications, insulin therapy, and frequent glucose monitoring.
- Hypertension:
  - Systolic blood pressure of >140 mmHg or an increase from prepregnancy of >30 mmHg.
  - Diastolic blood pressure of >90 mmHg or an increase from prepregnancy of >15 mmHg.
  - If prepregnancy blood pressure is unknown, hypertension due to a rise in systolic or diastolic blood pressure that is still below 140/90 mmHg may go undiagnosed.
  - Hypertension is seen in 7–10% of all pregnancies. Because the reduction of complications in mild to moderate disease through pharmacologic treatment may not justify the possible endangerment to the fetus by such treatment, the management of hypertension in obstetrics is controversial.
  - There are several forms of pregnancy-related hypertension:
    - Chronic hypertension:
      - Presents before 20 weeks gestation
      - Typically well tolerated if diastolic levels do not exceed 100 mmHg
      - Increases the risk of complications
    - Gestational hypertension:
      - Presents after 20 weeks gestation without other signs of preeclampsia
      - Typically well tolerated if diastolic levels do not exceed 100 mmHg
      - Increases the risk of complications
    - Preeclampsia:
      - Presents after 20 weeks of gestation with other findings such as proteinuria and/or edema
      - Etiology unknown
      - Occurs in approximately 5% of all pregnancies
      - Risk factors: primigravidas, preexisting hypertension (preeclampsia superimposed with chronic hypertension), diabetes, obesity, and age less than 20 or over 35 years
      - Pathophysiologic abnormalities: inadequate maternal vascular response to placenta development, endothelial dysfunction, generalized vasospasm, activation of platelets, and abnormal hemostasis
      - Maternal and perinatal mortality/morbidity: decreased uteroplacental blood flow, separation of the placenta from the uterine wall, and preterm delivery
      - Treatment: magnesium sulfate for seizure prophylaxis, hydralazine for blood pressure control, and delivery
      - Untreated sequelae: HELLP (hemolysis, elevated liver enzymes, low platelets) and progression to a convulsive phase (eclampsia)
    - Pregnancy-induced hypertension includes both gestational hypertension and preeclampsia.
- Eclampsia:
  - Convulsive seizures or coma without other etiology occurring concurrently with preeclampsia.

- More than 80% of patients with this condition are young primigravidas.
- May result in cerebral hemorrhage, aspiration pneumonia, hypoxia, encephalopathy, and thromboembolic events.
- This is the most life-threatening antepartum complication.
- Maternal death: aspiration of gastric contents.
- Fetal death: hypoxia.
- Seizures: 25% before labor, 50% during labor, 25% up to 7 to 10 days postpartum. This medical emergency likely to require immediate delivery.

PROGNOSIS

- Patients with preeclampsia are also at increased risk for complications that include morbidity/mortality of both the fetus and the mother.
- The risk of preterm or low birth weight deliveries may increase 6- to 11-fold with the presence of untreated periodontal disease.

DENTAL SIGNIFICANCE

ORAL CHANGES

Etiology: increase in progesterone and estrogen that increases sensitivity to bacterial irritants.

- Pregnancy gingivitis:
  - Occurs in 50–100% of all pregnancies.
  - Usually identified around the second month, peaking in approximately the eighth month.
  - Impeccable oral hygiene is necessary to reduce the plaque irritant and to prevent the exacerbation of any preexisting periodontal disease. Generalized tooth mobility without evidence of periodontal disease is a result of mineral changes in the lamina dura, attachment apparatus, or underlying pathology and has been reported to occur in some pregnancies. It usually resolves spontaneously.
- Pregnancy tumors (pyogenic granulomas):
  - Reported in nearly 5% of pregnant females.
  - Painless and appear in the second trimester.
    - Treatment: although the granuloma typically resolves spontaneously upon delivery, it can be removed if it causes the patient pain or interferes with function.

MATERNAL ORAL INFECTION (including periodontal disease)

- May result in neonatal mortality, preterm birth, and low birth weight.
- It is important to provide dental treatment to pregnant mothers to promote a healthy pregnancy outcome.

- With healthy pregnancies, most obstetricians prefer to have the source of the dental problem resolved (with proper consultation) rather than delaying treatment. Because obstetricians may not be familiar with routine dental procedures, however, dentists should be clear when consulting with them regarding the anticipated invasiveness of a procedure (including the possibility of bacteremia in patients with heart murmurs), the amount and type of anesthetic to be used (local, etc.), the anticipated postoperative pain, and the necessary postoperative medication.

DENTAL MANAGEMENT

FETAL HEALTH CONCERNS AND DELIVERY OF DENTAL CARE

- Goal: maintain fetal and maternal health during delivery of dental care
- Major concerns:
  - Induction of fetal hypoxia as evidenced by decreased fetal heart rate and avoided through correct patient positioning.
  - Exposure of the fetus to teratogens.
    - Examples: drugs, ionizing radiation, and infections.
    - Effects vary from minor alveolus clefting to spontaneous abortion.
    - Determination of effect: genetic predisposition, developmental stage, and route and level of exposure from the agent. The developmental stage at the time of exposure is critical in determining the effect.
    - After fertilization but prior to implantation, the ovum generally responds in an "all or none" fashion, either attaching or dying.
    - Major organogenesis occurs during the embryonic period (2 to

8 weeks), and the developing embryo is most sensitive to the teratogenic insult. Major developmental disturbances result in classic congenital malformations such as anencephaly and heart/limb defects.
  - During the fetal period (8 weeks until term), insults may result in cleft lip and palate, poor fetal growth, and more subtle developmental disturbances.

DRUG THERAPY

- The U.S. Food and Drug Administration (FDA) has created a pregnancy risk classification, or PRC, for all approved drugs (Table I-18). Unfortunately, less than 20% of all FDA-classified drugs are in PRC A or B. Nearly all drugs cross the placenta and are secreted into the breast milk to some extent. Whenever possible, if systemic medication is necessary, patients should take the medication immediately after breastfeeding to avoid peak levels at the time of nursing. Sustained-release formulas should be avoided (Table I-19).
- Prenatal fluoride supplementation
  - Evidence has not clearly demonstrated beneficial effects.
  - Currently, the ADA does not recommend any supplementation prior to 6 months of age.

DENTAL TREATMENT PLANNING CONSIDERATIONS/TREATMENT TIMING

- The initial evaluation is best performed early in the pregnancy so that any elective treatment may be planned for during the second trimester. Of course, if a patient initially presents during the later stages of the pregnancy, a thorough dental evaluation as discussed following is still recommended.

TABLE I-18 FDA Drug Pregnancy Risk Category (PRC) Descriptions

Pregnancy Risk Category	Description	Application in Dentistry
A	▪ Drug has been studied in humans. ▪ Evidence supports its safe use. ▪ Remote possibility of fetal harm.	May be appropriately administered during pregnancy.
B	▪ Animal studies demonstrate no fetal risk. ▪ Inadequate studies in pregnant women. ▪ Slightly increased fetal risk.	
C	▪ Teratogenic risk cannot be ruled out. ▪ Animal studies show potential adverse fetal effects. ▪ Potential benefits may outweigh risks.	May be used with caution.
D	▪ Drug demonstrates risk in humans. ▪ Potential benefits may outweigh risks.	Should be avoided.
X	▪ Drug demonstrates harm in mother or fetus. ▪ Risk clearly outweighs benefit.	

TABLE I-19 FDA Drug Pregnancy Risk Category (PRC) and Use During Breastfeeding

Generic Name	Brand Name(s)	FDA PRC	Use During Breastfeeding
ANTIMICROBIALS			
Amoxicillin	Amoxil; Polymox	B	Yes
Cephalexin	Keflex	B	Yes
Clindamycin	Cleocin	B	Yes
Doxycycline	Doryx; Vibramycin; Atridox; Periostat	D	No
Tetracycline	Actisite; Achromycin	D	No
Erythromycin*	Ery-Tab; E-Mycin; E.E.S.; PCE	B	Yes
Metronidazole	Flagyl	B	Caution
Penicillin V Potassium	V-Cillin K; V-Pen	B	Yes
Amoxicillin + Clavulanic Acid	Augmentin	B	Yes
Azithromycin	Zithromax	B	Yes
Nystatin	Mycostatin	B	Yes
Ketoconazole	Nizoral	C	No
Fluconazole	Diflucan	C	No
Chlorhexidine	Peridex	B	Yes
ANALGESICS			
Acetaminophen	Tylenol	B	Yes
Aspirin	Bayer	C/D3	No
Ibuprofen	Advil; Motrin	B/D3	Yes
Celecoxib/Valdecoxib	Celebrex/Bextra	C/D3	Unknown
Naproxen	Aleve; Anaprox	B/D3	Unknown
Codeine	Various combinations	C/D*	Yes
Hydrocodone	Various combinations	C/D*	Caution
Oxycodone	Various combinations	C/D*	Caution
SEDATIVES			
Hydroxyzine	Atarax/Vistaril	C	Unknown
Midazolam	Versed	D	No
Diazepam	Valium	D	No
Lorazepam	Ativan	D	No
Triazolam	Halcion	X	No
Chloral Hydrate	Somnote	C	Yes
Nitrous Oxide	n/a	None[t]	Controversial
LOCAL ANESTHETICS			
Lidocaine	Xylocaine	B	Yes
Etidocaine	Duranest	B	Yes
Prilocaine	Citanest	B	Yes
Mepivacaine	Carbocaine	C	Yes
Bupivacaine	Marcaine	C	Yes
Articaine	Septocaine	C	Unknown
VASOCONSTRICTORS			
Epinephrine 1:100,000; 1:200,000	n/a	C*	Yes
Levonordephrin 1:20,000	Neo-Cobefrin	None	Yes
TOPICAL ANESTHETICS			
Benzocaine	Anbesol; Hurricaine	C	Yes
Lidocaine	Xylocaine; DentiPatch	B	Yes
Tetracaine	Pontocaine	C	Yes

C/D3 = PRC D during the third trimester.
C/D* = PRC D in high doses at term or with prolonged use.
C* = PRC C in high doses.
* = Avoid estolate form.
t = Best used in the second and third trimesters and for < 30 minutes with at least 50% O_2; consult physician.
Adapted from Hilgers K, Douglass J, Mathieu G. Adolescent pregnancy: a review of dental treatment guidelines. *Pediatr Dent* 2003;25:459–467.

○ First Trimester:
- Assess the patient's current dental health and dental awareness.
- Chief complaint.
- Inform her of expected oral changes.
- Susceptibility to plaque (pregnancy gingivitis).
- Pyogenic granulomas.
- Discuss how to avoid maternal dental problems.
- Oral hygiene instructions.
- Objectives of treatment with respect to the fetus are to avoid fetal hypoxia, premature labor/abortion, and teratogenic effects.
- Record a thorough medical history:
  - History of hypertension, diabetes, heart murmur, and morning sickness
  - Pregnancy complications
  - Obstetrician concerns
  - Previous pregnancies, outcomes, and complications
  - Medications
  - Systemic disorders
  - Drug allergies
- Record blood pressure and refer those who are hypertensive.
- Physical appearance.
- Edema.
- Obesity.
- General appearance.
- When a patient is not under the care of an obstetrician, she should receive the proper referral.
- Record a dental history, including previous treatment complications.
- Untreated oral disease.
- Pain.
  - Type, duration, and frequency
  - What makes it better or worse?
- With no additional medical concerns, a thorough exam and dental prophylaxis should be performed. Look for:
  - Pregnancy gingivitis
  - Pyogenic granulomas or other pathology
  - Untreated caries or oral infection
- Necessary radiographs should be taken of teeth that are symptomatic or are suspected as having caries. In the absence of suspected dental disease, avaoid radiographs.
- If a patient presents with an abscess or multiple, large, carious lesions, the patient's obstetrician should be consulted, and the source of the infection removed as soon as possible (in uncomplicated pregnancies). Often, this requires either endodontic therapy or extraction of the offending tooth.
- There is no specific medical justification to defer elective treatment in a healthy pregnancy. However, approximately one in five pregnancies end in spontaneous abortion (with 85% occurring in the first trimester), and delaying elective treatment other than prophylaxis and examinations to the second trimester may avoid a correlation being made between dental treatment and a spontaneous abortion.

○ Second trimester:
- Perform elective restorative and periodontal treatment to prevent dental infection or complications during the third trimester.
- If the patient will not be returning during the third trimester, she should receive oral health counseling for her newborn. This should include information regarding the prevention of early childhood caries (ECC) and the recommendation that the baby's first dental visit be with the eruption of the first tooth and no later than 1 year of age. Encourage the mother to maintain her own dental health because preschool children whose mothers have low or suppressed *Mutans streptococci* levels may have significantly reduced caries experience.

○ Third trimester:
- Perform a second dental prophylaxis if there has been a lack of oral home care or if pregnancy gingivitis or a pregnancy tumor has occurred. Typically, in the third trimester pregnant females are in some form of generalized discomfort and oral home care may not be at its best.

• Dental Radiographs
○ There are two major risks to a developing fetus from radiation exposure:
- Induction of cancer
- Development of mental retardation
○ From studies of atomic bomb survivors and other irradiated populations, it appears that 10 μSv of radiation is required for a significant risk of either effect to occur. The fetus or embryo is the most sensitive to the neurogenic effects of radiation between the eighth and fifteenth weeks after conception during neuronal migration and organogenesis.
○ The average gonadal doses to females for a full-mouth radiographic series using 18 E-speed films is less than 0.005 μSv.
○ When compared to environmental background radiation, a full-mouth radiographic series, using 18 E-speed films and a rectangular collimated beam, results in a background radiation equivalency of 1 day; for four bitewing films, 7 hours.
○ Panoramic radiographic techniques have a background radiation equivalency of 12 hours, although some newer panoramic x-ray machines are equivalent to only 7 hours.
○ F-speed film has been shown to be of comparable diagnostic quality to E-speed film, and the exposure level is only 77%.
○ Digital radiographic imaging has recently gained popularity, and it has also been shown to decrease radiographic exposure by at least 50% of the fastest current film-based images while offering comparable diagnostic quality.
○ With the following proper radiographic techniques, radiation exposure to the fetus is actually so low that it cannot be measured by conventional dosimetric techniques:
- Rectangular collimation.
- Lead shielding (abdominal and thyroid).
- Use of the fastest available receptor (E- or F-speed film or digital).
- Use of a long cone, time/temperature controlled processing and the avoidance of retakes.
○ Reluctant patients should be educated that the risk of complications (mental retardation and cancer induction) is so low that it is almost impossible to measure. The risk of reaching a teratogenic threshold dosage of radiation related to dental radiographs is < 0.1%, which is more than 1000 times less than the anticipated risk of spontaneous abortion and malformation.
○ Recent studies suggest that the fetus may be at more risk from a lack of dental care when dental disease is present than from receiving treatment that includes dental radiographs.
○ Failing to utilize radiographs for certain procedures such as extractions or root canal therapy may be considered substandard care.
○ In summary, the use of dental radiographs (with proper techniques) is encouraged if potentially beneficial.

SUGGESTED REFERENCES

Briggs GG, Freeman RK, Yaffe SJ. *Drugs in Pregnancy and Lactation: A Reference Guide to Fetal and Neonatal Risk.* Philadelphia, Lippincott Williams & Wilkins, 2002.

Gajendra S, Kumar JV. Oral health and pregnancy: a review. *NY State Dent J* 2004;70(1):40–44.

Hilgers KK, Douglass J, Mathieu GP. Adolescent pregnancy: a review of dental treatment guidelines. *Ped Dent* 2003;25(5):459–467.

Lakshmanan S, Radfar L. Pregnancy and lactation. *Oral Surg Oral Med Oral Path Oral Radiol Endod* 2004;97:672–682.

Rayburn WF. Recommending medications during pregnancy: an evidence-based approach. *Clin Obstetrics and Gynecol* 2002;45(1):1–5.

Turner M, Aziz SR. Management of the pregnant oral and maxillofacial surgery patient. *J Oral Maxillofac Surg* 2002;60:1479–1488.

White SC. Assessment of radiation risks from dental radiography. *Dentomaxillofac Radio* 1992;21:118–126.

AUTHOR: **KELLY K. HILGERS, DDS, MS**

SYNONYM(S)

Primary Raynaud's phenomenon or Raynaud's disease
Secondary Raynaud's phenomenon

ICD-9CM/CPT CODE(S)

443.0 Raynaud's syndrome, Raynaud's disease, Raynaud's phenomenon (secondary)

OVERVIEW

Raynaud's phenomenon (RP) is a vasospastic disorder associated with an abrupt onset of a triphasic color response that includes a well-demarcated pallor of the digits progressing to cyanosis with pain and often numbness followed by reactive hyperemia on rewarming. Discoloration is usually seen in the digits and toes and occasionally in the nose and tongue. This reaction is precipitated by exposure to cold temperatures or emotional stress.

EPIDEMIOLOGY & DEMOGRAPHICS

INCIDENCE/PREVALENCE IN USA: Surveys note 4–20% of the general population have symptoms of RP. Primary RP is more common than secondary RP.
PREDOMINANT AGE: Primary PR usually first appears between ages 15 and 45 years. When the onset is after 30 years of age, there is a greater chance that RP is secondary to an underlying medical condition.
PREDOMINANT SEX: Female > male (4:1).
GENETICS: One-quarter of patients have a family history of RP in a first-degree relative.

ETIOLOGY & PATHOGENESIS

- Primary RP is referred to as Raynaud's disease when the etiology is not known or cannot be found.
  - Approximately 5–15% of patients with primary RP can develop a secondary cause such as scleroderma or CREST (calcinosis, Raynaud's phenomenon, esophageal dysmotility, sclerodactyly, telangiectasias) syndrome. Approximately 90% of patients with scleroderma experience Raynaud's phenomenon.
- In contrast to uncomplicated (primary) RP, secondary RP refers to arterial insufficiency of the extremities caused by various conditions, including CREST, scleroderma, systemic lupus erythematosus (SLE), mixed connective tissue disease, rheumatoid arthritis, drug-induced thromboangiitis obliterans, polycythemia, obstructive arterial disease, occupational trauma, carpal tunnel syndrome, and other conditions.
- The initial manifestations of RP occur when digits turn white due to vaso-

constriction or spasms of the digital arteries. Thus, with cessation of blood flow the digits become numb. The constrictions leave the blood in the veins and capillaries to become deoxygenated, thus resulting in a cyanotic appearance. With rewarming, blood flow restarts, producing reactive hyperemia.

- No single pathophysiologic mechanism adequately explains cold-induced vasospasm in all forms of the syndrome; in fact, there is no single form of RP for which the pathophysiology is entirely understood.
  - Possible mechanisms for cold-induced vasospasm in RP include aberrant endothelium-dependent vasoregulation, low levels of calcitonin gene-related peptide, abnormal α-adrenergic receptor response, and abnormal platelet activation.

CLINICAL PRESENTATION / PHYSICAL FINDINGS

- The classic manifestation of RP is a triphasic color response to cold exposure:
  - This response occurs in 4–65% of the afflicted patients. Exposure to cold and emotional instability, in some cases, present the signs and symptoms. Pallor of digit(s) results from vasospasm. Cyanosis is secondary to desaturated venous blood. The color changes are delineated, symmetric, and usually bilateral. Mild discomfort, paresthesias, numbness, and trace edema often accompany the color changes. Attacks favor the fingers, but vasospasms can occur in the toes, nose, ears, lips, and other parts of the body. Ulcerations and gangrene are rare in primary RP.
- In primary RP, the physical examination is normal between attacks.
- In secondary RP, pits or ulcerations may be found in fingers of patients with scleroderma, CREST syndrome, and/or thromboangiitis obliterans.

DIAGNOSIS

- The diagnosis of primary RP is based on the patient's description of the attacks and clinical findings. If there is a persistence of cyanosis and hyperemia, then secondary RP should be considered with entities such as scleroderma, CREST syndrome, mixed connective tissue disease, SLE, rheumatoid arthritis, drug-induced reactions, and related connective tissue diseases.
- Laboratory tests should include CBC, BUN, ESR, ANA, C-reactive protein, and urinalysis.
- Specific serological testing includes extractable nuclear antigens, anti-DNA, cryoglobulins, complement, anticen-

tromere antibodies, and Scl 70 antibodies.
- Appropriate questionnaires and color photographs may be helpful.

MEDICAL MANAGEMENT & TREATMENT

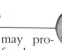

NONPHARMACOLOGIC

- The goal is to prevent ulcers and gangrene.
  - Patients should avoid cold exposure and emotional encounters and dress appropriately for cold weather (e.g., mittens and other garments).
  - Avoid medications such as β-blockers, vinblastine, bleomycin, ergotamine, methysergide, oral contraceptives, estrogen replacement therapy (ERT) without progesterone, nicotine, caffeine, and over-the-counter decongestants.

ACUTE AND CHRONIC CARE

- Dihydropyridine calcium channel-blocking agents are the drugs of choice. Nifedipine, 10 to 20 mg given 30 minutes to 1 hour before cold exposure, is the most frequent and effective treatment. Dosage is increased when vasospasm occurs more frequently. Other drugs that may be tried include amlodipine and diltiazem.
- Low-dose aspirin (81 mg per day) should be used for its antiplatelet effects. Additional antiplatelet treatment with dipyridamole (Persantine) at 50 to 100 mg three times per day can be helpful.
- When patients develop digital ulcers, the application of nitroglycerin ointment (Nitro-Bid) three times per day at the base of the affected finger is helpful. More resistant ulcers can respond to intravenous prostaglandin such as epoprostenol (Flolan).
- Surgical palmar digital sympathectomy has been used with good results in many patients with recurrent and medically resistant digital ischemia.

COMPLICATIONS

- Ischemic changes may progress with possible focal gangrene on the tips of digits, toes, ear lobes, cheeks, and chin.

PROGNOSIS

The prognosis of patients with primary Raynaud's is very good; there is no mortality reported. Secondary Raynaud's, associated with various underlying conditions, dictates the general control and outcomes of this health state. Primary preventive measures should be initiated to control ischemic/gangrene, allay symptoms, and prevent debilitating changes.

DENTAL SIGNIFICANCE

- If secondary collagen-vascular disease is diagnosed, rheumatology consult is indicated. Vascular surgery consult should be obtained regarding complications of ulcers and/or gangrene.
- Possible spasms of lips and tongue may occur.
- Tooth extraction site (sockets) may be slow to heal, compounded by susceptibility to infections in patients with secondary RP.
- Signs of underlying disease in secondary RP may need modification for oral/dental care as well as nutritional uptake.

DENTAL MANAGEMENT

- Consultation with a rheumatologist is a prime obligation.
- With appropriate medication, the control of oral, lips, and tongue spasms is possible. Therefore, general dental/ oral and hygiene care is possible with a limited compromise.
- The office cubicle and/or suite should have temperature control to prevent patient vasospasms.
- Consider the use of perioperative prophylactic antibiotics (see Appendix A, Box A-2, "Presurgical and Postsurgical Antibiotic Prophylaxis for Patients at Increased Risk for Postoperative Infections") for oral surgical procedures in patents with secondary RP.
- Counsel patient on tobacco cessation due to nicotine exposure and avoid caffeine and over-the-counter decongestants that can precipitate vasospasms.

SUGGESTED REFERENCES

Kleppel JH (ed): *Primer on the Rheumatic Diseases*, ed 12. Atlanta, The Arthritis Foundation, 2001.

Olin JW. Other peripheral arterial diseases, in Goldman L, Ansiello D (eds): *Cecil Textbook of Medicine*, ed 22. Philadelphia, WB Saunders, 2004, pp 471–477.

AUTHOR: **NORBERT J. BURZYNSKI, SR., DDS, MS**

SYNONYM(S)

Reiter's disease
Reactive arthritis
Seronegative spondyloarthropathy

ICD-9CM/CPT CODE(S)

099.3 Reiter's disease—complete

OVERVIEW

- Reiter's syndrome is one of the seronegative spondyloarthropathies (i.e., where the serum rheumatoid factor is not present) that also include ankylosing spondylitis, juvenile-onset ankylosing spondylitis, psoriatic arthritis, and arthropathy of inflammatory bowel disease.
- It is an asymmetric polyarthritis that mainly affects the lower extremities and is associated urethritis, cervicitis, dysentery, conjunctivitis, and mucocutaneous lesions.
- Two forms of Reiter's syndrome are recognized: sexually transmitted and postdysentery.

EPIDEMIOLOGY & DEMOGRAPHICS

INCIDENCE/PREVALENCE IN USA:
0.24–1.5% incidence after epidemics of bacterial dysentery; complicates 1–2% cases of nongonococcal urethritis.
PREDOMINANT AGE: 20 to 40 years.
PREDOMINANT SEX:
- Sexually transmitted form: male > female (5 to 10:1).
- Postdysenteric form: male = female.
GENETICS: HLA-B27 tissue antigen is present in 63–96% of patients; they are at increased risk for developing Reiter's syndrome after sexual contact or exposure to certain enteric bacterial infections.

ETIOLOGY & PATHOGENESIS

- Exact etiology unknown.
- Two patterns are noted:
  - The sexually transmitted form, which is the most common type in the U.S. and the U.K.
  - The postdysenteric form, which is the most common type in continental Europe and North Africa
- Genetically susceptible, HLA-B27-positive individuals are subject to Reiter's syndrome after being exposed to *Shigella, Salmonella, Yersinia,* or *Campylobacter* as well as the *Chlamydia*-associated diseases.

CLINICAL PRESENTATION / PHYSICAL FINDINGS

- Typically, urethritis develops 7 to 14 days after sexual contact or dysentery; low grade fever, conjunctivitis, and arthritis over the next few weeks.
  - Not all features need occur, so incomplete forms need to be considered.

- Musculoskeletal:
  - Oligoarthritis affecting mainly lower extremities with low-grade inflammation.
    - The distinctive arthropathy of Reiter's syndrome includes local enthesopathy (inflammation of the insertion of muscle tendons and ligaments into bones or joint capsules) common in insertions into calcaneus, talar, and subtalar joints.
  - Sausage-shaped finger (dactylitis) or toe, caused by uniform inflammation.
  - Knee(s) may become markedly edematous.
- Genitourinary:
  - Meatal edema and erythema and clear, mucoid discharge.
  - Prostatic tenderness (up to 80%) and vulvovaginitis.
- Dermatologic:
  - Balanitis circinata (shallow, painless ulcers at meatus and glans penis).
  - Keratoderma blennorrhagica [hyperkeratotic skin, which begins as clear vesicles on erythematous bases and progress to macules, papules, and nodules (found on soles of feet, toes, palms, scrotum, trunk, and scalp)].
  - Nail thickening and ridging.
- Oral:
  - Aphthous-like mucosal lesions.
- Ophthalmologic:
  - Conjunctivitis (most common), with mucopurulent discharge, chemosis, lid edema, and iritis.
- Cardiovascular:
  - Aortic regurgitation caused by inflammation of aortic wall and valve, similar to that seen in ankylosing spondylitis.

DIAGNOSIS

A scoring system for diagnostic points in Reiter-like spondyloarthropathies exists. Two or more of the following points establishes diagnosis (one of which must pertain to the musculoskeletal system):
- Asymmetric oligoarthritis, predominantly of the lower extremity
- Sausage-shaped finger (dactylitis), toe or heel pain, or other enthesitis
- Cervicitis or acute diarrhea within 1 month of the arthritis
- Conjunctivitis or iritis
- Genital ulceration or urethritis
LABORATORY
- No specific tests; ESR possibly elevated
- Synovial fluid examination and culture
- Cultures for gonococcus (urethral, cervical, stool)
IMAGING
- Radiographs of affected joints for erosion and/or joint space narrowing, especially in advanced cases

MEDICAL MANAGEMENT & TREATMENT

NONPHARMACOLOGIC
- Physical therapy to maintain mobility and motion
GENERAL CARE
- NSAIDs are recommended for arthritis/arthralgias (indomethacin, 25 to 50 mg PO tid).
- Enteric or urethral infection should be treated with appropriate antibiotics.
- Uveitis should be treated with steroid eye drops in consultation with an ophthalmologist.
- Enthesopathy (e.g., tendinitis, plantar fasciitis) to be treated with methylprednisolone injections (40 to 80 mg).
- Persistent and uncontrolled disease may warrant cytotoxic drugs as methotrexate or azathioprine in consultation with a rheumatologist.

COMPLICATIONS

- Recurrent arthritis (15–50%)
- Chronic arthritis or sacroiliitis (15–30%)
- Ankylosing spondylitis (30–50% of HLA-B27-positive patients)
- Aortic regurgitation
- Infection with HIV is associated with particularly severe cases of Reiter's syndrome

PROGNOSIS

- Signs and symptoms usually remit within 6 months.
- Poor prognosis is associated with hip arthritis, oligoarthritis, sausage finger or toe, ESR > 30, poor efficacy of NSAIDs, and onset in patients less than 16 years old.

DENTAL SIGNIFICANCE

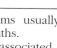

Oral lesions are seen in less than 20% of patients with Reiter's syndrome and are described as shallow, painless, aphthous-like ulcers or painless erythematous papules occurring on the tongue, buccal mucosa, palate, and gingiva.

DENTAL MANAGEMENT

- Systemic infection, eye, and arthritic components need the involvement of the primary care physician, rheumatologist, and/or ophthalmologist.
- Oral lesions are usually mild and require limited care. Corticosteroid rinses or topical applications may be utilized if needed.
- Preventive oral and dental care must be instituted and reinforced.

SUGGESTED REFERENCES

Arnett FC, in Klipel JH (ed): *Primer on the Rheumatic Diseases*, ed 12. Atlanta, The Arthritis Foundation, 2001, pp 245–250.

Reiter's syndrome, in Fitzpatrick TB, Johnson RA, Wolff K, Suurmond D (eds): *Color Atlas and Synopsis of Clinical Dermatology*, ed 4. New York, McGraw-Hill, pp 400–402.

See also "Reiter's Syndrome" in Section II, p 314.

AUTHOR: **NORBERT J. BURZYNSKI, SR., DDS, MS**

SYNONYM(S)

Chronic renal disease
Chronic renal failure (CRF)
End-stage renal disease (ESRD)
Kidney disease
Kidney transplant

ICD-9CM/CPT CODE(S)
585 Chronic renal failure—complete
55.6 Transplant of kidney—incomplete

OVERVIEW

Renal disease results in the kidney's inability to function as a filter to eliminate metabolic (nitrogenous) waste via the urine; maintain the body's fluid, acid/base, and electrolyte balance; reabsorb protein; and secrete the hormones renin and angiotensin (which are responsible for the control of blood pressure) and erythropoietin (which modulates red blood cell maturation).

Chronic renal failure (CRF) [or end-stage renal disease (ESRD)] is a progressive decrease in renal function, typically characterized by a glomerular filtration rate (GFR) < 60 mL/min for ≥ 3 months, with subsequent accumulation of nitrogenous waste products in the blood, electrolyte abnormalities, and anemia.

EPIDEMIOLOGY & DEMOGRAPHICS

INCIDENCE/PREVALENCE IN USA: Incidence is 308 per million; prevalence of ESRD is 1160 per million. The number of patients with ESRD is increasing at the rate of 7–9% per year in the U.S., with approximately 58,000 deaths annually related to ESRD.
PREDOMINANT AGE: While ESRD can affect children, the incidence and prevalence increase dramatically above the age of 40 years.
PREDOMINANT SEX: Slight male predilection.
GENETICS: Some etiologies of ESRD have known genetic patterns of inheritance, including autosomal dominant polycystic kidney disease, autosomal recessive polycystic kidney disease, and Alport's syndrome. Also, when compared to the general population, African-Americans are approximately five more likely to have ESRD.

ETIOLOGY & PATHOGENESIS

- Renal disease may be either acute or chronic.
- Acute renal failure is defined as a sudden decrease in renal function.
  - Causes include trauma, ischemia, septicemia, or adverse reaction to medications or toxic chemicals.
- End-stage renal disease occurs as a result of any condition that destroys nephrons and decreases renal excretory and regulatory function chronically.

- Causes include conditions that result from either malfunction of the kidney or systemic disease, including diabetes mellitus (responsible for approximately 37% of cases of ESRD), hypertension (approximately 30% of cases), chronic glomerulonephritis (approximately 12% of cases), autosomal dominant polycystic kidney disease (approximately 10% of cases), systemic lupus erythematosus, and drug-induced (nephrotoxic) nephropathies.

CLINICAL PRESENTATION / PHYSICAL FINDINGS

- A healthy kidney is capable of compensatory hypertrophy that allows it to carry out normal function by increasing in size to compensate for the loss, damage, or disease of the other kidney. Therefore, the ill effects of renal failure typically require dysfunction of both kidneys with less than 30% total intact renal function.
- The clinical presentation of ESRD varies with the degree of renal failure and its underlying etiology. Individuals can remain asymptomatic until renal failure is far advanced (GFR < 10 to 15 mL/min). Presenting signs and symptoms include:
- Skin:
  - Pallor due to anemia and/or accumulation of carotene-like, yellow-brown pigments along with uncomfortable pruritus.
  - Easily bruised with petechia and ecchymoses.
  - Uremic "frost" due to residual urea crystals left on the skin when perspiration evaporates.
- Cardiovascular:
  - Hypertension is present or develops in 90% of ESRD patients due to sodium overload and extracellular fluid expansion.
  - Congestive heart failure: patients with end-stage renal disease tend toward a high cardiac output state. They often have extracellular fluid overload, shunting of blood through an arteriovenous fistula for dialysis, and anemia. In addition to hypertension, these abnormalities cause increased myocardial work and oxygen demand.
  - Pericarditis: when the BUN concentration exceeds 100 mg/dL, pericarditis may develop. The cause is believed to be retention of metabolic toxins. Pericarditis may exacerbate (or precipitate) congestive heart failure.
- Pulmonary:
  - Pulmonary edema ("uremic lung") causing dyspnea and orthopnea.
- Gastrointestinal:
  - Anorexia, nausea, and occult gastrointestinal bleeding.

- Hematologic:
  - Normochromic, normocytic hemolytic anemia that responds to treatment with erythropoietin, iron, and/or folate deficiency anemias are also possible.
  - Impaired hemostasis resulting from:
    - Thrombocytopathia (possibly due to a decrease in Platelet Factor 3)
    - Mild to moderate thrombocytopenia decreased platelet production
    - Impaired prothrombin consumption
      - Lymphopenia with neutrophils demonstrating chemotactic and phagocytic defects
- Neurologic:
  - Development of symmetric sensory polyneuropathy similar to that found in diabetic patients.
  - Severe uremia can result in a "uremic delirium" characterized by impaired cognitive function, confusion, disorientation, lethargy, and coma.
- Bone:
  - A variety of bone disorders occurs in CRF, collectively referred to as renal osteodystrophy. Renal osteodystrophy is essentially a form of secondary hyperparathyroidism that results from increased serum phosphate levels and decreased serum calcium levels brought on by decreased glomerular filtration in CRF. The clinical manifestations of renal osteodystrophy include:
    - Osteitis fibrosa (bone resorption and osteolytic lesions)
    - Osteomalacia (increased unmineralized bone matrix)
    - Osteosclerosis (increased bone density)
      - With renal osteodystrophy, there is also a tendency for spontaneous fractures of bone with slow healing, myopathy, aseptic necrosis of the hip, and extraosseous calcifications.

DIAGNOSIS

- CBC: normochromic, normocytic anemia.
- Glomerular filtration rate (GFR): markedly decreased.
- Blood glucose: elevated.
- Blood urea nitrogen (BUN): markedly elevated.
- Serum creatinine: elevated, gives good estimate of degree of renal insufficiency.
- Electrolytes: elevated potassium, and phosphate, and depressed or normal serum calcium.
- Urinalysis: proteinuria, casts of red cells and white cells, hyaline. Twenty-four-hour urine collections are used to gauge creatinine clearance, protein, and electrolyte loss.

- Vitamin D levels: decreased when parathyroid hormone levels are elevated.
- Renal biopsy: definitive test for exact histopathologic diagnosis; may reveal glomerulonephritis and/or interstitial nephritis.
- Renal imaging: intravenous pyelogram (IVP), CT, tomograms, retrograde pyelograms, angiography, and/or ultrasound.
- Dental radiographs: may show signs of renal osteodystrophy that include loss of lamina dura, scanty or fine trabeculation, thinning of the inferior mandibular cortex, and/or thinning of the cortices surrounding the inferior alveolar canal. Evaluating serial radiographs may reveal a decrease in bone density.

MEDICAL MANAGEMENT & TREATMENT

PHARMACOLOGIC THERAPY

- Hypertension controlled with antihypertensives: angiotensin-converting enzyme (ACE) inhibitors, angiotensin receptor blockers, and nondihydropyridine calcium channel blockers (e.g., diltiazem or verapamil)
- Diuretics for significant fluid overload (loop diuretics are preferred)
- Vitamin D and calcium to manage secondary hyperparathyroidism (renal osteodystrophy)
- Vitamin E or quinine for muscle cramps.
- Erythropoietin (EPO) for anemia
- Desmopressin acetate (DDAVP), cryoprecipitate, platelets, dialysis for problems related to excessive or spontaneous bleeding
- Antihistamines and skin moisturizers for pruritus
- Insulin for glucose intolerance

NONPHARMACOLOGIC

- Hemodialysis: metabolic waste products are removed from the patient by passing their blood through a thin, semipermeable membrane. The patient's blood is then heparinized and returned back to them. This process is accomplished by the hemodialysis machine. Vascular access for hemodialysis can be accomplished by a native vein arteriovenous fistula (in about 30% of patients) or a foreign (bovine) or synthetic arteriovenous graft (in about 70% of patients). Patients typically require hemodialysis three times a week. Sessions last 3 to 4 hours depending on patient size, type of dialyzer used, and other factors.
- Peritoneal dialysis: this procedure is slower as the abdominal peritoneum serves as the semipermeable membrane. The most common kind of peritoneal dialysis is chronic (or continuous) ambulatory peritoneal dialysis (CAPD). Patients exchange the dialysate four or five times a day. The dialysate remains in the peritoneal cavity between exchanges.

SURGERY

- Renal transplantation is a means of improving the quality of life for the recipient. Renal transplants are ideally procured from a close relative with a good histocompatibility profile; however, cadaver kidneys are also used. Immunosuppressive drugs such as cyclosporine-A, corticosteroids (e.g., prednisone), azathioprine, cyclophosphamide, mycophenolate mofetil, and/or tacrolimus are employed to prevent rejection.

COMPLICATIONS

- Systemic complications of advanced renal disease develop uremia that is fatal if not treated.
- The failing kidney does not excrete sodium properly, which results in fluid retention, edema, hypertension, and cardiovascular disease.
- The inability of the kidney to eliminate nitrogenous waste products results in azotemia, metabolic acidosis, and electrolyte imbalances.
- Decreased erythropoietin production and a propensity toward bleeding due to decreased platelet aggregation and adhesiveness result in anemia.
- Host defenses may be compromised due to decreased production of white blood cells, nutritional deficiencies, and immunosuppressive therapy.
- Bone disorders (renal osteodystrophy) resembling hyperparathyroidism may be noted in the skeleton and mandible.
- Oral complications are related to uremic odor, mucosal ulceration and pain, xerostomia, secondary infection, and bleeding.

PROGNOSIS

- The prognosis of ESRD depends on the underlying disease process and the presence of comorbid conditions. The annual mortality rate for patients with ESRD requiring hemodialysis is approximately 20–25%.
- Kidney transplantation in certain patients with ESRD improves survival. The 2-year kidney graft survival rate for living, related-donor transplantations is > 80%, while the 2-year graft survival rate for cadaveric donor transplantation is approximately 70%.
- Graft vs host disease is an ominous prognostic sign and generally portends the ultimate rejection of a renal transplant.
- The oral cavity usually reflects the control of the renal disease. Therefore, more oral problems will be expected with the poorly controlled ESRD patient, indicating a poorer prognosis.

DENTAL SIGNIFICANCE

- Intraoral symptoms: the dentist should take a careful history of patients at risk for or with suspected or known renal disease. The review of systems and evaluation of the patient's blood pressure and sun-exposed skin for signs of renal disease as described previously will provide invaluable diagnostic information. If undiagnosed renal disease is suspected, evaluation of the patient's medication list may provide information related to drugs known to cause acute renal failure. Patients may complain of:
  ○ Anorexia
  ○ Dysgeusia
  ○ Intraoral pain or discomfort
  ○ Nausea
  ○ Xerostomia
- Intraoral signs: the dentist should examine the patient with renal disease for the following intraoral changes:
  ○ Halitosis: breath may smell like ammonia.
  ○ Gingival bleeding from impaired platelet function.
  ○ Acute necrotizing ulcerative gingivitis (ANUG).
  ○ Graft vs host disease: lichen planus-like lesions of the buccal mucosae noted in patients who are rejecting a renal transplant.
  ○ Uremic stomatitis: nonspecific, aphthous-like lesions of the oral mucosa. These lesions tend to be painful and are often covered by a pseudomembrane or uremic frost (urea crystal deposition).
  ○ Lip and oral mucous membranes: patients with renal transplants have increased incidence of squamous cell carcinoma of the lip, leukoplakia, and oral mucosal dysplasia.
  ○ Parotid inflammation and enlargement.

DENTAL MANAGEMENT

- The patient's physician should be consulted to ascertain the patient's systemic health pertaining to:
  ○ Hypertension
  ○ Anemia
  ○ Bleeding abnormalities (determination of bleeding times and platelet count prior to elective surgery is necessary)
  ○ The need for preoperative antibiotic prophylaxis to prevent:
    ■ Vascular access infections in either an indwelling catheter or AV fistula for hemodialysis

- Graft anastomosis endarteritis in renal transplantation patients
  - The need for corticosteroid augmentation therapy for renal transplant patients.
  - The infectious disease status for HIV and hepatitis C if the renal transplantation was performed prior to 1985 and 1987, respectively.
  - Referral to the patient's physician is necessary if undiagnosed renal disease is suspected or if the patient with a known renal disorder presents with signs of uncontrolled renal disease.
- The best time to provide dental care is the day after dialysis. Try to avoid dental treatment immediately after hemodialysis due to potential prolonged bleeding tendencies from the residual effect of heparin used during hemodialysis.
- Blood pressure must not be taken on the arm of the renal transplant patient who has an AV fistula. The resultant increase in intravenous pressure may cause the fistula to rupture.
- Attention must be paid to prescription of medications that might build up in the bloodstream due to impaired excretion such as narcotic analgesics (see Appendix A, Table A-2, "Drug Therapy in Chronic Renal Disease").
- Avoidance of nephrotoxic medications such as streptomycin, neomycin, and gentamicin is mandatory. Oral potassium-containing penicillins may be satisfactory for prophylactic use but should be used with caution for extended courses because they may lead to high levels of potassium that can cause cardiac dysrhythmias. The aminoglycosides, tetracyclines, and cephalosporins should usually be avoided owing to their nephrotoxicity; they can cause marked elevation of BUN. Salicylate and NSAID medications should also be avoided since they can be nephrotoxic and result in bleeding and fluid retention (see Appendix A, Table A-2, "Drug Therapy in Chronic Renal Disease").

- As a general guide, a 50% drop in creatinine clearance theoretically represents a twofold increase in the elimination half-life of a drug removed from the body solely via renal excretion.
- Consider the need for antibiotic prophylaxis to prevent postoperative infections, especially in renal transplant patients with immunosuppression secondary to antirejection and corticosteroid drugs. The need for and selection of prophylactic antibiotics in patients with ESRD requires careful consideration and should be done in consultation with the patient's physician. Antibiotic drug levels may be affected by altered excretion through the kidneys or the dialysis process, requiring dosage adjustments to avoid adverse effect. Vancomycin (typically 1 gram administered IV over the last hour of dialysis) can be given to the patient and will remain effective until their next dialysis appointment.
- Supplemental corticosteroid therapy (e.g., prednisone) may be necessary for patients on an immunosuppressive regimen following renal transplantation (see Appendix A, Box A-4, "Dental Management of Patients at Risk for Acute Adrenal Insufficiency").
- Treatment of mucous membrane ulceration is dependant on the cause. Discontinuance or adjusting the dose of an offending medication (such as cyclophosphamide in the transplant patient), if identified, will usually resolve the ulcerative stomatitis. If the lesions are not found to be of infectious origin (i.e., bacterial, viral, or fungal), a burst of systemic corticosteroids may be appropriate. Topical anesthetics such as 2% viscous lidocaine or 0.5% dyclonine hydrochloride may be applied prior to meals to allow the patient to eat more comfortably. Sucralfate suspension may be used between meals as a means of covering the ulceration(s), thereby providing relief from pain and irritation.
- Consider hospitalization for patients with severe infection or those requiring significant surgical dental procedures.
- Patients can be instructed to contact the National Kidney Foundation for useful patient information at (202) 244-7900.

SUGGESTED REFERENCES

De Rossi SS, Glick M. Dental considerations for the patient with renal disease. *J Am Dent Assoc* 1996;127(2):211–219.

Kerr AR. Update on renal disease for the dental practitioner. *Oral Surg Oral Med Oral Pathol Oral Radiol Endod* 2001;92(1):9–16.

Naylor GD, Hall EH, Terezhalmy GT. The patient with chronic renal failure who is undergoing dialysis or renal transplantation: another consideration for antimicrobial prophylaxis. *Oral Surg Oral Med Oral Pathol* 1989;65:116–121.

Sampson E, Meister Jr F. Dental complications in the end-stages of renal disease. *Gen Dent* 1984;32:297–299.

Sonis ST, Fazio RC, Fang L. Chronic renal failure, dialysis and transplantation, in *Principles and Practice of Oral Medicine*, ed 2. Philadelphia, WB Saunders, 1994, pp 293–304.

AUTHOR: **MICHAEL A. SIEGEL, DDS, MS**

SYNONYM(S)

None

ICD-9CM/CPT CODE(S)

714.0 Rheumatoid arthritis—complete

OVERVIEW

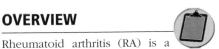

Rheumatoid arthritis (RA) is a chronic, systemic, inflammatory disease of unknown etiology characterized by a predilection for joint involvement. The disease involves cartilaginous destruction, bony erosions, and joint deformation. Extraarticular manifestations of RA include rheumatoid nodules, arteritis, neuropathy, pericarditis, scleritis, and splenomegaly.

EPIDEMIOLOGY & DEMOGRAPHICS

INCIDENCE/PREVALENCE IN USA: Prevalence is approximately 0.3–1.5%.
PREDOMINANT AGE: Age of onset is usually between 25 and 50 years of age.
PREDOMINANT SEX: Female > male (approximately 3:1).
GENETICS: Seropositive RA exhibits a well-defined familial predisposition. The concordance rate for RA averages approximately 15–20% for monozygotic twins and approximately 5% for dizygotic twins. Multiple gene loci are believed to be responsible for susceptibility to the disease, but most of these have not been identified yet. HLA-DR4 is found in 70% of Caucasian seropositive patients compared to 25% of controls. Increased relative risk is four to five times greater for DR4-positive persons, although a minority are affected. African-Americans tend not to exhibit this predilection. However, genetic factors vs their interaction with environmental facilitators is uncertain.

ETIOLOGY & PATHOGENESIS

- The specific etiology of RA remains unknown; however, it appears to require the complex interaction of genetic and environmental factors with the immune system and ultimately the synovial tissues throughout the body.
- In addition to genetics, proposed triggers have included bacteria (e.g., *Mycobacteria, Streptococcus, mycoplasma, Escherichia coli, Helicobacter pylori*), viruses (e.g., rubella, Epstein-Barr virus, parvovirus), superantigens, and others.
  - Rheumatic fever, reactive arthritis (Reiter's syndrome), and, more recently, Lyme arthritis are examples of arthritic syndromes where infectious triggers have clearly been demonstrated.
- Both the cellular and humoral immune systems appear to play a role in initiation and perpetuation of RA to some degree.

- T cells, particularly of the activated Th1 type, appear to predominate in synovial tissues and are presumably activated by some yet unknown antigen presented by macrophages.
  - B cells, or synoviocytes in the context of DR, secrete cytokines that drive further synovial proliferation.
  - Macrophage-derived cytokines, particularly interleukin-1 (IL-1) and TNF-α, play central roles in this ongoing inflammatory process.
- The synovial tissues are the primary target of the autoimmune inflammatory process that is RA. The pathologic findings in the joint include chronic synovitis with pannus formation. The synovitis results in the destruction of cartilage and bone and the stretching or rupture of tendons and ligaments. Joint deformities and disability result from the erosion and destruction of synovial membranes and articular surfaces.
  - In the acute phase, effusion and other manifestations of inflammation are common.
  - In the late stage, organization may result in fibrous ankylosis; true bony ankylosis is rare.
  - In both acute and chronic phases, inflammation of soft tissues around the joints may be prominent and is a significant factor in joint damage.
- Rheumatoid nodules can occur subcutaneously at sites of chronic irritation. Histologically, this is a granuloma with a central zone of fibrinoid necrosis, a surrounding palisade of radially arranged elongated connective tissue cells, and a periphery of chronic granulation tissue.
- Vasculitis can be found in skin, nerves, and visceral organs in severe cases of RA.

CLINICAL PRESENTATION / PHYSICAL FINDINGS

- Usually the disease starts in the small joints of the hands and the toes, followed by the larger joints including the wrists, knees, elbows, ankles, hips, and shoulders. Later, the temporomandibular, cricoarytenoid, and sterno-clavicular joints can be affected. The cervical spine at C1–C2 articulation follows.
- RA patients are at an increased risk of osteoporosis. The hands are a major site of involvement, as well as the feet and wrists. Involvement of large joints is common.
- The triad of immune neutropenia associated with seropositive nodular RA and splenomegaly is classified as Felty's syndrome.

SIGNS AND SYMPTOMS

- Constitutional: generalized pain, fatigue, anorexia, weight loss.
- Joint involvement: characteristically symmetric joint swelling with associ-

ated stiffness, warmth, tenderness (aggravated by movement), and pain; joint held in flexion; joint stiffness is more prominent in the morning and tends to subside during the day.
  - Hand and wrist: proximal interphalangeal and metacarpophalangeal.
  - Elbow: flexion contractures, nodules, bursitis.
  - Shoulder: rotator cuff.
  - Hip: groin discomfort.
  - Knee: popliteal cysts.
  - Cervical spine: subluxation, compression with possible spinal cord damage.
  - Ankle and foot: tenderness, swelling.
  - Temporomandibular joint (TMJ): affected approximately 75% of the time in RA; signs and symptoms mimic those of other joints.
- Extraarticular manifestations:
  - Dermatologic: rheumatoid (subcutaneous) nodules most commonly situated over bony prominences but also observed in the bursas and tendon sheaths; noted in 25% of RA patients.
  - Eye: episcleritis and scleromalacia may occur; xerophthalmia and keratoconjunctivitis sicca occur in approximately 25% of patients with RA and can be associated with Sjogren's syndrome.
  - Cardiovascular: usually asymptomatic but may develop carditis or pericarditis; rheumatoid vasculitis affects skin and visceral organs.
  - Pulmonary: pleuritis, intrapulmonary nodules, interstitial fibrosis.
  - Neurologic: peripheral neuropathy, entrapment neuropathies (particularly entrapment of the median nerve at the carpal tunnel of the wrist).
  - Hematologic: anemia, thrombocytosis.
  - Musculoskeletal: skeletal muscle weakness, osteoporosis.
- After months or years, deformities may occur; the most common are ulnar deviation of the fingers, boutonniere deformity (hyperextension of the distal interphalangeal joint with flexion of the proximal interphalangeal joint), "swan-neck" deformity (flexion of the distal interphalangeal with extension of the proximal interphalangeal joint), and valgus deformity of the knee.

DIAGNOSIS

LABORATORY

No specific laboratory tests are diagnostic for RA.

- Complete blood count (CBC): indicates the presence of a normocytic and normochromic anemia in approximately 80% of patients with RA. Thrombocytosis may be present.
- Erythrocyte sedimentation rate (ESR) is elevated in approximately 90% of patients with RA. This test usually is not performed in the acute setting.

- Serum rheumatoid factor (RF): positive (> 1:80) in approximately 70–80% of patients with RA.
- Antinuclear antibodies (ANA): positive in approximately 30% of patients with RA.
- Synovial fluid analysis: usually reveals a WBC count of 2,000 to 50,000/mm³ with no crystals or bacteria.
- C-reactive protein (CRP): when elevated, correlates with the development of erosive disease.

IMAGING
- Conventional radiography:
  - Joints: typical findings occur later in the disease course and include bony erosions, cysts, osteopenia, joint space swelling, calcifications, narrowed joint space, deformities, separations, and fractures.
  - Cervical spine: RA can affect the cervical spine with inflammation and destruction of cartilage, bone, and ligaments. This most commonly occurs in the upper cervical spine.
- CT and/or MRI:
  - Can further define the pathology of joints and cervical spine seen with conventional radiography; MRI may be necessary to demonstrate cord compression.

SPECIAL DIAGNOSTIC CRITERIA
- American College of Rheumatology criteria for the diagnosis of RA (five of the seven criteria must be present; criteria numbers 1 through 4 must be continuous with > 6 weeks' duration):
  1. Morning stiffness > 1 hour's duration
  2. Arthritis of at least three joint groups with soft tissue swelling or fluid
  3. Swelling involving at least one of the following joint groups: proximal interphalangeal, metacarpophalangeal, or wrists
  4. Symmetrical joint swelling
  5. Subcutaneous nodules
  6. Positive rheumatoid factor test
  7. Radiographic changes consistent with RA
- Functional classification of RA: grading of functional ability as measured by restriction of normal activities [i.e., activities of daily living (ADL)] due to RA:
  - Class I: Complete function; able to perform usual duties without handicap.
  - Class II: Moderate restriction; adequate function for normal activities, despite presence of pain or limited range of motion in one or more joints.
  - Class III: Marked restriction; inability to perform most of the patient's usual occupation or self-care; some assistance required.
  - Class IV: Incapacitation or confinement to a bed or wheelchair; largely or wholly incapacitated and dependent on assistance.

MEDICAL MANAGEMENT & TREATMENT

OVERVIEW
- Early recognition and diagnosis and timely introduction of therapy is the primary goal for patients with RA. Once a diagnosis has been made, key elements in the management and treatment of RA include:
  - Ongoing evaluation and control of disease activity, extent of synovitis, and structural damage
  - Minimizing pain, stiffness, inflammation, and complications
  - Improving functional status and quality of life

NONPHARMACOLOGIC
- Early intervention before joint damage presents itself.
- Exercise and mobility need emphasis; avoid joint stress.
- Cooperative efforts by professional medical staff.
- Patient education.
- Appropriate diet and avoid excessive body weight.

PHARMACOLOGIC
- Goal is to place disease in remission and maintain this state by continuing therapy.
- Initial drug therapy:
  - Aspirin or other NSAIDs (e.g., ibuprofen, naproxen, diclofenac):
    - Relieve pain and inflammation but do not modify disease progression.
    - No one drug has been found to be consistently superior to others; individual responses may vary.
    - Increased risk of upper gastrointestinal ulceration, hepatotoxicity, and nephrotoxicity.
  - COX-2 inhibitors [celecoxib (Celebrex)]:
    - COX-2 inhibitors compared to nonspecific NSAIDs have a decreased risk of upper gastrointestinal side effects and nephrotoxicity and an increased risk of potentially fatal cardiovascular events.
  - Corticosteroids (e.g., prednisone 5 to 15 mg per day):
    - Used in severe disease or to minimize disease activity while awaiting disease-modifying antirheumatic drugs (DMARDs) to act, decrease disease activity for a short period of time, or control active disease when NSAIDs/DMARDs have failed.
    - Generally to be used only for short periods. Long-term adverse effects include hyperglycemia, edema, osteonecrosis, myopathy, peptic ulcer disease, hypokalemia, osteoporosis, psychosis, immunosuppression, and increased risk of infections.
  - DMARDs (Table I-20) are given to control the disease process and should be started early since irreversible damage occurs within 1 to 2 years of diagnosis. Early intervention (< 3 months after diagnosis) improves most markers and outcome measures at 1 to 5 years compared with patients in whom treatment was delayed.

SURGICAL
Possible surgery (e.g., arthroplasty, synovectomy, prosthetic joint replacement) for severe mechanical symptoms (need to consider the long-term outcomes, risk/benefits, and cumulative effects of medical therapies when making surgical decisions with the RA patient).

COMPLICATIONS

- Joint degeneration and deformity that can lead to disability.
- Toxic effects of drug therapy (see Table I-20) and upper gastrointestinal ulceration and bleeding related to long-term use of aspirin or NSAIDs.
- Intracardiac rheumatoid nodules causing valvular and/or conduction abnormalities.
- Pleural, subpleural disease; interstitial fibrosis.
- Mononeuritis multiplex, median nerve entrapment.
- Systemic amyloidosis and vasculitis, which can involve vessels of all sizes including the aorta.
- Sjogren's syndrome, scleral rheumatoid nodules.
- Patients with Felty's syndrome are prone to serious bacterial infections that result in higher rates of morbidity and mortality than for other patients with RA.

PROGNOSIS

- Most patients with RA have progressive disease for life; however, approximately 15–20% of patients have intermittent disease with periods of exacerbations and relatively good prognosis.
- Approximately 50% of patients will be disabled or unable to work within 10 years of diagnosis.
- Overall, life expectancy is reduced by a mean of 3 to 7 years. The fatalities are usually due to the complications of RA.
- Factors correlated with increased morbidity include degree of functional state, severity of disease, concurrent disorders, tobacco smoking, advanced age, corticosteroid use, and high RF and ESR.
- Complete remission of RA is defined as the absence of:
  - Symptoms of active inflammatory joint pain (in contrast to mechanical joint pain)

TABLE I-20 Selected Disease-Modifying Antirheumatic Drugs

Type Generic (Trade) Name	Recommended Dosages	Toxic Effects
Gold Compounds		
Gold sodium thiomalate (Myochrysine)	IM: 10 mg followed by 25 mg 1 week later, then 25–50 mg weekly until there is toxicity, major clinical improvement, or cumulative dose = 1 g. If effective, interval between doses is increased.	Pruritus, dermatitis (frequent, one-third of patients), stomatitis, nephrotoxicity, blood dyscrasias, "nitritoid" reaction: flushing, weakness, nausea, dizziness 30 min after injection.
Aurothioglucose (Solganal)	IM: 10 mg; 2nd and 3rd doses 25 mg; 4th and subsequent 50 mg. Interval between doses: 1 week; if improvement or no toxicity, decrease dose to 25 mg or increase interval between doses.	Dermatitis, stomatitis, nephrotoxicity, blood dyscrasias.
Auranofin (Ridaura)	Oral: 3 mg bid or 6 mg qd. May increase to 3 mg tid after 6 months.	Loose stools, diarrhea (up to 50%), dermatitis.
Antimalarial		
Hydroxychloroquine (Plaquenil)	Oral: 400–600 mg qd with meals, then 200–400 mg qd.	Retinopathy, dermatitis, muscle weakness, hypoactive DTRs, CNS toxicity.
Cystine-depleting Agents		
Penicillamine (Cuprimine, Depen)	Oral: 125–250 mg qd, then increasing (at monthly intervals) doses to max. 750–1000 mg by 125–250 mg.	Pruritus, rash/mouth ulcers, bone marrow depression proteinuria, hematuria, hypogeusia, myasthenia, myositis, GI distress, pulmonary toxicity, teratogenic.
Antimetabolites and Immunosuppressives		
Methotrexate (Rheumatrex)	Oral: 7.5–15 mg weekly.	Pulmonary toxicity, ulcerative stomatitis, leukopenia, thrombocytopenia, GI distress, malaise, fatigue, chills, fever, CNS acute neurologic syndrome, elevated LFTs/liver disease, lymphoma, infection.
Azathioprine (Imuran)	Oral: 50–100 mg qd, increase at 4-week intervals by 0.5 mg/kg/d up to 2.5 mg/kg/d.	Leukopenia, thrombocytopenia, GI, neoplastic if previous Rx with alkylating agents.
Cyclosporine (Sandimmune)	Oral 2.5–5 mg/kg/d.	Nephrotoxicity, tremor, hirsutism, hypertension, gingival hyperplasia.
Alkylating-agent Antineoplastics		
Cyclophosphamide (Cytoxan)	Oral: 50–100 mg daily up to 2.5 mg/kg/d.	Leukopenia, thrombocytopenia, hematuria, GI, alopecia, rash, bladder cancer, non-Hodgkin's lymphoma, infection.
Chlorambucil (Leukeran)	Oral: 0.1–0.2 mg/kg/d.	Bone marrow suppression, GI or CNS infection.
5-Aminosalicylic Acid Derivative		
Sulfasalazine (Azulfidine)	Oral: 500 mg daily, then increase up to 3 g daily.	GI, skin rash, pruritus, blood dyscrasias, oligospermia.
Immunomodulator: Pyrimidine Synthesis Inhibitor		
Leflunomide (Arava)	Loading dose: 100 mg/d for 3 days. Maintenance therapy: 20 mg/d; if not tolerated, 10 mg/d.	Hepatotoxicity, carcinogenesis, immunosuppression, anemia, blood dyscrasias.
Immunomodulator: Tumor Necrosis Factor Modulators		
Etanercept (Enbrel)	25 mg given twice weekly as a subcutaneous injection 72–96 hours apart.	Immunosuppression, infections.
Adalimumab (Humira)	40 mg SC every 2 weeks; may increase to 40 mg SC weekly in some patients not taking concomitant methotrexate.	Immunosuppression, infections.
Infliximab (Remicade)	3 mg/kg given as an IV infusion followed with additional similar doses at 2 and 6 weeks after the first infusion, then every 8 weeks thereafter.	Immunosuppression, infections, nausea, urticaria, headache.
Immunomodulator: Interleukin Receptor Antagonist		
Anakinra (Kineret)	100 mg SC qd.	Immunosuppression, infections, leukopenia.

Bid, twice a day; CNS, central nervous system; DTR, deep tendon reflex; GI, gastrointestinal; IM, intramuscular; IV, intravenous; qd, every day; SC, subcutaneously; tid, three times a day.
Adapted in part from Rakel RE (ed): *Textbook of Family Practice*, ed 6. Philadelphia, WB Saunders, 2002, p 966.

- Morning stiffness
- Fatigue
- Synovitis on joint examination
- Progression of radiographic damage on sequential x-ray films
- Elevation of ESR or CRP level

DENTAL SIGNIFICANCE

- Active inflammatory joint pain and/or disability places patient at risk for maintenance of acceptable oral hygiene.
- TMJ involvement, such as limited oral opening, could limit nutritional intake, mastication, and oral hygiene.
- Patient's impaired mobility and ability to walk, sit, or hold objects could hinder the deliverance of dental care.
- Juvenile rheumatoid arthritis may impact on mandibular growth resulting in micrognathia, apertognathia, and possibly joint ankylosis.
- Dental management may be complicated by neutropenia, thrombocytopenia of Felty's syndrome, as well as immunosuppressive effects of multidrug therapy.
- Attitudinal behavior may need to be addressed regarding benefits of oral hygiene and nutrition. The health-compromised status of the patient can have an undesirable impact on dental and oral care.

DENTAL MANAGEMENT

The general evaluation of the dental patient with RA should include determining:

- The functional ability of the patient, especially in regard to any impairment of their ability to perform oral hygiene tasks
- The presence of TMJ involvement/dysfunction secondary to RA
- The presence of systemic manifestations and/or complications of RA (e.g., Felty's or Sjogren's syndrome)

- The patient's current medications and dosage (evaluate the patient for any significant side effects or toxic reactions associated with these drugs)
- The patient's history of surgical treatment for RA, especially prosthetic joint replacement(s)

Specific management considerations for the dental patient with RA would include:

- Short appointments as indicated; ensure physical comfort:
  - Frequent position changes
  - Comfortable chair position
  - Physical supports as needed (pillows, towels, etc.)
- Drug considerations:
  - Aspirin and NSAIDs: impaired hemostasis may become clinically significant with higher doses of aspirin (> 2 grams) or NSAIDs. Bleeding time (BT) or closure time (CT) can be used to assess hemostasis prior to surgical dental procedures as indicated.
  - Gold compounds, penicillamine, antimalarials, immunosuppressives (methotrexate, azathioprine), immunomodulators, antineoplastics: obtain complete blood cell count with differential (including platelet count).
    - Consider the use of antibiotic prophylaxis to prevent postoperative wound infection if immunosuppression is present (see Appendix A, Box A-2, "Presurgical and Postsurgical Antibiotic Prophylaxis for Patients at Increased Risk for Postoperative Infections").
    - Treat stomatitis symptomatically if present.
  - Corticosteroids: assess the risk for adrenal suppression and insufficiency (see Appendix A, Box A-4, "Dental Management of Patients at Risk for Acute Adrenal Insufficiency"). Patients being treated with systemic corticosteroids may also have an increased risk of infection due to immunosuppression and may require periop-

erative prophylactic antibiotics (see Appendix A, Box A-2, "Presurgical and Postsurgical Antibiotic for Patients at Increased Risk for Postoperative Infections").

- Patients with prosthetic joints may require antibiotic prophylaxis prior to invasive dental treatment for the prevention of late prosthetic joint infection.
- The Class III- or IV-functioning RA patient may have significant difficulty cleaning their teeth. Cleaning aids such as floss holders, toothpicks, irrigating devices, and mechanical toothbrushes may be recommended. Manual toothbrushes can be modified by adding a custom-molded acrylic handle to improve the grip.
- For patients with TMJ pain/dysfunction:
  - Decrease jaw function
  - Soft, nonchallenging diet
  - Moist heat or ice to face/jaw
  - Occlusal appliance to decrease joint loading
  - Consider surgery for persistent pain or dysfunction

SUGGESTED REFERENCES

Guidelines for the management of rheumatoid arthritis: 2002 Update. *Arthritis Rheum* 2002;46(2):328–346.

Klippel JH (ed): *Primer on the Rheumatic Diseases*, ed 12. Atlanta, The Arthritis Foundation. 2001.

O'Dell JR. Rheumatoid arthritis, in Goldman L, Ansiello D (eds): *Cecil Textbook of Medicine*, ed 22. Philadelphia, WB Saunders, 2004, pp 1644–1654.

O'Dell JR. Therapeutic strategies for rheumatoid arthritis. *N Engl J Med* 2004;350(25): 2591–2602.

AUTHORS: **NORBERT J. BURZYNSKI, SR., DDS, MS; F. JOHN FIRRIOLO, DDS, PHD**

SYNONYM(S)

Boeck's sarcoid

ICD-9CM/CPT CODE(S)
135.0 Sarcoidosis—complete

OVERVIEW

Sarcoidosis is a chronic, multisystem, granulomatous disease characterized by histopathology revealing noncaseating granulomas.

EPIDEMIOLOGY & DEMOGRAPHICS

INCIDENCE/PREVALENCE IN USA: Age-adjusted annual incidence is 35.5 per 100,000 African-Americans and 10.9 per 100,000 Caucasians.
• Seen with greater incidence in the winter and early spring months.
PREDOMINANT AGE: Usually seen in patients from the second to fourth decade.
PREDOMINANT SEX: Female > male (approximately 2:1).
GENETICS:
• Familial and racial clustering of cases.
• Association with certain HLA genotypes (e.g., class I HLA-A1 and HLA-B8).

ETIOLOGY & PATHOGENESIS

The etiology of sarcoidosis remains unknown.
• Both genetics and environmental factors play a role; there are geographic, ethnic, and racial differences in the mode of presentation and the clinical manifestations of sarcoidosis.
• Several immunologic abnormalities seen in sarcoidosis suggest the development of a cell-mediated response to an unidentified antigen:
  ○ Intraalveolar and interstitial accumulation of CD4+ T cells.
  ○ Tumor necrosis factor (TNF) is released at high levels by activated alveolar macrophages, and the TNF level in the bronchoalveolar fluid is a marker of disease activity.
• Bacteria, viruses, and fungi have been investigated as playing a role but without confirmation.
  ○ Several possible microbes that have been suggested as the inciting agent for sarcoidosis include mycobacteria, *Propionibacterium acnes*, and *Rickettsia* species.

CLINICAL PRESENTATION / PHYSICAL FINDINGS

• Sarcoidosis has a variable presentation based on stage of the disease and degree of organ involvement.
  ○ Pulmonary symptoms include a dry, nonproductive cough, dyspnea, and chest discomfort, with 90% of patients demonstrating intrathoracic involvement on a chest radiograph (CXR).
  ○ Approximately one-third of patients may have constitutional symptoms, including fever, weight loss, malaise, and fatigue.
  ○ Ten to 20% of patients present with a syndrome of bilateral hilar adenopathy and erythema nodosum, a constellation of findings that is called Löfgren's syndrome; fever and/or arthralgias may also accompany this form of presentation.
  ○ Fifteen to 25% of patients have some form of ocular involvement including blurred vision, xerophthalmia, conjunctivitis, uveitis, and iritis.
  ○ Five to 10% of patients have significant cardiac involvement including conduction defects (e.g., first-, second-, or third-degree heart block or a bundle branch block), ventricular or supraventricular dysrhythmias, and heart failure.
  ○ Other clinical manifestations include arthralgias, neurologic symptoms including cranial nerve palsies, xerostomia, and parotid enlargement.
• As many as 30–60% of patients have no symptoms at the time of presentation; the disease is identified because of abnormalities on a CXR.

DIAGNOSIS

• CXR frequently reveals adenopathy of the hilar and paratracheal nodes. CXRs are staged using Scadding's classification:
  ○ Stage 0 = normal
  ○ Stage 1 = hilar adenopathy alone
  ○ Stage 2 = hilar adenopathy plus parenchymal infiltrates
  ○ Stage 3 = parenchymal infiltrates alone
  ○ Stage 4 = advanced pulmonary fibrosis with evidence of honeycombing, hilar retraction, bullae, cysts, and emphysema
• Angiotensin-converting enzyme (ACE) is elevated in approximately 60% of patients with the disease. This is not a good predictor of the course of the disease.
• Hypercalcemia or hypercalciuria may occur in approximately 10–15% of the patients.
• Elevated alkaline phosphatase level suggests liver involvement.
• Biopsy of accessible tissues suspected of sarcoid involvement (e.g., conjunctiva, skin, lymph nodes) for diagnostic confirmation; bronchoscopy for a bronchial biopsy may also be indicated.
• Gallium-67 scan will localize in areas of granulomatous inflammation, including the lacrimal and parotid glands, but has little correlation with clinical status.
• Electrocardiogram to evaluate for possible dysrhythmias.

MEDICAL MANAGEMENT & TREATMENT

• Corticosteroids are the mainstay of treatment in patients with symptoms.
  ○ For example, prednisone 40 mg qd for 8 to 12 weeks with gradual tapering of the dose to 10 mg qod over 8 to 12 months.
• Patients refractory to corticosteroids are usually treated with methotrexate.
• Hydroxychloroquine is used for cutaneous lesions.
• Alternative therapies include cyclosporin, azathioprine, infliximab, and pentoxifylline.

COMPLICATIONS

• Complications from corticosteroid usage are possible.
• Untreated ocular involvement could lead to blindness.
• Sudden death from cardiac dysrhythmia could occur but is rare.
• Cranial nerve palsies and hypothalamic/pituitary dysfunction may occur.

PROGNOSIS

The majority of patients have spontaneous remission within 2 years. Functional impairment occurs in only 15–20% of patients, and overall mortality is at 5% for those untreated, usually due to lung disease or right-sided heart failure.

DENTAL SIGNIFICANCE

• Sarcoidosis can be associated with parotid enlargement and/or cervical node lymphadenopathy.
  ○ Heerfordt's syndrome (or uveoparotid fever) is a form of acute sarcoidosis and consists of parotid enlargement, anterior uveitis, facial paralysis, and fever.
  ○ Consider sarcoidosis in differential diagnosis of a patient with parotid enlargement.
• Cutaneous manifestations of sarcoidosis [chronic violaceous indurated plaques (lupus pernio)] occur about 25% of the time and frequently affect the nose, ears, lips, and face.
• Intraoral soft tissue and intraosseous lesions associated with sarcoidosis have been infrequently reported.
• The dentist should be aware of xerostomia if the parotid is involved, as well as the implications of long-term steroid therapy causing immunosuppression and/or adrenal suppression.

DENTAL MANAGEMENT

- Ophthalmologic referral and examination is indicated in all patients with suspected sarcoidosis.
- Treatment of xerostomia if salivary glands are involved.
- For patients being treated with systemic corticosteroids, assess the risk for adrenal suppression and insufficiency (see Appendix A, Box A-4, "Dental Management of Patients at Risk for Acute Adrenal Insufficiency").

- Patients being treated with systemic corticosteroids may also have an increased risk of infection and may require perioperative prophylactic antibiotics (see Appendix A, Box A-2, "Presurgical and Postsurgical Antibiotic Prophylaxis for Patients at Increased Risk for Postoperative Infections").

SUGGESTED REFERENCES

Batal H, Chou LL, Cottrell DA. Sarcoidosis: medical and dental implications. *Oral Surgery Oral Med Oral Pathol Oral Radiol & Endod* 1999;88(4):386–390.

Emedicine: www.emedicine.com Sarcoidosis. See also "Sarcoidosis" in Section II, p 315.

Ferri FF. Sarcoidosis, in Ferri FF (ed): *Ferri's Clinical Advisor: Instant Diagnosis and Treatment.* Philadelphia, Elsevier Mosby, 2005, pp 730–731.

Thomas KW, Hunninghake GW. Sarcoidosis. *JAMA.* 2003;289(24):3300–3303.

AUTHOR: **THOMAS P. SOLLECITO, DMD**

SYNONYM(S)

Epilepsy

ICD-9CM/CPT CODE(S)

345.0 Generalized nonconvulsive disorders
345.1 Generalized convulsive epilepsy

OVERVIEW

- A disorder characterized by a sudden, uncontrolled paroxysmal disturbance of central nervous system (CNS) function secondary to aberrant cerebral cortical electrical activity that is characterized by varying combinations of impaired consciousness, abnormal motor function, and/or inappropriate behavior, sensory disturbances, and autonomic dysfunction.
- The term "epilepsy" is used to describe any disorder characterized by recurrent seizures.

EPIDEMIOLOGY & DEMOGRAPHICS

PARTIAL SEIZURES

INCIDENCE/PREVALENCE IN USA:
20 cases/100,000 persons through age 65 years, then rises sharply; 6.5 cases/1000 persons for all types of epilepsy.
PREDOMINANT SEX: Males are affected slightly more often than females.

GENERALIZED TONIC CLONIC SEIZURES

INCIDENCE/PREVALENCE IN USA:
50 to 70 cases per 100,000 persons/year, with highest rates during early childhood and persons over 65 years of age; same as partial seizures.
PREDOMINANT SEX: Same as partial seizures.
GENETICS: Predisposition exists for the idiopathic generalized epilepsies.

ABSENCE SEIZURES

INCIDENCE/PREVALENCE IN USA:
11 cases/100,000 persons from ages 1 through 10 years old, rare after age 14. Peak incidence at 6 to 7 years; accounts for 2–15% of the cases of childhood epilepsy.
PREDOMINANT AGE: 4 to 8 years.
GENETICS: Clear genetic predisposition.

ETIOLOGY & PATHOGENESIS

- The etiologies of recurrent seizures (epilepsy) are classified into two broad categories as being either symptomatic (secondary to some identifiable cause) or idiopathic (not attributable to any detectable cause).
- Symptomatic epilepsy etiologies include:
  - Congenital abnormalities and perinatal injuries: epilepsy may be the result of a microscopic scar in the brain as a result of childbirth or other congenital or developmental brain defects.
  - Metabolic disorders: include hypoglycemia, hypoparathyroidism, phenyl-

ketonuria, hypocalcemia, pyridoxine deficiency, and withdrawal symptoms such as those seen with chronic use of alcohol, hypnotics, or tranquilizers.
  - Head trauma: an important cause of seizures in general and the most common cause of seizures in young adults. More than 90% of seizures secondary to head trauma will arise within 2 years following the injury.
  - CNS neoplasms: tend to affect patients in middle and later life.
  - Vascular diseases and expanding vascular lesions: include intracranial or cerebral hemorrhage, cerebral infarcts, and cerebral hypoxia resulting from carotid sinus hypersensitivity or Adams-Stokes syndrome; represent the most common causes of seizures that arise in patients who are age 60 or older.
  - Infectious diseases: include bacterial meningitis, herpetic encephalitis, neurosyphilis, rabies, tetanus, and cysticercosis. In patients with AIDS, seizures may result secondary to cryptococcal meningitis, viral encephalitis, or toxoplasmosis of the central nervous system.
  - Degenerative diseases: (e.g., Alzheimer's disease) are causes of seizures in older adults.
- Idiopathic (or constitutional) epilepsy usually starts between the ages of 2 to 14 with no identifiable cause or other neurologic abnormality.

CLINICAL PRESENTATION / PHYSICAL FINDINGS

- Partial (focal, local) seizures originate from one cerebral hemisphere of the brain and affect the contralateral side of the body.
  - Simple partial seizures are typically characterized by specific, isolated, or multiple neurologic aberrations. Consciousness is not impaired during a simple partial seizure.
  - Complex partial seizures (i.e., psychomotor seizures, temporal lobe seizures) will demonstrate impaired consciousness preceding, accompanying, or following the same type of neurologic symptoms seen in simple partial seizures. The period of clinical symptoms and impaired consciousness will last 1 to 2 minutes in most instances, with mental confusion persisting for an additional 1 to 2 minutes after apparent resolution of the seizure.
- Generalized seizures involve the entire brain and affect the body bilaterally.
  - Tonic-clonic (previously referred to as grandmal) seizures are characterized by a sudden loss of consciousness followed by muscular rigidity wherein the patient will fall to the ground and respiration may be temporarily compromised. The tonic phase usually

lasts for less than 1 minute. Next, the patient enters the clonic phase which lasts for 2 to 3 minutes and is characterized by arrhythmic jerking contractions of the muscles of the extremities, trunk, and head. During the clonic phase, urinary and fecal incontinence may occur, as well as bite injuries to the tongue, lips, or buccal mucosa. Immediately after the resolution of the clonic phase, the patient will enter a postictal stage wherein they may regain consciousness, with possible complaints of headache, disorientation, confusion, nausea, drowsiness, and muscle soreness, or they may enter a deep sleep.
    - Tonic-clonic seizures occur in 90% of patients with a seizure disorder, with 60% of patients exhibiting this form of seizure exclusively.
  - Absence (previously referred to as petit mal) seizures are characterized by an alteration or impairment of consciousness with minimal motor or autonomic disturbances. Absence seizures demonstrate an abrupt onset and resolution and typically last 5 to 10 seconds with a maximum duration usually no longer than 30 seconds; the patient is almost always unaware that the seizure has occurred. Clinically, the patient will exhibit a sudden cessation of activity and stares blankly. If an absence seizure occurs during a conversation, the patient may miss a few words or may break off in midsentence for a few seconds. Rapid blinking of the eyelids (at 3 times per second), slight deviation of the eyes and head, or brief minor movements of the hands or lips may also accompany the seizure.
    - Absence seizures occur in 25% of patients with a seizure disorder, with only 4% of patients exhibiting this form of seizure exclusively.
  - Myoclonic seizures will consist of sudden, involuntary contractions of single or multiple muscle groups resulting in arrhythmic jerking movements (myoclonic jerks) without any loss or impairment of consciousness.
  - Atonic (akinetic, astatic, "drop attack") seizures are most frequently seen in children and are characterized by a brief, complete loss of muscle tone and consciousness. Typically, the child will fall to the ground; therefore, this type of seizure carries the risk of serious physical trauma, especially head injury.
- Patients with recurrent seizures (particularly tonic-clonic seizures) may experience a prodrome which precedes the actual seizure by hours or even days. Typical seizure prodromes are characterized by nonspecific changes such as mood or behavioral alterations, headaches, lethargy, or myoclonic jerking.

- Seizure prodromes are distinct from the aura that may precede a seizure by a few seconds or minutes and are actually early focal manifestations of the seizure itself. Typical auras can include a visceral rising sensation from the epigastrium to the throat, overwhelming feelings of familiarity (déjà vu), paresthesias, and olfactory, visual, auditory, or gustatory hallucinations.
- Approximately 7% of patients will report that their seizures occur following exposure to a specific stimulus (or trigger). Examples of seizure triggers include flickering lights or visual patterns, reading, monotonous sounds, music, or loud noise.

DIAGNOSIS

LABORATORY
- Serum tests: including glucose, sodium, potassium, calcium, phosphorus, magnesium, BUN, and ammonia.
- Anticonvulsant drug levels: inadequate level of anticonvulsant medication is the most common cause of recurrent seizures in children and many adults.
- Drug and toxic screens: including alcohol.
- Complete blood count: helpful in evaluating infection.
- Additional blood studies and lumbar puncture as indicated by history and physical examination.
- Electroencephalogram (EEG): the most valuable diagnostic tool for identifying seizure type and predicting the likelihood of recurrence; however, a negative EEG does not rule out a seizure disorder.

IMAGING
- MRI: the imaging modality of choice in the evaluation of a seizure disorder.

MEDICAL MANAGEMENT & TREATMENT

GENERAL MEASURES
- In patients with symptomatic seizures, treatment would consist of elimination or control of the underlying causative pathology whenever possible. This would include treatments such as the correction of metabolic imbalances, treatment of CNS infections, or surgical removal of neoplasms.

PHARMACOLOGIC
- In patients with idiopathic and/or recurrent seizures that cannot be corrected through other means, drug therapy is usually initiated with the goal of preventing further seizure activity. Figure I-4 shows the primary indications for drugs used in the treatment of seizures, while Table I-21 lists the adverse effects of some of the drugs most commonly used in the treatment of seizures.

SURGICAL
- Stereotactic surgery involving resection of epileptogenic brain tissue has been advocated for seizures that cannot be adequately controlled by traditional pharmacologic therapy (e.g., complex partial seizures of temporal lobe origin).

- Vagus nerve stimulator:
  - This implanted electronic pulse generating device was approved by the FDA for adjunctive treatment (in combination with antiseizure medications) of partial seizures in adults and adolescents older than 12 years (subsequent postmarketing data also suggest its effectiveness in generalized seizures, especially drop attacks).
  - As with dental patients with implanted cardiac pacemakers, patients with implanted vagus nerve stimulators do not require antibiotic prophylaxis to prevent metastatic infections associated with this device prior to bacteriemia-producing dental procedures.

COMPLICATIONS

- Patients may injure themselves during a generalized tonic-clonic seizure; maxillofacial or dental injuries, lacerations, shoulder dislocations, and even fractures may result.
- *Status epilepticus* is the term used to describe a seizure that lasts longer than 30 minutes or a series of seizures in rapid succession such that the patient does not regain consciousness between seizures.
  - Tonic-clonic status epilepticus is the most common and serious form of this condition and is considered to be a life-threatening emergency.

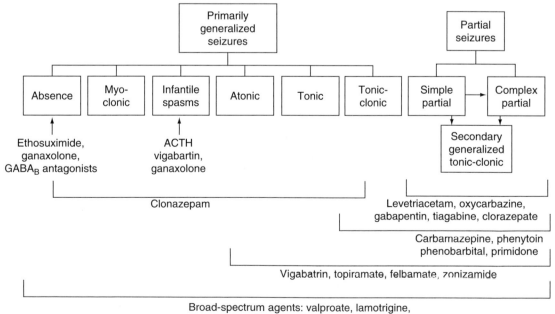

FIGURE I-4 Therapeutic spectra of anticonvulsant drugs. Anticonvulsant agents need to be matched to the convulsive disorder being treated. Phenytoin, phenobarbital, carbamazepine, oxycarbazine, vigabatrin, gabapentin, and tiagabine are not effective in but can aggravate absence and myoclonic seizures. Benzodiazepines and acetazolamide have broad spectra, but tolerance develops to their actions; so they cannot be used for maintenance therapy. (From Yagiela JA, Dowd FJ, Neidle EA. *Pharmacology and Therapeutics for Dentistry*, ed 5. St Louis, Mosby, 2004.)

- Patients with seizures secondary to developmental abnormalities or acquired brain injury may have impaired cognitive function and other neurologic defects.
- Patients often develop short-term memory loss that may progress over time.
- Patients with epilepsy are at risk of developing a variety of psychiatric problems including anxiety and depression.

PROGNOSIS

- The prognosis in patients with symptomatic seizures (epilepsy) is dependent on underlying causative pathology.
- For patients with an idiopathic seizure disorder:
  - Approximately 60–70% of all patients enter prolonged remission (> 5 years) with anticonvulsant drug therapy. About half of these patients eventually become seizure-free.
  - Approximately 30% of patients, usually with severe epilepsy starting in early childhood, continue to have seizures and never achieve remission.

DENTAL SIGNIFICANCE

- Consideration of dental treatment venue based on pretreatment evaluation and assessment of seizure control.
  - Modifications to dental treatment may be required depending on level of seizure control.
- Oral conditions associated with seizure medications include gingival hypertrophy and/or xerostomia (see Table I-21).

DENTAL MANAGEMENT

Determine:
- Etiology of seizures (e.g., history of head trauma, neoplasms, idiopathic)
- Current medication(s) and dose used to control seizures
- Type(s) of seizures (e.g., tonic-clonic, absence)
- Frequency of seizures under current medication and date of last seizure
- If patient has a known seizure prodrome and/or aura
- If patient has known factors that precipitate or trigger a seizure
- History of seizure-related injuries (injuries that occurred due to the patient's seizures, especially maxillofacial or dental injuries)

PHYSICAL AND DENTAL EXAMINATION

- Evaluate the patient for any adverse effects secondary to anticonvulsant medications:
  - Gingival hyperplasia: 40–50% of patients taking phenytoin for more than 3 months will exhibit some degree of gingival hyperplasia.
  - Blood dyscrasias (leukopenia and anemia): a complete blood count (CBC) with differential will identify clinically significant leukopenia that can result in an increased risk of infections, delayed wound healing, and/or anemia in patients taking phenytoin, carbamazepine, and valproic acid (valproate sodium).
  - Impaired hemostasis: in patients secondary to thrombocytopenia and inhibition of platelet aggregation in patients taking valproic acid:

- Valproic acid inhibits the secondary phase of platelet aggregation, which may be reflected in prolonged bleeding time and/or frank hemorrhaging.
- In addition, the leukopenic and thrombocytopenic effects of valproic acid may result in an increased incidence of microbial infection, delayed healing, and gingival bleeding. If leukopenia or thrombocytopenia occurs, dental work should be deferred whenever possible until blood counts have returned to normal. Patients should be instructed in proper oral hygiene, including caution in use of regular toothbrushes, dental floss, and toothpicks.
- Surgical considerations: because of the thrombocytopenic effects of valproic acid as well as its inhibition of the secondary phase of platelet aggregation and production of abnormal coagulation parameters (e.g., low fibrinogen), monitoring of platelet counts and coagulation tests (bleeding time or closure time) are recommended in patients prior to scheduled surgery.
  - CNS effects: ataxia, dizziness, confusion, sedation, headaches, behavioral changes.
  - Gastrointestinal effects: nausea, vomiting, anorexia.
  - Allergic signs: carbamazepine, ethosuximide, and phenytoin can cause intraoral lupus erythematosus-like intraoral lesions as well as skin rashes.
  - Evaluate the patient for any signs of previous seizure-related perioral or intraoral injury such as fractured teeth

TABLE I-21 Drugs Used in the Treatment of Seizure Disorders

Drug	Pharmacologic Category	Adverse Effects
Carbamazepine (Epitol, Tegretol)	Tricyclic	Sedation, dizziness, fatigue, confusion, ataxia, nausea, blood dyscrasias, hepatotoxicity
Clonazepam (Klonopin)	Benzodiazepine	Tachycardia, drowsiness, fatigue, anxiety, ataxia, headache, dizziness, blurred vision, xerostomia
Ethosuximide (Zarontin)	Succinimide	Ataxia, sedation, dizziness, hallucinations, behavioral changes, headache, Stevens-Johnson syndrome, systemic lupus erythematosus, nausea, anorexia
Gabapentin (Neurontin)	Neurotransmitter	Somnolence, dizziness, ataxia, fatigue, nystagmus
Phenobarbital (Barbita, Luminal, Solfoton)	Barbiturate	Dizziness, lightheadedness, sedation, ataxia, impaired judgement, skin rashes
Phenytoin (Dilantin)	Hydantoin	Dizziness, drowsiness, confusion, ataxia, nausea, gingival hyperplasia, megaloblastic anemia, leukopenia
Primidone (Mysoline)	Barbiturate derivative	Drowsiness, vertigo, ataxia, behavioral changes, headache, nausea
Topiramate (Topamax)	Sulfamate-substituted monosaccharide	Acidosis (may decrease serum bicarbonate concentrations), increased risk of kidney stones, hyperthermia, paresthesias, sedation, confusion, psychomotor slowing, mood disturbances
Valproic acid, sodium valproate (Depakene, Depakote)	Carboxylic acid	Anorexia, diarrhea, nausea, drowsiness, ataxia, irritability, confusion, headache, hepatotoxicity leukopenia, thrombocytopenia resulting in prolonged bleeding time

See related topics in Section IV, Drugs for more information.

or soft tissue scars due to lacerations or trauma.

DENTAL MANAGEMENT

- Avoid any factors known to precipitate (trigger) the patient's seizure (e.g., stress).
- Patients with poorly controlled seizures (i.e., more frequent than one per month) or those with stress-triggered seizures may require additional anticonvulsant or sedative medications (e.g., benzodiazepines) prior to treatment as determined after consultation with the patient's physician. (Nitrous oxide sedation has been known to induce seizures in some patients and should be used with caution.)
- Do not treat patients who are experiencing any of their known prodromal seizure symptoms.
- Minimize the risk of aspiration and injury if a seizure occurs during dental treatment:
  - Rubber mouth props may prove useful in preventing aspiration of foreign objects and/or injury to the patient if a seizure occurs during dental treatment.
  - A rubber dam is preferable to multiple intraoral cotton rolls for isolation.
  - Any instruments placed in the mouth (e.g., rubber dam clamps, rubber mouth props) should all have dental floss leads attached to prevent or assist in recovery if aspirated.

TREATMENT PLANNING CONSIDERATIONS

- Management of gingival hyperplasia (if present):
  - Surgical excision of hyperplastic gingival tissue as indicated.
  - Maintain an optimum level of plaque control and oral hygiene in the patient; reinforce a meticulous home oral hygiene program as well as an effective periodontal recall maintenance schedule.
- Fixed restorations are preferred to removable prostheses where feasible. Loose and defective restorations, poorly retained crowns and bridges, partial dentures (especially unilateral, "Nesbitt-type" partial dentures), as well as grossly carious or extremely mobile teeth all present a significant aspiration risk during a seizure.
- Laboratory-processed, metal-reinforced temporary crowns and bridges are preferred over all-acrylic, office-cured temporary prostheses.
- Metal major connectors and metal denture bases are considered mandatory in the fabrication of removable prostheses for patients with a seizure disorder.

SUGGESTED REFERENCES

Blume WT. Diagnosis and management of epilepsy. *CMAJ* 2003;168:441.

Chang BS, et al. Mechanisms of disease: epilepsy. *N Engl J Med* 2003;349:1257.

Croom JE. Seizures, febrile. Seizure disorder, partial. Seizure disorder, generalized tonic-clonic. Seizure disorder, absence, in Ferri FF (ed): *Ferri's Clinical Advisor: Instant Diagnosis and Treatment.* Philadelphia, Elsevier Mosby, 2005, pp 741–744.

Emedicine: www.emedicine.com

Nguyen DK, et al. Recent advances in the treatment of epilepsy. *Arch Neuro* 2003;60:929.

Stoopler ET, et al. Seizure disorders: update of medical and dental considerations. *Gen Dent* 2003;51:361.

AUTHORS: **ERIC T. STOOPLER, DMD; F. JOHN FIRRIOLO, DDS, PHD**

SYNONYM(S)

Obstructive sleep apnea (OSA)
Obstructive sleep apnea syndrome (OSAS)
Apneic sleep
Central sleep apnea (CSA)
Sleep-disordered breathing (SDB)

ICD-9CM/CPT CODE(S)

ICD-9CM
780.51 Insomnia with sleep apnea
780.53 Hypersomnia with sleep apnea
786.09 Snoring
780.57 Other and unspecified sleep apnea
CPT
E0601 Continuous Airway Pressure (CPAP) device
42145 Uvulopalatopharyngoplasty

OVERVIEW

Obstructive sleep apnea (OSA) is characterized by recurrent episodes of upper airway collapse and obstruction during sleep. These episodes of obstruction are associated with recurrent oxygen desaturations and arousals from sleep. OSA associated with excessive daytime sleepiness (EDS) is commonly called OSA syndrome. Despite being a common disease, OSA is underrecognized by most primary care physicians in the U.S.; an estimated 80% of Americans with OSA are not diagnosed. There are three general classifications of sleep apnea:

- Obstructive apnea is the cessation of airflow with persistent respiratory effort.
- Central apnea is the cessation of airflow with no respiratory effort.
- Mixed apnea is an apnea that begins as a central apnea and ends as an obstructive apnea.

EPIDEMIOLOGY & DEMOGRAPHICS

INCIDENCE/PREVALENCE IN USA: It is estimated that about 9–24% of all U.S. men and 4% of women between ages 30 and 60 suffer from sleep apnea.
PREDOMINANT AGE: As people age, the potential for sleep apnea increases. It must be stressed, however, that children also can suffer from obstructive sleep apnea, mostly due to enlarged tonsils or adenoids.
PREDOMINANT SEX: In an extensive study done by Madani, the ratio of men vs women was 9:1. The ratio in previously reported literature was 4:1.
GENETICS: Although no exact genetic factor has been identified as the cause for obstructive sleep apnea, clearly patients who suffer from congenital forms of dentofacial deformity (including retrognathism or micrognathism) are at greater risk of having this problem. Other inherited features also play important roles in genetic transfer of apnea, including the

size of various structures in the airway as well as the patient's body weight.
- Mortality: it is estimated that 38,000 people die each year in the U.S. as a consequence of complications caused by obstructive sleep apnea.

ETIOLOGY & PATHOGENESIS

Turbulent airflow and subsequent progressive vibratory trauma to the soft tissues of the upper airway are important factors contributing to snoring as well as to sleep apnea. Anatomic obstruction leads to greater negative inspiratory pressure, propagating further airway collapse and partial airway obstruction (hypopnea) or complete obstruction (apnea). Obstructive sleep apnea occurs in at least eight different sites in the head and neck region:

- Tongue (collapse of tongue in the pharynx)
- Jaws and chin position (retrognathism and micrognathism)
- Soft palate and uvula (enlargement and elongation)
- Nasal (deviated septum, enlarged nasal turbinates)
- Tonsils (obstructive tonsils, kissing tonsils) and enlarged adenoids
- Narrowing lateral pharyngeal walls (pharyngeal muscle hypertrophy); this is an independent predictor of OSA in men but not in women
- Position of hyoid
- Position of epiglottis

Besides the upper airway anatomy, there are two other factors involved in the development of obstructive sleep apnea: decreased dilating forces of the pharyngeal dilators and negative inspiratory pressure generated by the diaphragm.

CLINICAL PRESENTATION / PHYSICAL FINDINGS

Symptoms generally begin insidiously and are often present for years before the patient is referred for evaluation. Most common signs and symptoms are:

- Snoring, usually loud, habitual, and bothersome to others.
- Witnessed apneas, which often interrupt the snoring and end with a snort.
- Gasping and choking sensations that arouse the patient from sleep.
- Restless sleep, with patients often experiencing frequent arousals and tossing or turning during the night.
- Not feeling refreshed upon awakening.
- Morning headache, dry or sore throat.
- Personality changes, problems with memory or concentration.
- Falling asleep easily during the day (usually begins during quiet activities such as reading or watching television).
- As the severity of daytime sleepiness worsens, patients begin to feel sleepy during activities that generally require alertness such as driving or being at school or at work.

- Apnea is most frequently assessed by using the Epworth sleepiness scale (ESS). This questionnaire is used to help determine how frequently the patient is likely to doze off in eight frequently encountered situations. An ESS score greater than 10 is generally considered an indication that patient may be suffering from sleep apnea.
- It is well established that overweight patients with a neck size of greater than 16.5 inches and body mass index (BMI) of greater than 30 have far greater potential for having obstructive sleep apnea.

DIAGNOSIS

- The initial diagnosis could be made by careful analysis of the patient's medical and social history as well as assessment of the total body mass index (BMI). The likelihood of sleep apnea could be predicted based on Epworth scale as described previously.
- The most accurate diagnostic tool to evaluate an individual suspected of having obstructive sleep apnea is polysomnography (PSG), which is an overnight sleep study. During polysomnography, multiple body functions are monitored:
  - Sleep stages are recorded via an electroencephalogram (EEG), electrooculogram (EOG), and chin electromyogram (EMG).
  - Heart rhythm is monitored with electrocardiogram (ECG).
  - Leg movements are recorded via an anterior tibialis electromyogram.
  - Breathing is monitored, including airflow at nose and mouth, effort, and oxygen saturation.
  - The breathing pattern is analyzed for the presence of apneas and hypopneas.
  - The definition of a hypopnea varies significantly between sleep centers. However, a consensus statement defined a hypopnea as a 30% or more reduction in flow associated with a 4% drop in oxygen saturation.
  - Respiratory event-related arousal is an event in which patients have a series of breaths with increasingly negative pleural pressure that terminates with an arousal.
- The apnea hypopnea index (AHI) is derived from the total number of apneas and hypopneas divided by the total sleep time. It is considered abnormal if there are more than 5 episodes per hour of sleep.
  - Mild apnea: 5 to 15 episodes per hour
  - Moderate apnea: 15 to 30 episodes per hour
  - Severe apnea: more than 30 episodes per hour

MEDICAL MANAGEMENT & TREATMENT

- The treatment of sleep apnea partly depends on the severity of the problem. People with mild apnea have a wider variety of options, while people with moderate to severe apnea should be treated with nasal continuous positive airway pressure (CPAP). CPAP is the most effective treatment for OSA, and it has become the standard of care. CPAP works by gently blowing pressurized room air into the nose via a specially designed nasal mask or nasal pillows at a pressure high enough to keep the airway open. This pressurized air acts as a "splint." The air pressure is set according to the patient's needs at a level that eliminates the apneas and hypopneas that cause awakenings and sleep fragmentation. Frequent complaints from patients using CPAP for the treatment of sleep apnea include discomfort and/or skin irritation caused by the mask or nasal pillows, difficulty sleeping while wearing the mask or nasal pillows, and nasal congestion and/or drying ("stuffy" or "blocked-up" nasal passages). Unfortunately, long-term compliance in the use of CPAP is poor, and a reported 60% of patients do not continuously use this device.
- Conservative measures include weight loss, avoidance of alcohol for 4 to 6 hours prior to bedtime, and sleeping on one's side rather than on the stomach or back.
- Long-term studies by Madani suggest that laser-assisted uvulopalatopharyngoplasty (LA-UPPP) is a successful surgical treatment for patients who suffer from mild sleep apnea as well as snoring. In the same study, it was observed that this procedure could reduce the OSA by up to 50% and that in more severe cases CPAP must be used in addition to the surgery.
- Orthognathic surgery to reconstruct the micrognathism or other dentofacial deformities has been reported to produce similar results as CPAP in certain cases and is an excellent option available to the patient by the dental team. Finally, for extremely obese individuals when all other options have failed, tracheostomy can provide a definitive correction of apnea.

COMPLICATIONS

- Mood and anxiety disorders may develop from untreated obstructive sleep apnea and other sleep-related disturbances.
- Current medical literature supports the theory that these brain-based mental status changes are risk factors for morbidity and mortality from a host of medical conditions, including an increased risk of heart attack and stoke.

PROGNOSIS

The prognosis depends on the severity of the sleep apnea and, more importantly, the patient's compliance. Surgical procedures such as LA-UPPP are most effective in mild cases, but CPAP, if properly used, is effective in all cases of OSA.

DENTAL SIGNIFICANCE

- Evaluate the patient's oral cavity and recognize any facial deformities. Inquire about the patient's history of snoring or gasping for air while asleep and recommend additional care by a sleep specialist or a surgeon specializing in these conditions.
- Pediatric dentists should also check for an obstructive tonsil and refer the patients for evaluation or surgery if patients are reporting daytime sleepiness or having difficulty breathing while asleep.

DENTAL MANAGEMENT

- Oral appliances have been used as an adjunct for treatment of snoring and obstructive sleep apnea. They act by moving the tongue or mandible forward, enlarging the posterior airspace. Oral appliances have been shown to decrease the AHI in most patients. However, they are most effective for patients with AHI of less than 40 episodes per hour. Long-term compliance with oral appliances is poor, and alternative surgical options must be discussed with patients. Potential side effects on the temporomandibular joint (TMJ) such as pain and TM derangements also must be assessed and treated.
- Surgical treatments such as laser-assisted uvulopalatopharyngoplasty (LA-UPPP) as well as palatal and/or nasal radioablations, performed by trained oral and maxillofacial surgeons and otolaryngologists, could help reduce the signs and symptoms of obstructive sleep apnea.

SUGGESTED REFERENCES

Center For Corrective Jaw Surgery: www. snorenet.com

Isono S, Remmers JE, Tanaka A, Sho Y, Sato J, Nishino T. Anatomy of pharynx in patients with obstructive sleep apnea and in normal subjects. *J Appl Physiol* 1997;82:1319–1326.

Madani M. Complications of laser-assisted uvulopalatopharyngoplasty (LA-UPPP) and radiofrequency treatment of snoring and chronic nasal congestion: a 10-year review of 5600 patients. *J Oral Maxillofac Surg* 2004;62:1351–1362.

Madani M. Surgical treatment of snoring and mild sleep apnea. *Oral Maxillofac Surg Clin N Am* 2002;14:333–350.

Pack AI. *Sleep Apnea, Pathogenesis, Diagnosis, and Treatment*, vol 166. New York, Marcel Dekker, 2002, pp 575–605.

Yaggi HK, Concato J, Kernan WN, et al. Obstructive sleep apnea as a risk factor for stroke and death. *N Engl J Med* 2005;353: 2034–2041.

AUTHOR: **MANSOOR MADANI, DMD, MD**

SYNONYM(S)

Cerebrovascular accident
Brain attack

ICD-9CM/CPT CODE(S)

430 Subarachnoid hemorrhage—complete
431 Intracerebral hemorrhage—complete
434.1 Cerebral embolism—incomplete
435 Transient cerebral ischemia—incomplete
436 Acute, but ill-defined, cerebrovascular disease—complete

OVERVIEW

Cerebrovascular accident (CVA), or stroke, is defined as an acute onset of neurological deficit lasting more than 24 hours or culminating in death caused by a sudden impairment of cerebral circulation. Four neurological phenomena have been defined for stroke based on their duration:

- Transient ischemic attack (TIA): sudden, short-lasting, focal neurological deficit or "mini" stroke caused by transient and localized brain ischemia. These neurological deficits are reversible within 24 hours but often signal an impending stroke within days.
- Reversible ischemic neurologic defect (RIND): neurological impairment that is reversible but recovery from it will exceed 24 hours.
- Stroke in evolution: stroke-associated symptoms that progressively worsen over time.
- In contrast, neurological signs and symptoms that have been stable for more than 24 hours define a completed stroke.

EPIDEMIOLOGY & DEMOGRAPHICS

INCIDENCE/PREVALENCE IN USA: 160 per 100,000 (age 50 to 65, 1000 per 100,000; age > 80, 3000 per 100,000). Prevalence is 135 per 100,000. Stroke is the third-leading cause of death in the U.S. More prevalent in nonwhite races.
PREDOMINANT AGE: Risk increases over age 45 with the majority of ischemic strokes occurring in people over 65.
PREDOMINANT SEX: Affects males 3:1 over females.
GENETICS: Inheritance is polygenic with a tendency to clustering of risk factors within families.

ETIOLOGY & PATHOGENESIS

- Blood flow and delivery of essential oxygen and glucose to the brain tissue is interrupted, causing prolonged ischemia that results in irreversible cerebral tissue damage with neurological symptoms within minutes.

- The pathologic changes associated with stroke result from cerebral ischemia/infarction (constitute ~ 80% of strokes), intracerebral hemorrhage (~ 15% of strokes), or subarachnoid hemorrhage (~ 5% of strokes):
  - Cerebral infarctions are most commonly are caused by either atherosclerotic thrombi or emboli of cardiac origin:
    - Atherosclerotic thrombi are usually due to carotid artery atherosclerotic disease.
    - Emboli of cardiac origin may result secondary to:
      - Valvular (mitral valve) pathology
      - Acute anterior myocardial infarctions or congestive cardiomyopathies resulting in cardiac mural hypokinesias or akinesias with thrombosis
      - Cardiac dysrhythmias (typically atrial fibrillation)
  - The extent of a cerebral infarction is determined by a number of factors, including site of the occlusion, size of the occluded vessel, duration of the occlusion, and collateral circulation.
  - Neurologic abnormalities depend on the artery involved and the area it supplies.
  - Comorbid conditions such as hypertension, diabetes mellitus, and hypercholesterolemia are also risk factors for ischemic stroke.
  - The most common cause of intracerebral hemorrhage is hypertensive atherosclerosis, which results in microaneurysms of the arterioles. The vessels within the circle of Willis often are affected. Rupture of these microaneurysms within brain tissue leads to extravasation of blood, which displaces brain tissue and causes increased intracranial volume until the resulting tissue compression halts the bleeding.
  - The most common cause of subarachnoid hemorrhage is rupture of a saccular aneurysm at the bifurcation of a major cerebral artery.
  - Additional risk factors for hemorrhagic stroke include hypertensive encephalopathy, advanced age, abuse of alcohol or illicit drugs, strenuous exercise, and head injury.
- Hypercoagulable states, prior stroke, unhealthy diet, sedentary life style, oral contraceptive use, smoking, and psychological stress may also increase risk of stroke.

CLINICAL PRESENTATION / PHYSICAL FINDINGS

- Clinical manifestations are numerous and may include:

  - Sensory-motor dysfunctions (e.g., hemiplegia, hemiparesis, hypesthesia, compromised eye movements, visual defects, deafness, and language problems)
  - Memory disturbance, headache, altered mental status
  - Dizziness, nausea, and vomiting
- Clinical manifestations vary depending on the site and size of the brain lesion and type of stroke.
- In general, neurological symptoms of thrombotic strokes develop slowly.
- Sudden, multifocal, and maximal neurological deficits at the onset, early seizures, and hemorrhagic transformation often indicate embolic strokes.

DIAGNOSIS

Diagnostic tests that may help confirm a diagnosis of cerebrovascular disease include:

- Duplex carotid ultrasonography for evaluation of carotid artery atherosclerotic disease.
- Cerebral angiography or transcranial Doppler ultrasonography to detect site of cerebrovascular stenosis or obstruction.
- MRI (which is superior to CT) scan of head to detect acute intracerebral hemorrhage.
- Transthoracic echocardiogram; if normal and a cardiac source is suspected, follow up with transesophageal echocardiogram (both will aid in the diagnosis of valvular or myocardial pathology resulting in emboli).
- ECG and/or Holter monitoring (will help exclude a cardiac arrhythmia or recent myocardial infarction that might be serving as a source of embolization).
- EEG to evaluate seizure disorder that might result poststroke.
- CBC with platelet count (to evaluate for polycythemia, thrombocytosis, severe anemia).
- Prothrombin time (PT/INR) and partial thromboplastin time (PTT) to evaluate for hyper- or hypocoagulable states.
- Antiphospholipid antibodies (e.g., lupus anticoagulants and anticardiolipin antibodies promote thrombosis and are associated with an increased incidence of stroke).
- Lipid panel (elevated levels may indicate an increased risk of thrombotic stroke).
- ESR (may help exclude vasculitis).
- Additional tests:
  - BUN, creatinine, glucose, serum electrolytes, urinalysis
  - VDRL (for persons at increased risk of syphilis)

MEDICAL MANAGEMENT & TREATMENT

PREVENTION

- Primary prevention of the first stroke through lifestyle modification and screening for comorbid conditions (e.g., hypertension, diabetes, atherosclerosis, hyperlipidemia, cigarette smoking) and then attempting to reduce or eliminate as many of these as possible.
- Prophylactic antiplatelet [aspirin, dipyridamole/aspirin (Aggrenox), clopidogrel, or ticlopidine] or anticoagulant therapy (warfarin) in patients at risk for thromboembolism (e.g., chronic atrial fibrillation, previous myocardial infarction, congestive heart failure, mechanical heart valves) or a prior history of TIA/stroke.
- Carotid endarterectomy (CEA) plus optimal drug therapy and risk factor modification are highly effective in preventing stroke and death in symptomatic patients with carotid stenosis greater than 60–70%.

If a patient has a stroke, treatment is generally threefold:

1. Sustain life during the period immediately following the stroke. General measures include:
   - Maintain oxygenation
   - Monitor cardiac rhythm
   - Control hyperglycemia
   - Control of hypertension
   - Prevent hyperthermia
2. Prevent further thrombosis or hemorrhage: specific measures are dependent on the etiology, vascular regions involved, risk factors, and elapsed time from symptom onset to arrival at hospital, but can include:
   - Intravenous thrombolytic therapy with recombinant tissue plasminogen activator (tPA) to reduce neurologic deficit in selected patients with thromboembolic stroke.
   - Heparin therapy may be considered if atrial fibrillation and/or a cardiac mural thrombus is found on echocardiography.
   - Surgical intervention:
     ○ Intracerebral hemorrhage: surgical repair of structures causing the bleeding (repair of aneurysm, arteriovenous malformation) may be appropriate in some cases. Surgical evacuation of hematomas may also be indicated in some patients.
     ○ Subarachnoid hemorrhage: vascular ligation or occlusion either via a craniotomy and (metal surgical) clipping of the aneurysm or endovascular occlusion using a platinum coil device. Surgical evacuation of hematomas may also be indicated.

- Drugs such as diazepam or phenytoin are prescribed to manage seizures that may accompany the postoperative course of stroke.
3. Rehabilitation: including physical therapy, occupational therapy, and speech therapy as needed.

COMPLICATIONS

- Increased intracranial pressure (intracranial bleeding and edema)
- Poststroke seizures
- Secondary infections
- Deep vein thrombosis and pulmonary embolism
- Aspiration pneumonia
- Decubitus ulcers
- Disability
- Neurovascular deconditioning
- Poststroke sleep disordered breathing
- Poststroke depression
- Vascular dementia
- Poststroke sexual dysfunction

PROGNOSIS

- One-third of stroke victims die within 1 year of the event.
- Prognosis for survival after cerebral infarction is better than after cerebral or subarachnoid hemorrhage.
- One-third of recurrences occur within 1 month of the initial event.
- More than 50% of stroke survivors have temporary or permanent neurological impairment.
- The extent of the infarct governs the potential for rehabilitation.

DENTAL SIGNIFICANCE

- Loss of sensation in oral tissues
- Unilateral weakness and paralysis of orofacial muscles
- Impaired voluntary movements of oral structures
- Reduced gag reflex predisposing to aspiration pneumonia
- Difficulty managing oral secretions
- Pocketing food in different areas of the oral cavity predisposing patients to halitosis
- Unilateral oral atrophy and one-sided neglect opposite to the side of brain lesion
- Difficulty maintaining a reproducible jaw posture for functional occlusion
- Difficulty performing oral hygiene procedures and predisposition to periodontal and dental problems
- Dysphagia and secondary dietary changes leading to dental caries
- Poorly fitting prosthesis as a consequence of weight loss caused by dysphagia and inadequate food intake

- Hearing, speech, vision, and memory impairments leading to communication difficulties
- Medication-induced xerostomia and predisposition to caries
- Medication-induced impaired hemostasis after invasive oral procedures

DENTAL MANAGEMENT

The general evaluation of the dental patient with a history of cerebrovascular disease should include:

- Establish the specific diagnosis (e.g., TIA, RIND, CVA) and timing (dates) of the patient's cerebrovascular disease, including hospitalizations.
- Obtain an assessment of the patient's poststroke current status and stability. This would entail a summary of any residual neurologic deficits or disability, including motor, sensory, cognitive, memory, and behavioral deficits. This will usually require a medical consultation with the patient's physician.
- Identify the presence of continued risk factors for stroke (e.g., hypertension, diabetes, smoking, hyperlipidemia, chronic atrial fibrillation).
- Preoperative assessment of patients taking medication with adverse effect on hemostasis.
   ○ Antiplatelet agents: if bleeding-time > than 20 minutes, consult physician.
   ○ Anticoagulants (warfarin): if PT > 2.5 times normal or INR > 3.5, consult physician (see Appendix A, Box A-5, "Dental Management of Patients Taking Coumarin Anticoagulants").
- Radiographic findings: atherosclerotic lesions at the carotid bifurcation frequently are calcified and have been shown to be detectable on the panoramic dental radiographs of neurologically asymptomatic patients. Identifying a calcified carotid artery atheroma on a panoramic radiograph is of major clinical importance. Patients with such calcifications may be at a significantly increased risk of experiencing stroke and should be referred to an appropriate physician for confirmation of the findings and determination of the extent of disease.

Specific management considerations for the dental patient with a history of stroke would include:

- Defer elective dental care during the first 6 months after the stroke.
- Do not offer elective dental care to patients currently experiencing TIAs or RINDs.
- Arrange for short, midmorning dental appointments.
- Record pretreatment vital signs. Continuous (automated) monitoring of blood pressure, pulse, and blood oxygen saturation during dental treatment is advantageous.

- Reduce stress and anxiety prior to and during dental treatment: consider the use of N_2O-O_2 inhalation sedation and/or premedication with oral antianxiety medications such as benzodiazepines (e.g., triazolam, 0.125 to 0.5 mg the night before appointment and 0.125 to 0.5 mg 1 hour before treatment).
- Achieve profound anesthesia with minimum amount of local anesthetic with vasoconstrictor.
- Employ facilitative head positioning and effective suctioning to minimize risk of aspiration.
- Use atraumatic technique and local measures to minimize hemorrhage; administer nonadrenergic hemostatic agents and devices.
- Prescribe acetaminophen for postoperative analgesia if patient is taking aspirin, antiplatelet, or anticoagulant drugs.
- Evaluate patient's ability to perform effective oral hygiene; individualize oral hygiene aids and instructions, as necessary; educate personal caregiver on proper oral care of stroke patients.
- Recommend frequent recall appointments, regular fluoride applications, and saliva substitutes as indicated.

- Easily cleansable fixed dental prostheses are preferable to removable ones.
- Avoid fabrication of porcelain occlusal surface dental restorations.
- Take a compassionate and supportive approach in understanding patient's physical limitations.
- Allocate extra time for communication and clinical procedures.
- Recognize sign and symptoms of an impending stroke and react appropriately.

SUGGESTED REFERENCES

American Heart Association Scientific Statement: Primary prevention of ischemic stroke: a statement for health care professionals from the stroke council of the American Heart Association. *Circulation* 2001;103:167.

August M. Cerebrovascular and carotid artery disease. *Oral Surg Oral Med Oral Pathol Oral Radiol Endod* 2001;92:253–256.

Broderick JP, Hacke W. Treatment of acute ischemic stroke, part II: neuroprotection and medical management. *Circulation* 2002;106:1736–1740.

Cohen SN, et al. Carotid calcification on panoramic radiographs: an important marker for vascular risk. *Oral Surg Oral Med Oral Pathol Oral Radiol Endod* 2002;94:510–514.

Gorelick PB, Sacco RL, Smith DB, et al. Prevention of a first stroke. A review of guidelines and a multidisciplinary consensus statement from the National Stroke Association. *JAMA* 1999;281:1112–1120.

Ingall TJ. Preventing ischemic stroke: current approaches to primary and secondary prevention. *Postgrad Med* 2000;107(6):34–50.

Meschia JF, et al. Thrombolytic treatment of acute ischemic stroke. *Mayo Clin Proc* 2002;77:542.

Ostuni E. Stroke and the dental patient. *JADA* 1994;125:721–727.

Petty GW, Brown RD, Whisnant JP, et al. Ischemic stroke subtypes. A population-based study of functional outcome, survival, and recurrence. *Stroke* 2000;31:1062–1068.

Straus SE, Majumdar SR, McAlister FA. New evidence for stroke prevention: scientific Review. *JAMA* 2002;288(11):1388–1395.

Warlow C, Sudlow C, Dennis M, et al. Stroke. *Lancet* 2003;362:1211–1224.

AUTHOR: **MAHNAZ FATAHZADEH, DMD**

SYNONYM(S)

Lues
Lues venerea
"The great imitator"

ICD-9CM/CPT CODE(S)

097.9 Syphilis, acquired—unspecified

OVERVIEW

Syphilis is a complex infectious disease caused by *Treponema pallidum*, a spirochete capable of infecting almost any organ or tissue. It presents as a painless ulcer or chancre at the site of inoculation associated with regional lymphadenopathy. Postinoculation, syphilis becomes a systemic infection with secondary and tertiary stages. Approximately 30% of untreated patients show late disease of the heart, central nervous system, other organs, skin, and bone.

See "Syphilis" in Section II, p 326 for more information.

EPIDEMIOLOGY & DEMOGRAPHICS

INCIDENCE/PREVALENCE IN USA: In 2003, primary and secondary (P&S) syphilis cases reported to the Centers for Disease Control increased to 7177 from 6862 in 2002, an increase of 4.6% Although the rate of P&S syphilis in the United States declined by 89.7% during 1990–2000, the rate of P&S syphilis remained unchanged between 2000 and 2001 and increased in 2002 and 2003. Overall increases in rates during 2001–2003 were observed only among men.

PREDOMINANT AGE: Most common during the years of peak sexual activity. Most new cases occur in persons 15 to 40 years old, with the highest infection rates occurring in 20- to 29-year-olds.

PREDOMINANT SEX: The male:female ratio in 2002 was 3.4:1; in 2003 it was 5.2:1.

GENETICS: Not applicable.

ETIOLOGY & PATHOGENESIS

- The infection is caused by the spirochete *Treponema pallidum*, which does not live or cause disease outside the human body. It is spread through direct contact with an infectious lesion or by intrauterine transfer.
- Primary syphilis is the most contagious stage of the disease. It is carried by the blood to all organs in the body. Late in its course, syphilis becomes a vascular disease. *T. pallidum* is not known to produce toxins. Primary syphilis has an incubation period range of 10 to 90 days prior to a clinical chancre.
- Secondary syphilis appears 2 to 6 months after primary infection, with clinical dermal signs of exanthema and/or generalized papulopustular eruptions.

- Tertiary signs have a range of 2 to 60 years. Gummas develop by the fifteenth year.

CLINICAL PRESENTATION / PHYSICAL FINDINGS

- Primary syphilis: a localized infection at site of inoculation. The chancre occurs at the site of inoculation as a painless, clean-based, indurated ulcer. Most chancres are single but multiple sites are possible. Usually there is a degree of regional lymphadenopathy. The chancre usually resolves in 3 to 6 weeks without treatment.
- Secondary syphilis: diffused exanthematous, papulopustular and/or condylomata lata lesions are seen at this state. Generalized lymphadenopathy is noted. Most patients have cutaneous lesions. Lesions may be difficult to delineate on dark-skinned individuals. Differential diagnosis includes pityriasis rosea, drug eruption, psoriasis, lichen planus, acute febrile exanthems, and infectious mononucleosis.
- Relapsing syphilis: up to 30% of patients experience cutaneous lesions postprimary and secondary syphilis.
- Latent syphilis: represents a period between resolution of primary and secondary syphilis, and tertiary manifestations of disease with no clinical signs or symptoms of infection. Late latent syphilis (more than 1 year after the resolution of primary or secondary syphilis) is not infectious; however, women in this stage can spread the disease in utero.
- Tertiary syphilis: considered the destructive and crippling stage. There are cutaneous (e.g., lues maligna, gummas), neurologic (e.g., meningovascular disease, general paresis, and tabes dorsalis), and cardiovascular (e.g., syphilitic aortitis leading to aortic regurgitation and/or aortic aneurysm) manifestations. The disease is generally not thought to be infectious at this stage.
- Congenital syphilis: congenital infection may lead to fetal death in utero and stillbirths, fetal growth retardation, and severe infection in the neonate. Most children who survive the first 6 to 12 months of life untreated progress to latent syphilis followed by neurosyphilis later in life. Skeletal and soft tissue manifestations of congenital syphilis are permanent.

DIAGNOSIS

- Nontreponemal serologic tests:
  - Venereal Disease Reference Laboratory (VDRL) test.
  - Rapid plasma reagin (RPR) test.
    - Measures nonspecific nontreponemal reaginic antibody in the patient's serum and is used to make a presumptive diagnosis of syphilis in conjunction with a treponemal test.
- Treponemal serologic tests:
  - Microhemagglutination test for *T. pallidum* (MHA-TP).
  - Fluorescent treponemal antibody absorption (FTA-ABS) test.
    - Measures specific antitreponemal antibody in the patient's serum and is used to confirm a positive nontreponemal test.
- Dark field microscopy: a direct laboratory test for the detection of *T. pallidum* from serous exudate from a primary chancre, mucous patch, or condyloma latum.
  - Examination of specimens from mouth or anal lesions is worthless because nonpathogenic treponemes are always present (normal flora) and cannot be distinguished with certainty from *T. pallidum*.

MEDICAL MANAGEMENT & TREATMENT

- *T. pallidum* is inhibited by less than 0.01 μg/mL of penicillin G. Recommended regimen is 2.4 million units IM in one dose. Alternative antimicrobial therapy is doxycycline, 100 mg PO bid for 2 weeks. Other substitutes include erythromycin and ceftriaxone. Dosages vary according to stage of syphilis.
- Cases should be reported to local or state health department for referral, follow-up, and partner notification.
- The catastrophic consequences of congenital syphilis are entirely preventable by adequate prenatal care, screening, and treatment for syphilis in early pregnancy.

COMPLICATIONS

- Complications of tertiary syphilis include:
  - Cardiovascular syphilis: in the form of syphilitic aortitis, leads to slowly progressive dilation of the aortic root and arch, which causes aortic valve insufficiency and aneurysms of the proximal aorta.
  - Meningovascular syphilis: obliterative endarteritis and perivascular inflammation in the brain producing symptoms including chronic meningitis (headache, irritability), cranial nerve palsies (basilar meningitis), and unequal reflexes.
  - Paretic syphilis: results from widespread parenchymal CNS invasion characterized by progressive dementia with major frontal lobe signs and evidence of involvement of the motor cortex and the parietal and temporal lobes. Tremors and a parkinsonian

presentation may also result from basal ganglion involvement.

- o Tabes dorsalis: the result of damage to the sensory nerves in dorsal roots, producing ataxia and loss of pain sensation, proprioception, and deep tendon reflexes in joints.
- o Syphilitic gummas: may be single or multiple and occur most commonly in bone, skin, and the mucous membranes of the upper airway and mouth, although any organ may be affected. If they occur intracerebrally, they may mimic a brain tumor. If they are multiple and involve the meninges, the patient may present with dementia and focal neurologic signs.
- Children with congenital syphilis suffer with physical anomalies:
  - o Classic manifestations of untreated congenital syphilis include the Hutchinson triad: notched central incisors, interstitial keratitis with blindness, and deafness from eighth cranial nerve injury.
  - o Syphilitic osteochondritis and periostitis affect all bones, although lesions of the nose (i.e., the characteristic saddle nose deformity) and lower legs are most distinctive.

PROGNOSIS

The prognosis for patients with primary, secondary, and latent syphilis is excellent, providing adequate treatment is given.

DENTAL SIGNIFICANCE

- The characteristic lesion is a painless chancre appearing on lips or mouth in about 3 weeks postexposure.
- More than 50% of patients have mucosal lesions (pharyngitis, tonsillitis, mucous patch on the oral mucosa and/or tongue); the palate may be inflamed.
- Condylomata lata may be present.
- Transmission is possible with contact involving wet mucosa of a syphilitic patient.

DENTAL MANAGEMENT

- Referral is mandatory to primary care physician, infectious disease specialist, or local health department.
- Patients who are being treated or have a positive serological test results for syphilis should be viewed as potentially infectious. However, necessary dental treatment may be provided unless oral lesions are present.
- Untreated syphilis has a variable course of acute exacerbations followed by periods of remission over weeks, months, and/or years. It is a treatable disease if therapy is initiated prior to irreversible cardiovascular and/or neurologic damage. However, with congenital syphilis patients physical anomalies present depending on the level of fetal development when the infection occurs.

SUGGESTED REFERENCES

Centers for Disease Control and Prevention. Sexually transmitted diseases treatment guidelines. *MMWR Morb Mortal Wkly Rep* 2002;51(RR-6).

Fitzpatrick TB, Johnson RA, Wolff K, Suurmond D (eds). Syphilis, in *Color Atlas and Synopsis of Clinical Dermatology*. New York, McGraw-Hill, 2001, pp 889–900.

Hook III EW. Syphilis, in Goldman L, Ansiello D (eds): *Cecil Textbook of Medicine*, ed 22. Philadelphia, WB Saunders, 2004, pp 1923–1932.

AUTHOR: **NORBERT J. BURZYNSKI, SR., DDS, MS**

SYNONYM(S)

SLE

Disseminated lupus erythematosus

ICD-9CM/CPT CODE(S)

710.0 Systemic lupus erythematosus

OVERVIEW

This autoimmune disease is based on polyclonal B-cell immunity that involves connective tissue and blood vessels. It is a life-threatening disease, as opposed to the limited skin involvement in chronic cutaneous lupus erythematosus.

EPIDEMIOLOGY & DEMOGRAPHICS

INCIDENCE/PREVALENCE IN USA: SLE is the most common major connective tissue disease of children, with a prevalence of 5 to 10 per 100,000. In the general population, SLE affects about 1 in 2000 individuals. It is more common in African-Americans, Asians, and Hispanics.
PREDOMINANT AGE: SLE is primarily a disease of young women, with peak incidence between ages 15 and 40.
PREDOMINANT SEX: The ratio of female to male is 6 to 10:1.
GENETICS: Genetic markers are HLA-B8, HLA-DR2, and HLA-DR3.

ETIOLOGY & PATHOGENESIS

- The causes of the immune abnormalities are unknown.
- It is a chromic inflammatory connective tissue disorder that can involve joints, kidneys, serous surfaces, and blood vessel walls.
- Pathologic findings are manifested by inflammation, blood vessel abnormalities that encompass blood vasculopathy and vasculitis, and immune complex depositions. Studies of SLE imply an etiology by genetically determined immune abnormalities that can be triggered by indigenous and exogenous factors.

CLINICAL PRESENTATION / PHYSICAL FINDINGS

- Skin: erythematosus rash over the malar eminences, generally with sparing of the nasolabial folds (butterfly rash); alopecia; raised erythematosus patches with subsequent edematous plaques and adherent scales; leg, nasal, or oropharyngeal ulcerations; livedo reticularis; pallor (from anemia); petechiae (from thrombocytopenia).
- Cardiac: pericardial rub (in patients with pericarditis), heart murmurs (valvular dysfunction, Libman-Sacks vegetations).
- Respiratory: decreased breath sounds.
- Joints: tenderness, swelling, or effusion, generally involving peripheral joints.
- Neurologic: psychosis and seizure.

- Kidney: glomerular disease (hematuria or proteinuria), kidney failure.
- Hematologic: reduction in circulating blood cells.
- Oral: sicca syndrome, ulcers in purpuric necrotic lesions on palate, mucosa, gingival tissue.
- Other: splenomegaly, peripheral neuropathy, hepatomegaly, neuropathy, gastrointestinal pathology, photosensitivity.

DIAGNOSIS

The American Rheumatism Association accepts four or more of the listed criteria for a diagnosis:
- Discoid rash
- Butterfly rash
- Photosensitivity; hyper- or hypopigmentation, telangiectasia
- Oral mucosal ulcers; possible candidiasis
- Arthritis: multiple joints, migratory, nonerosive
- Serositis (e.g., pleuritis, pericarditis, peritonitis)
- Renal disorders: persistent proteinuria and/or casts
- Neurologic disorders of the CNS, such as seizures, headache, psychosis
- Hematologic disorders: hemolytic anemia, thrombocytopenia
- Immunologic disorder
- Abnormal titer of ANA by immunofluorescence
- Other signs and symptoms:
  - Raynaud's phenomenon
  - Chronic fatigue
  - Depression
  - Anxiety
  - Dermatitis

LABORATORY TESTS

- Immunologic evaluation: antinuclear antibody (ANA) in the serum is positive for 96–100% of patients with SLE. Additional autoantibodies may be positive in patients with SLE, including anti-native DNA (60% of patients), rheumatoid factor (20% of patients), antibody to Smith (Sm) antigen (10–25% of patients), antibody to Ro (SS-A) antigen (15–20% of patients), and antibody to La (SS-B) antigen (5–20% of patients). A patient with elevated ANA and anti-native DNA most likely has lupus.
- CBC with differential, platelet count, urinalysis for protein and casts, erythrocyte sedimentation rate, PTT and anticardiolipin antibodies in patients with thrombotic events, creatinine and blood urea nitrogen (BUN) to evaluate renal function. (Patients with SLE will demonstrate a false-positive serologic test for syphilis.)
- Biopsy of skin and/or oral mucosal lesions. Shows collagenous and fibrinoid changes, cellular necrosis, granulomatous reaction, and periarterial sclerosis.

IMAGING/SPECIAL TESTS

- Chest for pulmonary involvement
- Pulmonary function tests
- Echocardiogram for valvular heart disease, thickening, and dysfunction

MEDICAL MANAGEMENT & TREATMENT

NONPHARMACOLOGIC

- Avoid sunlight and use high-factor sun screen
- Refer patient to primary care physician and/or dermatologist

ACUTE TREATMENT

- Joint pain, serositis: NSAIDs, hydroxychloroquine
- Cutaneous: corticosteroids, antimalarials
- Renal: prednisone, immunosuppressive
- CNS: corticosteroids, anticonvulsants, antipsychotics
- Hemolytic anemia: corticosteroids
- Thrombocytopenia: corticosteroids, vincristine, immunoglobulins
- Infections: appropriate medications

CHRONIC TREATMENT

- Monitor exacerbations, frequent follow-up and review of laboratory data
- Monitor remissions
- Dialysis or renal transplantation in kidney failure

COMPLICATIONS

- The leading cause of death in SLE is infection (one-third of all deaths); active nephritis causes approximately 18% of deaths and CNS disease causes 7%.
- Symptomatic pericarditis occurs in more than 25% of patients.
- Renal function monitoring is needed in predicting disease outcome.

PROGNOSIS

- Most patients with SLE experience remissions and exacerbations (flare-ups). The initial acute phase merits serious control.
- Five-year survival is 93%; 10-year survival rate is around 85%. African-Americans and Hispanics have a worse prognosis. The more severe the disease, the greater the risk of iatrogenic drug-induced complications that further add to morbidity and mortality.

DENTAL SIGNIFICANCE

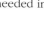

Oral manifestations and complications of SLE include:
- Characteristic oral lesions:
  - Lip lesions often have a central, atrophic, and occasionally ulcerated area with small white dots surrounded by a keratinized border

- composed of small, radiating white striae (lines).
  - Intraoral mucosal lesion presentation includes a central, depressed, red atrophic area surrounded by a 2- to 4-mm elevated keratotic zone that dissolves into small, radiating white striae.
  - Angular cheilosis, mucositis, ulcerations, and glossitis.
- Xerostomia secondary to Sjögren's syndrome that can significantly increase the occurrence of dental caries and candidiasis, especially when patients are being treated with corticosteroids or other immunosuppressive drugs.
- Temporomandibular disorders may cause pain and mechanical dysfunction.

DENTAL MANAGEMENT

- Patient should be referred to primary care physician, rheumatologist, and/or dermatologist. Specialists in dermatology and nephrology should be utilized.
- Maintain general oral/dental care as needed. Proceed with caution in performing elective surgery or dental procedures, especially in patients who have a history of postsurgery lupus flare-ups.
- Oral lesions can be treated with corticosteroids. Both topical and oral rinse can be administered. Advise patient that oral ulcers cannot be cured but can be controlled.
- For patients being treated with systemic corticosteroids, assess the risk for adrenal suppression and insufficiency (see Appendix A, Box A-4, "Dental Management of Patients at Risk for Acute Adrenal Insufficiency").
- Patients who are taking cytotoxic or immunosuppressive drugs, including systemic corticosteroids, are at an increased risk of infection and may require perioperative prophylactic antibiotics (see Appendix A, Box A-2, "Presurgical and Postsurgical Antibiotic Prophylaxis for Patients at Increased Risk for Postoperative Infections").
- Patients with SLE can frequently develop normochromic normocytic anemia, hemolytic anemia, leukopenia, thrombocytopenia, and impaired hemostasis (lupus anticoagulant). Prior to any intensive dental procedures, a preoperative CBC with differential, platelet count, and PT/INR and PTT should be performed to assess for the presence of any of these conditions.
- Patients with SLE should be referred to a physician (cardiologist) to assess for the presence of cardiac valvular pathology, including Libman-Sacks vegetations under the mitral valve leaflets that represent an increased risk for bacterial endocarditis. Presence would require the use of antibiotic prophylaxis prior to dental treatment that is likely to cause bacteremia [see Appendix A, Box A-1, "Antibiotic Prophylaxis Recommendations by the American Heart Association (AHA) for the Prevention of Bacterial Endocarditis"].
- In SLE patients with secondary renal disease, the patient's renal function (including creatinine clearance, serum creatinine, and BUN) should be assessed prior to dental treatment. Additional precautions would be required for patients with severe renal function impairment, chronic renal disease, and/or who are receiving hemodialysis.
- Drugs that have been related to acute lupus flare-ups include penicillin, sulfonamides, and nonsteroidal antiinflammatory drugs (NSAIDs) with photosensitizing potential. Any of these should be used with caution.

SUGGESTED REFERENCES

Al, Attia, Haider M et al. Associate autoimmune disorders in patients with classic lupus erythematosus. *J Clin Rheum* 2005; 11(1):63–64.

Greenspun B. SLE. www.emedicine.com/pmr/topic.135.htm

Lupus erythematosus, in Fitzpatrick TB, Johnson RA, Wolff K, Suurmond D (eds): *Color Atlas and Synopsis of Clinical Dermatology*, ed 4. New York, McGraw-Hill, 2001, pp 361–367.

Marx R, Stern D. *Oral and Maxillofacial Pathology: A Rationale for Diagnosis and Treatment*, Chicago, Quintessence Publishing Co., Inc., 2003.

Piselsky DS, Bunyons JP, Manzu S. Systemic lupus erythematosus, in Klippel JH (ed): *Primer on the Rheumatic Diseases*, ed 12. Atlanta, Arthritis Foundation, 2001, pp 329–352.

AUTHORS: **NORBERT J. BURZYNSKI, SR., DDS, MS; LAWRENCE T. HERMAN, DMD, MD; SARA H. RUNNELS, DMD, MD; PAUL R. WILSON, DMD**

SYNONYM(S)

Lockjaw

ICD-9CM/CPT CODE(S)

037 Tetanus

OVERVIEW

- Nervous system disorder characterized by increased muscle tone and spasms caused by tetanospasmin (tetanus toxin), which is produced by *Clostridium tetani*.
- Four clinical patterns of tetanus: generalized (most common), local, cephalic, and neonatal.

EPIDEMIOLOGY & DEMOGRAPHICS

INCIDENCE/PREVALENCE IN USA:

- 0.16 cases/million population annually (43 cases per year, on average).
- Older patients with diabetes are at higher risk for developing tetanus, with an annual incidence of 0.70 cases/million population.
- Decrease of about 25% compared to the 1980s.

PREDOMINANT AGE: 60 years of age (0.35 cases/million population). Older patients with diabetes are also at higher risk for developing tetanus, with an annual incidence of 0.70 cases/million population. The increased incidence in older individuals is consistent with decreasing proportion with age of patients who have received tetanus toxoid in the previous 10 years.

PREDOMINANT SEX: No predominant sex.

GENETICS: Not applicable.

ETIOLOGY & PATHOGENESIS

- The etiologic agent of tetanus is the spore-forming anaerobe *Clostridium tetani*, which is normally present in the gut of mammals and in soil.
- Once the organism gains access to the human host as a spore (usually via a traumatic event), the organism transforms into a vegetative, rod-shaped bacterium. The organism then produces the tetanus toxin, a metalloproteinase known as tetanospasmin. The mean incubation period before development of symptoms is 7 days.
- The traumatic event is usually a penetrating injury, such as a puncture wound. Common types of puncture wounds to produce tetanus include piercing splinters and intravenous drug use.
- While contamination of a wound with spores of *Clostridium tetani* is probably common, germination and toxin production are rare. This usually requires a wound with low oxygen tension, such as devitalized tissue, infected tissue, or wounds with a foreign body. The low oxygen tension is

necessary since *C. tetani* is an anaerobic organism.

- Once tetanospasmin is formed, it binds to nerve terminals, becomes internalized, and then is transported to the spinal cord and brain via retrograde axonal transport.
- Once in the central nervous system, tetanospasmin irreversibly binds to a receptor on the presynaptic membrane and causes cleavage of membrane proteins on presynaptic neurons involved in exocytosis of the inhibitory neurotransmitter γ-aminobutyric acid (GABA), resulting in an irreversible block of the release of GABA.
- The effect of blocking GABA release results in disinhibition of excitatory impulses from the motor cortex, anterior horn cells of the spinal cord, and autonomic neurons.
- The result of the disinhibition is increased muscle tone, painful muscle spasms, and widespread autonomic instability.

CLINICAL PRESENTATION / PHYSICAL FINDINGS

- Generalized tetanus, the most common form of tetanus, usually initially presents with increased tone in the masseter muscles with the patient noticing progressive trismus. More than half of patients initially present with trismus.
- Shortly after trismus presents, the patient will often develop dysphagia due to spasm of pharyngeal muscles and neck, shoulder, and back stiffness.
- Progressive involvement of other muscle groups produces the classic findings in tetanus.
- Abdominal muscle spasm produces a rigid, board-like abdomen.
- The disease then progresses to proximal limb muscles and back muscles, resulting in an arched back (opisthoclonus).
- Contraction of the muscles of facial expression results in *risus sardonicus* (a sardonic smile).
- Generalized tetanus is also characterized by periods of generalized, painful muscle spasms. These spasms are characterized by fist clenching, arched back, and flexing and abducting of the arms while extending the legs. Patients can often become apneic during these violent spasms due to sustained contraction of pharyngeal and/or laryngeal muscles, thoracic muscles, and the diaphragm.
- These spasms are often spontaneous but can be provoked by a sensory stimulus such as light or sound.
- The severity of generalized tetanus varies from mild muscle rigidity to severe paroxysms of spasm resulting in apnea. The severity has been linked to the duration of the incubating period,

with longer periods resulting in a less severe disease. The presence of an up-to-date tetanus toxoid vaccination has also been shown to prevent or decrease the severity of the disease.

- Autonomic instability is also a part of the disease process. Autonomic instability is characterized by labile or sustained hypertension, tachycardia, cardiac dysrhythmias, fevers, diaphoresis, and peripheral vasoconstriction.
- Local and cephalic tetanus are two uncommon forms of tetanus. Cephalic tetanus occurs after an injury to the head and neck region or an ear infection. This involves trismus and at least one other cranial nerve (mostly the facial nerve), although any cranial nerve can be involved.
- Local tetanus is restricted to muscles that are in proximity to the wound, with prognosis being excellent.
- Neonatal tetanus is very rare in developed countries. This usually occurs in children born to poorly vaccinated mothers and after the umbilical cord stump is treated in an unsterile fashion. The child presents in the first 2 weeks of life with rigidity, spasms, and poor feeding.

DIAGNOSIS

- The diagnosis of tetanus is based on clinical presentation, with laboratory testing providing adjunctive information.
- The leukocyte count may be elevated in cases where an infected wound is the initiating event.
- Creatinine kinase levels are likely to be elevated in cases with sustained muscle spasm.
- Serum antitoxin levels are likely to be low since levels greater than 0.01 U/mL are considered protective.
- An electrocardiogram should be obtained, monitoring for dysrhythmias and ischemia.
- Evaluation of the cerebrospinal fluid is normal.
- Radiographs may be helpful if a fracture is suspected.

MEDICAL MANAGEMENT & TREATMENT

- The five general tetanus treatment goals are halting toxin production, neutralizing unbound toxin, controlling muscle spasms, management of autonomic dysfunction, and supportive measures.
- Once tetanus is diagnosed, the patient is admitted to an intensive care unit for close cardiopulmonary monitoring with emphasis on respiratory status. Early endotracheal intubation for airway protection and mechanical ventilation is

usually warranted. If prolonged intubation is foreseen, a tracheostomy is usually done early, providing for better tracheal suctioning.

- Since energy demands are high in tetanus, nutritional support via enteral feeding is usually started early. Prophylaxis against stress ulceration and thromboembolism is also an important supportive measure in tetanus treatment.
- Halting toxin production involves adequate wound management and antimicrobial therapy. Aggressive wound debridement is essential to remove necrotic tissue and spores, thus preventing further germination. Antimicrobial therapy is recommended even though it is generally believed to have a minor role. The drug of choice against *C. tetani* is intravenous or intramuscular penicillin G. For penicillin-allergic patients, clindamycin is an alternate drug. Metronidazole is also gaining credence as an effective treatment. In one study, patients receiving metronidazole required fewer muscle relaxants and sedatives than those who received penicillin. This is thought to be a result of the GABA antagonist effect of penicillin, which may lead to CNS excitability.
- Neutralizing unbound toxin is a mainstay of treatment of tetanus and has been shown to reduce mortality. Human tetanus immune globulin (HTIG) is the antitoxin of choice and should be given immediately. HTIG functions by binding to and inactivating tetanus toxin.
- Control of muscle spasms is also essential since generalized muscle spasms are life-threatening. The patient should be placed in a quiet, dark room to avoid stimulation.
- Benzodiazepines are the first line of therapy. Diazepam is usually used in doses starting at 10 to 30 mg intravenously up to 120 mg/kg/day; it functions by increasing GABA release, which is an inhibitory neurotransmitter. Other benzodiazepines can also be used with equal efficacy. Barbiturates and propofol are other agents that can be used. Ventilatory support is often necessary with the high doses required for adequate control of spasms.
- Neuromuscular blocking agents are used when sedation is inadequate. A long-acting, nondepolarizing agent, such as pancuronium, is the drug of choice. Obviously, ventilatory support is required with neuromuscular blockers.
- In a few small studies, intrathecal baclofen has shown promise. Baclofen stimulates postsynaptic GABA receptors, thus decreasing muscle excitability.
- The autonomic instability of tetanus is managed pharmacologically with α- and β-blockade, with labetalol being the

drug most often employed. Morphine and magnesium also play a role in autonomic instability. If hypotension or bradycardia develops, these are managed with atropine, vasopressors, chronotropic agents, and/or volume expansion with intravenous fluids.
- Active immunization should also be administered since the disease does not induce immunity.
- Perhaps the best treatment of tetanus is to prevent the disease. The primary vaccination series for adults consists of three doses of tetanus-diphtheria toxoid (Td). A booster dose is then given every 10 years.
- All children should be immunized against tetanus. Children usually receive the tetanus vaccine in a preparation including the diphtheria toxoid, tetanus toxoid, and acellular pertussis vaccine (DTaP). They should receive doses at 2, 4, and 6 months of age with booster doses at 15 to 18 months and 4 to 6 years of age. At 11 to 12 years of age, children should receive the Td toxoid and then every 10 years after that (Box I-4).
- For patients presenting with a clean or minor wound, it is recommended that the patient receive Td toxoid if they are not adequately immunized or have not received a booster in 10 years. Patients who have a severe or contaminated wound should receive Td toxoid if they have not had a booster in the last 5 years. These patients should also be passively immunized with human tetanus immune globulin (Table I-22).

COMPLICATIONS

- Complications of tetanus include airway compromise, respiratory disturbances, autonomic instability, cardiac dysrhythmia, and death.

PROGNOSIS

- With adequate treatment and supportive measures in a timely fashion, mortality rates have been reported as low as 10% compared to as high as 50–60% without adequate treatment.

- In neonates and elderly patients, the prognosis is worse.
- Prior immunization improves prognosis.
- The usual time course of the disease is about 4 to 6 weeks, with ventilatory support needed for about 3 weeks.
- Increased tone and minor muscle spasms can be expected to last for months, with complete recovery eventually occurring.

DENTAL SIGNIFICANCE

- Dental implications of tetanus include the importance of an up-to-date immunization of patients with any injury, including avulsed or subluxed teeth, dentoalveolar fractures, lacerations, and jaw fractures. Patients with any of these injuries should receive appropriate treatment for tetanus prophylaxis.
- Rarely, a patient with trismus due to an odontogenic infection can mimic the trismus seen initially with tetanus. With tetanus, this trismus will progress rapidly.

DENTAL MANAGEMENT

- Dental management in these patients is limited. During active tetanus, proper oral care should be provided, including routine hygiene.
- Following recovery from tetanus, patients should be evaluated for any dental trauma that may have occurred during masseter spasms.

SUGGESTED REFERENCES

Abrutyn E. Tetanus, in Braunwald E, et al. (eds): *Harrison's Principles of Internal Medicine*, ed 15. New York, McGraw-Hill, 2001, pp 918–920.

Ahmadsyah I, Salim A. Treatment of tetanus: an open study to compare the efficacy of procaine penicillin and metronidazole. *BMJ* 1985;291:648.

Cook TM, et al. Tetanus: a review of the literature. *Br J Anaesth* 2001;87:477.

Pascual FB, et al. Tetanus surveillance—United States, 1998–2000. *MMWR Surveillance Summary* 2003;52:1.

AUTHORS: **DAVID C. STANTON, DMD, MD; DOUGLAS SEEGER, DMD, MD**

BOX I-4   Vaccination Schedule for Children

DTaP (diphtheria toxoid, tetanus toxoid, acellular pertussis)
2, 4, and 6 months of age
15 to 18 months of age
4 to 6 years of age

Td (tetanus-diphtheria toxoid)
11 to 12 years of age

TABLE I-22 Tetanus Prophylaxis

	Previously received 3 or more doses of Td	Never received 3 doses of Td
Clean or minor wounds	Td if last dose more than 10 years ago	Start primary series, first Td now, second in 1 month, third in 12 months
Contaminated or severe wounds	Td if last dose more than 5 years ago	Tetanus IG (250 U IM) and start primary series

Thrombocytopathies (Congenital and Acquired)

SYNONYM(S)

Abnormal platelet function
Qualitative platelet disorder

ICD-9CM/CPT CODE(S)

287.1 Qualitative platelet defects—complete

OVERVIEW

Thrombocytopathia refers to a disorder of platelet function (a qualitative platelet disorder) characterized by a prolonged bleeding time (BT) or closure time (CT) in conjunction with a (characteristically) normal platelet count. Thrombocytopathia may be congenital (hereditary) or acquired. In either case, platelets exhibit defects of adhesion, aggregation, or release.

EPIDEMIOLOGY & DEMOGRAPHICS

INCIDENCE/PREVALENCE IN USA: Varies due to underlying etiology.
PREDOMINANT AGE: Varies due to underlying etiology.
PREDOMINANT SEX: Varies due to underlying etiology.
GENETICS: Some thrombocytopathies (e.g., von Willebrand's disease, Glanzmann's thrombasthenia, Bernard-Soulier syndrome, storage pool disease) have established familial patterns of inheritance.

ETIOLOGY & PATHOGENESIS

ACQUIRED THROMBOCYTOPATHIES

- Drugs are the most common cause of thrombocytopathia and include:
  - Aspirin: causes a mild bleeding tendency by irreversibly acetylating cyclooxygenase, an enzyme that participates in platelet aggregation. The effects of aspirin on platelet function are irreversible and occur within 1 hour and last for the duration of the affected platelets' life span (approximately 1 week). The effect is not entirely dose-dependent, and as little as 40 to 80 mg of aspirin may produce a detectable alteration in platelet function resulting in a detectable increased BT for up to 96 hours. As little as 325 mg of aspirin may double the normal BT for several days.
  - Non-COX-selective, nonsteroidal antiinflammatory drugs (NSAIDs): can also inhibit platelet cyclooxygenase, thereby blocking the formation of thromboxane A2. These drugs produce a systemic bleeding tendency by impairing thromboxane-dependent platelet aggregation and thus prolonging the BT. However, these drugs inhibit cyclooxygenase reversibly, and the duration of their action depends on the specific drug dose, serum level, and elimination half-life.

- It is important to note that the clinical risk of impaired hemostasis with aspirin or nonaspirin, nonselective NSAIDs is enhanced by the use of alcohol or anticoagulants and associated conditions such as advanced age, liver disease, and other coexisting coagulopathies.
  - Other platelet inhibitor drugs such as clopidogrel (Plavix), dipyridamole (Persantine), and ticlopidine (Ticlid) affect platelet function through various mechanisms. The effects of these drugs on platelet function are irreversible and last for the duration of the affected platelets' life span. Their clinical effect on hemostasis is dose-dependent and is similar to that seen with aspirin.
  - Antibiotics: certain antibiotics [including β-lactam antibiotics (e.g., penicillin, amoxicillin, cephalosporins)] cause a mild bleeding tendency (which is not usually clinically significant), presumably by coating the surface of platelets and interfering with their function.
- Renal failure: when resulting in uremia causes abnormal platelet function by uncertain mechanisms but is believed to possibly be related to a decease in platelet factor 3. The severity of the bleeding tendency is roughly proportionate to the degree of renal insufficiency, and patients may present with clinically significant bleeding when blood urea nitrogen (BUN) is > 50 mg/dL and creatinine is > 4 mg/dL. Bleeding is most commonly mucosal and gastrointestinal and may occasionally be severe.
- Hepatic failure: thrombocytopathia occurs secondary to liver disease, but the exact mechanism and the extent to which it contributes to bleeding are unclear, as impaired hemostasis in hepatic failure is largely a result of deficiencies of coagulation factors. The BT may be prolonged in moderately severe liver disease when the platelet count is greater than 90,000/mm³.
- Myeloproliferative disorders: all the myeloproliferative disorders (e.g., leukemia, polycythemia vera, myelofibrosis) can produce abnormalities in platelet function. A number of biochemical abnormalities are present in these platelets, but the cause of the bleeding tendency is unclear.
- Autoimmune: patients with autoantibodies against platelets may have prolonged bleeding times even in the absence of thrombocytopenia. Platelet-associated IgG levels are correspondingly high.

CONGENITAL THROMBOCYTOPATHIES

- Von Willebrand's disease (vWD): transmitted in an autosomal dominant pattern. It is a group of disorders characterized by a compound defect involving platelet function and the coagulation pathway. In vWD, there is deficient or defective von Willebrand factor (vWF), a protein synthesized in megakaryocytes and endothelial cells and circulated in plasma, that mediates platelet adhesion. Von Willebrand factor has a separate function of binding the Factor VIII coagulant protein (Factor VIII:C) and protecting it from degradation; therefore, a deficiency of vWF gives rise to a secondary decrease in Factor VIII levels. See "Von Willebrand's Disease" in Section I, p 220 for additional information.
- Glanzmann's thrombasthenia is a rare, autosomal recessive intrinsic platelet disorder causing bleeding. Platelets are unable to aggregate because of lack of receptors (containing glycoproteins IIb and IIIa) for fibrinogen, which form the bridges between platelets during aggregation. Clinically, it is manifested chiefly as mucosal (e.g., epistaxis, gingival bleeding, menorrhagia) and postoperative bleeding.
- Bernard-Soulier syndrome (giant platelet disease) is a rare, autosomal recessive intrinsic platelet disorder in which the platelets vary widely in shape and size and demonstrate defective adherence to subendothelial collagen owing to deficient membrane glycoprotein Ib. Severe bleeding may be observed.
- Storage pool disease: encompasses a group of mild hereditary bleeding disorders of platelet function characterized by defective secretion of platelet granule contents (especially ADP) that stimulate platelet aggregation. Mild thrombocytopenia may also be present. Most patients are mildly affected and have increased bruising and postoperative bleeding.
  - There is also an acquired form of storage pool disease which refers to the circulation of "exhausted platelets" that have been stimulated to release their granule contents and hence are no longer functional. Such granule release occurs in response to cardiopulmonary bypass and severe vasculitis.

CLINICAL PRESENTATION / PHYSICAL FINDINGS

- Hemorrhage can be mild to severe after surgery, dental extraction, or other trauma; some patients may have spontaneous epistaxis.
  - With uremia, hemorrhage can be spontaneous and severe.
- Easy bruising or prolonged bleeding after minor trauma to skin or mucous membranes.
- Menorrhagia is a common presenting complaint in women.

DIAGNOSIS

Laboratory tests used in the diagnosis and monitoring of a qualitative platelet disorder include:

- Bleeding time (BT): used to evaluate the platelet and vascular phases of hemostasis from a functional standpoint (Table I-23).
- Closure time (CT) (PFA-100® test): has gained acceptance as a useful screen for platelet dysfunction and is sensitive to platelet adherence and aggregation abnormalities and may also be useful to monitor the response of therapeutics, such as desmopressin acetate (DDAVP) infusions, renal dialysis, and platelet and antiplatelet drug therapy (see Table I-23).

MEDICAL MANAGEMENT & TREATMENT

- Prolonged bleeding due to thrombocytopathies ordinarily responds to platelet transfusions except when it is secondary to uremia or hepatic failure or when a causative drug remains present in the circulation. For some causes of thrombocytopathia, other treatment measures may be effective:
  - Drugs: discontinue use of causative drug (see following Dental Management section).
  - Renal failure: dialysis is effective in reducing the bleeding tendency but may not completely eliminate it. Patients respond to desmopressin acetate (DDAVP).
  - Hepatic failure: DDAVP has been reported to improve the bleeding time.
  - Myeloproliferative disorders: bleeding decreases when the platelet count is controlled with myelosuppressive therapy. In cases of life-threatening bleeding with high platelet counts, plateletpheresis may be necessary.
  - Autoimmune: bleeding tendency responds quickly to modest doses of corticosteroids (e.g., prednisone, 20 mg/day).
  - Von Willebrand's disease: see "Von Willebrand's Disease" in Section I, p 220 for additional information.

COMPLICATIONS

- Bleeding diatheses: gastrointestinal, genitourinary, intracranial bleeding; hematomas
- Development of antibodies to transfused platelets
- Viral hepatitis, HIV infection secondary to transfusions (now rare)

PROGNOSIS

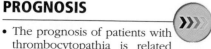

- The prognosis of patients with thrombocytopathia is related to the underlying disease or condition.

- The use of sterile platelet replacement transfusions has reduced the risk of bloodborne diseases.

DENTAL SIGNIFICANCE

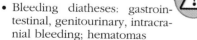

- Excessive bleeding after invasive dental treatment or oral surgery.
  - See Dental Significance in "Coagulopathies (Clotting Factor Defects, Acquired)," Section I, p 58 for additional information.
- Aggressive treatment of oral infections and establishment of good oral hygiene is necessary.

DENTAL MANAGEMENT

- Consultation with physician:
  - Determine/confirm underlying etiology of thrombocytopathia.
    - Patients with thrombocytopathia are at potential risk from both the underlying (causative) disorder and resultant impaired hemostasis. Both factors must be considered in relation to dental treatment.
  - Rule out the presence of a comorbid hemostatic pathology (e.g., thrombocytopenia, coagulation factor defect/deficiency).
  - Obtain results of current BT or CT prior to invasive dental treatment.
- Platelet replacement may be necessary for those patients with moderate to severe thrombocytopathia, especially for block injections, extractions, or periodontal surgery.
- Local hemostatic measures [e.g., absorbable gelatin sponges (Gelfoam®), oxidized cellulose (SURGICEL™), microfibrillar collagen (Avitene®), topical thrombin, tranexamic acid, epsilon-aminocaproic acid (EACA), sutures, and surgical splints and stents].
- Examine patient 24 hours after dental procedure for hemostasis and signs of infection.
- Avoid use of aspirin or NSAIDs.
- Additional considerations for patients with drug-induced thrombocytopathia:
  - Aspirin:
    - Clinically significant (i.e., in most dental surgical situations) prolonged bleeding usually does not occur until the patient is using aspirin at therapeutic doses of 2 g or more per day for a prolonged period (i.e., more than 1 week). However, lower doses of aspirin may result in clinically significant prolonged bleeding by exacerbating previously undiagnosed bleeding disorders such as mild vWD or mild thrombocytopenia.
    - The best screening test for aspirin's effect on hemostasis is the CT; if

this is not available, then the BT can be used. Although aspirin affects platelets and the coagulation process through its effect on platelet release, it does not usually lead to a significant bleeding problem unless the BT is greater than two to three times the upper limit of the control value for the test (this is probably true for CT as well).

- For patients taking aspirin who require moderate-risk dental procedures and have a BT less than two to three times the upper limit of the control value, local hemostatic measures can be used to control bleeding and any postoperative oozing resulting from treatment.
- As an additional consideration for patients requiring moderate-* to high-risk† elective (nonemergent) dental procedures, with approval from the physician, the aspirin can be discontinued for 3 to 7 days prior to surgery, which allows for a sufficient number of new platelets to arrive into the circulation and should result in a BT within normal limits.
- If moderate-* or high-risk† dental treatment must be performed under emergency conditions and the BT exceeds two to three times the upper limit of the control value, DDAVP infusion can be used to shorten the BT. This should be done in consultation with the patient's physician or hematologist.
  - Other platelet inhibitor drugs such as clopidogrel (Plavix), dipyridamole (Persantine), and ticlopidine (Ticlid):
    - These drugs interfere with platelet function irreversibly, and their effect lasts for the duration of the affected platelets' life span. Their clinical effect on hemostasis is dose-dependent and similar to that seen with aspirin. These drugs are typically used prophylactically in the prevention of thromboembolic disease (e.g., myocardial infarction, stroke) at a dose that has an overall anticoagulant effect analogous to that of low-dose (325 mg) daily aspirin therapy.
    - In most circumstances, it is unnecessary to discontinue use of one of these platelet inhibitors in a patient who is going to receive surgical dental treatment, and any minor increased bleeding should be manageable with local hemostatic measures.
    - If a patient is to undergo elective dental treatment or surgery and an antiplatelet effect is not desired for some reason, the platelet inhibitor drug should be discontinued 5 days prior to surgery in consultation with the patient's physician.

Thrombocytopathies (Congenital and Acquired)

○ Non-COX-selective, nonsteroidal anti-inflammatory drugs (NSAIDs):

■ These drugs inhibit cyclooxygenase reversibly, and the duration of their action in affecting platelet function depends on the specific drug dose, serum level, and elimination half-life. Generally, once the drug is discontinued and the clinician waits three serum (elimination) half-lives of the drug, levels will be sufficiently eliminated to allow for normal platelet function to return.

- For example, ibuprofen has a serum half-life of 2 to 4 hours; therefore, platelet function should return to normal in 6 to 12 hours after the patient has stopped taking ibuprofen.

---

* Moderate-risk procedures include subgingival scaling and root planing; subgingival restorations; uncomplicated forceps extraction of one to three teeth that are amenable to primary closure; endodontic procedures; injections of local anesthetics that are not confined to well-defined areas over bone, including regional infiltrations and blocks.

† High-risk procedures include periodontal surgical procedures; insertion of osseointegrated implants; extensive (i.e., more than three teeth) or complex oral surgery procedures including those involving removal of bone (e.g., extraction of impacted or unerupted third molars, preprosthetic alveoloplasty, or tuberosity reduction).

SUGGESTED REFERENCES

Catalano PM. Platelet and vascular disorders, in Rose LF, Kaye D (eds): *Internal Medicine for Dentistry,* ed 2. St Louis, Mosby, 1990, pp 346–353.

Patrono C. Aspirin as an antiplatelet drug. *N Engl J Med* 1994;330:1287–1294.

AUTHORS: **WENDY S. HUPP, DMD; F. JOHN FIRRIOLO, DDS, PHD**

TABLE I-23 Laboratory Tests for the Diagnosis and Evaluation of Thrombocytopathia

Laboratory Test	Factors or Functions Measured	Normal Values
Bleeding Time (BT)	Platelet function and vascular integrity	Duke method: 1–5 minutes Ivy method: 1–9 minutes Template (Mielke) method: 2.5–10 minutes
Closure Time (CT)	Platelet function	CEPI[1]: 85–165 seconds CADP[2]: 71–118 seconds

1. CEPI = Collagen and epinephrine
2. CADP = Collagen and adenosine diphosphate

SYNONYM(S)

Thrombopenia
Plastocytopenia
Low platelet count
Decreased platelet count
Low platelets

ICD-9CM/CPT CODE(S)

287.3 Primary thrombocytopenia—complete
287.4 Secondary thrombocytopenia—complete
287.5 Thrombocytopenia, unspecified—complete

OVERVIEW

A congenital or acquired disorder of platelet production, distribution, or destruction in which the number of circulating platelets is decreased but their function is normal.

EPIDEMIOLOGY & DEMOGRAPHICS

INCIDENCE/PREVALENCE IN USA: Varies due to underlying etiology.
PREDOMINANT AGE: Varies due to underlying etiology.
PREDOMINANT SEX: Varies due to underlying etiology.
GENETICS: Not established.

ETIOLOGY & PATHOGENESIS

- Hypoplasia of hematopoietic stem cells (megakaryocytes):
  - Aplastic anemia
  - Marrow damage from drugs (e.g., thiazide diuretics, methotrexate and other antineoplastic drugs), ethanol, toxins, ionizing radiation, infection
  - Congenital and hereditary thrombocytopenias
  - Thrombocytopenia with absent radii (TAR) syndrome
  - Wiskott-Aldrich syndrome
  - May-Hegglin anomaly
- Replacement of normal marrow:
  - Leukemias
  - Metastatic tumor (e.g., prostate, breast, lymphoma)
  - Myelofibrosis
- Ineffective thrombocytopoiesis (with normal or increased numbers of megakaryocytes):
  - Cobalamin (vitamin B_{12}) or folate deficiency
  - Hematopoietic dysplastic syndromes
- Increased destruction of platelets:
  - Immune disorders:
    - Idiopathic thrombocytopenic purpura
    - Secondary causes:
      - Cancer, such as chronic lymphocytic leukemia, lymphoma, systemic autoimmune disorders [systemic lupus erythematosus (SLE), polyarteritis nodosa]
      - Infectious diseases such as infectious mononucleosis, cytomegalovirus (CMV), and human immunodeficiency virus (HIV)
      - Drugs such as quinidine, quinine, heparin, aspirin, sulfonamides, rifampin, thiazides, methyldopa, gold salts, digitoxin, carbamazepine, aminosalicylic acid, and others
  - Nonimmune disorders:
    - Disseminated intravascular coagulation (DIC)
    - Cavernous hemangioma
    - Thrombotic microangiopathies such as thrombotic thrombocytopenic purpura (TTP)
    - Hemolytic-uremic syndrome
    - Sepsis
    - Malaria
    - Paroxysmal nocturnal hemoglobinuria
    - Congenital cyanotic heart disease
    - Prosthetic heart valves and other prosthetic intravascular devices
    - Acute renal transplant rejection
- Disorders of distribution:
  - Hypersplenism/splenomegaly: results in splenic platelet sequestration
- Dilutional:
  - Secondary to transfusion with packed erythrocytes or nonfresh whole blood

(Modified from Goldman L, Ausiello D (eds): *Cecil Textbook of Medicine*, ed 22. Philadelphia, WB Saunders, 2004.)

CLINICAL PRESENTATION / PHYSICAL FINDINGS

PATIENT HISTORY

- The location and severity of bleeding (if any):
  - History of spontaneous bleeding and/or prolonged bleeding after surgery, dental extraction, or other trauma (Table I-24).
  - Menorrhagia is a common presenting complaint in women.
- The temporal profile of the hemostatic defect (acute, chronic or relapsing).
- Presence of symptoms of a secondary illness (e.g., neoplasm, infection, autoimmune disorder).
- A history of recent medication use, ethanol ingestion, or transfusion.
- Presence of risk factors for certain infections (e.g., particularly HIV, viral hepatitis).
- Family history of thrombocytopenia.

SIGNS AND SYMPTOMS

- Petechiae and purpura (spontaneous or secondary to trauma).
- Spontaneous mucous membrane bleeding, epistaxis, and gastrointestinal bleeding.
- Lymphadenopathy: may indicate a viral infection, such as infectious mononucleosis or HIV infection, or a neoplastic lymphoproliferative disorder.

DIAGNOSIS

- Platelet count (PC) (normal adult: 140,000 to 400,000/μL)
- Bleeding time (BT) is prolonged when the platelet count goes below 90,000/μL or when a functional platelet abnormality exists.

MEDICAL MANAGEMENT & TREATMENT

- Treat underlying condition:
  - For example, splenectomy for splenomegaly; bone marrow transplant for aplastic anemia or myelofibrosis.
  - Chronic ITP is often treated with splenectomy and corticosteroids.
- Platelet replacement transfusions are effective for thrombocytopenia only when the cause is decreased production. Thrombocytopenia due to increased peripheral platelet destruction or sequestration is usually refractory to platelet transfusion.

COMPLICATIONS

- Bleeding diatheses: gastrointestinal, genitourinary, intracranial bleeding; hematomas
- Development of antibodies to transfused platelets
- Viral hepatitis, HIV infection secondary to transfusions (now rare)

TABLE I-24 Platelet Count Effects on Bleeding

Platelet Count	Effect on Bleeding
≥ 100,000/μL	No abnormal bleeding even with major surgery.
50,000 to 100,000/μL	May bleed longer than normal with severe trauma.
20,000 to 50,000/μL	Prolonged bleeding occurs with minor trauma, but spontaneous bleeding is unusual.
< 20,000/μL	May experience spontaneous bleeding.
< 10,000/μL	Spontaneous bleeding is likely; high risk for severe, prolonged bleeding.

PROGNOSIS

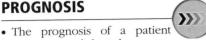

- The prognosis of a patient with acquired thrombocytopenia is related to the underlying disease or condition.
- The use of sterile platelet replacement transfusions has reduced the risk of bloodborne diseases.

DENTAL SIGNIFICANCE

- Excessive bleeding after invasive dental treatment or oral surgery.
  - See Dental Significance in "Coagulopathies (Clotting Factor Defects, Acquired)," Section I, p 58 for additional information.
- Aggressive treatment of oral infections and establishment of good oral hygiene is necessary.

DENTAL MANAGEMENT

- Consultation with physician:
  - Determine/confirm underlying etiology of thrombocytopenia.
    - Patients with thrombocytopenia are at potential risk from both the underlying (causative) disorder and resultant impaired hemostasis. Both factors must be considered in relation to dental treatment.
  - Rule out the presence of a comorbid hemostatic pathology (e.g., thrombocytopenia, coagulation factor defect/deficiency).
  - Obtain results of current PC prior to invasive dental treatment.
- Prophylactic platelet transfusion prior to surgical dental procedures (e.g., extractions, periodontal surgery) is usually indicated when the PC is below 50,000/μL (i.e., the PC should be above 50,000/μL before surgery is attempted).
- Local hemostatic measures [e.g., absorbable gelatin sponges (Gelfoam®), oxidized cellulose (SURGICEL™), microfibrillar collagen (Avitene®), topical thrombin, tranexamic acid, epsilon-aminocaproic acid (EACA), sutures, and surgical splints and stents].
- Examine patient 24 hours after dental procedure for hemostasis and signs of infection.
- Avoid use of aspirin or NSAIDs.

SUGGESTED REFERENCE

Wagner JD, Moore DL. Preoperative laboratory testing for the oral and maxillofacial surgery patient. *J Oral Surg* 1991;49:177–182.

AUTHOR: **WENDY S. HUPP, DMD**

SYNONYM(S)

Toxoplasma gondii

ICD-9CM/CPT CODE(S)
130 Toxoplasmosis—incomplete
130.7 Toxoplasmosis of other specified sites—complete
130.8 Multisystemic disseminated toxoplasmosis—complete
130.9 Unspecified toxoplasmosis—complete
771.2 Toxoplasmosis (congenital)

OVERVIEW

Toxoplasmosis is a relatively common zoonotic infection caused by *Toxoplasma gondii*, an obligate intracellular parasite (similar to the pathogen that causes malaria). This parasitic infection is typically classified as either acquired or congenital toxoplasmosis and affects humans and other warm-blooded animals. Most infections acquired after birth are asymptomatic but result in the chronic persistence of tissue cysts within host tissues.

EPIDEMIOLOGY & DEMOGRAPHICS

INCIDENCE/PREVALENCE IN USA: It is estimated that one-quarter to one-half of the U.S. population (serologic evidence of infection in healthy adults ranges from 3–70% depending on the population group and geographic location studied) may be infected but few have symptoms of disease. Geographic distribution of *T. gondii* is worldwide but infections are more common in cooler climates at lower altitudes. Four hundred to 4000 congenital cases of toxoplasmosis are diagnosed per year in the U.S.
PREDOMINANT AGE: The prevalence of positive serologic reaction increases with age. Studies report that 6–21% of children and 10–67% of adults over the age of 50 show serologic evidence of prior infection with toxoplasmosis.
PREDOMINANT SEX: There is no sexual predilection for this infection. However, in pregnant women the risk of congenital toxoplasmosis is higher during the first two trimesters but severity of disease declines as gestation proceeds. Women planning to become pregnant should be tested and, if serology is negative, they should take the necessary precautions.

ETIOLOGY & PATHOGENESIS

- *T. gondii* tissue cysts are present in birds, mice, or raw meat eaten by cats.
  - In the cat's intestine, the parasites invade intestinal mucosa, replicate and complete a sexual cycle, and are then excreted in the animal's feces as oocysts.
- Oocysts can survive in soil for up to one year. Thus, infection can occur by ingesting parasitic cysts or oocysts directly from contaminated soil (present on unwashed fruits and vegetables) or infected meat.
- The parasite is also transmitted to humans by:
  - Inhalation and ingestion of oocysts while cleaning a cat's litter box.
  - Transplacentally (55% in untreated mothers).
  - Through organ transplantation, blood transfusion, needlestick injuries, or laboratory accident (more rare).
- Single cyst is all that is needed for infection.
- In an infected person the oocysts are digested, releasing parasites that are then picked up by macrophage and spread throughout the body.
- The parasite may live inside the macrophage or infect other cells (except RBCs).
- In healthy individuals, humoral and cell-mediated immunity contain the parasite in a calcified pseudocyst where it remains dormant as long as host defenses remain intact.
- Congenital infection can occur when a previously nonimmune woman becomes infected during pregnancy, leading to transplacental transmission. Approximately 15–60% of such infections are transmitted to the fetus but only a small percentage result in miscarriage or active disease. Fetal infection is typically more severe early in pregnancy.

CLINICAL PRESENTATION / PHYSICAL FINDINGS

ACQUIRED TOXOPLASMOSIS
- Eighty to 90% of infections in healthy adults are asymptomatic.
- Ten to 20% of cases develop acute, mild illness that resembles infectious mononucleosis.
- Patients may develop fever, lymphadenopathy, malaise, myalgia, and a skin rash that spares the palms and soles.
- Other organs may also be affected in the immunosuppressed: eyes (chorioretinitis), heart (myocarditis), lungs (pneumonia), and muscles (myositis).
- After the initial infection phase, pseudocysts disperse to other organ tissue and proliferation of the organism ceases with the host response. The cysts that form lie dormant and intact within the host unless the patient's immune system becomes suppressed. Reactivated toxoplasmosis occurring in immunocompromised individuals can be life-threatening.

CONGENITAL TOXOPLASMOSIS
- The classic clinical triad of intracerebral calcifications, convulsions, and retinochoroiditis defines congenital toxoplasmosis.
- Other sequelae include mild, nonspecific disease, failure to thrive, lymphadenopathy, and myocarditis.
- May cause intrauterine death, growth retardation, mental retardation, ocular defects, or blindness
- May be present subclinically at birth, which may evolve later in life or range in severity from mild to severe at birth.

RISK FACTORS
- Immunodeficiency (i.e., AIDS).
- Immunosuppression (i.e., organ transplantation, malignancy).
- Exposure to cats.
- Ingestion of raw or partially cooked meat.

DIAGNOSIS

DIFFERENTIAL DIAGNOSIS
- Mononucleosis
- Lymphoma
- Myocarditis
- Tuberculosis
- Sarcoidosis
- Pneumonia
- Leukemia
- Herpes encephalitis
- Cat scratch disease
- Fungal disease

LABORATORY
- Part of TORCH [toxoplasmosis, other (*T. pallidum*, varicella-zoster virus VZV, parvovirus B19), rubella virus, cytomegalovirus (CMV), and herpes simplex virus (HSV)] prenatal screening serology.
- In adults, rising antibody titers to *T. gondii* may be seen 10 to 14 days after an infection.
- Sabin-Feldman dye test, fluorescent antibody testing, and ELISA are used.
- Immunosuppressed patients may not be able to mount an immune response and may not demonstrate antibodies.
- Biopsy of the involved lymph node may be suggestive of an infection but should be confirmed with serology.
- Parasites may also be visible in patient specimens including bronchoalveolar lavage samples, CSF, or brain biopsy.
- Parasite genetic material may be detected by PCR screening, which is especially useful in detecting in utero infections (via amniocentesis).

IMAGING
- MRI or cranial CT if CNS involvement is suspected (may see single or multiple ring-enhancing lesions).

MEDICAL MANAGEMENT & TREATMENT

- In healthy, nonpregnant adults no treatment other than supportive therapy is necessary as symptoms are usually mild and self-limited.
- In pregnant patients, sulfadiazine, pyrimethamine, and folinic acid are used for 4 weeks. Early treatment can reduce the incidence of fetal infection

and congenitally infected newborns are usually treated aggressively.

- In immunosuppressed patients the same treatment regimen is used as for pregnant patients.
- Immunosuppressed patients must be stabilized with treatment for seizures, respiratory failure, and cardiovascular compromise.
- In patients allergic to sulfa medications, clindamycin substituted for sulfadiazine.
- Bone marrow suppression may be seen with pyrimethamine, so CBC must be followed.
- Consider lymph node biopsy if diagnosis unclear.
- HIV patients with a low CD4 count (< 200) are given suppressive therapy to prevent reactivation of toxoplasmosis. Bactrim (trimethoprim/sulfamethoxazole), which is often used as *Pneumocystis carinii* pneumonia prophylaxis, is also effective in preventing toxoplasmosis. Alternatively, dapsone is given in combination with weekly pyrimethamine and leucovorin (folinic acid).

COMPLICATIONS

- In congenital toxoplasmosis, complications can be severe. Infection can lead to mental retardation, epilepsy, and impaired vision.
- In acquired toxoplasmosis of immunocompetent individuals, acute infection typically resolves with no complications. Rarely, infections may cause chorioretinitis, myositis, and heart, lung, liver, or CNS symptomatic involvement.

- In immunocompromised patients, complications can involve multiorgan systems. Toxoplasmosis can cause pneumonitis, carditis, hepatitis, myositis, and encephalitis. In patients with AIDS, CNS dysfunction, or ocular lesions are more common.

PROGNOSIS

In healthy individuals, the infection is benign and self-limited. Since toxoplasmosis in immunocompromised individuals has the potential to reactivate, suppression therapy should be used when appropriate. Individuals with recurrent disease are more likely to have permanent complications from toxoplasmosis. Untreated disease is rapidly fatal in immunocompromised patients with CNS involvement.

DENTAL SIGNIFICANCE

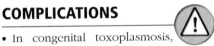

Infection with *T. gondii* is not known to cause oral sequelae. Dental clinicians may suspect toxoplasmosis if a patient presents with sore throat and cervical lymphadenopathy and reports symptoms of fever, malaise, rash, myalgia, or headache. A thorough history should include assessment of risk factors for toxoplasmosis and history of exposure to the parasite. Medications used to treat toxoplasmosis may cause adverse effects including diarrhea, nausea, abdominal pain, and rash. Pyrimethamine has been reported to cause atrophic glossitis, while clarithromycin can the adverse oral effect of abnormal taste.

DENTAL MANAGEMENT

If toxoplasmosis is suspected based on history or signs and symptoms, the dental clinician should refer the patient to their physician, an infectious disease specialist, neurologist, or ophthalmologist (for CNS and ocular involvement, respectively) for evaluation.

Dental treatment may be rendered with minimal risk of infection from patient to clinician. The infection cannot be transmitted through casual contact. Personal protective equipment and standard precautions are highly recommended since the infection may be transmitted by blood. However, it is important to remember that up to one-half of the population has already been exposed to the parasite in the past and very likely have immunity to it.

SUGGESTED REFERENCES

Centers for Disease Control: http://www.cdc.gov/ncidod/dpd/parasites/toxoplasmosis/factsht_toxoplasmosis.htm

Hill D, Dubey JP. Toxoplasma gondii: transmission, diagnosis and prevention. *Clin Microbio Infect* 2002;8(10):634–640.

Kravetz JD, et al. Toxoplasmosis in pregnancy. *Am J Med* 2005;118(3)212–216.

Montoya JG. Opportunistic parsitic infections: *Toxoplasma gondii*, in Cohen J, Powderly WG, Berkley SF, et al. (eds): *Infectious Diseases*, ed 2. St Louis, Mosby, 2004, pp 1183–1187.

Sciammarella J. Toxoplasmosis, on www.eMedicine.com

AUTHORS: **ERNESTA PARISI, DMD; LAWRENCE T. HERMAN, DMD, MD; SARA H. RUNNELS, DMD, MD; PAUL R. WILSON, DMD**

SYNONYM(S)

TB
Consumption

ICD-9CM/CPT CODE(S)

010.00 Primary tuberculous infection, unspecified
011   Pulmonary tuberculosis

OVERVIEW

- Tuberculosis (TB) is a chronic, recurrent infection most commonly caused by *Mycobacterium tuberculosis* that most commonly manifests itself as pulmonary disease.
- Infection with *M. tuberculosis* may also result in extrapulmonary disease, which can affect the pleura, lymph nodes, genitourinary tract, skeleton, meninges, peritoneum, or pericardium.

EPIDEMIOLOGY & DEMOGRAPHICS

INCIDENCE/PREVALENCE IN USA:

- Approximately 5.1 cases per 100,000 (14,874 cases reported in 2003, lowest in reported history).
- Estimated 10 to 15 million people are infected in the U.S.
  - Although the TB case rate has decreased, there remains a huge reservoir of individuals who are infected with *M. tuberculosis*.
  - New cases of TB can be expected to develop from this group if effective treatment for latent TB is not effectively administered.
- In 2003, 82% of new TB cases occurred in racial and ethnic minority groups.
- The incidence of TB has increased among persons infected with HIV, particularly African-American and Hispanic IV drug users, most commonly city-dwelling men 25 to 44 years old.

PREDOMINANT AGE:

- Primary infection: any age, especially pediatric patients.
- Latent TB infection: adults and the elderly.

PREDOMINANT SEX:

- No specific predilection.
- Disproportionate male incidence due to male predominance in shelters, prisons, and persons with AIDS.

GENETICS:

- None established; however:
  - Populations with widespread low native resistance have been intensely infected when initially exposed to TB; following statistical elimination of those with least native resistance, incidence and prevalence of TB tend to decline.

ETIOLOGY & PATHOGENESIS

ETIOLOGY

- *Mycobacterium tuberculosis*, sometimes referred to as the tubercle bacillus, is the principal causative organism of TB in the U.S.

  - *M. tuberculosis* and four related species, *Mycobacterium bovis, Mycobacterium africanum, Mycobacterium microti,* and *Mycobacterium canetti* comprise what is known as the *M. tuberculosis* complex.
  - *M. bovis* and *M. africanum* cause TB in rare cases.
  - *M. tuberculosis* is a slow-growing, aerobic, nonspore-forming, nonmotile bacillus with a lipid-rich layer; it has no known endotoxins or exotoxins.
  - Humans are the only reservoir for *M. tuberculosis*.

PATHOGENESIS

Tuberculosis Infection (Primary Tuberculosis)

- Spread primarily person-to-person by tiny, airborne particles (droplet nuclei).
  - When an infectious person with active pulmonary TB coughs, sneezes, speaks, or sings, droplet nuclei are expelled into the air. Transmission may occur if another person inhales the droplet nuclei, which may contain fewer than 10 bacilli.
  - Transmission occurs depending on four factors:
    - The infectiousness of the person with TB
    - The environment in which the exposure occurred
    - The duration of exposure
    - The virulence of the organism
- Tubercle bacilli that reach the alveoli are ingested by alveolar macrophages. Infection follows if the inoculum escapes alveolar macrophage microbicidal activity.
- Once infection is established, lymphatic and hematogenous dissemination of *M. tuberculosis* typically occurs before cell-mediated immunity develops over period of 3 to 6 weeks and *M. tuberculosis* is arrested, though small numbers of viable bacilli may remain within the resultant granulomas.
- In 90% of normal, immunocompetent adults, infection is self-limited. The inflammatory and cellular immune response is sufficient to control the disease.
- As a result of primary infection with *M. tuberculosis,* two TB-related conditions exist:
  - Active TB disease: resulting from the inability of the immune system to limit the disease
  - Latent TB infection: resulting from infection that is controlled by the immune response but may develop into active TB disease at some time in the future
    - Ten percent of individuals who acquire primary TB infection and are not given preventive drug therapy will develop active TB.

Active Tuberculosis Disease

- TB bacilli overcome the immune system and multiply resulting in progression from TB infection to TB disease.
- Of the 10% of individuals who develop active TB, about 5% develop the disease in the first 2 years after infection, and about 5% progress later in their lives.
- Clinical manifestations vary depending on host factors such as immune status, coexisting diseases, and immunization with bacillus Calmette-Guerin (BCG); microbial factors such as the virulence of the organism and predilection for specific tissue; and the host-microbe interaction.
  - In primary progressive pulmonary tuberculosis, the primary granuloma containing viable bacilli in the lung enlarges rapidly, erodes the bronchial tree, and spreads, a sequence that results in adjacent "satellite" lesions.
  - This process is accompanied by caseous enlargement of the hilar lymph nodes, which may erode through the wall of a bronchus and discharge bacilli, thereby producing tuberculous pneumonia.
  - These highly active lesions may seed the bloodstream with tubercle bacilli and result in life-threatening dissemination of the bacilli.

Latent Tuberculosis Infection

- Latent TB infection (LTBI) is the presence of *M. tuberculosis* organisms without symptoms or radiographic evidence of TB disease.
  - Bacilli are inactive.
  - The tuberculin skin test is positive.
  - Infected persons do not feel sick. Those with latent TB infection are not infectious and cannot spread TB infection to others.
  - Treatment of latent TB infection is required to prevent progression to active disease.
- Targeted tuberculin testing is used to focus on groups at the highest risk for TB. It detects persons who would benefit from treatment and deemphasizes testing of groups that are not at high risk for TB.

Reactivation Tuberculosis (Secondary Tuberculosis)

- Reactivation TB results from reactivation of dormant, endogenous tubercle bacilli in a patient with latent TB infection.
- May develop any time after the primary infection, even decades later.
- Reactivation typically begins in the apical or posterior segments of one or both upper lobes ("Simon's foci") where the organisms were seeded during the primary infection.
- A fibrous capsule surrounds a caseous, acellular center that contains numerous tubercle bacilli.

- From these cavitary nodules the organisms can spread through the lungs and be discharged into the air during bouts of coughing.

Multiple Drug-Resistant Tuberculosis

- Strains of *M. tuberculosis* have emerged that are resistant to the drugs normally used to treat TB.
- About 15% of all TB cases tested involved strains resistant to at least one antituberculosis drug, and 4% were resistant to two of the most effective antituberculosis drugs.

CLINICAL PRESENTATION / PHYSICAL FINDINGS

- Signs and symptoms of pulmonary tuberculosis include:
  - Cough
    - Nearly universal; typically, it is initially dry but then progresses with increasing volumes of purulent secretions and the variable appearance of blood streaking or gross hemoptysis.
  - Fever and night sweats
    - Fever peaks as high as 104.0 to 105.8°F, typically occurring in the evening; however, although most patients with TB complain of feeling feverish, a substantial proportion does not have fever when measured.
  - Weight loss
  - Malaise
  - Lymphadenopathy
  - Nonpleuritic chest pain
  - Localized rales
    - Rales are early findings; coarse rhonchi evolve as secretions become more voluminous and tenacious; signs of lung consolidation are rarely heard.
      - Wheezing and/or regionally diminished breath sounds may be heard in cases with peri- or endobronchial airway compression.
- See Table I-25 for clinical classifications of tuberculosis.

DIAGNOSIS

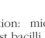

LABORATORY

- Sputum examination: microscopy with acid-fast bacilli (AFB) staining.
  - Recovery of *M. tuberculosis* from a patient's three consecutive morning sputum specimens is advised when attempting to recover *M. tuberculosis* organisms.
- Sputum culture:
  - Definitive diagnosis depends on recovery of *M. tuberculosis* from cultures.
  - Culture is more sensitive than microscopy and can detect much lower numbers of bacilli and allows identification of mycobacterial species and drug susceptibility testing.
  - Disadvantage: culture takes time (1 to 3 weeks for broth cultures and 3 to 8 weeks for solid media).
- Direct identification of mycobacteria by nucleic acid amplification:
  - Ribosomal RNA probes or DNA polymerase chain reaction allow identification within 24 hours.
    - The polymerase chain reaction (PCR) permits rapid detection of mycobacterial DNA and differentiation of *M. tuberculosis* from other mycobacteria.

SPECIAL TESTS

- Tuberculin skin test (TST):
  - Purified protein derivative (PPD) of tuberculin (antigenic culture extracts) is injected intradermally into the volar or dorsal aspect of the forearm; dose is 0.1mL of 5 tuberculin units (intermediate-strength PPD).
  - Within 2 to 10 weeks after infection with *M. tuberculosis* the person develops a positive reaction to the TST.
  - The TST identifies individuals who have been infected at some time with *M. tuberculosis* but does not distinguish between current disease and past infection.
  - A positive TST is commonly the only indication that infection with *M. tuberculosis* has taken place; the majority of pulmonary TB infections are clinically and radiographically inapparent.
  - Both false-positive and false-negative TST reactions occur.
    - The TST will be false-negative in 20-25% of patients at the time of diagnosis.

DIAGNOSTIC IMAGING

- Chest radiograph (CXR) examination:
  - Primary pulmonary TB
    - Small homogeneous infiltrates (usually in the upper lobe)
    - Hilar and paratracheal lymph node enlargement
    - Segmental atelectasis
    - Pleural effusion may be present, especially in adults, sometimes as the sole radiographic abnormality
  - Reactivation pulmonary TB
    - Necrosis
    - Cavitation (especially on apical lordotic views)
    - Fibrosis and hilar retraction
    - Bronchopneumonia
    - Interstitial infiltrates
    - Diffuse miliary pattern possible
- Additional considerations:
  - TB activity is often not established by single CXR examination.

TABLE I-25 Diagnostic Standards and Classification of Tuberculosis (TB) in Adults and Children

Class 0: No TB exposure, not infected	• No history of exposure and a negative tuberculin skin test (if tested).
Class 1: TB exposure, no evidence of infection	• History of exposure but a negative reaction to tuberculin skin test. • Action depends on the degree of exposure and how recent it was. • Significant exposure in the past 3 months warrants a follow-up tuberculin skin test 10 weeks after the last exposure.
Class 2: Latent TB infection, no disease	• Positive reaction to the tuberculin skin test, negative bacteriologic studies (if done), and no clinical or radiographic evidence of active TB.
Class 3: TB, clinically active	• Person must have clinical, bacteriologic and/or radiographic evidence of current TB to fit in this class. • If diagnosis is still pending, the person should be classified as a TB suspect (class 5).
Class 4: TB, not clinically active	• History of previous episode(s) of TB or abnormal stable radiographic findings in a person with a positive tuberculin skin test, negative bacteriologic studies (if done), and no clinical and/or radiographic evidence of current disease.
Class 5: TB suspect (diagnosis pending)	• Diagnosis of TB is being considered (whether or not treatment has been started), and diagnostic procedures have not been completed. • A person should not remain in this class for more than 3 months.

Source: The American Thoracic Society/Centers for Disease Control and Prevention/Infectious Diseases Society of America. *Am J Respir Crit Care Med* 2000;161:1376–1395.

○ Serial CXR examinations are excellent indicators of TB progression or regression.

MEDICAL MANAGEMENT & TREATMENT

PHARMACOLOGIC
Primary TB

- In most circumstances, the treatment regimen for all adults with previously untreated TB should consist of a 2-month initial phase of isoniazid (INH), rifampin (RIF), pyrazinamide (PZA), and ethambutol (EMB). If (when) drug susceptibility test results are known and the organisms are fully susceptible, EMB need not be included.
- The continuation phase of treatment is given for either 4 or 7 months. The 4-month continuation phase should be used in the large majority of patients. The 7-month continuation phase is recommended only for three groups:
  ○ Patients with cavitary pulmonary TB caused by drug-susceptible organisms and whose sputum culture obtained at the time of completion of 2 months of treatment is positive.
  ○ Patients whose initial phase of treatment did not include PZA.
  ○ Patients being treated with once per week INH and rifapentine and whose sputum culture obtained at the time of completion of the initial phase is positive.

Latent TB

- Treatment of latent TB infection for patients infected with *M. tuberculosis* but without active disease (i.e., patients with positive tuberculin skin test results but without signs or symptoms of TB):
  ○ If clinical suspicion for active TB is low, the options are to begin treatment with combination chemotherapy or to defer treatment until additional data have been obtained to clarify the situation (usually within 2 months). Even when the suspicion of active TB is low, treatment for latent TB infection with a single drug should not be initiated until active TB has been excluded.
  ○ Preferred options are INH for 9 months or RIF (with or without INH) for 4 months. RIF and PZA for a total of 2 months can be used for patients not likely to complete a longer regimen and who can be monitored closely.
- Special treatment considerations for TB would include children; patients with HIV/AIDS, extrapulmonary TB, culture-negative TB, or hepatic or renal disease; and women who are pregnant or are breastfeeding.
- Vaccines for tuberculosis:
  ○ A number of live TB vaccines are available and are known collectively

as BCG after the original strain of bacterium used in the vaccine (bacillus Calmette-Guérin).
  ○ A vaccine for the prevention of TB has not been approved in the U.S.

COMPLICATIONS

PRIMARY TB
- Primary progressive TB
  ○ Risk for reactivation TB

REACTIVATION TB
- Miliary TB is the disseminated form of TB and is caused by seeding of the bacilli through lymphatics or blood vessels to produce minute, yellow-white lesions resembling millet seeds (hence "miliary").
- The lung, lymph nodes, kidneys, adrenals, bone marrow, spleen, liver, meninges, brain, eyes, and genitalia are all common sites of miliary lesions.

PROGNOSIS

- Almost all properly treated patients with TB are cured.
  ○ Relapse rates are less than 5% with current regimens.
  ○ The main cause of treatment failure is noncompliance with drug therapy.

DENTAL SIGNIFICANCE

ORAL MANIFESTATIONS
- Oral lesions of TB are uncommon but can occur as nodular, granular, ulcerated, or (rarely) firm, leukoplakic areas; they may occur at any age.
  ○ The reported prevalence of clinically evident oral lesions varies from 0.5–1.5%.
  ○ The classic mucosal lesion is a painful, deep, irregular ulcer on the dorsum of the tongue.
    ▪ The palate, lips, buccal mucosa, and gingiva may also be affected.
  ○ Most of the lesions represent secondary infection from the initial pulmonary lesions.
- The discovery of pulmonary TB as a result of the investigation of oral lesions is unusual but not rare.
  ○ Primary oral TB without pulmonary involvement is rare. The oral involvement of primary TB usually involves the gingiva, mucobuccal fold, and areas of inflammation adjacent to teeth or in extraction sites and is usually associated with enlarged regional lymph nodes.
- Tuberculous osteomyelitis has been reported in the jaws and appears as ill-defined areas of radiolucency.
- Enlargement of the oropharyngeal lymphoid tissues with involvement of the cervical lymph nodes is termed scrofula.

○ This form of TB is rare in North America.
- Biopsy of oral lesions in addition to culture can be diagnostic.
- Lesions that are painful should be managed symptomatically.
- Oral lesions resolve secondary to appropriate TB therapy for active disease.

INFECTION CONTROL ISSUES
- Due to the potential for transmission of *M. tuberculosis* that exists in outpatient settings, dental practices should develop a TB control program appropriate for their level of risk according to the Centers for Disease Control (CDC) guidelines for infection control. See Suggested References following for specific information.
  ○ A community risk assessment should be conducted periodically, and TB infection-control policies for each dental setting should be based on the risk assessment.
  ○ The policies should include provisions for detection and referral of patients who might have undiagnosed active TB and management of patients with active TB who require urgent dental care.
  ○ Staff education, counseling, and tuberculin skin test (TST) screening should be included in the policy.
  ○ Staff who have contact with patients should have a baseline TST, preferably by using a two-step test at the beginning of employment.
  ○ The facility's level of TB risk will determine the need for routine, follow-up TST.

DENTAL MANAGEMENT

- Dental evaluation is directed at the identification of patients with active TB.
- Assess each patient for a history of TB as well as symptoms suggestive of active TB during all initial medical histories and at periodic updates.
  ○ The medical history should include questions regarding the presence of TB in family members as well as other (i.e., occupational) sources of exposure to TB.
  ○ The patient should be questioned about the presence of signs and symptoms suggestive of TB (i.e., fever, chills, night sweats, bloody sputum production, weight loss).
  ○ Record dates and results of prior TSTs.
  ○ Patients with a history of TB should be asked about:
    ▪ The degree of disease involvement
    ▪ The type and duration of therapy received
    ▪ The current status of disease activity
      - A medical consult with the patient's physician will usually be necessary to obtain and/or confirm this information.

- Patients with a medical history or symptoms indicative of undiagnosed active TB should be referred promptly for medical evaluation to determine possible infectiousness.
  - Such patients should not remain in the dental care facility any longer than required to evaluate their dental condition and arrange a referral.
  - While in the dental office, the patient should be isolated from other patients and staff, wear a surgical mask when not being evaluated, or be instructed to cover their mouth and nose when coughing or sneezing.
  - Elective dental treatment should be deferred until a physician confirms that a patient does not have infectious TB or, if the patient is diagnosed with active TB disease, until it is confirmed that the patient is no longer infectious.
- If urgent dental care is provided for a patient who has or is suspected of having active TB disease, the care should be provided in a facility (e.g., hospital) that provides airborne infection isolation (i.e., using such engineering controls as TB isolation rooms, negatively pressured relative to the corridors, with air either exhausted to the outside or HEPA-filtered if recirculation is necessary).
  - Standard surgical face masks do not protect against TB transmission.
- Patients with recently diagnosed, clinically active TB may be treated in the office after receiving therapy for several weeks and have been confirmed by their physician to be noninfectious.
- Patients reporting a past history of TB should be followed up with complete medical history, including diagnosis, dates of treatment, and type of treatment.
  - Treatment duration of less than 18 months, if treated in the past, or of 9 months, if treated recently, would require consultation with the physician to determine the patient's status.
- Patients with a positive TST (recent conversion to positive tuberculin skin test) should be viewed as having been infected with TB.
  - The patient should give a history of being evaluated for active disease.
  - Once the patient is under medical treatment and confirmed by a physician to be absent of clinically active disease, they can be treated in a normal manner. No special precautions are required.

SUGGESTED REFERENCES

Centers for Disease Control and Prevention: guidelines in infection control in dental health-care settings—2003. *MMWR* 2003; 52(RR-17):1–68.

Centers for Disease Control and Prevention, National Center for HIV, STD, and TB Prevention, Division of Tuberculosis Elimination: www.cdc.gov/nchstp/tb/default.htm

Iseman M. Tuberculosis, in Goldman L, Ausiello D (eds): *Cecil Textbook of Medicine*. Philadelphia, WB Saunders, 2004, pp 1894–1902.

Little J, Falace D, Miller C, Rhodus N. *Dental Management of the Medically Compromised Patient*. St Louis, Mosby, 2002, pp 136–144.

Miller C, Palenik C. *Infection Control & Management of Hazardous Materials for the Dental Team*. St Louis, Elsevier Mosby, 2005, pp 98–103.

Official statement of the American Thoracic Society and the Centers for Disease Control: diagnostic standards and classification of tuberculosis in adults and children. *Am J Respir Crit Car Med* 2000;161:1376–1395.

AUTHOR: **THERESA G. MAYFIELD, DMD**

SYNONYM(S)

Ulcerative enteritis
Colitis
Inflammatory bowel disease

ICD-9CM/CPT CODE(S)

556.9 Ulcerative colitis, unspecified

OVERVIEW

A chronic, inflammatory condition of the colon or rectal mucosa.

EPIDEMIOLOGY & DEMOGRAPHICS

INCIDENCE/PREVALENCE IN USA: The annual incidence in the U.S. is approximately 10 to 12 cases per 100,000 individuals. The prevalence rate is 35 to 100 cases per 100,000 individuals. The incidence of ulcerative colitis has been reported to be two to four times higher in Jewish people, but not in the U.S. Ulcerative colitis occurs more frequently among Caucasians and less often in those of South American, Asian, and African descent.
PREDOMINANT AGE: There is a bimodal distribution of the incidence in patients aged 15 to 25 years and 55 to 65 years old; however, it can occur at any age.
PREDOMINANT SEX: Ulcerative colitis affects 30% more females than males.
GENETICS: Genetic susceptibility has been identified as associated with chromosomes 12 and 16. A family history of ulcerative colitis is associated with a higher risk for developing the condition.

ETIOLOGY & PATHOGENESIS

- Although the etiology remains unclear, ulcerative colitis is believed to be an autoimmune phenomenon. Both serum and mucosal autoantibodies are detectable against intestinal epithelial cells. There is an imbalance of humoral and cell-mediated immunity, which may be related to enhanced reactivity against intestinal bacterial antigens. The central event that appears to be the pathogenesis of ulcerative colitis is the loss of tolerance against indigenous enteric flora. Environmental factors and genetics may also play a role in the etiology of ulcerative colitis.
- In ulcerative colitis, the inflammatory response is largely confined to the mucosa and submucosa. It usually affects the colon or rectal mucosa and extends in a confluent and contiguous manner, generally with clearly demarcated borders between normal and abnormal areas.

CLINICAL PRESENTATION / PHYSICAL FINDINGS

- The hallmark of ulcerative colitis is bloody diarrhea with each bowel movement. It may be accompanied by abdominal pain, weight loss, and anemia. Rectal symptoms such as urgency and frequency may also be present.
- Extracolonic manifestations may include synovitis, ankylosing spondylitis, sacroiliitis, erythema nodosum, pyoderma gangrenosum, iritis, aphthous stomatitis, renal stones, and primary sclerosing cholangitis.
- Physical findings may include mild fever, tachycardia, dehydration, malnutrition, abdominal tenderness, and blood on rectal digital examination.

DIAGNOSIS

- Serologic testing can help obtain a diagnosis. A negative ASCA and positive p-ANCA antigen is strongly suggestive of ulcerative colitis. Ten to 15% of patients with inflammatory bowel disease cannot be clearly defined as having either ulcerative colitis or Crohn's disease. These patients are said to have "indeterminate colitis."
- Laboratory, radiologic, endoscopic, and histologic findings can all contribute to the diagnosis of ulcerative colitis. Laboratory studies often reveal anemia due to chronic blood loss. Elevated sedimentation rate and elevated C-reactive protein both correlate with disease activity. Other nonspecific laboratory findings in ulcerative colitis include thrombocytosis, hypoalbuminemia, hypokalemia, hypomagnesemia, and elevated alkaline phosphatase.
- Imaging studies such as plain abdominal radiographs may demonstrate colonic dilation or toxic megacolon in some cases. Barium enemas are used only in mild cases since their use may precipitate complications. A CT scan may help detect biliary dilation, which is suggestive of primary sclerosing cholangitis. Radionucleotide scans may be used when colonoscopy or barium enemas are contraindicated.
- Colitis can be diagnosed using flexible sigmoidoscopy. During a colonoscopy, a biopsy can confirm the diagnosis of ulcerative colitis. Colonoscopy can also detect the extent of disease involvement, monitor disease activity, and detect potentially malignant lesions.

MEDICAL MANAGEMENT & TREATMENT

- Therapy for ulcerative colitis is based on severity of disease. The goals of pharmacotherapy are to reduce morbidity and prevent complications.
- Sulfasalazine (Azulfidine) and other 5-amino salicylic acid agents are administered to reduce inflammation.
- In severe cases, immunosuppressants such as azathioprine, cyclosporine, and 6-mercaptopurine are used to inhibit activity of the immune system.
- Corticosteroids are used in severe active cases to induce remission. Long-term use of corticosteroids can lead to many adverse effects.
- Severe colitis is treated with ciprofloxacin or metronidazole.
- Approximately 25% of patients with refractory ulcerative colitis require surgical intervention, which is usually colectomy. This surgical procedure is curative.

COMPLICATIONS

- Toxic megacolon occurs in approximately 2–3% of cases of ulcerative colitis.
- In patients with ulcerative colitis, there is an increased risk of developing colon carcinoma. The risk of cancer is highest in patients with pancolitis of 10 or more years' duration, in whom it is twentyfold to thirtyfold higher than in a control population. Colonoscopies are recommended every 1 to 2 years in patients with extensive colitis, beginning 8 to 10 years after diagnosis.

PROGNOSIS

- Most cases of ulcerative colitis are controlled with pharmacotherapy; however, response to treatment is highly variable.
- Prognosis is worse when there is involvement of the entire colon.
- The patient will typically experience periods of remission and exacerbation.
- In severe cases, colectomy is curative.

DENTAL SIGNIFICANCE

- Oral manifestations of ulcerative colitis are less common than in Crohn's disease. Oral lesions generally do not present in undiagnosed disease.
  - Aphthous ulcers and angular cheilitis develop in 5–10% of patients and may arise during the active phase of disease and disappear as the colitis resolves.
  - Pyostomatitis vegetans is also known to affect patients with ulcerative colitis and often aids in the diagnosis. This condition produces raised, erythematous, papillary, or vegetative projections of the labial mucosa, gingiva, and palate. The tongue rarely is involved.

DENTAL MANAGEMENT

- Aside from potential drug interactions and adverse effects, patients with ulcerative colitis are not at greater risk for infection or bleeding from the disease.

- Medications used for treatment should be carefully assessed (consultation with the patient's physician is recommended if the patient is taking immunosuppressive medications).
  - Assess the risk for adrenal suppression and insufficiency in patients being treated with systemic corticosteroids (see Appendix A, Box A-4, "Dental Management of Patients at Risk for Acute Adrenal Insufficiency").
  - Patients who are taking cytotoxic or immunosuppressive drugs, including systemic corticosteroids, may have an increased risk of infection and may require perioperative prophylactic antibiotics (see Appendix A, Box A-2, "Presurgical and Post-surgical Antibiotic Prophylaxis for Patients at Increased Risk for Postoperative Infections").
- Broad-spectrum antibiotics such as clindamycin should be avoided in patients taking sulfasalazine because they could reduce the bacterial flora of the colon, leading to diminished cleavage of sulfasalazine.

SUGGESTED REFERENCES

Chutkan RK. Inflammatory bowel disease. *Primary Care* 2001;28(3):539–556.

Jewell DP. Ulcerative colitis, in Feldman M, Friedman LS, Sleisenger MH (eds): *Sleisinger & Fordtran's Gastrointestinal and Liver Disease*, ed 7. St Louis, WB Saunders, 2002, pp 2039–2067.

AUTHOR: ERNESTA PARISI, DMD

SYNONYM(S)

Chicken pox
Shingles
Herpes zoster

ICD-9CM/CPT CODE(S)

052.9 Varicella/chicken pox
053.9 Herpes zoster/shingles

OVERVIEW

- Varicella is a common viral illness characterized by acute onset of generalized vesicular rash and fever.
- Herpes zoster is caused by a reactivation of the varicella-zoster virus. Following the primary infection (varicella), the virus remains latent in the dorsal root ganglia and reemerges when there is a weakening of the immune system (secondary to disease or advanced age).

EPIDEMIOLOGY & DEMOGRAPHICS

VARICELLA

INCIDENCE/PREVALENCE IN USA:
Varicella is extremely contagious. More than 90% of unvaccinated contacts become infected. Peak incidence is in the springtime.
PREDOMINANT AGE: 5 to 10 years old.
PREDOMINANT SEX: Male = female.
GENETICS: None established.

ZOSTER

INCIDENCE/PREVALENCE IN USA:
215 per 100,000 per year; occurs in 10–20% of the population at some time. There is an increased incidence in immunocompromised patients, the elderly, and children who acquired varicella when younger than 2 months old.
PREDOMINANT AGE: Incidence increases with age. Eighty percent of cases occur in persons over age 20 years (2 to 3 per 1000, age 20 to 50; 10 per 1000, > 80 years).
PREDOMINANT SEX: Male = Female.
GENETICS: None established.

ETIOLOGY & PATHOGENESIS

VARICELLA

- Varicella-zoster virus (VZV) is the human herpes virus III (HHV-3) that can manifest as varicella or herpes zoster.

ZOSTER

- Reactivation of VZV.

CLINICAL PRESENTATION / PHYSICAL FINDINGS

VARICELLA

Findings vary with clinical course.
- The incubation period of varicella ranges from 9 to 21 days.
- Initial symptoms consist of fever, chills, backache, generalized malaise, and headache.
- Symptoms are generally more severe in adults.

- Initial lesions generally occur on the trunk and occasionally on the face; these lesions consist primarily of 3- to 4-mm red papules with an irregular outline and a clear vesicle on the surface.
- Intense pruritus generally accompanies this stage.
- New lesion development generally stops by the fourth day with subsequent crusting by the sixth day.
- Lesions generally spread to the face and the extremities.
- Infectious period begins 2 days before onset of clinical symptoms and lasts until all the lesions have crusted.
- Crusts generally fall off within 5 to 14 days.
- Fever is usually highest during the eruption of vesicles; temperature generally returns to normal following disappearance of vesicles.
- Excoriations may be present if scratching is prominent.

ZOSTER

- Pain generally precedes skin manifestation by 3 to 5 days and is generally localized to the dermatome that will be affected by the skin lesions.
- Constitutional symptoms are often present (e.g., fever, malaise, headache).
- The initial rash consists of erythematous maculopapules generally affecting one dermatome (thoracic region in a majority of cases); some patients (< 50%) may have scattered vesicles outside of the affected dermatome.
- The initial maculopapules evolve into vesicles and pustules by the third or fourth day.
- The vesicles have an erythematous base, are cloudy, and are of various sizes.
- The vesicles subsequently become umbilicated and then form crusts that generally fall off within 3 weeks; scarring may occur.
- Pain during and after the rash is generally significant.

DIAGNOSIS

VARICELLA

- Diagnosis is usually made based on patient's history and clinical presentation.
- CBC may reveal leukopenia and thrombocytopenia.
- Direct fluorescent assay (DFA) and viral culture will be positive for virus if infection is present.
- Serum varicella titers will show significant rise in serum varicella IgG antibody level if infection is present.

ZOSTER

- Diagnosis is usually made on patient's history and clinical presentation.
- DFA and viral culture will be positive for virus if infection is present.

MEDICAL MANAGEMENT & TREATMENT

VARICELLA

- Nonpharmacologic:
  - Antipruritic lotions, antihistamines for symptomatic relief.
  - Avoid scratching to prevent excoriations.
  - Use a mild soap for bathing.
- Pharmacologic:
  - Use of acetaminophen for fever and myalgias; aspirin should be avoided because of the increased risk of Reye's syndrome.
  - Oral acyclovir initiated at the earliest sign (within 24 hours of illness) is useful in healthy, nonpregnant individuals 13 years of age or older to decrease the duration and severity of signs and symptoms. Immunocompromised patients should be treated with IV acyclovir for 7 to 10 days.
  - Varicella-zoster immunoglobulin (VZIG) is effective in preventing varicella in susceptible individuals. May repeat dose 3 weeks later if the exposure persists. VZIG must be administered as early as possible after presumed exposure.
  - Varicella vaccine is available for children and adults; protection lasts at least 6 years. Patients with HIV or other immunocompromised patients should not receive the live, attenuated vaccine.

ZOSTER

- Nonpharmacologic:
  - Wet compresses applied for 15 to 30 minutes, 5 to 10 times a day are useful to break vesicles and remove serum and crust.
- Pharmacologic:
  - Gabapentin is effective in the treatment of pain and sleep interference associated with postherpetic neuralgia (PHN).
  - Lidocaine patch 5% is also effective in relieving PHN. Patches are applied to intact skin to cover the most painful area for up to 12 hours within a 24-hour period.
  - Oral antiviral agents can decrease acute pain, inflammation, and vesicle formation when treatment is begun within 48 hours of onset of rash. Treatment options include:
    - Acyclovir 800 mg, 5 times daily, for 7 to 10 days
    - Valacyclovir 1000 mg, 3 times daily for 7 days
    - Famciclovir 500 mg, 3 times daily, for 7 days
  - Immunocompromised patients should be treated with IV acyclovir for 7 days, with close monitoring of renal function and adequate hydration; vidarabine is also an effective treat-

ment of disseminated herpes zoster in immunocompromised patients.

○ Patients with AIDS and transplant patients may develop acyclovir-resistant varicella-zoster; these patients can be treated with foscarnet continued for at least 10 days or until lesions are completely healed.

○ Capsaicin cream can be useful for treatment of PHN. It is generally applied 3 to 5 times daily for several weeks after the crusts have fallen off.

○ Sympathetic blocks with 0.25% bupivicaine and rhizotomy are reserved for severe cases unresponsive to conservative treatment.

○ Corticosteroids should be considered in older patients if there are no contraindications. When used, there is a decrease in the use of analgesics and time to resumption of usual activities, but there is no effect on the incidence and duration of PHN.

COMPLICATIONS

VARICELLA
- Bacterial skin infections
- Neurologic complications
- Pneumonia
- Hepatitis

ZOSTER
- Secondary bacterial infection with *S. aureus* or *S. pyogenes*
- Postherpetic neuralgia

PROGNOSIS

VARICELLA
- The course is generally benign in immunocompetent adults and children.
- Infants who develop varicella and are incapable of controlling the infection should be given VZIG.

ZOSTER
- The incidence of PHN (defined as pain that persists more than 30 days after onset of rash) increases with age (30% by age 40, > 70% by age 70).
- The incidence of disseminated herpes zoster is increased in immunocompromised hosts.
- Immunocompromised hosts are more prone to neurologic complications. The mortality rate is 10–20% in immunocompromised patients with disseminated zoster.
- Motor neuropathies occur in 5% of all cases of zoster; complete recovery occurs in > 70% of patients.

DENTAL SIGNIFICANCE

VARICELLA
- Vesicles attributed to varicella may appear on the face and in the perioral region but are not common in the oral cavity.

ZOSTER
- Zoster infections commonly appear on the face and in the perioral region as well as in the oral cavity.
- The ophthalmologic branch of the trigeminal nerve is most commonly affected, followed by the maxillary and mandibular branches, respectively. Intraoral vesicles appear unilaterally, which is pathognomonic for a zoster infection. Postherpetic neuralgia involving the affected branch of the trigeminal nerve is relatively common.
- Herpes zoster may involve the geniculate ganglion of cranial nerve VII. This can cause facial palsy and a painful ear, with the presence of vesicles in the mouth, on the pinna and external auditory canal (Ramsay-Hunt syndrome).

DENTAL MANAGEMENT

VARICELLA
- Evaluate for intraoral vesicles due to varicella infection (rare). If vesicles are present, consider performing DFA/viral culture to confirm diagnosis.
- Consider deferring elective dental treatment for patients with active varicella infection to avoid reinoculation with virus.

ZOSTER
- If the patient has intraoral lesions, complete DFA/viral culture to determine if VZV is present.
- Consider deferring elective dental treatment for patients with active zoster lesions on exposed surfaces to avoid reinoculation with virus.
- Manage patients with antivirals and corticosteroids to reduce possibility of PHN; refer to specialist for management, if necessary.

SUGGESTED REFERENCES

Ferri FF. Chickenpox, in Ferri FF (ed): *Ferri's Clinical Advisor: Instant Diagnosis and Treatment*. St Louis, Mosby, 2005, p 184.

Ferri FF. Herpes zoster, in Ferri FF (ed): *Ferri's Clinical Advisor: Instant Diagnosis and Treatment*. St Louis, Mosby, 2005, p 384.

Gnann JW, Whitley RJ. Herpes zoster. *N Engl J Med* 2002;347:340.

Stoopler ET. Oral herpetic infections (HSV-1–8). *Dent Clin North Am* 2005;49:15.

Stoopler ET, Pinto A, DeRossi SS, Sollecito TP. Herpes simplex and varicella-zoster infections: clinical and laboratory diagnosis. *Gen Dent* 2003;51:281.

AUTHOR: **ERIC T. STOOPLER, DMD**

SYNONYM(S)

Angiohemophilia
Constitutional thrombopathy
Factor VIII deficiency with vascular defect
Pseudohemophilia type B
Vascular hemophilia
Von Willebrand's-Jurgens' disease

ICD-9CM/CPT CODE(S)

286.4 Von Willebrand's disease complete

OVERVIEW

Von Willebrand's disease (vWD) is characterized by a quantitative or qualitative deficiency of von Willebrand factor (vWF) that leads to a compound problem of both a qualitative platelet defect and a deficiency of coagulation Factor VIII. The platelet disorder appears as a reduction of the adhesion of platelets to the vascular subendothelium and to each other.

EPIDEMIOLOGY & DEMOGRAPHICS

INCIDENCE/PREVALENCE IN USA: Clinically significant vWD affects approximately 125 persons per million population, with severe disease affecting approximately 0.5 to 5 persons per million population.
PREDOMINANT AGE: Bleeding symptoms may occur at any age, even just after or during birth.
PREDOMINANT SEX: Male = Female.
GENETICS: Most cases (75–80%) are believed to have an autosomal dominant inheritance pattern, although some cases appear recessive. The vWF gene is located near the tip of the short arm of chromosome 12.

ETIOLOGY & PATHOGENESIS

- In vWD, there is deficient or defective von Willebrand factor (vWF), a protein that mediates platelet adhesion. Von Willebrand factor is synthesized in megakaryocytes and endothelial cells and circulates in plasma. Von Willebrand factor has a separate function of binding the Factor VIII coagulant protein (Factor VIII:C) and protecting it from degradation; therefore, a deficiency of vWF gives rise to a secondary decrease in Factor VIII levels.
- More than 20 variants of vWD have been described, which can be grouped into three major categories:
  - Type I: generally characterized mild to moderate quantitative deficiency in vWF (i.e., approximately 20–50% of normal levels) resulting in relatively mild abnormal bleeding. It accounts for approximately 75% of the cases of vWD.
  - Type II: characterized by qualitative defects in vWF and is further divided into four variants (IIA, IIB, IIN, and

IIM) based on the characteristics of the dysfunctional vWF. Types II accounts for 20–25% of the cases of vWD and is associated with mild to moderate bleeding.
  - Type III: the most rare variant of vWD with an incidence of 0.5 to 5.3 per million and appears to result from the inheritance of a mutant vWF gene from both parents. It is also the most severe and is associated with very little or no detectable plasma or platelet vWF, resulting in a profound bleeding disorder.

CLINICAL PRESENTATION / PHYSICAL FINDINGS

- Familial history of prolonged bleeding/vWD.
- Patient history of:
  - Easy bruising.
  - Menorrhagia (affects 50–75% of women and may be the initial symptom).
  - Mucosal bleeding (e.g., gingival, epistaxis); gastrointestinal bleeding is rare.
  - Prolonged bleeding after minor trauma to skin or mucous membranes (characteristic of vWD).
  - Heavy bleeding is common after tooth extraction or other oral surgery such as tonsillectomy and adenoidectomy.
  - Severe hemorrhage after major surgery is less common, but delayed bleeding may occur up to several weeks after surgery.
- Most patients with vWD have mild disease that may go undiagnosed until trauma or surgery.
- Bleeding tendency increases with use of antiplatelet aggregation drugs (e.g., aspirin, NSAIDs, clopidogrel).
- Bleeding tendency decreases during pregnancy and estrogen or oral contraceptive use.

DIAGNOSIS

- Bleeding time (BT): usually prolonged; however, a prolonged BT is not specific for vWD.
- Closure time (CT) (PFA-100® test): will be abnormally elevated with both collagen/epinephrine (CEPI) and collagen/adenosine-diphosphate (CADP) membranes.
- Partial thromboplastin time (PTT): mildly prolonged in approximately 50% of patients with vWD.
- Platelet count (PC): usually normal.

MEDICAL MANAGEMENT & TREATMENT

- Desmopressin acetate (DDAVP) is administered prophylactically prior to minor surgical proce-

dures or with posttraumatic bleeding in mild type I vWD.
  - Dose is 0.3 µg/kg in 100 mL of normal saline solution IV infused > 20 minutes.
  - DDAVP is also available as a nasal spray (dose of 150-µg spray administered to each nostril).
  - Typically, a maximal rise of vWF and Factor VIII is observed within 30 to 60 minutes for both IV- and intranasally-administered DDAVP.
  - DDAVP is not effective in type IIA vWD and is potentially dangerous in type IIB (increased risk of bleeding and thrombocytopenia).
- In patients with severe vWD, replacement therapy in the form of cryoprecipitate is the method of choice.
  - The standard dose is 1 bag of cryoprecipitate per 10 kg of body weight.
- Factor VIII concentrate rich in vWF (Humate-P, Armour) is useful to correct bleeding abnormalities.
- Life-threatening hemorrhage unresponsive to therapy with cryoprecipitate or Factor VIII concentrate may require transfusion of normal platelets.

COMPLICATIONS

- Spontaneous bleeding is rare.
- Soft tissue bleeding can occur after trauma or infection.
- Viral hepatitis, HIV infection secondary to contaminated cryoprecipitates (now rare).

PROGNOSIS

- Most patients have minor bleeding complications and are able to lead a normal life.
- The use of recombinant or sterile factor replacement transfusions has reduced the risk of bloodborne diseases. The reduction of fear of becoming infected has led to better management of the disease.
- Genetic counseling has helped to educate patients on the risks to their children.

DENTAL SIGNIFICANCE

- Excessive bleeding after invasive dental treatment or oral surgery.
  - See Dental Significance in "Coagulopathies (Clotting Factor Defects, Acquired)," Section I, p 58 for additional information.
- Aggressive treatment of oral infections and establishment of good oral hygiene is necessary.

DENTAL MANAGEMENT

- Consultation with physician:

○ Obtain results of current PTT, BT, or CT prior to invasive dental treatment; however, results of BT or CT do not always correlate with bleeding propensity after replacement therapy.

- See the preceding Medical Management & Treatment section for use of DDAVP prior to oral surgical procedures.

- Local hemostatic measures [e.g., absorbable gelatin sponges (Gelfoam®), oxidized cellulose (SURGICEL™), micro-fibrillar collagen (Avitene®), topical thrombin, tranexamic acid, epsilon-aminocaproic acid (EACA), sutures, and surgical splints and stents].

- Examine patient 24 hours after dental procedure for hemostasis and signs of infection.

- Avoid use of aspirin or NSAIDs.

SUGGESTED REFERENCE

Camm JH, Murata SM. Emergency dental management of a patient with von Willebrand's disease. *Endod Dent Traumaltol* 1992;8: 176–181.

AUTHORS: **WENDY S. HUPP, DMD;** **F. JOHN FIRRIOLO, DDS, PHD**

SYNONYM(S)

None

ICD-9CM/CPT CODE(S)
446.4 Wegener's granulomatosis

OVERVIEW

Wegener's granulomatosis (WG) is a granulomatous, necrotizing vasculitis of small arteries, arterioles, and capillaries involving the upper and lower respiratory tract and kidneys and, less commonly, the eyes, joints, skin, and neurologic and cardiac tissue.

EPIDEMIOLOGY & DEMOGRAPHICS

INCIDENCE/PREVALENCE IN USA: Incidence estimated at approximately 0.4/100,000; prevalence 3/100,000.
PREDOMINANT AGE: Mean age at diagnosis is 20 to 40 years but can occur in all age groups; the reported age range is 8 to 99 years.
PREDOMINANT SEX: Occurs predominantly in males (3:2).
GENETICS: WG may have a possible genetic association with higher prevalences reported among small numbers of patients expressing HLA-DR1 and HLA-DQw7; however, larger studies have failed to identify any unique genetic markers.

ETIOLOGY & PATHOGENESIS

- The etiology of WG remains unknown; however, clinical and histopathologic features of WG support an autoimmune origin for the disease. See "Wegener's Granulomatosis" in Section II, p 337 for more information on action of antibodies.
- The characteristic histopathology in WG is necrotizing, granulomatous vasculitis involving small arteries and veins, most reliably found on biopsies of the lung. Specific pathologic findings in WG include:
  - Lung: granulomatous arteritis involving vessels of all sizes, classically medium-sized arteries.
  - Upper airways: granulomatous inflammation frequently seen, although not specific unless showing actual vasculitis.
  - Kidney: necrotizing and crescentic glomerulonephritis without immunofluorescent staining (pauci-immune) is common; granulomatous vasculitis rarely seen.
  - Skin: vasculitic lesions from leukocytoclastic vasculitis of small vessels; granulomatous arteritis seen occasionally.

CLINICAL PRESENTATION / PHYSICAL FINDINGS

WG is classically associated with a triad of pulmonary, renal, and head and neck manifestations; however, the clinical manifestations of WG often vary with the stage of the disease and degree of organ involvement. Clinicopathologic findings in WG include:

- Upper airway (90–95%): sinusitis, serous otitis media, rhinitis, nasal ulcerations/septal perforation, epistaxis, oral ulcerations, "saddle nose" deformity (later), headaches.
- Lower airway (90–95%): cough, dyspnea, hemoptysis, pulmonary infiltrates (may be fleeting or persistent), nodules, cavities, pleural effusions/pleuritis, subglottic stenosis, endobronchial lesions, interstitial lung disease.
- Kidneys (75%): urinary sediment abnormalities (microscopic hematuria, casts, proteinuria), with or without renal insufficiency, nephrotic syndrome, hypertension.
- Musculoskeletal (70–90%): polyarthalgias; myalgias; monoarthritis, oligoarthritis, or polyarthritis (may be in a rheumatoid pattern); myositis; muscle weakness.
- Eye (50–65%): conjunctivitis, scleritis/episcleritis, uveitis, proptosis, nasolacrimal duct obstruction, orbital mass lesions, retinal vasculitis, corneoscleral ulceration.
- Skin (50%): palpable purpura, subcutaneous nodules, petechiae, vesicles, ulcers, Raynaud's phenomenon, digital ischemia, livedo reticularis, necrotic papules, pyoderma gangrenosum-type lesions (rare).
- Neurologic (20–25%): mononeuritis multiplex, peripheral neuropathy, cranial neuropathy, central nervous system vasculitis (cerebral hemorrhage, cerebritis, syncope, diabetes insipidus).
- Cardiac (20%): pericarditis, pancarditis, cardiomyopathy, dysrhythmias, coronary arteritis.
- Gastrointestinal (15–30%): alkaline phosphatase and/or aminotransferase elevations, granulomatous hepatitis/triaditis, small bowel vasculitis, ascites, splenic granulomatous vasculitis.
- Miscellaneous (< 1–5%): involvement of the breast, prostate, testicle, pinnae, urethra, ureter, lymph nodes, parotid, pulmonary or temporal artery, vagina, other.
- Constitutional: fatigue, weight loss, fever, malaise, anorexia.

(From Goldman L, et al. (eds): *Cecil Textbook of Medicine*, ed 21. Philadelphia, WB Saunders, 2000, p 1530.)

DIAGNOSIS

LABORATORY TESTS

- Positive indirect immunofluorescence for serum antibodies directed against cytoplasmic components of neutrophils with a cytoplasmic pattern of staining (c-ANCA) is detected in a majority (60–90%) of patients with WG and is highly specific (+90%).
- Biopsy of one or more affected organs should be attempted, with the lung as the most reliable source for tissue diagnosis. Lesions in the nasopharynx (if present) can be easily biopsied.
- See "Wegener's Granulomatosis" in Section II, p 337 for information on complete blood count (CBC), urinalysis, serum chemistry, and rheumatologic tests.

IMAGING STUDIES

- Chest radiograph may reveal bilateral nodular pulmonary densities often with central necrosis and cavitation. Local infiltrates or more diffuse interstitial involvement may also be seen, as are radiographic findings of pulmonary hemorrhage.
- Radiographs of the upper airways may reveal chronic otitis and sinusitis, often with evidence of erosion into bony structures.
- CT scans of sinuses are useful in demonstrating mucosal and bony involvement.

MEDICAL MANAGEMENT & TREATMENT

GENERAL MEASURES

- Ensure proper airway drainage.
- Give nutritional counseling.

PHARMACOLOGIC THERAPY

- Prednisone 60 to 80 mg/day and cyclophosphamide 2 mg/kg/day are generally effective and are used to control clinical manifestations; once the disease comes under control, prednisone is tapered and cyclophosphamide is continued.
- Trimethoprim/sulfamethoxazole (TMP-SMX) therapy may represent a useful alternative in patients with lesions limited to the upper and/or lower respiratory tracts in absence of vasculitis or nephritis. Treatment with TMP-SMX (160 mg to 800 mg bid) also reduces the incidence of relapses in patients with WG in remission.
- See "Wegener's Granulomatosis" in Section II, p 337 for more information on treatment.

COMPLICATIONS

- Renal failure
- Interstitial lung disease
- Deafness from refractory otitis
- Necrotic pulmonary nodules with hemoptysis
- Foot drop from peripheral nerve disease
- Destructive nasal lesions with saddle nose deformity
- Skin ulcers; digital and limb gangrene from peripheral vascular involvement
- Treatment-related drug toxicity is significant in WG, especially from the typical therapy of daily oral cyclophosphamide continued for 12 months

after the patient achieves remission that has resulted in severe toxicity, including:

- A 2.4-fold increased risk of all malignancies
- A 33-fold increase in bladder cancer
- An 11-fold increase in the likelihood of lymphoma or leukemia
- A 60% chance of ovarian failure

PROGNOSIS

Without treatment, WG is almost uniformly fatal, with a 10% 2-year survival and mean survival of 5 months. With aggressive treatment, survival improves to 75–90% at 5 years.

DENTAL SIGNIFICANCE

While oral manifestations of WG are not seen in the majority of patients with the disease, multiple oral findings have been reported in some patients and include:

- Oral mucosal ulcerations (ulcerative stomatitis): nonspecific, deep ulcerations on any surface of the oral and oropharyngeal mucosa are the most common oral manifestation of WG, occurring in 26% of patients. The oral ulcerations are usually seen in the later stages of WG, with more than 60% of patients also demonstrating renal involvement.
- Florid granular gingival hyperplasia ("strawberry gingivitis"): the most char-

acteristic (pathognomonic) manifestation of WG, even though it is less common than oral mucosal ulcerations. It may be an early manifestation of WG and occurs before renal involvement in most cases. These gingival lesions are characterized by multiple, short bulbous or granular projections that are red to purplish in color, friable, and hemorrhagic. The buccal attached gingival surfaces are more frequently affected, beginning in the interdental papilla and spreading laterally to the adjacent areas. Destruction of the periodontium, including alveolar bone loss, tooth mobility, and tooth loss have been reported.

- Unilateral or bilateral enlargement of the submandibular or parotid glands (leading to decreased salivary function) due to primary involvement of the granulomatous process may occur early in the course of WG or in limited forms of the disease, although it is a relatively rare manifestation.
- Other less common oral manifestations of WG include labial mucosal nodules, oral-antral fistulae, delayed healing of tooth extraction sites, and osteonecrosis and ulceration of the palate from nasal extension.
- Neuropathy of the facial nerve may be present.

DENTAL MANAGEMENT

There are no unique measures for the dental management of a patient with

WG; however, some general guidelines would include:

- Coordinating any dental treatment with the patient's physician and addressing any systemic complications secondary to WG, such as renal failure.
- Remaining watchful for any drug toxicities and complications associated with treatment, including those related to immunosuppression such as infections.
- Understanding that the underlying vasculitic properties of WG combined with the use of corticosteroids in its treatment frequently results in poor wound healing, especially when the disease is in its active state.
- Sialogogues and fluoride treatment should be considered if salivary hypo function is present.

See also "Wegener's Granulomatosis" in Section II, p 337.

SUGGESTED REFERENCES

Gubbels SP. Head and neck manifestations of Wegener's granulomatosis. *Otolaryngol Clin North Am* 2003;36(4):685–705.

Hoffman GS, et al. Wegener's granulomatosis: an analysis of 158 patients. *Ann Intern Med* 1992;115:488–498.

Regan MJ, et al. Treatment of Wegener's granulomatosis. *Rheum Dis Clin North Am* 2001;27:863.

AUTHORS: **F. JOHN FIRRIOLO, DDS, PHD; THOMAS P. SOLLECITO, DMD**

Oral and Maxillofacial Pathology

SYNONYM(S)

"Lumpy jaw"
Cervicofacial actinomycosis
Actinomycetes
Actinomyces

ICD-9CM/CPT CODE(S)

039.9 Actinomycotic infections
CPT General Exam or Consultation
(e.g., 99243 or 99213)

OVERVIEW

An acute, deep, suppurative abscess of the upper neck, perioral area, and/or jaws with an associated draining sinus tract containing sulfur granules. The process is most commonly caused by the filamentous, branching, facultative, anaerobic, gram-positive bacteria *Actinomyces israelii*.

EPIDEMIOLOGY & DEMOGRAPHICS

INCIDENCE/PREVALENCE: Approximately 1 case per 300,000; no racial predilection.
PREDOMINANT AGE: Young adults.
PREDOMINANT SEX: Men affected 3:1 over women.
GENETICS: No genetic predilection.

ETIOLOGY & PATHOGENESIS

Causative organisms include:
- *A. naeslundii*
- *A. viscosus*
- *A. odontolyticus*
- *A. meyeri*

Risk factors include:
- Extensive tooth decay
- Maxillofacial trauma
- Oral surgical procedures
- Periodontal surgical procedures

CLINICAL PRESENTATION / PHYSICAL FINDINGS

- Signs include swelling, induration, and firm nodularity on the cheek or neck, subperiosteal jaw, or oral cavity due to fibrosis. Nodules often observed as being "woody hard."
- Spontaneously occurring abscesses and drainage tracts with surrounding granulations that discharge yellow-gold granules containing the organism.
- Limited jaw opening many months following trauma or tooth removal.
- Pyrexia.
- Osteolysis is a common feature in patients with actinomycosis.

DIAGNOSIS

- Histopathologic examination can confirm the presence of *Actinomyces*.
- Lytic bone destruction surrounded by areas of increased bone density seen on plain films.
- CT and MR images show a soft tissue mass with inflammatory changes and an infiltrative nature in the cervicofacial region.

MEDICAL MANAGEMENT & TREATMENT

- Surgical debridement
- Gram staining and aerobic and anaerobic cultures prior to antibiotic administration
- Susceptible to a wide range of antibiotics, including penicillin G (most preferred), tetracycline, erythromycin, clindamycin, and ciprofloxacin

COMPLICATIONS

- Include pulmonary and abdominal infections spreading to the brain, nearby bones, and soft tissues.
- Oral infection may spread to the major salivary glands, tongue, hypopharynx, larynx, trachea, salivary glands, and paranasal sinuses.
- Bony involvement originating from an adjacent soft tissue infection may lead to osteomyelitis and necrosis.

PROGNOSIS

- Usually a full recovery with appropriate long-term antibiotic treatment

DENTAL SIGNIFICANCE

- Extensive surgical and medical management procedures, including debridement and curettage, may need to be initiated as well as continued.

DENTAL MANAGEMENT

- Oral hygiene status will need to be improved in order to prevent a recurrence.

SUGGESTED REFERENCES

Hirshberg A, Tsesis I, Metzger Z, Kaplan I. Periapical actinomycosis: a clinicopathologic study. *Oral Surg Oral Med Oral Pathol Oral Radiol Endod* 2003;95:614.

Maurer P, Otto C, Eckert AW, Schubert J. Actinomycosis as a rare complication of orthognathic surgery. *Int J Adult Orthodon Orthognath Surg* 2002;17:230.

Miller M, Haddad AJ. Cervicofacial actinomycosis. *Oral Surg Oral Med Oral Pathol Oral Radiol Endod* 1998;85:496.

Oostman O, Smego RA. Cervicofacial actinomycosis: diagnosis and management. *Curr Infect Dis Rep* 2005;7:170.

AUTHOR: **JAMES T. CASTLE, DDS, MS**

SYNONYM(S)

None

ICD-9CM/CPT CODE(S)

213.0–213.1   Benign neoplasm—bones of skull and face, lower jaw bone

CPT   General Exam or Consultation (e.g., 99243 or 99213)

OVERVIEW

Adenomatoid odontogenic tumor is a relatively uncommon odontogenic tumor. It has been designated in the past as adenoameloblastoma or ameloblastic adenomatoid tumor. It appears that the tumor derives from the enamel organ epithelium.

EPIDEMIOLOGY & DEMOGRAPHICS

The tumor most often involves the anterior portions of the jaw, with the maxilla being twice as affected as the mandible. **PREDOMINANT AGE:** Younger age incidence than ameloblastoma; most cases of adenomatoid odontogenic tumor occur in the second decade. It is unusual in patients over 30 years of age. **PREDOMINANT SEX:** More common in females than males (2:1 ratio).

ETIOLOGY & PATHOGENESIS

No known genetic or environmental factors that increase the likelihood of this benign neoplasm.

CLINICAL PRESENTATION / PHYSICAL FINDINGS

- Most adenomatoid odontogenic tumors are asymptomatic.
- Impacted teeth are frequently associated with the tumor, but some lesions

also arise in the periphery or outside the bone and may be found in soft tissue. These lesions can present as small masses on the maxillary gingiva.
- Usually unilocular radiolucencies with sharp, sclerotic-circumscribed borders associated with an uninterrupted tooth, frequently a maxillary canine. Given this radiographic feature, they frequently can be confused radiographically with a dentigerous cyst. Some authors have described a fine type of radiopacity described as "snowflake," which is said to be helpful in differentiating an adenomatoid odontogenic tumor from a dentigerous cyst. This radiographic feature is dependent upon the amount of mineralized material produced by the neoplasm.

DIAGNOSIS

The tumor consists predominantly of spindle-shaped epithelial cells that form whorled masses or rosettes in a scant, fibrous stromal background (Figure II-1). Duct-like structures lined by cuboidal or columnar epithelial cells with nuclei polarized away from the lumen may be found in abundance but can be scant or even absent in some tumors. Foci of amyloid as well as varying amounts of dentin or cementum-like material may be present.

MEDICAL MANAGEMENT & TREATMENT

Adenomatoid odontogenic tumor is best treated with conservative surgical removal; frequently the tumor can be easily curetted.

COMPLICATIONS

As with most other odontogenic tumors, therapeutic management characteristically consists of conservative surgical removal.

PROGNOSIS

The prognosis is excellent because recurrence rates are very low.

DENTAL SIGNIFICANCE

If an AOT is diagnosed in association with an enervated tooth, an attempt should be made to preserve the tooth.

DENTAL MANAGEMENT

Postsurgical management may include a need for fixed or removable prosthodontics to replace missing teeth.

SUGGESTED REFERENCES

Curran AE, Miller EJ, Murrah VA. Adenomatoid odontogenic tumor presenting as periapical disease. *Oral Surg Oral Med Oral Pathol Oral Radiol Endod* 1997;84:557–560.

Hicks MJ, Flaitz CM, Batsakis JG. Adenomatoid and calcifying epithelial odontogenic tumors. *Ann Otology, Rhinology Laryngology* 1993;102(2):159–161.

Toida M, Hyodo I, Okuda T, Tatematsu N. Adenomatoid odontogenic tumors: report of two cases and survey of 126 cases in Japan. *J Oral Maxillofac Surg* 1990;48:404–408.

AUTHOR: **STEVEN D. VINCENT, DDS, MS**

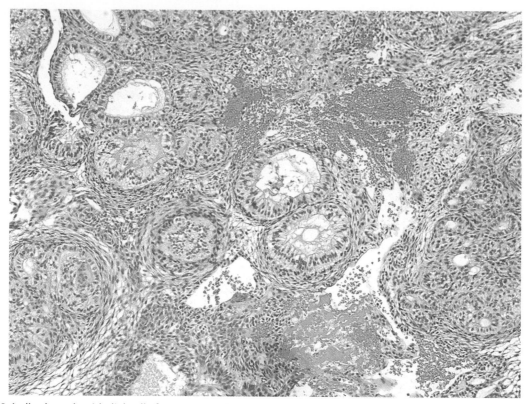

FIGURE II-1 Spindle-shaped epithelial cells forming whorled masses and rosettes in a scant, fibrous, stromal background. Duct-like structures are lined by cuboidal and columnar epithelial cells with nuclei polarized away from the lumen. Foci of eosinophilic amorphous amyloid is also noted (hematoxylin and eosin stain, original magnification 40×).

SYNONYM(S)

None

ICD-9CM/CPT CODE(S)

709.09 Amalgam tattoo
CPT   General Exam or Consultation
       (e.g., 99243 or 99213)

OVERVIEW

Pigmented lesion resulting from implantation of dental amalgam into the oral mucosa or alveolar bone.

EPIDEMIOLOGY & DEMOGRAPHICS

Amalgam tattoo is a common oral lesion.

ETIOLOGY & PATHOGENESIS

- Amalgam may be introduced into the tissues in several ways:
  - Particles entering laceration or area of abrasion
  - Fragments falling into extraction site
  - Particles driven in by high-speed hand piece
  - Dental floss contaminated with amalgam particles
  - Endodontic retrofill procedures
- Macrophage activity may result in lateral spread of lesion.
- Foreign body response or fibrosis may develop.

CLINICAL PRESENTATION / PHYSICAL FINDINGS

HISTORICAL FEATURES

- History of dental procedures.
- Question patient about history of trauma to rule out implantation of other materials, such as pencil graphite, which may produce a similar lesion.

CLINICAL FEATURES

- Usually a solitary lesion but may be multiple.
- Usually a gray, black, or blue macule but may be slightly raised and palpable if associated with fibrosis.
- May have well-defined or irregular borders.
- Size varies and may increase laterally over time.
- Most common on gingiva, alveolar mucosa, and buccal mucosa, but any mucosal surface may be involved.

DIAGNOSIS

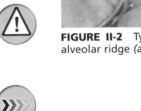

Periapical radiograph may demonstrate metallic particles. If no metallic particles are demonstrated on the radiograph, biopsy is required to establish diagnosis and rule out melanocytic neoplasia.

MEDICAL MANAGEMENT & TREATMENT

No treatment necessary

COMPLICATIONS

Potential complications of biopsy procedure, if required to establish diagnosis

PROGNOSIS

Excellent; does not lead to serious sequelae.

DENTAL SIGNIFICANCE

- Intraoral nevi and early melanoma may mimic amalgam tattoo.
- Risk of amalgam tattoo may be decreased by use of rubber dam and careful irrigation of surgical sites.

DENTAL MANAGEMENT

Establish diagnosis by means of radiograph or biopsy.

SUGGESTED REFERENCE

Neville BW, Damm DD, Allen CM, Bouquot JE. *Oral and Maxillofacial Pathology*. Philadelphia, WB Saunders, 2002, pp 269–272.

AUTHOR: **CYNTHIA L. KLEINEGGER, DDS, MS**

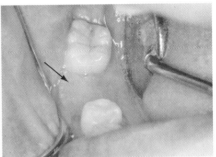

FIGURE II-2 Typical amalgam tattoo on alveolar ridge *(arrow)*.

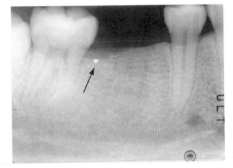

FIGURE II-3 This radiograph is a similar case as seen in Figure II-2 but shows radiographic evidence of metallic fragments *(arrow)*.

SECTION II

SYNONYM(S)

None

ICD-9CM/CPT CODE(S)
213.0–213.1 Benign neoplasm—bones of skull and face, lower jaw bone
CPT General Exam or Consultation (e.g., 99243 or 99213)

OVERVIEW

The ameloblastic fibroma is a benign odontogenic neoplasm characterized by proliferation of immature mesenchymal and ameloblastic cells, both of which are characteristic of developing teeth. Unlike the ameloblastic fibroodontoma or the variants of odontoma (complex vs compound), an ameloblastic fibroma does not have the capacity of producing enamel, dentin, or cementum.

EPIDEMIOLOGY & DEMOGRAPHICS

The tumor can be found in any tooth-bearing site. However, the tumor is most often seen in the premolar-molar region of the mandible.
PREDOMINANT AGE: Lesion is usually identified in patients under 20 years of age.
PREDOMINANT SEX: No gender predilection.
GENETICS: None established.

ETIOLOGY & PATHOGENESIS

No known genetic or environmental factors that increase the likelihood of this benign neoplasm.

CLINICAL PRESENTATION / PHYSICAL FINDINGS

- The ameloblastic fibroma, similar to other odontogenic neoplasms, appears radiographically as a well-demarcated, well-corticated radiolucency. Depending on the size of the tumor, the radiolucency may be unilocular or multilocular. It may be associated with the crown of an unerupted tooth.
- As with other odontogenic neoplasms, the lesion is slow-growing and asymptomatic unless secondarily inflamed.
- A firm expansion of the buccal cortical plate of the mandible or maxilla is the most common clinical finding.

DIAGNOSIS

The histopathologic features of an ameloblastic fibroma are characterized by the proliferation of both epithelial and mesenchymal elements. The mesenchymal component presents as a relatively cellular young, basophilic fibromyxoid tissue suggestive of a developing tooth pulp or dental papillae. The cells appear stellate or spindled. Admixed within this mesenchymal background are islands, cords, and strands of cuboidal and occasionally columnar epithelium. Small islands may show a peripheral rim of cuboidal or columnar cells with a central area of stellate epithelial cells characteristic of stellate reticulum. Mitosis is very uncommon. Occasional islands may show a peripheral rim of eosinophilic acellular material representing an induction effect. However, there will be no evidence of mineralization.

MEDICAL MANAGEMENT & TREATMENT

Conservative surgical enucleation of the tumor is the treatment of choice. The tumor does not have the infiltrative margins characteristic of an ameloblastoma, and therefore recurrence rates are very low.

COMPLICATIONS

Complications are related primarily to the location and size of the neoplasm and the type of surgery necessary.

PROGNOSIS

With early detection and removal, the long-term prognosis is very favorable.

DENTAL SIGNIFICANCE

Loss of dentition during treatment for ameloblastic fibroma will increase the necessity of consultation prior to the planned surgical procedure.

DENTAL MANAGEMENT

Postsurgical management may include a need for fixed or removable prosthodontics to replace missing teeth.

SUGGESTED REFERENCES

Dallera P, Bertoni F, Marchetti C, et al. Ameloblastic fibroma: a follow-up of six cases. *Int J Oral Maxillofacial Surg* 1996; 25:199–202.
Sawyer DR, Nwoku AL, Mosadomi A. Recurrent ameloblastic fibroma: report of two cases. *Oral Surg Oral Med Oral Pathol* 1982;53:19–24.
Takeda Y. Ameloblastic fibroma and related lesions: current pathologic concept. *Oral Oncol* 1999;35:535–540.
Trodahl JN. Ameloblastic fibroma: a survey of cases from the Armed Forces Institute of Pathology. *Oral Surg Oral Med Oral Pathol* 1972;33:547–558.

AUTHOR: **STEVEN D. VINCENT, DDS, MS**

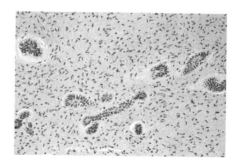

FIGURE II-4 Ameloblastic fibroma. Epithleial islands and cords showing ovoid, cuboidal, and in some areas collumnar morphology with nuclei polarized toward the center of the islands. The adjacent connective tissue is loose and very cellular with numerous, plump, spindle-shaped fibroblasts (hematoxylin and eosin stain, original magnification 40×).

SYNONYM(S)

Follicular ameloblastoma

ICD-9CM/CPT CODE(S)

213.0–213.1 Benign neoplasm—bones of skull and face, lower jaw bone
CPT   General Exam or Consultation (e.g., 99243 or 99213)

OVERVIEW

Ameloblastoma is a neoplasm, the cells of which recapitulate ameloblastic development that may arise from the lining of an odontogenic cyst. In the soft tissues of the oral cavity (e.g., gingiva), ameloblastomas may arise from the basal cell layer.

Three main clinical types exist: solid, unicystic, and peripheral. Of these three, unicystic and peripheral have a much better clinical outcome after a conservative removal.

Note: The term "follicular" is used as a descriptor of solid ameloblastomas. Some authors denote solid ameloblastomas as "follicular ameloblastoma."

EPIDEMIOLOGY & DEMOGRAPHICS

Solid intraosseous ameloblastomas occur in the mandible and maxilla, with the former five times as likely to be involved. Ameloblastomas may involve the maxillary sinus and nasal cavity.

PREDOMINANT AGE: The reported age range of ameloblastoma is 4 to 92 years, with a median age of 35.
PREDOMINANT SEX: The distribution among males and females is approximately equal (47% female, 53% male).
GENETICS: None established.

ETIOLOGY & PATHOGENESIS

No known genetic or environmental factors that increase the likelihood of this benign neoplasm.

CLINICAL PRESENTATION / PHYSICAL FINDINGS

- A painless swelling or expansion of the buccal cortical plate is the most common clinical presentation.
- As with other odontogenic cysts and tumors, ameloblastomas are usually asymptomatic unless secondarily inflamed.

DIAGNOSIS

Small ameloblastomas appear as unilocular radiolucencies with well-demarcated, corticated borders, indistinguishable from other cysts or benign tumors of the jaws. Larger lesions may show a "soap bubble" or honeycomb appearance when loculations are small. Roots of adjacent teeth may be resorbed. Ameloblastomas frequently displace unerupted and erupted teeth.

HISTOLOGY

- Although multiple microscopic subtypes of the solid, intraosseous ameloblastoma exist, it is most critical to recognize the lesion as ameloblastoma because the subtype has no bearing on the prognosis. In addition, many tumors will show a variety of histopathologic patterns.
- The specific types of patterns are:
  - Follicular
  - Plexiform
  - Granular cell
  - Acanthomatous
  - Desmoplastic
  - Basal cell type

The following is a description of the various histologic patterns.

- Follicular pattern (Figure II-5)
  - Most common variant of ameloblastomas. The epithelium is arranged with a peripheral column of cells that resemble ameloblasts with the nucleus oriented away from the surrounding connective tissue and pointing inward to the epithelial proliferation. These peripheral cells also show cytoplasmic

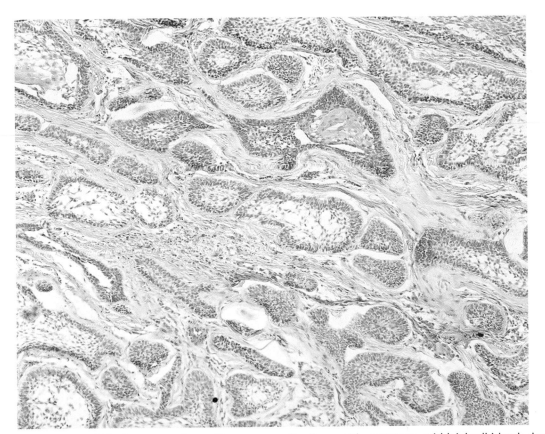

FIGURE II-5 Ameloblastoma, follicular variant. Dense fibrous connective tissue with numerous epithleial cell islands showing peripheral columnar and cuboidal cells with nuclei polarized away from the adjacent connective tissue. Centrally, the islands show myxomatous stellate, reticulum-like foci, and areas of squamous metaplasia (hematoxylin and eosin stain, original magnification 40×).

basal vacuolization. The central portions of these epithelial nests show stellate, reticulum-like cells. Microcyst formation is common in this subtype.

- Plexiform pattern
  - Second most common after the follicular pattern. The plexiform type shows long plexiform or anastomosing columns and sheets of cuboidal or columnar epithelium with little or no evidence of stellate reticulum. Cyst formation is less common in this type.
- Granular cell pattern
  - The granular cell pattern shows eosinophilic granules in the cytoplasm of tumor cells usually found centrally within the epithelial islands. Peripheral columnar and cuboidal cells retain their reverse polarity.
- Acanthomatous pattern
  - In the acanthomatous cell pattern, large areas of squamous metaplasia and keratin formation are present. The critical distinction to be made in this pattern is to not mistake acanthomatous ameloblastoma for squamous carcinoma. Lack of marked nuclear atypia and the presence of a peripheral columnar cell arrangement should help differentiate the two lesions.
- Desmoplastic pattern
  - The desmoplastic pattern shows only small nests of tumor cells within a very sclerotic and densely collagenized background. This relatively rare variant is more often found in the anterior segments of the mandible. Islands of ameloblastic epithelium show less peripheral palisading and may appear more squamous, often making evaluation of additional sections necessary to confirm the diagnosis.
- Basal cell pattern
  - Least common of the histologic variants of ameloblastoma. Nests of basaloid cells with peripheral cuboidal to columnar cells are seen. Unfortunately, little or no stellate reticulum is seen.

MEDICAL MANAGEMENT & TREATMENT

Gardner (see Suggested References following) has pointed out two main factors that explain the behavior of ameloblastomas:

1. Their ability to infiltrate cancellous bone but relative inability to infiltrate compact bone; and
2. The location of the tumor.

Those tumors near vital structures such as the orbit and cranium are much more difficult to control and remove and pose greater clinical problems. Free margins of excision are difficult to obtain in ameloblastomas arising in the posterior maxilla. Dense, compact bone such as that of the inferior border of the mandible or ramus acts as an effective barrier in preventing tumor spread. In the maxilla, only a thin cortical plate exists, and it is a poor barrier to the spread of ameloblastoma.

Ameloblastoma is well-known to recur after curettage. This is possibly because ameloblastomas infiltrate the trabeculae of cancellous bone. This infiltration frequently extends beyond the apparent radiographic margin. Some clinicians are tempted to curette only to the corticated clinical or radiographic margins; this increases the likelihood of recurrence.

COMPLICATIONS

Complications are related primarily to the location and size of the neoplasm and the type of surgery necessary.

PROGNOSIS

- The location of the tumor is a very important factor in the long-term prognosis. Those tumors that are in the anterior maxilla or body of the mandible are less likely to cause significant problems than those of the posterior mandible/ramus and those of the posterior maxilla.
- As attempts to remove the tumor by curettage can leave small bits of tumor within the bone, it is thought that resection with adequate margin is the best treatment. Nevertheless, recurrence rates up to 10–15% have been reported even after enblock resection. Some surgeons advocate the margin of resection should be at least 1 cm past the radiographic limits of the tumor.

DENTAL SIGNIFICANCE

Loss of dentition during treatment for ameloblastoma will increase the necessity of consultation prior to the planned surgical procedure.

DENTAL MANAGEMENT

Postsurgical management may include a need for fixed or removable prosthodontics to replace missing teeth.

SUGGESTED REFERENCES

Daramola JO, Ajagbe HA, Oluwasannii JO. Recurrent ameloblastoma of the jaws— a review of 22 cases. *Plast Reconstr Surg* 1980;65:577–579.

Gardner DG. Some current concepts on the pathology of ameloblastomas. *Oral Surg Oral Med Oral Pathol* 1996;82:660–669.

Kaffe I, Buchner A, Taicher S. Radiologic features of desmoplastic variant of ameloblastoma. *Oral Surg Oral Med Oral Pathol* 1993; 76:525–529.

Lolachi CM, Madan SK, Jacobs JR. Ameloblastic carcinoma of the maxilla. *J Laryngol Otol* 1995;109:1019–1022.

Mintz S, Anavi Y, Sabes WR. Peripheral ameloblastoma of the gingiva. A case report. *J Periodontol* 1990;61:649–652.

Ng KH, Siar CH. Peripheral ameloblastoma with clear cell differentiation. *Oral Surg Oral Med Oral Pathol* 1990;70:210–213.

Pogrel MA. The management of lesions of the jaws with liquid nitrogen cryotherapy. *J Calif Dent Assoc* 1995;23(12):54–57.

Williams TP. Management of ameloblastoma: a changing perspective. *J Oral Maxillofac Surg* 1993;51:1064–1070.

AUTHOR: **STEVEN D. VINCENT, DDS, MS**

SYNONYM(S)

None

ICD-9CM/CPT CODE(S)
526.20 Aneurysmal bone cyst
CPT   General Exam or Consultation
(e.g., 99243 or 99213)

OVERVIEW

The aneurysmal bone cyst is an intraosseous lesion that is generally seen in young individuals. It can be seen in any bone in the body, but overall, the jaws are relatively uncommon sites for this lesion to occur. However, when appearing in the jaws, this type of cyst occurs most often in the posterior mandible.

EPIDEMIOLOGY & DEMOGRAPHICS

PREDOMINANT AGE: Seen most commonly in teenagers, although they have been seen in older adults.
PREDOMINANT SEX: Appears to be no gender predilection.

ETIOLOGY & PATHOGENESIS

These are often seen in association with other lesions such as giant cell lesions or benign fibroosseous lesions. In fact, the aneurysmal bone cyst may actually be a variation of a central giant cell granuloma.

CLINICAL PRESENTATION / PHYSICAL FINDINGS

- Relatively rapidly enlarging lesion of the mandible; often painful.
- Lesions may be multilocular, although they are generally not well-corticated.
- Copious amounts of blood are often encountered upon entering the lesion. The bleeding is profuse but not a high-pressure type of bleeding. The hemorrhage often results in the inability for the surgeon to clear the area.

DIAGNOSIS

The diagnosis is generally a combination of clinical, radiographic, and histopathologic features. Upon histopathologic exam, multiple nonendothelial-lined, blood-filled cavities will be noted. This may be associated with either multinucleated giant cells and/or a benign fibroosseous lesion.

MEDICAL MANAGEMENT & TREATMENT

- Although the lesions can be enucleated, application of sclerosis agents to the area may be effective.
- Intralesional steroids may also help resolve the lesions.
- In addition, there may be some indication that treatment similar to a central giant cell granuloma with systemic calcitonin could result in resolution of the lesion. This remains experimental.
- Because of the clinical risks of entering into a hemorrhage-filled cavity and the possibility that not enough tissue is secured for diagnosis, interventional angiograms are sometimes indicated.
- If an angiogram is performed, no flow characteristics suggesting "feeding" vessels will be noted.

COMPLICATIONS

The lesions can become large and perforate the mandible. They can also result in tooth loss. Intraoperative hemorrhage may also be a source of complications.

PROGNOSIS

Prognosis of the lesions is good, although recurrence upon attempts at enucleation would not be unexpected.

DENTAL SIGNIFICANCE

Lesions can expand rapidly and cause pain simulating a toothache or abscess.

DENTAL MANAGEMENT

No specific alterations in dental management are necessary except for proper diagnosis and treatment. Occasionally, the size of the lesion and enucleation will result in loss of teeth.

SUGGESTED REFERENCES

Auclair P, Arendt D, Hellstein J. Giant cell lesions of the jaws. *Oral and Maxillofacial Surg Clin No Am* 1997;9(4):655–680.
Neville BW, Damm DD, Allen CM, Bouquot JE. *Oral and Maxillofacial Pathology*, ed 2. Philadelphia, WB Saunders, 2002, pp 551–552.

AUTHOR: **JOHN W. HELLSTEIN, DDS, MS**

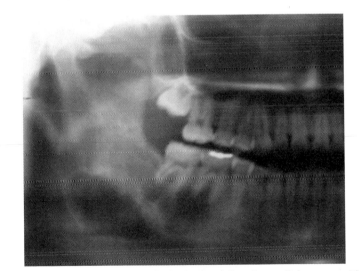

FIGURE II-6 Panoramic radiograph displaying multilocular radiolucency with thinning and probable erosion of the cortex *(arrow)*. (From Auclair P, Arendt D, Hellstein J. Giant cell lesions of the jaws. *Oral and Maxillofacial Surg Clin No Am* 1997;9(4):655–680, Figure 6, p 664.)

SECTION II

SYNONYM(S)

Angular cheilosis
Perlèche

ICD-9CM/CPT CODE(S)

528.5 Angular cheilitis
CPT General Exam or Consultation
(e.g., 99243 or 99213)

OVERVIEW

Lesion of the skin surface of the labial commissure, most often as a result of infection with *Candida albicans* and/or *Staphylococcus aureus*

EPIDEMIOLOGY & DEMOGRAPHICS

Occurs more commonly in older patients with decreased vertical dimension of occlusion.

ETIOLOGY & PATHOGENESIS

Decreased vertical dimension of occlusion results in fold of skin in which saliva may pool at the labial commissure. The moist environment promotes growth of yeast and/or bacteria. This may also occur in patients who habitually lick the labial commissures. Angular cheilitis may be a component of chronic mucocutaneous candidosis or a manifestation of immunosuppression or anemia. Patients with angular cheilitis may also exhibit intraoral candidosis.

CLINICAL PRESENTATION / PHYSICAL FINDINGS

- The corners of the mouth appear erythematous with fissuring, cracking, scaling, and/or weeping.
- The patient may report variably intense soreness, burning, or irritation.

DIAGNOSIS

- Diagnosis is typically made based on clinical and historical features.
- Cytologic preparations stained with periodic acid-Schiff stain modified for fungi may be used to confirm fungal infection.
- Culture may be used to evaluate for infection or coinfection with *Staphylococcus aureus*.

MEDICAL MANAGEMENT & TREATMENT

- Antifungal cream such as ketoconazole 2% or clotrimazole 1%; apply thin film to corners of mouth qid (PC and HS), NPO one-half hour after.
- For severe cases, antifungal cream may be mixed with an equal part of topical steroid cream such as triamcinolone 0.1% to reduce inflammation.
- For cases not responsive to antifungal therapy alone, antifungal cream may be mixed with an equal part of mupirocin ointment 2%.
- Maintenance therapy may be required if predisposing factors cannot be eliminated or controlled.

COMPLICATIONS

Chronic angular cheilitis may result in scarring or hyperpigmentation.

PROGNOSIS

Very good with appropriate management

DENTAL SIGNIFICANCE

- Deficient vertical dimension of occlusion is the most common cause for angular cheilitis.
- Dentures should be fabricated with and periodically evaluated for adequate vertical dimension of occlusion to prevent angular cheilitis.

DENTAL MANAGEMENT

- Evaluate for and correct deficiency in vertical dimension of occlusion.
- Evaluate for intraoral candidosis.
- Refer for medical evaluation if underlying systemic disease is suspected.

SUGGESTED REFERENCE

Neville BW, Damm DD, Allen CM, Bouquot JE. *Oral and Maxillofacial Pathology*, ed 2. Philadelphia, WB Saunders, 2002, pp 192–197.

AUTHOR: **CYNTHIA L. KLEINEGGER, DDS, MS**

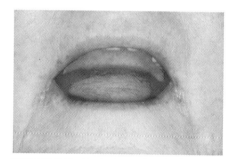

FIGURE II-7 Typical angular cheilitis presentation.

SYNONYM(S)

Aphthous ulcers
Canker sores

ICD-9CM/CPT CODE(S)
528.2 Aphthous stomatitis
CPT General Exam or Consultation
(e.g., 99243 or 99213)

OVERVIEW

Aphthous ulcers are among the most frequently encountered disease processes of the oral cavity. In most people, these ulcers will be at times irritating but so infrequent that they have little disruption of their normal life. The disease may be divided into three different subgroups:

- Aphthous minor
- Aphthous major (also known as Sutton's disease)
- Herpetiform aphthous stomatitis

Generally, the people who are afflicted with herpes major or herpetiform aphthous seek treatment in the clinical setting. Some aphthous minor patients may also enter the practice with this as a chief complaint or a related question.

EPIDEMIOLOGY & DEMOGRAPHICS

INCIDENCE/PREVALENCE IN USA: Wide variation in the estimated prevalence of aphthous ulcers, although most would consider the prevalence as 20–30% in most populations.

PREDOMINANT AGE: Seen in the first decade of life as well as in old age. Many patients' first indication of the disease is seen in the early elementary school age, although onset may be later in life.

GENETICS: There may be a genetic predisposition to the disease, with some indication that this genetic predisposition is a dominant pattern. Variations in expression and penetrance could explain some of the variability in the presentation of the disease.

ETIOLOGY & PATHOGENESIS

- Although the definitive pathogenesis remains uncertain, the disease is immunologically based with antigen exposure producing a hypersensitivity reaction. The antigen exposure may be related to minor trauma, altered mucosal irritation, bacteria, or variations in the endocrine system.
- Nutritional deficiencies as well as hematologic abnormalities have also been cited as possibly predisposing reasons for an outbreak.
- Many authors also cite stress as a possible predictive predisposing agent.

CLINICAL PRESENTATION / PHYSICAL FINDINGS

- Presents as an acute-onset disease with ulcers generally being less than 1 cm in diameter.
- No evidence of systemic manifestations and no evidence of lymphadenopathy unless other causes of lymphadenopathy are concurrently present.
- The ulcers in aphthous minor are generally single, but patients presenting for exam are often those who experience multiple concurrent ulcers.
- In aphthous major, multiple ulcers are common, with some of the ulcers potentially being greater than 1 cm in diameter.
- Ulcers are somewhat concave with a raised erythematous border generally on the order of 1 mm in width.
- Limited to nonkeratinized oral mucosa, although in reality almost all areas of the oral mucosa have some evidence of keratin formation.
- The areas of the soft palate, buccal mucosa, lateral ventral tongue, floor of mouth, and vestibular mucosa below the mucogingival line are generally less keratinized; it is in these areas of less keratinized mucosa where aphthous ulcers will always occur. This is in stark contrast to recurrent herpes where the hard palate, gingiva, and vermilion–skin interface are the areas involved.
- In aphthous minor, the individual ulcers will usually heal without scarring in 7 to 14 days.
- In aphthous major (which also may be known as Sutton's disease), these ulcers may take as long as 6 weeks to heal. In addition, in some cases of Sutton's disease, the ulcers will heal with scarring.

DIAGNOSIS

- In some cases of aphthous major, the diagnosis may be problematic.
- Laboratory tests or biopsies are generally not indicated for the diagnosis of aphthous.
- The diagnosis is generally based on the clinical signs and symptoms, the recurrent nature of the problem, and a periodicity in the rate of healing.
- Other diseases to eliminate from the differential diagnosis include Behçet's syndrome, Reiter's syndrome, and erythema multiforme.

MEDICAL MANAGEMENT & TREATMENT

- To decrease the antigenic exposure of the immune system underlying the thin mucosa, it is thought that maintenance of the salivary pellicle is essential. For this reason, patients should avoid toothpastes containing sodium lauryl sulphate, which is disruptive to the salivary pellicle. Popular brands of toothpastes such as Biotene®, Rembrandt for Canker Sores™, or Rembrandt Naturals™ are examples of toothpastes that do not contain sodium lauryl sulphate. Many other brands may be available locally. At least one study has shown a 40–50% reduction in the number of aphthous ulcers over a period of time.
- Topical steroids applied to the ulcer may be beneficial in decreasing the duration of the ulcers and may have some preventive effect in some patients. Perhaps the most easily available steroid rinse is dexamethasone 0.5 mg per 5 mL.
  - Dispense: 240 mL.
  - Significant: if the patient only has occasional or single ulcers, topical steroids are probably not indicated.
  - The rinse should only be used by patients who are experiencing ulcers for more than 15 days in any given month.
- Topical steroid ointments may also be used, such as clobetasol 0.05% ointment; dispense 15 g and apply 2 to 3 times daily to the area of ulceration.
- Fluocinolone and triamcinolone are other popular steroids that may provide some relief.
- Over-the-counter numbing products such as Ora-Gel™, which contains benzocaine, may also be preferred by some patients for minor outbreaks.
- Rinses for patients experiencing ulcerations for more than 15 days in any given month are generally administered by using the rinse at bedtime only when ulcers are not present and then 4 times per day when ulcers are present.
- Systemic medications such as colchicine or pentoxifylline have been utilized by some practitioners. Note: Use of these systemic medications is best left to the specialist.

COMPLICATIONS

Steroid treatments may predispose the patient to an outbreak of oral candidosis. If such an outbreak occurs, antifungals will need to be administered.

PROGNOSIS

For the minor aphthous patient, the disease is generally not a major factor in their life. However, patients with aphthous major or herpetiform aphthous may find it difficult to cope with the disease process and will need close follow-up and help from their healthcare specialists. The disease can be managed but not cured, and this is very difficult for some patients to accept.

DENTAL SIGNIFICANCE

Many dental procedures may produce trauma to the oral mucosal surfaces or create stress in the patient. Because of this, some outbreaks are often associated with a recent dental procedure. In some patients, this can be predicted, and prophylactic measures prior to and after dental appointments may be implemented. Steroid rinses may be beneficial in such cases.

DENTAL MANAGEMENT

When treating patients in whom mucosal trauma is a factor, rubber dams and care to decrease any trauma to the nonkeratinized mucosa may be beneficial. Drying agents such as cotton rolls may be particularly problematic.

SUGGESTED REFERENCES

Neville BW, Damm DD, Allen CM, Bouquot JE. *Oral and Maxillofacial Pathology*, ed 2. Philadelphia, WB Saunders, 2002, pp 285–290.

Porter SR, Kingsmill V, Scully C. Audit of diagnosis and investigations in patients with recurrent aphthous stomatitis. *Oral Surg Oral Med Oral Pathol* 1993;76:449.

AUTHOR: **JOHN W. HELLSTEIN, DDS, MS**

SYNONYM(S)

Basal cell epithelioma
Rodent ulcer

ICD-9CM/CPT CODE(S)

173.0–173.9 Malignant neoplasm of skin. See code book for specific site.

CPT   General Exam or Consultation (e.g., 99243 or 99213)

OVERVIEW

Basal cell carcinoma is the most common cutaneous skin malignancy in humans. It has a clinical course characterized by slow growth, minimal soft tissue invasiveness, and a high cure rate. These tumors, which show a reduplication of the epidermal basal cell layer, show a predilection for the head and neck, and most often appear in individuals 40 to 60 years of age. The primary etiologic route is increased time and degree of solar exposure, particularly UVB.

EPIDEMIOLOGY & DEMOGRAPHICS

INCIDENCE/PREVALENCE IN USA:
Lifetime risk of 30% to develop a basal cell carcinoma. In the U.S., about 150 cases per 100,000 population; in Australia, incidence is approximately 726 cases per 100,000 population. Depending on the country, reporting figures range between 40 and > 700 per 100,000 population per year.
PREDOMINANT AGE: Peak incidence 50 to 60 years of age, ranging from 40 to 75 years or older. More common in those with a history of severe sunburns in childhood, overexposure to ultraviolet rays, and exposure to arsenic.
PREDOMINANT SEX: 2:1 male-to-female predilection.
GENETICS:
- Low incidence in the African-American, Asian, and Hispanic populations.

- High incidence in:
  - Persons with Fitzpatrick skin type I (always burns, never tans)
  - Caucasians with fair skin, red hair, green eyes
- Associated development in conjunction with albinism, xeroderma pigmentosa, and nevoid basal cell carcinoma syndrome.

ETIOLOGY & PATHOGENESIS

- Patched receptor of the Sonic hedgehog (Shh) signaling pathway is implicated in association with multiple basal cell carcinomas seen in nevoid basal cell carcinoma syndrome.
- Ultraviolet radiation-induced alterations resulting in inactivation of tumor suppressor gene p53 and cytochrome P-45-CYP2D6.

CLINICAL PRESENTATION / PHYSICAL FINDINGS

- Pearly or translucent papule
- White, light pink, flesh-colored, or brown coloration
- Waxy or translucent surface with overlying telangiectasias
- Central ulceration with raised, rolled border
- Flat or slightly raised
- Friable, nonhealing lesions that bleed frequently and will not heal
- Indolent, slowly progressive growth

DIAGNOSIS

- Skin shave, excisional or punch biopsy techniques
- Diagnostic imaging only for advanced tumors with questionable invasion of bone or soft tissue

MEDICAL MANAGEMENT & TREATMENT

- Electrodesiccation and curettage

- Full thickness (en bloc) excisional surgery for deep, diffuse lesions
- Cryosurgery
- Mohs' micrographic surgery
- Topical photodynamic therapy
- Radiation therapy in rare cases
- Topical fluorouracil
- Topical imiquimod

COMPLICATIONS

- Invasion of adjacent tissues or structures
- Recurrence
- Loss of skin graft in advanced cases
- Scarring

PROGNOSIS

- Recurrences related to depth of invasion and location.
- Cure rate of more than 95%.
- If tumor cells are found at the surgical margin, recurrence rate increases to 30%.
- Sclerosing/morpheaform type shows increased rate of recurrence due to lateral and deep spread.

DENTAL SIGNIFICANCE

No specific dental implications

SUGGESTED REFERENCES

Miller SJ. Etiology and pathogenesis of basal cell carcinoma. *Clin Dermatol* 1995;13:527.
Rubin AI, Chen EH, Ratner D. Basal-cell carcinoma: *N Eng J Med* 2005;353:2262–2269.
Telfer N, Colver G, Bowers P. Guidelines for the management of basal cell carcinoma. *Br J Dermatol* 1999;141:415.
Wong CS, Strange RC, Lear JT. Basal cell carcinoma. *BMJ* 2003;327:794.

AUTHOR: **JAMES T. CASTLE, DDS, MS**

SYNONYM(S)

Branchial cleft cysts
Oral lymphoepithelial cysts

ICD-9CM/CPT CODE(S)

528.4 Lymphoepithelial cyst of the oral cavity
744.42 Branchial cleft cyst
CPT General Exam or Consultation (e.g. 99243 or 99213)

OVERVIEW

Branchial cleft cysts may occur along the anterior edge of the sternocleidomastoid muscle from the clavicle up to the area of the tragus of the ear. They are generally thought to be developmental and thought to arise from epithelial inclusions within the branchial arches.

Oral lymphoepithelial cysts will generally be in the region of Waldeyer's ring. These are also seen in other areas of the ral mucosa, especially in the floor of the mouth and ventral surface of the tongue.

EPIDEMIOLOGY & DEMOGRAPHICS

Both the branchial cleft cyst and the oral lymphoepithelial cyst may be noted at any age but are most common in the third and fourth decades of life.

ETIOLOGY & PATHOGENESIS

Developmental from epithelial remnants derived from the branchial arches

The oral lymphoepithelial cysts are thought to evolve from entrapped epithelial crypts during development.

CLINICAL PRESENTATION / PHYSICAL FINDINGS

- Secondarily infected cysts may present with pain. In general, these lesions will be relatively soft and well-formed with an ovoid to spherical shape.
- Branchial cleft cysts may get relatively large, while the oral lymphoepithelial cysts are generally less than 1 cm in diameter.
- The oral lymphoepithelial cysts generally present with a yellow or white hue and are often thought to be a lipoma.

DIAGNOSIS

Diagnosis is microscopic, with a central cystic lumen being associated with lymphoid aggregates.

MEDICAL MANAGEMENT & TREATMENT

Condition can be treated by simple excision of the cyst.

COMPLICATIONS

- Pain
- Mass effect
- Nerve damage

Secondary infection of branchial cleft cysts may be problematic. In addition, large branchial cleft cysts (those near the ear) may provide surgical problems due to proximity to vital structures, especially nerves.

PROGNOSIS

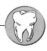

The prognosis is excellent, although risk to vital structures such as facial nerves, jugular vein, and submandibular duct may complicate surgical removal.

DENTAL SIGNIFICANCE

Although oral lesions are generally small, early diagnosis will enhance management.

DENTAL MANAGEMENT

No altered dental therapy except for the necessity of proper oral exam to establish a differential diagnosis and ensure excision.

SUGGESTED REFERENCES

Flaitz CM. Oral lymphoepithelial cyst in a young child. *Pediatr Dent* 2000;22(5): 422–423.
Glosser JW, Pires CA, Feinberg SE. Branchial cleft or cervical lymphoepithelial cysts: etiology and management. *JADA* 2003;134(1): 81–86.
Neville BW, Damm DD, Allen CM, Bouquot JE. *Oral and Maxillofacial Pathology*, ed 2. Philadelphia, WB Saunders, 2002, pp 34–35.

AUTHOR: JOHN W. HELLSTEIN, DDS, MS

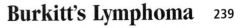

SYNONYM(S)

B-cell lymphoma, small cell, Burkitt's type Endemic or African Burkitt's lymphoma

ICD-9CM/CPT CODE(S)
200.2   Burkitt's tumor or lymphoma
200.20 Burkitt's tumor or lymphoma, unspecified site
200.21 Burkitt's tumor or lymphoma involving lymph nodes of head, face, and neck
200.28 Burkitt's tumor or lymphoma involving lymph nodes of multiple sites
CPT   General Exam or Consultation (e.g., 99243 or 99213)

OVERVIEW

This is a non-Hodgkin's lymphoma of B-cell origin, first described by Dennis Burkitt in young African children in Uganda in 1958. It is generally thought to occur in two forms:

- The endemic or African form is most predominant in Africa, but the endemic form is also seen in South America. In some areas of Africa, 50% of all cancers are of the Burkitt's lymphoma type. The African form will present in extranodal sites most often as a rapidly growing mass. Although it may occur in only one jaw quadrant, it may involve all four jaw quadrants. Almost all patients with the African or endemic form have high levels of Epstein-Barr virus antibodies.
- The nonendemic or American form may also be labeled sporadic. This form occurs worldwide, not just in America, and generally occurs in an older age group. It will usually be intranodal with the abdominal lymph nodes most often affected. Antibodies to Epstein-Barr virus are also elevated in the American form but not to the levels seen in the endemic form.

A third recognizable type occurs as an immunodeficiency type associated with HIV disease.

EPIDEMIOLOGY & DEMOGRAPHICS

INCIDENCE/PREVALENCE IN USA: Incidence of endemic Burkitt's lymphoma is 10/100,000, while the sporadic type is 0.9/100,000.

PREDOMINANT AGE: African Burkitt's lymphoma is more common in children and represents about 30% of childhood non-Hodgkin's lymphomas. The younger the child is, the more commonly it presents in the vicinity of the jaws. The peak incidence of the African form is at 3 to 8 years of age. In the American form, the tumor occurs in older children or young adults. Sporadic Burkitt's lymphoma is more common in adults but represents less than 1% of non-Hodgkin's lymphomas.

PREDOMINANT SEX: Eighty-nine percent of affected individuals are males.
GENETICS: It is associated with translocations of the long arm of chromosome 8. Several known translocations are t(8;14), t(2;8), and t(8;22).

ETIOLOGY & PATHOGENESIS

- In North America, 15% of cases are associated with Epstein-Barr virus (EBV) compared to 90% in young African children.
- EBV containing Burkitt's lymphoma has also been associated with certain HIV-related lymphomas.
- Chromosome 8 translocations in Burkitt's lymphoma directly affect tumor cell proliferation, making Burkitt's lymphoma the highest-proliferating human tumor. It has a population doubling time of 24 hours and a growth fraction that may be as high as 100%.
- The chromosome 8 breakpoint in the endemic type is upstream of c-*myc* locus, while it is within the c-*myc* locus in the sporadic type.

CLINICAL PRESENTATION / PHYSICAL FINDINGS

- Endemic or African Burkitt's lymphoma commonly affects the jaws (58%), abdomen (58%), central nervous system (19%), orbit (11%), and bone marrow (7%).
- Sporadic Burkitt's lymphoma commonly presents as peripheral lymphadenopathy affecting the abdomen (91%), central nervous system (14%), jaws (7%), orbit (1%), and bone marrow (20%).
- Jaw involvement is age-related; 90% of 3-year-old patients have jaw involvement, while 25% of patients older than age 15 have jaw lesions.
- Jaw lesions tend to peak at age 7.
- Jaw involvement more commonly affects the maxilla rather than the mandible (usually located in the posterior segments).
- Endemic Burkitt's lymphoma usually affects the four quadrants of the jaw, while jaw involvement in the sporadic type is more localized.
- Usually presents with rapidly expanding intraoral mass, pain, lip paresthesia, proptosis, tooth mobility and migration, and alveolar bone destruction.

DIAGNOSIS

- Diagnosis is based on histopathologic findings, although immunohistochemical and fluoride cytometric studies may be beneficial.
- Demonstration of a highly proliferative B cell immunophenotype in addition to chromosomal translocation.
- There are elevated antibody titers to EBV.

- Histopathology demonstrates proliferation of undifferentiated B lymphocytes, including abundant histiocytic cells, giving the characteristic "starry sky" appearance.
- Radiographic imaging displays patchy, radiolucent bony destruction with ragged border.

MEDICAL MANAGEMENT & TREATMENT

- This is managed best through the use of chemotherapy with cyclophosphamide; the resolution of lesions following chemotherapy is often dramatic.
- Treatment should commence within 48 hours of diagnosis.

COMPLICATIONS

- Complications, including mucositis, are associated with treatment with high-dose chemotherapy.
- Tumor lysis syndrome and renal failure may develop due to the burden caused by rapid destruction of rapidly proliferating tumor cells.
- Tumor lysis syndrome is characterized by presence of any combinations of hyperphosphatemia, hyperkalemia, hyperuricemia, hypercalcemia, and lactic acidosis.

PROGNOSIS

Even with modern chemotherapy, Burkitt's lymphoma still has a mortality rate of 15–25%. However, the 5-year survival rate can be as high as 95%.

DENTAL SIGNIFICANCE

- Jaw involvement more commonly affects the maxilla rather than the mandible and is usually located in the posterior segments.
- Endemic Burkitt's lymphoma usually affects the four quadrants of the jaw, while jaw involvement in the sporadic type is more localized.
- Expanding intraoral mass, pain, and lip paresthesias are usual complaints.
- Chemotherapy-induced complications (e.g., mucositis, xerostomia).
- Restoration of dentition following chemotherapy; loss of teeth due to extreme bone destruction may happen in some cases.

DENTAL MANAGEMENT

- Management is generally not altered, although prechemotherapeutic extraction may be suggested, and chemotherapy may produce infection, mucosal ulcerations, or erythema.

- While the body is immunosuppressed, elective dental procedures should be avoided.
- See "Non-Hodgkin's Lymphoma" in Section I, p 155 for more information.

SUGGESTED REFERENCES

Kasamon YL, Swinnen LJ. Treatment advances in adult Burkitt lymphoma and leukemia. *Curr Opin Oncol* 2004;16(5):429–435.

Neville BW, Damm DD, Allen CM, Bouquot JE. *Oral and Maxillofacial Pathology,* ed 2. Philadelphia, WB Saunders, 2002, pp 523–524.

Tsui SH, Wong MH, Lam WY. Burkitt's lymphoma presenting as mandibular swelling—report of a case and review of publications. *Br J Oral Maxillofac Surg* 2000;38(1):8–11.

AUTHORS: **JOHN W. HELLSTEIN, DDS, MS; SUNDAY O. AKINTOYE, BDS, DDS, MS**

SYNONYM(S)

Stomatodynia
Glossodynia
Burning tongue

ICD-9CM/CPT CODE(S)

529.6 Glossodynia
CPT General Exam or Consultation
(e.g., 99243 or 99213)

OVERVIEW

Burning mouth syndrome is generally a poorly understood disease that presents with clinical symptoms of burning without any evidence of clinical abnormalities.

EPIDEMIOLOGY & DEMOGRAPHICS

INCIDENCE/PREVALENCE IN USA: The population prevalence is debatable but may range from approximately 0.5–2.5%.

PREDOMINANT SEX: The overwhelming preponderance of patients with burning mouth syndrome are female, but males may be seen with this affliction.

PREDOMINANT AGE: In females, usually occurs after menopause.

ETIOLOGY & PATHOGENESIS

Burning mouth syndrome has been associated with a number of factors including gingivitis, psychogenic factors, xerostomia, candidosis, gastroesophageal disease, periodontitis, iron deficiency, hormonal factors, and nutrition.

CLINICAL PRESENTATION / PHYSICAL FINDINGS

By definition, no clinical abnormalities are noted. Occasionally, the patient may present with a concomitant geographic tongue. However, this is often only a coincidental finding.

DIAGNOSIS

Definitive laboratory tests and diagnostic tests are often limited. However, various laboratory tests may be helpful with individual patients and may be ordered as needed. Such tests include:

- Cytology for candidosis
- Evaluation of salivary flow
- Evaluation of xerostomia-causing medications
- Hormonal changes
- Nutritional/vitamin deficiencies
- Allergies
- Autoimmune conditions
- Depression
- Anemia
- Sjögren's syndrome
- Diabetes

MEDICAL MANAGEMENT & TREATMENT

- Medical management is usually very difficult.
- Initially, topical antibiotics such as chlorhexidine or antifungal therapy with clotrimazole troches may be beneficial although they are rarely curative. It must be stressed to the patient at the beginning that burning mouth symptoms are generally managed rather than cured. Previously mentioned studies may help direct a possible course of therapy. See preceding Diagnosis section (e.g., positive cytology for candidosis, anemia, diagnosis of autoimmune conditions).
- Trials of tricyclic antidepressants in low doses may also be beneficial. These low-dose antidepressants, in conjunction with a sialogogue such as buffered citrate, are often the most clinically beneficial. Buffered citrate is usually obtained as the over-the-counter product Saliva-Sure™. Nortriptyline (initial dose 25 mg at bedtime) is a medication that may show benefit without too many side effects. Clonazepam and gabapentin are often necessary, but side effects and dependency issues indicate their use is best left to specialists. Other prescription sialogogues include pilocarpine (Salagen™) or cevimeline (Evoxac™).

COMPLICATIONS

- Pilocarpine may induce sweating or other side effects that are undesirable to the patient.
- The tricyclic antidepressants or benzodiazepine such as clonazepam may produce drowsiness as well as a number of other potential drug side effects.

PROGNOSIS

These patients are often very difficult to treat successfully. The symptoms are often long-term and only marginally manageable.

DENTAL SIGNIFICANCE

Symptoms sometimes ensue shortly after dental treatment, and patients may erroneously consider this a causative relationship.

DENTAL MANAGEMENT

No special dental management considerations

SUGGESTED REFERENCES

Allen CM, Blozis GG. Oral mucosal reactions to cinnamon-flavored chewing gum. *JADA* 1988;116:664.

Buchanan J, Zakrzewska J. Burning mouth syndrome. *Clin Evid* 2004;11:1774–1780.

Gibson J, Lamey PJ, Lewis M, Frier B. Oral manifestations of previously undiagnosed non-insulin dependent diabetes mellitus. *J Oral Pathol Med* 1990;19:284.

Lamey PJ, Freeman R, Eddie SA, Pankhurst C, Rees T. Vulnerability and presenting symptoms in burning mouth syndrome. *Oral Surg Oral Med Oral Pathol Oral Radiol Endod* 2005;99(1):48–54.

Lauria G, Majorana A, Borgna M, Lombardi R, Penza P, Padovani A, Sapelli P. Trigeminal small-fiber sensory neuropathy causes burning mouth syndrome. *Pain* 2005;115(3): 332–337.

Neville BW, Damm DD, Allen CM, Bouquot JE. *Oral and Maxillofacial Pathology*, ed 2. Philadelphia, WB Saunders, 2002, pp 752–753.

AUTHOR: JOHN W. HELLSTEIN, DDS, MS

SECTION II

SYNONYM(S)

Pindborg tumor
Calcifying odontogenic tumor

ICD-9CM/CPT CODE(S)

213.0–213.1	Benign neoplasm—bones of skull and face, lower jaw bone
CPT	General Exam or Consultation (e.g., 99243 or 99213)

OVERVIEW

The calcifying odontogenic tumor (Pindborg tumor) is an unusual odontogenic neoplasm characterized by sheets of hyperchromatic, pleomorphic cells with foci of mineralization.

EPIDEMIOLOGY & DEMOGRAPHICS

Calcifying epithelial odontogenic tumors occur more often in the mandible vs the maxilla with a ratio of approximately 2:1. They are most often located in the molar-premolar region. As with other odontogenic tumors, they may or may not be associated with unerupted tooth crowns.
INCIDENCE/PREVALENCE IN USA: These tumors are rare.
PREDOMINANT SEX: They have been reported more often in males.
PREDOMINANT AGE: They show an unusual bimodal age pattern with a slight increase in tumors reported during the twenties and again during the forties.
GENETICS: None established.

ETIOLOGY & PATHOGENESIS

There are no known genetic or environmental factors that increase the likelihood of this benign neoplasm.

CLINICAL PRESENTATION / PHYSICAL FINDINGS

- A painless swelling or expansion of the buccal cortical plate is the most common clinical presentation. As with other odontogenic cysts and tumors, calcifying odontogenic tumors are usually asymptomatic unless secondarily inflamed.
- Calcifying odontogenic tumors present most often as a well-circumscribed, corticated, unilocular or multilocular radiolucency. Some tumors produce enough mineralization that small radiopacities may be detected within the radiolucent area.
- Rare tumors have been reported outside of cortical bone. In these instances, the underlying cortical bone may show evidence of resorption.

DIAGNOSIS

The tumor is characterized by islands and sheets of epithelial cells dispersed throughout a nonspecific, fibrous stroma. In many instances, the polygonal, epithelial cells show remarkable pleomorphism and nuclear hyperchromasia. Borders of the epithelial cells are well-defined, and prominent intracellular bridges are characteristic. Some tumors will show a prominent clear cell component. Foci of homogenous eosinophilic material shown to be amyloid based on crystal violet, and Congo red stains are found within the tumor. Also noted are small, round globules of mineralized material exhibiting a Liesegang ring phenomenon.

MEDICAL MANAGEMENT & TREATMENT

As with most other odontogenic tumors, therapeutic management characteristically consists of conservative surgical removal.

COMPLICATIONS

Complications are related primarily to the location and size of the neoplasm and the type of surgery necessary.

PROGNOSIS

Recurrence rates are most often listed at less than 10%; therefore, the long-term prognosis is favorable.

DENTAL SIGNIFICANCE

Loss of dentition during treatment for calcifying odonto-genic tumors will increase the necessity of consultation prior to the planned surgical procedure.

DENTAL MANAGEMENT

Postsurgical management may include a need for implants or fixed or removable prosthodontics to replace missing teeth.

SUGGESTED REFERENCES

Fulciniti F, Vetrani A, Zeppa P, Califano L, Palombini L. Calcifying epithelial odontogenic tumor (Pindborg's tumor) on fine-needle aspiration biopsy smears: a case report. *Diagnostic Cytopathology* 1995;12(1):71–75.

Hicks MJ, Flaitz CM, Wong ME, McDaniel RK, Cagle PT. Clear cell variant of calcifying epithelial odontogenic tumor: case report and review of the literature. *Head Neck* 1994;16(3):272–277.

Houston GD, Fowler CB. Extraosseous calcifying epithelial odontogenic tumor: report of two cases and review of the literature. *Oral Surg Oral Med Oral Path Oral Radiol Endodon* 1994;83(5):577–583.

Takata T, Ogawa 1, Miyauchi M, Ijuhin N, Nikai H, Fujita M. Non-calcifying Pindborg tumor with Langerhans cells. *J Oral Pathol Med* 1993;22(8):378–383.

AUTHOR: **STEVEN D. VINCENT, DDS, MS**

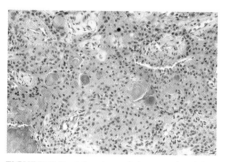

FIGURE II-8 Islands and sheets of epithelial cells dispersed throughout a nonspecific fibrous stroma. The polygonal, epithelial cells show remarkable pleomorphism and nuclear hyperchromasia. Borders of the epithelial cells are well-defined with prominent intracellular bridges. Several small, rounded islands of mineralized material exhibiting a Liesegang ring phenomenon are noted (hematoxylin and eosin stain, original magnification 40×).

SECTION II

SYNONYM(S)

Candidiasis
"Thrush"

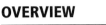

ICD-9CM/CPT CODE(S)
112.0 Candidiasis of mouth
CPT General Exam or Consultation
(e.g., 99243 or 99213)

OVERVIEW

Oral candidosis is a fungal infection usually caused by *Candida albicans*, which is present as a commensal organism in approximately 50% of people. Most infections are superficial.

EPIDEMIOLOGY & DEMOGRAPHICS

Candidosis is a common oral fungal infection.

ETIOLOGY & PATHOGENESIS

- Development of infection primarily depends on the immune status of host and the oral mucosal environment.
- Local and systemic factors that predispose an individual to develop candidosis:
  - Xerostomia
  - Intraoral prosthetic devices
  - Other mucosal diseases
  - Broad-spectrum antibiotic use
  - Immunocompromising diseases and medical treatments
  - Nutritional deficiencies
  - Metabolic disorders

CLINICAL PRESENTATION / PHYSICAL FINDINGS

CLINICAL VARIANTS

- Pseudomembranous candidosis ("thrush")
  - White, curd-like material on mucosa
  - Erythematous underlying mucosa
  - May be associated with burning
  - May be associated with metallic taste
- Acute atrophic candidosis
  - Erythematous mucosa
  - Localized or generalized
  - Often painful
  - May be associated with antibiotic use
- Chronic atrophic candidosis
  - Most common type of candidosis
  - Often denture-related (may also be seen with acrylic orthodontic appliances)
  - Limited to denture-bearing area
  - Often related to poor denture hygiene or wearing denture 24 hours a day
  - Erythematous mucosa
  - Usually asymptomatic
- Chronic hyperplastic candidosis
  - White lesion that does not wipe off
  - Increased incidence in tobacco users
  - Often found on the buccal mucosa
  - Yeast hyphae invade epithelium
  - Associated with increased epithelial atypia
  - Resolves with antifungal therapy

- Angular cheilitis
  - Tenderness, erythema, and fissuring at the labial commissures
  - Usually caused by *Candida albicans* but can be caused by other factors
  - Often associated with intraoral candidosis
- Cheilitis/perioral dermatitis
  - Diffuse involvement of vermilion border and/or perioral epidermis
  - May be associated with intraoral candidosis

DIAGNOSIS

Clinical diagnosis of candidosis may be confirmed with cytologic preparations stained with periodic acid-Schiff stain modified for fungi. Lesions suspected to represent chronic hyperplastic candidosis that do not respond to antifungal therapy must be biopsied to evaluate for other possible diseases such as epithelial dysplasia or squamous cell carcinoma.

MEDICAL MANAGEMENT & TREATMENT

- Identification and, if possible, elimination or control of systemic predisposing factors
- Antifungal therapy (Table II-1)

COMPLICATIONS

- In severely immunocompromised patients, candidosis may progress to invasive disease.
- Drug interactions and side effects associated with systemic antifungal medications.

PROGNOSIS

Good; however, maintenance therapy may be required to prevent recurrent infection if predisposing factors cannot be eliminated or controlled.

DENTAL SIGNIFICANCE

- Patients receiving dental prostheses should be educated in proper use and care to prevent chronic atrophic candidosis.
- Dentures should be fabricated with and periodically evaluated for adequate vertical dimension of occlusion to prevent angular cheilitis.
- Thorough oral soft tissue examination will identify asymptomatic forms of candidosis.

TABLE II-1	**Management of Oral Candidosis**
Medication	**Dosage and Directions[1]**
Chlorhexidine 0.12% oral rinse (Peridex, PerioGard)[2] or 0.2% alcohol-free aqueous[3]	15 mL mouthrinse and expectorate tid. NPO ½ hr after use.
Nystatin oral suspension 100,000 units/mL[4]	5 mL mouthrinse 1 min and expectorate[5] qid (PC and HS). NPO ½ hr after use.
Clotrimazole 10 mg/mL suspension[6]	Swab 1–2 mL on affected area qid (PC and HS). NPO ½ hr after use.
Ketoconazole 2% cream (Nizoral) or clotrimazole 1% cream (Lotrimin)	Apply thin film to inner surface of denture(s) and/or corners of mouth qid (PC and HS). NPO ½ hr after use.
Clotrimazole 200 mg vaginal tablets (Gyne Lotrimin)	Dissolve ½ tablet slowly in mouth bid. NPO ½ hr after use.
Clotrimazole 10 mg oral troches (Mycelex)	Dissolve 1 troche slowly in mouth 5x daily. NPO ½ hr after use.
Ketoconazole 200 mg tablets (Nizoral)	1 tablet PO qd for 7 to 10 days. Do not take antacids within 2 hours of this medication.[7]
Fluconazole 100 mg tablets (Diflucan)	1 tablet PO bid for first day, then 1 tablet PO QD for 10 to 14 days.

[1] In most patients, decreased frequency and dosages may be used if maintenance therapy is required.
[2] High alcohol content (11.6%) will irritate mucosa and enhance xerostomia. Should not be prescribed for recovering alcoholics.
[3] Must be prepared by experienced compounding pharmacist. Many formulas include flavorings that decrease efficacy.
[4] High sucrose content. Not first-line choice.
[5] May be swallowed for pharyngeal involvement.
[6] Compounded in confectioner's glycerin.
[7] Acidic environment is required for absorption.
Source: Kleinegger CL. Diseases of the mouth, in Rakel RE, Bope ET (eds): *Conn's Current Therapy.* Philadelphia, WB Saunders, 2002, p 831, Table 2.

DENTAL MANAGEMENT

- Identification and, if possible, elimination or control of local predisposing factors.
- Patients with denture-related candidosis should be educated regarding proper denture use and care.

- Medical consultation regarding possible systemic predisposing factors.
- Consideration of possible side effects and drug interactions for patients taking systemic antifungal medication.

SUGGESTED REFERENCES

Kleinegger, CL. Diseases of the mouth, in Rakel RE, Bope ET (eds): *Conn's Current Therapy*. Philadelphia, WB Saunders, 2002, pp 831, 833–834.

Neville BW, Damm DD, Allen CM, Bouquot JE. *Oral & Maxillofacial Pathology*. Philadelphia, WB Saunders, 2002, pp 189–197.

AUTHOR: **CYNTHIA L. KLEINEGGER, DDS, MS**

SECTION II

SYNONYM(S)

Central giant cell reparative granuloma
Central giant cell lesion
Giant cell tumor

ICD-9CM/CPT CODE(S)

526.3 Central giant cell granuloma
CPT General Exam or Consultation
(e.g., 99243 or 99213)

OVERVIEW

A benign osteolytic lesion arising centrally within the jaws.

EPIDEMIOLOGY & DEMOGRAPHICS

INCIDENCE/PREVALENCE IN USA: The mandible is more frequently involved than the maxilla. Some serial studies report an increased incidence of CGCG affecting the anterior mandible with a tendency to cross the midline.

PREDOMINANT AGE: The central giant cell granuloma (CGCG) occurs over a wide patient age spectrum with a majority of cases occurring before age 30 years.

PREDOMINANT SEX: Females are more commonly affected than males.

ETIOLOGY & PATHOGENESIS

- The etiology and pathogenesis of the CGCG has yet to be fully understood.
- Since the CGCG has been associated with a variety of other primary diseases of bone and odontogenic tumors, some believe the CGCG represents an exuberant reactive or reparative process.
- A subset of clinically aggressive CGCGs behaves more like a true neoplasm than a reparative process.

CLINICAL PRESENTATION / PHYSICAL FINDINGS

- Two clinical subtypes of CGCG exist: nonaggressive lesions and aggressive lesions.

- Both subtypes present as a well-delineated unilocular or multilocular radiolucent lesion with noncorticated borders.
- The nonaggressive subtype is more common, exhibiting few clinical symptoms and demonstrating slow growth with a lack of root resorption or perforation of the cortical plate.
- The aggressive subtype is characterized by pain and swelling with rapid growth; usually causes root resorption and cortical perforation.
- Serum calcium and parathormone are within normal limits.

DIAGNOSIS

- Histologic examination shows numerous, multinucleated (osteoclast-like) giant cells arrayed within a cellular background stroma composed of plump to spindle-shaped mesenchymal cells. Erythrocyte extravasation with subsequent hemosiderin deposition in the background stroma is often a prominent finding.
- The diagnosis of CGCG generally requires the exclusion of underlying hyperparathyroidism.

MEDICAL MANAGEMENT & TREATMENT

- Since the CGCG is histologically and radiographically indistinguishable from the brown tumor seen in hyperparathyroidism, it is imperative that all hyperparathyroidism be excluded in all cases of CGCG.
- The nonaggressive subtype of CGCG is generally treated with surgical curettage.
- The aggressive subtype is prone to recurrence following curettage and may require resection.

- Alternative therapy using corticosteroids or calcitonin has been reported with varying results.

COMPLICATIONS

The aggressive subtype may require radical surgery.

PROGNOSIS

- Recurrence rates following surgical curettage are reportedly as high as 20%.
- Metastases have not been reported.

DENTAL SIGNIFICANCE

Root resorption of affected teeth may necessitate their removal.

DENTAL MANAGEMENT

See preceding.

SUGGESTED REFERENCES

Carlos R, Sedano HO. Intralesional corticosteroids as an alternative treatment for central giant cell granuloma. *Oral Surg Oral Med Oral Pathol Oral Radiol Endod* 2002;93:161–166.

Gungormus M, Akgul HM. Central giant cell granulomas of the jaws: a clinical and radiographic study. *J Contemp Dent Pract* 2003;4:87–97.

Pogrel MA. Calcitonin therapy for central giant cell granuloma. *J Oral Maxillofac Surg* 2003;61:649–653.

Whitaker SB, Waldron CA. Central giant cell lesions of the jaws: a clinical, radiographic, and histopathologic study. *Oral Surg Oral Med Oral Pathol* 1993;75:199–208.

AUTHOR: CHRISTOPHER G. FIELDING, DDS, MS

SYNONYM(S)

Cervical adenitis
Cervical lymphadenopathy
Specific types of lymphadenitis (i.e., mycobacterial lymphadenitis, granulomatous)
Lymphadenitis

ICD-9CM/CPT CODE(S)

683 Acute lymphadenitis
041.1 Use additional code to identify organism such as Staphylococcus
785.6 Excludes enlarged glands NOS
289.1 Chronic or subacute lymphadenitis
289.3 Unspecified lymphadenitis
CPT General Exam or Consultation (e.g., 99243 or 99213)

OVERVIEW

Cervical lymphadenitis indicates reactive inflammatory involvement of the lymph nodes of the neck. The term lymphadenopathy refers more generally to any enlargement of the lymph nodes. The majority of cases include tenderness and enlargement of the affected nodes. The condition most commonly represents a transient response to a localized or general inflammatory insult such as an upper respiratory tract or odontogenic infection, but occasionally it results from a more serious disorder or infection. If a specific cause is known for the lymphadenitis, then that diagnosis can be used to indicate the type of lymphadenitis. The condition may be chronic or acute, depending on the type of stimulus.

EPIDEMIOLOGY & DEMOGRAPHICS

INCIDENCE/PREVALENCE IN USA: Cervical lymphadenitis is a nonspecific diagnostic term and, due to the ubiquitous nature of antigenic challenges in the head and neck region, cervical lymphadenitis is a very common condition affecting a broad range of patients.
PREDOMINANT AGE: Pediatric patients are particularly sensitive to these stimuli and represent the most commonly affected group. Pediatric patients are also at risk for atypical mycobacterial lymphadenitis.

ETIOLOGY & PATHOGENESIS

- Reactive or inflammatory cervical lymphadenitis results from exposure of the lymph nodes to antigenic elements, typically viral, bacterial, or chemical in nature, through the relevant lymphatic drainage. In response the lymph nodes become enlarged and tender. Common sources of inflammation include upper respiratory infections, systemic viral infections, pharyngitis/tonsillitis, and odontogenic infections.
- Acute bacterial cervical lymphadenitis is most commonly the result of streptococcal or staphylococcal infection.
- Chronic infectious lymphadenitis results from direct infection of cervical lymph nodes. Common infectious agents include tuberculosis, atypical mycobacteria, toxoplasmosis, and cat scratch disease.
- Less commonly, cervical lymphadenitis is the result of drug reactions, autoimmune diseases, or malignancy.

CLINICAL PRESENTATION / PHYSICAL FINDINGS

- Enlargement of cervical lymph nodes.
- Tenderness to palpation with overlying cutaneous erythema.
- Draining sinus tracts may develop.
- Onset and duration may be acute or chronic.
- Examination should include dental evaluation.

DIAGNOSIS

- The clinical diagnosis of cervical lymphadenitis may be based on the history and physical examination.
- Lymphadenitis that persists or fails to respond to conservative therapy requires additional evaluation, including fine-needle aspiration biopsy or lymph node biopsy followed by microscopic examination.
- Microbial culture results provide the gold standard for the diagnosis of infectious agents; however, polymerase chain reaction analysis and evaluation of special stains can provide an acceptable level of diagnostic accuracy.
- Computed tomography (CT) images can be valuable in determining the extent of nodal involvement and the presence of necrosis.

MEDICAL MANAGEMENT & TREATMENT

Transient cases of cervical lymphadenitis require no specific intervention. Infectious cases are managed with antibiotic therapy, surgery, or both.

COMPLICATIONS

Suppurative lymphadenitis may result in drainage through cutaneous sinus tracts. Involved nodes may become fibrotic.

PROGNOSIS

Cervical lymphadenitis is generally self-limited. When properly diagnosed and appropriately treated, cases that require antibiotic therapy or surgery respond excellently.

DENTAL SIGNIFICANCE

Cervical lymphadenitis may result from chronic or acute odontogenic infections. Any potentially contributory dental conditions should be evaluated and corrected.

DENTAL MANAGEMENT

Teeth noted to have potential sources of infection, such as untreated periapical lesions, may be treated in standard fashion.

SUGGESTED REFERENCES

Albright JT, Pransky SM. Nontuberculous mycobacterial infections of the head and neck. *Pediatr Clin No Am* 2003;50:503–514.

Goel MM, Ranjan V, Dhole TN, Srivastava AN, Mehrotra A, Kushwaha MR, Jain A. Polymerase chain reaction vs. conventional diagnosis in fine needle aspirates of tuberculous lymph nodes. *Acta Cytol* 2001;45(3):333–340.

Leung AK, Robson WL. Childhood cervical lymphadenopathy. *J Pediatr Health Care* 2004;18:3-7.

Neville BW, Damm DD, Allen CM, Bouquot JE. *Oral & Maxillofacial Pathology*, ed 2. Philadelphia, WB Saunders, 2002.

AUTHOR: ROBERT D. FOSS, DDS, MS

SYNONYM(S)

Familial fibrous dysplasia

ICD-9CM/CPT CODE(S)

526.89 Cherubism
CPT   General Exam or Consultation
       (e.g., 99243 or 99213)

OVERVIEW

Cherubism is a rare developmental and inherited disease affecting the jaws that usually manifests in early childhood. Multilocular, radiolucent, expansile lesions are generally seen affecting both maxilla and mandible in a symmetric fashion, causing the characteristic cherubic facial appearance.

EPIDEMIOLOGY & DEMOGRAPHICS

PREDOMINANT SEX: No predominance.
PREDOMINANT AGE: Clinical manifestations of cherubism are seen in early childhood with the disease progressing until puberty when the condition begins to slowly resolve.
GENETICS: Cherubism is an autosomal dominant inherited disorder with complete penetrance seen in males and reduced penetrance in females. The genetic mutation has been found on the *SH3BP2* gene that is mapped to chromosome 4p16.

ETIOLOGY & PATHOGENESIS

- Autosomal dominant inherited disorder
- Multilocular, radiolucent lesions affecting the jaws consisting of fibrovascular connective tissue containing a variable number of multinucleated giant cells
- Rare association of cherubism with syndromic conditions (Noonan syndrome, Ramon syndrome, neurofibromatosis)

CLINICAL PRESENTATION / PHYSICAL FINDINGS

- Symmetrical enlargement of the mandible and/or maxilla
- Multiloculated radiolucent lesions of the jaws (mandible > maxilla)
- Upward gaze
- Delayed eruption and development of the dentition
- Impacted teeth
- Root resorption
- Malocclusion
- V-shaped palatal vault

DIAGNOSIS

- Diagnosis requires histopathologic and radiographic correlation.
- Histologic examination shows a benign, multinucleated giant cell lesion that is histomorphologically identical to a central giant cell granuloma.
- Radiographic correlation showing multiquadrant or jaw involvement is essential for definitive diagnosis.

MEDICAL MANAGEMENT & TREATMENT

- Many cases spontaneously resolve following puberty.
- Surgical correction is recommended for extreme cases and those that show lasting disfigurement.

COMPLICATIONS

Psychosocial problems caused by facial disfigurement and functional impairment caused by loss of dentition and/or malocclusion.

PROGNOSIS

- Prognosis is case-dependent.
- Some individuals show complete resolution following puberty, while others exhibit varying degrees of permanent facial deformity.

DENTAL SIGNIFICANCE

Loss of dentition and or malocclusion with resulting functional impairment

DENTAL MANAGEMENT

Extensive dental rehabilitation may be required in extreme cases.

SUGGESTED REFERENCES

Beaman FD, Bancroft LW, Peterson JJ, Kransdorf MJ, Murphey MD, Menke DM. Imaging characteristics of cherubism. *AJR Am J Roentgenol* 2004;182(4):1051–1054.

Kozakiewicz M, Perczynska-Partyka W, Kobos J. Cherubism: clinical picture and treatment. *Oral Dis* 2001;7(2):123–130.

Schultze-Mosgau S, Holbach LM, Wiltfang J. Cherubism: clinical evidence and therapy. *J Craniofac Surg* 2003;14(2):201–206.

AUTHOR: **CHRISTOPHER G. FIELDING, DDS, MS**

SYNONYM(S)

Enchondroma

ICD-9CM/CPT CODE(S)

756.4 Enchondromatosis
CPT General Exam or Consultation
(e.g., 99243 or 99213)

OVERVIEW

A benign neoplasm of mature cartilaginous tissue that rarely occurs in the jawbones.

EPIDEMIOLOGY & DEMOGRAPHICS

PREVALENCE/INCIDENCE IN USA: The chondroma is one of the most common bone tumors, representing about 10% of all benign bone tumors; however, they are uncommon in the jaws. Up to 60% of chondromas are found in the tubular bones of the hands and feet.
PREDOMINANT AGE: The majority of cases are diagnosed in the third or fourth decade, but tumor growth tends to cease after adolescence.
PREDOMINANT SEX: Chondromas do not display any sex predilection.

ETIOLOGY & PATHOGENESIS

- Chondroma is a true benign neoplasm of chondrocytes associated with hyaline cartilage.
- Cartilaginous lesions of the jaws arise from embryologic cartilage rests.
- Chondroma should be distinguished from the more frequent chondromatous (or chondroid) metaplasia of soft tissue, most commonly occurring in the anterior maxilla and the tongue. Chondromatous metaplasia also occurs in the mandibular posterior alveolar ridge region of edentulous patients due to denture trauma.

CLINICAL PRESENTATION / PHYSICAL FINDINGS

- Chondroma is the most common tumor of the hand, with about 35% of chondromas occurring in the small tubular bones of the hands.
- Chondroma can cause tooth mobility and root resorption.
- Usually presents as a painless, slow-growing mass lesion.
- It may cause bony expansion.

- Maxillofacial examples most commonly affect the condyle.
  - Rarer cases occur in the anterior maxilla.
- Root resorption and tooth mobility may be present in affected teeth.
- Radiolucency with central radiopacity.
- Chondroma usually occurs as a solitary lesion, but it can occur as multiple lesions in two systemic diseases:
  - Maffucci's syndrome: soft tissue angiomas in association with skeletal chondromatosis.
  - Ollier's disease: multiple, diffusely located chondromas, usually unilateral.

DIAGNOSIS

- Radiographically, it appears as a well-circumscribed, radiolucent lesion with variable central radiopaque areas.
- Diagnosis is by biopsy and histopathologic examination of tissue.
- Microscopically, chondroma consists of a well-circumscribed tumor mass of mature hyaline cartilage demonstrating small chondrocytes with small, round lacunae.
- Histopathologic distinction between chondroma and low-grade chondrosarcoma is subtle and difficult.

MEDICAL MANAGEMENT & TREATMENT

- Chondrosarcoma of the jaws is more common than chondroma; a microscopic diagnosis of chondroma should be viewed initially with skepticism. Histopathologic consultation and/or a second opinion are recommended.
- Recommended treatment is complete surgical removal. Some surgeons treat chondroma as a low-grade chondrosarcoma. Lesions of the condyle are usually treated by condylectomy.

COMPLICATIONS

- Misdiagnosis of chondrosarcoma as chondroma results in delay of appropriate treatment.

- Irradiation of chondromas is contraindicated because of potential for transformation into sarcoma.

PROGNOSIS

Prognosis is good once an accurate diagnosis is obtained.

DENTAL SIGNIFICANCE

The dentist should seek a second opinion if a jaw lesion is histopathologically diagnosed as chondroma.

DENTAL MANAGEMENT

- Teeth involved by or adjacent to the chondroma may be removed to ensure adequate surgical control. Restoration of the area may proceed following an acceptable disease-free interval.
- Complete surgical removal of the tumor.

SUGGESTED REFERENCES

Chandu A, Spencer JA, Dyson DP. Chondroma of the mandibular condyle: an example of a rare tumour. *Dentomaxillofac Radiol* 1997;26:242–245.

Huvos AG. Solitary enchondroma, in *Bone Tumors. Diagnosis, Treatment, and Prognosis,* ed 2. Philadelphia, WB Saunders, 1991, pp 268–276.

Lazow SK, Pihlstrom RT, Solomon MP, Berger JR. Condylar chondroma: report of a case. *J Oral Maxillofac Surg* 1998;56:373–378.

Neville BW, Damm DD, Allen CM, Bouquot JE. *Oral & Maxillofacial Pathology*, ed 2. Philadelphia, WB Saunders, 2002.

Potdar GG, Srikhande SS. Chondrogenic tumors of the jaws. *Oral Surg Oral Med Oral Pathol* 1970;30:649–658.

Waldron CA (author of original version in ed 1). Bone pathology, in Neville BW, Damm DD, Allen CM, Bouquot JE (eds): *Oral & Maxillofacial Pathology*, ed 2. Philadelphia, WB Saunders, 2002, p 571.

AUTHORS: **MICHAEL W. FINKELSTEIN, DDS, MS; ROBERT D. FOSS, DDS, MS**

SYNONYM(S)

Cleidocranial dysostosis
Marie-Sainton syndrome
Osteodental dysplasia

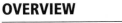

ICD-9CM/CPT CODE(S)
755.59 Cleidocranial dysostosis
CPT   General Exam or Consultation
       (e.g., 99243 or 99213)

OVERVIEW

Cleidocranial dysplasia is a congenital, generalized bone dysplasia characterized by a variety of dental and skeletal abnormalities. In general, the skeletal abnormalities are seen affecting the skull and the pectoral and pelvic girdles. Delayed eruption of the permanent dentition and supernumerary teeth are the most common dental abnormalities.

EPIDEMIOLOGY & DEMOGRAPHICS

INCIDENCE/PREVALENCE IN USA:
Reported at 0.5 per 100,000 live births.
PREDOMINANT SEX: Males and females are equally affected.
GENETICS: Cleidocranial dysplasia is a congenital autosomal dominant inherited disorder with variable expressivity. Spontaneous mutation reported in over one-third of cases.

ETIOLOGY & PATHOGENESIS

- Autosomal dominant inheritance
- Caused by a mutation in the *CBFA1* gene mapped to chromosome 6p21 that normally controls bone formation

CLINICAL PRESENTATION / PHYSICAL FINDINGS

- Oral cavity: delayed eruption of permanent teeth, which is often permanent, leading to dentigerous cyst formation around the unerupted teeth; supernumerary teeth and high, arched palate
- Skull: delayed closure of fontanels, open cranial sutures, wormian bones filling suture lines, brachycephaly, hypoplasia of the maxilla, hypoplasia of the paranasal sinuses and mastoids
- Pectoral girdle: aplasia (or, more commonly, hypoplasia) of the clavicles permitting the shoulders to approximate each other in front of the chest
- Pelvic girdle: delayed closure of the pubic symphysis
- Other: conduction hearing deficit, hypertelorism, abnormalities of the extremities, and mental retardation in some cases

DIAGNOSIS

Diagnosis is made on the constellation of clinical findings that can be supported by radiographic studies.

MEDICAL MANAGEMENT & TREATMENT

- Patients generally function well despite skeletal abnormalities.
- Treatment is often directed toward orthopedic correction.

COMPLICATIONS

- Respiratory distress due to chest wall defects.
- Frequent ear and sinus infections due to hypoplastic paranasal sinuses.
- Conduction hearing deficit due to structural abnormalities of the ossicles.
- Gait abnormalities due to pelvic and femoral abnormalities.

PROGNOSIS

The life span of individuals with cleidocranial dysplasia is normal.

DENTAL SIGNIFICANCE

- Multiple unerupted and/or supernumerary teeth, leading to malocclusion
- Dentigerous cyst formation in unerupted teeth

DENTAL MANAGEMENT

Multidisciplinary approach utilizing a combination of surgical, orthodontic, and prosthetic treatments.

SUGGESTED REFERENCES

Butterworth C. Cleidocranial dysplasia: modern concepts of treatment and a report of an orthodontic resistant case requiring a restorative solution. *Dent Update* 1999;26: 458–462.

Feldman VB. Cleidocranial dysplasia: a case report. *J Can Chiropr Assoc* 2002;46:185–191.

Golan I, Baumert U, et al. Dentomaxillofacial variability of cleidocranial dysplasia: clinicoradiological presentation and systematic review. *Dentomaxillofac Radiol* 2003;32: 347–354.

Tan S, Papandrikos A, et al. Dental management of cleidocranial dysostosis. *Columbia Dental Review* 2000;5:8–10.

AUTHOR: **CHRISTOPHER G. FIELDING, DDS, MS**

SYNONYM(S)
Venereal wart

ICD-9CM/CPT CODE(S)
078.11 Condyloma acuminatum
CPT   General Exam or Consultation
      (e.g. 99243 or 99213)

OVERVIEW

- Condyloma acuminatum is a reactive, papillary epithelial soft tissue enlargement caused by human papilloma virus (HPV) (see "Human Papilloma Virus Diseases" in Section I, p 112).
- It can occur on oropharyngeal mucosa as well as the anogenital region and is considered a sexually transmitted disease.

EPIDEMIOLOGY & DEMOGRAPHICS
PREDOMINANT AGE: Condyloma acuminatum can occur at any age but is most common in teens and young adults. In one study, 81% of patients were between the ages of 21 and 40.
PREDOMINANT SEX: Lesions are more common in males (95% in one study).

ETIOLOGY & PATHOGENESIS
- Condyloma acuminatum is caused by an infection from a variety of human papilloma virus (HPV) types, including types 2, 6, 11, 53, and 54. Anogenital lesions are sometimes associated with types 16 and 18, which have been associated with development of squamous cell carcinoma. There has been no association with transformation to squamous cell carcinoma in oral lesions.
- Oral condylomas are often a sexually transmitted disease. They often occur simultaneously with genital warts in the patient or sexual partners.
- Nonsexual transmission and autoinoculation have been reported. Also, perinatal transmission from mother to child has been documented.

CLINICAL PRESENTATION / PHYSICAL FINDINGS
- Lesions may be solitary, but in one study approximately one-third of patients with oral condyloma had multiple oral lesions.
- The most common locations for oral lesions are the lips, floor of mouth, tongue, and gingiva.
- Lesions are pink to white, raised, well-circumscribed, with a pebbly or papillary surface. They have the general appearance of a warty lesion. The base of the lesion is more commonly sessile rather than pedunculated.
- Most lesions are asymptomatic, although occasionally patients report tenderness.
- In terms of size, condyloma tends to be larger than squamous papilloma and is characteristically clustered with other condylomata. The average size of condyloma is 1.0 to 1.5 cm, but oral lesions as large as 3.0 cm have been reported.
- Clinical differential diagnosis most commonly includes squamous papilloma and verruca vulgaris.

DIAGNOSIS

Lesions are diagnosed by histopathologic examination of biopsy specimens.

MEDICAL MANAGEMENT & TREATMENT

Since condyloma is a sexually transmitted disease, treatment of anogenital lesions in the patient and sexual partners is necessary.

COMPLICATIONS

- Autoinoculation of lesions is possible.
- Transformation of anogenital condylomata of HPV types 16 and 18 into squamous cell carcinoma is possible. The exact role of HPV in oral carcinogenesis remains to be elucidated. Oral condylomata do not appear to be a precursor to squamous cell carcinoma at this time.
- The presence of oral condylomata in young children may indicate sexual abuse.

- Patients with anogenital condyloma acuminatum are at risk for other sexually transmitted diseases such as chlamydia, syphilis, and gonorrhea.

PROGNOSIS

Recurrence of oral lesions is common. Removal of all oral and anogenital lesions in the patient and sexual partners is mandatory.

DENTAL SIGNIFICANCE

Patient education regarding the sexually transmitted nature of condyloma acuminatum is an important aspect of patient management. Referral of the patient for treatment of anogenital lesions is important.

DENTAL MANAGEMENT

- Complete surgical removal is the most common treatment.
- Since lesions are contagious they should be removed.
- Topical applications of podophyllum resin have been used in conjunction with surgery in recurrent cases.

SUGGESTED REFERENCES

Butler S, et al. Condyloma acuminatum in the oral cavity: four cases and a review. *Rev Infect Dis* 1988;10:544–550.
Epithelial pathology, in Neville BW, Damm DD, Allen CM, Bouquot JE (eds): *Oral & Maxillofacial Pathology,* ed 2. Philadelphia, WB Saunders, 2002, pp 318–319.
Marquard JV, Racey GL. Combined medical and surgical management of intraoral condyloma acuminata. *J Oral Maxillofac Surg* 1981;39:459–461.
Panici PB, et al. Oral condyloma lesions in patients with extensive genital human papillomavirus infection. *Am J Obstet Gynecol* 1992;167:451–458.
Zunt SL, Tomich CE. Oral condyloma acuminatum. *J Dermatol Surg Oncol* 1989;15: 591–594.

AUTHOR: **MICHAEL W. FINKELSTEIN, DDS, MS**

SYNONYM(S)

Giant cell arteritis
Temporal arteritis

ICD-9CM/CPT CODE(S)

446.5 Giant cell arteritis
CPT General Exam or Consultation
(e.g., 99243 or 99213)

OVERVIEW

Cranial arteritis is an inflammatory disease that primarily affects medium and large cranial arteries and which, if left untreated, may result in sudden, permanent blindness. It is often referred to as *temporal arteritis* because of its propensity to involve the temporal arteries. The term *giant cell arteritis* is also commonly used due to the fact that multinucleated giant cells are often observed in biopsies of the involved vessels.

EPIDEMIOLOGY & DEMOGRAPHICS

INCIDENCE/PREVALENCE IN USA:
Prevalence increases with age, rising from 50 cases per 100,000 population age 50 or older to 850 cases per 100,000 population age 85 or older.
PREDOMINANT AGE:
Primarily affects individuals over the age of 50 (average age at diagnosis is 70 years).
PREDOMINANT SEX: Affects women approximately twice as often as men.
GENETICS:
- May occur in any racial group but is most common in Caucasians.
- May affect any ethnic group but is most common in those of European descent.
- There appears to be a genetic predisposition as evidenced by an increased prevalence of the HLA-DR4 haplotype in effected patients and occasional familial clustering.

ETIOLOGY & PATHOGENESIS

- The cause of the condition is unknown, although evidence tends to support an immunologic pathogenesis.
- The morphologic alterations suggest an immunologic reaction to the elastin in the arterial wall.
- The elevation of serum proteins, particularly gamma globulin, and the rapid response to treatment with steroids are consistent with an immune-mediated process.
- The majority of the clinical features associated with cranial arteritis are due to ischemia of tissues supplied by the involved arteries.

CLINICAL PRESENTATION / PHYSICAL FINDINGS

HISTORY

- Throbbing headache (usually unilateral, often coincides with heartbeat)
- May have retroorbital pain, visual disturbance, or loss of vision
- May have fever, malaise, fatigue, nausea, anorexia, or vomiting
- May have scalp tenderness
- May have ear pain
- May have pain on mastication
- May have muscle ache and stiffness

Up to 50% of cranial arteritis cases are associated with polymyalgia rheumatica, a clinical syndrome that involves pain and stiffness of the shoulders and pelvic girdle, often accompanied by fever, night sweats, malaise, anorexia, and weight loss.

CLINICAL FEATURES

- Involved arteries may be:
  - Painful to palpation
  - Erythematous, swollen, tortuous
  - Firm and pulseless
- Rarely, lingual or labial tissue necrosis.

DIAGNOSIS

LABORATORY

- Erythrocyte sedimentation rate (ESR): usually greater than 80 mm/hr but may be normal
- C-reactive protein (CRP): used for diagnosis and for assessing response to treatment

BIOPSY

- Temporal artery biopsy provides definitive diagnosis. "Skip lesions" that represent alternating areas of diseased and normal vessel wall are a hallmark of cranial arteritis. It is important that an adequate length of artery be examined, and in some cases, bilateral biopsies may be necessary.
- In cases where there is a high clinical suspicion of cranial arteritis, treatment should not be delayed pending the biopsy procedure since biopsies obtained up to 2 weeks after initiation of therapy will still be diagnostic.

MEDICAL MANAGEMENT & TREATMENT

- Referral to ophthalmologist or neurophthalmologist
- Long-term, high-dose corticosteroid therapy

COMPLICATIONS

Side effects of corticosteroid therapy

PROGNOSIS

- Untreated, 25–50% result in blindness.
- Rarely, vascular involvement is widespread and fatal even with treatment.

DENTAL SIGNIFICANCE

- May mimic toothache or temporomandibular joint (TMJ) dysfunction
- Oral side effects of corticosteroid therapy (e.g., candidosis, dry mouth, poor wound healing, petechiae)
- Systemic side effects of corticosteroid therapy

DENTAL MANAGEMENT

In consideration of corticosteroid therapy:
- Monitor vital signs at each appointment due to cardiovascular side effects.
- Avoid aspirin-containing products.
- Assess salivary flow as a factor for caries, periodontal disease, and candidosis.
  - Manage salivary insufficiency.
- Seek medical consultation regarding possible blood dyscrasia, immunosuppression, need for antibiotic prophylaxis, or need for supplemental steroids.

SUGGESTED REFERENCE

Kleinegger CL, Lilly GE. Cranial arteritis. A medical emergency with orofacial manifestations. *J Am Dent Assoc* 1999;130: 1203–1209.

AUTHOR: CYNTHIA L. KLEINEGGER, DDS, MS

SYNONYM(S)

Pituitary adamantinoma
Rathke's pouch tumor

ICD-9CM/CPT CODE(S)

237.0 Pituitary gland and craniopharyngeal duct
CPT Exam codes (possibly cephalometric radiograph) but needs full neurologic workup.
General Exam or Consultation (e.g., 99243 or 99213)

OVERVIEW

Craniopharyngioma is a benign, slow-growing, mainly intracranial epithelial tumor that predominantly involves the intrasellar or suprasellar space. Although benign, such tumors can behave in an aggressive fashion and have an extremely low incidence of metastasis. In rare instances, these tumors can enter the nasal cavity.

EPIDEMIOLOGY & DEMOGRAPHICS

INCIDENCE/PREVALENCE IN USA: Overall incidence is 0.13 per 100,000 population per year. Represents 3–5% of intracranial tumors (5–10% in children).
PREDOMINANT AGE: Can develop at any time from birth to old age, with peaks at 5 to 10 years of age and 40 to 60 years of age.
PREDOMINANT SEX: Equal sex predilection.

ETIOLOGY & PATHOGENESIS

- Originates from remnants of the craniopharyngeal duct and/or the resultant cleft of Rathke's pouch.
- May also originate from residual squamous epithelial remnants following involution of Rathke's duct.

CLINICAL PRESENTATION / PHYSICAL FINDINGS

- Can present as a single large cyst or multiple cysts filled with a brown fluid that contains floating yellow flecks of cholesterol crystals
- Headache, nausea, vomiting, nasal obstruction
- Visual disturbances including oculomotor palsy, amblyopia, and blindness
- Pituitary hypofunction (growth failure)
- Adrenal hypofunction resulting in hypoglycemia, hyperkalemia, cardiac arrhythmias, lethargy, confusion, and/or anorexia
- Diabetes insipidus and symptoms of hypothyroidism (weight gain, fatigue, cold intolerance, constipation)
- Obesity, seizures, and coma

DIAGNOSIS

- On CT and MRI, typically presents as a tumor with calcifications along the rim (more often seen in children).
- The papillary variant will show on CT and MRI as a noncalcified mass or cystic mass that can show peripheral nodules.
- Imaging may show extension into the third ventricle.
- Angiography may be helpful in characterizing the displacement of the cerebral vasculature.
- Complete endocrinologic and ophthalmologic examinations are necessary.

MEDICAL MANAGEMENT & TREATMENT

- Total tumor resection
- Initial surgical procedure followed by radiotherapy

COMPLICATIONS

- Compression of nearby structures such as the optic chiasm or hypothalamus.
- Displacement of the circle of Willis.
- Adhesion to surrounding vascular structures may lead to incomplete tumor removal.
- Recurrences can present from implantation of tissue along the surgical field as well as from the primary site.
- Potential for seizures, and blindness.

PROGNOSIS

- Five-year survival rate of more than 80%.
- Recurrence rate approaches 20%.
- Many patients show permanent, endocrinologic disturbances.
- Temporary visual disturbances.

DENTAL SIGNIFICANCE

May mimic the histologic appearance of odontogenic tumors such as ameloblastoma and calcifying odontogenic cyst.

DENTAL MANAGEMENT

No specific dental management is indicated for this condition.

SUGGESTED REFERENCES

Bunin GR, Surawicz TS, Witman PA. The descriptive epidemiology of craniopharyngioma. *J Neurosurg* 1998;89:547.
Curtis J, Daneman D, Hoffman HJ. The endocrine outcome after surgical removal of craniopharyngiomas. *Pediatr Neurosurg* 1994;21(Suppl 1):24.
Fujimoto Y, Matsushita H, Velasco O, et. al. Craniopharyngioma involving the infrasellar region: a case report and review of the literature. *Pediatr Neurosurg* 2002;37:210.
Hayward R. The present and future management of childhood craniopharyngioma. *Childs Nerv Syst* 1999;15:764–769.

AUTHOR: **JAMES T. CASTLE, DDS, MS**

SYNONYM(S)

Teratoid cyst
Epidermoid cyst

ICD-9CM/CPT CODE(S)
528.4 Dermoid cyst
CPT General Exam or Consultation
(e.g., 99243 or 99213)

OVERVIEW

Dermoid cysts are uncommon cystic malformations or developmental lesions that represent a benign, cystic form of teratoma.

EPIDEMIOLOGY & DEMOGRAPHICS
INCIDENCE/PREVALENCE IN USA: Dermoid cysts are uncommon entities; they predominantly (approximately 7%) occur in the head and neck. They represent approximately 0.01% of oral cysts.
PREDOMINANT SEX: Males and females are equally affected.
PREDOMINANT AGE: The age at diagnosis ranges from birth (congenital presentation) to middle age with most cases diagnosed in the second and third decade of life.

ETIOLOGY & PATHOGENESIS
Dermoid cysts are presumed to be derived from entrapped embryological rests in the affected area.

CLINICAL PRESENTATION / PHYSICAL FINDINGS
- Classically, a sublingual mass located in the midline.
  ○ The tongue may be displaced in a posterior-superior direction.
- Cysts below the geniohyoid may present as a submental mass.
- Compressible with a doughy or rubbery consistency.
- Asymptomatic unless secondarily infected.

DIAGNOSIS

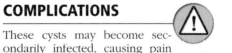

- The diagnosis of a dermoid cyst is based on microscopic examination of the surgical specimen. Histologically, dermoid cysts are lined by orthokeratotic stratified. The lumen is filled by keratinaceous debris while the cyst wall is fibrous and contains dermal appendages such as sebaceous glands, apocrine glands, or hair follicles. Similar cysts that lack the dermal appendages are referred to as epidermoid cysts.
- CT and MRI imaging studies can be valuable adjuncts for confirming the cystic nature and extent of the dermoid cyst.

MEDICAL MANAGEMENT & TREATMENT

Dermoid cysts are readily treated by complete surgical removal.

COMPLICATIONS

These cysts may become secondarily infected, causing pain or discomfort and complicating surgical removal. Rare examples of squamous cell carcinoma developing in a dermoid cyst have been reported.

PROGNOSIS

Complete surgical removal is typically curative, and recurrence is unlikely.

DENTAL SIGNIFICANCE

The teeth are not affected by dermoid cysts.

DENTAL MANAGEMENT

No special dental considerations are required.

SUGGESTED REFERENCES

Howell CJ. The sublingual dermoid cyst. Report of five cases and review of the literature. *Oral Surg Oral Med Oral Pathol* 1985;59:578–580.

King RC, Smith BR, Burk JL. Dermoid cyst in the floor of the mouth. Review of the literature and case reports. *Oral Surg Oral Med Oral Pathol* 1994;78:567–576.

Longo F, Maremonti P, Mangone GM, De Maria G, Califano L. Midline (dermoid) cysts of the floor of the mouth: report of 16 cases and review of surgical techniques. *Plast Reconstr Surg* 2003;112:1560–1565.

Neville BW, Damm DD, Allen CM, Bouquot JE (eds): *Oral & Maxillofacial Pathology*, ed 2. Philadelphia, WB Saunders, 2002.

AUTHOR: **ROBERT D. FOSS, DDS, MS**

SYNONYM(S)

Discoid lupus erythematosus refers to the skin lesions of chronic cutaneous lupus erythematosus (CCLE).

ICD-9CM/CPT CODE(S)
695.4 Lupus erythematosus (discoid)
CPT General Exam or Consultation (e.g., 99243 or 99213)

OVERVIEW

- Lupus erythematosus is an immune-mediated disease that occurs in several forms, including systemic lupus erythematosus and several types of cutaneous lupus erythematosus.
- Unlike systemic lupus erythematosus, discoid lupus does not have systemic manifestations such as arthritis, anemia, leukopenia, thrombocytopenia, and kidney disease. Skin lesions of chronic cutaneous lupus erythematosus are termed discoid lupus erythematosus.

EPIDEMIOLOGY & DEMOGRAPHICS

INCIDENCE/PREVALENCE IN USA: Estimated as between 500,000 to 1.5 million cases. Cutaneous (discoid) lupus erythematosus is two to three times more common than systemic lupus erythematosus (SLE).
PREDOMINANT SEX: More common in women, with one report giving the female to male ratio as 4.5:1.
PREDOMINANT AGE: Lesions of discoid lupus can occur at any age. The peak incidence is in the fourth decade.
GENETICS: Genetics may be a factor in predisposing individuals to discoid lupus (see following).

ETIOLOGY & PATHOGENESIS

- Factors that have been mentioned as predisposing an individual to discoid lupus erythematosus include genetic factors, dysfunction of the immune system, and environmental factors, particularly sun exposure.
- Autoantibodies are deposited in the basement membrane of skin and mucosa.

CLINICAL PRESENTATION / PHYSICAL FINDINGS

- Skin lesions of discoid lupus most commonly involve the face, scalp, ears, neck, and other sun-exposed areas. Skin of the head and neck area is involved in approximately 80% of discoid lupus cases.
- The characteristic skin lesions of discoid lupus are erythematous plaques, often covered with a scale. The lesions tend to heal with scarring.
- Older lesions or lesions that are healing may have central, atrophic scarring

and hyperkeratosis at the periphery. Hyperpigmentation or hypopigmentation and telangiectasia may occur. Alopecia is common.
- Mucosal lesions have been reported in 24% of patients with discoid lupus. Oral mucosal lesions are typically painful ulcers and erythematous erosions centrally with white rough epithelial thickening or white striae at the periphery.
- Oral mucosal lesions clinically most closely resemble lichen planus.
- Oral lesions of discoid lupus can resolve spontaneously, but the lesions often persist for months to years. Lesions may heal in one area and develop in another area.

DIAGNOSIS

- Diagnosis of lesions of discoid lupus requires incisional biopsy of skin and/or oral mucosal lesions for histopathologic diagnosis.
- Direct immunofluorescence studies of active lesions can be helpful. Tissue for direct immunofluorescence should be placed in Michel's solution rather than formalin.
- To exclude systemic lupus erythematosus, the following tests are performed: serum antinuclear antibodies, complete blood count and differential, and urinalysis for proteinuria and cellular casts.

MEDICAL MANAGEMENT & TREATMENT

- Patients should be educated that discoid lupus cannot be cured but can usually be controlled with medications.
- Patients should minimize exposure to ultraviolet radiation by using sunscreens and protective clothing.
- Clinicians should understand that some patients with classic discoid lupus lesions will already have, or will develop, systemic lupus. Patients with discoid lupus should be evaluated for systemic lupus.
- Medications can be helpful in the management of discoid lupus lesions.
  - For skin lesions, topical steroids, intralesional injection of steroids, systemic steroids, and antimalarial drugs are useful.
  - For oral mucosal lesions, topical and/or systemic steroids are used.

COMPLICATIONS

- Medications used in treatment can result in complications. Systemic corticosteroids can cause immunosuppression and adrenal corti-

cal suppression. Antimalarial drugs can occasionally cause diffuse pigmentation of oral mucosa and skin.
- Atrophy of skin and alteration of pigmentation can occur with skin lesions.
- Development of oral candidiasis following treatment for oral mucosal lesions can occur.
- More than 5% of patients with discoid lupus already have, or will develop, systemic lupus erythematosus.

PROGNOSIS

- Lesions of discoid lupus tend to be chronic and have exacerbations and remissions but can usually be managed with medications.
- About half of the patients with discoid lupus have resolution of the disease after several years.

DENTAL SIGNIFICANCE

For patients with chronic, painful oral mucosal ulcers and erosions, consider discoid lupus in the clinical differential diagnosis, especially when lesions have the appearance of lichen planus.

DENTAL MANAGEMENT

- Be aware of immunosuppressive medication, such as corticosteroids, that the patient may be taking.
- Consider referring a patient with discoid lupus to a physician for management of skin lesions and evaluation for systemic lupus erythematosus.
- Oral mucosal lesions can be effectively managed with topical and/or systemic steroids. Antifungal medications will be necessary if candidiasis develops.

SUGGESTED REFERENCES

Brennan MT, Valerin MA, Napenas JJ, Lockhart PB. Oral manifestations of patients with lupus erythematosus. *Dent Clin N Am* 2005; 49:127–141.
Brown RS, Flaitz CM, Hays GL, Trejo PM. The diagnosis and treatment of discoid lupus erythematosus with oral manifestations only: a case report. *Compend Contin Educ Dent* 1994;15:724–734.
Burge SM, Frith PA, Juniper RP, Wojnarowska F. Mucosal involvement in systemic and chronic cutaneous lupus erythematosus. *Br J Dermatol* 1989;121:727–741.
Neville BW, Damm DD, Allen CM, Bouquot JE (eds). *Oral & Maxillofacial Pathology*, ed 2, Philadelphia, WB Saunders, 2002, pp 689–692.

AUTHOR: MICHAEL W. FINKELSTEIN, DDS, MS

SECTION II

SYNONYM(S)

Fibrous dysplasia is one of the diseases in the category of bone diseases termed benign fibroosseous lesions of the jaws.

Polyostotic fibrous dysplasia with endocrinopathy (McCune-Albright syndrome)

Polyostotic fibrous dysplasia

Craniofacial fibrous dysplasia

Monostotic fibrous dysplasia

ICD-9CM/CPT CODE(S)

756.54 Polyostotic fibrous dysplasia of bone

526.89 Fibrous dysplasia of jaw

CPT General Exam or Consultation (e.g., 99243 or 99213)

OVERVIEW

- Fibrous dysplasia (FD) is a nonneoplastic developmental overgrowth of bone in which normal bone is replaced by cellular, fibrous connective tissue containing scattered trabeculae of bone.
- The extent of the disease varies from involvement of one bone (monostotic fibrous dysplasia) to involvement of numerous bones of the skeleton (polyostotic fibrous dysplasia), sometimes with extraskeletal systemic manifestations.

EPIDEMIOLOGY & DEMOGRAPHICS

PREDOMINANT AGE:

- Because fibrous dysplasia is a developmental abnormality, the initial diagnosis most commonly occurs during the first two decades of life.
- Occasionally monostotic fibrous dysplasia is first diagnosed in an older patient, but the patient usually has a history that the lesion began during the first two decades of life.
- The median age for onset of symptoms in polyostotic FD has been reported as young as 8 years; two thirds of patients had symptoms before age 10.

PREDOMINANT SEX: There is no sex predilection.

GENETICS:

- Fibrous dysplasia arises as a result of an activating mutation in the GNAS1 gene. Activation of this gene results in abnormal bone and fibrous growth in the affected bones (see following).
- Degree of involvement depends on the point during fetal or postnatal life at which the mutation occurs.

ETIOLOGY & PATHOGENESIS

- Fibrous dysplasia occurs as a result of sporadic mutation in the guanine nucleotide-binding protein, α-stimulating activity polypeptide 1 (GNAS1) gene.
- Mutation of the GNAS1 gene early in embryonic development leads to involvement of osteoblasts, melanocytes, and endocrine system cells resulting in multiple bone lesions, pigmented lesions of skin, and endocrine abnormalities (McCune-Albright syndrome).
- Mutation at a later stage in embryonic development results in development of multiple bony lesions.
- Mutation of the GNAS1 gene following birth leads to involvement of one bone.

CLINICAL PRESENTATION / PHYSICAL FINDINGS

MONOSTOTIC FIBROUS DYSPLASIA

- Monostotic fibrous dysplasia of the jaws is considerably more common than the polyostotic form, comprising 80–85% of cases.
- The most common clinical manifestation is a slow growing, painless enlargement of the bone.
- The jaws are some of the most common sites of involvement in monostotic fibrous dysplasia.
- Involvement of the maxilla is more common than the mandible.
- Craniofacial fibrous dysplasia: when fibrous dysplasia involves the maxilla, it also commonly involves the maxillary sinus and may involve adjacent bones, such as the zygoma, sphenoid, temporal, orbital, nasal, frontal, and occipital bones. Although multiple bones are involved, the disease is still classified as monostotic because of the contiguous distribution of the lesions.
- Despite the number of bones affected in craniofacial fibrous dysplasia, it is typically a unilateral disease.
- When the mandible is involved, it typically is the only bone involved.
- Typically, patients do not experience paresthesia or dysesthesia.

POLYOSTOTIC FIBROUS DYSPLASIA

- The extent of skeletal involvement in polyostotic fibrous dysplasia is highly variable and ranges between 5–60%.
- The jaws may be involved in polyostotic fibrous dysplasia, but this disease primarily involves the long bones.
- The long bones are more susceptible to fracture, resulting in bony deformities such as decreased length.
- The most common initial signs and symptoms of polyostotic fibrous dysplasia include a limp, pain, or fracture.
- About 3–5% of patients with polyostotic fibrous dysplasia have extraskeletal manifestations.
- Jaffe-Lichtenstein disease is a polyostotic fibrous dysplasia accompanied by pigmented melanotic macules called café au lait pigmentation.
  - The café au lait pigmentations are large, flat, tan to brown, freckle-like lesions with irregular borders as opposed to the smooth-bordered café au lait spots found in neurofibromatosis.
- McCune-Albright syndrome (also known simply as Albright's syndrome) is polyostotic fibrous dysplasia with café au lait pigmentation and endocrine abnormalities.
  - The most common endocrinopathies in McCune-Albright syndrome include precocious puberty in females, pituitary adenoma, accelerated skeletal growth, and hyperthyroidism.

DIAGNOSIS

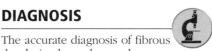

The accurate diagnosis of fibrous dysplasia depends on close cooperation between the clinician and the pathologist. Correlation of biopsy results, clinical presentation, and the lesion's radiographic presentation is required. Histologically, fibrous dysplasia is composed of haphazardly arranged, irregular, C-shaped or "Chinese character" trabeculae of bone that feather into an abundant, fibrous component.

- Radiographically, the lesions are fusiform in shape with a ground-glass texture and are not well demarcated; the typical lesion blends into the surrounding, uninvolved bone.
- Some lesions may demonstrate foci of irregular or denser calcification superimposed on the typical ground-glass appearance.
- Early lesions can be radiolucent or radiolucent with scattered radiopaque areas, but this presentation is less common in the jaws than the ground-glass appearance.
- Painless expansion of the cortical plates is common, but perforation of the cortex should not occur.
- Displacement of normal anatomical structures such as the inferior alveolar canal can occur. Teeth are often displaced by the lesion but remain firm.
- The most characteristic radiographic appearance of craniofacial fibrous dysplasia is increased density of the base of the skull, including occiput, sphenoids, sella turcica, and roof of orbit and frontal bone, as well as displacement of the floor and/or obliteration of the maxillary sinus.

MEDICAL MANAGEMENT & TREATMENT

- Management of fibrous dysplasia is directed at correcting any cosmetic deficits that may have resulted from bony expansion and facial asymmetry. Surgical recontouring can be effective in establishing a satisfactory cosmetic result, but the lesion may regrow.
- Radiation therapy is contraindicated.
- Polyostotic fibrous dysplasia is a disease that may require the efforts of a

team of specialists, including orthopedic surgery, neurosurgery, head and neck surgery, and endocrinology.

COMPLICATIONS

- Involvement of bones at the base of the skull can cause narrowing of the cranial foramina, leading to impaired vision and hearing.
- Skeletal growth disturbances due to numerous fractures can occur in polyostotic fibrous dysplasia.
- Significant craniofacial deformity and disfigurement can occur.
- Endocrine abnormalities can complicate growth and development in McCune-Albright's syndrome.
- Regrowth of the affected bone occurs in up to 50% of cases following cosmetic contouring. Fibrous dysplasia is not considered a premalignant condition, but rare examples of malignant transformation have been reported. Radiation therapy should be avoided due to the risk of development of osteosarcoma. Most cases of osteosarcoma developing in patients with fibrous dysplasia have occurred in irradiated patients.

PROGNOSIS

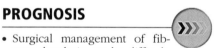

- Surgical management of fibrous dysplasia can be difficult, but the disease rarely interferes with a normal lifespan.
- The extent of bony involvement in fibrous dysplasia is highly variable.
  - For most patients, the lesions are recognized in childhood, grow slowly, and stabilize in early adult life.
  - The time at which the lesions stabilize is unpredictable, usually occurring by the end of skeletal growth but not necessarily by puberty.
- For many patients, surgical recontouring or debulking of the lesion after the lesion stops growing will provide acceptable cosmetic and functional results.
- Lifelong monitoring of the lesions is necessary.

DENTAL SIGNIFICANCE

- Fibrous dysplasia is often associated with dental anomalies such as rotated teeth, oligodontia, and displacement of teeth leading to malocclusion, but the curvilinear pattern of the dental arch tends to remain preserved.
- Teeth displaced by fibrous dysplasia are typically firm and not mobile.
- Most patients with fibrous dysplasia have normal development and eruption of teeth.

DENTAL MANAGEMENT

- Patients with fibrous dysplasia of the jaws generally do not require special dental management and are able to receive routine dental treatment without exacerbation of the lesions of fibrous dysplasia.
- Patients with fibrous dysplasia of the jaws who receive orthodontic treatment may expect treatment time to be increased, but orthodontic treatment has not been associated with exacerbation of the lesions of fibrous dysplasia.
- Since the bony lesions are poorly defined, complete surgical removal is usually not feasible.

- If the jaw lesions of monostotic fibrous dysplasia are causing minimal cosmetic or functional problems, then no treatment is necessary.
- If the lesions result in facial asymmetry, bony recontouring to improve the aesthetics is often performed.
- Continued growth of the lesions occurs, especially in younger patients, in one-fourth to one-half of the patients.
- In most cases, the lesions stop growing when skeletal maturation is reached. It is preferable to delay surgery until the active growth phase of the lesion has slowed.

SUGGESTED REFERENCES

Akintoye SO, et al. Dental characteristics of fibrous dysplasia and McCune-Albright syndrome. *Oral Surg Oral Med Oral Pathol Oral Radiol Endod* 2003;96:275–282.

Alawi F. Benign fibro-osseous diseases of the maxillofacial bones. A review and differential diagnosis. *Am J Clin Pathol* 2002; 118(Suppl 1)S50–S70.

Brannon RB, Fowler CB. Benign fibro-osseous lesions: a review of current concepts. *Adv Anat Pathol* 2001;8:126–143.

Neville BW, Damm DD, Allen CM, Bouquot JE (eds): *Oral & Maxillofacial Pathology*, ed 2. Philadelphia, WB Saunders, 2002, pp 553–557.

Posnick JC. Fibrous dysplasia of the craniomaxillofacial region: current clinical perspectives. *Br J Oral Maxillofac Surg* 1998;36: 264–273.

Waldron CA. Fibro-osseous lesions of the jaws. *J Oral Maxillofac Surg* 1985;43: 249–262.

AUTHORS: **ROBERT D. FOSS, DDS, MS; MICHAEL W. FINKELSTEIN, DDS, MS**

SYNONYM(S)

Bald tongue of pernicious anemia
Atrophic glossitis
Hunter's glossitis
Moeller's glossitis
Glossodynia exfoliativa

ICD-9CM/CPT CODE(S)

529.0 Glossitis
CPT General Exam or Consultation
(e.g., 99243 or 99213)

OVERVIEW

Atrophic glossitis (AG) is a clinical manifestation of numerous nutritional deficiencies often leading to an absence or flattening of the filiform papillae of the tongue, leaving a smooth-surfaced, "beefy red tongue." An altered sense of taste and an occasionally painful, burning sensation can be encountered.

EPIDEMIOLOGY & DEMOGRAPHICS

INCIDENCE/PREVALENCE IN USA: In general terms, AG primarily affects elderly, debilitated patients. Folate deficiency can be seen in those patients taking sulphonamide antibiotics or antifolate chemotherapeutic agents such as methotrexate or azathioprine.
PREDOMINANT AGE: More common in those 40 to 70 years of age.
PREDOMINANT SEX: Equal predilection in both sexes. In Plummer-Vinson syndrome (see Etiology & Pathogenesis following), 90% of those affected are women.
GENETICS: In pernicious anemia, elderly patients of northern European descent are the target population; it is rarely seen in African- or Asian-Americans.

ETIOLOGY & PATHOGENESIS

- Results from numerous nutritional deficiencies including:
  - Iron deficiency
  - Vitamin B_6 (pyridoxine) deficiency
  - Folate deficiency
  - Vitamin B_{12} deficiency
  - Niacin deficiency
  - Thiamine deficiency
  - Riboflavin deficiency (vitamin B_2)
  - Zinc deficiency
- Included as an element in, Plummer-Vinson syndrome (postcricoid dysphagia, upper esophageal webs, and iron deficiency anemia) (see "Plummer-Vinson Syndrome" in Section II, p 306).
- In Plummer-Vinson syndrome, pathogenic mechanisms include iron and nutritional deficiencies, genetic predisposition, and autoimmunity. The underlying cause of iron deficiency anemia (e.g., gastrointestinal blood loss, celiac sprue) should be investigated.

- In vitamin B_6 (pyridoxine) deficiency, intake is reduced in cases of severe malnutrition, and absorption is reduced in elderly persons and patients with intestinal disease or surgery.
- Pyridoxine clearance is enhanced by liver disorders such as hepatitis and several medications.
- Pyridoxine breakdown is enhanced in conditions associated with increased alkaline phosphatase levels.
- Pernicious anemia results from poor absorption of vitamin B_{12} (cobalamin, extrinsic factor) usually through a loss of binding with intrinsic factor (see "Anemia: Pernicious" in Section I, p 15).
- Intrinsic factor may be lacking due to autoimmune destruction of the parietal cells of the stomach or following gastric bypass operations.
- Autosomal dominant, with variable expressivity or congenitally present in autosomal recessive cases.
- Folate deficiency via decreased ingestion, impaired absorption via celiac sprue or disorders affecting the small intestine, impaired utilization, or increased requirements such as in pregnancy.

CLINICAL PRESENTATION / PHYSICAL FINDINGS

- Significant erythema of the dorsal surface of the tongue, leaving a beefy red color.
- Atrophy or flattening of the filiform papillae, leaving a smooth dorsal tongue surface.
- In pernicious anemia, systemic symptoms of weakness, fatigue, and vague burning sensation of the tongue and possibly lips.
- Macrocytic anemia.

DIAGNOSIS

- CBC counts.
- Peripheral blood smears to evaluate for macrocytic anemia.
- Iron studies to include serum iron, total iron-binding capacity (TIBC), ferritin, and saturation percentage to confirm an iron deficiency.
- Levels of 4-pyridoxic acid can be measured in the urine since it is the major inactive metabolite of pyridoxine metabolism.

MEDICAL MANAGEMENT & TREATMENT

- Treat iron deficiency and its underlying cause.
  - Iron replacement.
  - Dysphagia in Plummer-Vinson syndrome may improve with iron

replacement; advanced webs managed with mechanical dilation.
- Supplementation of vitamin B_6 (pyridoxine hydrochloride) (meats, particularly liver, fish, and chicken; vegetables, particularly beans, peas, and tomatoes; fruits such as oranges, bananas, and avocados; and grains such as enriched breads, cereals, and grains).
- In pernicious anemia, intramuscular injections of cyanocobalamin.
- Complete resolution of atrophic glossitis following oral multivitamin supplementation has not been conclusively documented to diminish this condition, although this treatment should be initiated following a complete patient evaluation.
- Folate supplements.

COMPLICATIONS

- In Plummer-Vinson syndrome, prevalence of esophageal carcinoma is more evident.
- Potential for an increase of 1–2% for gastric carcinoma in patients with pernicious anemia.
- Neurologic problems associated with vitamin B_{12} deficiency.

PROGNOSIS

- Noticeable change in lingual mucosa following administration of appropriate nutritional supplement or cofactor.
- No long-term oral complications following resolution.

DENTAL SIGNIFICANCE

- May lead to transient neurological deficits of the tongue if vitamin B_{12} deficiency is left unchecked.

DENTAL MANAGEMENT

- Glossodynia (burning sensation) needs to be monitored and evaluated for fungal infections, with administration of oral antifungal suspensions.

SUGGESTED REFERENCES

Byrd JA, Bruce AJ, Rogers RS. Glossitis and other tongue disorders. *Dermatol Clin* 2003;21:123.
Field EA, Speechley JA, Rugman FR, Varga E, Tyldesley WR. Oral signs and symptoms in patients with undiagnosed vitamin B12 deficiency. *Oral Pathol Med* 1995;24:468.
Schmitt RJ, Sheridan PJ, Rogers RS. Pernicious anemia with associated glossodynia. *JADA* 1988;117:838.

AUTHOR: JAMES T. CASTLE, DDS, MS

SECTION II

SYNONYM(S)

Vagoglossopharyngeal neuralgia

ICD-9CM/CPT CODE(S)
784.0 Pain, facial
CPT General Exam or Consultation
(e.g., 99243 or 99213)

OVERVIEW

Neuralgia of the ninth cranial nerve that is similar to trigeminal neuralgia except in anatomic location.

EPIDEMIOLOGY & DEMOGRAPHICS

INCIDENCE/PREVALENCE IN USA: Occurs only once for every 100 cases of trigeminal neuralgia.
PREDOMINANT AGE: Peak onset 40 to 60 years, with a predilection for the left side in females.
PREDOMINANT SEX: No gender predilection.

ETIOLOGY & PATHOGENESIS

Unknown etiology; various theories include vascular compression of the ninth cranial nerve, neural ischemia, neoplasms, infections/inflammation.

CLINICAL PRESENTATION / PHYSICAL FINDINGS

- Rarely bilateral.
- Intense, paroxysmal pain may be felt in the infraauricular area, tonsil, base of tongue, posterior mandible, or lateral wall of the pharynx.
- Abrupt onset and short duration (30- to 60-second bursts that may occur for up to 1 hour).
- May be triggered by swallowing (especially cold items), chewing, yawning, talking, or coughing.
- Difficult to identify trigger zones.

DIAGNOSIS

DIFFERENTIAL DIAGNOSIS
- Eagle's syndrome
- Neoplasm
- Atypical facial pain
- Geniculate neuralgia
- Trigeminal neuralgia

WORKUP
- Application of topical or local anesthetic to the tonsil or pharynx provides rapid relief.

IMAGING
- MRI or CT with contrast to evaluate for neoplasm.

MEDICAL MANAGEMENT & TREATMENT

- Conservative treatment with medication versus surgical intervention.
- Surgery consists of intracranial section of the rootlets of the ninth cranial nerve and the upper two rootlets of the tenth cranial nerve.
- Drug of choice is carbamazepine, but other anticonvulsants may be tried.
- Carbamazepine 200 to 1600 mg/day. Side effects include drowsiness, anemia, thrombocytopenia, and agranulocytosis.
- Serum levels and CBC with differential must be obtained at regular intervals with chronic therapy.

COMPLICATIONS

Up to 10% of patients may lose consciousness, possibly due to bradycardia or asystole.

PROGNOSIS

The prognosis is guarded for complete relief of symptoms since there can be unpredictable remission and recurrence.

DENTAL MANAGEMENT

Patients may be referred to neurologist or neurosurgeon.

SUGGESTED REFERENCES

Neville BW, Damm DD, Allen CM, Bouquot JE (eds): *Oral & Maxillofacial Surgery*, ed 2. Philadelphia, WB Saunders, 2002, pp 744–745.
Rozen TD. Trigeminal neuralgia and glossopharyngeal neuralgia. *Neurol Clin No Am* 2004;22:185–206.

AUTHOR: **DARYL E. BEE, DDS, MS**

SYNONYM(S)

None

ICD-9CM/CPT CODE(S)
274.0 Gout
CPT General Exam or Consultation
(e.g., 99243 or 99213)

OVERVIEW

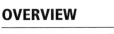

Painful and potentially disabling inflammatory arthritis caused by accumulation of uric acid. Urate crystals are deposited in various tissues, organs, and joints. Can lead to destructive arthropathy; urolithiasis can lead to kidney failure. See "Gout" in Section I, p 89.

EPIDEMIOLOGY & DEMOGRAPHICS

INCIDENCE/PREVALENCE IN USA: Gout affects 2.1 million people in the U.S. **PREDOMINANT AGE:** Rare in children and young adults. Most common inflammatory arthritis in men over 40 years of age. In women, the incidence increases after menopause. **PREDOMINANT SEX:** Male gender is a risk factor.

ETIOLOGY & PATHOGENESIS

- Caused by an excessive blood level of uric acid, a waste product formed from the breakdown of purines.
- Hyperuricemia can be due to increased urate production, decreased excretion, or both.
- Urate crystals rather than urate in solution.
- Ten percent of patients are overproducers of urate secondary to errors of metabolism.
- In the majority of patients, renal function is normal, but reduced clearance of urate results in hyperuricemia.
- Causes of secondary hyperuricemia include drugs (diuretics, cyclosporine, toxins including lead), acquired chronic renal insufficiency, chronic hemolysis, and endogenous metabolic products (lactate, ketoacids, B-hydroxybutyrate).

- Greatest risk factor is hyperuricemia.
- Other risk factors include obesity, hypertension, hyperlipidemia, thiazide diuretic use, renal insufficiency, lead exposure, and alcohol use.

CLINICAL PRESENTATION / PHYSICAL FINDINGS

- Seventy-five percent of initial attacks are monoarticular, with 50% involving the metatarsophalangeal joint of the great toe.
- The affected joint becomes hot, dusky red, and is exquisitely painful and tender.
- See "Gout" in Section I, p 89 for more common signs and symptoms.

DIAGNOSIS

DIFFERENTIAL DIAGNOSIS

- Pseudogout (calcium pyrophosphate dihydrate deposition)
- Septic arthritis
- Rheumatoid arthritis
- Bursitis
- Cellulitis
- Tendonitis
- Acute rheumatic fever
- Thrombophlebitis

WORKUP

- Diagnosis is established by demonstrating brilliant, negatively birefringent, needle-shaped monosodium urate crystals with polarized light microscopy in the leukocytes of synovial fluid.

LABORATORY

- Gram stain and culture of synovial fluid to rule out infection that may be coexistent
- 24-hour urinary excretion of uric acid (> 600 mg/day suggests overproduction)

MEDICAL MANAGEMENT & TREATMENT

- Lifestyle changes: moderate protein/low-fat diet, avoid

excessive alcohol use, treat hypertension, and avoid excess weight gain.
- NSAIDs: avoid salicylates because of their effects on urate excretion.
- Intraarticular corticosteroid injection.
- Oral colchicine is effective but has a low therapeutic index with gastrointestinal side effects. The IV form has many serious side effects and is to be used with caution.
- Allopurinol 300 mg/day.
- Probenecid 0.5 to 1 g twice daily.

COMPLICATIONS

See "Gout" in Section I, p 89.

PROGNOSIS

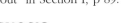

See "Gout" in Section I, p 89.

DENTAL SIGNIFICANCE

Gout may present in the temporomandibular joint (TMJ) and needs to be considered in the evaluation of the painful joint.

DENTAL MANAGEMENT

Patients may be referred to a rheumatologist or their primary care physician. See Dental Management in "Gout," Section I, p 89 for more tips.

SUGGESTED REFERENCE

Schlesinger N. Management of acute and chronic gouty arthritis: present state of the art. *Drugs* 2004;64(21):2399–2416.

AUTHOR: **DARYL E. BEE, DDS, MS**

SYNONYM(S)

Black hairy tongue

ICD-9CM/CPT CODE(S)

529.3 Hairy black tongue
CPT General Exam or Consultation
(e.g., 99243 or 99213)

OVERVIEW

Hairy tongue is a clinical descriptive term referring to either a marked accumulation of keratin or hypertrophy of the filiform papillae; involves the dorsal surface of the tongue; gives the tongue a hairy or coated appearance.

ETIOLOGY & PATHOGENESIS

- Unknown etiology.
- Possibly related to an alteration in microbial flora with an overgrowth of fungi and chromogenic bacteria. Many organisms, including *Candida*, may be cultured, but there is no proof of a cause-and-effect relationship.
- Possible risk factors include heavy smoking, antibiotic therapy, poor oral hygiene, general debilitation, radiation therapy, and use of oxidizing mouth rinses.

CLINICAL PRESENTATION / PHYSICAL FINDINGS

- Patients may complain of burning or painful tongue, halitosis, and a gagging sensation.
- Elongated papillae with a matted, thick appearance that may have varying degrees of staining as a result of pigment-producing bacteria or from tobacco and food. Color may range from white to brown or black.
- Most commonly involves the midline just anterior to the circumvallate papillae; not usually on the lateral border, as is seen in hairy leukoplakia.

DIAGNOSIS

DIFFERENTIAL DIAGNOSIS

- Hairy leukoplakia caused by the Epstein-Barr virus (usually associated with AIDS)

WORKUP

- This is a clinically recognizable process, and no specific tests are indicated.

MEDICAL MANAGEMENT & TREATMENT

Elimination of possible etiologic agents. See Dental Management following.

COMPLICATIONS

Other than appearance, there are no complications of this condition.

PROGNOSIS

This process is totally benign with no serious sequelae.

DENTAL MANAGEMENT

- Good oral hygiene, including brushing of the tongue
- Peridex mouth rinse

SUGGESTED REFERENCES

Marx RE, Stern DS (eds): *Oral and Maxillofacial Pathology. A Rationale for Diagnosis and Treatment.* Carol Stream, IL, Quintessence Publishing Company, 2003, pp 79–80.

Neville B, Damm D, Allen C, Bouquot J (eds): *Oral & Maxillofacial Pathology*, ed 2. Philadelphia, WB Saunders, 2002, pp 13–14.

AUTHOR: **DARYL E. BEE, DDS, MS**

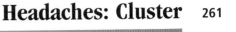

SECTION II

SYNONYM(S)

Migrainous neuralgia
Sphenopalatine neuralgia
Histamine cephalgia
Histamine headache
Horton headache

ICD-9CM/CPT CODE(S)

346.2 Variants of migraine headache including cluster headache
CPT General Exam or Consultation (e.g., 99243 or 99213)

OVERVIEW

An excruciating, unilateral orbital, supraorbital, or temporal pain that typically lasts 15 to 180 minutes and occurs several times per day. Cluster refers to grouping of the headaches. These clusters can go on for several months and then go into remission for several months. The cluster headache is called "suicide headache" because of its severity and "alarm clock headache" because of its periodicity.

See "Headaches: Cluster" in Section I, p 92.

EPIDEMIOLOGY & DEMOGRAPHICS

INCIDENCE/PREVALENCE IN USA: Affects 1% of population. Circadian regularity in 47% of cases.
PREDOMINANT AGE: Peak onset in males in forties and females in sixties.
PREDOMINANT SEX: Strong male predilection.
GENETICS: Family history of headaches, smoking, and/or head injury may be associated with cluster headaches.

ETIOLOGY & PATHOGENESIS

- Unknown etiology but PET scan and MRI imaging indicate the basic pathophysiology is in the hypothalamic gray matter.
- Possibly a neurovascular event.
- Triggers seem to be hypoxia (which may be seen in sleep apnea), vasodilators such as alcohol and nitroglycerin.
- Eighty percent of patients are heavy smokers.

CLINICAL PRESENTATION / PHYSICAL FINDINGS

- Severe headache pain usually around orbital, supraorbital, and temporal area.

- Unilateral, with pain recurring on the same side during the clusters; however, can occur on different sides in later attacks.
- Usually no aura, as in migraine.
- Often occurs during sleep and wakes the patient up.
- Headache lasts 15 to 180 minutes and can occur several times in 1 day; may occur daily for 1 to 4 months.
- May be accompanied by ipsilateral conjunctival injection or lacrimation, ipsilateral nasal congestion or rhinorrhea, ipsilateral eyelid edema, ipsilateral forehead and facial sweating, ipsilateral miosis, or ptosis.
- May see facial flushing or pallor, nausea, tenderness of the ipsilateral carotid artery, bradycardia, restlessness, or agitation.
- Episodic cluster headache is defined as at least two cluster periods lasting 7 to 365 days and separated by pain-free remissions of 1 month or longer.
- Chronic attacks recur over more than 1 year without remission or with remission of less than 1 month.

DIAGNOSIS

DIFFERENTIAL DIAGNOSIS

- Orbital myositis
- CNS neoplasm
- Paroxysmal hemicranial headaches
- Giant cell arteritis
- Sinusitis
- Subarachnoid hemorrhage
- Trigeminal neuralgia

WORKUP

- Cluster headaches are diagnosed by history; the key feature is a pattern of recurrent bouts of near-daily attacks lasting for days, weeks, or months.

IMAGING

- Imaging studies are not diagnostic but can be used to rule out other pathology.

MEDICAL MANAGEMENT & TREATMENT

- Oxygen inhalation with face mask at a 7 to 8 L/min flow for 10 to 15 minutes.
- Patients with severe snoring should be evaluated for sleep apnea.
- Surgical decompression of the trigeminal nerve or rhizotomy of the

sphenopalatine ganglion for refractive cluster headaches has been tried in limited cases.
- Sumatriptan, subcutaneous or nasal spray, 6 mg SC, 20 mg nasal spray.
- Intranasal dihydroergotamine 0.5 mg nasal spray.
- Intranasal lidocaine.
- Intranasal capsaicin.
- Prophylactic: verapamil 120 to 160 mg tid; oral sumatriptan not effective; prednisone 50 to 80 mg/day tapered over 12 days; topiramate 25 mg/day for 7 days, increased gradually to maximum dose of 200 mg/day.
- Chronic headaches: verapamil 120 mg, tid; lithium 300 mg, tid (adjust according to therapeutic blood levels).

COMPLICATIONS

See "Headaches: Cluster" in Section I, p 92.

PROGNOSIS

Recurrent attacks likely, with prolonged remissions; avoiding possible triggers may lessen attacks.

DENTAL MANAGEMENT

Patients may be referred to a neurologist or their primary care physician. See Dental Management in "Headaches: Cluster," Section I, p 92 for more tips.

SUGGESTED REFERENCES

Beck E, Sieber W, Trejo R. Management of cluster headache. *Am Fam Phys* 2005;71(4):717–724.
Freitag FG. Cluster headache. *Prim Care Clin Off Prac* 2004;31:313–329.

AUTHOR: DARYL F. REE, DDS, MS

SYNONYM(S)

Hemicrania

ICD-9CM/CPT CODE(S)

346.9 Migraine
CPT General Exam or Consultation
(e.g., 99243 or 99213)

OVERVIEW

Recurrent headache disorder, often with nausea and vomiting, that may be unilateral or bilateral and may occur with or without prodromal symptoms (aura). Approximately 20% of migraines are preceded by an aura, which can consist of dizziness, photophobia, tinnitus, scotomas, or visual scintillations.

See "Headaches: Migraine" in Section I, p 93.

EPIDEMIOLOGY & DEMOGRAPHICS

INCIDENCE/PREVALENCE IN USA: Ten to 20% of U.S. population (6% of men and 15–17% of women).
PREDOMINANT AGE: First attack often in childhood, rarely later than age 30. Migraines continue through the thirties and forties, decreasing in severity and frequency with age.
PREDOMINANT SEX: Female to male ratio 3:1.
GENETICS: Demonstrated familial disposition.

ETIOLOGY & PATHOGENESIS

- Unknown.
- Seventy percent family history of migraines.
- Growing evidence of serotonin and dopamine receptor activity as being involved.

- Attacks may be precipitated by certain foods such as red wine, aged cheeses, chocolate, citrus fruits, or nuts and by emotional stress, menses, and by certain medications such as birth control pills and vasodilators.

CLINICAL PRESENTATION / PHYSICAL FINDINGS

- Moderately severe headache with or without a prodrome or aura, unilateral or bilateral (30–40%); may last 4 to 72 hours.
- Systemic manifestations may include nausea, vomiting, photophobia, phonophobia, and lightheadedness.
- Temporary neurological findings may include hemiparesis, aphasia, and third nerve paralysis in ophthalmoplegic migraine with ocular muscle paralysis, and ptosis.

DIAGNOSIS

DIFFERENTIAL DIAGNOSIS

- Cluster headache
- Tension headache
- Stroke
- Sinusitis
- Meningitis
- Temporal arteritis
- Subarachnoid hemorrhage

LABORATORY

- CBC, sedimentation rate, other lab studies as indicated to rule out diagnoses in the differential

IMAGING

- CT if atypical case

MEDICAL MANAGEMENT & TREATMENT

- Minimize visual and auditory stimulation.

- Avoid known triggering agents (may include dietary changes).
- Sumatriptan (5-HT1 serotonin receptor agonist) 25 mg PO, additional doses every 2 hours up to 300 mg/day. 6 mg SC can be followed by one additional injection after 1 hour.
- Frovatriptan (serotonin agonist).
- Eletriptan (serotonin agonist).
- Naratriptan (serotonin agonist).

COMPLICATIONS

See "Headaches: Migraine" in Section I, p 93.

PROGNOSIS

Recurrent attacks likely, with prolonged remissions; avoiding possible triggers may lessen attacks.

DENTAL MANAGEMENT

Patients may be referred to a neurologist or their primary care physician. See Dental Management in "Headaches: Migraine," Section I, p 93 for more tips.

SUGGESTED REFERENCES

Blanda M. Headache, migraine. www.eMedicine.com.
Lawrence EC. Diagnosis and management of migraine headache. *Southern Med J* 2004;97(11):1069–1078.

AUTHOR: **DARYL E. BEE, DDS, MS**

SYNONYM(S)

Capillary hemangioma
Cavernous hemangioma
Arterial venous (AV) malformation

ICD-9CM/CPT CODE(S)

228.00–228.09 Hemangioma
CPT   General Exam or Consultation (e.g., 99243 or 99213). Multiple surgical procedures could also apply if needed.

OVERVIEW

These vascular malformations of the oral and maxillofacial region are generally divided into soft tissue and intrabony varieties. Also important is whether the lesion is congenital and whether it is enlarging out of proportion to the patient's growth if the patient is a child. The flow characteristics of the lesion are important from a clinical and treatment standpoint. In general, AV malformations are defined as having both arterial and venous components. These are always high-flow lesions. Cavernous and capillary hemangiomas that are large or intrabony may often require treatment even if they are relatively low-flow. Other low-flow vascular malformations, although potentially life-threatening, are normally of less emergent concern than the AV malformations. The head and neck region is a common area for hemangiomas and vascular malformations in general.

See "Hemangioma (Soft Tissue)" in Section II, p 264 for more information.

EPIDEMIOLOGY & DEMOGRAPHICS

INCIDENCE/PREVALENCE IN USA: Because of the wide variation and presentation of vascular malformations in general, it is somewhat difficult to give specific demographics.
PREDOMINANT SEX: Much more common in females, with perhaps a 3:1 ratio.
PREDOMINANT AGE: Hemangiomas are generally most common at birth.

ETIOLOGY & PATHOGENESIS

These are best thought of as congenital lesions, though developmental and proliferative stages are also possible in some lesions.

CLINICAL PRESENTATION / PHYSICAL FINDINGS

- When seen at birth, they are generally bosselated and presented as raised lesions.
- Intrabony lesions generally present as mixed radiolucent and radiopaque lesions.
- The wide range of presentations (from a pure radiolucent lesion to one that would be thought of as almost sclerotic) makes the definitive diagnosis of intrabony vascular malformations very difficult on standard radiographs.
- On those lesions that can be palpated, a thrill may be felt. A thrill is simply the feeling of flowing liquid through tissue.
- A bruit may also be heard by auscultation.

DIAGNOSIS

Determining the flow characteristics of the particular lesion may be necessary. This is generally done through arteriograms performed by interventional radiologists.

MEDICAL MANAGEMENT & TREATMENT

- All intrabony lesions should be first aspirated to assess for the possibility of vascular malformations. This preventive step is extremely important in clinical practice.
- If an emergency is encountered due to an unexpected vascular lesion during tooth extraction or other intrabony procedure, it may be advisable to briefly put the tooth back into the socket while materials are gathered. In general, the tooth is not a good tool to leave in to apply direct pressure except during the brief time frame for gathering material.
- Packing of hemostatic agents such as Gelfoam® or Surgicel™ into the defect should be accomplished first; then digital pressure with gauze should be applied. Depending on the amount of hemorrhage, transport to emergency facilities may be appropriate.
- Once the hemorrhage is controlled, releasing incisions of the surrounding soft tissue would be helpful to allow for tight suture closure over the socket or defect.
- Definitive therapy for hemangiomas and arterial venous malformations should be well-planned and accomplished in a very specialized setting. Although sclerosing agents, hypotensive anesthesia, ligation, resection, or simple follow-up all have their place, the decision on which to use is highly dependent upon the individual characteristics of the malformation.
- Soft tissue lesions may be addressed by a simple excision and ligation but this also depends on size and flow characteristics. Like the intrabony lesion, the intervention radiology, sclerosing agents, and so forth may also be appropriate depending on the size of the lesion. Congenital soft tissue lesions often resolve spontaneously and are most often left for clinical follow-up instead of seeking active treatment.

COMPLICATIONS

Extreme hemorrhage and even death have occurred following tooth extractions and intrabony lesions. The soft tissue lesions are easily controlled through use of direct pressure. With that said, these should also be approached with appropriate planning and a risk–benefit assessment.

PROGNOSIS

Although most small lesions may never cause a problem, at times they must be addressed. However, the overall prognosis is that the congenital lesions will generally resolve over time; for larger and higher-flow lesions, the consequences may be grave.

DENTAL SIGNIFICANCE

Being well aware of the intrabony characteristics and soft tissue characteristics of the hemangioma will allow the dentist to avoid trauma to these potentially hazardous lesions. All intrabony lesions should be aspirated prior to creation of a large access opening.

DENTAL MANAGEMENT

Extreme care, differential diagnosis, and avoidance of trauma to the area is advised. Aspiration of all intrabony lesions is essential, and hemangiomas are the prime reason why radiographic evaluation of the jaws is advised prior to tooth extraction. See Medical Management & Treatment, preceding, for more information.

SUGGESTED REFERENCES

Giaoui L, Princ G, Chiras J, Guilbert F, Bertrand JC. Treatment of vascular malformations of the mandible: a description of 12 cases. *Int J Oral Maxillofac Surg* 2003;32(2):132–136.

Neville B, Damm D, Allen C, Bouquot J (eds): *Oral & Maxillofacial Pathology*, ed 2. Philadelphia, WB Saunders, 2002, pp 467–468.

Perugini M, Renzi G, Gasparini G, Cerulli G, Becelli RJ. Intraosseous hemangioma of the maxillofacial district: clinical analysis and surgical treatment in 10 consecutive patients. *Craniofac Surg* 2004;15(6):980–985.

Prochazkova L, Machalka M, Prochazka J, Tecl F, Klimovic M. Arteriovenous malformations of the orofacial area. *Acta Chir Plast* 2000;42(2):55–59.

AUTHOR: JOHN W. HELLSTEIN, DDS, MS

SYNONYM(S)

Port wine stain
Vascular nevus
Strawberry nevus

ICD-9CM/CPT CODE(S)

228.0   Hemangioma, any site
228.01 Hemangioma, skin and subcutaneous tissue
CPT   General Exam or Consultation (e.g., 99243 or 99213)

OVERVIEW

Vascular lesion that is a true neoplasm of endothelial cells and is characterized by hyperplasia and cellular proliferation. Must be distinguished from a vascular malformation, which has normal endothelial cell turnover and does not demonstrate cellular hyperplasia. Vascular malformations are structural malformations that are present at birth and grow proportionately with the child. They can be categorized by the type of vessel and according to the flow characteristics.

EPIDEMIOLOGY & DEMOGRAPHICS

PREDOMINANT AGE: Usually appear early in infancy and undergo rapid growth during the first years of life followed by gradual involution. Most common tumors of infancy.
PREDOMINANT SEX: Female to male ratio 3:1.

ETIOLOGY & PATHOGENESIS

- Neoplastic origin

- The hemangioma is described as a neoplasm, however may be in many cases a hamartoma or malformation
- Head and neck regions are most common sites (60%)

CLINICAL PRESENTATION / PHYSICAL FINDINGS

- Fully developed hemangiomas rarely present at birth.
- Hemangiomas of oral soft tissue are similar to those of the skin and may appear as flat or raised lesions, usually deep red or bluish-red, depending on the depth of the lesion.
- Firm and rubbery to palpation and will blanch to pressure, but cannot be totally evacuated.

DIAGNOSIS

DIFFERENTIAL DIAGNOSIS

- Vascular malformations
- Lymphatic malformations
- Telangiectasia
- Pyogenic granuloma

IMAGING

- CT with contrast can help differentiate lesion from vascular malformation.
- MRI.
- Angiography rarely indicated.

MEDICAL MANAGEMENT & TREATMENT

- Watchful neglect: most resolve spontaneously.
- Surgical intervention rarely indicated during infancy.
- Sclerosing agents into the lesion.
- For problematic or life-threatening lesions, systemic steroids may help reduce the size of the lesion.
- Interferon-α has been used in treatment of severe lesions that do not respond to steroids and are potentially life-threatening.

COMPLICATIONS

Most common complication is ulceration of the overlying skin due to rapid growth, with resultant bleeding that is usually not life-threatening.

PROGNOSIS

Most resolve spontaneously; 90% will resolve by adolescence.

DENTAL MANAGEMENT

Practitioners may refer patients to an oral and maxillofacial surgeon, plastic surgeon, vascular surgeon, or interventional radiologist.

SUGGESTED REFERENCES

Neville B, Damm D, Allen C, Bouquot J (eds): *Oral & Maxillofacial Pathology*, ed 2. Philadelphia, WB Saunders, 2002, pp 467–468.
Selected Readings in Oral and Maxillofacial Surgery 2004;12(3):21–23. Dallas, TX.

AUTHOR: DARYL E. BEE, DDS, MS

SYNONYM(S)

Aphthous pharyngitis
Vesicular pharyngitis

ICD-9CM/CPT CODE(S)

074.0 Herpangina
CPT General Exam or Consultation
(e.g., 99243 or 99213)

OVERVIEW

Acute viral infection that usually affects the tonsillar fossa region and the soft palate in children and youth.

EPIDEMIOLOGY & DEMOGRAPHICS

INCIDENCE/PREVALENCE IN USA:
Frequently occurs in epidemics or generalized outbreaks; occurs most frequently in the summer or early fall months.
PREDOMINANT AGE: Children affected more frequently than adults.

ETIOLOGY & PATHOGENESIS

- Caused by Coxsackie virus A and B (usually A1–A6, A8, A10, A22, and unspecified B).
- Transmitted by contaminated saliva and possibly oral-fecal contamination.
- Incubation period is 2 to 10 days, with mild to moderate symptoms lasting 1 week or less.

CLINICAL PRESENTATION / PHYSICAL FINDINGS

- Sore throat
- Fever
- Dysphasia
- Malaise
- Vesicles 1 to 2 mm on soft palate and tonsillar fossa that quickly rupture, forming 2- to 4-mm grey, fibrinous ulcers on erythematous mucosa

DIAGNOSIS

DIFFERENTIAL DIAGNOSIS

- Primary herpetic stomatitis.
- Hand, foot, and mouth disease.
- Acute lymphonodular pharyngitis.
- Streptococcal pharyngitis.
- Varicella.
- Aphthous stomatitis.
- Generally, a diagnosis can be made from clinical signs and symptoms.

WORKUP

- Laboratory confirmation can be made by viral isolation or detection of serum antibodies.

MEDICAL MANAGEMENT & TREATMENT

No specific treatment required other than supportive care, rest, antipyretics, and analgesics.

PROGNOSIS

Usually resolution of acute symptoms within 5 to 7 days, with resolution of ulcerations within 2 weeks

DENTAL MANAGEMENT

See preceding Medical Management & Treatment.

SUGGESTED REFERENCES

Marx R, Stern D. (eds): *Oral and Maxillofacial Pathology: A Rationale for Diagnosis and Treatment.* Carol Stream, IL, Quintessence Publishing Company, 2003, p 122.
Neville B, Damm D, Allen C, Bouquot J (eds): *Oral & Maxillofacial Pathology,* ed 2. Philadelphia, WB Saunders, 2002, pp 227–230.
Regezi J, Sciubba J. *Oral Pathology, Clinical Pathologic Correlations,* ed 3. Philadelphia, WB Saunders, 1999, pp 11–12.

AUTHOR: DARYL E. BEE, DDS, MS

SYNONYM(S)

Cold sore
Fever blister
Herpes labialis
Acute gingivostomatitis

ICD-9CM/CPT CODE(S)

054.0 Eczema herpeticum
054.1 Genital herpes
054.2 Primary herpes gingivostomatitis
054.9 Recurrent herpes, herpes labialis
079.9 Viral infection
528.0 Stomatitis
529.0 Glossitis
CPT   General Exam or Consultation (e.g., 99243 or 99213)

OVERVIEW

There are eight human herpes viruses (HHVs): herpes simplex I and II (HHV-1 and HHV-2); varicella-zoster (HHV-3, see "Herpes Zoster" in Section II, p 267); Epstein-Barr virus (HHV-4); cytomegalovirus (HHV-5); human herpes virus 6 (HHV-6); human herpes virus 7 (HHV-7); and human herpes virus 8 (HHV-8, associated with Kaposi's sarcoma). All contain a DNA core surrounded by a capsid and an envelope. Herpes simplex I is associated with oral, perioral, and occasionally genital infections. Herpes simplex II is associated with genital infections and occasionally oral and perioral infections.

EPIDEMIOLOGY & DEMOGRAPHICS

PREDOMINANT AGE: Primary infection of herpes I (HSV-1) usually involves infants and children but can occur in adolescents and adults.

ETIOLOGY & PATHOGENESIS

- Spread by direct physical contact of the virus.
- Secondary herpes is a result of latent virus residing in the trigeminal ganglion that activates and travels down the nerve branches to the epithelial surface to infect the basal and parabasal cells in a localized area.
- Can be triggered by stress, exposure to cold or sunlight, fever, trauma, or immunosuppression.

CLINICAL PRESENTATION/PHYSICAL FINDINGS

SYMPTOMATIC PRIMARY HSV-1

- Fever
- Malaise
- Headache
- Nausea
- Anorexia
- Lymphadenopathy
- Generalized vesicles turning to ulcers involving all oral mucosa
- Extremely painful lesions (1 to 3 mm) that can coalesce to form larger areas

- Drooling
- Foul breath
- Sore throat

SECONDARY HSV-1

- Occurs at the site of primary inoculation or areas of epithelium supplied by the involved ganglion. There is usually a brief prodromal period (1 to 2 hours) with some mild discomfort or altered sensation of the affected area.
- The vermillion border of the lips (herpes labialis) is the most frequent site of reoccurrence, followed by any keratinized oral mucosa (attached gingiva and the palate).
- Clusters of several to multiple small vesicles filled with active virus rupture and crust within 1 to 2 days.
- Intraoral vesicles rupture, forming an area of ulceration with a white, fibrinous surface with a red, peripheral mucosal margin.
- Herpetic eczema: herpetic infection superimposed upon a preexisting eczema.
- HSV encephalitis.
- Disseminated herpes simplex of the newborn.

DIAGNOSIS

DIFFERENTIAL DIAGNOSIS

- Aphthous stomatitis
- Herpes zoster
- Impetigo
- Erythema multiforme/drug reaction
- Pemphigus
- Epidermolysis bullosa
- Necrotizing ulcerative periodontitis
- Chemical burns
- Streptococcal pharyngitis
- Contact allergy

LABORATORY

- Viral identification from tissue culture can take up to 2 weeks.
- Serological tests for HSV antibodies are positive 4 to 8 days after the initial exposure; useful in identifying a primary infection.
- Cytologic smears may identify viral particles and multinucleated giant cells.

MEDICAL MANAGEMENT & TREATMENT

Management involves reducing the duration of symptoms and severity of the disease. All medications are viralstatic, not viralcidal.

PRIMARY HSV-1

- Primary measures are mostly supportive/palliative unless early treatment (< 72 hours) can be initiated. These include topical anesthetics, use of acetaminophen or NSAIDs, and maintaining fluid hydration.
- Acyclovir: 200 mg, 5× daily for 10 days.

- Valacyclovir: 1000 mg, 2× daily for 10 days.
- Famciclovir (not FDA-approved for HSV-1).

SECONDARY HSV-1

- Does not necessarily warrant treatment. Oral and topical agents can aid if started early enough. The course of existing lesions will not be altered, but new lesions can be prevented.
- Valacyclovir preferred: 2000 mg, 2× daily for 1 day.
- Topical agents for recurrent HSV: acyclovir ointment, penciclovir cream, and doconazole cream.

COMPLICATIONS

- Herpetic whitlow (infections of the nails or fingers) may occur.
- Herpetic keratoconjunctivitis: conjunctivitis, keratitis, and corneal ulceration.

PROGNOSIS

- No cure for HSV.
- Untreated primary HSV-1 usually runs its course in 14 to 21 days.
- Untreated recurrent HSV usually runs its course in 10 to 14 days.

DENTAL SIGNIFICANCE

The virus can be transmitted to skin surfaces; prior to dentists wearing gloves, it was not uncommon for HSV-1 infections to form on dental professionals' fingers, known as herpetic whitlow.

DENTAL MANAGEMENT

- Patient may require referral to primary care physician.
- Instruct patients to wash hands; take general precautions for a contact-contagious disease; avoid immunosuppressed individuals, infants, or pregnant women while active disease present.

SUGGESTED REFERENCES

Marx RE, Stern D (eds): *Oral and Maxillofacial Pathology. A Rationale for Diagnosis and Treatment.* Carol Stream, IL, Quintessence Publishing Company, 2003, pp 110–114.

Neville B, Damm D, Allen C, Bouquot J (eds): *Oral & Maxillofacial Pathology,* ed 2. Philadelphia, WB Saunders, 2002, pp 213–220.

Stooper ET. Oral herpetic infections (HSV 1–8). *Dent Clin No Am* 2005;49:15.

AUTHOR: DARYL E. BEE, DDS, MS

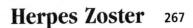

SYNONYM(S)

Shingles

ICD-9CM/CPT CODE(S)
053.0   Herpes zoster with meningitis
053.12 Postherpetic trigeminal neuralgia
053.13 Postherpetic polyneuropathy
053.9   Herpes zoster without mention of complication
CPT   General Exam or Consultation (e.g., 99243 or 99213)

OVERVIEW

There are eight kinds of human herpes viruses (HHVs). Herpes zoster, caused by the reactivation of the latent varicella zoster virus (HHV-3 or VZV), is a painful, vesiculoulcerative disease affecting cutaneous or mucosal surfaces. VZV virus becomes dormant in dorsal root or cranial nerve ganglia after a primary infection of chicken pox. When reactivated, the virus follows a peripheral sensory nerve distribution precisely and stops abruptly at the midline.

EPIDEMIOLOGY & DEMOGRAPHICS

INCIDENCE/PREVALENCE IN USA: Herpes zoster affects 10–20% of the population, mostly the older population or the immunocompromised population such as those with lymphoid or hematopoietic malignancies, those on cytotoxic or immunosuppressive drugs, those on steroids or receiving high-dose radiation, and AIDS patients.

ETIOLOGY & PATHOGENESIS

- Varicella zoster virus (VZV) is a human herpes virus (HHV-3). It is a DNA virus composed of a nucleocapsid surrounded by a proteinaceous compartment and an outer lipid envelope.
- The initial infection in man is known as varicella or chicken pox. The virus is not completely eradicated; it enters sensory nerve ganglia and remains dormant for a variable period of time. A cutaneous or mucosal vesiculoulcerative eruption follows the reactivation of the virus.

CLINICAL PRESENTATION / PHYSICAL FINDINGS

- Prodromal symptoms of extreme pain and itching are the result of virus replication in the nerve ganglia causing necrosis and inflammation. As the virus travels down the nerve, the pain may intensify in the area enervated by the affected sensory nerve.
- Typically, one dermatome is affected, but two or more can become involved.
- The dermatomes of the chest wall are the most common site involved, followed by the trigeminal nerve distributions, particularly the ophthalmic division.
- Ten percent of affected individuals will have no prodromal pain.
- Fever, malaise, and headache may be present 1 to 4 days before the development of lesions.
- Acute phase begins with formation of clusters of vesicles that within 3 to 4 days become pustular and ulcerated, with crusts developing 7 to 10 days later.
- Remission usually occurs in several weeks, often with scarring or changes in pigmentation.
- Involvement of the facial and auditory nerves produces the Ramsey-Hunt syndrome with facial paralysis, vesicles of the ipsilateral external ear, tinnitus, deafness, and vertigo.
- Chronic phase occurs when the pain persists longer than 3 months after the initial rash, called postherpetic neuralgia. Pain is described as burning, itching, throbbing, or aching. Light touch or even the presence of clothing can aggravate the discomfort.

DIAGNOSIS

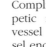

DIFFERENTIAL DIAGNOSIS
- Herpes zoster can usually be diagnosed by its characteristic unilateral distribution along specific dermatomes.
- Herpes simplex.

LABORATORY
- Viral cultures: take 24 hours
- Cytological smears: direct staining with fluorescent monoclonal antibodies for VZV
- Dot-blot hybridization and polymerase chain reaction (PCR)

MEDICAL MANAGEMENT & TREATMENT

- Supportive and symptomatic measures include antipruritics and nonaspirin antipyretics.
- Capsaicin topical cream for postherpetic neuralgia.
- Acyclovir: 800 mg 5× daily for 7 days,
- Valacyclovir: 1000 mg 3× daily for 7 days.
- Famciclovir: 500 to 750 mg 3× daily for 7 days.
- No consensus on steroid use.
- Immunocompromised patients exposed to herpes zoster may benefit from varicella zoster immune globulin.
- Carbamazepine: 200 mg 1× to 3× daily for postherpetic neuralgia.
- Gabapentin: 1800 to 3600 mg daily for postherpetic neuralgia.

COMPLICATIONS

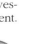

Complications include postherpetic neuralgia, myelitis, large vessel granulomatous arteritis, small vessel encephalitis, and ocular involvement.

PROGNOSIS

Success of treatment can vary from patient to patient.

DENTAL SIGNIFICANCE

Oral lesions may be associated with significant bone necrosis and loss of teeth in the involved areas. Oral lesions are unilateral, extending to the midline and abruptly stopping.

DENTAL MANAGEMENT

Patients may require referral to a neurologist, ophthalmologist (mandatory with any eye symptoms), or their primary care physician.

SUGGESTED REFERENCES

Chakrabarty A, Beutner K. Therapy of other viral infections: herpes to hepatitis. *Derm Ther* 2004;17:465–490.

Marx RE, Stern D (eds): *Oral and Maxillofacial Pathology. A Rationale for Diagnosis and Treatment.* Carol Stream, IL, Quintessence Publishing Company, 2003, pp 115–117.

Neville B, Damm D, Allen C, Bouquot J (eds): *Oral & Maxillofacial Pathology,* ed 2. Philadelphia, WB Saunders, 2002, pp 222–224.

AUTHOR: DARYL E. BEE, DDS, MS

SYNONYM(S)

Darling's disease

ICD-9CM/CPT CODE(S)

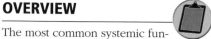

115.9 Histoplasmosis
CPT General Exam or Consultation
(e.g., 99243 or 99213)

OVERVIEW

The most common systemic fungal infection found in the U.S.; it is caused by the organism *Histoplasma capsulatum*. It is dimorphic, growing as a yeast in the human host and as a mold in the natural environment.

EPIDEMIOLOGY & DEMOGRAPHICS

INCIDENCE/PREVALENCE IN USA:
Estimated that over 40 million people have been infected in the U.S., with 500,000 new cases each year. Endemic in the Mississippi and Ohio River basins but found in temperate zones of the world.

ETIOLOGY & PATHOGENESIS

- Mycelial form of the fungus is found in the soil, especially in areas contaminated with bird or bat droppings.
- Infections typically caused by inhalation of windborne spores from point sources such as bird roosts, old barns, or activities disrupting the soil such as farming or excavation.
- Not transmissible from person-to-person contact.
- People whose vocation could potentially expose them to histoplasmosis should take precautions as outlined by the Centers for Disease Control and Prevention.

CLINICAL PRESENTATION / PHYSICAL FINDINGS

- Majority of people with normal immune systems have an asymptomatic infection or mild, flu-like symptoms for 1 to 2 weeks.
- Acute pulmonary histoplasmosis following heavy exposure can cause diffuse pulmonary involvement with high fever, chills, headache, fatigue, weight loss, malaise, nonproductive cough, and chest pain.
- Chronic pulmonary histoplasmosis may produce tuberculosis-like symptoms and is usually associated with preexisting abnormal lung architecture, such as emphysema.
- In immunosuppressed individuals, productive cough, weight loss, fever, dyspnea, chest pain, hemoptysis, weakness, and fatigue occur.
- Disseminated histoplasmosis is the progressive spread of infection to extrapulmonary sites, usually in older, debilitated, or immunodeficient patients. Symptoms vary depending on the area of infection, but fever is the most common finding.
- Oral lesions usually found in the chronic or disseminated forms present as nodular, vegetative, or ulcerative lesions on the buccal mucosa, gingival, tongue, palate, or lips.

DIAGNOSIS

DIFFERENTIAL DIAGNOSIS

- Oral differential
  - Other deep fungal infections
  - Squamous cell carcinoma/oral malignancy
  - Oral TB
  - Syphilitic chancre
  - Sarcoidosis
- Tuberculosis and other chronic pulmonary diseases
- Pulmonary malignancy

WORKUP

- Culture of tissue specimen
- Tissue biopsy with histopathologic identification, including special stains

LABORATORY

- Serologic tests

IMAGING

- Chest radiograph may show hilar or mediastinal lymph nodes and patchy infiltrates.
- Chronic disease may show fibrotic apical infiltrates with cavitation.

MEDICAL MANAGEMENT & TREATMENT

- Treatment depends on the severity of the clinical symptoms. Mild cases may require only supportive care; however, chronic or disseminated disease and severe or prolonged acute pulmonary infections require antifungal therapy.
- Itraconazole: 200 to 400 mg PO daily for 6 to 12 months.
- For severe manifestations or disseminated disease, amphotericin B (IV), 0.7 to 1.0 mg/kg per day and prednisone, 60 mg daily for 2 weeks followed by itraconazole, 200 mg 2× daily.

PROGNOSIS

- Severe acute and chronic histoplasmosis: 20% mortality if untreated.
- Disseminated histoplasmosis: 90% mortality if untreated, 7–23% mortality even when treated.

DENTAL MANAGEMENT

If suspicious oral lesions are found, refer to infectious disease specialist or primary care physician.

SUGGESTED REFERENCES

Kurowski R, Ostapchuk M. Overview of histoplasmosis. *Am Fam Phys* 2002;66(12): 2247–2252.

Marx RE, Stern D (eds): *Oral and Maxillofacial Pathology. A Rationale for Diagnosis and Treatment.* Carol Stream, IL, Quintessence Publishing Company, 2003, pp 97–99.

Neville B, Damm D, Allen C, Bouquot J (eds): *Oral & Maxillofacial Pathology*, ed 2. Philadelphia, WB Saunders, 2002, pp 197–201.

Wheat LJ, Kauffman CA. Histoplasmosis. *Infect Dis Clin North Am* 2003;17(1):1–19.

AUTHOR: DARYL E. BEE, DDS, MS

SYNONYM(S)

Hodgkin's lymphoma
Malignant lymphoma
Lymph node cancer

ICD-9CM/CPT CODE(S)

ICD-9CM
201.4x Hodgkin disease, lymphocyte predominance
201.5x Hodgkin disease, nodular sclerosis
201.6x Hodgkin disease, mixed cellularity
201.7x Hodgkin disease, lymphocyte depleted
201.9x Hodgkin disease, unspecified
Fifth digit: in place of ×
0: unspecified site
1: head and neck, facial
4: axillary and arm nodes
5: inguinal enlarged nodes
8: multiple site nodes
CPT General Exam or Consultation (e.g., 99243 or 99213)
38500 Superficial lymph node biopsy
38510 Deep jugular lymph node biopsy

OVERVIEW

Uncommon malignancy of lymphoid tissue.

- Classification is important and is dependent upon background cells and ratios.
  - Lymphocyte predominance
  - Nodular sclerosis most common
  - Mixed cellularity second-most common
  - Lymphocyte depleted

See "Hodgkin's Disease" in Section I, p 108 for more information on all areas of this topic.

EPIDEMIOLOGY & DEMOGRAPHICS

PREDOMINANT AGE: A bimodal age distribution with peaks at 20 and 70 years of age.
PREDOMINANT SEX: More common in males in developed vs undeveloped countries.
GENETICS: No genetic patterns have been identified.

ETIOLOGY & PATHOGENESIS

- Generally unknown.
- Risk factors include autoimmune diseases and acquired and inherited immunodeficiency syndromes.
- Epstein-Barr virus (EBV) has been implicated as a possible contributory agent.

CLINICAL PRESENTATION / PHYSICAL FINDINGS

- The initial presentation is painless swelling of lymph nodes in the neck, axilla, and groin.

- Other organs of the hemic and lymphatic systems can also be involved, including spleen, bone marrow, and liver.
- Because of the intimate association, the immune system also becomes compromised.
- The disease usually commences in a single lymph node group and spreads in an orderly fashion from one contiguous nodal group to another.
- Most begin about the diaphragm.
- The spleen is frequently involved early and the liver and bone marrow only in advanced disease.
- The GI tract is involved by direct tumor extension rather than primary disease.

Signs & Symptoms

- Systemic symptoms may include weight loss, unexplained fever, and night sweats.
- Enlarged, painless lymph nodes and splenomegaly.
- Advanced disease can show extralymphatic extension in skin, lungs, GI tract, and other soft tissues surrounding nodal areas.

DIAGNOSIS

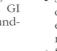

DIFFERENTIAL DIAGNOSIS

- Non-Hodgkin's lymphomas
- Cat scratch disease
- Tuberculosis
- Other inflammatory disease
- Metastatic tumors
- Sarcoid
- AIDS
- Drug reaction
- Reactive adenopathy

LABORATORY

- CBC with differential, ESR, electrolytes, renal, and liver profiles

IMAGING/SPECIAL TESTS

- Chest radiograph, CT scans of the chest, abdomen, pelvis; bipedal lymphangiogram and gallium scanning are useful.
- Technician bone scanning is less informative.
- Lymph node biopsy: entire node, fresh to pathologist for evaluation; do not send in fixative.
- The pathognomic Reed-Sternberg cells must be identified to confirm the diagnosis of Hodgkin's disease.
- Fine-needle aspirates and true-cut biopsies can be suggestive but not conclusive.
- Flow cytometry is critical on evaluation and cannot be done if specimen has been placed in formalin or alcohol.
- Staging laparotomy with splenectomy and liver biopsy.
- Bone marrow biopsy/aspiration.
- Staging:
  - Subclass A: asymptomatic.

- Subclass B: symptomatic.
- Stage I: single nodal group.
- Stage II: two or more nodal groups on the same side of diaphragm or localized involvement of extranodal tissue.
- Stage III: nodal groups on both sides of the diaphragm or extranodal involvement.
- Stage IV: disseminated disease involving one or more extralymphatic organs.
- Subclass "X": bulky disease, node greater than 10 cm, or widened mediastinum.

MEDICAL MANAGEMENT & TREATMENT

- General: aimed at complete remission in all cases. Factors influencing success include extensive extranodal disease, anemia, age, elevated ESR, and bone marrow involvement.
- Stage I and II: typically, radiation or chemotherapy alone unless bulky disease is present; then combined treatment should be advocated.
- Stage IIIA: primarily radiation but the combined treatment is becoming more popular.
- Stage IIIB and IV:
  - Chemotherapy (with or without radiation).
  - High-dose chemotherapy with bone marrow transplant for treatment failures.
  - Psychological therapy.
  - The patient education for long-term effects of treatment as well as the risk of future malignancies (recurrent and secondary).
- Medications
  - Combination chemotherapy regimen, the most common being MOPP (nitrogen mustard, Oncovin, procarbazine, and prednisone) and ABVD (Adriamycin, bleomycin, Velban, dacarbazine).

COMPLICATIONS

See "Hodgkin's Disease" in Section I, p 108 for information on potential complications.

PROGNOSIS

- Overall success rates are about 75%.
- "A" groups do better than "B" groups.
- Patients with combined therapy have slightly improved complete remission compared to those with single therapy.
- Generally accepted survival by stage:
  - Stages I and II: +90% 5-year survival.

SECTION II

○ Stage III: 80% 5-year; 75% 10-year survival.
○ Stage IV: 75% 5-year; 66% 10-year survival.

SUGGESTED REFERENCES

Rabel RE, Bope ET (eds): *Conn's Current Therapy 2005*. Philadelphia, Elsevier, 2005, pp 492–500.

Urba WJ, Longo DL. Hodgkin disease. *N Engl J Med* 1992;326:678–687.

AUTHORS: **TERESA BIGGERSTAFF, DDS, MD; DALE J. MISIEK, DMD**

SECTION II

SYNONYM(S)

None

ICD-9CM/CPT CODE(S)

252.00 Hyperparathyroidism, unspecified
CPT   General Exam or Consultation (e.g., 99243 or 99213)

OVERVIEW

In general, four parathyroid glands are situated posterior to the thyroid gland. Parathormone (PTH) is the only hormone secreted by the parathyroid glands and is one of the major regulators of calcium metabolism and homeostasis. PTH is normally secreted in response to low serum calcium levels. Excess secretion of PTH (hyperparathyroidism) causes increased bone resorption from the skeleton, increases renal tubular reabsorption and retention of calcium, and increases the renal synthesis of a vitamin D analog that enhances the absorption of calcium from the gastrointestinal system.

See "Hyperparathyroidism" in Section I, p 114 for more information.

EPIDEMIOLOGY & DEMOGRAPHICS

INCIDENCE/PREVALENCE IN USA:

- The prevalence of primary hyperparathyroidism reportedly occurs in 1 out of every 1000 people over the age of 50.
- Approximately 100,000 new cases of primary hyperparathyroidism are reported in the U.S. each year.
- The frequency of secondary hyperparathyroidism depends on the frequency of the underlying disease.

PREDOMINANT AGE: The incidence of hyperparathyroidism increases with age.
PREDOMINANT SEX: It is 3 to 4 times more common in females than males.
GENETICS: Primary hyperparathyroidism is associated with rare, genetically transmissible conditions (i.e., familial hypocalciuric hypercalcemia and multiple endocrine neoplasias).

ETIOLOGY & PATHOGENESIS

- Primary hyperparathyroidism is generally the result of a parathyroid adenoma (80%), primary parathyroid hyperplasia (15%), and, less commonly, parathyroid carcinoma (< 5%) resulting in increased serum PTH and calcium levels.
- Secondary hyperparathyroidism is the result of prolonged stimulation of the parathyroid gland due to decreased serum calcium; it is generally the result of chronic renal failure. Other causes of secondary hyperparathyroidism include vitamin D deficiency and malabsorption states.

- Tertiary hyperparathyroidism is the result of long-standing secondary hyperparathyroidism and is characterized by the development of autonomous hypersecretion of PTH after correction of low serum calcium levels.

CLINICAL PRESENTATION / PHYSICAL FINDINGS

- Skeletal: decreased bone density, loss of lamina dura, subperiosteal resorption of the phalanges, brown tumors, and osteitis fibrosa cystica; renal osteodystrophy associated with secondary hyperparathyroidism
- Muscular: generalized weakness
- Renal: renal calculi and metastatic calcifications involving other soft tissues
- Gastrointestinal: nausea, vomiting, peptic ulcers, and pancreatitis
- Central nervous system: depression, seizures, dementia

DIAGNOSIS

- Primary hyperparathyroidism:
  - Increased serum calcium
  - Increased serum PTH
  - Decreased serum phosphorus
  - Increased alkaline phosphatase
- Secondary hyperparathyroidism:
  - Increased PTH
  - Increased alkaline phosphatase
  - Variable serum calcium levels
- Technetium scanning is the most accurate technique for localizing abnormal parathyroid glands.
- Plain film radiographs show a loss of bony trabeculation, producing a ground-glass appearance, loss of cortical bone, loss of lamina dura, subperiosteal resorption of phalanges, and osteolytic bone lesions.
- Bone biopsy shows prominent peritrabecular fibrosis (osteitis fibrosa cystica) and increased bone resorption with increased number of osteoclasts (brown tumors).

MEDICAL MANAGEMENT & TREATMENT

- Intravenous hydration is the most critical treatment for a patient with an acute presentation of hyperparathyroidism.
- Primary hyperparathyroidism is definitively treated by parathyroidectomy; bone lesions may resolve if normal calcium levels are restored.
- Secondary hyperparathyroidism is treated by identifying and treating the underlying disease.
  - The goal of medical management is to normalize calcium levels.
  - Supplementation of vitamin D and calcium as necessary.

- Parathyroidectomy may be necessary in patients who develop tertiary hyperparathyroidism and metabolic bone disease.

COMPLICATIONS

- Bone fractures due to osteoporosis.
- Kidney damage may be permanent.
- Changes in mental status may be permanent.
- Hypercalcemia enhances the action of some drugs (i.e., cardiac glycosides) and therefore increases their toxic potential.

PROGNOSIS

- Prognosis for treated primary hyperparathyroidism is excellent.
  - Approximately 5% of patients with primary hyperparathyroidism that is treated by parathyroidectomy experience persistent hypercalcemia.
- Prognosis of secondary hyperparathyroidism is dependent on control of underlying disease.

DENTAL SIGNIFICANCE

- Brown tumors of bone causing pain and expansion of the jaws.
- Brown tumors and central giant cell granulomas display identical histopathologic features; therefore, hyperparathyroidism must be ruled out in all cases of central giant cell granuloma.
- Pulp stones.
- Risk for sialolithiasis may be increased.

DENTAL MANAGEMENT

Patients with secondary hyperparathyroidism due to chronic renal failure may require special dental management related to dialysis and the use of potentially nephrotoxic drugs. Consultation with patient's nephrologist is critical.

SUGGESTED REFERENCES

Antonelli JR, Hottel TL. Oral manifestations of renal osteodystrophy: case report and review of the literature. *Spec Care Dentist* 2003;23:28–34.
Taniegra ED. Hyperparathyroidism. *Am Fam Physician* 2004;69:333–339.
www.emedicine.com

AUTHOR: **CHRISTOPHER G. FIELDING, DDS, MS**

SYNONYM(S)

Mono
Glandular fever
Monocytic angina
Pfeiffer's disease
Kissing disease

ICD-9CM/CPT CODE(S)

075 Infectious mononucleosis
CPT General Exam or Consultation
(e.g., 99243 or 99213)

OVERVIEW

- Viral infection due to the Epstein-Barr virus (EBV) that generally involves persons in the range of ages 15 to 35 years old.
- Affects the lymphoreticular system and is earmarked by fever, pharyngitis, cervical lymphadenopathy, splenomegaly, and fatigue.
- Infection is self-limited and leads to carrier state, which confers lifelong immunity.
  See "Epstein-Barr Virus Diseases: Infectious Mononucleosis" in Section I, p 83 for more information.

EPIDEMIOLOGY & DEMOGRAPHICS

INCIDENCE/PREVALENCE IN USA:
Unknown.
PREDOMINANT AGE: The peak age for males occurs slightly later than for females, 18 to 23 and 15 to 16 years of age, respectively.

ETIOLOGY & PATHOGENESIS

- EBV belongs to the DNA group of herpes viruses. It was first identified in 1964 and was etiologically linked to mononucleosis in 1973.
- The virus is shed in oropharyngeal secretions, which is also the main route of entry.
- It replicates in the oropharyngeal and nasopharyngeal epithelial tissues, salivary tissues, and B lymphocytes.

SYSTEMS AFFECTED

- Oropharynx: sore throat, edematous uvula, and palatal petechiae; at risk for tonsillar enlargement resulting in airway obstruction.
- Lymphatics: generalized lymphadenopathy from the lymphocytosis, including marked cervical lymphadenopathy, enlarged tonsils.
- Cardiac: pericarditis and ECG changes.
- Spleen: splenomegaly; at risk for rupture, either spontaneously or secondary to trauma.
- Liver: hepatitis, hepatomegaly, and jaundice.
- Renal: nephrotic syndrome, glomerular nephritis.
- Hematologic: thrombocytopenia, lymphocytosis, and hemolytic anemia (rare).
- Skin: nonspecific rash, urticaria.

- Neurologic: altered mentation, Guillain-Barré syndrome, Bell's palsy, encephalitis, optic neuritis, cerebellar ataxia, and Reye's syndrome.
- Ophthalmic: periorbital edema, dry eyes, keratitis, uveitis, conjunctivitis, retinitis, and ophthalmoplegia.
- Pulmonary (rare): hilar mediastinal lymphadenopathy and interstitial pneumonia.

CLINICAL PRESENTATION / PHYSICAL FINDINGS

- Onset occurs within 4 to 7 weeks after exposure.
- Prodrome: lasts approximately 5 to 7 days with malaise, fatigue, headache, arthralgias, fever/chills, dysphagia, and anorexia.
- In persons over the age of 40, the presentation is commonly atypical without many of the symptoms listed previously. Instead, such patients present with fever, jaundice, and hepatomegaly leading to diagnostic confusion.
- Fever: lasting for 3 or more weeks.
- Pharyngitis: results in sore throat, difficulty swallowing, and possible dehydration.
- Lymphadenopathy: generalized and cervical, in particular.
- Splenomegaly: tender and enlarged in the left upper quadrant of the abdomen.
- Hepatomegaly: tender and enlarged in the right upper quadrant of the abdomen.
- Skin: nonspecific rash or urticaria.
- Ophthalmic: periorbital edema, dry eyes, conjunctivitis, and ophthalmoplegia.
- Hematologic:
  - During active infection, there is an increase in IgG, IgM antibodies to viral capsid antigens (VCA) and transient antibodies to diffuse antigen, and no antibodies to EBV-nuclear antigen (EBNA).
  - Because patients do not present early enough in the course of the disease prior to the VCA-IgG levels decreasing, the most accurate hallmark during the active phase is the VCA-IgM antibodies.
  - When the disease progresses beyond the active phase, the antibody most sensitive as marker of recent infection is the VCA-IgG.
  - The VCA-IgM and anti-EBNA are not present.
  - In the carrier state, only moderate levels of VCA-IgG and anti-EBNA are found.
  - If the patient is immunosuppressed, there is different radiation in the timing of the antibodies formed.

DIAGNOSIS

DIFFERENTIAL DIAGNOSIS

- Strep throat
- Diphtheria
- Hodgkin's disease
- Leukemias
- Lymphomas
- CMV
- Rubella
- HIV
- Hepatitis A/B
- Toxoplasmosis

LABORATORY

- CBC with differential: lymphocytosis secondary to increased numbers of B and T cells
- Thrombocytopenia: occurs in 50% of patients

IMAGING/SPECIAL TESTS

- Monospot test: evaluate heterophile antibodies via latex agglutination.
  - Is only about 80% sensitive in adults
  - Has poor sensitivity in children less than 4 years old; infants do not produce heterophile antibodies.
  - In adults, false positive rate of approximately 15% secondary to other viruses such as adenovirus, CMV, and toxoplasmosis.
- ELISA, Western blot.

MEDICAL MANAGEMENT & TREATMENT

GENERAL

- Supportive, bed rest, no strenuous exercise for 3 to 4 weeks (particularly with splenomegaly)

MEDICATIONS

- Acetaminophen or ibuprofen for pain. Avoid aspirin due to possibility of Reye's syndrome.
- May give gamma globulin for cases not responsive to corticosteroids in preceding situations.
- Acyclovir is not routinely recommended because it does not lessen the time of infection.
- No antibiotics indicated.
- In severe, life-threatening airway obstruction due to tonsillar hyperplasia, may elect to give corticosteroid as adjunct treatment with intubation. Other indications for corticosteroids are neurologic changes, hemolytic anemia, thrombocytopenic purpura, myocarditis, or pericarditis.

COMPLICATIONS

- If splenic rupture occurs, this is a life-threatening emergency requiring splenectomy due to internal hemorrhage. This is the most common fatal complication.

See "Epstein-Barr Virus Diseases: Infectious Mononucleosis" in Section I, p 83 for more information on complications.

PROGNOSIS

- Generally, if the patient recovers without fatal or disabling organ system damage, the prognosis is excellent.

- Splenic rupture occurs in 0.1–0.5% of proven infectious mononucleosis.

DENTAL SIGNIFICANCE

See "Epstein-Barr Virus Diseases: Infectious Mononucleosis" in Section I, p 83 for more information on dental implications and management.

SUGGESTED REFERENCES

Neville B, Damm D, Allen C, Bouquot J (eds): *Oral & Maxillofacial Pathology*, ed 2. Philadelphia, WB Saunders, 2002, pp 224–226.

Rakel RE, Bope ET (eds): *Conn's Current Therapy 2005*. Philadelphia, Elsevier, 2005, pp 128–133.

AUTHOR: **TERESA BIGGERSTAFF, DDS, MD**

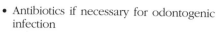

SYNONYM(S)

Odontogenic cysts
Nonodontogenic cysts

ICD-9CM/CPT CODE(S)

ICD-9CM
522.8 Radicular/periapical cyst
526.0 Developmental odontogenic cyst
(dentigerous, lateral periodontal,
odontogenic keratocyst)
526.1 Fissural cyst of jaw (globulomaxillary, incisive canal)
CPT
20220 Biopsy bone; needle aspiration;
superficial
20240 Biopsy bone; superficial
21030 Excision of cyst of facial bone
other than mandible
21040 Excision of cyst of mandible;
simple
21041 Excision of cyst of mandible;
complex

OVERVIEW

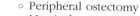

An epithelial-lined, pathologic
cavity that may contain fluid or
debris from degenerating cells.

EPIDEMIOLOGY & DEMOGRAPHICS

ODONTOGENIC CYSTS

- Radicular/periapical cyst
  ○ Most common
  ○ Usually occurs in anterior maxilla
- Dentigerous cyst
  ○ Associated with crown of unerupted
  tooth
  ○ Most common in mandibular third
  molars
- Lateral periodontal cyst
  ○ Rare
  ○ Usually in mandibular premolars or
  maxillary lateral incisor
  ○ Teeth usually vital
- Odontogenic keratocyst
  ○ Sixty percent occurs between ages of
  10 and 40
  ○ Slight male predilection
  ○ Usually in posterior mandible
  ○ Often perforates cortex and extends
  into soft tissue

NONODONTOGENIC CYSTS

- Globulomaxillary cyst

  ○ Occurs between the maxilla and pre-
  maxilla
- Incisive canal cyst
  ○ Occurs in the incisive foramen

ETIOLOGY & PATHOGENESIS

RADICULAR/PERIAPICAL CYST

- Develops within an existing periapical
granuloma
- Secondary to inflammation or infection

DENTIGEROUS CYST

- Caused by fluid accumulation between
the follicle and enamel of unerupted
tooth

CLINICAL PRESENTATION / PHYSICAL FINDINGS

- Slow expansion of alveolar process
- Facial swelling
- Loosening or displacement of teeth
- Odontogenic infection

DIAGNOSIS

DIFFERENTIAL DIAGNOSIS

- Odontogenic cyst
- Nonodontogenic cyst
  ○ Ameloblastoma
  ○ Central giant cell granuloma
  ○ Arteriovenous malformation
  ○ Periapical cemental dysplasia
  ○ Odontogenic myxoma
  ○ Adenoid odontogenic tumor
  ○ Idiopathic bone cavity

WORKUP

- Tooth vitality testing

LABORATORY

- Histopathologic examination necessary
to rule out tumors or cysts with high
recurrence potential
- Aspiration of luminal contents

IMAGING

- CT scan: accurate determination of
extent of lesion and possible cortical
perforation
- Panorex

MEDICAL MANAGEMENT & TREATMENT

ACUTE TREATMENT

- Extraction
- Curettage of cyst contents and histopathologic evaluation

- Antibiotics if necessary for odontogenic
infection
- Odontogenic keratocyst
  ○ Chemical curettage with Carnoy's
  solution
  ○ Peripheral ostectomy
  ○ Marginal resection with removal of
  soft tissue if cortical perforation found
- Marsupialization with large cysts to
shrink, followed by curettage

CHRONIC TREATMENT

- Odontogenic keratocyst: long-term follow-up due to high recurrence rates

PROGNOSIS

- Odontogenic keratocyst has a
high recurrence rate (greater
than 50%); long-term follow-up with
radiographs necessary; recurrence
requires retreatment.
- Curettage is usually curative; excellent
for odontogenic and nonodontogenic
cysts.

DENTAL SIGNIFICANCE

Panorex is a primary screening
tool since most cysts are found
on routine radiograph examination.

DENTAL MANAGEMENT

See preceding Medical Management &
Treatment for information on managing
these conditions.

SUGGESTED REFERENCES

Neville B, Damm D, Allen C, Bouquot J (eds):
Oral & Maxillofacial Pathology, ed 2.
Philadelphia, WB Saunders, 2002, pp
590–608.
Regezi, JA, Sciubba, JJ (eds): *Oral Pathology:
Clinical Pathologic Correlations*, ed 4.
Philadelphia, WB Saunders, 2003.

AUTHOR: **DALE J. MISIEK, DMD**

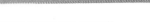

SYNONYM(S)

Endothelial cell sarcoma

ICD-9CM/CPT CODE(S)

ICD-9CM
176   Kaposi sarcoma
176.0 Skin
176.1 Soft tissue
       Includes: blood vessel, connective tissue, fascia, ligament, lymphatics, and muscle
       Excludes: lymph glands and nodes (176.5)
176.2 Palate
176.3 Gastrointestinal sites
176.4 Lung
176.5 Lymph nodes
176.8 Other specified sites
       Includes: oral cavity
176.9 Unspecified; viscera
CPT
11440 Excision face/lip/mucosa up to 5 cm
40490 Biopsy of lip
40808 Biopsy vestibule of mouth
41100 Biopsy anterior two-thirds of tongue
41105 Biopsy posterior one-third of tongue
41108 Biopsy floor of mouth
42100 Biopsy of palate, uvula
42104 Excision lesion palate, uvula; without closure

OVERVIEW

A malignant neoplasm of capillary origin, generally presenting in three varying clinical patterns:

- First: a rare, indolent skin tumor involving the lower extremities of older men of Mediterranean heritage, reddish brown to blue in color and found in various locations.
- Second: endemic in Africa, seen in blacks with preference for the extremities.
- Third: oral lesions found in patients suffering from immunodeficiency (i.e., AIDS).

EPIDEMIOLOGY & DEMOGRAPHICS

The first pattern is seen predominantly in older men of Mediterranean origin. The second pattern is seen primarily on the extremities of African blacks.

ETIOLOGY & PATHOGENESIS

- Endothelial cells and dermal and submucosal dendrocytes are considered to be the cells of origin.
- Etiology is generally considered to be unknown; the following factors play a role in the genesis of these lesions:
  - Genetic predisposition
  - Environmental factors
  - Viral infections
  - Immune system breakdown

SYSTEMS AFFECTED

- Cutaneous: primary system affected, with the skin of the extremities the most common site. To a lesser extent, the face and other locations can be involved, depending upon the pattern of the disease.
- Oral mucosa: frequently associated with acquired immunodeficiency syndrome (AIDS).
- Lymph node and visceral: involvement may occur in advanced cases.

CLINICAL PRESENTATION / PHYSICAL FINDINGS

SIGNS & SYMPTOMS

- Skin:
  - Usually painless but can be uncomfortable when ulceration or cellulitis occurs.
  - Typically are reddish brown to blue patches, plaques, and nodules on the distal lower extremities.
  - Initially unilateral or bilateral with gradual coalescence and proximal spread.
  - Ulceration may occur.
  - Upper extremity and facial lesions may be seen in certain forms of the disease.
- Oral mucosa:
  - Usually asymptomatic but can be uncomfortable and disruptive, especially when exophytic in nature.
  - Reddish brown to blue, flat or exophytic lesions seen often in the patients with AIDS.
  - When ulceration occurs, these lesions can clinically resemble squamous cell carcinoma.
- Lymph nodes: nonpainful lymphadenopathy.
- Visceral:
  - Asymptomatic gastrointestinal lesions present in 50% of AIDS patients.
  - Gastric outlet obstruction and occasional GI bleeding have been reported.
- Pulmonary:
  - Dyspnea and hemoptysis; seen in advanced cases of AIDS.

DIAGNOSIS

DIFFERENTIAL DIAGNOSIS

- Kaposi's sarcoma
- Hemangioma
- Pyogenic granuloma
- Melanoma
- Erythroplakia
- Squamous cell carcinoma

LABORATORY

- HIV testing: to positively identify patients with acquired immunodeficiency syndrome (AIDS)
- Stain and culture for oral candidiasis (often seen in AIDS patients)

IMAGING/SPECIAL TESTS

- Chest radiograph: reveals infiltrates, mediastinal enlargement and pleural effusion
- Biopsy: colon
  - Histology reveals bland-appearing spindle cells and multiple vascular canals.
  - Advanced lesion may show atypical vascular channels with red blood cells, hemosiderin, and inflammatory cells in stroma.

MEDICAL MANAGEMENT & TREATMENT

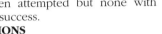

GENERAL

- Various forms of treatment have been attempted but none with uniform success.

MEDICATIONS

- Chemotherapy: often employed in patients with disseminated disease who have not been helped by radiotherapy; especially useful in patients with lymph node or visceral involvement or surgery

EXCISION

- Often used with success on small and localized lesions
  - In AIDS patients, perform hematologic evaluation prior to elective surgery.

RADIATION

- Low-dose application useful for larger, multifocal lesions
- Hopeful to reduce pain and improve appearance

PATIENT INSTRUCTIONS

- Diagnosis of Kaposi's sarcoma mandates immediate investigation of HIV status.

PROGNOSIS

- Varies markedly depending upon the pattern of the disease (three forms):
  - First pattern: the lesions are usually multifocal and on the skin of the lower extremities; oral lesions are rare. The clinical course is long with a fair to good prognosis.
  - Second pattern: skin lesions are typical; oral lesions are rare. The clinical course is long with a fair prognosis.
  - Third pattern: skin lesions can be found over the entire body and/ or often multifocal. Oral lesions are often seen and can be the initial site of involvement. Visceral and lymph node lesions can also be encountered. The clinical course can be rapid and aggressive and prognosis poor.

SECTION II

SUGGESTED REFERENCES

Chor PJ, Santa Cruz DJ. Kaposi's sarcoma. A clinical pathologic review and differential diagnosis. *J Cutan Pathol* 1992;19: 6–20.

Neville B, Damm D, Allen C, Bouquot J (eds): *Oral & Maxillofacial Pathology*, ed 2. Philadelphia, WB Saunders, 2002, pp 213, 235–237, 242–243, 248, 484–486.

Rakel RE, Bope ET (eds): *Conn's Current Therapy 2005*. Philadelphia, Elsevier, 2005, pp 51, 65, 964.

Regezi JA, Sciubba J. *Oral Pathology*, ed 4. Philadelphia, WB Saunders, 2003.

Zurrida S, et al. Classic Kaposi sarcoma: a review of 90 cases dermatology. *J Dermatol* 1992;19:548–552.

AUTHORS: **TERESA BIGGERSTAFF, DDS, MD; DALE J. MISIEK, DMD**

SYNONYM(S)

Squamous cell carcinoma
Solar keratosis
Verruca vulgaris

ICD-9CM/CPT CODE(S)

ICD-9CM
078.10 Viral warts, unspecified type
140.0 Malignant neoplasm of upper lip, vermilion border
140.1 Malignant neoplasm of lower lip, vermilion border
238.2 Keratoacanthoma
CPT
11440 Excision benign lesion, lips 0.5 cm or less
11441 Excision of benign lesion, lips 0.6 to 1.0 cm
11442 Excision benign lesion, lips 1.1 to 2.0 cm
11443 Excision benign lesion, lips 2.1 to 3.0 cm
40490 Biopsy of the lip

OVERVIEW

- A self-limiting, rapidly growing, benign epithelial proliferation, occurring secondary to sun exposure
- Strong clinical and histopathological similarity to well differentiated squamous cell carcinoma
- Occurs mainly on sun-exposed skin and/or lips

EPIDEMIOLOGY & DEMOGRAPHICS

INCIDENCE/PREVALENCE IN USA:

- Ninety five percent of solitary lesions were found on sun-exposed skin.
- Eight percent of all lesions were found on the outer edge of the vermilion border of the lips.
- Equal frequency on upper and lower lips.
- In the immunocompromised patient and those with Muir-Torre syndrome, there is an increased frequency.

PREDOMINANT AGE: Rarely seen in patients less than 45 years of age.

PREDOMINANT SEX: Male predilection.

GENETICS: Genetic previous position for multiple lesions

ETIOLOGY & PATHOGENESIS

- Originates from squamous cells within the infundibulum of the hair follicles.
- Cause is unknown, although sun damage and human papillomavirus (HPV) subtypes 26 or 37 have been proposed.
- Keratoacanthoma-like lesions have been produced in animals by the cutaneous application of carcinogens.
- Other possible induction factors include trauma, chemical agents, and genetic or hereditary factors.

CLINICAL PRESENTATION / PHYSICAL FINDINGS

- There is a firm, nontender, well-demarcated, sessile, dome-shaped nodule with a central core of keratin.
- When found intraorally, there is a lack of the keratin central core.
- The central keratin plug is yellowish to brownish black, irregular, and crusted often with a verruca form surface.
- The outer portion of the nodule often demonstrates normal texture and color, although may be erythematous at the borders.
- Rapid enlargement is typical.
- Diameter often seen between 1 and 2 cm within 6 weeks.
- Most lesions spontaneously regress within 6 to 12 months of onset, frequently leaving scarring in the area of the lesion.

DIAGNOSIS

- Histologically, a keratin plug surrounded by squamous epithelium.
- Marked pseudoepitheliomatosis hyperplasia present with mixed inflammatory infiltrates.
- Often confused with well-differentiated squamous cell carcinoma.

- Antigens such as involucrin are possible histologic markers for keratoacanthoma.

MEDICAL MANAGEMENT & TREATMENT

- Medications include intralesional methotrexate.
- Oral retinoid therapy.
- From a surgical perspective, observation only with biopsy; if lesion fails to regress, consider well-differentiated squamous cell carcinoma.
- Excisional biopsy recommended with thorough curettage at the base of the lesion.
- Irradiation is not indicated in these lesions. Despite the self-limiting nature of the keratoacanthoma, the surgical excision of a large lesion is indicated for optimal aesthetic results secondary to the lesion's nature of scarring.

PROGNOSIS

- With adequate treatment, less than 2% recurrence rates are to be expected.
- Lesions left untreated usually spontaneously involute.
- Aggressive behavior and malignant transformation into carcinoma has been reported in a small population. The close histologic similarities between keratoacanthomas and squamous cell carcinoma makes it difficult to rule out the possibility of misinterpretation from a microscopic examination.
- All lesions should be followed closely.

SUGGESTED REFERENCE

Neville B, Damm D, Allen C, Bouquot J (eds): *Oral & Maxillofacial Pathology*, ed 2. Philadelphia, WB Saunders, 2002, pp 354–355.

AUTHOR: **ROBERT M. LAUGHLIN, DMD**

SECTION II

SYNONYM(S)

Solar keratosis
Solar cheilitis

ICD-9CM/CPT CODE(S)

ICD-9CM
370.24 Actinic conjunctivitis
702.0 Actinic keratosis
692.72 Actinic cheilitis
692.74 Solar elastosis
701.1 Hyperkeratosis
CPT
11100 Biopsy, skin
13131 Mouth, repair, complex
17340 Cryotherapy, skin
40500 Vermilionectomy with mucosal advancement
40490 Biopsy, lip
41116 Excision, lesion, floor of mouth
99000 Handling and transport of specimens

OVERVIEW

Common, cutaneous, premalignant lesion caused by accumulative ultraviolet radiation to sun-exposed skin

EPIDEMIOLOGY & DEMOGRAPHICS

INCIDENCE/PREVALENCE IN USA: Skin lesions found in > 50% of Caucasian adults with significant sun exposure. It is estimated that 1 in 1000 individual lesions will become invasive.
PREDOMINANT SEX: 15% for males > 40 years old and 6% for females > 40 years old.
PREDOMINANT AGE: Prevalence increases with age. Rare in patients < 40 years old.
GENETICS: Those with fair skin and red to strawberry-blond hair have greater incidence.

ETIOLOGY & PATHOGENESIS

- Excessive sun exposure.
- Increased recreational sun exposure decreases age of first appearance of lesions.
- UV radiation (artificial or natural) may cause actinic keratosis.

CLINICAL PRESENTATION / PHYSICAL FINDINGS:

- Generally asymptomatic.
- Face, neck, dorsum of hands, forearms, and scalp of bald-headed men are most common sites.
- Irregular, scaly plaques.
- Color ranges from normal to white, gray, or brown, superimposed on an erythematous background.
- Sandpaper-roughened texture on palpation.
- Typically, the lesion is smaller than 7 mm in diameter but may reach larger than 2 cm in diameter.
- Usually minimal elevation.
- A hyperkeratotic "horn" may be seen arising from the central aspect of the lesion.
- Other clinical types in addition to the classic papular lesion include:
  ○ Lichenoid actinic keratosis
  ○ Actinic cheilitis
  ○ Hypertrophic actinic keratosis
  ○ Pigmented actinic keratosis
  ○ Actinic conjunctiva

DIAGNOSIS

HISTOPATHOLOGY

- Characterized by hyperparakeratosis and acanthosis.
- Some degree of epithelial dysplasia is present.
- Full-thickness epithelial dysplasia is termed bowenoid actinic keratosis.
- Suprabasilar acantholysis, melanosis, and lichenoid inflammatory infiltrates may also be seen. The dermis exhibits a band of pale, basophilic changes, which represent sun-damaged collagen and elastic fibers.
- Chronic inflammatory cells are typical.

MEDICAL MANAGEMENT & TREATMENT

- Because these are precancerous, destruction by cryotherapy with liquid nitrogen is recommended.
- Topical application of 5-fluorouracil, curettage, electrodesiccation, or surgical excision.

COMPLICATIONS

At least 13% of the high-risk population of affected individuals will develop squamous cell carcinoma from at least one of the actinic keratotic lesions. Frequency of malignant transformation is unknown.

PROGNOSIS

Recurrence is rare, but additional lesions frequently arise in adjacent sun-damaged skin. Long-term follow-up is recommended.

DENTAL SIGNIFICANCE

No specific dental implications.

SUGGESTED REFERENCES

Neville B, Damm D, Allen C, Bouquot J (eds): *Oral & Maxillofacial Pathology*, ed 2. Philadelphia, WB Saunders, 2002, pp 351–352.
Rakel RE, et al. (eds): *Conn's Current Therapy 2005*. Philadelphia, Elsevier, 2005, pp 941–942.
Regezi JA, et al. (eds): *Oral Pathology: Clinical-Pathologic Correlations*, ed 4. Philadelphia, WB Saunders, 2003.

AUTHOR: **ROBERT M. LAUGHLIN, DMD**

SYNONYM(S)

Glottic carcinoma

Carcinoma of the supraglottis, glottis, or subglottis

True/false vocal cord carcinoma

ICD-9CM/CPT CODE(S)

ICD-9CM

161.9 Neoplasm, laryngeal, malignant

CPT

21085 Oral surgical splint

21089 Unlisted maxillofacial prosthetic procedure, by report

OVERVIEW

- Laryngeal carcinoma is usually squamous cell carcinoma.
- Lesions involving the free edge of the vocal cords are frequently detected early, secondary to the patient's complaint of hoarseness or other vocal complaints.
- Lesions arising in areas adjacent to the larynx may remain silent until disease is significantly advanced.

EPIDEMIOLOGY & DEMOGRAPHICS

ETIOLOGY & PATHOGENESIS

- Primary etiologic factor: long-term tobacco abusc/use.
- Alcohol likely not a significant cofactor, unlike with oral and pharyngeal cancers.
- Laryngeal tumors may obstruct the airway.
- Laryngeal carcinomas metastasize first to the cervical lymphatic chains.

CLINICAL PRESENTATION / PHYSICAL FINDINGS

- Persistent hoarseness
- Recurrent sore throat
- Hemoptysis
- Dysphagia and/or dysphonia
- Slow onset of painless neck masses
- Weight loss
- Airway obstruction in advanced disease
- Painless neck masses secondary to cervical metastasis

DIAGNOSIS

IMAGING/SPECIAL TESTS

- Direct laryngoscopy with biopsy
- Flexible fiberoptic laryngoscopy

LARYNGEAL CARCINOMA

- CT with and without contrast
- MRI scan

MEDICAL MANAGEMENT & TREATMENT

- Generally, radiation therapy alone is used for T1 and T2 lesions without metastasis.
- Advanced lesions are often treated with chemotherapy and subsequent radiation with or without surgery. Medications are *cis*-platinum and 5-fluorouracil.
- Analgesics.
- Liquid nutritional supplements.
- Surgery may involve partial or complete removal of the larynx.

PROGNOSIS

- Dependent on stage; small lesions have better prognosis than larger lesions.
- Cervical metastasis is an unfavorable prognostic sign.
- Recurring or persistent lesions following radiation therapy are often successfully salvaged by laryngectomy. Patients who have undergone laryngectomy are known as neck breathers; they breathe entirely through the tracheal stoma.
- Speech in laryngectomy patients is possible by means of esophageal speech or through sound-producing devices placed against the skin of the neck.

DENTAL MANAGEMENT

- Preradiation evaluation to determine unsalvageable dentition. Extractions and periodontal therapy should precede radiation
- Therapeutic radiation fields frequently involve the oral cavity and/or neck. It is therefore advisable prior to any oral surgical endodontic or periodontic procedures that consultation with radiation oncology is performed.
- The fabrication of fluoride carrying trays should be requested by the radiation oncologist for those patients whose radiation fields involve the oral cavity and teeth-bearing bony structures.

SUGGESTED REFERENCES

Bailey BJ. Early glottic carcinoma, in Bailey BJ (ed): *Head & Neck Surgery Otolaryngology.* Philadelphia, JP Lippincott, 1993, pp 1337–1360.

Fried MP, Girdhar-Gopal, HV. Advanced cancer of the larynx, in Bailey BJ (ed): *Head & Neck Surgery Otolaryngology.* Philadelphia, JP Lippincott, 1993, pp 1361–1372.

AUTHOR: **ROBERT M. LAUGHLIN, DMD**

SECTION II

SYNONYM(S)

Hyperkeratosis
Leukokeratosis
Erythroleukoplakia
Oral leukoplakia

ICD-9CM/CPT CODE(S)

ICD-9CM
528.6 Leukoplakia
CPT
11100 Biopsy of mucous membrane
11101 Each additional lesion
11440 Excision, benign lesion 0.5 cm or less
11441 Lesion 0.6 cm to 1 cm
11442 Lesion 1.1 cm to 2 cm
11443 Lesion 2.1 cm to 3 cm
40490 Biopsy of lip
40808 Biopsy, vestibule of mouth
40820 Destruction of lesion vestibule of mouth by physical method (laser, cryo)
41100 Biopsy of tongue
42100 Biopsy of palate, uvula
42104 Excision, lesion of palate without closure

OVERVIEW

- Leukoplakia is a clinical term that encompasses a group of diseases.
- A white plaque or patch of oral mucosa that does not rub off and cannot be diagnosed clinically as any other disease.
- Excluded are diseases that can be diagnosed, such as lichen planus and candidiasis.
- Microscopic examination of leukoplakia will reveal hyperkeratosis, epithelial dysphagia, carcinoma in situ, or superficially invasive squamous cell carcinoma.

ETIOLOGY & PATHOGENESIS

- Many leukoplakias are idiopathic.
- Use of combustible or smokeless tobacco can produce leukoplakia; lesion may resolve if tobacco is discontinued.
- *Candida albicans* is associated with many leukoplakias, although its role as an etiologic agent is not proven.
- Mechanical trauma from dentures, restorations, or habits.
- Ultraviolet radiation on vermilion border of lower lip.

SYSTEMS AFFECTED

- Leukoplakia can occur on any oral mucosal surface.

CLINICAL PRESENTATIONS / PHYSICAL FINDINGS

SIGNS & SYMPTOMS

- Asymptomatic thickening of oral epithelium, not a soft tissue tumor. The surface is white, yellow, or gray. Some lesions have interspersed red areas ("speckled leukoplakia").
- Wrinkled, fissured, nodular, or smooth, and typically rough to palpation.
- Cannot be removed by rubbing or scraping.

DIAGNOSIS

DIFFERENTIAL DIAGNOSIS

- Lichen planus: multiple lesions bilaterally distributed; often has striations.
- Candidiasis: white plaques rub off, leaving an erythematous base; usually symptomatic.
- White sponge nevus (familial epithelial hyperplasia): familial history, present from childhood, multiple diffuse lesions.
- Nicotinic stomatitis: located on hard palate of smokers.
- Discoid lupus erythematosus: painful ulcers often associated with white areas; skin lesions common.
- Verrucous carcinoma: indurated, folded, attached to underlying structures.

LABORATORY

- Brush biopsy as a screening tool to determine presence of dysplasia.
- Biopsy with histopathologic examination is necessary for definitive diagnosis.

IMAGING/SPECIAL TESTS

- Toluidine blue vital staining may be helpful in determining whether an incisional biopsy would be diagnostic, but it should never be used as a screening tool.

MEDICAL MANAGEMENT & TREATMENT

GENERAL

- Location of lesion is important in determining treatment.
- If located on keratinized oral mucosa (including gingiva, attached alveolar mucosa, hard palate, and dorsum of tongue) and appears to be the result of chronic mechanical irritation, the lesion probably represents a callus (hyperkeratosis).
- Lesion can be observed rather than performing immediate biopsy.
- If associated with a tobacco habit, discontinue tobacco and then reevaluate in several weeks; if the lesion is still present, then incisional biopsy should be performed.

SURGICAL

- If an incisional biopsy is performed on a leukoplakia and the microscopic diagnosis is hyperkeratosis, no further surgery is necessary; if the diagnosis is dysplasia, carcinoma in-situ, or squamous cell carcinoma, a complete surgical removal of the lesion is necessary.
- Leukoplakia located on nonkeratinized mucosa in high-risk areas such as floor of the mouth, ventral-lateral tongue, soft palate, and retromolar trigone are more likely to represent epithelial dysplasia, carcinoma in situ, or superficial squamous cell carcinoma; these lesions should be biopsied.
- Lesions with speckled, erythematous, or nodular areas are especially serious and should be biopsied.
- Large areas of leukoplakia may require multiple biopsies to adequately examine the lesion.

IRRADIATION

- Not indicated

PROGNOSIS

- The clinical course and prognosis of leukoplakia depend upon the microscopic diagnosis and removal of etiology.
- Smoking cessation is necessary for resolution.
- Hyperkeratosis: the lesion is benign, at least in the short term; persistent hyperkeratosis, especially on nonkeratinized mucosal surfaces; will rarely progress to a more serious lesion.
- Dysplasia: some dysplastic lesions regress spontaneously, while others progress to invasive squamous cell carcinoma; they should be considered premalignant.
- Carcinoma in situ: surgical excision should be curative. If untreated, this lesion will progress to invasive squamous cell carcinoma.
- Squamous cell carcinoma: excision of superficial lesions should be curative. Prognosis of more deeply invasive lesions depends upon microscopic differentiation and clinical staging.

COMPLICATIONS

Dysplasia lesions may progress to squamous cell carcinoma.

SUGGESTED REFERENCES

Brightman VJ. Red and white lesions of the oral mucosa, in Lynch MA (ed): *Burkett's Oral Medicine*, ed 9. Philadelphia, JB Lippincott, 1994, pp 51–120.

Neville B, Damm D, Allen C, Bouquot J (eds): *Oral & Maxillofacial Pathology*, ed 2. Philadelphia, WB Saunders, 2002, pp 337–345.

Silverman S, Gorsky M, Lozada F. Oral leukoplakia and malignant transformation. A follow-up study of 257 patients. *Cancer* 1984;53:563–568.

WHO Collaborating Center for Oral Precancerous Lesions. Definition of leukoplakia and related lesions: an aid to studies on oral precancer. *Cancer* 1978;46:518–539.

AUTHORS: **TERESA BIGGERSTAFF, DDS, MD; DALE J. MISIEK, DMD**

SECTION II

SYNONYM(S)

None

ICD-9CM/CPT CODE(S)

ICD-9CM

054.2	Primary herpes
054.9	Recurrent herpes
079.9	Viral infection
112.0	Candidiasis of mouth
136.9	Bacterial infection
141.2	Squamous cell carcinoma
141.3	Carcinoma in situ
400.0	Burn
528.0	Stomatitis
528.2	Aphthous
528.9	Ulcer
529.0	Glossitis
694.6	Cicatricial pemphigoid
694.4	Pemphigus
695.1	Erythema multiforme
695.4	Lupus erythematous
697.0	Lichen planus

CPT

11900	Intralesional injection
40812	Incisional biopsy, mouth with simple repair
87252	Culture isolation
88160	Cytologic preparation
99000	Transport specimen to outside laboratory

OVERVIEW

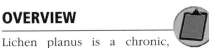

Lichen planus is a chronic, recurrent, noninfectious, inflammatory disease affecting the mucosa and/or skin.

SYSTEMS AFFECTED

- Oral mucosa: hyperkeratotic striations (lacy pattern) and plaques, mucosal atrophy resulting in clinical erythema, and ulceration.
- Skin: erythematous macules with overlying keratotic crusts.

EPIDEMIOLOGY & DEMOGRAPHICS

INCIDENCE/PREVALENCE IN USA:

Seen in 0.1–2.2% of the general population.

PREDOMINANT SEX: Ratio of females to males is 3:2.

ETIOLOGY & PATHOGENESIS

- The cause of lichen planus is unknown.
- CD4 and CD8 T cells account for the inflammatory infiltrate noted microscopically and account for the basal cell liquefaction degeneration of the epithelium.
- The same reaction is noted in lichenoid, drug, and skin eruptions and in graft vs host disease.
- Associated with systemic disease including diabetes mellitus, rheumatic disease, and hypertension.

- Some investigators believe lichen planus is premalignant and report malignant transformation rates of 2–10%.

CLINICAL PRESENTATION / PHYSICAL FINDINGS

SIGNS & SYMPTOMS

- Recurrent oral discomfort, usually with exacerbations and partial or complete remissions.
- Sensitivity to hot, spicy, and citric foods and beverages.
- Pruritus in extensor surfaces of extremities and on palms and soles.
- Hyperkeratotic striations, usually widespread orally involving buccal, glossal, labial, palatal, and gingival mucosa, unilaterally or bilaterally; the pattern of mucosal involvement will change over the course of days or weeks.
- Mucosa associated with or underlying the striations will be relatively erythematous.
- During exacerbations, ulcerations will characteristically be found associated with the erythematous and hyperkeratotic mucosa.

DIAGNOSIS

DIFFERENTIAL DIAGNOSIS

- Lichenoid mucositis (drug induced)
- Graft vs host disease
- Lupus erythematosus
- Epithelial dysplasia

LABORATORY

- No clinical laboratory tests or values.
- An incisional biopsy may be indicated to establish the diagnosis; a biopsy should be considered for any area not responsive to therapy.

IMAGING/SPECIAL TESTS

- Microscopic features include areas of surface epithelial hyperkeratosis, atrophy, and sometimes ulceration; liquefaction degeneration of the basal cell area replaced by a band of fibrin is noted. A band-like, superficial infiltrate of lymphocytes is found in the underlying connective tissue.

MEDICAL MANAGEMENT & TREATMENT

- Avoid hot and spicy foods during exacerbation.
- Avoid exacerbation "triggers" if identified.

MEDICATIONS

- Topical steroid gel: fluocinonide, betamethasone, clobetasol in a 0.5% gel applied tid or qid during flare-up, reducing to qd or qod for maintenance.

- Topical steroid suspension: triamcinolone acetonide 0.1% aqueous suspension, dispensed 20 mL, sid 5-mL oral rinse and expectorate qid, pc, and hs nod 1 hour. (Directions to the pharmacist: Injectable triamcinolone qs into water for irrigation, add 5 mL of ethanol to increase solubility). May alter suspension to include viscous lidocaine as a topical anesthetic.
- Prednisone burst therapy, 40 mg qd in the morning 30 minutes after waking for 5 days, then 20 mg qod also 30 minutes after arising for an additional 1 to 2 weeks.

SURGERY

- Incisional biopsy

PATIENT INSTRUCTIONS

- Patient education is important because therapy may promote healing of current ulcers and atrophic mucosa and, if used as subtherapeutic doses, can prevent recurrences but cannot cure the patient of the disease.
- Lesions may have malignant potential; so monitoring is important.

PROGNOSIS

- Long-term management is aimed at finding the minimum amount of therapy that will keep the ulcers from recurring.
- This can usually be accomplished by using the topical triamcinolone tid, bid, od, qod, or even prn. Those patients in remission (asymptomatic) will continue to show hyperkeratotic striations.
- The most common complication/side effect of long-term topical triamcinolone is oral candidiasis.
- In these cases, an antifungal such as nystatin can be used in a topical triamcinolone suspension (replacing the water).

SUGGESTED REFERENCES

Neville B, Damm D, Allen C, Bouquot J (eds): *Oral & Maxillofacial Pathology*, ed 2. Philadelphia, WB Saunders, 2002, pp 680–685.

Regezi JA, Sciubba JJ. Ulcerative conditions, in *Oral Pathology: Clinical Pathologic Correlations*, ed 4. Philadelphia, WB Saunders, 2003.

Silverman S, Gorsky M, Lozada-Nur F. A prospective follow-up study of 570 patients with oral lichen planus—persistence, remission in malignant association. *Oral Surg Oral Med Oral Path* 1985;60:30–34.

Vincent SD, Fotos PG, Baker KA, Williams TP. Oral lichen planus: the clinical, historical, and therapeutic features of 100 cases. *Oral Surg Oral Med Oral Path* 1990;70:165–171.

AUTHORS: **TERESA BIGGERSTAFF, DDS, MD; DALE J. MISIEK, DMD**

SYNONYM(S)

Pharyngitis
Odontogenic infection

ICD-9CM/CPT CODE(S)

ICD-9CM
528.3 Ludwig's angina
CPT
21501 IND, soft tissues, neck
31500 Emergency endotracheal intubation
31600 Tracheostomy, planned
31603 Tracheostomy, emergency procedure
41015 Extraoral IND, sublingual
41016 Extraoral IND, submental
41017 Extraoral IND, submandibular
41800 Drainage of abscesses from dentoalveolar structure
70350 Cephalogram
70355 Panorex
70360 Radiographic exam, soft tissue of neck
87040 Blood culture
87070 Culture and source other than nose-throat blood
87205 Smear, primary source of interpretation
99000 Transport specimen to outside laboratory

OVERVIEW

Acute, toxic, aggressive, diffuse, and rapidly spreading cellulitis (phlegman) with involvement of the sublingual, submandibular, and submental spaces bilaterally

EPIDEMIOLOGY & DEMOGRAPHICS

No predominant sex, age, or genetics.

ETIOLOGY & PATHOGENESIS

- Spread of acute infection from the lower molar teeth, usually the second or third molar in approximately 70% of cases.
- Can arise from peritonsillar oropharyngeal abscesses, oral lacerations, fractures of the mandible, or submandibular sialadenitis.
- Increased prevalence in immunocompromised patients such as those with diabetes mellitus, organ transplantation, AIDS, or aplastic anemia.

CLINICAL PRESENTATION / PHYSICAL FINDINGS

- Massive swelling/neck swelling.
- Sublingual space causes a "woody tongue"—elevation, posterior enlargement, and protrusion of tongue.
- Drooling, trismus, and fetor oris.
- Submandibular space cellulitis causes a "bull" neck—enlargement and tenderness of the neck above the level of the hyoid bone.
- Typically, infection is initially unilateral with spread to the contralateral neck.
- Pain in the neck and floor of the mouth may also be seen along with restriction of neck movement, dysphagia, dysphonia, dysarthria, drooling, and sore throat.
- Respiratory obstruction secondary to laryngeal edema.
- Malaise, fever, chills, and tachypnea.
- Classically, collections of pus are not present.

DIAGNOSIS

LABORATORY

- Leukocytosis on complete blood chemistry
- Stain and culture aspirate or drainage from infected bacteria, including anaerobic and fungal
- Monitor electrolytes

IMAGING/SPECIAL TESTS

- CT scan of neck with and without contrast
- Panorex
- Lateral soft tissue of neck

MEDICAL MANAGEMENT & TREATMENT

See following Dental Management for treatment information.

COMPLICATIONS

- Death occurs in fewer than 10% of the patient population secondary to pneumonia, mediastinitis, sepsis, empyema, and respiratory obstruction.
- Incomplete therapy can lead to reinfection or spread to masseteric and pharyngeal spaces.

PROGNOSIS

- Prior to the advent of modern antibiotics, the mortality rate associated with Ludwig's angina exceeded 50%. This mortality rate has been reduced to less than 10% with modern antibiotics.

DENTAL MANAGEMENT

- Primary concerns:
  - Maintenance of the airway
  - Incision and drainage
  - Antibiotic therapy
  - Elimination of the original focus of infection
- If signs and symptoms indicate airway obstruction development, endotracheal intubation or tracheostomy or cricothyroidotomy should be performed.
- High-dose IV penicillin is the antibiotic of choice.
- Antibiotic therapy is tailored and adjusted according to the culture and sensitivity results.
- Incision and drainage of bilateral sublingual, submandibular, and submental spaces. Placement of drains in the sublingual, submental, and submandibular spaces with access for irrigation.
- Aminoglycosides are given for resistant organisms.
- Clindamycin or chloramphenicol used in the penicillin-sensitive patient.
- Extraction of diseased teeth.

SUGGESTED REFERENCES

Fritsch DG, Klein DG. Ludwig's angina. *Heart Lung* 1992;21:39–46.

Goldberg MH, Topazian RG. Odontogenic infections and deep fascial space infections of dental origin, in Topazian RG, Goldberg MH, Hupp JR (eds): *Oral and Maxillofacial Infections*, ed 4. Philadelphia, WB Saunders, 2002, pp 177–181.

Neville B, Damm D, Allen C, Bouquot J (eds): *Oral & Maxillofacial Pathology*, ed 2. Philadelphia, WB Saunders, 2002, pp 124–125.

Owens BM, Shuman NJ. Ludwig's angina. *Gen Dent* 1994;42:84–87.

AUTHOR: **ROBERT M. LAUGHLIN, DMD**

SYNONYM(S)

Lung cancer
Mesothelioma
Bronchoalveolar carcinoma

ICD-9CM/CPT CODE(S)

ICD-9CM
162.9 Neoplasm, lung
CPT
38510 Biopsy of deep cervical nodes
38520 Biopsy of deep cervical nodes with scalene fat pad

OVERVIEW

- Malignant neoplasm originating in lung tissue.
- Primary carcinoma of the lung is increasing annually.
- It has long been the leading cause of cancer-related death in men and recently has become one of the principal causes of cancer in women.
- At the time of diagnosis, more than 50% have distant metastasis and only 20% have only local disease.
- Most patients die within 1 year.
- The common malignancies of the lung can be divided into two major calcifications:
  o Small cell carcinoma (oat cell).
  o Nonsmall cell carcinoma, which includes epidermoid (squamous cell) carcinoma (most common), adenocarcinoma, and large cell carcinoma.
- Other malignancies (sarcoma, lymphoma, carcinoid, melanoma, and mesothelioma) are uncommon.

EPIDEMIOLOGY & DEMOGRAPHICS

PREDOMINANT AGE: Peak incidences between age 55 and 65. Prevalence increases with age, rising from 50 cases per 100,000 population age 50 or older to 850 cases per 100,000 population age 85 or older.
PREDOMINANT SEX: Males predominate with an incidence of 70 in 100,000.

ETIOLOGY & PATHOGENESIS

- Cigarette smoking; benzopyrene is a major carcinogen in tobacco smoke.
- Environmental pollutants.
- Industrial pollutants.
- Radioisotopes.
- Asbestos exposure.
- Inorganic arsenic.
SYSTEMS AFFECTED
- Pulmonary.
- Brain, bone, and liver are predominant sites of metastasis with resultant seizures, neurologic deficits, pathologic fractures, liver dysfunction, and pain.

CLINICAL PRESENTATION / PHYSICAL FINDINGS

SIGNS & SYMPTOMS
- Asymptomatic: 5–15% of diagnosis result from routine chest radiograph.

- General: weakness, malaise, shortness of breath, dyspnea on exertion, clubbing (hypertrophic pulmonary osteoarthropathy), anorexia, cachexia, and weight loss.
- Central or endobronchial lesion: cough, dyspnea, hemoptysis, fever, productive sputum, and wheezing.
- Peripheral growth lesion: cough, pleuritic pain, and restrictive shortness of breath.
- Regional spread: hoarseness, cervical or axillary adenopathy, Horner's syndrome, superior vena cava syndrome, pleural effusion, cardiac dysrhythmia or tamponade, and shoulder bone or chest pain.

DIAGNOSIS

DIFFERENTIAL DIAGNOSIS
- Metastatic carcinoma
- Granulomatous disease
- Fungal infection
- Hematoma
- Lung abscess
LABORATORY
- CBC: anemia secondary to chronic disease or bone marrow involvement
- Calcium: increased secondary to bone metastases or ectopic parathyroid hormone production (epidermoid cancer)
- Coagulation: disseminated intravascular coagulation (DIC) and migratory venous thrombophlebitis (Trousseau's syndrome)
- Sodium: decreased for syndrome of inappropriate secretion of antidiuretic hormone (SIADH) from small cell cancer
- Liver profile: increased bilirubin, transaminases, and alkaline phosphatase with metastases
IMAGING/SPECIAL TESTS
- Chest radiograph: basic study to detect lung cancer.
- CT scan of chest: to confirm presence and extent of pulmonary mass.
- Bone scan: to document metastasis of symptomatic.
- PET scan with 2-FDG: to evaluate extent of disease including hilar/mediastinal extension and for staging.
- Other CT scans: brain and abdomen to document metastases.
- Ventilation/perfusion lung scan: evaluation of functional lung parenchyma.
- Barium swallow: for esophageal symptoms.
- Special diagnostic procedures: pulmonary function test (PFTs), fiberoptic bronchoscopy with brushings and biopsy, mediastinoscopy, fine-needle biopsy (accessible or CT-guided), and lymph node biopsy (scalene, axillary, or mediastinal).

MEDICAL MANAGEMENT & TREATMENT

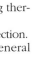

GENERAL
- Supportive care including respiratory care, nutritional supplementation, and correction or treatment of laboratory abnormalities.
- Encourage the patient to stop smoking.
- Avoid occupational and environmental toxins (e.g., asbestos).
- Small cell carcinoma: most have spread and are not resectable at time of diagnosis. Treatment would consist of combination chemotherapy and radiotherapy or radiotherapy alone.
- Nonsmall cell carcinoma:
  o Pulmonary resection is the treatment of choice for operable tumors.
  o Radiotherapy for unresectable and node positive tumors.
  o Radiotherapy for inoperable tumors and metastases to extrathoracic sites.
- Chemotherapy for inoperable tumors in patients with good performance status in extrathoracic disease.
MEDICATION
- Analgesics: pain control.
- Antibiotics: pulmonary infection.
- Chemotherapy: combination drug therapy.
- Surgery: see preceding General section.
- Irradiation: see preceding General section.

PROGNOSIS

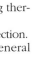

SMALL CELL CARCINOMA:
- Cure rate of 15–25% for limited disease and 1–5% for extensive disease.
- Ninety to 95% will show objective tumor shrinkage.
NONSMALL CELL CARCINOMA:
- Operable stage 1 tumors resected for cure have 55% 5-year survival and 15% 10-year survival.
- Stage II and stage III tumors vary between 35% and 10% 5-year survival, varying with cell type and extent of nodal involvement.
- The majority of patients thought to have had a curative resection die in 2 years, indicating need for adjunctive therapy.

DENTAL MANAGEMENT

If patients are taking bisphosphonate medications for metastatic disease, the dentist should be alert to the onset of osteonecrosis.

SUGGESTED REFERENCE
Rakel RE, Bope ET (eds): *Conn's Current Therapy 2005.* Philadelphia, Elsevier, 2005, pp 265–272.

AUTHOR: **TERESA BIGGERSTAFF, DDS, MD**

SYNONYM(S)

Lyme borreliosis
Lyme arthritis
Bannwarth's syndrome
Acrodermatitis chronica atrophicans

ICD-9CM/CPT CODE(S)

ICD-9CM
088.81 Lyme disease
CPT
86618 *Borrelia burgdorferi* immunologic identification

OVERVIEW

Multi-system illness caused by a
tickborne spirochete that produces a wide range of atypical arthritic,
dermal, neurologic, cardiovascular, and
ocular signs and symptoms usually
occurring over a period of many months

EPIDEMIOLOGY & DEMOGRAPHICS

Widespread throughout the U.S.; can
occur at any age without sexual predilection.

ETIOLOGY & PATHOGENESIS

- First recognized in 1975, is caused by a
  spiral-shaped bacterium called the
  Borrelia burgdorferi spirochete. It is
  carried and transmitted by several
  species of the tiny *Ixodes* (deer ticks),
  which are predominantly located in
  the northeastern, midwestern, and
  western United States as well as other
  Asian and European countries.
- Transmission to humans most often
  occurs in June or July (May to
  November range) when the tick attaches
  to the host and regurgitates midgut contents into the wound site. Studies suggest that tick attachment of 24 hours or
  more are necessary for spirochetal transmission to the host.
- Following inoculation, the spirochete
  spreads laterally in the dermis, eventually reaching regional lymphatics and
  disseminating in the blood to the internal organs, distant skin, and musculoskeletal sites. The organism can be
  cultured from the blood within weeks
  of infection.
- An apparent immunosuppression
  occurs initially following infection with
  an increase in T suppressor cell activity and poor mononuclear cell responsiveness to *Borrelia* antigens. This
  early hyporesponsiveness to these anti-

gens is later supplanted by B lymphocyte hyperactivity resulting in elevated
serum IgM, cryoprecipitates, and circulating immune complexes. Over a
period of months to years, a specific
antibody response to the spirochete
gradually develops, although the
organism is phagocytosed by PMNs and
activated macrophages in vitro. It has
been suggested that the organism may
be capable of surviving intracellularly.

SYSTEMS AFFECTED

- Skin: characterized as erythema chron-
  icum migrans (macular, intensely red
  migrating rings, hot to touch, but nontender), which initially occur at the site
  of the tick bite.
- Musculoskeletal: within several weeks
  to 2 years after onset, most patients
  develop intermittent arthritis or chronic
  synovitis.
- Neurologic: early in the disease, the
  patients develop severe headaches or
  neck pain and stiffness typically lasting
  for hours. Within months, abnormalities such as meningitis, encephalitis,
  chorea, myelitis, and fascial palsy
  (Bell's palsy) can develop. These
  abnormalities typically last for months,
  can recur, or become chronic.
- Cardiac: invasion of heart muscle can
  result in myocarditis leading to varying
  degrees of heart block.
- Ocular: involvement of the deeper eye
  tissues can result in panophthalmitis
  and blindness with spirochetal invasion of the vitreous humor.

CLINICAL PRESENTATION / PHYSICAL FINDINGS

SIGN & SYMPTOMS

- Malaise, fatigue, lethargy, headaches,
  fever, arthralgias, nausea, photophobia, vertigo, cough, chest and abdominal pain, diarrhea, and backache
- Regional or generalized lymphadenopathy, conjunctivitis, and periorbital
  edema, neck pain on flexion, malar
  rash, chronic dermal erythema migrans
  or annular lesions, muscular tenderness,
  and abdominal tenderness
- Migratory arthritis, joint swelling and
  effusions

DIAGNOSIS

DIFFERENTIAL DIAGNOSIS

- Rheumatic collagen disorders
- Epstein-Barr virus
- Cytomegalovirus

LABORATORY

- Culture of *Borrelia*
- Detection of *Borrelia*-specific serum
  IgM or IgG (ELISA)
- Elevated serum AST, APT, and LDH

MEDICAL MANAGEMENT & TREATMENT

MEDICATIONS

- Tetracycline, 250 mg to 500 mg
  po qid (oral); penicillin V 500 mg po
  qid (oral); doxycycline 100 mg po bid
  for 2 to 4 weeks depending on stage of
  infection.
- Established Lyme disease may require
  repeated course of therapy given a frequent incidence of relapse.

FIRST STEPS TO TAKE IN AN EMERGENCY

- If acute arthritis appears, immediately
  confer with infectious disease specialist
  and/or rheumatologist.

PATIENT INSTRUCTIONS

- Examine children for attached ticks
  and telltale characteristic rash of
  exposed areas.

COMPLICATIONS

Fifty percent of all patients
treated experience late complications of disease (i.e., chronic headache, myalgia, arthralgia, lethargy)
lasting hours to days.

PROGNOSIS

The development of complicating cardiac conduction block-
age, meningitis, or peripheral or cranial
neuropathies indicates the need for intravenous antimicrobial therapy.

SUGGESTED REFERENCES

A new test for Lyme disease. *Johns Hopkins
Med Letter* 1994;6(6):3.
Rakel RE, Bope ET (eds): *Conn's Current
Therapy 2005*. Philadelphia, Elsevier, 2005,
pp 154–160.
Steere AC. Proceedings of the First Inter-
national Symposium on Lyme Disease. *Yale
J Biol Med* 1984;57.

AUTHORS: **TERESA BIGGERSTAFF, DDS, MD;
DALE J. MISIEK, DMD**

SYNONYM(S)

Jaw cancer

ICD-9CM/CPT CODE(S)

ICD-9CM
170.0 Malignant tumor maxilla
170.1 Malignant tumor mandible
198.5 Secondary metastasis maxilla/mandible
200.2 Burkitt's lymphoma
203.0 Multiple myeloma
CPT
21034 Excision of malignant tumor of maxilla
21044 Excision of malignant tumor of mandible
21045 Radical resection of malignant tumor of mandible
20220 Biopsy bone
31225 Maxillectomy without orbital enucleation

OVERVIEW

Primary or metastatic malignancies found within or involving the jaws

EPIDEMIOLOGY & DEMOGRAPHICS

OSTEOSARCOMA
- Six to 8% of all osteosarcomas
- Slight male predominance

CHONDROSARCOMA
- Wide range of age at diagnosis
- No sex predilection

EWING'S SARCOMA
- Peak prevalence in second decade
- Slight male predominance

METASTATIC TUMORS
- Peak prevalence in fifth through seventh decades
- No sex predilection

ETIOLOGY & PATHOGENESIS

OSTEOSARCOMA
- Increased prevalence associated with Paget's disease and/or radiation
- Maxilla/mandible equal frequency
- Mandibular tumors more common in posterior bodies and horizontal ramus
- Maxillary tumors more common in alveolus, sinus floor, and palate

CHONDROSARCOMA
- Ten percent of all primary tumors but rare in jaws
- One to 3% of chondrosarcomas found in head and neck
- Most frequent in maxilla, rare in mandible

EWING'S SARCOMA
- One to 2% occurs in jaws

METASTATIC TUMORS
- Primarily noted in breast, lung, thyroid, prostate, and kidney
- Usually occurs by hematogenous route

CLINICAL PRESENTATION / PHYSICAL FINDINGS

OSTEOSARCOMA
- Swelling and pain
- Loosening of teeth
- Paresthesia
- Nasal obstruction

CHONDROSARCOMA
- Painless masseter swelling
- Separation or loosening of teeth
- Nasal obstruction, congestion, epistaxis, photophobia, or visual loss

EWING'S SARCOMA
- Pain, intermittent, ranging from dull to severe
- Fever and leukocytosis
- Paresthesia
- Loosening of teeth

METASTATIC TUMOR
- Variety of symptoms including pain, swelling, loosening of teeth, and/or paresthesia
- Nonhealing extraction site

DIAGNOSIS

DIFFERENTIAL DIAGNOSIS
- Osteomyelitis or osteoradionecrosis
- Infected jaw cyst
- Odontogenic tumor
- Primary bone malignancy
- Primary soft tissue malignancy
- Metastatic malignancy

WORKUP
- Clinical examination
- History of primary malignancy of breast, lung, thyroid, prostate, and kidney
- Biopsy

LABORATORY
- Serum electrophoresis
- Urinalysis for Bence-Jones proteins in multiple myeloma
- Epstein-Barr titer in Burkitt's lymphoma
- Chromosomal analysis in Burkitt's lymphoma
- Histopathologic evaluation

IMAGING
- Plain radiographs
  - Radiopacity, moth-eaten radiolucency, or mixed
  - "Sunray" appearance in osteosarcomas (rare)
  - Widened periodontal ligament space
  - "Onion skin" appearance in Ewing's sarcoma
  - "Punched-out" lesions in multiple myeloma
- CT Scans
  - Shows lesions in better detail
  - Better to determine extent of lesions
- Metastatic workup
  - Thyroid scan
  - Chest radiograph
  - Mammogram
  - Barium enema
  - Abdominal CT scan

MEDICAL MANAGEMENT & TREATMENT

- Osteosarcoma: radical resection
- Chondrosarcoma: radical resection
- Ewing's sarcoma: combination radical resection, radiation, and chemotherapy
- Burkitt's lymphoma: chemotherapy
- Multiple myeloma: chemotherapy
- Metastatic tumor: radical resection with radiation and/or chemotherapy dictated by primary lesion

DISPOSITION/REFERRAL
- Referral for oncologic evaluation

PROGNOSIS

OSTEOSARCOMA
- Usually low-grade with few metastases
- Depends on completeness of tumor removal
- Four-year survival rates approach 80%
- Local, uncontrolled disease is usual cause of death

CHONDROSARCOMA
- Related to size, location, and grade of lesion
- Slow-growing with low metastatic potential
- 5-, 10-, and 15-year survival rates are 67.6%, 53.7%, and 43.9%, respectively

EWING'S SARCOMA
- Forty to 80% 5-year survival
- Frequently metastasizes to lungs, liver, lymph nodes, and other bones

METASTATIC TUMORS
- Poor because by definition jaw metastasis places patient in stage IV disease
- Five-year survival rare; most patients do not survive 1 year

SUGGESTED REFERENCES
Arlen M, et al. Chondrosarcoma of the head and neck. *AMS Surg* 1970;120:456–460.
Gamington G, et al. Osteosarcomas of the jaw. Analysis 56 cases. *Cancer* 1967;20:377 391.
Neville B, Damm D, Allen C, Bouquot J (eds): *Oral & Maxillofacial Pathology*, ed 2. Philadelphia, WB Saunders, 2002, pp 574–584.
Zarbo RJ. Malignancies of the jaws, in Regezi JA, Sciubba J (eds): *Oral Pathology: Clinical-Pathologic Correlations*, ed 4. Philadelphia, WB Saunders, 2003, pp 321–338.

AUTHOR: DALE J. MISIEK, DMD

SYNONYM(S)

Central papillary atrophy of the tongue

ICD-9CM/CPT CODE(S)

ICD-9CM

250.00 Type II non-insulin-dependent, adult onset, or unspecified, not stated as uncontrolled

250.01 Type I insulin-dependent, juvenile- type onset, not stated as uncontrolled

250.02 Type II, non-insulin-dependent, adult onset, or unspecified, uncontrolled

250.03 Type I, insulin-dependent, juvenile-type, uncontrolled

529.2 Median rhomboid glossitis

CPT

41100 Biopsy, tongue, anterior 2/3

99000 Transport specimen to outside laboratory

OVERVIEW

Well-demarcated, ovoid, diamond/rhomboid-shaped, nonulcerated, flat or slightly raised pink area of the central middle third of the dorsum of the tongue

EPIDEMIOLOGY & DEMOGRAPHICS

INCIDENCE/PREVALENCE IN USA: Incidence less than 1%

PREDOMINANT SEX: 3 to 4:1 female to male predominance

ETIOLOGY & PATHOGENESIS

- Evidence is suggestive of a relationship with a localized, chronic *Candida albicans* infection.

- Fungal hyphae seen in 85% of histologic sections associated with a significant decrease in the number and function of specialized macrophages (Langerhans cells in the epithelium of the lesion).
- Particularly common in the diabetic patient.

CLINICAL PRESENTATION / PHYSICAL FINDINGS

- Lesion is generally painless, appears innocuous.
- Burning sensation or pain may be present if a *Candida* infection is diagnosed.
- Loss of papillae with varying degrees of hyperparakeratosis gives area a distinct appearance from the rest of the tongue.

DIAGNOSIS

LABORATORY

- If the patient is diabetic, accumulation of ketones, acetone, β-hydroxybutyrate and acetoacetate, and hyperglycemia; recommend arterial blood gas.
- Depleted bicarbonate levels and decreased pH.
- Acetone and ketones in urine.
- Standing culture for candidiasis (PAS stand).

IMAGING/SPECIAL TESTS

- Loss of histology reveals loss of papilla and hyperparakeratosis. There is elongation, branching, and anastomosis of rete pegs within the spinous layer. Increased vascularity, increased lymphocytic infiltration in connective tissue.

- Degenerative and hyalinization within muscular layer.

MEDICAL MANAGEMENT & TREATMENT

- Treatment is necessary only if the patient is symptomatic.
- Control of systemic disease (diabetes).
- Management of chronic candidiasis and *Candida* infections.
- Modification of drug regimen to control diabetes.
- Oral/topical clotrimazole/ketoconazole, nystatin. Biopsy is only necessary if needed for diagnosis.

PROGNOSIS

- Lesions in some cases will regress spontaneously without treatment.
- Antifungal agents may cause lesions to regress.
- Control of underlying systemic disturbances will occasionally result in resolution of the lesion.

SUGGESTED REFERENCES

Carter LC. MRG: a puzzling entity. *Compend Cont Educ Dent* 1990;11:446–451.

Farman AG, et al. Central papillary atrophy of the tongue. *Oral Surg Oral Med Oral Path* 1977;43:48–58.

Walsh LJ, et al. Quantitative evaluation of Langerhans cells in median rhomboid glossitis. *J Oral Path Med* 1992;21:28–33.

AUTHOR: ROBERT M. LAUGHLIN, DMD

SECTION II

SYNONYM(S)

Malignant melanoma
Melanocarcinoma

ICD-9CM/CPT CODE(S)

ICD-9CM
143.9 Malignant neoplasm, gingiva
145.0 Malignant neoplasm, buccal mucosa
145.2 Malignant neoplasm, hard palate
145.3 Malignant neoplasm, soft palate
145.9 Malignant neoplasm, mouth, unspecified
172.0 Melanoma, lip
172.3 Melanoma, unspecified parts of the face
172.4 Melanoma, neck and scalp
CPT
11100 Biopsy, skin
13131 Mouth, repair, complex
40808 Biopsy, mouth intraoral
41116 Floor of mouth, excision, lesion

OVERVIEW

- Malignancy of melanocytes
- Five major forms:
  - Superficial spreading melanoma (70%)
  - Nodular melanoma (15%)
  - Lentigo maligna melanoma (4–10%)
  - Acral-lentiginous melanoma (2–8%)
  - Mucosal melanoma

EPIDEMIOLOGY & DEMOGRAPHICS

PREDOMINANT AGE: Mucosal melanoma is predominately found in those over age 50 years; cutaneous melanoma is more common in those under age 50 years.
GENETICS: White-complexioned individuals have a higher predisposition to development of melanoma than those with darker complexions.

ETIOLOGY & PATHOGENESIS

- Melanocytes are one type of dendritic cell found in epidermis and in various mucosal epithelia. When malignant transformation of these cells occurs, the tumor is called a melanoma. Melanocytic nevi are also composed of melanocytes and can undergo malignant transformation.
- Increased sun exposure plays a direct role; the history of even a single severe, blistering sunburn may be as significant as chronic exposure.
- Dysplastic nevi, especially in conjunction with familial history of melanoma, display an increased relative risk.
- People having a total body count of more than 20 melanocytic nevi (larger than 2 mm) may begin to show an increased risk; more than 50 total nevi is considered to greatly increase the risk of melanoma.
- Familial history is important.

- Congenital nevi display an increased risk.
- Lentigo maligna lesions should be closely followed due to possible malignant transformation.
- Mucosal lesions do not follow increased predilection of skin melanomas.
- Darker-complexioned individuals may have a slightly increased risk for mucosal, palmar, and plantar lesions.

SYSTEMS AFFECTED

- Skin: all surfaces at risk, with sun-exposed at greater risk than nonsun-exposed.
- Oral mucosa: all mucosal surfaces may be affected. Gingiva and palate are the most common sites.
- Eye: conjunctiva, retina.
- Nasal mucosa.
- Any upper aerodigestive tract mucosa can be involved.

CLINICAL PRESENTATION / PHYSICAL FINDINGS

SYMPTOMS & SIGNS

- Lesions are generally black, blue black, or brown. Can be hypopigmented.
- Generally flat with or without visible spread beneath superficial epithelium. Can be raised.
- Nasal congestion.
- Epistaxis/bleeding mucosa.
  Remember this ABCDE eponym:
A = asymmetry; lesion cannot be divided into mirror images.
B = border; edges display notches or other irregularities.
C = color; there is variation in color within the lesion.
D = diameter; should be able to cover the lesion with the pencil eraser.
E = evolution; if it is changing, it needs to be biopsied.

LABORATORY

No specific laboratory tests are available.

IMAGING/SPECIAL TESTS

- Biopsy.
- Regional node assessment must be performed and recorded prior to biopsy.
- All oral nevi should be excised.
- Periapical radiographs can be of help in confirming the diagnosis of amalgam tattoos if the metallic fragments are radiographically evident.
- Remember that deciduous teeth long since exfoliated may have had amalgam restorations.

DIAGNOSIS

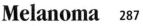

DIFFERENTIAL DIAGNOSIS

- Amalgam tattoo
- Melanocytic nevus
- Peutz-Jeghers syndrome
- Vascular/blood-derived lesion
- Pigmented seborrheic keratosis
- Dysplastic nevus
- Pigmented actinic keratosis

- Lentigo maligna
- Sebaceous carcinoma

MEDICAL MANAGEMENT & TREATMENT

MEDICATIONS

- Chemotherapy is generally aimed at palliation and quality of life. Various regimens have been used.
- Specific active immunotherapy continues to show promise for the future.

SURGERY

- Surgical excision is the therapy of choice with the general consensus being 1-cm margins; 3-cm margins have also been recommended in areas where feasible. In lesions less than 1 mm in thickness, it appears that simply clear margins do not improve prognosis versus larger margins.
- Excisions to limiting anatomic barrier, if applicable.
- Elective node dissections do not aid in survivability, though it may be done when imaging studies display evidence of single chain involvement.
- Mohs surgery not indicated.

RADIATION

Not indicated

PATIENT INSTRUCTIONS

- Visit physician frequently for careful examinations to detect recurrences or new lesions.
- Contact National Cancer Institute for helpful literature: (301) 496-5583.

PROGNOSIS

- Most studies agree that oral lesions have a 10–25% 5-year survival.
- One MD Anderson Cancer Center study showed a 45% survival rate for head and neck mucosal melanomas.
- Overall skin survival at 10 years is 75%, with histologic depth of invasion and histologic type being important prognostic factors.
- Presence of metastatic lesions is a dire predictor, with most patients only surviving 6 months.

SUGGESTED REFERENCES

Breslow A. Thickness and cross-sectional areas and depth of invasion in the prognosis of cutaneous melanoma. *Ann Surg* 1970;1782: 902.

Cochran AJ, et al. Malignant melanoma of the skin, in Haskell CM (ed): *Cancer Treatment*, ed 4. Philadelphia, WB Saunders, 1995, pp 810–824.

Moschella SL, Hurley HJ. *Dermatology*, ed 3. Philadelphia, WB Saunders, 1991, pp 1745–1763.

Neville B, Damm D, Allen C, Bouquot J (eds): *Oral & Maxillofacial Pathology*, ed 2. Philadelphia, WB Saunders, 2002, pp 376–380.

Rakel RE, Bope ET (eds): *Conn's Current Therapy 2005*. Philadelphia, Elsevier, 2005, pp 936–941, 962.

Regezi JA, Sciubba J. *Oral Pathology: Clinical Pathologic Correlations*, ed 4. Philadelphia. WB Saunders, 2003, pp 137–139.

Rhodes AR, Weinstock MA, Fitzpatrick TV, et al. Risk factors for cutaneous melanoma. A practical method of recognizing predisposed individuals. *JAMA* 1987;258: 3146–3154.

AUTHOR: **TERESA BIGGERSTAFF, DDS, MD**

SYNONYM(S)

Mucus extravasation phenomena
Mucus escape reaction
Mucus retention cyst

ICD-9CM/CPT CODE(S)

ICD-9CM
527.6 Mucocele
CPT
40810 Excision lesion of mucosa and submucosal, vestibule of mouth; without repair
40812 with simple repair
41116 Excision, lesion of floor of mouth
42100 Biopsy of palate, uvula
42104 Excision, lesion of palate uvula; without closure
42106 with simple, primary closure

OVERVIEW

A benign, raised lesion consisting of a collection of mucin into the surrounding soft tissues

EPIDEMIOLOGY & DEMOGRAPHICS

Common occurrence most often in first through third decades

ETIOLOGY & PATHOGENESIS

- Mucus extravasation phenomena: trauma to a minor salivary expiatory duct, with collection of mucus in the adjacent connective tissue stroma.
- Retention cyst: excretory duct obstruction of a minor salivary gland resulting in blockage of salivary flow.
- Superficial mucocele: no known etiologic or precipitating factors. Some appear to be related to various foods or beverages.

CLINICAL PRESENTATION / PHYSICAL FINDINGS

- Mucus retention phenomenon
  - Painless, movable swelling with bluish/pink hue
  - Mucus-filled vesicles raised above the adjacent mucosa
  - Ulceration with associated pain and inflammation
- Mucus retention cyst
  - Painless, moveable swelling with color of adjacent mucosa
  - Mucus-filled cystic cavity lined with ductal epithelium
- Superficial mucocele
  - Clear, tense vesicles which may ulcerate leaving a pseudo membrane

DIAGNOSIS

DIFFERENTIAL DIAGNOSIS

- Pleomorphic adenoma
- Monomorphic adenoma
- Mucoepidermoid carcinoma
- Adenocystic carcinoma
- Traumatic fibroma
- Ranula
- Vesiculobullous lesions

WORKUP

- Clinical examination
- Observation if nonpainful

LABORATORY

- Histopathologic evaluation

MEDICAL MANAGEMENT & TREATMENT

ACUTE GENERAL TREATMENT

- Excisional biopsy

CHRONIC TREATMENT

- Observation

PATIENT INSTRUCTIONS

- Will recur even if they spontaneously drain

PROGNOSIS

Complete excision is curative.

SUGGESTED REFERENCES

Bodner L, Tal H. Salivary gland cysts of the oral cavity: clinical observation and surgical management. *Compendium* 1992;12:150–156.

Everson JW. Superficial mucocele: pitfalls in clinical and microscopic diagnosis. *Oral Surg Oral Med Oral Path* 1998;66:318–322.

Jenson JL. Recurrent intraoral vesicles. *JADA* 1990;120:569–570.

Neville B, Damm D, Allen C, Bouquot J (eds): *Oral & Maxillofacial Pathology*, ed 2. Philadelphia, WB Saunders, 2002, pp 389–391.

Praetorius F, Hammarstrom L. A new concept of the pathogenesis of oral mucocysts based on a study of 200 cases. *J Dent Assoc S Afr* 1992;47:226–231.

Regezi JA, Sciubba J (eds): *Oral Pathology: Clinical-Pathologic Correlations,* ed 4. Philadelphia, WB Saunders, 2003, pp 183–184.

Yamasoba T, Tayama N, Syoji M, Fukuta M. Clinicostatistical study of lower lip mucoceles. *Head Neck* 1990;12:316–320.

AUTHOR: **DALE J. MISIEK, DMD**

SECTION II

SYNONYM(S)

Mucoepidermoid tumor

ICD-9CM/CPT CODE(S)

142.0 Malignant neoplasm, parotid
142.1 Malignant neoplasm subman-dibular gland
142.2 Malignant neoplasm, sublingual gland
142.8 Malignant neoplasm of con-tiguous or overlapping sites of salivary glands and ducts whose point of origin cannot be deter-mined
142.9 Malignant neoplasm of major salivary gland not otherwise specified
145.9 Malignant neoplasm of minor salivary glands
145.0 Buccal mucosa
145.2 Hard palate
145.3 Soft palate
145.9 Not otherwise specified
CPT General Exam or Consultation (e.g., 99243 or 99213)

OVERVIEW

One of the most common sali-vary gland malignancies. Ranges in aggressiveness from low- to high-grade.

EPIDEMIOLOGY & DEMOGRAPHICS

PREDOMINANT AGE: Can occur at any age. Most common in the third through fifth decades.

PREDOMINANT SEX: May be a slight female predilection.

ETIOLOGY & PATHOGENESIS

Unknown

CLINICAL PRESENTATION / PHYSICAL FINDINGS

- Palate: asymptomatic swelling for low-grade; ulcerated swelling for high-grade.
- Parotid: asymptomatic swelling.
- High-grade in parotid can cause facial n. palsy.
- In minor salivary glands can be blue-tinged and fluctuant, resembling mucous retention phenomenon.

DIAGNOSIS

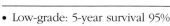

DIFFERENTIAL DIAGNOSIS

- Benign or malignant salivary gland tumors.
- High-grade (which is ulcerative and destructive of bone) includes squamous cell carcinoma.

LABORATORY

- Incisional biopsy of nonparotid lesions

IMAGING

- CT or MRI to evaluate bone involve-ment and margins

MEDICAL MANAGEMENT & TREATMENT

- Parotid: superficial parotidec-tomy for lesion in superficial lobe; complete parotidectomy if in deep lobe.

- Submandibular gland: removal of gland.
- Sublingual gland: removal of gland.
- Minor salivary gland (low-grade): 1-cm margins.
- High grade: resection. If neck nodes involved, neck dissection and radiation.

COMPLICATIONS

- Clinical course correlates with the histopathologic grade.
- Can have a central mucoepidermoid carcinoma; most are low-grade and require resection for treatment.

PROGNOSIS

- Low-grade: 5-year survival 95%
- High-grade: 5-year survival 35%; 10-year survival 25%

DENTAL SIGNIFICANCE

No specific implications.

SUGGESTED READINGS

Marx RE, Stern D (eds): *Oral and Maxillofacial Pathology. A Rationale for Diagnosis and Treatment.* Carol Stream, IL, Quintessence Publishing Company, 2003, pp 543–550.
Neville B, Damm D, Allen C, Bouquot J (eds): *Oral & Maxillofacial Pathology*, ed 2. Philadelphia, WB Saunders, 2002, pp 420–423.

AUTHOR: **MICHAEL J. DALTON, DDS**

SYNONYM(S)

Wermer's syndrome (MEN-1)
Sipple syndrome (MEN-2)

ICD-9CM/CPT CODE(S)

258.0 MEN-1
193 MEN-2
CPT General Exam or Consultation
(e.g., 99243 or 99213)

OVERVIEW

Multiple endocrine neoplasia (MEN) syndromes encompass a group of disorders inherited as autosomal dominant traits. They are characterized by synchronous or, more often, metachronous proliferative lesions involving different endocrine glands and sometimes nonendocrine tissues of nervous system and/or mesenchymal origin. They are subdivided into two main varieties according to the type of affected endocrine glands.

MEN-1 is a combination of tumors of the pituitary parathyroids and pancreatic islets.

MEN-2 is further divided into:

- MEN-2A: medullary thyroid cancer, pheochromocytoma, and hyperparathyroidism
- MEN-2B: medullary thyroid cancer, pheochromocytoma, multiple mucosal neuromas, and familial medullary thyroid cancer (FMTC)

EPIDEMIOLOGY & DEMOGRAPHICS

INCIDENCE/PREVALENCE IN USA:

- MEN-1: incidence is between 0.02 to 0.2/1000 inhabitants in clinical studies; to 0.25% in autopsy series.
- MEN-2: 500 to 1000 affected kindreds reported in the literature.

ETIOLOGY & PATHOGENESIS

MEN syndromes have autosomal dominant transmission.

CLINICAL PRESENTATION / PHYSICAL FINDINGS

MEN-1

- Hyperparathyroidism
- Anterior pituitary
- Endocrine pancreas
- Adrenal cortex
- Thymus
- Cutaneous proliferations (lipomas, collagenomas, café au lait macules, primary malignant melanoma)

MEN-2A

- Medullary thyroid cancer: occurs in 95% of cases
- Pheochromocytoma: occurs in 50% of cases
- Hyperparathyroidism: occurs in 19–35% of cases

MEN-2B

- Medullary thyroid cancer
- Pheochromocytoma
- Multiple mucosal neuromas of the lips, tongue, and buccal mucosa
- Marfanoid appearance: thin, elongated limbs, thin face, but the lips are thick and protuberant due to mucosal neuromas

FMTC

- Families who have autosomal dominant transmission of only medullary carcinoma of the thyroid without the presence of other endocrinopathies

DIAGNOSIS

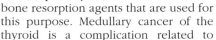

- Basal serum calcitonin levels can usually confirm the etiology of thyroid carcinoma.
- Serum calcitonin after pentagastrin stimulation should be performed in all first-degree relatives.
- Measurements of the RET protooncogene mutations in family members of affected individuals have allowed preclinical diagnosis of this disorder.
- Genetic analysis identifies more than 95% of responsible mutations.
- Serum immunoreactive calcitonin before and after a provocative test with the infusion of calcium or of pentagastrin.
- CT studies of neck and abdomen.

MEDICAL MANAGEMENT & TREATMENT

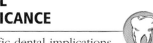

SURGERY

- Medullary thyroid cancer: surgical resection is the only curative treatment or preventive treatment for medullary thyroid cancer in patients with MEN-2.
- Pheochromocytoma: the only potentially curative treatment for patients with MEN-2 with pheochromocytoma is surgical resection.
- Hyperparathyroidism: patients with MEN-2 should have annual screening for hyperparathyroidism by serum calcium and intact parathyroid hormone level measurements. Parathyroidectomy should be considered in all patients with biochemical evidence of hyperparathyroidism. Surgery is the only effective, long-term therapy for primary hyperparathyroidism.

COMPLICATIONS

Hyperparathyroidism: while surgery is the only effective, long-term therapy for primary hyperparathyroidism, pharmacologic therapy is necessary when patients present with hypercalcemic crisis. Etidronate, pamidronate, plicamycin, and calcitonin are bone resorption agents that are used for this purpose. Medullary cancer of the thyroid is a complication related to MEN-2A and MEN-2B.

PROGNOSIS

Guarded if medullary cancer is present.

DENTAL SIGNIFICANCE

No specific dental implications.

DENTAL MANAGEMENT

- Refer to endocrinologist, general surgeon, or geneticist.
- Genetic counselling is very important for the whole family of an affected individual. Clinically important primary hyperparathyroidism presents in at least half of patients by age 20. Penetrance is more than 80% by age 50, although blood and urine tests could detect 90% by this age.

SUGGESTED REFERENCES

Adreoli TE, Bennett JC, Carpenter CCJ, Plum F. The thyroid gland, in *Cecil Essentials of Medicine,* ed 4. Philadelphia, WB Saunders, 1997, pp 495–496.

Bordi C. Multiple endocrine neoplasia (MEN)-associated tumours. *Digestive Liver Dis* 2004;36(Suppl 1):S31–S34.

Calender A, et al. New insights in genetic testing of multiple endocrine neoplasia type 1 (MEN1). *Pathologica* 2003;95:268–274.

Gertner ME, et al. Multiple endocrine neoplasia type 2. *Curr Treatment Options Oncol* 2004;5:315–325.

AUTHOR: **ANDREW M. DEWITT, DDS**

SYNONYM(S)

None

ICD-9CM/CPT CODE(S)

205.1 Chronic myelogenous leukemia
238.4 Polycythemia vera
238.7 Essential thrombocytosis, chronic lympha proliferative disease, chronic myeloproliferative disease, idiopathic thrombocythemia, mega karyocytic myelosclerosis, myelodysplastic syndrome, myelosclerosis with myeloic/metaplasia
289.89 Agnogenic myeloid metaplasia/myelofibrosis
CPT General Exam or Consultation (e.g., 99243 or 99213)

OVERVIEW

- Neoplastic diseases of the multipotent hematopoietic stem cell.
- The four major diseases are chronic myelogenous leukemia (CML), polycythemia vera (PV), agnogenic myeloid metaplasia with myelofibrosis (AMM/MF), and essential thrombocytosis (ET).
- These diseases arise as clone expansions of single, transformed stem cells.
- Nearly all the myeloid cells are derived from the neoplastic clone at the time of diagnosis.

CML

- Increased production of neutrophils and marked splenomegaly.
- Divided into chronic and blastic or Q-phase. The chronic phase is typified by hyperplasia of mature marrow elements.
- The blastic phase evolves into proliferation of immature marrow elements (i.e., blasts and promyelocytes).
- Blast crisis can develop into acute myelogenous leukemia.

PV

- Increased production of all myeloid cells that dominated by increased RBCs with splenomegaly.

AMM/MF

- Neoplastic stem cells proliferate and lodge in multiple sites outside the bone marrow.
- Splenomegaly and fibrosis at the marrow spaces occur.

ET

- Markedly elevated platelet count in the absence of a recognizable stimulus.

EPIDEMIOLOGY & DEMOGRAPHICS

PREDOMINANT SEX: Incidences are equal in males and females.
GENETICS: Possible familial connection.

ETIOLOGY & PATHOGENESIS

- Etiology is unknown for general population, although familial cases have been identified.
- Increased incidence of CML following atomic radiation and radiation therapy for cervical cancer and ankylosing spondylosis.

SYSTEMS AFFECTED

- Hematopoietic: proliferation of myeloid clone
- Lymphatic: lymphadenopathy
- Renal: urate stones secondary to hyperuricemia due to increased cellular turnover; uric acid nephropathy

CLINICAL PRESENTATION / PHYSICAL FINDINGS

SIGNS & SYMPTOMS

- General: most patients are asymptomatic at the time of diagnosis or have a vague complaint of malaise.
- CML: symptomatic splenomegaly, anemia, weight loss, fever, and arthralgias may be severe.
- PV: thrombotic or hemorrhagic event, arterial or venous insufficiency, headache, tinnitus, syncope, vertigo, scatomas secondary to decreased cerebral perfusion; splenomegaly develops late.
- AMM/MF: symptomatic splenomegaly followed by hepatomegaly; petechia and bleeding in 10–20% of cases; occasional ascites, jaundice, and lymphadenopathy.
- ET: spontaneous bleeding and easy bruising; venous or arterial thrombosis, transient ischemic attacks or strokes may occur.

DIAGNOSIS

DIFFERENTIAL DIAGNOSIS

- CML: leukemoid reaction secondary to infections, neoplasm, or stress; blastic phase can resemble acute myelogenous leukemia.
- Paroxysmal nocturnal hemoglobinuria.
- AMM/MF: difficult to differentiate between other stages of CML, PV, and ET, metastatic carcinoma, leukemia or lymphoma, tuberculosis, Paget's disease, metabolic toxins exposure (benzene), Gaucher's disease, and toxic exposure to radiographs.
- PV: secondary polycythemia, chronic cardiac or pulmonary disease, hypernephroma or other renal disease (increased erythropoietin production), decreased plasma volume (dehydration), and hemoglobinopathy.
- ET: secondary thrombocytosis.

LABORATORY

- General:
  - Basophilia
  - Increased serum vitamin B_{12} and vitamin B_{12} binding capacity
  - Hyperuricemia

- CML: marked granulocytosis, low or absent leukocyte alkaline phosphatase, near-normal platelet morphology.
- PV: marked hemoglobin elevation, normochromic and normocytic RBC, leukocytosis in more than 60%, normal ESR, thrombocytosis in more than 50%, and increased leukocyte alkaline phosphatase.
- AMM/MF: anemia, leukocytosis in 50%, leukopenia in 20%, thrombocytosis to thrombocytopenia as disease progresses, abnormal liver function test (increased bilirubin and alkaline phosphatase).
- ET: thrombocytosis (which is polymorphic) abnormality in platelet aggregation.

IMAGING/SPECIAL TESTS

- Skeletal radiograph: identifies marrow sclerosis and increased bone density in axial skeleton and proximal long bones.
- Bone marrow biopsy: essential to the diagnosis of AMM/MF.
- Philadelphia chromosome (Ph1): present in 95% of CML; red cell mass determination with 51 Cr labeled autologous blood for PV.

MEDICAL MANAGEMENT & TREATMENT

GENERAL

- Measures to maintain hydration, relieve arthralgias, prevent thrombotic episodes, and prevent infections.
- With massive splenomegaly, splenectomy will not prolong survival but can provide some symptomatic relief.

MEDICATIONS

- Chronic phase of CML treated with hydroxyurea (Hydrea) or busulfan (Myleran) (alkylating agent) does not alter inexorable progression to acute phase. Intense therapy only provides transient remission with no prolongation of survival.
- Bone marrow transplant (BMT): syngenic or allogenic transplant provides increased disease-free interval in 40–50% of patients; long-term survival in the patients younger than 20 years of age is 70%; older patients, 40%. Hydroxyurea is a first-line drug, followed by other alkylating agents (busulfan, cyclophosphamide, and melphalan).
- Interferon-α provides better long-term results.
- Allopurinol for hyperuricemia and after chemotherapy.
- Polycythemia vera; phlebotomy alone has extended survival 10 to 12 years, reduced hematocrit to approximately 45%, myelosuppressive therapy with radioactive 32P or chemotherapy with alkylating agents.

- Can also use hydroxyurea and allopurinol and give cyproheptadine for pruritus.
- Agnogenic myeloid metaplasia with myelofibrosis: there is no definitive therapy, transfusions or androgens with or without corticosteroids to improve anemia; myelosuppressive therapy with alkylating agents is rarely indicated except for splenomegaly or thrombocytosis; splenectomy only for hemolysis, severe thrombocytopenia, and intractable symptoms of splenomegaly; androgens with or without glucocorticoids may be tried.
- Essential thrombocytosis: indications for treatment are unsettled; with severe bleeding or thrombotic episodes, hydroxyurea is indicated. Alkylating agents or radioactive phosphorus can be used if hydroxyurea fails; aspirin and dipyridamole may prevent symptoms; platelet phoresis can manage acute crisis; use nonsteroidal antiinflammatory drugs to prevent vasoocclusive syndrome secondary to thrombocytosis.

COMPLICATIONS

- Infections in neutropenic patients are common, which require hospitalization for intravenous antibiotics.
- Hematologic/infectious complications from removal of the spleen can occur.

PROGNOSIS

CML
- Dependent upon progression to blastic phase.
- Ten percent progress within the first 2 years after diagnosis, with 20% per year thereafter.
- BMT provides patients younger than 20 years of age with 70% long-term survival and older patients with 40% long-term survival.
- Median survival is 5 years after diagnosis, decreasing to 1½ years after blastic stage and to 3 months after blast crisis, 85% die in blast crisis.

PV
- Median survival without treatment is only 1 year.
- Phlebotomy alone group had increased risk of death from hemorrhage or thrombosis in first 4 years.
- Similar survival rates for all treatment modalities until the seventh year.
- Alkylating agents predispose to acute leukemia later in course.
- Statistically significant incidence of second hematologic malignancy (lymphoma or leukemia.)
- Occasional asymptomatic survivor for more than 20 years.

AMM/MF
- Generally a prolonged course with median survival of 5 years from diagnosis; 25% live up to 15 years.

- Transformation to acute leukemia occurs in 5–10% of cases.
- Major causes of death include congestive heart failure, renal failure, hemorrhage, portal hypertension, and infection.

ET
- Median survival is not well-defined.
- Less than 10% transformation to acute leukemic phase.

DENTAL SIGNIFICANCE

Unusual bleeding after minor dental procedure may be a sign of ET. Patients who are neutropenic are more at risk for infections such as herpes simplex. Consultation with a hematologic oncologist is recommended prior to treatment.

SUGGESTED REFERENCES

Dolin R. Myeloproliferative disorders, in Dambrow M (ed): *Griffith's 5-Minute Clinical Consult*, Baltimore, Lippincott Williams & Wilkins, 1995, pp 696-697.

Lichtman MA. Classification and clinical manifestations of the hematopoietic stem cell disorders, in Beutler E, et al. (eds): *Williams Hematology*, ed 5, New York, McGraw-Hill, 1995, pp 229-238.

AUTHOR: **TERESA BIGGERSTAFF, DDS, MD**

SECTION II

SYNONYM(S)

Salivary gland tumor
Squamous cell carcinoma of the tongue
Squamous cell carcinoma of the floor of
  mouth
Hyperthyroidism
Tuberculosis
Parotid swellings
Brachial cleft cyst
Thyroglossal cyst
Cat scratch disease
Mononucleosis
Cystic hygroma
Ranula
Carotid body tumor

ICD-9CM/CPT CODE(S)

ICD-9CM

017.2	Tuberculosis cervical gland
196.0	Metastatic cervical node
200.1	Hodgkin granuloma
202.1	Lymphomas depending on classification
202.8	Lymphoma (malignant)
204.9	Thyromegaly
245.9	Thyroiditis
527.2	Submandibular sialadenitis
528.4	Oral dermoid cyst
744.42	Branchial cyst
759.2	Thyroglossal cyst

CPT

10021	Fine needle aspiration, thyroid, lymph node, or salivary gland
38500	Biopsy of lymph nodes
38550	Excision of cystic hygroma
38700	Suprahyoid neck dissection
38720	Radical neck dissection
38724	Modified radical neck dissection
42440	Submandibular gland excision
42810	Excision, branchial cyst
60200	Excision, thyroid cyst or tumor
60280	Excision, thyroglossal cyst

OVERVIEW

Neck masses can be divided into four anatomic sites:
- Masses of the midline
- Masses of the anterior triangle
- Masses of the posterior triangle
- Masses of the submandibular triangle

See entries on specific neck masses in Sections I and II for more information.

EPIDEMIOLOGY & DEMOGRAPHICS

See entries on specific neck masses in Sections I and II for specific information.

ETIOLOGY & PATHOGENESIS

MIDLINE
- Developmental dermoid and thyroglossal cyst
- Thyroid swellings, which can be cystic, neoplastic, autoimmune, or goiter
- Submental nodes, both inflammatory and neoplastic

SUBMANDIBULAR
- Submandibular gland may become enlarged secondary to infection, obstruction, and/or neoplasm (rare).
- Submandibular nodes may be inflammatory, neoplastic, or cystic hygroma (hamartoma).

ANTERIOR TRIANGLE
- Developmental brachial cyst
- Inflammatory lymph nodes and neoplastic lymph nodes
- Parotid tail masses of neoplastic and/or cystic origin
- Carotid body tumor

POSTERIOR TRIANGLE
- Reactive lymph nodes, inflammatory lymph nodes, and neoplastic lymph nodes

CLINICAL PRESENTATION / PHYSICAL FINDINGS

PHYSICAL DIAGNOSIS
- Painless: neoplastic or cystic
- Painful: infective

MIDLINE MASSES
- Dermoid cyst: doughy to palpation; floor of mouth elevation.
- Thyroglossal cyst: cystic with movement on swallowing or protrusion of tongue.
- Thyroid swelling: unilateral and/or bilateral with involvement of the entire thyroid; may be indurated or soft, moves on swallowing.

SUBMANDIBULAR TRIANGLE MASSES
- Submandibular gland: firm, bimanually palpable
- Palpable stone in submandibular ducts: lack of salivary flow, inability to milk saliva from Wharton duct or purulent discharge on manual manipulation
- Submandibular node: unilateral palpation

ANTERIOR TRIANGLE MASSES
- Brachial cleft cyst: round and partially anterior to sternomastoid
- Sternomastoid cyst: painful swelling following injury from cat or other domestic animal; cat scratch disease
- Carotid body tumor: firm, in line with carotid; has no inferior-superior movement but has anterior-posterior or medial-lateral movement

POSTERIOR TRIANGLE MASSES
- Usually node masses; matted, shoddy nodes may indicate tuberculosis.

LYMPH NODES
- Tender, shoddy nodes, usually inflammatory, areas of drainage for odontogenic infections, and tonsillitis need to be examined. Generally, bilateral tender nodes indicate tonsillitis or glandular fever.
- Examine junction of hard and soft palate for ecchymosis.
- Nontender nodes may indicate autoimmune disease.

- Firm, rubbery nodes with no primary site noted in the young or old may be due to a lymphoma.
- Firm nodes on palpation in older populations frequently are neoplastic.
- For nodes involved in the upper neck, one needs to examine the mouth, pharynx, nasopharynx, and larynx for possible primary site.
- For firm nodes in the supraclavicular region, one should suspect lung or stomach cancer.

DIAGNOSIS

LABORATORY
- Complete blood chemistry, Monospot, HIV testing, and viral titers may be used for suspected infective etiology for lymphadenopathy.
- If lupus or other rheumatologic causes are suspected, use antibody titer screening.
- Thyroid function test with midline masses.

IMAGING/SPECIAL TESTS
- CT scans or MRI for lymphoma, metastatic nodes, thyroid masses, thyroglossal cyst, or carotid body tumors
- Ultrasounds for cystic and cystic lesions and thyroid masses
- Thyroid nuclear scans for solitary nodules
- Carotid angiogram for possible carotid body tumor
- Sialogram and/or CT with and without contrast for submandibular gland involvement
- Fine-needle aspiration biopsy
- Panendoscopy to rule out head and neck as a primary site before biopsy when enlarged nodes are present
- Node biopsy for culture and histologic evaluation

MEDICAL MANAGEMENT & TREATMENT

GENERAL
- Treatment will be dictated by diagnosis.
- Developmental lesions require surgical excision such as thyroid gland cyst, dermoid cyst, and brachial cleft cyst.
- Lymphadenopathy of infective nature is treated with antibiotics as indicated for bacterial infections.
- Thyroid diseases may be treated surgically and/or medically depending on the nature.
- Autoimmune disease requires medical therapy.
- Lymphomas are treated with chemotherapy and/or radiation.
- Metastatic nodes can be treated with surgery and/or radiation depending on the primary site.

COMPLICATIONS

Complications vary depending on condition. See entries on specific neck masses in Sections I and II for more information.

PROGNOSIS

- Developmental lesions are curable with surgery.
- Bacterial infections and/or tuberculosis treated with specific antibiotics are usually curative.

- Neoplastic disease prognosis depends on staging. The presence of a metastatic node is an ominous prognostic sign for head and neck cancer, which reduces expected survival by approximately 50%.

DENTAL MANAGEMENT

See entries on specific neck masses for information on specific dental significance and dental management.

SUGGESTED REFERENCES

Bland KI. Neck masses, in Polk HC, et al. (eds): *Basic Surgery*, ed 4. St Louis, Quality Medical Publishing, 1993, pp 212–188.

Neville B, Damm D, Allen C, Bouquot J (eds): *Oral & Maxillofacial Pathology*, ed 2. Philadelphia, WB Saunders, 2002.

Rakel RE, et al. (eds): *Conn's Current Therapy 2005*. Philadelphia, Elsevier, 2005.

AUTHOR: **ROBERT M. LAUGHLIN, DMD**

SECTION II

SYNONYM(S)

Stomatitis nicotina
Pipe smoker's palate
Nicotinic stomatitis
Nicotine palatinus

ICD-9CM/CPT CODE(S)

ICD-9CM
528.7 Leukokeratosis nicotina palati
CPT
42100 Biopsy of palate, uvula

OVERVIEW

Heat-induced type of mucosal keratosis secondary to tobacco smoke; usually associated with pipe smoking. In South American and Southeast Asian cultures, reverse smoking (lit and held in mouth) produces a pronounced palatal keratosis or reverse smoker's palate.

EPIDEMIOLOGY & DEMOGRAPHICS

PREDOMINANT SEX: Most commonly found in men
PREDOMINANT AGE: Greater than 45 years of age

ETIOLOGY & PATHOGENESIS

- Keratotic changes develop in response to heat from the tobacco smoke rather than the chemicals.
- Pipe smoking generates a greater amount of heat on the palate than other forms of smoking, with the exception of reverse smoking.
- Similar changes have been produced by long-term use of extremely hot beverages such as coffee and hot teas.
- The white keratotic changes do not appear to have a premalignant nature.
- Reverse smoker's palate has been demonstrated to have a significant potential to develop dysplasia or carcinoma.

CLINICAL PRESENTATION / PHYSICAL FINDINGS

- Typically asymptomatic.
- With long-term exposure to heat, the palatal mucosa becomes diffusely gray and/or white.

- Numerous elevated plaques or papules are noted with red, punctate centers.
- Such papules represent inflamed minor salivary glands and their ductal apparatus.
- The palatal keratin may become so thickened that a fissured or cobblestone appearance is imparted on the palate.
- The whiteness may extend and involve the marginal gingiva and interdental papilla.
- Leukoplakia of the buccal mucosa is occasionally seen.
- Heavy brown or black tobacco stains may also be present on teeth.

DIAGNOSIS

- Histologic features.
- Hyperkeratosis and acanthosis of the palatal epithelium and mild, patchy, chronic inflammation of the subepithelial connective tissue and mucosal glands.
- Squamous metaplasia of the excretory ducts.
- Inflammatory exudate noted within the ductal lamina.
- With papular elevation, hyperplastic ductal epithelium is seen near the orifice.
- The degree of epithelial hyperkeratosis and hyperplasia correlates positively with the duration and level of heat exposure.
- Epithelial dysplasia is rarely seen.

MEDICAL MANAGEMENT & TREATMENT

See Complications and Dental Management following.

COMPLICATIONS

Any white lesion of the palatal mucosa that persists after 1 month of smoking cessation should be considered a true leukoplakia and managed accordingly.

PROGNOSIS

- No evidence to support pre-malignant potential of nicotine stomatitis.
- Nicotine stomatitis is completely reversible. Palate returns to normal within 1 to 2 weeks of smoking cessation.

DENTAL SIGNIFICANCE

Lesion only occurs in persons with significant tobacco usage; therefore, the entire oral mucosa should be examined thoroughly on a regular basis for erythroplakia and/or leukoplakia-like lesions occurring elsewhere in the oral cavity.

DENTAL MANAGEMENT

Encourage smoking cessation and treat leukoplakias or other lesions as necessary (see Complications preceding).

SUGGESTED REFERENCES

Neville B, Damm D, Allen C, Bouquot J (eds): Oral & Maxillofacial Pathology, ed 2. Philadelphia, WB Saunders, 2002, pp 350–351.
Regezi JA, Sciubba J. Oral Pathology: Clinical-Pathologic Correlations, ed 4. Philadelphia, WB Saunders, 2003.

AUTHOR: **ROBERT M. LAUGHLIN, DMD**

SYNONYM(S)

None

ICD-9CM/CPT CODE(S)

213.0 Benign neoplasm of maxilla
213.1 Benign neoplasm of mandible
CPT   General Exam or Consultation
      (e.g., 99243 or 99213)

OVERVIEW

The odontogenic myxoma is a relatively uncommon, benign neoplasm apparently arising from the mesenchymal portion of the tooth-forming unit, the dental papillae. Odontogenic myxomas have been identified most often in the posterior tooth-bearing areas of both upper and lower jaws and, more often, in the mandible vs the maxilla.

EPIDEMIOLOGY & DEMOGRAPHICS

PREDOMINANT AGE: Most tumors are identified during the second or third decade of life.
PREDOMINANT SEX: There has been no identified gender predilection.

ETIOLOGY & PATHOGENESIS

There are no known genetic or environmental factors that increase the likelihood of this benign neoplasm.

CLINICAL PRESENTATION / PHYSICAL FINDINGS

- As with other odontogenic neoplasms, clinical findings usually consist of a smooth, bony, hard expansion of the buccal aspect of the alveolus. In some instances, odontogenic myxomas have been identified as forming outside the body of the mandible, in which case they would present as a smooth-surfaced, soft tissue enlargement.
- Radiographically, an odontogenic myxoma will show a unilocular or multilocular radiolucency. Most lesions show a well-demarcated, corticated border.

DIAGNOSIS

Odontogenic myxomas are characterized by a relatively acellular, acid mucopolysaccharide, pale basophilic mesenchymal matrix with prominent, thin-walled vascular channels. The cells are well-demarcated and show a spindle or stellate morphology. Nuclei are small and uniform in size. Mitosis is very rare. Occasional strands and cords of odontogenic epithelium may be noted in many but not all neoplasms. Occasionally macrophages are found in the tumors. The ultrastructural features suggest that many lesional cells are very similar to myofibroblasts (Fig. II-9).

MEDICAL MANAGEMENT & TREATMENT

Due to the loose, gelatinous nature of the tumor, surgical enucleation can be difficult. Some surgeons recommend enucleation followed by chemical cauterization as the therapeutic management of choice. Larger tumors have been managed via resection.

COMPLICATIONS

Complications are related primarily to the location and size of the neoplasm and the type of surgery necessary.

PROGNOSIS

Recurrence rates can vary significantly from case to case and often show a direct correlation with the size of the lesion at initial diagnosis.

DENTAL SIGNIFICANCE

Loss of dentition during treatment for odontogenic myxoma will increase the necessity of consultation prior to the planned surgical procedure.

DENTAL MANAGEMENT

Postsurgical management may include a need for fixed or removable prosthodontics to replace missing teeth.

SUGGESTED REFERENCES

Barker BF. Odontogenic myxoma. *Semin Diagn Pathol* 1999;16:297–301.

Chiodo AA, Strumas N, Gilbert RW, et al. Management of odontogenic myxoma of the maxilla. *Otolaryngol Head Neck Surg* 1997;117:S73–S76.

Kaffe I, Naor H, Buchner A. Clinical and radiological features of odontogenic myxoma of the jaw. *Dentomaxillofac Radiol* 1997;26:299–303.

Lo Muzio L, Nocini PF, Favia G, et al. Odontogenic myxoma of the jaws: a clinical, radiologic, immunohistochemical and ultrastructural study. *Oral Surg Oral Med Oral Pathol Oral Radiol Endod* 1996;82: 426–433.

AUTHOR: **STEVEN D. VINCENT, DDS, MS**

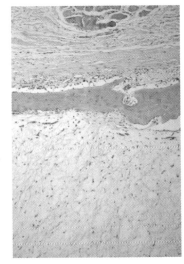

FIGURE II-9 Odontogenic myxoma. Incisional biopsy of an odontogenic myxoma shows foci of skeletal muscle and fibrous connective tissue (*top*) overlying an expanded buccal cortical plate of lamellar bone. The trabecular bone has been replaced (*bottom*) with loose, myxomatous connective tissue with spindle- and stellate-shaped cells and thin-walled vascular channels (hematoxylin and eosin stain; original magnification 40×).

SYNONYM(S)
None

ICD-9CM/CPT CODE(S)
213.0 Benign neoplasm of maxilla
213.1 Benign neoplasm of mandible
CPT General Exam or Consultation
(e.g., 99243 or 99213)

OVERVIEW

Odontomas are the most commonly diagnosed odontogenic tumors. They are considered by many to be a hamartoma rather than a true neoplasm. Odontomas are subdivided into two subtypes: complex and compound odontomas. Complex odontomas, when fully developed, consist almost entirely of sheets of enamel, dentin, and cementum arranged in a haphazard manner. Compound odontomas consist of enamel matrix, dentin, and cementum with the overall appearance suggestive of multiple small, malformed teeth.

Complex and compound odontomas occur with equal frequency and some lesions show features of both subtypes. They may cause morphologic problems with developing teeth and may delay eruption (Figures II-10 and II-11).

EPIDEMIOLOGY & DEMOGRAPHICS

PREDOMINANT AGE: Most odontomas are initially diagnosed within the first two decades of life.
GENETICS: Unknown.

ETIOLOGY & PATHOGENESIS

There are no known genetic or environmental factors that increase the likelihood of this benign neoplasm or hamartoma. Odontomas occur somewhat more frequently in the maxilla compared to the mandible. The compound variant is found more often in the anterior maxilla with the complex variant occurring more often in the posterior maxilla.

CLINICAL PRESENTATION / PHYSICAL FINDINGS

- Complex and compound odontomas are always asymptomatic unless secondarily inflamed by trauma or continuity with the surface.
- They range in size from less than 1 cm to more than 6 cm in diameter.
- Both show a well-demarcated radiolucency with a uniform, corticated border delineating the lesion from surrounding bone.
- Centrally, the lesion will show increasing evidence of homogenous radiopaque material as mineralization of the tooth matrix material progresses.
- In compound odontomas, the radiopaque material will eventually appear multilobular, coinciding with the formation of multiple, poorly formed, tooth-like structures.

DIAGNOSIS

Complex odontomas, when mature, consist almost entirely of a conglomeration of dentin, cementum, and enamel. Compound odontomas consist of the same three mineralized products but are arranged so as to suggest the formation of teeth. During the demineralization process necessary for routine microscopic sectioning, the enamel portion of complex and compound odontomas will be reduced to a retracted and fragmented, homogenous, basophilic material. This is because enamel is roughly 95% mineralized in its natural state.

MEDICAL MANAGEMENT & TREATMENT

Complex and compound odontomas are treated by removal.

COMPLICATIONS

Complications are related primarily to the location and size of the neoplasm/hamartoma and the type of surgery necessary.

PROGNOSIS

Recurrence is very rare.

DENTAL SIGNIFICANCE

Loss of dentition during treatment for odontomas will increase the necessity of consultation prior to the planned surgical procedure.

DENTAL MANAGEMENT

Postsurgical management may include a need for fixed or removable prosthodontics to replace missing teeth.

SUGGESTED REFERENCES

Budnick SD. Compound and complex odontomas. *Oral Surg Oral Med Oral Pathol* 1976;42:501–506.

Hirshberg A, Kaplan I, Buchner A. Calcifying odontogenic cyst associated with odontoma: a possible separate entity (odontocalcifying odontogenic cyst). *J Oral Maxillofac Surg* 1994;52(6):555–558.

Mosqueda-Taylor A, Ledesma-Montes C, Caballero-Sandoval S, Portilla-Robertson J, Ruiz-Godoy Rivera LM, Meneses-Garcia A. Odontogenic tumors in Mexico: a collaborative retrospective study of 349 cases. *Oral Surg Oral Med Oral Pathol Oral Radiol Endod* 1997;84:672–675.

Philipsen HP, Reichart PA, Praetorius F. Mixed odontognic tumours and ondontomas. Considerations on interrelationship. Review of the literature and presentation of 134 new cases of odontomas. *Oral Oncol* 1997;33:86–99.

Sapp JP, Gardner DG. An ultrastructural study of the calcifications in calcifying odontogenic cysts and odontomas. *Oral Surg Oral Med Oral Pathol* 1977;44:754–766.

AUTHOR: **STEVEN D. VINCENT, DDS, MS**

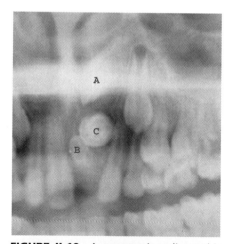

FIGURE II-10 A panoramic radiographic view of the anterior maxilla in a 12-year-old boy showing (*A*) an impacted left central incisor, (*B*) a mesiodens, and (*C*) a 1.5 cm × 1.5 cm homogenous radiopacity found at the time of surgical removal to be a complex odontoma.

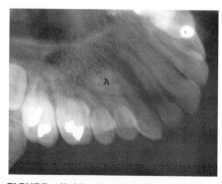

FIGURE II-11 An anterior maxillary occlusal radiograph showing a multilobular radiopacity (*A*) adjacent to the roots of the premolars, characteristic of a compound odontoma.

SYNONYM(S)

Ossifying fibromas
Cementifying fibromas

ICD-9CM/CPT CODE(S)

213.0 Benign neoplasm of maxilla
213.1 Benign neoplasm of mandible
CPT General Exam or Consultation
(e.g., 99243 or 99213)

OVERVIEW

A relatively rare, true mesenchymal neoplasm of odontogenic origin. It is generally agreed that ossifying fibromas, cementifying fibromas, and ossifying/cementifying fibromas of the jaws represent variants of the same neoplasm.

EPIDEMIOLOGY & DEMOGRAPHICS

INCIDENCE/PREVALENCE IN USA: Fibromas are prevalent in any tooth-bearing site, with the most common location being the mandibular molar and premolar region.
PREDOMINANT AGE: Most tumors are identified during the third and fourth decades of life.
PREDOMINANT SEX: Definite female predilection

ETIOLOGY & PATHOGENESIS

No known genetic or environmental factors that increase the likelihood of this benign neoplasm.

CLINICAL PRESENTATION / PHYSICAL FINDINGS

CLINICAL FINDINGS: The neoplasms are usually asymptomatic unless secondarily inflamed. Small tumors are usually noted only on radiographs made for other reasons. Larger lesions may cause noticeable enlargements and, in extreme cases, facial asymmetry.
RADIOGRAPHIC FINDINGS: As with other benign neoplasms of the jaws, ossifying/cementifying fibromas will show a unilocular or multilocular radiolucency or combination radiolucency/radiopacity depending on the degree of mineralization within the tumor. Lesions show a well-demarcated, corticated border.

DIAGNOSIS

The neoplasm consists of relatively cellular fibrous connective tissue with plump, spindle-shaped fibroblasts and few vascular channels. There will be varying amounts of bony trabeculae and cementum-like spherules. While it is generally agreed that the progenitor cells for these mineralized foci are the same and are of odontogenic origin in the jaws, microscopically identical cementum-like material has been reported in tumors of the orbital, frontal, sphenoid, and ethmoid bones.

MEDICAL MANAGEMENT & TREATMENT

These neoplasms are very slow-growing and therefore well circumscribed. They are characteristically enucleated from their bony crypts with ease. This ease of enucleation is a feature that can be used to distinguish cementifying/ossifying fibromas, which are true neoplasms, from other fibroosseous lesions with identical microscopic features such as periapical cemental dysplasia and focal or florid cementoosseous dysplasia. These dysplasias of bone will not be well-demarcated from the surrounding normal bone and will therefore be difficult to enucleate.

COMPLICATIONS

Complications are related primarily to the location and size of the neoplasm and the type of surgery necessary.

PROGNOSIS

Recurrence is very rare and there is no evidence of malignant transformation.

DENTAL SIGNIFICANCE

Loss of dentition during treatment for ossifying/cementifying fibromas will increase the necessity of consultation prior to the planned surgical procedure.

SECTION II

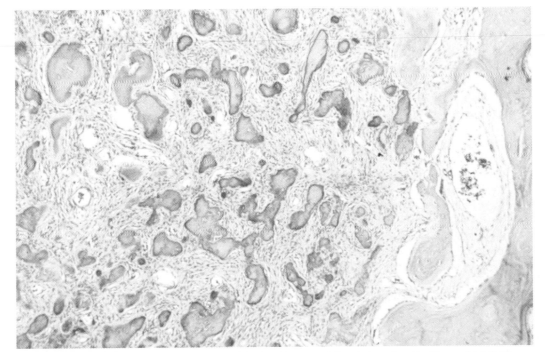

FIGURE II-12 Ossifying/cementifying fibroma of the mandible showing a peripheral rim of cortical bone *(right)*. The neoplasm consists of cellular fibrous connective tissue with irregular-shaped trabeculae of vital bone and islands of relatively acellular, cementum-like mineralized material (hematoxylin and eosin staining; original magnification 40×).

DENTAL MANAGEMENT

Postsurgical management may include a need for fixed or removable prosthodontics to replace missing teeth.

SUGGESTED REFERENCES

Macdonald-Jankowski DS. Cemento-ossifying fibromas in the jaws of Hong Kong Chinese. *Dentomaxillofacial Radiol* 1998; 27:298–304.

Su L, Weathers DR, Waldron CA. Distinguishing features of focal cemento-osseous dysplasias and cemento-ossifying fibromas I. A pathologic spectrum of 316 cases. *Oral Surg Oral Med Oral Pathol Oral Radiol Endod* 1997;84:301–309.

Waldron CA, Giansanti JS. Benign fibro-osseous lesions of the jaws II. Benign fibro-osseous lesions of periodontal ligament origin. *Oral Surg Oral Med Oral Pathol* 1973;35:340–350.

AUTHOR: **STEVEN D. VINCENT, DDS, MS**

SYNONYM(S)

Osteoid osteoma (closely related to, but not synonymous with)

Cementoblastoma (related entity)

ICD-9CM/CPT CODE(S)

213.0 Bones of skull and face
213.1 Lower jaw bone
CPT General Exam or Consultation (e.g., 99243 or 99213)

OVERVIEW

- Osteoblastoma is a benign neoplasm of bone arising from osteoblasts.
- Osteoblastoma and osteoid osteoma are similar bony tumors. The two lesions are distinguished primarily on the basis of size and the characteristics of the pain symptoms.
- Osteoid osteoma is less than 2 cm in diameter, and osteoblastoma is typically larger than 2 cm in diameter.

EPIDEMIOLOGY & DEMOGRAPHICS

INCIDENCE/PREVALENCE IN USA:
Osteoblastomas are uncommon benign tumors of bone, representing 1% of bone tumors.

PREDOMINANT AGE: The mean age at diagnosis is approximately 20 years and 85% of cases occur under age 30.

PREDOMINANT SEX: Males are affected two to three times more often than females.

ETIOLOGY & PATHOGENESIS

- Osteoblastoma is a true, benign neoplasm of osteoblasts.
- The histopathologic features are very similar, if not identical, to cementoblastoma; however, cementoblastoma is distinguished by its fusion to a tooth.

CLINICAL PRESENTATION / PHYSICAL FINDINGS

- The most common locations for osteoblastoma are vertebrae, sacrum, calvaria, long bones, and small bones of the hands and feet.
- Jaw lesions are more common in the mandible (especially posterior mandible) than in the maxilla.

- A typical osteoblastoma is 2 to 4 cm in diameter but may be as large as 10 cm.
- Most common presenting clinical signs and symptoms are bony expansion and swelling, usually painful.
- Spontaneous pain and/or tenderness are often present with osteoblastoma. Unlike osteoid osteoma, the pain is not well controlled with salicylates.
- Aggressive osteoblastoma is a variant that occurs in older patients (usually over age 30) and is usually painful.
- Compared to conventional osteoblastoma, these lesions tend to be larger and more locally aggressive.
- Lesions have been described in the mandible.

DIAGNOSIS

- Radiographic features of osteoblastoma include a radiolucent lesion with patchy radiopaque areas within it. The borders vary from well-defined to poorly-defined and a corticated border is not evident.
- Diagnosis is by biopsy and histopathologic examination that reveals mineralized material with a prominent rim of plump osteoblasts and numerous osteoclasts.
- Aggressive osteoblastoma may be more cellular, with osteoblasts that are larger and have mitotic activity; the mineralized material is less likely to be well-formed trabeculae.

MEDICAL MANAGEMENT & TREATMENT

Usual treatment is local surgical excision or curettage.

COMPLICATIONS

- Aggressive osteoblastoma may be locally aggressive, and 50% will recur. They do not metastasize, although rare cases have caused death of the patient.
- Rare cases of transformation into osteosarcoma have been reported, and it may be difficult to histopathologically distinguish some cases from osteosarcoma.

- Local mass effects on involved teeth may result in root resorption or loosening.

PROGNOSIS

- Conventional osteoblastoma has a good prognosis with complete excision or curettage.
- Occasionally lesions will recur.

DENTAL SIGNIFICANCE

Lesions occurring in areas of the teeth can cause tooth mobility and pain, resembling odontogenic inflammatory disease.

DENTAL MANAGEMENT

Usual treatment is local surgical excision or curettage.

SUGGESTED REFERENCES

Alvares Capelozza AL, Giao Dezotti MS, Casati Alvares L, Negrao Fleury R, Sant'Ana E. Osteoblastoma of the mandible: systematic review of the literature and report of a case. *Dentomaxillofac Radiol* 2005;34:1–8.

Gordon SC, et al. A review of osteoblastoma and case report of metachronous osteoblastoma and unicystic ameloblastoma. *Oral Surg Oral Med Oral Pathol Oral Radiol Endod* 2001;91:570–575.

Ohkubo T, et al. "Aggressive" osteoblastoma of the maxilla. *Oral Surg Oral Med Oral Pathol Oral Radiol Endod* 1989;68:69–73.

Slootweg PJ. Cementoblastoma and osteoblastoma: a comparison of histologic features. *J Oral Pathol Med* 1992;21:385–389.

Waldron CA (author of original version in ed 1). Bone pathology. In Neville BW, Damm DD, Allen CM, Bouquot JE (eds): *Oral & Maxillofacial Pathology*, ed 2. Philadelphia, WB Saunders, 2002, pp 568–570.

Weinberg S, et al. Osteoblastoma of the mandibular condyle: review of the literature and report of a case. *J Oral Maxillofac Surg* 1987;45:350–355.

AUTHORS: **MICHAEL W. FINKELSTEIN, DDS, MS; ROBERT D. FOSS, DDS, MS**

SECTION II

SYNONYM(S)

None

ICD-9CM/CPT CODE(S)

695.3 Rosacea
CPT General Exam or Consultation
(e.g., 99243 or 99213)

OVERVIEW

By definition, perioral dermatitis should spare the area immediately surrounding the vermilion of the lip. Multiple papules are the hallmark of the disease, though these often produce confluent lesions within the multipapular pattern.

EPIDEMIOLOGY & DEMOGRAPHICS

PREDOMINANT AGE: Most of these women will be relatively young (in their twenties or thirties), although any age may be affected.
PREDOMINANT SEX: The overwhelming preponderance of cases will be in women, with an approximately 9:1 female to male ratio.

ETIOLOGY & PATHOGENESIS

Although contact allergies or microfloral elements are often implicated, idiosyncratic responses to unknown antigens are often suspected as the primary etiologic agent. Similar types of reactions resembling perioral dermatitis may also occur. In most of these, either the area immediately adjacent to the vermilion is involved or the reaction extends outside the perioral region. In such cases, other disease processes should be considered. For instance, reactions to pyrophosphates in tartar reducing toothpastes usually involve the skin contiguous with the vermilion border. Simple removal of the pyrophosphate toothpaste is sufficient treatment for this malady. Perioral candidosis is also usually contiguous with the vermilion.

CLINICAL PRESENTATION / PHYSICAL FINDINGS

The perioral erythematous of papules may occur over the course of several days to several weeks. These may be somewhat pyretic. Pustular changes are uncommon. If pustules are present, impetigo should be considered and ruled out.

DIAGNOSIS

Diagnosis is made on clinical exam and historical features. Laboratory tests and biopsy are usually not necessary.

MEDICAL MANAGEMENT & TREATMENT

- The application of potent steroids actually worsens this disease. Therefore, steroids should be avoided in any case of perioral dermatitis.
- Topical antibiotics such as metronidazole cream are often effective. These may be combined with the use of nonsteroidal antiinflammatories such as tacrolimus or pimecrolimus.
- Mupirocin may also be used as a topical antibiotic.
- If there is some question of an additional angular cheilitis or fungal element, metronidazole, mupirocin, and ketoconazole may all be combined. This is usually only necessary if the area immediately adjacent to the vermilion is also concomitantly involved.

COMPLICATIONS

The use of topical steroids confusion worsens the disease and may predispose the patient to perioral candidal dermatitis.

PROGNOSIS

Although the overall prognosis is good, treatment can be of several weeks or more in duration. Cosmetic considerations may be the patient's chief concern. Lesions caused by antigenic response to such things as cosmetics are particularly problematic and often recur. In addition, some patients may have obsessive-compulsive disorders with extreme lip-licking. This is not true perioral dermatitis but is often treated similarly.

DENTAL SIGNIFICANCE

No dental implications, although occasionally contact allergies to latex and rubber dams create a similar perioral distribution.

DENTAL MANAGEMENT

No change in dental management is necessary unless sensitivities to latex or pyrophosphates are elucidated by history and physical exam.

SUGGESTED REFERENCES

Hafeez ZH. Perioral dermatitis: an update. *Int J Dermatol* 2003;42(7):514–517.
Neville B, Damm D, Allen C, Bouquot J (eds): *Oral & Maxillofacial Pathology*, ed 2. Philadelphia, WB Saunders, 2002, pp 304–305.
Weber K, Thurmayr R. Critical appraisal of reports on the treatment of perioral dermatitis. *Dermatology* 2005;210(4):300–307.

AUTHOR: **JOHN W. HELLSTEIN, DDS, MS**

SYNONYM(S)

None

ICD-9CM/CPT CODE(S)

523.8 Peripheral giant cell granuloma
CPT General Exam or Consultation
(e.g., 99243 or 99213)

OVERVIEW

Relatively common lesion of the oral cavity. Regarded as a reactive, nonneoplastic lesion, it appears as a localized, tumor-like enlargement of the gingival and alveolar mucosa.

EPIDEMIOLOGY & DEMOGRAPHICS

PREDOMINANT AGE: Wide age range; 50% of cases are in patients 40 to 59 years old.

ETIOLOGY & PATHOGENESIS

Underlying cause is unclear, even though the disorder is often associated with local irritation.

CLINICAL PRESENTATION / PHYSICAL FINDINGS

- Mandible involved more frequently than maxilla.
- Sessile or pedunculated.

- Deep red to purple.
- Rarely larger than 20 mm in diameter.
- Features may vary considerably.

DIAGNOSIS

DIFFERENTIAL DIAGNOSIS

- Peripheral ossifying fibroma
- Pyogenic granuloma
- Central giant cell granuloma
- Primary hyperparathyroidism
- Malignant or metastatic lesions

LABORATORY

- Blood chemistry (when indicated for recurrent lesions or signs of hypercalcemia)
  - Parathormone, serum calcium, and phosphate levels (elevated in HPT). Alkaline phosphatase assay is a less reliable indicator.

IMAGING

- Periapical radiographs of affected area. Teeth directly related may show complete or partial loss of lamina dura.

MEDICAL MANAGEMENT & TREATMENT

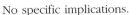

Excision including periosteum reduces the likelihood of recurrence.

COMPLICATIONS

Because of the possibility of recurrence, patients should be reviewed regularly.

PROGNOSIS

In almost all cases, removal of adjacent teeth is not required with excision of the lesion.

DENTAL SIGNIFICANCE

No specific implications.

DENTAL MANAGEMENT

Refer to oral and maxillofacial surgeon.

SUGGESTED REFERENCES

Junquera LM, et al. Multiple and synchronous peripheral giant cell granulomas of the gums. *Ann Otol Rhinol Laryngol* 2002;111: 751–753.
Shields JA. Peripheral giant-cell granuloma: a review. *J Irish Dent Assoc* 1994;40:239–241.

AUTHOR: **ANDREW M. DEWITT, DDS**

SECTION II

SYNONYM(S)

Calcifying fibrous epulis

ICD-9CM/CPT CODE(S)
213.1 Peripheral odontogenic fibroma
CPT   General Exam or Consultation
       (e.g., 99243 or 99213)

OVERVIEW

Benign focal overgrowth of oral soft tissue occurring in the oral mucosa

EPIDEMIOLOGY & DEMOGRAPHICS

PREDOMINANT AGE: Mean age 40 years; range 4 to 80 years
PREDOMINANT SEX: Slight female predilection

ETIOLOGY & PATHOGENESIS

Unknown; some investigators believe this lesion to arise from the periodontal ligament.

CLINICAL PRESENTATION / PHYSICAL FINDINGS

- Attached gingival; usually the molar/premolar are the most common locations.
- Even distribution between the maxilla and mandible.
- Uncommon, benign, focal unencapsulated exophytic gingival mass composed of fibrous connective tissue associated with various amounts of calcifications and islands of odontogenic epithelium.

DIAGNOSIS

DIFFERENTIAL DIAGNOSIS
- Pyogenic granuloma
- Peripheral giant cell granuloma
- Peripheral ameloblastoma
- Peripheral calcifying odontogenic cyst
- Peripheral calcifying epithelial odontogenic tumor

IMAGING
- Periapical radiograph is indicated to evaluate underlying bone prior to biopsy.

MEDICAL MANAGEMENT & TREATMENT

Excisional biopsy

COMPLICATIONS

None

PROGNOSIS

This lesion has a recurrence rate of up to 39%.

DENTAL SIGNIFICANCE

No specific dental implications.

SUGGESTED REFERENCES
Daley TD, et al. Peripheral odontogenic fibroma. *Oral Surg Oral Med Oral Path* 1994;78:329–336.

Dunlap CL. Odontogenic fibroma. *Sem Diagn Path* 1999;16:4,293–296.

Manor Y, et al. Peripheral odontogenic tumours-differential diagnosis in gingival lesions. *Int J Oral Maxillofac Surg* 2004;33: 268–273.

AUTHOR: **ANDREW M. DEWITT, DDS**

SYNONYM(S)

Benign mixed tumor

ICD-9CM/CPT CODE(S)

210.2   Benign tumors of major salivary glands
210.2   Parotid, submandibular, sublingual
210.4   Benign tumors of minor salivary glands
210.0   Lips
210.4   Oral cavity and pharynx
CPT   General Exam or Consultation (e.g., 99243 or 99213)

OVERVIEW

The most common salivary neoplasm, composed of a mixture of ductal and myoepithelial cells

EPIDEMIOLOGY & DEMOGRAPHICS

PREDOMINANT AGE: Most common between 30 and 50 years of age but can occur at any age
PREDOMINANT SEX: Slight female predilection

ETIOLOGY & PATHOGENESIS

Unknown

CLINICAL PRESENTATION / PHYSICAL FINDINGS

- May occur in parotid gland, 90% in superficial lobe.
- Palate is the most common oral site but can be found in lips and buccal mucosa.
- Typically firm, painless, slow-growing mass.
- If overlying mucosa is moveable, the mass is usually moveable. On the palate it will not be moveable.

DIAGNOSIS

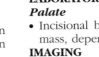

DIFFERENTIAL DIAGNOSIS
Parotid
- Basal cell adenoma
- Malignant salivary gland tumors
- Hemangioma
- Lymphangioma
- Lipoma
- Lymphoma
- Warthin's tumor

Palate
- Salivary gland neoplasms (benign and malignant)
- Non-Hodgkin's lymphoma

LABORATORY
Palate
- Incisional biopsy at the center of the mass, dependent upon size

IMAGING
Parotid
- CT or MRI

Palate
- CT

MEDICAL MANAGEMENT & TREATMENT

Parotid (superficial lobe)
- Superficial parotidectomy
Other locations (1-cm margins)
- On palate, remove overlying normal mucosa and periosteum

COMPLICATIONS

"Shelling out" lesion may lead to recurrences.

PROGNOSIS

Ninety-five percent cure rate (i.e., low recurrences).

DENTAL SIGNIFICANCE

No specific dental implications.

SUGGESTED REFERENCES

Marx RE, Stern D (eds): *Oral and Maxillofacial Pathology. A Rationale for Diagnosis and Treatment.* Carol Stream, IL, Quintessence Publishing Company, 2003, pp 528–533.
Neville B, Damm D, Allen C, Bouquot J (eds): *Oral & Maxillofacial Pathology,* ed 2. Philadelphia, WB Saunders, 2002, pp 410–413.

AUTHOR: MICHAEL J. DALTON, DDS

SECTION II

SYNONYM(S)

Paterson-Kelly syndrome
Paterson-Brown-Kelly syndrome
Waldenström's disease
Sideropenia dysphagia

ICD-9CM/CPT CODE(S)

280.8 Other specified iron deficiency
    anemias
CPT General Exam or Consultation
    (e.g., 99243 or 99213)

OVERVIEW

Plummer-Vinson syndrome (PVS) is a rare, pathologic condition consisting of iron deficiency anemia, esophageal webbing with resultant progressive dysphagia, and atrophic glossitis.

EPIDEMIOLOGY & DEMOGRAPHICS

INCIDENCE/PREVALENCE IN USA: Not established (now uncommon because of improved nutrition)
PREDOMINANT AGE: Adults
PREDOMINANT SEX: PVS is more frequently observed in women.
GENETICS: Not established

ETIOLOGY & PATHOGENESIS

- The specific etiology of Plummer-Vinson syndrome is unknown but has been attributed to esophageal innervation disturbances (impaired esophageal motility), iron deficiency anemia and other nutritional deficiencies, and autoimmune conditions (e.g., rheumatoid arthritis, pernicious anemia, celiac disease, and thyroiditis).
- In addition, esophageal webs may be congenital but can also arise with pemphigoid, epidermolysis bullosa, and pemphigus vulgaris. When esophageal webs from these etiologies are present concurrently with iron deficiency anemia, they are sometimes diagnosed as PVS.

CLINICAL PRESENTATION / PHYSICAL FINDINGS

- Fatigue
- Dyspnea on exertion
- Dizziness
- Brittle hair
- Possible splenomegaly
- Eyes
  ○ Visual changes
  ○ Conjunctiva pale
  ○ Conjunctivitis
  ○ Keratitis, blepharitis
- Oral cavity
  ○ Soreness of the tongue
  ○ Erythematous tongue with atrophy of the lingual papillae (similar in appearance to that seen in megaloblastic anemia)
  ○ Glossitis
  ○ Angular cheilitis
  ○ Dry, pale mucous membranes
  ○ Progressive dysphagia with choking and regurgitation; typically intermittent and limited to solids and usually felt in the throat
  ○ Degenerative changes in oropharynx and esophagus; increased risk for and tissue breakdown and ulcer production
- Integument: seborrheic dermatitis, hyperkeratosis and koilonychia (spoon nails)
- Gynecologic: inflammation, infection associated with iron deficiency anemia
- Hematologic: hypochromic microcytic anemia present

DIAGNOSIS

DIFFERENTIAL DIAGNOSIS

- Esophageal neoplasia/cysts
- Achalasia
- Barrett's esophagitis
- Peptic esophagitis
- Benign stricture of the esophagus
- Lower esophageal ring
- Raynaud's phenomenon
- Scleroderma
- Systemic lupus erythematosus
- Esophageal diverticula

HISTORY

- Fatigue, decreased exercise tolerance, mild dyspnea (see Clinical Presentation/Physical Findings preceding).

LABORATORY

- Serum iron studies (serum iron, ferritin, total iron-binding capacity) confirm the presence of iron deficiency while anemia may or may not be present.
- CBC counts and peripheral blood smears are also helpful.

IMAGING

- Esophagram combined with videocinematography are very sensitive methods for the detection of esophageal webs.
- Barium esophagram.

MEDICAL MANAGEMENT & TREATMENT

- Esophageal endoscopy with biopsy and lysis of esophageal webbing/dilation.
- Treat iron deficiency and its underlying cause:
  ○ The anemia is a critical sign of an underlying lesion that may be benign or as threatening as an occult malignancy. Identifying its cause is imperative.
  ○ Iron replacement is necessary to correct the anemia, if present, and to resolve most of the physical signs of iron deficiency. The most commonly administered preparation is ferrous sulfate 325 mg PO qd, frequently prescribed with meals for improved tolerance.
- Dysphagia may improve with iron replacement alone, particularly in patients whose webs are not substantially obstructive. Dysphagia caused by more advanced webs is unlikely to respond to iron replacement alone and may require mechanical esophageal dilation and/or surgery.

COMPLICATIONS

Patients with PVS seem to be at an increased risk for hypopharyngeal and esophageal cancers, but evidence is inconsistent.

PROGNOSIS

- Following iron supplementation and surgical treatment of the esophageal webs, dysphagia, glossitis, and iron deficient anemia improve.
- There is an increased incidence of carcinoma involving the oral mucosa, hypopharynx, and esophagus. Regular, long-term follow-up is indicated.

DENTAL SIGNIFICANCE

Iron deficiency anemia commonly leads to pallor of the face, lips, mucosa, and tongue; when chronic, can lead to atrophic glossitis, glossodynia, and angular cheilitis.

DENTAL MANAGEMENT

- Palliative care for oral discomfort/pain.
- Refer to primary care physician and/or gastroenterologist. Following diagnosis and appropriate treatment for iron deficiency anemia, the oral/facial structures should return to a normal clinical status.
- The treating dentist should update medical status on all subsequent visits.

SUGGESTED REFERENCES

Chen TN, et al. Rise and fall of the Plummer-Vinson syndrome. *J Gastroenter and Hepat* 1994;9:654–658.

Duffy TP. Microcytic and hypochromic anemias, in Goldman L, Ansiello D (eds): *Cecil Textbook of Medicine,* ed 22. Philadelphia, WB Saunders, 2004, pp 1003–1008.

Hoffman RM, et al. Plummer-Vinson syndrome: a case report and literature review. *Arch Intern Med* 2005;155:2008–2011.

AUTHORS: **ANDREW M. DEWITT, DDS; NORBERT J. BURZYNSKI, SR., DDS, MS**

SYNONYM(S)

None

ICD-9CM/CPT CODE(S)

446.0 Polyarteritis nodosa
CPT General Exam or Consultation
(e.g., 99243 or 99213)

OVERVIEW

A connective tissue disorder characterized by necrotizing inflammation of small and medium-sized arteries in any organ system in the body. The vascular effect results in secondary ischemia of tissues supplied by the involved arteries.

EPIDEMIOLOGY & DEMOGRAPHICS

PREDOMINANT AGE: Mean age 45
PREDOMINANT SEX: Male to female ratio 2.5:1

ETIOLOGY & PATHOGENESIS

- Etiology is unclear. It is thought to be an immune complex-mediated process. The process begins with increased vascular permeability and activation of complement. Immune complexes then deposit along the vessel wall with excess antigen, thus attracting platelets to the site of injury.
- Destruction of the media and internal elastic lamina, which produces aneurysms, is a classic feature of polyarteritis nodosa.

CLINICAL PRESENTATION / PHYSICAL FINDINGS

- Fever, malaise, weakness, abdominal pain, and myalgias.

- Cutaneous findings are seen in 20–50% of cases, ranging from erythema and bullae to ulcers and livedo reticularis.
- Peripheral neuropathy and cardiovascular and renal involvement are also seen.
- Aneurysms, which range in size from 1 to 5 mm, occur in the mesenteric, hepatic, and renal arteries in 90% of cases.

DIAGNOSIS

DIFFERENTIAL DIAGNOSIS

- Giant cell arteritis
- Temporal arteritis
- Wegener's granulomatosis
- Churg-Strauss syndrome
- Drug-induced vasculitis
- Henoch-Schönlein purpura

WORKUP

- Excisional biopsy of the skin demonstrates necrotizing arteritis in the subcutaneous tissue or lower dermis.

IMAGING

- An arteriogram revealing an aneurysm of the hepatic, renal, or vascular arteries is pathognomonic for polyarteritis nodosa.

MEDICAL MANAGEMENT & TREATMENT

- Removal of offending antigen (i.e., drugs or infection).
- Prevention of deposition of immune complexes through plasmapheresis.
- Suppression of the inflammatory response with the use of nonsteroidal antiinflammatory drugs.

- Corticosteroids are effective in modulation of the underlying immune mechanism involved in the vasculitis.
- Cyclophosphamide has been found to facilitate disease control and decrease recurrence and relapse.
- Methotrexate has been suggested for patients unresponsive to systemic corticosteroids.

PROGNOSIS

If untreated, the disease is usually fatal due to failure of one or more vital organs.

DENTAL MANAGEMENT

Refer to rheumatologist.

SUGGESTED REFERENCES

Crowson AN, et al. Cutaneous vasculitis: a review. *J Cutan Pathol* 2003;30:161–173.
Herbert CR, et al. Polyarteritis nodosa and cutaneous polyarteritis nodosa. *Skin Med* 2003;2:277–285.

AUTHOR: **ANDREW M. DEWITT, DDS**

SECTION II

SYNONYM(S)

None

ICD-9CM/CPT CODE(S)

238.4 Polycythemia vera
CPT General Exam or Consultation
(e.g., 99243 or 99213)

OVERVIEW

Polycythemia vera (PV) constitutes a variety of disorders characterized by excess red blood cell production. They are chronic, clonal blood stem cell disorders characterized by excessive proliferation of erythroid, myeloid, and megakaryocytic elements within bone marrow. There is a resultant increase in red blood cell mass and potentially elevated peripheral granulocyte and platelet counts.

EPIDEMIOLOGY & DEMOGRAPHICS

INCIDENCE/PREVALENCE IN USA: PV is a rare disorder with an incidence of 2.3 per 100,000.
PREDOMINANT AGE: While rarely seen in individuals younger than 40 years of age, the disorder can occur in children and young adults.
PREDOMINANT SEX: Occurs more frequently in men.
GENETICS: Risk factors are unknown but incidence is highest among people of eastern European Jewish ancestry.

CLINICAL PRESENTATION / PHYSICAL FINDINGS

- The evolution of PV begins with an asymptomatic phase that can include splenomegaly and erythrocytosis and thrombocytosis.
- Symptoms begin during the erythrocytotic phase secondary to excessive proliferations of red blood cells and platelets.
- Symptoms include:
  - Pruritus (especially after a hot bath)
  - Headache
  - Weakness
  - Dyspnea
  - Visual disturbances
  - Paresthesias
  - Epigastric complaints

DIAGNOSIS

DIFFERENTIAL DIAGNOSIS

- Primary erythrocytosis
- Stress erythrocytosis (Gaisböck's syndrome)
- Secondary polycythemia
  - Generalized hypoxia
  - High altitude
  - Chronic obstructive pulmonary disease
  - Cardiovascular shunt
  - Pickwickian syndrome
  - High-oxygen-affinity hemoglobin
  - Smoking
  - Local hypoxia
  - Renal cysts
  - Hydronephrosis
  - Renal artery stenosis
  - Autonomous erythropoietin production
  - Renal carcinoma
  - Hepatoma
  - Cerebellar hemangioblastoma
  - Uterine fibroid tumors
  - Recessive familiar polycythemia

LABORATORY

Diagnostic criteria for PV are as follows:
- A1: raised red cell mass (> 25% above mean normal predicted value of > 60 in males or 56 in females)
- A2: absence of cause of secondary erythrocytosis
- A3: palpable splenomegaly
- A4: clonality marker
- B1: thrombocytosis (platelet count > 400×10^9/l)
- B2: neutrophil leucocytosis (neutrophil count > 10×10^9/l; > 12.5×10^9/l in smokers)
- B3: splenomegaly demonstrated on isotope or ultrasound scanning
- B4: characteristic BFU-E growth or reduced serum erythropoietin or polycythemia rubra vera-1 overexpression (BRU-E: burst-forming units-euthyroid)

Note: Diagnosis of PV is acceptable if the following combinations are present: A1 + A2 + A3 or A4; A1 + A2 + two of B.

MEDICAL MANAGEMENT & TREATMENT

- Phlebotomy: remove 500 to 2000 mL of blood per week until the hematocrit reaches 45% and repeat phlebotomy whenever hematocrit rises 4–5%.
- Iron supplements are contraindicated.
- Radioactive phosphorous is indicated when periodic phlebotomy is inadequate to control the hematocrit.
- Hydroxyurea may produce remission. Intermittent maintenance therapy is usually required.
- Pipobroman is an alternative in patients with high risk of thrombosis.

PROGNOSIS

- In treated patients, the survival period is about 13 years.
- About 5% of all patients die of acute leukemia.

DENTAL SIGNIFICANCE

No specific dental implications.

DENTAL MANAGEMENT

Refer to hematologist.

SUGGESTED REFERENCES

Golden C. Polycythemia vera: a review. *Clin J Onc Nurs* 2003;7(5):552–556.

Pahl H. Diagnostic approaches to polycythemia vera in 2004. *Expert Rev Mol Diagn* 2004;4(4):495–502.

Passamonti F, et al. Treatment of polycythemia vera and essential thrombocythemia: the role of pipobroman. *Leukemia Lymphoma* 2003;44(9):1483–1488.

AUTHOR: **ANDREW M. DEWITT, DDS**

Polymorphous Low-Grade Adenocarcinoma

SYNONYM(S)

None

ICD-9CM/CPT CODE(S)

145.9 Malignant neoplasm of minor salivary glands
145.0 Buccal mucosa
145.2 Hard palate
145.3 Soft palate
145.9 Not otherwise specified
CPT General Exam or Consultation (e.g., 99243 or 99213)

OVERVIEW

The polymorphous, low-grade adenocarcinoma is a low-grade malignancy of the minor salivary glands. It is characterized by slow growth, small size, and limited metastatic potential.

EPIDEMIOLOGY & DEMOGRAPHICS

PREDOMINANT AGE: Usually occurs in patients 50 years of age and older
PREDOMINANT SEX: A slight female predilection

ETIOLOGY & PATHOGENESIS

Unknown

CLINICAL PRESENTATION / PHYSICAL FINDINGS

- Usually occurs in minor salivary glands.
- The palate is the most common site, followed by buccal mucosa and upper lip.
- Firm, painless mass, rarely ulcerated on its surface.

DIAGNOSIS

DIFFERENTIAL DIAGNOSIS

- Other slow-growing masses; pleomorphic adenoma
- Benign salivary gland tumors
- Adenoid cystic carcinoma, low-grade mucoepidermoid carcinoma, canalicular adenoma

LABORATORY

- Incisional biopsy, dependent upon size

IMAGING

- CT or MRI to differentiate the extent of the lesion.

MEDICAL MANAGEMENT & TREATMENT

Wide (1.5 cm) margins, sometimes including bone if involved

PROGNOSIS

Metastasis is rare; local recurrences can occur and are treated with reexcision. Ten-year survival rate is 80%.

DENTAL SIGNIFICANCE

No specific dental implications.

SUGGESTED REFERENCES

Marx RE, Stern D (eds): *Oral and Maxillofacial Pathology. A Rationale for Diagnosis and Treatment*. Carol Stream, IL, Quintessence Publishing Company, 2003, pp 554–556.
Neville B, Damm D, Allen C, Bouquot J (eds): *Oral & Maxillofacial Pathology*, ed 2. Philadelphia, WB Saunders, 2002, pp 428–430.

AUTHOR: **MICHAEL J. DALTON, DDS**

SECTION II

SYNONYM(S)

Postherpetic trigeminal neuralgia
Shingles
Zona
Postherpetic neuropathy

ICD-9CM/CPT CODE(S)

ICD-9CM
053.12 Postherpetic trigeminal neuralgia
053.13 Postherpetic polyneuropathy
053.79 Herpes zoster with nervous system complication
CPT
64400 Anesthetic agent injection, trigeminal nerve
64450 Anesthetic agent injection, peripheral nerve branch NOS
64510 Anesthetic agent injection, stellate ganglion

OVERVIEW

- Self-limiting infection by varicella zoster virus causing unilateral eruptions and neuralgia along affected nerves.
- Severe pain persisting or reemerging following the healing of the cutaneous rash seen with reactivation of varicella zoster virus infection (herpes zoster, shingles).
- Pain may be spontaneous or triggered by light touch; affected area is usually insensitive to pinprick and local heat or cold.
- Pain may be persistent or reemergent, developing 1 to 6 months after healing of the rash.
- Incidence, severity, and duration all increase with age.
  See "Varicella-Zoster Virus Diseases" in Section I, p 218 for more information.

EPIDEMIOLOGY & DEMOGRAPHICS

- Herpes is a condition of the older adult population and those with compromised immune responses.
- Nine to 14% of patients with herpes zoster develop postherpetic neuralgia.

ETIOLOGY & PATHOGENESIS

- Primary infection with varicella zoster virus, causing chicken pox.

- After skin lesions heal, the virus can pass from cutaneous sensory nerves to the dorsal root ganglia and lie dormant until reactivated; reactivation produces the clinical condition known as shingles.
- Herpes zoster results in cell degeneration, death, and scarring in the spinal cord, sensory ganglia, and peripheral nerves; these changes result in cells and the afferent sensory pathway becoming hyperexcitable and prone to spontaneous discharge.
- Risk factors include ophthalmic herpes zoster, diabetes mellitus, cancer, severity of herpes zoster, and immunocompromise.

SYSTEMS AFFECTED

- Nervous: intense pain in affected dermatome.
- Skin: the patient may avoid cleaning affected area, resulting in localized accumulation of dirt, sebum, or debris; this may lead to lichenification, inflammation, and ulceration.
- Mental state: impacted by severe and chronic pain.

CLINICAL PRESENTATION / PHYSICAL FINDINGS

SIGNS & SYMPTOMS

- Spontaneous pain described as burning, throbbing, stabbing, shooting, sharp, or aching; may be continuous with fluctuating intensity or paroxysmal. Intense pain may also be triggered by normally nonpainful stimuli such as the light touch of clothing; symptoms may be worsened by cold weather or stress.
- Skin: unilateral, dermatomal, hypopigmented band of skin, often with residual scarring.
- Nervous system: affected area usually insensitive to pinprick and local heat or cold; mild, normally nonpainful stimuli may trigger pain (allodynia).

DIAGNOSIS

DIFFERENTIAL DIAGNOSIS

- Trigeminal neuralgia
- Atypical facial pain
- Ramsay Hunt syndrome

MEDICAL MANAGEMENT & TREATMENT

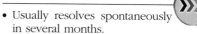

GENERAL

- Avoidance of stimulation of trigger areas

MEDICATIONS

- Somatic or sympathetic nerve blockade during herpes zoster attack may reduce acute pain and decrease likelihood of postherpetic neuralgia.
- Acyclovir therapy during herpes zoster attacks substantially reduces risk of developing postherpetic neuralgia.
- Tricyclic antidepressants relieve postherpetic neuralgia: amitriptyline 75 mg per day; side effects include constipation, sedation, and urinary retention.
- Topical capsaicin cream applied to affected area may help some individuals; side effects include burning sensation after application.
- Lidocaine 5% prilocaine cream (EMLA) and 5–10% Lidocaine gels applied topically have been shown to be effective.

PROGNOSIS

- Usually resolves spontaneously in several months.
- Some patients suffer for years or permanently.

SUGGESTED REFERENCES

Loeser JD. Herpes zoster and postherpetic neuralgia, in Bonica JJ (ed): *The Management of Pain*, ed 2. Philadelphia, Lea & Febiger, 1990, pp 257–263.

Pasqualucci V, et al. The early treatment of herpes zoster with continuous neural blockade prevents postherpetic neuralgia. American Pain Society 13th annual meeting abstracts. Abstract no. 94657:A-50, 1994.

Rakel RE, Bope ET (eds): *Conn's Current Therapy 2005*. Philadelphia, Elsevier, 2005, pp 947–953.

Watson CPN. Herpes zoster and postherpetic neuralgia, in *Pain Research and Clinical Management*. New York, Elsevier, 1993.

AUTHOR: **TERESA BIGGERSTAFF, DDS, MD**

SYNONYM(S)

None

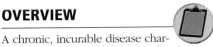

ICD-9CM/CPT CODE(S)
696.1 Psoriasis
CPT General Exam or Consultation
(e.g., 99243 or 99213)

OVERVIEW

A chronic, incurable disease characterized most commonly by symmetrical skin rashes that spontaneously resolve and exacerbate. Associated arthropathy may occur.

EPIDEMIOLOGY & DEMOGRAPHICS

INCIDENCE/PREVALENCE IN USA: Psoriasis affects 1–3% of the population. Psoriatic arthritis affects about 1% of the population (7–42% of those with psoriasis). **PREDOMINANT AGE:** Onset usually occurs between 30 and 55 years of age. **PREDOMINANT SEX:** Affects men and women equally. **GENETICS:** A genetic predisposition that is most likely due to multiple loci.

ETIOLOGY & PATHOGENESIS

Unknown; however, precipitating factors include infection, hormonal influences, medications, trauma, and psychogenic causes.

CLINICAL PRESENTATION / PHYSICAL FINDINGS

- Thick scaling, well-demarcated symmetrical lesions.
- Pruritus.
- Nail pitting.
- Joint involvement: pain, swelling, stiffness. May involve the TMJ.
- Red, raised scaly patches on scalp, extensor surfaces of the knee or elbows.

- Flaking of skin.
- Rare oral lesions consisting of plaques.

DIAGNOSIS

DIFFERENTIAL DIAGNOSIS

- Seborrheic eczema
- Lichen planus
- Lichen simplex
- Discoid eczema
- Intraepidermal carcinoma
- Mycosis fungoides
- Pityriasis rubra pilaris
- Basal cell carcinoma

WORKUP

- Biopsy: epidermis reveals microabscesses, parakeratosis, lack of a granular layer, thinning of the suprapapillary plate, clubbing, and elongation of the rete ridges.

LABORATORY

- HLA antigens
- Rheumatoid factor (negative)
- Leukocytosis and increased sedimentation rate

MEDICAL MANAGEMENT & TREATMENT

- Solar radiation in conservative amounts
- Skin moisturizers
- Oatmeal bath for pruritus
- Cool compresses
- Primary topical:
  - Topical corticosteroids
  - Tar compounds
  - Dithranol
  - UV radiation
  - Keratolytic agents: topical salicylates
- Secondary systemic:
  - Etretinate alone
  - Psoralen plus ultraviolet light (PUVA)
  - Etretinate with PUVA

- Tertiary systemic:
  - Methotrexate
  - Cyclosporine
  - Azathioprine (Imuran)
  - Isotretinoin
  - Corticosteroids
  - Sulfasalazine
  - Antimalarials
  - Gold
  - Etanercept (Enbrel)
  - Infliximab (Remicade)
  - Alefacept

COMPLICATIONS

If a patient shows pustule formation he or she should be sent for immediate emergency care.

PROGNOSIS

Psoriasis is a chronic, incurable disease.

DENTAL SIGNIFICANCE

A small percentage of patients can develop psoriatic arthritis of the temporomandibular joint.

DENTAL MANAGEMENT

Refer to dermatologist and/or rheumatologist.

SUGGESTED REFERENCES

Goffe B. Etanercept (Enbrel)—an update. *Skin Therapy Letter* 2004;9:10.
Langley R, et al. The use of alefacept in the treatment of psoriasis. *J Cut Med Surg* 2004;3 Aug:14–18.
Tam A, et al. Psoriatic arthritis. *Orthopaedic Nur* 2004;23(5):311–314.

AUTHOR: **ANDREW M. DEWITT, DDS**

SECTION II

SYNONYM(S)

Pregnancy tumor
Pregnancy epulis
Granuloma pyogenicum

ICD-9CM/CPT CODE(S)

528.9 Pyogenic granuloma

OVERVIEW

A small, elevated proliferation of reactive granulation tissue on the oral mucosa. The lesion is friable and often has a hemorrhagic or ulcerated appearance.

EPIDEMIOLOGY & DEMOGRAPHICS

- Seventy-five percent occurs in gingival, with the majority seen in the maxillary anterior facial gingiva. Hemorrhage may be spontaneous or easily provoked, but rarely is there dental pain, mobility, or loss of teeth.
- Ten percent occurs in the lips.
- Five percent occurs in the tongue. In this region, the lesion may have an effect on speech and mastication.
- Four percent occurs in the buccal mucosa.

ETIOLOGY & PATHOGENESIS

- A reactive lesion produced in response to some chronic irritation, which provides a pathway for the invasion of microbes.
- Lesions are often noted during pregnancy when the levels of circulating estrogens are high, subsequently shrinking postpartum.

CLINICAL PRESENTATION / PHYSICAL FINDINGS

- Lesions are pedunculated or sessile with smooth, lobulated, or rough surface.
- Lesions may have a red or purple color, depending on the vascularity; hemorrhage is usually spontaneous or easily provoked.

DIAGNOSIS

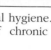

DIFFERENTIAL DIAGNOSIS

- Peripheral giant cell granuloma
- Peripheral odontogenic fibroma
- Hemangioma
- Traumatic fibroma
- Benign or malignant mesenchymal neoplasms
- Kaposi's sarcoma
- Melanoma
- Bacillary angiomatosis

MEDICAL MANAGEMENT & TREATMENT

Skin lesions may be treated by excision, shave excision, laser surgery, sclerotherapy, electrodesiccation, curettage, ligation, or a combination of these methods.

PROGNOSIS

Recurrence is rare but can be expected if incomplete removal was performed.

DENTAL MANAGEMENT

- Improve oral hygiene.
- Removal of chronic gingival irritants.
- Chlorhexidine.
- If the lesion does not resolve quickly, excisional biopsy is indicated to remove and accurately diagnose the lesion.

SUGGESTED REFERENCES

Lin RL, Janniger CK. Pyogenic granuloma. *Cutis* 2004;74(4):229–233.

Ong MAH, et al. Recurrent gigantic pyogenic granuloma disturbing speech and mastication: a case report and literature review. *Ann Acad Med Singapore* 1998;27:258–261.

AUTHOR: **ANDREW M. DEWITT, DDS**

SYNONYM(S)

None

ICD-9CM/CPT CODE(S)
527.6 Ranula

OVERVIEW

A mucous retention or mucous extravasation phenomenon located in the floor of the mouth. Often it is a unilateral, fluid-filled swelling with a bluish appearance, but can be midline.

EPIDEMIOLOGY & DEMOGRAPHICS

Unknown

ETIOLOGY & PATHOGENESIS

- A ranula occurs when mucin accumulates in the tissues of the floor of the mouth. It is thought to be due to a complete or partial blockage in the ducts of the sublingual glands.
- Usually no sialolith is demonstrated.
- Ranula can be due to rupture of a salivary duct or from dilation of a salivary duct.
- The plunging ranula is a rare variant that herniates through the mylohyoid musculature and presents as a swelling in the upper neck (more common in children).

CLINICAL PRESENTATION / PHYSICAL FINDINGS

- Asymptomatic swelling in the floor of the mouth.
- Unilateral fluctuant swelling in the floor of the mouth, usually located near the submandibular duct.
- Overlying mucosa is usually normal but with a bluish appearance.

DIAGNOSIS

DIFFERENTIAL DIAGNOSIS

- Floor of mouth swelling
  - Dermoid cyst
- Neck swelling
  - Branchial cleft cyst
  - Thyroglossal duct cyst
  - Cystic hygroma

WORKUP

- Aspiration of fluid to test for amylase and total protein. This will differentiate between ranula and cystic hygroma.

MEDICAL MANAGEMENT & TREATMENT

- Marsupialization can be used as initial treatment; packing the cavity with gauze may be useful.
- In refractory cases, removal of the sublingual gland is necessary.

PROGNOSIS

- Occasionally recurs even if excision is performed.
- Even if lesion spontaneously drains, it will recur if not surgically managed.
- Multiple recurrences may necessitate removal of the sublingual gland.

DENTAL SIGNIFICANCE

No specific dental implications.

SUGGESTED REFERENCES

Bodner L, Tal H. Salivary gland cysts of the oral cavity: clinical observation and surgical management. *Compendium* 1991;12(3):150, 152, 154–156.

Herschaft E, Waldron C. Salivary gland pathology, in *Oral & Maxillofacial Pathology*. Philadelphia, WB Saunders, 1996, pp 323–324.

Langlois NE, Kolhe P. Plunging ranula: a case report and a literature review. *Hum Pathol* 1992;23(11):1306–1308.

AUTHOR: **ANDREW M. DEWITT, DDS**

SECTION II

SYNONYM(S)

Reiter's disease
Reactive arthritis
Seronegative spondyloarthropathy

ICD-9CM/CPT CODE(S)
099.3 Reiter's syndrome

OVERVIEW

Reiter's syndrome is an aseptic, inflammatory polyarthritis that includes arthritis, urethritis, conjunctivitis, skin lesions, and oral mucosal lesions similar to aphthous ulcers.

EPIDEMIOLOGY & DEMOGRAPHICS

PREDOMINANT SEX: Predilection for males in the third decade. It is the most common cause of arthritis in young men.

ETIOLOGY & PATHOGENESIS

Reiter's syndrome usually occurs following an infection in a genetically susceptible person. Over two-thirds of these patients are HLA-B27-positive. Patients who are HLA-B27-negative frequently are positive for cross-reacting agents such as B7, B22, B40, and B42.

CLINICAL PRESENTATION / PHYSICAL FINDINGS

- Urogenital: urethritis is typically asymptomatic. May have intermittent urethral discharge.
- Eyes: itching, erythema, and burning of conjunctiva or may be asymptomatic.
- Arthritis: joints are painful, warm, and erythematous and accompanied by fever and malaise. An acute episode will last from days up to several months.
- Skin lesions: nonpainful, crusted, scaling papules on palms, soles, and glans penis. Keratin buildup under nails.
- Oral mucosa: aphthous-like ulcers are relatively painless and may appear anywhere on oral mucosa.

DIAGNOSIS

DIFFERENTIAL DIAGNOSIS
- Aphthous ulcers of oral mucosa
- Gonococcal urethritis
- Viral conjunctivitis
- Psoriasis of skin
- Rheumatoid or psoriatic arthritis

LABORATORY
- Rheumatoid factor and antinuclear antibodies are negative

MEDICAL MANAGEMENT & TREATMENT

- No cure is available. Goal of treatment is relief of symptoms. When joint problems occur, bed rest, physical therapy, and NSAIDs are needed.
- Patient education, physical therapy, and NSAIDs for arthritis.

- Acute general Rx
  - Indomethacin (Indocin)
  - Doxycycline (Vibramycin)
  - Intraarticular corticosteroid injections
- Chronic Rx
  - Sulfasalazine (Azulfidine)
  - Methotrexate
  - Azathioprine (Imuran)

PROGNOSIS

Chronic; no cure is available.

DENTAL SIGNIFICANCE

Oral lesions are mild and usually require no treatment.

SUGGESTED REFERENCES

Barth WF, et al. Reactive arthritis (Reiter's syndrome). *Am Fam Phy* 1999;60:2.

Keat A. Reactive arthritis, in Fitzgerald R, Goutier H, Lahiri S (eds): *Advance in Experimental Medicine and Biology*. New York, Plenum Press, 1999, pp 201–206.

Parker CT, Thomas D. Reiter's syndrome and reactive arthritis. *JAOA* 2000;100(2): 101–104.

See also "Reiter's Syndrome" in Section I, p 178.

AUTHOR: **ANDREW M. DEWITT, DDS**

SYNONYM(S)

None

ICD-9CM/CPT CODE(S)
135 Sarcoidosis
CPT General Exam or Consultation
(e.g., 99243 or 99213)

OVERVIEW

Sarcoidosis is a multisystem, granulomatous disorder resulting in noncaseating granulomatous inflammation.

EPIDEMIOLOGY & DEMOGRAPHICS

INCIDENCE/PREVALENCE IN USA:
African-Americans are afflicted 10 to 17 times more often than Caucasians.
PREDOMINANT AGE: Typically arises in people between ages 20 and 40
PREDOMINANT SEX: Females more prone than males

ETIOLOGY & PATHOGENESIS

- Improper degradation of antigenic material
- Possibly mycobacteria

CLINICAL PRESENTATION / PHYSICAL FINDINGS

- Symptoms occur acutely and are variable. Common symptoms include dyspnea, dry cough, chest pain, fever, malaise, arthralgia, and weight loss.

- Twenty percent of cases are asymptomatic and are found on routine chest radiographs.
- Lupus pernio: purple indurated lesions on the lips or cheeks.
- Erythema nodosum: tender erythematous nodules frequently on lower legs.
- Salivary gland enlargement (bilateral parotid): can mimic Sjögren's syndrome (see "Sjögren's Syndrome" in Section II, p 319).

DIAGNOSIS

DIFFERENTIAL DIAGNOSIS

- Bilateral parotid enlargement (Sjögren's syndrome)
- Lymphoma
- Cat scratch disease
- Lymphadenopathy (stage of HIV)

LABORATORY

- Kveim test can be performed (not often done any more).
- Biopsy of parotid, 93% accurate.
- Transbronchial biopsy.
- Serum angiotensin-converting enzyme.

IMAGING

- Chest radiograph: bilateral hilar lymphadenopathy.

MEDICAL MANAGEMENT & TREATMENT

Corticosteroids if symptoms are severe, especially pulmonary fibrosis

PROGNOSIS

- Some patients undergo spontaneous resolution.
- If symptoms are more severe, patients will require corticosteroids.
- Patients with pulmonary fibrosis have the poorest prognosis.
- Five to 8% of patients die of respiratory failure.

DENTAL SIGNIFICANCE

Depending on the patient's medications, the disease treatment may be altered. For example, steroids require changes in dosing depending on the extent of the procedure. Check with the patient's physician to determine any special needs.

SUGGESTED REFERENCES

Marx RE, Stern D (eds): *Oral and Maxillofacial Pathology. A Rationale for Diagnosis and Treatment.* Carol Stream, IL, Quintessence Publishing Company, 2003, pp 47–50.
Neville B, Damm D, Allen C, Bouquot J (eds): *Oral & Maxillofacial Pathology*, ed 2. Philadelphia, WB Saunders, 2002, pp 292–29.

AUTHOR: **MICHAEL J. DALTON, DDS**

SECTION II

SYNONYM(S)

None

ICD-9CM/CPT CODE(S)

072.9 Mumps
527.2 Sialadenitis
527.5 Sialolithiasis
527.8 Sialosis
CPT General Exam or Consultation (e.g., 99243 or 99213)

OVERVIEW

Inflammation of the salivary glands

EPIDEMIOLOGY & DEMOGRAPHICS

PREDOMINANT AGE: Can occur at any age depending on underlying cause

ETIOLOGY & PATHOGENESIS

- Viral: mumps most common.
- Bacterial: due to stones, obstruction, or decreased salivary flow.
- Adjacent tumors causing blockage of salivary ducts.
- *Staphococcus aureus* is the most common bacterium.

CLINICAL PRESENTATION / PHYSICAL FINDINGS

- Most common in the parotid.
- The affected gland is swollen, painful, and the overlying skin may be erythematous.
- Low-grade fever may be present.
- Purulent discharge from the duct may be seen.

DIAGNOSIS

DIFFERENTIAL DIAGNOSIS

- Salivary tumors
- Sialolithiasis
- Odontogenic infection

LABORATORY

- Culture and sensitivity of purulence to help choose appropriate antibiotics

IMAGING

- Radiographs to ascertain if sialolith is present

MEDICAL MANAGEMENT & TREATMENT

- Antibiotics based on culture
- Rehydration
- Stimulate salivary flow

COMPLICATIONS

Infection and sepsis in debilitated patients can lead to death.

PROGNOSIS

If chronic, may require removal of salivary gland.

DENTAL SIGNIFICANCE

No specific implications.

SUGGESTED REFERENCES

Marx RE, Stern D (eds): *Oral and Maxillofacial Pathology. A Rationale for Diagnosis and Treatment.* Carol Stream, IL, Quintessence Publishing Company, 2003, pp 522–524.

Neville B, Damm D, Allen C, Bouquot J (eds): *Oral & Maxillofacial Pathology,* ed 2. Philadelphia, WB Saunders, 2002, pp 395–397.

AUTHOR: **MICHAEL J. DALTON, DDS**

SYNONYM(S)

Calculi
Salivary stones

ICD-9CM/CPT CODE(S)

527.2 Sialadenitis
527.5 Sialolithiasis
CPT General Exam or Consultation
(e.g., 99243 or 99213)

OVERVIEW

Sialoliths are calcified structures that develop within the salivary ductal system.

EPIDEMIOLOGY & DEMOGRAPHICS

PREDOMINANT AGE: Can occur at any age but most common in middle-aged and young adults.

ETIOLOGY & PATHOGENESIS

- Stones usually form around a nidus in concentric layers.
- Submandibular gland is more likely to be affected due to the course of duct and thickened secretions.

CLINICAL PRESENTATION / PHYSICAL FINDINGS

- Episodic pain and swelling of the affected gland, especially at mealtime
- May be purulence at duct opening
- May be fibrosis of gland itself
- Most common in submandibular gland

DIAGNOSIS

DIFFERENTIAL DIAGNOSIS

- Need to differentiate sialolith versus calcified lymph node or tonsillith

IMAGING

- Panoramic film
- Occlusal radiographs
- CT to pinpoint radiopacity if posterior or in or near the gland

MEDICAL MANAGEMENT & TREATMENT

- If distal enough, can remove sialolith surgically. May need Silastic tubing to keep duct open.
- May require removal of affected gland.
- Rehydration and salivary stimulants may cause stone to pass.

PROGNOSIS

- Removal of gland has no long-term effects.
- Even with removal of stone, gland may be painful and require removal.

DENTAL SIGNIFICANCE

No specific implications.

SUGGESTED REFERENCES

Marx RE, Stern D (eds): *Oral and Maxillofacial Pathology. A Rationale for Diagnosis and Treatment.* Carol Stream, IL, Quintessence Publishing Company, 2003, pp 519–522.

Neville B, Damm D, Allen C, Bouquot J (eds): *Oral & Maxillofacial Pathology*, ed 2. Philadelphia, WB Saunders, 2002, pp 393–395.

AUTHOR: MICHAEL J. DALTON, DDS

SECTION II

SYNONYM(S)

Sinus infection

ICD-9CM/CPT CODE(S)

461.0 Acute maxillary sinusitis
461.9 Acute sinusitis, unspecified
473.0 Chronic maxillary sinusitis
473.9 Chronic sinusitis, unspecified
CPT   General Exam or Consultation
      (e.g., 99243 or 99213)

OVERVIEW

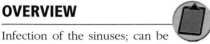

Infection of the sinuses; can be acute or chronic. Secondary to viral infection, allergic rhinitis, or dental infection.

EPIDEMIOLOGY & DEMOGRAPHICS

Sinusitis is one of the most common health problems in the U.S.

ETIOLOGY & PATHOGENESIS

Thought to be blockage of the ostial-meatal complex; can be secondary to a viral infection or allergies

CLINICAL PRESENTATION / PHYSICAL FINDINGS

- Acute sinusitis: headache, fever, facial pain, nasal discharge, toothache, or peri-orbital pain
- Chronic sinusitis: less specific pressure, sensation of obstruction, headache, sore throat
- Fetid breath or odor
- Tender over anterior wall of the sinus

DIAGNOSIS

DIFFERENTIAL DIAGNOSIS

- Viral illness: cold or flu
- Acute dental infection
- Headache from another cause
- Atypical facial pain

LABORATORY

- Cultures, nasal endoscopy

IMAGING

- CT scan
- Water's view radiograph
- Panorex

MEDICAL MANAGEMENT & TREATMENT

- Antibiotics: First-line treatment is amoxicillin; if not successful, use clavulanate, trimethoprim, sulfamethoxazole, cefaclor
- Antihistamines
- Topical decongestants
- Nasal endoscopy
- Meatal surgery

COMPLICATIONS

Pansinusitis may occur and involue multiple sinuses.

PROGNOSIS

Chronic sinusitis may be difficult to eradicate.

DENTAL SIGNIFICANCE

Can be confused with dental pain. If several teeth are painful in maxillary posterior, at least consider maxillary sinusitis as a possible cause.

SUGGESTED REFERENCE

Marx RE, Stern D (eds): *Oral and Maxillofacial Pathology. A Rationale for Diagnosis and Treatment*. Carol Stream, IL, Quintessence Publishing Company, 2003, pp 184–186.

AUTHOR: **MICHAEL J. DALTON, DDS**

SYNONYM(S)

Sjögren syndrome
Sjögren disease
Sjögren's disease
Gougerot-Sjögren disease
Sicca syndrome
Sicca complex
Dry eye syndrome
Dry mouth syndrome
Keratoconjunctivitis sicca

ICD-9CM/CPT CODE(S)

710.2 Sicca syndrome—complete
CPT General Exam or Consultation
(e.g., 99243 or 99213)

OVERVIEW

- Sjögren's syndrome (SS) is an autoimmune disorder characterized by lymphocytic and plasma cell infiltration and destruction of salivary, lacrimal, and other exocrine glands, causing diminished secretions with resulting xerostomia (dry mouth) and xerophthalmia (dry eyes).
  - This triad of xerostomia, xerophthalmia, and lymphocytic infiltration of the exocrine glands is also known as the sicca complex.
- SS occurs as:
  - Primary disease where xerostomia and xerophthalmia develop as isolated entities.
  - Secondary disease in association with any of several other autoimmune diseases [e.g., systemic lupus erythematosus (SLE), rheumatoid arthritis (RA), scleroderma, systemic sclerosis, cryoglobulinemia, polyarteritis nodosa].

EPIDEMIOLOGY & DEMOGRAPHICS

INCIDENCE/PREVALENCE IN USA:

- Primary SS: incidence is 4 per 100,000 new cases per year; prevalence is 1 case per 2500 persons.
- Secondary SS is just as common and can affect up to one-third of SLE patients and nearly 20% of RA patients.

PREDOMINANT AGE: Forty to 60 years of age, with peak incidence in the sixth decade. It is rare in children, but it can occur.

PREDOMINANT SEX: Female > male (9:1).

GENETICS: None confirmed. Possible associations with HLA-B8, HLA-DR3, and DRW52 as well as HLA-DQA1 and HLA-DQB1 loci in patients with anti-SS-A or anti-SS-B antibodies.

ETIOLOGY & PATHOGENESIS

- SS is a chronic autoimmune disease of unknown etiology characterized by lymphocytic infiltration of the exocrine glands.
  - The infiltrate contains predominantly activated CD4f helper T cells and some B cells, including plasma cells that secrete antibody locally.
  - Lacrimal and salivary glands are involved as well as glands in the stomach, pancreas, and intestines. Dryness is extended to nose, throat, airways, and skin.
- SS is also considered a rheumatic disease as well as a disorder of connective tissue.
  - Among the associated disorders, RA is the most common, but some patients have systemic lupus erythematous (SLE), Raynaud's phenomenon, cryoglobulinemia, polyarteritis nodosa, Hashimoto's thyroiditis, antiphospholipid antibody syndrome, scleroderma (SCL), systemic sclerosis, polymyositis and dermatomyositis (PM/DM), reflex undifferentiated connective tissue disease, and mixed connective tissue disease.
  - Approximately 70–90% of patients with SS test positive for antibodies directed against two ribonucleoprotein antigens, SS-A (Ro) and SS-B (La).
  - Antinuclear antibodies (ANAs) are detected in 50–80% of patients with SS.
  - Patients have an elevated total serum IgG and circulating rheumatoid factors.
- Some circumstantial evidence links viruses (e.g., EBV, hepatitis C virus) as initiating agents in SS.

CLINICAL PRESENTATION / PHYSICAL FINDINGS

Highly variable clinical presentation

EYES

- Keratoconjunctivitis sicca: xerophthalmia, blurring of vision, burning, and itching, and thick secretions accumulate in the conjunctival sac.
- Dry eyes are usually worse at night or upon wakening.

ORAL

- Xerostomia: fissures on tongue and lips (cheilosis); dry, erythematous, parchment-like tongue and oral mucosa; atrophy of filiform papillae on lingual dorsum
- Absence of salivary flow from Stensen's duct
  - Secondary to xerostomia:
    - Increased incidence of dental caries (especially cervical decay)
    - Possible candidiasis (may also be present in the vagina)
- Bilateral, parotid gland enlargement (25–66% of primary SS patients; rare in secondary SS), sometimes accompanied by erythema or superimposed infection

OTHER EXOCRINE GLAND INVOLVEMENT

Less frequent:

- Decreased mucous secretions in the respiratory tree may lead to dry cough, hoarseness, chronic/recurrent bronchitis, and pneumonitis.
- Decreased exocrine secretions in the gastrointestinal tract may lead to signs of atrophic gastritis or subclinical pancreatitis (acute or chronic pancreatitis is rare).
- Dry skin (40% of cases).
  Other signs include:
- Low-grade fever (frequent)
- Lymphadenopathy (approximately 14–20% of primary SS patients)

Extraglandular manifestations (generally mild or subclinical) are more common with primary SS; they are especially rare in secondary SS patients with RA and may include:

- Skin and vascular symptoms (occur in approximately 38% of primary SS patients)
  - Small vessel vasculitis (25%); photosensitivity; Raynaud's phenomenon
- Pulmonary symptoms (occur in approximately 14–20% of primary SS patients; usually mild)
  - Dyspnea; lymphocytic alveolitis; lymphocytic interstitial pneumonitis and fibrosis; COPD
- Neurologic symptoms (occur in 2–20% of primary SS patients)
  - Peripheral neuropathy and mononeuritis multiplex; hearing loss; carpal tunnel syndrome
- Renal symptoms (occur in approximately 9–12% of primary SS patients)
  - Type I renal tubular acidosis; tubular interstitial nephritis; hyposthenuria
- Hepatic involvement (occurs in approximately 5–6% of primary SS patients)
  - Hepatomegaly; primary biliary cirrhosis
- Musculoskeletal symptoms
  - Polyarthralgia; polyarthritis; myopathy/polymyositis
- Endocrine symptoms:
  - Hashimoto's thyroiditis with possible hypothyroidism

DIAGNOSIS

- Time from onset of first symptoms to diagnosis of SS ranges from 2 to 8 years.

PRIMARY SS

- Symptoms and objective signs of xerophthalmia:
  - Schirmer's test: < 8 mm wetting per 5 minutes
  - Positive rose bengal or fluorescein staining of cornea and conjunctiva to demonstrate keratoconjunctivitis sicca
- Symptoms and objective signs of xerostomia:
  - Unstimulated whole saliva collection or other quantitive assessment of saliva production
- Evidence of systemic autoimmune disorder:
  - Elevated titer of rheumatoid factor > 1:320
  - Elevated titer of ANA > 1:320
  - Presence of anti-SS A (Ro) or anti-SS B (La) antibodies

SECONDARY SS

- Characteristic signs and symptoms of SS (described in preceding Clinical Presentation/Physical Findings)
- Clinical features sufficient to allow a diagnosis of RA, SLE, polymyositis, scleroderma

DIFFERENTIAL DIAGNOSIS

- Sarcoidosis
- Mumps
- Dehydration
- Medication-induced xerostomia
- Previous radiation therapy to head and neck area

LABORATORY

- Positive ANA (>60% of patients) with autoantibodies anti-SS A and anti-SS B may be present.
- Complete blood count (CBC): mild normochromic normocytic anemia is present in 50% of SS patients; leukopenia occurs in up to 42% of SS patients.
- Additional laboratory abnormalities may include elevated ESR, abnormal liver function studies, elevated serum β_2 microglobulin levels, positive rheumatoid factor.
- A definite diagnosis of SS can be made with a salivary gland biopsy of one or more minor salivary glands in the inner lower lip. Criterion supportive for diagnosis is more than one focus of at least 50 round cells (lymphocytes or plasma cells) per 4-mm^2 area of glandular tissue.

MEDICAL MANAGEMENT & TREATMENT

- Usually, a rheumatologist will coordinate treatment among a number of specialists. These should include, allergy, dental, dermatology, gastroenterology, gynecology, neurology, ophthalmology, otolaryngology, pulmonology, and urology.
  - Frequent dental and ophthalmology evaluations are recommended to control negative aspects of syndrome.
- Treatment varies for each patient with SS depending on symptoms and organs systems affected:
  - Adequate fluid replacement.
  - Xerophthalmia:
    - Use of artificial tears as needed
    - Cyclosporine 0.05% ophthalmic emulsion (Restasis), one drop bid in both eyes, may also be of benefit
  - Xerostomia:
    - Salagen (pilocarpine), 5 mg PO qid
    - Evoxac (cevimeline), 30 mg PO tid
      - Use caution in patients with significant cardiovascular disease, including angina, myocardial infarction, or conduction distur-

bance; uncontrolled asthma, COPD, or chronic bronchitis; narrow-angle glaucoma; acute iritis.
  - Regular dental examinations and oral hygiene are crucial for reducing subsequent oral health issues (i.e., caries associated with xerostomia).

COMPLICATIONS

- Increased (>40 times) relative risk of lymphoproliferative disorders, including lymphadenopathy and non-Hodgkin's lymphoma (prevalence: 2.5–6%).
  - May occur after years of apparently benign disease is observed, mostly in patients with systemic disease with rapidly progressive lymphadenopathy.
  - Some noted symptoms include enlargement of salivary glands and lymph nodes.
- Ocular complications include corneal ulceration, vascularization, opacification, and perforation (rare).
- Extraglandular manifestations of SS (as described in Clinical Presentation/Physical Findings preceding).

PROGNOSIS

SS is usually benign and may be consistent with a normal life span; prognosis is influenced mainly by the nature of the associated disease.

DENTAL SIGNIFICANCE

- Dry mouth, may be with sticky or ropey saliva; dental decay and erosion; erythematous mucosa and tongue; cracked lips and angular cheilitis
- Difficulty in swallowing, chewing, and talking
- Need for salivary flow and quality to be examined
- Oral/dental relationship to other organs and body systems

DENTAL MANAGEMENT

- Dental visits are to be frequent and tailored to patient's need.
- Oral/dental hygiene is extremely important.
  - Prophylaxis, flossing, and tutorial nutrition need emphasis to control consequences.
  - Rinse mouth with water several times a day.
  - Avoid mouthwashes with alcohol, due to drying potential of alcohol.

  - Use fluoride toothpaste with a soft-bristle toothbrush. Brush teeth, tongue, and gums after each meal and before bedtime. Nonfoaming toothpaste is less drying. Toothpaste for dry mouths is available OTC.
  - Floss teeth after each meal.
- Nutritional counseling:
  - Avoid sugar (especially refined) in foods and fluids (soft drinks, juices). All consumed products should be sugar-free.
- Management of xerostomia:
  - Oral lubricants and lip balms containing water base, beeswax base, or vegetable oil base (e.g., Surgilube).
  - Sugarless lemon drops, sorbitol-based chewing gum, buffered solution of glycerin and water.
  - Gel-based saliva substitutes tend to give the longest relief, but all saliva products are limited since they all are swallowed.
  - Consider treatment with pilocarpine or cvimeline (if not contraindicated).
- Monitor for possible oral *Candida* infection and treat with Nystatin if necessary.

SUGGESTED REFERENCES

Abazan N, Torreti M, Milor M, Balsara G. The role of labial salivary gland biopsy in the diagnosis of Sjögren's syndrome. *J Oral Maxillofac Surg* 1993;51:574–580.

Anaya J, Talal N. Sjögren's syndrome and connective tissue diseases associated with other immunologic disorders, in Koopman WJ (ed): *Arthritis and Allied Conditions: A Textbook of Rheumatology*, ed 13. Baltimore, Lippincott Williams & Wilkins 1997, pp 1561–1580.

Aquavella JV. www.emedicine.com/oph/topic477.htm

Garcia-Carrasco M, et al. Primary Sjögren syndrome: clinical and immunologic disease patterns in a cohort of 400 patients. *Medicine (Baltimore)* 2002;81:270.

Marx RE, Stern D (eds): *Oral and Maxillofacial Pathology. A Rationale for Diagnosis and Treatment.* Carol Stream, IL, Quintessence Publishing Company, 2003.

Naguwa S, Gershwin ME. Sjögren's syndrome, in Goldman L, Ausiello D (eds): *Cecil Textbook of Medicine*, ed 22. Philadelphia, WB Saunders, 2004, pp 1677–1684.

Pillimer SR. Sjogren's syndrome, in Klippel JH (ed): *Primer on the Rheumatic Diseases*, ed 12. Atlanta, The Arthritis Foundation, 2001, pp 377–384.

Talal N. Sjögren's syndrome: historical overview and clinical spectrum of disease. *Rheum Dis Clin North Am* 1992;18(3):507–515.

AUTHORS: **NORBERT J. BURZYNSKI, SR., DDS, MS; F. JOHN FIRRIOLO, DDS, PHD; LAWRENCE T. HERMAN, DMD, MD; SARA H. RUNNELS, DMD, MD; PAUL R. WILSON, DMD**

SYNONYM(S)

Epidermoid carcinoma of the floor of the mouth

ICD-9CM/CPT CODE(S)
144.0 Anterior portion
144.1 Lateral portion
144.9 Floor of mouth unspecified
CPT General Exam or Consultation (e.g., 99243 or 99213)

OVERVIEW

- A malignant neoplasm that has morphologic characteristics of stratified squamous epithelium found on the floor of mouth.
- Accounts for approximately 15% of oral cancers.
- Risk factors include tobacco use (smoked and smokeless), alcohol abuse, HPV, HIV, *Candida albicans*, and betel nuts.

EPIDEMIOLOGY & DEMOGRAPHICS

INCIDENCE/PREVALENCE IN USA: Estimated 60,000 new cases of oral squamous cell carcinoma each year.
PREDOMINANT AGE: Generally, patients are over the age of 40.
PREDOMINANT SEX: Male to female ratio is 3:1.
GENETICS: Not known; African-Americans demonstrate higher prevalence.

ETIOLOGY & PATHOGENESIS

Smoking and alcohol use have been identified as potential risk factors.

CLINICAL PRESENTATION / PHYSICAL FINDINGS

- Squamous cell carcinoma presents with an ill-defined border.
- Tissue is raised, ulcerated, and firm to palpation.
- Lesion exhibits leukoplakia, erythroplakia, or a mixture of both.
- Often fast-growing and painless at first onset.
- Lesions can cross midline easily because of increased lymphatic drainage.
- Nodal involvement is a common finding.

DIAGNOSIS

Diagnosis usually based on incision biopsy containing both normal and abnormal tissue.

DIFFERENTIAL DIAGNOSIS
- Trauma
- Chemical burn
- Tuberculosis
- Lichen planus
- Aphthous ulcer
- Syphilis

WORKUP
- Head and neck exam
- Fiberoptic exam of oral pharynx and nasopharynx
- Histologic examination/confirmation
- CT/MRI/PET
- Chest radiograph
- TNM classification and staging
- Serum chemistry studies
- Ponograph

MEDICAL MANAGEMENT & TREATMENT

- Surgery, radiotherapy, or a combination of both depending on size of primary tumor, nodal involvement, metastasis, staging, patient's ability to survive such treatments, and tumor board/hospital philosophy.
  - Excision of tumor is usual with 1.5 cm margins.
  - Radiotherapy 5000 to 6000 cGy.
  - If nodal involvement, then bilateral neck dissection is usually indicated.
- Patients monitored monthly for first 18 months.
- Follow-up CT recommended in 6 months.
- Yearly chest radiograph.

PROGNOSIS

Squamous cell carcinoma of the floor of the mouth has a 50% 5-year survival rate.

DENTAL MANAGEMENT

If patient is to be radiated, he/she should have a thorough dental evaluation, questionable teeth removed, and flouride trays constructed. Artificial saliva should also be produced.

SUGGESTED REFERENCES

Harrison LB, Lee HJ, Pfister DG, et al. Long-term results of primary neck dissection for squamous cell cancer of the base of the tongue. *Head Neck* 1998;20(8):668–673.
Kelly DJ. www.emedicine.com/ent/topic264.htm
Marx RE, Stern D (eds): *Oral and Maxillofacial Pathology. A Rationale for Diagnosis and Treatment.* Carol Stream, IL, Quintessence Publishing Company, 2003.
www.emedicine.com/ent/topic258.htm

AUTHORS: **LAWRENCE T. HERMAN, DMD, MD; SARA H. RUNNELS, DMD, MD; PAUL R. WILSON, DMD**

SYNONYM(S)

Epidermoid carcinoma of the lip

ICD-9CM/CPT CODE(S)
140.0 Upper lip
140.1 Lower lip
CPT   General Exam or Consultation
      (e.g., 99243 or 99213)

OVERVIEW

- A malignant neoplasm that has morphologic characteristics of stratified squamous epithelium found on the lip.
- Risk factors include tobacco use (smoked and smokeless), alcohol abuse, HPV, HIV, *Candida albicans*, betel nuts, and increased UVB light exposure.

EPIDEMIOLOGY & DEMOGRAPHICS

INCIDENCE/PREVALENCE IN USA: Estimated 60,000 new cases of oral squamous cell carcinoma each year.
PREDOMINANT AGE: Generally, patients over age 40 are affected.
PREDOMINANT SEX: Male to female ratio is 3:1.
GENETICS: Not known; African-Americans demonstrate higher prevalence.

ETIOLOGY & PATHOGENESIS

Smoking and sun exposure are risk factors.

CLINICAL PRESENTATION / PHYSICAL FINDINGS

- Squamous cell carcinoma presents with an ill-defined border.
- Tissue is raised, ulcerated, and firm to palpation.
- Lesion exhibits leukoplakia, erythroplakia, or a mixture of both.
- Often fast-growing and painless at first onset.
- Lesions can cross midline easily because of increased lymphatic drainage.

DIAGNOSIS

Diagnosis usually based on incision biopsy containing both normal and abnormal tissue. Incision should be vertical rather than horizontal to avoid seeding of normal tissue.

DIFFERENTIAL DIAGNOSIS
- Upper lip: basal cell carcinoma
- Lower lip: keratoacanthoma (see "Keratoacanthoma" in Section II, p 277)

WORKUP
- Head and neck exam
- Fiberoptic exam of oral pharynx and nasopharynx
- Histological examination/confirmation
- CT/MRI/PET
- Chest radiograph
- TNM classification and staging
- Serum chemistry studies
- Ponograph

MEDICAL MANAGEMENT & TREATMENT

- If lesion is less than 40% of lip, then a V-shaped incision with 5-mm to 1-cm margins can be excised.
- If lesion is greater than 40% of lip, then use a Karapandzic flap.
- Prophylactic neck dissection if palpable nodes.
- Follow-up: patients should be monitored every 4 months for first 18 months.

PROGNOSIS

Squamous cell carcinoma of the lip has an 85% 5-year survival rate.

SUGGESTED REFERENCES

Harrison LB, Lee HJ, Pfister DG, et al. Long-term results of primary neck dissection for squamous cell cancer of the base of the tongue. *Head Neck* 1998;20(8):668–673.
Kelly DJ. www.emedicine.com/ent/topic264.htm
Marx RE, Stern D (eds): *Oral and Maxillofacial Pathology. A Rationale for Diagnosis and Treatment.* Carol Stream, IL, Quintessence Publishing Company, 2003. www.emedicine.com/ent/topic258.htm

AUTHORS: **LAWRENCE T. HERMAN, DMD, MD; SARA H. RUNNELS, DMD, MD; PAUL R. WILSON, DMD**

SYNONYM(S)

Epidermoid carcinoma of the tongue

ICD-9CM/CPT CODE(S)

141.9 Tongue—unspecified
141.0 Base of the tongue
141.1 Dorsal surface of the tongue
141.3 Ventral surface of the tongue
CPT General Exam or Consultation
(e.g., 99243 or 99213)

OVERVIEW

- A malignant neoplasm that has morphologic characteristics of stratified squamous epithelium found anterior to the circumvallate papillae of the tongue.
- Risk factors include tobacco use (smoked and smokeless), alcohol abuse, HPV, HIV, *Candida albicans*, and betel nuts.
- Accounts for 20–30% of oral cancers.

EPIDEMIOLOGY & DEMOGRAPHICS

INCIDENCE/PREVALENCE IN USA: Estimated 60,000 new cases of oral squamous cell carcinoma each year
PREDOMINANT AGE: Generally, patients over age 40 are affected.
PREDOMINANT SEX: Equal sex distribution
GENETICS: Not known; African-Americans demonstrate higher prevalence.

ETIOLOGY & PATHOGENESIS

Smoking and alcohol use are considered risk factors.

CLINICAL PRESENTATION / PHYSICAL FINDINGS

- Squamous cell carcinoma presents with an ill-defined border.

- Tissue is raised, ulcerated, and firm to palpation.
- Lesion exhibits leukoplakia, erythroplakia, or a mixture of both.
- Often fast-growing and painless at first onset.
- Most often found on the lateral border of the tongue.

DIAGNOSIS

Diagnosis usually based on incision biopsy containing both normal and abnormal tissue deep into the muscle layer.

DIFFERENTIAL DIAGNOSIS

- Trauma
- Chemical burn
- Tuberculosis
- Lichen planus

WORKUP

- Head and neck exam
- Fiberoptic exam of oral pharynx and nasopharynx
- Histological examination/confirmation
- CT/MRI/PET
- Chest radiograph
- TNM classification and staging
- Serum chemistry studies

MEDICAL MANAGEMENT & TREATMENT

- Surgery, radiotherapy, or a combination of both depending on size of primary tumor, nodal involvement, metastasize, staging, patient's ability to survive such treatments, and tumor board/hospital philosophy.
  - Excision of tumor is normal with 1.5-cm margins.
  - Radiotherapy 5000 to 6000 cGy.
  - If nodal involvement, then neck dissection is usually indicated.

- Patients should be monitored monthly for the first 18 months.
- Follow-up CT recommended in 6 months.
- Yearly chest radiograph.

PROGNOSIS

Squamous cell carcinoma of the lip has an 85% 5-year survival rate.

DENTAL MANAGEMENT

If the patient is to undergo radiation therapy, he/she should have a thorough dental evaluation, removal of questionable teeth, construction of flouride trays, and a prescribed salivary substitute.

SUGGESTED REFERENCES

Harrison LB, Lee HJ, Pfister DG, et al. Long-term results of primary neck dissection for squamous cell cancer of the base of the tongue. *Head Neck* 1998;20(8):668–673.
Kelly DJ. www.emedicine.com/ent/topic 264.htm
Marx RE, Stern D (eds): *Oral and Maxillofacial Pathology. A Rationale for Diagnosis and Treatment.* Carol Stream, IL, Quintessence Publishing Company, 2003.
www.emedicine.com/ent/topic258.htm

AUTHORS: **LAWRENCE T. HERMAN, DMD, MD; SARA H. RUNNELS, DMD, MD; PAUL R. WILSON, DMD**

SECTION II

SYNONYM(S)

None

ICD-9CM/CPT CODE(S)

213.0 Bones of skull and face
213.1 Lower jaw bone
CPT   General Exam or Consultation
      (e.g., 99243 or 99213)

OVERVIEW

The squamous odontogenic tumor (SOT) is a rare, benign, epithelial odontogenic neoplasm.

EPIDEMIOLOGY & DEMOGRAPHICS

INCIDENCE/PREVALENCE IN USA: Uncommon occurrence
PREDOMINANT AGE: The SOT has been reported in patients ranging in age from 8 to 74 years, with a peak incidence seen in the third decade of life.
PREDOMINANT SEX: No apparent sex predilection
GENETICS: A familial association has been reported.

ETIOLOGY & PATHOGENESIS

The SOT arises from the odontogenic rests of Malassez within the periodontal ligament or possibly surface gingival epithelium in rare, peripheral (extraosseous) cases.

CLINICAL PRESENTATION / PHYSICAL FINDINGS

- The SOT is found in a near-equal distribution between the mandible and maxilla and generally is found originating in the tooth-bearing areas of the jaws.
- Multiple jaw lesions are seen in approximately 25% of reported cases.
- Radiographic findings typically consist of a triangular or semicircular radiolucent defect adjacent to a root surface or occurring between the roots of adjacent teeth.

- Rare, peripheral SOTs located on the gingival mucosa have been reported.
- Signs and symptoms include tooth mobility associated with a painless or painful expansion of the alveolus.

DIAGNOSIS

- Histopathologic examination shows islands of bland-appearing, squamous epithelium of varying size arrayed within a mature, fibrous connective tissue stroma.
- Central microcystic degeneration and laminated calcified bodies are sometimes found within the squamous epithelial islands.
- The squamous epithelium lacks atypical or malignant features, exhibits defined intercellular bridging, and occasionally demonstrates vacuolization and keratinization.
- Ameloblastic features such as the presence of a stellate reticulum and peripheral columnar cells with polarized nuclei are not observed.

MEDICAL MANAGEMENT & TREATMENT

- Treatment consists of conservative surgical excision or curettage with extraction of involved teeth.
- Peripheral SOTs require simple excision to include a thin margin of clinically uninvolved tissue.
- Since multicentric lesions are not uncommon, close clinical follow-up is recommended.

COMPLICATIONS

- Maxillary lesions may behave more aggressively due to the porous nature of the maxillary bone.
- A rare case of malignant transformation in a SOT has recently been reported.

PROGNOSIS

- Recurrence after conservative treatment is unusual.
- The few instances of recurrence that have been reported subsequently responded well to further local excision.

DENTAL SIGNIFICANCE

- The potential exists for SOTs to be misdiagnosed as an ameloblastoma or squamous cell carcinoma leading to unnecessary and aggressive management with significant morbidity.
- Given the radiographic presentation, the SOT is often mistaken clinically for alveolar bone loss secondary to periodontal disease.

SUGGESTED REFERENCES

Batsakis JG, Cleary KR. Squamous odontogenic tumor. *Ann Otol Rhinol Laryngol* 1993;102:823–824.

Haghighat K, et al. Squamous odontogenic tumor: diagnosis and management. *J Periodontol* 2002;173:654–656.

Philipsen HP, Reichart PA. Squamous odontogenic tumor: a benign neoplasm of the periodontium. A review of 36 reported cases. *J Clin Periodontol* 1996;23:922–926.

AUTHOR: **CHRISTOPHER G. FIELDING, DDS, MS**

SYNONYM(S)

Erythema multiforme, major
Erythema multiforme exudativum

ICD-9CM/CPT CODE(S)

695.1 Erythema multiforme and Stevens-Johnson syndrome
CPT General Exam or Consultation (e.g., 99243 or 99213)

OVERVIEW

Stevens-Johnson syndrome (SJS) is a severe hypersensitivity reaction associated with erythema multiforme. This very acute disease manifests with very painful mucosal target or bull's eye lesions that involve the mouth, eyes, and genitalia. This syndrome can be very debilitating due to:

- Eye lesions causing blindness.
- Esophageal ulcerations preventing swallowing.
- Scar contracture of mouth, skin, and genitalia.

See "Erythema Multiforme (Stevens-Johnson Syndrome)" in Section I, p 85 for more information.

EPIDEMIOLOGY & DEMOGRAPHICS

INCIDENCE/PREVALENCE IN USA: 1.2 to 6 cases per million individuals; HIV-infected patients average 1 case per 1000 individuals.
PREDOMINANT AGE: Most often involves children under the age of 15 but median age is 48.
PREDOMINANT SEX: No gender predilection

ETIOLOGY & PATHOGENESIS

Fifty percent of SJS cases are a hypersensitivity autoimmune response to antigenic drug.

- Patients have an altered metabolism of certain drugs by Cytochrome P-450, which triggers an immune response by CD4 and CD8 cells.
- Immune response via cytokines IL4, TNF produces destruction of epithelial cells and represents classic skin lesions.
- Skin lesions present as erythematous maculates often in the form of a target-shaped lesion. Ulceration and necrosis then ensue, followed by scar formation.

CLINICAL PRESENTATION / PHYSICAL FINDINGS

- Onset of symptoms over a period of 1 to 2 weeks.
- Following administration of antigenic drug, lesions are seen on skin, oral mucosa, labial mucosa, and scrotum/genitalia.

DIAGNOSIS

DIFFERENTIAL DIAGNOSIS

- Pemphigoid
- Pemphigus vulgaris
- Toxic epidermal necrolysis

WORKUP

- Mucosal or skin biopsy is recommended to evaluate pattern of destruction and to rule out possibility of a viral disease.

MEDICAL MANAGEMENT & TREATMENT

- Due to its very serious nature, hospitalization and administration of systemic prednisone 100 to 160 mg per day for about 2 weeks is recommended.
- Hydration is usually needed because of poor intake secondary to pharyngeal and oral lesions.

- Antibiotics also recommended.
- Silvadene antimicrobial cream for skin.

COMPLICATIONS

Dehydration, blindness, and scarring.

PROGNOSIS

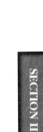

Disease is usually self-limited within a period of 4 to 6 weeks, but mortality is possible.

See "Erythema Multiforme (Stevens-Johnson Syndrome)" in Section I, p 85 for more information.

DENTAL SIGNIFICANCE

Refer patient to dermatologist, rheumatologist, ophthalmologist, and primary care physician. Burn center or ICU setting may be necessary.

See "Erythema Multiforme (Stevens-Johnson Syndrome)" in Section I, p 85 for more information on dental significance.

SUGGESTED REFERENCES

Marx RE, Stern D (eds): *Oral and Maxillofacial Pathology. A Rationale for Diagnosis and Treatment.* Carol Stream, IL, Quintessence Publishing Company, 2003
Revis, Don R. www.emedicine.com/med/topic272.htm

AUTHORS: **SARA H. RUNNELS, DMD, MD; LAWRENCE T. HERMAN, DMD, MD; PAUL R. WILSON, DMD**

SYNONYM(S)
Lues
Lues venerea
"The great imitator"

ICD-9CM/CPT CODE(S)
097.9 Syphilis, acquired—unspecified
095.8 Nose and tongue
091.3 Lip
CPT General Exam or Consultation
(e.g., 99243 or 99213)

OVERVIEW

A disease caused by a gram-negative spirochete called *Treponema pallidum* transferred sexually, bloodborne, and transplacentally.

See "Syphilis" in Section I, p 198 for more information on this topic.

EPIDEMIOLOGY & DEMOGRAPHICS

INCIDENCE/PREVALENCE IN USA: In 1996, around 52,000 documented cases were reported to the Centers for Disease Control, in contrast to only 7177 cases reported in 2003.

ETIOLOGY & PATHOGENESIS

There are three stages of syphilis (primary, secondary, and tertiary); see "Syphilis" in Section I, p 198 for description of etiology.

CLINICAL PRESENTATION / PHYSICAL FINDINGS

PRIMARY SYPHILIS
- Localized chancre/ulceration at point of contact after 21-day incubation period.
- Open wound contains numerous spirochetes.

SECONDARY SYPHILIS
- Manifests 3 to 10 years after initial infection following occasional long latency period of assumed successful treatment.

TERTIARY SYPHILIS
- Involves every organ, primarily central nervous system (CNS) and cardiovascular system.
- Destructive lesions called gummas can produce horrific damage to the palate, nose, and alveolus via osteomyelitis.
- Dizziness, blurred vision, dementia, and behavioral changes (neurosyphilis) caused by CNS lesions.
- Cardiovascular lesions in the walls of large blood vessels and heart tissue produce aneurysms and poor cardiac output.

CONGENITAL SYPHILIS
- Transferred from mother
- Seen at birth; often has latency period
- Hutchinson triad: blindness, deafness, and dental anomalies

DIAGNOSIS

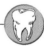

DIFFERENTIAL DIAGNOSIS
- TB, sarcoid/squamous cell carcinoma

LABORATORY
- ICE syphilis recombinant antigen test
- Fluorescent treponemal antibody-absorption (FTA-ABS) test
- Dark field microscopy via Warthin-Starry staining

IMAGING
- CT, MRI for tertiary disease detection and to assess the amount of destruction.
- Angiography, echocardiogram, and ECG may be useful in detection of cardiovascular destruction.

See "Syphilis" in Section I, p 198 for more information on diagnosis techniques.

MEDICAL MANAGEMENT & TREATMENT

Varies depending on stage of syphilis. Generally, penicillin G benzathine, 1.2 to 2.4 million units IM in the gluteal region three times at 7-day intervals.

COMPLICATIONS

See "Syphilis" in Section I, p 198 for information on complications.

PROGNOSIS

Lesions in primary syphilis generally heal with antibiotic treatment in 1 to 2 weeks; 4 to 8 weeks without treatment. Prognosis for other stages of syphilis varies.

DENTAL SIGNIFICANCE

Dental anomalies of congenital syphilis include peg-shaped lateral incisors and "mulberry molars," which lack cuspal development.

See "Syphilis" in Section I, p 198 for more information on dental significance.

SUGGESTED REFERENCE

Marx RE, Stern D (eds): *Oral and Maxillofacial Pathology. A Rationale for Diagnosis and Treatment.* Carol Stream, IL, Quintessence Publishing Company, 2003.

AUTHORS: **LAWRENCE T. HERMAN, DMD, MD; SARA H. RUNNELS, DMD, MD; PAUL R. WILSON, DMD**

SYNONYM(S)

Thyroglossal tract cyst
Thyrolingual duct cyst

ICD-9CM/CPT CODE(S)

759.2 Thyroglossal duct cyst
CPT General Exam or Consultation
(e.g., 99243 or 99213)

OVERVIEW

- Congenital defect that represents a slowly-expanding mass usually found at the midline of the anterior neck
- Most commonly found after an upper respiratory tract infection in which the cyst becomes fluid-filled and/or infected

EPIDEMIOLOGY & DEMOGRAPHICS

PREDOMINANT AGE: 60% are found in adults in their second decade.

ETIOLOGY & PATHOGENESIS

- Cysts develop from remnants of cells in the formation of the thyroid gland as it descends from the posterior tongue to its final position in the lower neck.

CLINICAL PRESENTATION / PHYSICAL FINDINGS

- Small, round, often painful mass in anterior neck.
- Sixty percent occur in midline of neck.
- Fifteen percent occur off midline of neck.
- Two percent occur within tongue.

DIAGNOSIS

Mass often moves superiorly upon extension of tongue.

DIFFERENTIAL DIAGNOSIS

- Lipoma
- Dermoid cyst
- Cat scratch disease
- Lymphoma

LABORATORY TESTS

- Thyroid function test, TSH, T3, T4

IMAGING/SPECIAL TESTS

- Ultrasound to evaluate size and location
- Thyroid scans to evaluate hyperactivity of thyroid gland
- CT or MRI to evaluate anatomic site and confirm cystic fluid-filled lesion

MEDICAL MANAGEMENT & TREATMENT

- Antibiotic therapy
- Sistrunk procedure with or without removal of the hyoid body

PROGNOSIS

Excellent following complete removal.

DENTAL MANAGEMENT

Refer to oral/maxillofacial surgeon, ear/ nose/throat (ENT) specialist.

SUGGESTED REFERENCES

Marx RE, Stern D (eds): *Oral and Maxillofacial Pathology. A Rationale for Diagnosis and Treatment.* Carol Stream, IL, Quintessence Publishing Company, 2003.
www.healthsystem.virginia.edu/uvahealth/peds_ent/thyrgduct.cfm

AUTHORS: **LAWRENCE T. HERMAN, DMD, MD; SARA II. RUNNELS, DMD, MD; PAUL R. WILSON, DMD**

SECTION II

SYNONYM(S)

Exostoses
Bony exostoses
Torus mandibularis
Torus palatinus
Mandibular tori
Palatal tori
Tubercles

ICD-9CM/CPT CODE(S)

526.81 Exostosis of jaw (torus mandibularis and torus palatinus)
CPT   General Exam or Consultation (e.g., 99243 or 99213)

OVERVIEW

Tori/exostoses are nonpathologic, localized osseous protuberances that vary in size, shape, and location and arise from the alveolar cortical plates of the jaw bones. Considered developmental anomalies (hamartomas) of generally little or no clinical concern, they are composed of cancellous bone covered with compact bone. Several variants exist:

- Palatal tori: a boney hard mass seen arising along the midline suture of the hard palate.
- Mandibular tori: bony protuberances seen along the lingual aspect of the mandible in the canine and premolar region above the mylohyoid line. Ninety percent are bilateral, may be single or multinodular, and can become so large as to "kiss" in the midline.
- Buccal exostoses: bilateral or unilateral rows of bony, hard nodules along the facial aspect of the maxillary and/or mandibular alveolar ridge.
- Palatal exostoses: bilateral or unilateral bony protuberances that develop along the lingual aspect of the maxillary tuberosities.
- Solitary exostoses: bony nodules that may occur in response to local irritation or may be seen under free gingival or skin grafts due to stimulation of the underlying periosteum.
- Reactive subpontine exostosis: rare, bony growth that may develop from alveolar crestal bone beneath the pontic of a posterior fixed bridge.

EPIDEMIOLOGY & DEMOGRAPHICS

INCIDENCE/PREVALENCE IN USA:
Approximate prevalence of torus palatinus in the U.S. is 20–35%, and torus mandibularis in 7–10% of the general population. Studies have reported anywhere from 10–60% prevalence depending upon population and methods used in studies. Tori are more common in dentate individuals.
PREDOMINANT AGE: Highest incidence in adults aged 35 to 65 years.
PREDOMINANT SEX:
- Palatal tori are twice as common in women; presence of large, palatal tori

in postmenopausal Caucasian women has been correlated with higher mean bone densities.
- Mandibular tori are equally distributed among the sexes.

GENETICS:
- Several studies indicate an autosomal dominant genetic transmission.
- Least common in Chileans (0.4%); most common in Asians and the Inuit (66–80%).
- Mandibular tori are slightly more common in African-Americans.
- Palatal tori are more common in Caucasians.

ETIOLOGY & PATHOGENESIS

Unknown but postulated to be dynamic lesions caused by an interplay of:
- Genetic influences
- Functional factors (masticatory forces, occlusal hyperfunction)
- Nutrition
- Behavior
- Climate

CLINICAL PRESENTATION / PHYSICAL FINDINGS

- First visible during the second or third decades of life but may occur at any age.
- Not usually noticed until middle age and patient may be alarmed upon finally noticing its presence.
- May increase in size throughout life but most are less than 2 cm in greatest dimension.
- Generally asymptomatic.
- Exostoses, by definition, occur on the facial aspect of the alveolar processes.
- Mandibular tori occur on the lingual aspect of the mandible; palatal tori on the palate.
- Thin, pale overlying mucosas are easily susceptible to ulceration from trauma.
- Shape of tori is variable but may be described as flat, spindle-shaped (most common), nodular, irregular, or lobular.
- Tori and exostoses may be grooved, sessile, or pedunculated.

DIAGNOSIS

Tori and exostosis are generally an easy clinical diagnosis.
DIFFERENTIAL DIAGNOSIS
- Large tori: osteoma, osteoblastomas, osteoid osteomas, odontomas, malignant bony tumors (osteosarcomas, metastatic tumors).
- Palatal tori may be confused with salivary gland tumors, palatal abscesses, lymphomas, infectious diseases, or sinus pathology.
IMAGING
- Tori and exostoses may be seen as relative radiopacities on dental radiographs.

- Radiopacities may be superimposed over the roots of teeth.
- Mandibular tori are easily visualized on occlusal radiographs.
- More sophisticated imaging and laboratory tests are unnecessary unless the diagnosis is uncertain.

MEDICAL MANAGEMENT & TREATMENT

Generally, tori do not need any treatment unless prosthetic appliances need to be placed in the area of the bony overgrowth. In such cases, the tori may be removed either through use of chisels or rotary instruments.

COMPLICATIONS

- Benign condition has infrequent complications (ulceration, pain).
- Due to the thin mucosa, overlying tori and exostoses are easily traumatized with the resulting ulceration sometimes taking a long time to heal.
- A new complication being reported in recent years has been the exposure of tori in patients taking bisphosphonate medications. These lesions may especially be problematic in healing. Sequestration and infection may occur in cases uncomplicated by the bisphosphonates but may be problematic if bisphosphonates are being administered to the patient.

PROGNOSIS

Condition is benign; generally tori are not problematic and can be removed if prosthetic devices must be made.

DENTAL SIGNIFICANCE

This is an oral/maxillofacial pathologic condition with direct dental implications.

DENTAL MANAGEMENT

- In patients being administered bisphosphonates, the tori should not be surgically manipulated, and the clinician should be aware that even in patients not on bisphosphonates the overlying mucosa is often easily traumatized.
  - If lesion is ulcerated, emphasize good hygiene and rinsing with warm salt water or chlorhexidine.
- Prostheses may need to be adjusted.
- Consider OTC pain medications as needed.
- Most tori and exostoses are slow-growing and clinically distinct; biopsy is usually unnecessary.

- If the diagnosis is unclear, biopsy to rule out other bony pathology.
- Surgical removal may be necessary if:
  - Mass is repeatedly exposed to trauma or becomes ulcerated or painful.
  - Needed to accommodate a dental prosthesis.
  - Necessary to allow proper flap adaptation during periodontal surgery.
  - Mass interferes with oral hygiene, speech, or mastication or if associated with adjacent periodontal disease.
  - Patient desires removal (cancerphobia).

SUGGESTED REFERENCES

Abrams S. Complete denture covering mandibular tori using three base materials: a case report. *J Can Dent Assoc* 2000;66: 494–496.

Antoniades DZ, et al. Concurrence of torus palatinus with palatal and buccal exostoses. *Oral Surg Oral Med Oral Pathol Oral Radiol Endod* 1998;85:552–557.

Belsky JL, et al. Torus palatinus: a new anatomical correlation with bone density in postmenopausal women. *J Clin Endocrinol Metab* 2003;88(5):2081–2086.

Echeverria JJ, et al. Exostosis following a free gingival graft. *J Clin Periodontol* 2002;29: 474–477.

Exostoses, torus palatinus, and torus mandibularis, in Neville B, Damm D, Allen C, Bouquot J (eds): *Oral & Maxillofacial Pathology*, ed 2. Philadelphia, WB Saunders, 2002, pp 18–21.

Gorsky M, et al. Genetic influence on the prevalence of torus palatinus. *Am J Med Gen* 1998;75:138–140.

Jainkittivong A, et al. Buccal and palatal exostoses: prevalence and concurrence with tori, *Oral Surg Oral Med Oral Pathol Oral Radiol Endod* 2000;90:48–53.

Komori T, et al. Time-related changes in a case of torus palatinus. *J Oral Maxillofac Surg* 1998;56:492–494.

Ruprecht A, Hellstein J, Bobinet K, Mattinson C. The prevalence of radiographically evident mandibular tori in the University of Iowa dental patients. *Dentomaxillofac Radiol* 2000;29:291–296.

Sonnier KE, et al. Palatal tubercles, palatal tori, and mandibular tori: prevalence and anatomical features in a U.S. population. *Periodontol* 1999;70:329–336.

AUTHORS: **JOHN W. HELLSTEIN, DDS, MS; LAWRENCE T. HERMAN, DMD, MD; SARA H. RUNNELS, DMD, MD; PAUL R. WILSON, DMD**

SECTION II

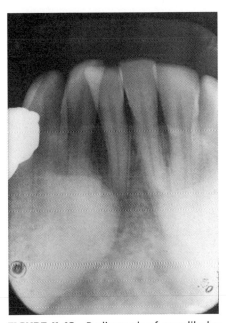

FIGURE II-13 Radiograph of mandibular tori.

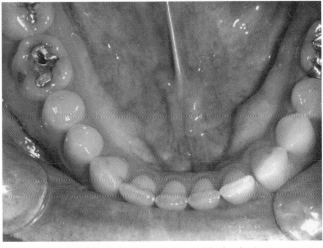

FIGURE II-14 Typical mandibular tori.

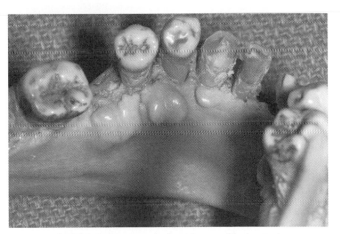

FIGURE II-15 Dry skull with mandibular tori.

Traumatic Fibroma

SYNONYM(S)

Irritation fibroma
Fibrous nodule
Hyperplastic scar
Fibroma
Focal fibrous hyperplasia

ICD-9CM/CPT CODE(S)

210.0 Benign neoplasm of lip
210.1 Benign neoplasm of tongue
210.4 Benign neoplasm, other oral site
CPT   General Exam or Consultation
       (e.g., 99243 or 99213)

OVERVIEW

The most common, benign tumor of the oral cavity.

EPIDEMIOLOGY & DEMOGRAPHICS

INCIDENCE/PREVALENCE IN USA: Frequency is 12 per 1000 adults.
PREDOMINANT AGE: Commonly seen in adults in the fourth to sixth decades of life.
PREDOMINANT SEX: Male to female ratio is 1:2.

ETIOLOGY & PATHOGENESIS

- Reactive (not neoplastic) growth of fibrous connective tissue in response to local irritation or trauma:
  - Cheek or tongue biting
  - Cheek sucking
  - Irritation from dentures, restorations, or subgingival calculus
- Trauma results in overexuberant fibrous scar tissue repair in the submucosa.

CLINICAL PRESENTATION / PHYSICAL FINDINGS

- Can occur anywhere but is most commonly seen along the bite line of the buccal mucosa, on the labial mucosa, lateral tongue, or gingival.
- Pink, smooth, firm nodule similar in color to surrounding tissues.
- Lesions may be gray-brown color in African-Americans.
- If continually traumatized, the surface may be white (due to excess keratin).
- May be broad-based (sessile) or on a stalk (pedunculated).
- Nodules do not blanch and are not painful to palpation.
- Average size is 1.5 cm or less.
- Slow-growing.
- Most are asymptomatic unless traumatized or ulcerated.

DIAGNOSIS

DIFFERENTIAL DIAGNOSIS

- Schwannoma, neurofibroma or granular cell tumor
- Lipoma
- Leiomyoma
- Mucocele
- Benign salivary gland tumor
- Malignant tumors (salivary, metastatic)

MEDICAL MANAGEMENT & TREATMENT

No specific medical management/treatment; see Dental Management following.

PROGNOSIS

- Excellent prognosis with complete excision
- Rarely recur unless the area continues to be traumatized
- No malignant potential

DENTAL SIGNIFICANCE

This is an oral/maxillofacial pathologic condition with direct dental implications.

DENTAL MANAGEMENT

- Smooth any sharp restorations and relieve dentures.
- Nonsteroidal pain medications as needed.
- Conservative surgical excision/biopsy to exclude more serious pathology.

SUGGESTED REFERENCES

Bouquot JE, et al. Oral exophytic lesions in 23,616 white Americans over 35 years of age. *Oral Surg Oral Med Oral Path* 1986;62(3):284–291.
Christopoulos P, et al. True fibroma of the oral mucosa: a case report. *Int J Oral Maxillofac Surg* 1994;23:98–99.
Neville B, Damm D, Allen C, Bouquot J (eds): *Oral & Maxillofacial Pathology*, ed 2. Philadelphia, WB Saunders, 2002, pp 438–439.

AUTHOR: **SARA H. RUNNELS, DMD, MD**

SYNONYM(S)

TN
Fothergill's disease
Tic douloureux ("painful jerking")
Hemifacial spasm
Trifacial neuralgia

ICD-9CM/CPT CODE(S)

350.1 Trigeminal neuralgia
350.2 Atypical facial pain
350.8 Other specified trigeminal disorder
350.9 Trigeminal neuralgia, unspecified
CPT General Exam or Consultation
(e.g., 99243 or 99213)

OVERVIEW

Trigeminal neuralgia is a peripheral neuropathic pain syndrome that occurs along one or more divisions of the trigeminal nerve. It is one of the most common and severe pain syndromes (also known as "suicide disease") and is generally recognized by history alone. Two major forms exist: primary (idiopathic) type (exam reveals no motor or sensory impairments) and secondary type (more common form caused by compression of the trigeminal root by an aberrant blood vessel). Trigeminal neuralgia is typical when a patient is pain-free between paroxysmal attacks but can also occur when a patient has constant, dull background pain between attacks (which may represent an evolution from the typical course).

EPIDEMIOLOGY & DEMOGRAPHICS

INCIDENCE/PREVALENCE IN USA:
Two to 5 per 100,000 people affected annually. No racial differences have been noted. Seasonal (fall and spring) exacerbations seen due to increase in temperature, humidity, or pollen.
PREDOMINANT AGE: Prevalence increases with age. Ninety percent benign after age 40 (mean age is 50) but may occur at any age. In younger patients, suspect multiple sclerosis.
PREDOMINANT SEX: Female preponderance (3:2).
GENETICS: Most cases are sporadic, but familial (autosomal dominant) cases have been reported.

ETIOLOGY & PATHOGENESIS

- Uncertain.
- Popular theory is that an aberrant vascular loop compresses a trigeminal nerve root a few millimeters from the exit from the pons (nerve root entry zone).
- Compression produces focal demyelination of axons, which allows for ectopic foci of nerve impulses to be generated or cross-talk between other axons and the thalamus.

- Nerve compression and TN may also be due to aneurysms, tumors, inflammatory disease, metabolic abnormalities, infections, trauma, or multiple sclerosis demyelinations.

CLINICAL PRESENTATION / PHYSICAL FINDINGS

- Initial onset of attacks is spontaneous.
- Pain in distribution of trigeminal branch described as burning, shooting, stabbing, lancinating, or electric-like in nature.
- Right side of face affected more often than left; 90% are unilateral.
- Always limited to the trigeminal nerve (usually the maxillary and mandibular divisions and, rarely, the ophthalmic division).
- Pain may provoke brief facial muscle spasm (tic), excess lacrimation, or skin flushing.
- Attacks are brief and paroxysmal (may last few seconds to a few minutes) and are repetitive with short intervals between attacks (may have hundreds during one day).
- Attacks can overlap.
- Attacks may be spontaneous or evoked by mild, nonpainful stimuli on specific areas of the scalp, face, or oral cavity (trigger zones).
- Common trigger zones include the skin of the nose, lips, eyes, and ears.
- Patients can often identify the trigger zone.
- Common triggers include facial sensory stimulation (light touch, vibration) or facial movement (during eating, talking, shaving, brushing teeth, or applying makeup).
- Attacks occur in bouts lasting weeks to months followed by periods of spontaneous remission of variable duration.
- Attacks rarely occur at night during sleep.
- Physical exam is usually normal (may see mild sensory loss in the distribution of one branch of the trigeminal nerve).

DIAGNOSIS

DIFFERENTIAL DIAGNOSIS

- Myofascial pain disorder
- Intracranial tumors
- Trigeminal neuropathy
- Vascular anomalies
- Atypical neuralgia
- Local disease of the sinus, jaw, throat, dentition or facial bones
- Neuralgia-inducing cavitational osteonecrosis (NICO)
- Temporomandibular joint disorders
- Multiple sclerosis
- Postherpetic neuralgia
- Cluster headaches
- Glossopharyngeal neuralgia
- Consider diagnostic nerve blocks

CRITERIA FOR DIAGNOSIS

- Severe, lancinating, paroxysmal pain
- Unilateral
- Limited to a division of the trigeminal nerve
- Trigger areas present
- No sensory deficit apparent

MEDICAL MANAGEMENT & TREATMENT

- Drug therapy is first-line therapy.
- Goal is to use monotherapy maintained at the lowest effective dose.
- First-line agents are carbamazepine (Tegretol), oxycarbezine (Trileptal), baclofen (Lioresal), and phenytoin (Dilantin).
- Dosage can be reduced slowly if patient is pain-free for 4 to 6 weeks.
- If monotherapy is unsuccessful, consider adding or using alternative medications: clonazepam (Klonopin), lamotrigine (Lamictal), gabapentin (Neurontin), topiramate (Topamax), or valproic acid (Depakote).
- Surgical therapy used for patients unable to tolerate or are unresponsive to medications or if MRI reveals area of compression.
- Most successful when applied early in course.
- Goal is to partially destroy the trigeminal ganglion or root or decompress it.
- Surgical options:
  - Percutaneous radiofrequency trigeminal gangliolysis
  - Percutaneous retrogasserian glycerol rhizolysis
  - Percutaneous balloon decompression of the ganglion
  - Gamma knife radiosurgery
  - Microvascular decompression of the trigeminal nerve root
- Complementary and alternative options include transcutaneous electrical nerve stimulation (TENS), hypnosis, and biofeedback.

COMPLICATIONS

- Morbidity due to fear of attacks, which then limits the patient's activity (stay at home, oral intake impaired, weight loss ensues).
- High rate of secondary depression.
- Infrequent sequelae of therapy include anesthesia dolorosa (painful numbness), corneal ulceration, reactivation of herpetic infections, and blood dyscrasias due to medications.

PROGNOSIS

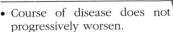

- Course of disease does not progressively worsen.

- Seventy percent of patients respond to initial drug therapy.
- In 50% of cases medical therapy ultimately fails, thus necessitating surgery.
- May recur, which then requires reinstating therapy.
- Clusters of attacks wax and wane, with shorter periods of remission with older age.
- Dull ache may persist between paroxysms later in course.

DENTAL SIGNIFICANCE

- Fear of contact with trigger zone causes patients to avoid cleaning the affected area (including the skin and oral cavity) leading to skin debris, ulceration, and intraoral caries and periodontal disease.
- Dental disease may exacerbate symptoms; it is important that patients maintain healthy dentition.

SUGGESTED REFERENCES

Ashkenazi A, Levin M. Three common neuralgias: how to manage trigeminal, occipital, and postherpetic pain. *Postgrad Med* 2004;116(3):16–32.

Bagheri S, et al. Diagnosis and treatment of patients with trigeminal neuralgia. *JADA* 2004;135:1713–1717.

Huff JS. Trigeminal neuralgia. *eMedicine online,* 2005.

Liu JK, Apfelbaum RI. Treatment of trigeminal neuralgia. *Neurosurg Clin N Am* 2004;15(5): 319–334.

Scrivani S, et al. Percutaneous stereotactic radiofrequency thermal rhizotomy for the treatment of trigeminal neuralgia. *J Oral Maxillofac Surg* 1999;57:104–111.

AUTHOR: **SARA H. RUNNELS, DMD, MD**

SECTION II

SYNONYM(S)

TB
Consumption
Scrofula

ICD-9CM/CPT CODE(S)

010.0–018.9 Tuberculosis

OVERVIEW

A disease caused by the slow-growing bacterium *Mycobacterium tuberculosis* that characteristically attacks the lungs, but may attack other areas of the body as well (kidney, spine, brain, lymph nodes, etc.). Once was the leading cause of death in the U.S. Multidrug-resistant form (MDR-TB) was first recognized in 1991; this has a more virulent course, is difficult to treat, and is often fatal (70%).

EPIDEMIOLOGY & DEMOGRAPHICS

INCIDENCE/PREVALENCE IN USA: Resurgence was seen from 1985 to 1992 due to rise in HIV-positive and indigent populations; indigent populations have a risk that is 300 times greater than the national risk and HIV-positive persons have a risk 200 to 400 times greater than the national risk. More than 14,000 reported cases in the U.S. in 2004; highest rates seen in California, Florida, Illinois, New York, and Texas. Worldwide prevalence is 2 billion, with 8 million new cases and mortality estimated at 3 million annually. Ninety percent of exposed people are clinically asymptomatic, 5% develop disease within the first year, and 5% develop disease later in life. Active TB is fatal in up to 50% of untreated individuals.

PREDOMINANT AGE: Two-thirds of cases occur among minorities (median age 39 years). Majority of cases are in the 25- to 44-year-old age bracket.

PREDOMINANT SEX: Risk is twice as high for men as women.

ETIOLOGY & PATHOGENESIS

- Spread via aerosolized droplets: an infected person with active TB coughs or sneezes expelling droplets that are then inhaled by others, leading to disease.
- A single cough may generate 3000 droplets.
- Mycobacterium then settle and grow in the lungs and throat and are easily spread to other people.
- Active disease occurs if the immune system is unable to control the growth of TB (10–30%).
- Disseminated infection to other organs occurs via hematogenous route (miliary TB).
- Most commonly, the immune system is able to prevent bacterial growth, causing inactivation of the bacterium and lack of symptoms but a positive PPD (latent TB).
- Reactivation of latent TB occurs in 1% per year of immunocompetent hosts and 10% in the immunocompromised.
- Less commonly, TB may also be acquired by consuming infected, unpasteurized cow's milk.

CLINICAL PRESENTATION / PHYSICAL FINDINGS

- Patients who develop an active infection usually have pulmonary symptoms (80%):
  ○ Cough lasting longer than 2 weeks
  ○ Productive cough
  ○ Dyspnea
  ○ Chest pain
  ○ Hemoptysis
- Other symptoms of active disease include:
  ○ Weakness or fatigue
  ○ Anorexia
  ○ Fever
  ○ Weight loss
  ○ Chills
  ○ Night sweats
- Most common extrapulmonary manifestation is asymptomatic cervical or supraclavicular lymphadenopathy (10%).
- Less than 1% exhibit primary TB of the head and neck (persistent, painful ulceration, discrete mass or swelling, intrabony involvement, or salivary gland enlargement).
- Scrofula is tuberculous lymphadenitis of the cervical lymph nodes acquired through drinking infected milk.
- People who have TB but do not feel sick and have no symptoms have latent TB.
- Patients with latent TB cannot spread TB to others but may themselves develop active disease.

DIAGNOSIS

DIFFERENTIAL DIAGNOSIS

- Lymphoma
- Bacterial or viral pneumonia
- Fungal infection
- Oral ulcers may be confused with:
  ○ Traumatic lesions
  ○ Squamous cell carcinoma
  ○ Syphilitic chancres

LABORATORY TESTS

- Tuberculin skin test (PPD) (5 units or 0.1 mL) intradermally injected, then read at least 48 hours later (for induration, not erythema)
- Positivity is:
  ○ 5 mm + induration if HIV-positive or recent active infection
  ○ 10 mm + induration for IV drug abusers, homeless persons, prisoners, nursing home residents, or other indigent populations
  ○ 15 mm + induration in young and healthy patients
- Immunosuppressed individuals may not be able to mount an immune response to this test; an anergy panel should also be injected to test their immunocompetence.
- Patients who received a bacille Calmette-Guérin (BCG) vaccine as children may have a positive PPD that may be difficult to interpret.
- QuantiFERON-TB Gold (QFT) is a blood test used to check for the presence of TB proteins but is not universally available.
- Mycobacterial bacteremia (bacillemia) is also detectable using specific blood cultures.
- Sputum samples should be obtained to check for the presence of mycobacterium (acid-fast bacilli).
- Lymph nodes or other oral lesions may be biopsied if diagnosis unclear.
- For disseminated infections, more specific testing is warranted (urinalysis, blood cultures, etc.).
- All patients with active TB who are not known to be HIV-positive should have HIV testing.
- Prior to beginning treatment, a battery of tests should be done (liver function tests, complete blood count, blood chemistry) to monitor for drug side effects.

IMAGING

- Patients with positive PPD or QFT should have a chest radiograph.
- In active disease, ipsilateral hilar adenopathy may be seen with atelectasis.
- In latent disease, calcified lesions (Ghon lesion) are seen classically in the apical portion of the lungs.

MEDICAL MANAGEMENT & TREATMENT

- Patients with active disease should be quarantined until no longer infectious (either at home or in negative-pressure rooms in the hospital).
- Multidrug therapy is used to treat active infections to kill a larger volume of mycobacterium and prevent resistance until drug susceptibilities are known.
- The most common drug regimen includes the following four medications for 6 months:
  ○ Isoniazid (INH)
  ○ Rifampin (RIF)
  ○ Ethambutol (ETB)
  ○ Pyrazinamide (PZA)
- Therapy for 2 weeks reduces bacterial load one hundredfold.
- Patients must be monitored for major side effects to the medications: anorexia, nausea, vomiting, jaundice, fever, abdominal pain, tingling in the extremities, rash, easy bleeding, arthralgias, circumoral tingling, visual changes, tinnitus, hearing loss, and seizures.

- Minor side effects include:
  - Photosensitivity
  - Orange discoloration of urine, saliva, or tears
  - Interaction with methadone treatment
  - Ineffectiveness of birth control pills (requiring the use of another form of birth control)
- Patients with latent TB (with a positive PPD or QFT) and are at high risk should be treated to prevent active infection. Patients at high risk include:
  - HIV-positive
  - Elderly
  - Those infected in the last 2 years
  - IV drug abusers
  - Babies and young children
  - Pregnant women
  - Other immunosuppressive states
- Patients with latent infections generally have a lower bacterial load; thus, many are successfully treated with only one medication, INH (Isoniazid).

PROGNOSIS

- Prognosis excellent if patient is complaint with drug therapy and monitored closely by their physician.
- Complications include development of cavitary lesions, spread to susceptible contacts, drug resistance, and side effects of medications.

DENTAL SIGNIFICANCE

All healthcare workers and caregivers should use respiratory precautions.

DENTAL MANAGEMENT

Patients presenting with suspected or proven cases of TB must be reported to the local public health department and quarantined until notified by their physician. Dental professionals who have been in close contact with such a patient should be tested for latent TB and treated prophylactically.

SUGGESTED REFERENCES

Alawi F. Granulomatous diseases of the oral tissues: differential diagnosis and update. *Den Clin N Am* 2005;49:203–221.

Centers for Disease Control Website: www.cdc.org for Questions and Answers About TB.

Li J. Tuberculosis, on www.eMedicine.com

Marx RE, Stern D (eds): *Oral and Maxillofacial Pathology. A Rationale for Diagnosis and Treatment.* Carol Stream, IL, Quintessence Publishing Company, 2003, pp 39–44.

Sezer B, et al. Oral mucosal ulceration: a manifestation of previously undiagnosed pulmonary tuberculosis. *JADA* 2004;135: 336–340.

AUTHOR: **SARA H. RUNNELS, DMD, MD**

SYNONYM(S)

See Clinical Presentation/Physical Findings following for the names of specific deficiencies.

ICD-9CM/CPT CODE(S)

264.9 Vitamin A deficiency
266.9 B complex deficiency
265.0 with beriberi
265.2 with pellagra
265.1 Vitamin B_1 deficiency
266.0 Vitamin B_2 deficiency
266.1 Vitamin B_6 deficiency
266.2 Vitamin B_{12} or folate deficiency
267 Vitamin C deficiency with scurvy
268.9 Vitamin D deficiency
268.2 with osteomalacia
268.0 with rickets
269.1 Vitamin E deficiency
269.0 Vitamin K deficiency
269.2 Multiple deficiency
CPT General Exam or Consultation (e.g., 99243 or 99213)

OVERVIEW

Vitamins are organic compounds needed in trace amounts for normal physiologic functions and for proper growth and development. They are not produced in sufficient amounts by the body; they must be obtained from external food sources. Vitamins are categorized as fat-soluble (A, D, E, K) or water-soluble (C, B vitamins, biotin, and folate). Fat-soluble vitamins are stored in body fat and can reach toxic levels whereas water-soluble vitamins are not stored, which means they need to be included in the diet daily. Deficiencies in these nutrients (especially water-soluble vitamins) can result in a wide variety of illnesses.

EPIDEMIOLOGY & DEMOGRAPHICS

INCIDENCE/PREVALENCE IN USA: Less common in the U.S. compared with developing countries.

ETIOLOGY & PATHOGENESIS

- Seen more commonly in patients with a history of malabsorptive syndromes, alcoholism, certain medications, pregnancy, hemodialysis, total parenteral nutrition, certain fad diets, unbalanced diets, eating disorders, or inborn errors of metabolism.
- Deficiencies are also more likely to occur as a component of general malnutrition.
- Deficiencies occur slowly over time, with specific symptoms seen late in the course of deficiency.
- Fat-soluble vitamin (A, D, E, K) absorption is dependent on the gut (ileum) and pancreas.
- Diseases that interfere with gut absorption (malabsorption syndromes such as celiac sprue, enteritis, or cystic fibrosis,

or bowel resection) or pancreatic disease (pancreatitis, tumors) can lead to fat-soluble vitamin deficiencies.
- Biotin and vitamin K can be manufactured by the intestinal flora and certain antibiotics may kill off the bacteria, resulting in a deficiency.
- Biotin absorption is also inhibited by the ingestion of raw eggs.
- Water-soluble vitamins are not stored in the body (except for B_{12}, which is stored in the liver); inadequate intake gradually results in deficiency.
- Intrinsic factor (IF) is necessary for absorption of B_{12}, and deficiency of IF results in pernicious anemia.
- Certain medications can also lead to deficiencies [isoniazid produces B_6 deficiency and warfarin (Coumadin) is a vitamin K antagonist].
- During winter months or if the skin is not adequately exposed to sunlight, vitamin D deficiency may occur.

CLINICAL PRESENTATION / PHYSICAL FINDINGS

- Vitamin A (retinol) is a constituent of visual pigments and aids in maintenance of epithelium. Deficiency can result in night blindness, dry eyes (xerophthalmia), corneal ulceration, and dry skin or mucous membranes.
- Vitamin B_1 (thiamine) functions as a cofactor in the citric acid cycle and associated pathways. Beriberi is a deficiency associated with "polished" rice diets and produces polyneuritis, cardiac failure, and edema. Wernicke-Korsakoff syndrome is seen in malnourished alcoholics, causing brain lesions that lead to psychosis, ophthalmoplegia, ataxia, confusion, anterograde amnesia, and confabulations.
- Vitamin B_2 (riboflavin) is a cofactor in oxidative-reductive reactions. Deficiency may result in angular stomatitis, cheilosis, mouth soreness, seborrheic dermatitis, corneal vascularization, and anemia.
- Vitamin B_3 (niacin) is derived from tryptophan and is a cofactor for oxidative-reduction reactions in the generation of adenosine triphosphate (ATP). Pellagra is the deficiency characterized by diarrhea, dermatitis, dementia, and glossitis.
- Vitamin B_5 (pantothenate) is a cofactor in fatty acid synthesis, with deficiency characterized by dermatitis, enteritis, alopecia, and adrenal insufficiency.
- Vitamin B_6 (pyridoxine) is a cofactor in several metabolic reactions. Deficiency is manifested by stomatitis, glossitis, cheilitis, weakness, hyperirritability, and convulsions if severe. May be caused by isoniazid use for treatment of tuberculosis.
- Biotin is a cofactor in carboxylation reactions, and deficiency may result in dermatitis or enteritis.

- Folic acid (folate) is a coenzyme in several reactions and is important in the synthesis of DNA and RNA. Deficiency in utero can result in neural tube defects and, in adults, macrocytic or megaloblastic anemia.
- Vitamin B_{12} (cobalamin) is synthesized by bacteria and is found only in animal products; it is important in several metabolic reactions. Deficiency may result in pernicious or megaloblastic anemia with neurologic sequelae (optic neuropathy, subacute combined degeneration syndrome, paresthesia) and glossitis.
- Vitamin C (ascorbic acid) cross-links collagen in collagen synthesis. Deficiency results in scurvy characterized by malaise, weakness, gingival hyperplasia, bleeding, easy bruising, anemia, petechiae, and delayed wound healing.
- Vitamin D (ergocalciferol, cholecalciferol) increases absorption of calcium and phosphate and resorption of these minerals from bone. Deficiency results in rickets in children (bones bend easily and enamel and dentin may be abnormal, leading to delayed eruption of teeth) or osteomalacia in adults (softening of bones to hypomineralized matrix).
- Vitamin E (alpha tocopherol) is an antioxidant that protects cell membranes, specifically protecting red blood cells from hemolysis. Deficiency results in increased fragility of erythrocytes. Other symptoms include areflexia, gait disturbances, ophthalmoplegia, and other neurologic deficits.
- Vitamin K is synthesized by intestinal flora and catalyzes the carboxylation of glutamic acid components of clotting factors II, VII, IX, X, and protein C and S. Deficiency can result in increased PT and PTT with increased bleeding (often of the gingiva).

DIAGNOSIS

Differential diagnosis depends on which organ system is affected, but may include:
- Congestive heart failure (CHF)
- Peripheral neuropathy
- Malnutrition
- Infection
- Allergy
- Neoplasm

MEDICAL MANAGEMENT & TREATMENT

- Deficiencies are generally replaced orally unless otherwise indicated.
- Niacin is replaced (along with tryptophan) at 10 mg per day.
- Thiamine should be given as 50 mg per day IM for several days, then 2.0 to 2.5 mg daily by mouth.

- Riboflavin is given orally as 30 mg per day then tapered to 2 to 4 mg per day.
- Niacin replacement is 300 to 500 mg per day.
- Pyridoxine may be supplemented at 30 mg per day (or higher with certain medications such as isoniazid).
- Vitamin C is given as 100 mg three to five times per day until a total of 4 g has been given, then 100 mg per day.
- Vitamin D may be supplemented orally as 600+ mg per day in sun-deprived patients.
- Night blindness and conjunctival dryness may be treated with 30,000 IU of vitamin A daily for 1 week; corneal ulcers are treated with higher daily doses.
- Vitamin E replacement is 50 to 100 IU per day by mouth.
- Vitamin K may be given as 10 mg IM or SC for emergent bleeding.

- Chronic treatment: daily multivitamin supplementation as well as a balanced diet.

PROGNOSIS

- Prognosis depends on whether replacement was undertaken expeditiously and to what extent the deficiency had progressed prior to diagnosis.
- Wernicke Korsakoff syndrome (B_1 deficiency) is unfortunately irreversible.

DENTAL SIGNIFICANCE

Signs of vitamin deficiencies may be noted during dental appointments with the presence of such conditions as cheilosis (vitamin B_2), cheilitis (vitamin B_6), mouth soreness (vitamin B_2), glossitis (vitamins B_3, B_6, B_{12}), gingival hyperplasia and bleeding (vitamin C, vitamin K), delayed wound healing (vitamin C), and delayed or deformed eruption of the teeth (vitamin D).

SUGGESTED READINGS

Moynihan P, Petersen P. Diet, nutrition and the prevention of dental disease. *Public Health Nutrition* 2004;7(1A):201–226.
Peckenpaugh, NJ. *Nutrition Essentials and Diet Therapy*. Philadelphia, WB Saunders, 2003, pp 101–113.

AUTHOR: **SARA H. RUNNELS, DMD, MD**

SECTION II

SYNONYM(S)

None

ICD-9CM/CPT CODE(S)
446.4 Wegener's granulomatosis
CPT General Exam or Consultation
  (e.g., 99243 or 99213)

OVERVIEW

Wegener's granulomatosis (WG) is an uncommon, immune-based, necrotizing vasculitis that affects the small arterioles, venules, and capillaries of several organ systems. The classic triad involves the upper airway, lungs, and kidneys, but virtually any organ system can be affected.

EPIDEMIOLOGY & DEMOGRAPHICS

INCIDENCE/PREVALANCE IN USA:
Majority of patients are Caucasian.
PREDOMINANT AGE: Affects adults between 30 and 50 years old
PREDOMINANT SEX: 3:2 male predilection.

ETIOLOGY & PATHOGENESIS

- Autoantibodies are created to cANCA (cytoplasmic pattern antineutrophil cytoplasmic antibodies) and pANCA (perinuclear antineutrophil cytoplasmic antibodies).
- cANCA and pANCA are both autoantibodies to normal components of the cytoplasm of neutrophils.
- These autoantibodies attack these intracellular components, leading to lysis of the cell and the release of enzymes and proteases that produce a localized vasculitis.
- The vasculitis can result in thrombosis and occlusion of vessel lumen, leading to tissue necrosis and destruction. See "Wegener's Granulomatosis" in Section I, p 222 for more information.

CLINICAL PRESENTATION / PHYSICAL FINDINGS

- Diagnosis preceded by several months of upper respiratory and systemic symptoms, which prompt the patient to seek care. See "Wegener's Granulomatosis" in Section I, p 222 for extensive information on signs and symptoms.

DIAGNOSIS

DIFFERENTIAL DIAGNOSIS
- Collagen vascular diseases
- Systemic fungal infections (histoplasmosis, coccidiomycosis, blastomycosis)
- Localized fungal infections (mucormycosis, aspergillosis)
- Granulomatous diseases (sarcoidosis, tuberculosis)
- Malignancy (squamous cell carcinoma, non-Hodgkin's lymphoma, midline lethal granuloma)
- Salivary gland disease (necrotizing sialometaplasia, benign and malignant tumors)

LABORATORY
- CBC (normochromic, normocytic anemia, leukocytosis, thrombocytosis)
- Serum chemistry (elevated BUN and creatinine, decreased creatinine clearance)
- Urinalysis (hematuria, proteinuria, red cell casts)
- Rheumatologic tests [elevated erythrocyte sedimentation rate (ESR) and C-reactive protein, immune complexes, rheumatoid factor present in low to moderate titers in up to 50% of patients with WG]
- Sputum for analysis and culture
- Accessible oral and nasal lesions should be cultured (aerobic, anaerobic, fungal)

IMAGING
- Posteroanterior and lateral chest radiographs
- Chest CT
- CT scan of the head to image sinuses, nasal, mastoid, and ear involvement

BIOPSY
- Necessary for definitive diagnosis.
- If oral lesions are present, these may be biopsied and tested for cANCA and pANCA.
- cANCA-positive specimens are more specific for Wegener's granulomatosis.

MEDICAL MANAGEMENT & TREATMENT

- Cyclophosphamide (Cytoxan) and prednisone daily to immediately control the disease and prevent potentially irreversible kidney damage.
- With this regimen, 90% of patients experience improvement, and 75% achieve a complete remission.
- Azathioprine and plasmapheresis are alternative treatments if cyclophosphamide is contraindicated.

- Sinus disease may be treated with topical corticosteroids, daily saline irrigations, and empiric antibiotics if superinfection is suspected.
- Arthralgia is treated with nonsteroidal antiinflammatory drugs.
- Methotrexate and trimethoprim sulfamethoxazole may be used to maintain remission.

COMPLICATIONS

See "Wegener's Granulomatosis" in Section I, p 222 for information on complications.

PROGNOSIS

- Fatal within 2 years without treatment.
- Most common cause of death results from renal failure.
- If treatment is provided expeditiously, most patients experience long remissions.
- Maintenance therapy may occasionally be necessary.
- All treatments require monitoring of blood counts and for toxic side effects of medications (cyclophosphamide can cause bladder cancer and sterility).

DENTAL MANAGEMENT

See "Wegener's Granulomatosis" in Section I, p 222 for information on dental implications.

Refer to primary care physician, rheumatologist, pulmonologist, otolaryngologist, or nephrologist.

SUGGESTED READINGS
Eufinger H, et al. Oral manifestations of Wegener's granulomatosis. *Int J Oral Maxillofac Surg* 1992;21:50–53.

Marx RE, Stern D (eds): *Oral and Maxillofacial Pathology A Rationale for Diagnosis and Treatment.* Carol Stream, IL, Quintessence Publishing Company, 2003, pp 199–201.

Shafiei K, et al. Wegener Granulomatosis: case report and brief literature review. *J Am Board Fam Pract* 2003;16(6):555–559.

Sneller M. Wegener's granulomatosis. *JAMA* 1995;273(16):1288–1291.

AUTHOR: SARA H. RUNNELS, DMD, MD

Emergencies

SYNONYM(S)

Acute adrenal insufficiency
Addisonian crisis
Adrenal crisis
Relative AI

ICD-9CM/CPT CODE(S)

255.4 Acute adrenal insufficiency
255.4 Corticoadrenal insufficiency
    Addisonian crisis
    Addison's disease NOS
    Adrenal
        Atrophy (autoimmune)
        Calcification
        Crisis
        Hemorrhage
        Infarction
        Insufficiency NOS
    Excludes: Tuberculosis
        Addison's disease (017.6)

OVERVIEW

Acute adrenal insufficiency (AAI) is a rare but life-threatening condition. AAI (also known as relative AI) can occur when the endogenous cortisol production or the exogenous corticosteroid administration is sufficient for the needs of the unstressed patient but insufficient to support the homeostatic needs of the clinically stressed patient. Cortisol is a hormone produced and released by the adrenal gland, but this release is suppressed by the replacement with exogenous corticosteroids, especially in high doses and over an extended period of time.

ETIOLOGY & PATHOGENESIS

- Fever
- Dehydration
- Injury
- Surgery
- Anesthesia
- Inadequate replacement therapy of adrenal insufficiency
- Noncompliance of replacement therapy
- Recent/abrupt stoppage of corticosteroid
- History of long-standing use of corticosteroid

CLINICAL PRESENTATION / PHYSICAL FINDINGS

SIGNS & SYMPTOMS

- Weakness
- Feeling extreme fatigue
- Hypotension from clinical/surgical stress
  - Pallor
  - Diaphoresis
  - Nausea
  - Tachycardia
- Abrupt mental changes
- Loss of consciousness, partial or complete
- Abdominal pain
- Myalgias
- Headache
- Slow/sluggish movement
- Dehydration
- High fever
- Shaking/chills
- Confusion or coma
- Darkening of skin
- Joint pain
- Unintentional weight loss
- Rapid respiratory rate (tachypnea)
- Unusual/excessive sweating of face/palms
- Skin rash may be present
- Loss of appetite

DIAGNOSIS

LABORATORY

- Low fasting blood sugar
- Elevated serum potassium (primary adrenal insufficiency)
- Decreased serum sodium (primary adrenal insufficiency)

TESTS

- ACTH (Cortrosyn) stimulation test shows low cortisol
- Baseline cortisol levels
- Fasting blood sugar is low
- Serum potassium is elevated
- Serum sodium is decreased

MEDICAL MANAGEMENT & TREATMENT

GENERAL

- Terminate procedure.
- Monitor vital signs (pulse, blood pressure, PaO_2, respirations).
- Trendelenburg if hypotensive (< 90/60 mmHg) and symptomatic.
- Activate 911.
- IV access.
- Medications:
  - Dexamethasone (Decadron®), 4mg IV/IM, or hydrocortisone, 100 mg IV
- Fluid replacement is necessary for hypotension.
- 5% dextrose with normal saline: 1 liter, rapid infusion.
- Monitor and record vital signs.
- Transport to medical facility.

SURGICAL MEASURES

- IV access
  - Hypotension: fluid replacement
    - 5% dextrose with normal saline.
    - Rapid infusion.
    - 1 liter.
    - Reevaluate.
    - Oral fluid replacement is not sufficient.
- Medications
  - Dexamethasone (Decadron®), 4mg IV/IM, or hydrocortisone 100 mg IV

MONITORING

- Monitor and record vital signs.
- Blood pressure monitoring before, during, and after stressful procedures.

PREVENTION/AVOIDANCE

- Identify patients at potential risk.
- Hypotension can signal impending adrenal crisis.
- Make patients aware of signs of potential stress.
- Advise patients to carry medical identification.
- Obtain profound local anesthesia and pain control.
- If patient is currently on corticosteroids:
  - Use stress reduction protocol.
  - Monitor pulse and blood pressure before, during, and after appointments.
  - Double daily dose of steroids the day before, the day of, and the day after procedures.
  - Have patient return to regular dose on the second postoperative day.
- If patient is not currently on corticosteroids but meets the "Rule of Twos" (has received at least 20 mg of hydrocortisone (cortisol or equivalent) for more than 2 weeks within the past 2 years):
  - Use stress reduction protocol.
  - Monitor pulse and blood pressure before, during, and after appointments.
  - Double daily dose of steroids the day before, the day of, and the day after procedures.

COMPLICATIONS

- Shock
- Coma
- Seizures
- Life-threatening condition: immediate treatment necessary

PROGNOSIS

Acute adrenal insufficiency is a medical condition that has serious implications for the dental patient. Medical consultation and risk evaluation will allow for a stress reduction protocol to attempt to avoid this situation. In the event that this condition arises, treatment needs to be initiated prior to the arrival of advanced medical support.

DENTAL MANAGEMENT

- Identification of the patient at potential risk for acute adrenal insufficiency and consultation with the patient's treating physician should be done in preparation for treatment of this type of patient. Following the guidelines given for supplemental corticosteroid therapy should be received and documented.
- Avoid hypotension precipitated by rapid patient repositioning from supine to upright position in the dental chair.

SUGGESTED REFERENCE

Bennett JD, Rosenberg MB. *Medical Emergencies in Dentistry*. Philadelphia, WB Saunders, 2002, pp 383–384.

AUTHOR: DONALD P. LEWIS, JR., DDS, CFE

SYNONYM(S)

Foreign body obstruction (FBO)

ICD-9CM/CPT CODE(S)

E912 Airway obstruction (foreign body)

E912 Inhalation and ingestion of other object causing obstruction of respiratory tract or suffocation

Aspiration and inhalation of foreign body except food (into respiratory tract) NOS

    Foreign object in nose

    Obstruction of pharynx by foreign body

    Compression

    Interruption of respiration—by foreign body

    Obstruction of respiration—in esophagus

    Excludes: Injury except asphyxia and obstruction of respiratory passage caused by foreign body (E915)

E915 Obstruction of esophagus by foreign body without mention of asphyxia or obstruction in respiratory passage

933   Foreign body in pharynx and larynx

933.0 Pharynx

    Nasopharynx

    Throat NOS

933.1 Larynx

    Asphyxia due to foreign body

    Choking due to:

        Food (regurgitated)

        Phlegm

934   Foreign body in trachea, bronchus, and lung

934.0 Trachea

934.1 Main bronchus

934.8 Other specified parts

    Bronchioles

    Lung

934.9 Respiratory tree, unspecified

    Inhalation of liquid or vomitus, lower respiratory tract NOS

935   Foreign body in mouth, esophagus, stomach

935.0 Mouth

OVERVIEW

An obstruction caused by soft tissues in the head and neck, bronchoconstriction, secretion, or solid material causing a decrease or absence of ventilatory movements.

ETIOLOGY & PATHOGENESIS

- Supraglottic
  - Posterior displacement of tongue
- Loss of tone of pharyngeal muscles from deep sedation/general anesthesia
- Foreign body: secretions/solid material
- Posterior swelling of tongue

CLINICAL PRESENTATION / FINDINGS

SIGNS & SYMPTOMS

- Choking, gagging
- Violent expiratory effort
- Substernal notch retraction
- Cyanosis
- Labored breathing
- Rapid pulse
- Hypoxia
- Respiratory arrest
- Cardiac arrest

MEDICAL MANAGEMENT & TREATMENT

EARLY TREATMENT

- Place patient in upright position
- Pack off operative/surgical site
- Suction oropharynx
- Traction of tongue anteriorly
- Gauze
- Tongue forceps
- Hemostat
- Suture

ADVANCED TREATMENT

- If no success at clearing airway:
  - Supine position
  - Chin lift, jaw thrust
  - Check for respiratory sounds
  - Ventilate
  - Abdominal thrust
- Continued airway obstruction:
  - Oral/pharyngeal airways
  - Positive pressure ventilation with bag-mask
  - Endotracheal intubation
  - Activate EMS

SWALLOWED OBJECTS

- Cough to attempt to remove
- Heimlich maneuver:
  - Stand behind patient.
  - Place fist slightly above patient's navel.
  - Grasp fist with other hand.
  - Give quick, upward thrust.
- Radiograph to determine if object was swallowed

CHOKING/UNCONSCIOUS

- Activate 911.
- Place patient on back.
- If object can be seen, perform finger sweep.

- Open airway.
- Attempt to ventilate.
- If obstructed, give five abdominal thrusts above navel with heel of hand.
- Repeat until obstruction is clear.

PREVENTION/AVOIDANCE

- Proper placement of mouth pack.
- Preoperative removal of potential foreign bodies.
- Adequate suctioning.
- Adequate visualization.
- Maintain proper head position.
- Training/equipment to deliver positive pressure ventilation (bag-mask-valve ventilation).
  - Must have proper size of mask for ventilation.
  - Rescue breaths need to be delivered slowly.
  - Prevent overbreathing causing gastric distention.

PROGNOSIS

- Breathing returns to normal.
- Foreign body is removed or swallowed.

DENTAL SIGNIFICANCE

- During operative procedures where there is even a remote possibility of having airway obstruction caused by a foreign body, all possible measures should be taken to avoid this potential medical emergency. Throat packs and securing of small dental instruments should be undertaken.
- In the event that the airway is obstructed by a foreign body, timely recognition and treatment are necessary.
- Foreign body airway obstruction is also a major cause of airway depression in pediatric dental patients. The position of the larynx, shape of the epiglottis, and angulation of the right main stem bronchus need to be evaluated, and the differences between the pediatric patient and adult patient need to be recognized.

SUGGESTED REFERENCE

Lewis DP, et al. *Advanced Protocols for Medical Emergencies: An Action Plan for Office Response.*

AUTHOR: DONALD P. LEWIS, JR., DDS, CFE

SECTION III

SYNONYM(S)

Anaphylactic reaction
Anaphylactic shock

ICD-9CM/CPT CODE(S)

995.0 Anaphylactic shock
Allergic shock— NOS or due to adverse effect
Anaphylactic reaction—of correct medicinal substances
Anaphylaxis—properly administered

OVERVIEW

- Anaphylaxis is an IgE-mediated, acute, allergic reaction that is characterized by a sudden and severe collapse of the cardiovascular system (severe hypotension) and respiratory compromise (bronchospasm). This is an acute, life-threatening, systemic reaction that is manifested by urticaria, angioedema, upper airway obstruction, bronchospasm, hypotension, and gastrointestinal disturbances.
- Anaphylactic shock can occur when an individual has been previously sensitized to a specific antigen. Parenteral-administered drugs, especially penicillin, cephalosporins, and iodine contrast media are common offenders. This condition can produce decreased blood pressure, decreased cardiac output, vasodilation, and peripheral edema. Rapid treatment requires epinepherine, fluid support, corticosteroids, and antihistamine. Upper airway obstruction is the most common cause of death in anaphylaxis.

ETIOLOGY & PATHOGENESIS

- When the body reacts to the allergen, it releases histamine and other substances. This causes the following reactions:
  - Constriction of the airway resulting in wheezing and difficulty in breathing.
  - Gastrointestinal symptoms including abdominal pain, cramps, vomiting, and diarrhea.
  - Blood vessels dilate and leak fluid from the bloodstream into the tissues, causing the blood volume to drop.
  - Pulmonary edema caused by the leaking of the fluid into the alveoli of the lung.
- Food allergy
- Environmental: insect bites/stings
- Latex allergies
- Medications
  - Penicillin
  - Cephalosporins
  - Iodated contrast media
  - Aspirin/nonsteroidal antiinflammatory drugs
  - Local anesthetics: methylparaben (preservative)
- Idiopathic

CLINICAL PRESENTATION / PHYSICAL FINDINGS

SIGNS & SYMPTOMS

- Onset:
  - Injected medications: 5 to 30 minutes.
  - Oral ingestion: up to 2 hours.
  - Can begin immediately.
  - The more immediate the reaction, the more severe it is.
- Skin:
  - Flushed face
  - Rash/hives
  - Urticaria (nose/hands):
    - Itching
    - Flushing
  - Tingling (lips, axilla, groin, hand, feet)
  - Angioedema
    - Swelling of lips/eyes/tongue
    - No warmth or erythema
- Respiratory:
  - Laryngeal edema:
    - Hoarseness
    - Dysphagia (difficulty in swallowing)
    - Lump in throat
    - Airway obstruction
    - Drooling
  - Apnea
  - Abnormal breath sounds
  - Coughing
  - Dysphonia
  - Inspiratory stridor
  - Bronchospasm:
    - Wheezing
    - Cough
    - Dyspnea (shortness of breath)
    - Difficult breathing
    - Chest tightness
- CNS:
  - Diaphoresis
  - Feeling of impending doom
  - Altered/loss of consciousness
  - Seizure
  - Incontinence
  - Confusion
  - Slurred speech
- Cardiovascular:
  - Cyanosis
  - Pallor
  - Dizziness
  - Pallor
  - Hypotension
  - Dysrhythmias
  - Tachycardia or bradycardia
  - Vascular collapse: hypovolemic shock
  - Myocardial infarction
  - Cardiac arrest
- Gastrointestinal disturbances:
  - Nausea
  - Vomiting
  - Diarrhea
  - Abdominal pain
- Rhinitis:
  - Nasal congestion
  - Itching
  - Sneezing

DIAGNOSIS

SPECIAL TESTS

- Examination of eyes or face showing hives and swelling
- Cyanosis due to lack of oxygen
- Angioedema of the throat, which may impair the airway
- Specific allergy testing prior to procedure or usage of drugs/medications

MEDICAL MANAGEMENT & TREATMENT

EARLY TREATMENT

- Activate EMS.
- Supine position.
- Begin basic life support (BLS).
- Administer 100% oxygen.
- Ventilate if necessary.
- Monitor pulse, blood pressure, and PaO_2.
- Monitor patient responsiveness.
- Document and record result (both response and time).
- Recheck/reevaluate patient's medical history and medications to have for EMS.

ADVANCED TREATMENT

- Epinephrine 0.3 to 0.5 mg (1:1000 solution) administered sublingual, subcutaneous, or intramuscular.
- Monitor vital signs.
- Communicate with EMS en route.
- Start IV fluids (1000 mL or 500 mL of NS or Ringer's lactate).
- Advanced cardiac life support (ACLS) when trained:
  - Epinephrine 3 to 5 mL (1:10,000 solution) IV.
  - May repeat in 10 to 20 minutes if necessary.

IF PATIENT IS INTUBATED

- Administer epinephrine:
  - Adults: 5 to 10 mL of 1:10,000 concentrations.
  - Children: 0.01 mg/kg.
- Treatment of bronchospasm:
  - Albuterol 2 to 4 puffs initially; may repeat after 10 to 20 minutes.
  - Dexamethasone (Decadron®), 4 mg IV or hydrocortisone, 100 mg IV push.
  - Transfer patient to medical facility for further treatment.

COMPLICATIONS

- Shock
- Cardiac arrest
- Respiratory arrest
- Airway obstruction

PROGNOSIS

Patients with mild reactions limited to urticaria, angioedema, or mild bronchospasm should be observed for a minimum of 6 hours. Patients with more severe reactions should be admitted to a hospital for close observation of possible biphasic reaction.

DENTAL
SIGNIFICANCE

Prevention of anaphylaxis requires a thorough medical history with updates at each patient visit to identify offending antigens for avoidance. Medical consultation and skin testing results should be completed with any suspected drug allergy for confirmation.

SUGGESTED REFERENCES

Ferri FF (ed): *Practical Guide to the Care of the Medical Patient.* St Louis, Mosby, 2004.

Lewis DP, et al. *Advanced Protocols for Medical Emergencies: An Action Plan for Office Response,* 2004.

The Washington Manual of Medical Therapeutics, ed 30. Philadelphia, Lippincott Williams & Wilkins, 2001.

AUTHOR: **DONALD P. LEWIS, JR., DDS, CFE**

SYNONYM(S)

Stable or common angina
Unstable angina
Variant angina
Coronary artery spasm
Acute coronary syndrome

ICD-9CM/CPT CODE(S)

413   Angina pectoris
413.0 Angina decubitus
       Nocturnal angina
413.1 Prinzmetal angina
       Variant angina pectoris
413.9 Other and unspecified angina
       pectoris
       Angina
         NOS   Anginal syndrome
         Cardiac Status anginosus
         Of effort Stenocardia
                  Syncope anginosa
413.2 Excludes: Preinfarction angina

OVERVIEW

- Angina pectoris is chest pain or discomfort due to coronary artery disease and is a symptom of myocardial ischemia. This discomfort occurs when the myocardial oxygen demand exceeds the supply. This usually happens because one or more of the heart's arteries is narrowed or blocked. The pain may also occur in the shoulders, arms, neck, jaw, or back and is frequently mistaken for indigestion. Most patients with angina have narrowed coronary arteries due to atherosclerosis.
- Angina pectoris can be classified as follows:
  - Class I: ordinary physical activity does not cause angina, but rapid or strenuous exertion does.
  - Class II: slight limitation of ordinary activity (e.g., walking, climbing stairs rapidly).
  - Class III: marked limitations of ordinary physical activity (e.g., walking one or two blocks on level ground).
  - Class IV: inability to perform any physical activity without angina appearing.

EPIDEMIOLOGY & DEMOGRAPHICS

Risk is higher in patients with certain uncontrollable factors such as advanced age, genetic predisposition, or coronary artery anomalies. Modifiable factors that increase risk include:
- Hypertension
- High cholesterol
- Obesity
- Smoking
- Diabetes
- Sedentary lifestyle
- Cocaine use

ETIOLOGY & PATHOGENESIS

- Insufficient blood supply to the myocardium
- Resultant decrease in blood supply

- Narrowing or constriction of the coronary arteries
- Increased cardiac demand for oxygen

CLINICAL PRESENTATION / PHYSICAL FINDINGS

SIGNS & SYMPTOMS

- Substernal pain:
  - Described as burning, pressure, squeezing, or tightness in the chest
- Early symptoms often mistaken for indigestion
- Usually starts in the chest from behind the sternum
- Feeling of heaviness in the chest
- Crescendo-decrescendo pattern
- Pain of short duration (30 seconds to 30 minutes)
- Shortness of breath
- Nausea
- Diaphoresis
- Numbness or discomfort in left arm, jaw, or shoulder

DIAGNOSIS

DIFFERENTIAL DIAGNOSIS

- Pulmonary disease
- Pulmonary hypertension
- Pulmonary embolism
- Pleurisy
- Pneumothorax
- Pneumonia
- Gastrointestinal disorders
  - Peptic ulcer disease
  - Indigestion
  - Pancreatitis
  - Esophageal reflux
- Musculoskeletal conditions
  - Costochondritis
  - Muscle strain
  - Myositis
- Acute aortic dissection
- Herpes zoster and its prodrome
- Mitral valve prolapse
- Anxiety

LABORATORY

- Fasting lipoprotein profile: check cholesterol levels.
- Fasting blood glucose: check blood sugar level.
- Hemoglobin: red blood cells' ability to carry oxygen.
- Lipid panel.
- Hematocrit.
- Thyroid stimulating hormone: older patients.

SPECIAL TESTS

- ECG (electrocardiogram) at rest
- Exercise stress test:
  - Evaluation of chest pain syndromes
  - Typical angina or effort-induced angina
  - Atypical chest pain
  - Evaluation of exercise intolerance
- Chest radiograph
- Echocardiogram
- Cardiac catheterization
  - Coronary angiography

MEDICAL MANAGEMENT & TREATMENT

- Terminate procedure.
- Monitor vital signs.
- Nitroglycerin sublingually (0.2 to 0.6 mg) every 5 minutes to maximum of 3 doses over 15 minutes.
- Upright/semireclining, comfortable position.
- Oxygen 100%.
- EKG monitoring.
- Set up and activate automatic external defibrillator (AED).
- Review medical history.
- After third dose of nitroglycerin, assume/treat myocardial infarction.
- Activate EMS.
- Aspirin, 325 mg PO.

COMMON SURGICAL MEASURES

- Angioplasty: to open blocked or narrowed coronary arteries.
- Coronary artery bypass surgery: bypass blocked coronary arteries.

KEY QUESTIONS FOR PATIENT

- What causes angina to occur?
- What does it feel like?
- How long does it last?
- What relieves the discomfort?
- Look for changes in patterns.

PREVENTION/AVOIDANCE

- Consult with patient's physician prior to treatment.
- Premedication for stress reduction.
- Consider preoperative use of nitroglycerin (0.2 to 0.6 mg sublingual 5 to 10 minutes prior to procedure).
- Use supplemental oxygen (100%).
- Monitor vital signs.
- Limit use of epinephrine.
- Reassure patient.

DENTAL MANAGEMENT

The management of acute angina should include identification and treatment. Specific treatment in the dental office should initially be directed toward improving the myocardial oxygen supply and reducing the oxygen demand. Prevention should include understanding the history of the patient's angina and developing a protocol to reduce stress and decrease cardiac oxygen demand.

SUGGESTED REFERENCES

Ferri FF (ed): *Practical Guide to the Care of the Medical Patient.* St Louis, Mosby, 2004.
Lewis DP, et al. *Advanced Protocols for Medical Emergencies: An Action Plan for Office Response,* 2004.
Schwartz GR, et al. *Principles and Practice of Emergency Medicine.* Baltimore, Lippincott Williams & Wilkins, 1999.
The Washington Manual of Medical Therapeutics, ed 30. Philadelphia, Lippincott Williams & Wilkins, 2001.

AUTHOR: **DONALD P. LEWIS, JR., DDS, CFE**

SYNONYM(S)

Hereditary angioneurotic edema (HAE, ANE)

ICD-9CM/CPT CODE(S)
995.1 Angioneurotic edema
   Giant urticaria
   Excludes: Urticaria due to serum
   (999.5)—other specified

OVERVIEW

- Hereditary angioneurotic edema is a limited subcutaneous or submucosal edema that can last at least 12 hours and can relapse with some frequency. It may be manifested by an acute upper airway obstruction, gastrointestinal symptoms, and angioedema of the skin that can mimic anaphylaxis. This is caused by a C1 esterase inhibitor deficiency, which is an autosomal dominant disorder.
- Hereditary angioneurotic edema is caused by a defective synthesis and/or functional impairment of the C1 inhibitor protein. This absence or deficiency in turn affects the blood vessels. In affected patients, this can lead to rapid swelling of the hands, feet, limbs, face, and intestinal cramping. It can also lead to airway problems with swelling of the larynx or trachea.
- Attacks can be precipitated by stress or trauma and will begin sometime in adolescence and continue throughout life on an intermittent basis.

EPIDEMIOLOGY & DEMOGRAPHICS

Hereditary, autosomal dominant

ETIOLOGY & PATHOGENESIS

- Trauma
- Stress, even minor

- Edema developing in a patient taking angiotensin-converting enzyme (ACE) inhibitor

CLINICAL PRESENTATION / PHYSICAL FINDINGS

- Itching or relapsing edema that does not respond to any antiallergic treatment
- Relapsing abdominal pain without any clear-cut, surgically treatable cause
- Subcutaneous/submucosal, white, soft, nonpruritic edema
- Occurs episodically
- Lasts 3 to 5 days

SIGNS & SYMPTOMS

- Swelling of arms, legs, lips, eyes, tongue, or throat
- Sudden hoarseness
- Airway obstruction
- Intestinal swelling
- Severe nausea/vomiting: resembles medical emergency
- Dehydration
- Pain
- Occasional shock
- Urticaria/hypotension is absent

DIAGNOSIS

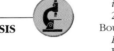

DIFFERENTIAL DIAGNOSIS

- Anaphylaxis

LABORATORY

- Decreased C1 inhibiting factor activity
- Decreased C4 and C2 levels

RISK FACTORS

- Contraindicated drugs:
  - Dextrans
  - ACE inhibitors

MEDICAL MANAGEMENT & TREATMENT

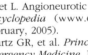

- Prevention by avoiding trauma.
- Avoid precipitating factors.

- Danazol, 50 to 600 mg/day (increases C1 inhibitor synthesis).
- Severe attacks: hospital admission for preoperative Danazol.

COMPLICATIONS

- Airway problems with swelling of the larynx
- Surgery for abdominal pain
- Fatal laryngeal swelling
- Shock

PROGNOSIS

Limited treatment options

DENTAL SIGNIFICANCE

A careful medical history will reveal this condition. All measures should be taken to avoid stress and to make the procedure as atraumatic as possible.

SUGGESTED REFERENCES

Bennet JD, Rosenberg MB. *Medical Emergencies in Dentistry.* Philadelphia, WB Saunders, 2002.
Bouillet L. Angioneurotic edema, in *Orphanet Encyclopedia* (www.orpha.net, accessed February, 2005).
Schwartz GR, et al. *Principles and Practice of Emergency Medicine.* Baltimore, Lippincott Williams & Wilkins, 1999.
The Washington Manual of Medical Therapeutics, ed 30. Philadelphia, Lippincott Williams & Wilkins, 2001.

AUTHOR: **DONALD P. LEWIS, JR., DDS, CFE**

SYNONYM(S)

Acute atrial tachycardia
Multifocal atrial tachycardia (MAT)

ICD-9CM/CPT CODE(S)
Cardiac dysrhythmias
427.0 Paroxysmal supraventricular tachycardia
Atrial (PAT) junctional
Atrioventricular nodal
427.3 Atrial fibrillation and flutter
427.31 Atrial fibrillation
427.32 Atrial flutter

OVERVIEW

- Atrial tachycardia is a rapid heart rate that is caused by inappropriate electrical impulses traveling to the ventricles of the heart from multiple locations in the atria. Most of these impulses are conducted to the ventricles, leading to a rapid heart rate. This rate can be anywhere from 100 to 250 bpm, causing the inability of the ventricles to refill with blood and therefore reducing the flow of blood to the brain and body.
- Different types of atrial tachycardia:
  - Sinus tachycardia:
    - Rate 100 to 200 bpm
    - Physiologic response to stresses:
      - Fever
      - Exercise
      - Anxiety
      - Anemia
  - Atrial flutter:
    - Rate 250 to 350 bpm
    - In patients with pericarditis or respiratory failure
    - Can deteriorate to atrial fibrillation if left untreated
  - Atrial fibrillation:
    - Rate 350 to 600 bpm
    - Most often associated with:
      - Congestive heart failure
      - Chronic lung disease
      - Thyrotoxicosis
      - Acute ethanol intoxication
      - Irregular heart rhythm
  - Paroxysmal supraventricular tachycardia:
    - Reentry-type abnormality
    - Produces prolonged PR interval
    - Rapid rhythm without P waves
    - See "Cardiac Dysrhythmias" in Section I, p 35

EPIDEMIOLOGY & DEMOGRAPHICS

Most common in patients over 50 years of age

ETIOLOGY & PATHOGENESIS

- Fever
- Exercise
- Anxiety
- Intravascular volume depletion
- Electrolyte abnormality
- Thyrotoxicosis

- Hypotension
- Heart failure
- Acute myocardial infarction
- Ischemic heart disease
- Medication reaction
- Pulmonary embolism
- Hyperthyroidism
- Pericarditis
- Chronic lung disease

CLINICAL PRESENTATION / PHYSICAL FINDINGS

- Tachycardia
- Blood pressure normal or low
- Signs of poor circulation
- Congestive heart failure
- Decreased level of consciousness

SIGNS & SYMPTOMS

- Sensation of increased heart rate: palpitations
- Lightheadedness
- Fainting
- Shortness of breath
- Chest tightness
- Chest pain
- Weakness
- Dizziness
- Difficulty in breathing when lying down

DIAGNOSIS

DIFFERENTIAL DIAGNOSIS

- Syncope
- Hypotension
- Acute myocardial infarction
- Angina
- Congestive heart failure
- Sick sinus syndrome
- Anxiety
- Anemia

LABORATORY

- Digoxin level
- Thyroid function studies
- Alcohol screening
- WBC
- Arterial blood gases

SPECIAL TESTS

- Electrocardiogram (ECG)
- Chest radiograph
- Thyroid scan
- Echocardiogram

DIAGNOSTIC IMAGING

- Electrocardiogram (ECG)
- Holter monitor
- Electrophysiologic study

MEDICAL MANAGEMENT & TREATMENT

- Initial treatment is aimed at underlying cause.
  - Determine specific rhythm.
  - Confirm unstable condition.
- If heart rate is > 150 bpm and unstable: cardioversion.
- Supplemental oxygen.
- Pulse oximeter.
- Suction.
- Intubation equipment.
- Establish IV access.

- Secure airway.
- Consider medication if blood pressure and condition allow.
  - Sedatives:
    - Midazolam (Versed®), 1 mg every 2 to 3 minutes, up to 5 mg.
  - Analgesics:
    - Meperidine (Demerol®), 25 to 50 mg IV every 10 to 20 minutes, up to 100 mg.
    - Fentanyl (Sublimaze®), 50 µg IV every 3 minutes as needed.
- Synchronized cardioversion.
- Successful cardioversion: adenosine, 6 mg rapid IV push.
  - May repeat every 30 seconds with 12 mg for two more doses.
  - Immediately flush with 10 mL of normal saline.

FOLLOW-UP

- Emergency facility
- Consult primary health care provider

MONITORING

- ECG
- Pulse oximeter
- Blood pressure

PREVENTION/AVOIDANCE

- Can be achieved by prompt treatment of disorders that cause atrial tachycardia

COMPLICATIONS

- Reduced pumping action of heart: hypoperfusion of end-target organs
- Heart failure
- Cardiomyopathy

PROGNOSIS

Patients with atrial tachycardia have a controllable situation if the underlying condition is controlled.

DENTAL SIGNIFICANCE

The heart beating too fast for the patient's cardiovascular condition can cause insufficient and inadequate blood flow through the heart. An unstable condition can arise that requires immediate diagnosis and treatment. When treating patients with a known history of an unstable tachydysrhythmia, care should be taken to prevent recurrence or prevent complications associated with the specific tachydysrhythmia.

SUGGESTED REFERENCES

Hupp JR, et al. (eds): *The 5-Minute Clinical Consult for Dental Professionals*. Philadelphia, Lippincott Williams & Wilkins, 1995.
Lewis DP, et al. *Advanced Protocols for Medical Emergencies: An Action Plan for Office Response*, 2004.
The Washington Manual of Medical Therapeutics, ed 30. Philadelphia, Lippincott Williams & Wilkins, 2001.

AUTHOR: **DONALD P. LEWIS, JR., DDS, CFE**

SYNONYM(S)

Acute bradycardia
Sinus bradycardia
Vagal tone

ICD-9CM/CPT CODE(S)

427.81   Other specified cardiac dys-
rhythmias
427.81.1 Sinoatrial node dysfunction
Sinus bradycardia
Syndrome
Sick sinus
Tachycardia-bradycardia
Excludes: Sinus bradycardia
NOS (427.89)

OVERVIEW

- Sinus bradycardia is defined as a sinus rhythm of a resting heart rate of 60 bpm or less. The pathophysiology of sinus bradycardia depends on the underlying cause. It is usually an incidental finding in patients who are otherwise healthy and asymptomatic, as seen in young, athletic patients. It can also be related to increase in vagal tone, drug effects, ischemia, and primary sinus node disease.
- Patients affected with acute bradycardias that are symptomatic may complain of fatigue, exercise intolerance, dyspnea, angina on exertion, or confusion in elderly patients.
- See "Cardiac Dysrhythmias" in Section I, p 35 for more information.

ETIOLOGY & PATHOGENESIS

- Sick sinus syndrome is one of the most common pathologic causes.
- Medication reaction:
  - Supratherapeutic doses of:
    - Digitalis glycosides
    - Beta blockers
    - Calcium channel blockers
- Vagal stimulation.
- Acute myocardial infarction: inferior wall myocardial infarction.
- Toxic/environmental exposure.
- Electrolyte disturbances.
- Sleep apnea.
- Infection.
- Hypoglycemia.
- Increased intracranial pressure.
- Hypothyroidism.
- Myocarditis.

CLINICAL PRESENTATION / PHYSICAL FINDINGS

- Previous cardiac history (myocardial infarction, congestive heart failure, valvular failure)
- Medications
- Toxic exposures
- Prior illness
- Peripheral pulses reveal a slow, regular pulse

- Clinical exam may reveal:
  - Decreased level of consciousness
  - Cyanosis
  - Peripheral edema
  - Dyspnea
  - Poor perfusion

SIGNS & SYMPTOMS

- Syncope
- History of chest pain
- Diaphoresis
- Pallor
- Nausea
- Shortness of breath
- Drowsiness
- Weakness
- Fatigue
- Dizziness
- Lightheadedness
- Hypotension
- Congestive heart failure
- Unstable angina
- Premature ventricular contractions (PVCs)

DIAGNOSIS

LABORATORY TESTS

- Helpful if cause is thought to be related to electrolytes, drugs, or toxins
  - Electrolytes
  - Glucose
  - Calcium
  - Magnesium
  - Thyroid function tests
  - Toxicologic screen

DIAGNOSTIC PROCEDURES

- 12-lead ECG to confirm diagnosis

MEDICAL MANAGEMENT & TREATMENT

- Not usually indicated for asymptomatic patients

SYMPTOMATIC PATIENTS

- Rate < 60 bpm and has:
  - Chest pain
  - Shortness of breath
  - Decrease/loss of consciousness
- Signs:
  - Low blood pressure
  - Pulmonary congestion
- Treatment to consider:
  - Evaluate airway/breathing/circulation (ABCs).
  - Secure airway as needed.
  - Provide supplemental oxygen (100%).
  - Establish IV access.
  - Monitor ECG.
  - Determine specific bradycardia rhythm.
  - Review patient history/medication: problem-focused.
  - Reevaluate patient.
  - Consider possible/probable causes.
  - Determine if bradycardia is symptomatic.
    - Atropine, 0.5 to 1 mg IV; repeat every 3 to 5 minutes to maximum dose of 3 mg (0.03 mg/kg).

- Activate EMS with diagnosis of ventricular tachycardia.
- Transport to medical facility.

FOLLOW-UP

- Patient to be seen by medical physician for follow-up and treatment

MONITORING

- Pulse
- Blood Pressure
- ECG

PREVENTION/AVOIDANCE

- Medical history
- Baseline vital signs

COMPLICATIONS

- Sick sinus syndrome may convert to atrial fibrillation.
- Sudden death.
- Cardiac arrest.

PROGNOSIS

- In patients with sinus bradycardia resultant from exposure to precipitating factors, the prognosis is good after the offending agent has been eliminated.
- Patients with sinus bradycardia due to sick sinus syndrome have a relatively poor prognosis.

DENTAL SIGNIFICANCE

- Vital signs need to be taken; patients with asymptomatic bradycardia require no treatment. Baseline vital signs should be recorded and updated at subsequent dental visits.
- In the symptomatic bradycardia patient, treatment should be directed toward the underlying etiology by referral to the primary care physician.
- Sinus bradycardia is harmless in an otherwise healthy patient, but bradycardia in cardiac-compromised patients can be life-threatening by causing a complete heart block.

SUGGESTED REFERENCES

Lewis DP, et al. *Advanced Protocols for Medical Emergencies: An Action Plan for Office Response*, 2004.
Livingston M. Sinus bradycardia, at www.emedicine.com/emerg/topic534.htm
Schwartz GR, et al. *Principles and Practice of Emergency Medicine*. Baltimore, Lippincott Williams & Wilkins, 1999.
The Washington Manual of Medical Therapeutics, ed 30. Philadelphia, Lippincott Williams & Wilkins, 2001.

AUTHOR: **DONALD P. LEWIS, JR., DDS, CFE**

SYNONYM(S)

Acute bronchospasm
Status asthmaticus

ICD-9CM/CPT CODE(S)

493   Asthma
         Excludes: Wheezing NOS
         (786. 07)
493.0   Extrinsic asthma
             Allergic with atopic
             children
             Hay
             Platinum
             Hay fever with asthma
493.1   Intrinsic asthma
493.2   Chronic obstructive asthma
             Asthma with COPD
             Chronic asthmatic bronchitis
         Excludes: Acute bronchitis
         (466.0) and chronic obstruc-
         tive bronchitis
493.8   Other forms of asthma
493.81   Exercise-induced bronchospasm
493.82   Cough variant asthma
493.9   Asthma—unspecified
             Asthma (bronchial, allergic
             NOS)
             Bronchitis (allergic, asthmatic)
             V17.5 Asthma (family history)
466   Acute bronchitis and bronchi-
         olitis
             Bronchospasm
             Obstruction
466.0   Acute bronchitis
             Bronchitis, acute or subacute
             Fibrinous
             Membranous
             Pneumococcal
             Purulent
             Septic
             Viral
             With tracheitis
             Croupous bronchitis

OVERVIEW

Asthma is a disease characterized
by the inflammation of the airway and an increased responsiveness to a
wide variety of stimuli. Bronchospasm is
a generalized condition involving the contraction of smooth muscle of the bronchi
and bronchioles of the lungs. This results
in a restriction of the flow of air during
inhalation and exhalation of the lungs.
The severity of the obstruction widely
varies and can manifest this condition as
cough, dyspnea, chest tightness, and
wheezing. Asthma is an episodic disease
with periods of acute exacerbation followed by symptom-free periods. Asthma
attacks (or acute bronchospasm) are
episodes of shortness of breath or wheezing that last minutes to hours.

ETIOLOGY & PATHOGENESIS

- Exercise
- Exposure to triggers: smoke, perfume,
  allergens
- Viral respiratory infection
- Changes in hormones
- Medications (aspirin or NSAIDs)

CLINICAL PRESENTATION / PHYSICAL FINDINGS

- Usually a history of progressively wors-
  ening dyspnea.
- Tachypnea: > 30 breaths/minute.
- Patient is usually sitting forward.
- Diaphoresis.
- Inability to speak.
- Use of accessory respiratory muscles.
- Changes in mental status.

SIGNS & SYMPTOMS

- Labored breathing or signs of diminish-
  ing respiratory status/shortness of breath
- Difficulty on expiration
- Cyanosis
- Decreased oxygen saturation
- Decreased ventilation patterns on
  capnograph
- Chest tightness
- Exercise intolerance
- Anxiety
- Bronchial spastic cough
- Wheezing
  Note: Absence of wheezing is an indi-
  cation of worsening condition.

DIAGNOSIS

DIFFERENTIAL DIAGNOSIS

- Pneumonia
- Atelectasis
- Pneumothorax

LABORATORY

- Arterial blood gases (ABGs):
  - Mild:
    - Decreased PaO_2
    - Decreased $PaCO_2$
    - Increased pH
  - Moderate:
    - Decreased PaO_2
    - Normal $PaCO_2$
    - Normal pH
  - Severe:
    - Markedly decreased PaO_2
    - Increased $PaCO_2$
    - Decreased pH
- Complete blood count (CBC)
  - Sputum: eosinophils
  - Chest radiograph: evidence of thoracic
    hyperinflation

SPECIAL TESTS

- Electrocardiogram (ECG) to show:
  - Tachycardia and nonspecific ST–T
    wave changes
  - Right bundle branch block
- Pulmonary function tests (PFTs)
  - Severe bronchospasm with have:
    - FEV1 < 1 liter

- Peak expiratory flow rate (PEFR)
  < 80 L/minute

MEDICAL MANAGEMENT & TREATMENT

EARLY TREATMENT

- Patient in upright position.
- Management of airway.
- Maximize oxygen delivery (100%).
- Minimize CO_2 buildup.

ADVANCED TREATMENT

- Activate EMS.
- CPR if indicated.
- Inhaled β-agonist drugs.
- Bronchodilating medications:
  - Albuterol (Ventolin®), 2 puffs STAT;
    repeat every 10 to 20 minutes; or
  - 0.5 mL nebulized solution mixed in
    3 to 6 mL NS; repeat every 20 minutes.
  - Ipratropium bromide (Atrovert®), 2
    puffs STAT; repeat every 20 minutes;
    or
  - 0.5 mL of 0.02% solution nebulized
    solution; repeat every 20 minutes.
  - Epinephrine, 0.3 to 0.5 mg (1:1000)
    subcutaneous (SC); repeat every
    20 minutes to maximum of 1 mg total.
  - Prednisone, 40 to 60 mg orally (PO),
    one-time dose.
  - Aminophylline, 50 mg per minute
    (alternative).
  Note: To administer medication, the
  patient must be awake (PO) or endotra-
  cheal intubation must be placed for
  delivery.

OBTUNDED PATIENTS

- Epinephrine (SC), 5 mL of 1:10,000 solution.
- Epinephrine (sublingual), 0.5 mL of
  1:1000 solution if anaphylaxis.

SPONTANEOUS BREATHING— INADEQUATE EXCHANGE

- 100% oxygen with full face mask
- Consider intubation if:
  - Hypoxemia
  - Worsening obtundation

FOLLOW-UP

Patient should be followed by primary
care physician regarding control of precipitating factors and medications.

MONITORING

- Precordial stethoscope
- Pulse oximeter
- Capnograph

PREVENTION

- Assessment of severity
- Physical examination
  - Presence/absence of wheeze
  - Distress at rest
  - Diaphoresis
  - Agitation
  - Tachypnea > 28 breaths/minute
  - Tachycardia >110 beats/minute
- Stress reduction

COMPLICATIONS

- Breathing does not improve
- Signs of cyanosis
- Patient appears to tire
- Breathing begins to slow
- Wheezing is interrupted
- Hospital admission for treatment/ observation

PROGNOSIS

Breathing returns to normal rate and sound.

DENTAL SIGNIFICANCE

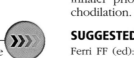

Proper patient history and physical exam are of utmost importance. Have the patient bring medications to the dental appointment. Consider having the patient use their inhaler prior to appointment for bronchodilation.

SUGGESTED REFERENCES

Ferri FF (ed): *Practical Guide to the Care of the Medical Patient*. St Louis, Mosby, 2004.

Lewis DP, et al. *Advanced Protocols for Medical Emergencies: An Action Plan for Office Response*. Hudson, Ohio, Lexi-Comp Inc.

The Washington Manual of Medical Therapeutics, ed 30. Philadelphia, Lippincott Williams & Wilkins, 2001.

AUTHOR: **DONALD P. LEWIS, JR., DDS, CFE**

SECTION III

SYNONYM(S)
Cardiac arrest
Sudden cardiac arrest
Sudden cardiac death
Sudden death

ICD-9CM/CPT CODE(S)
427.5 Cardiac arrest
Cardiorespiratory arrest
433 Occlusion and stenosis of precerebral arteries
Embolism—of basilar
Narrowing—carotid
Obstruction—vertebral
Thrombosis—arteries

OVERVIEW

- Cardiac arrest is the sudden and abrupt loss of heart function. It is also called sudden cardiac arrest or unexpected cardiac arrest; death can occur within minutes after symptoms appear. The most common underlying cause of death from cardiac arrest is coronary heart disease.
- Usually, cardiac arrest that leads to sudden death is from ventricular tachycardia or ventricular fibrillation. These dysrhythmias cause the heart to suddenly arrest. Occasionally, the slowing of the heart beat (bradycardia) can precipitate a cardiac arrest. (See "Cardiac Dysrhythmias" in Section I, p 35.)
- Sudden death is not synonymous with myocardial infarction.

EPIDEMIOLOGY & DEMOGRAPHICS
Patients with the following conditions are more at risk for cardiac arrest, though it can be spontaneous without known risk factors:
- Heart attack
- Coronary artery disease
- Diabetes
- Hypercholesterolemia
- Hypertension
- Cigarette smoking
- Drug/alcohol abuse
- Excess weight
- High-fat diet
- Lack of exercise
- Stress
- Family history
- Congenital heart disorders

CLINICAL PRESENTATION / PHYSICAL FINDINGS
- Prodromal symptoms:
  - Chest discomfort
  - Unusual fatigue
  - Shortness of breath
- Triggers:
  - Ischemia
  - Electrolyte imbalances
    - Hypokalemia
    - Hypomagnesemia

- Platelet abnormalities resulting in thrombosis
- Psychologic stress

SIGNS & SYMPTOMS
- Sudden loss of consciousness
- Agonal breathing
- Unresponsive
- Undetectable blood pressure/pulse
- Acute myocardial infarction
- Cardiomyopathy
- Medication reaction
- Hypoxia
- Electrolyte imbalance
- Hypothermia
- Electrocution
- Chest trauma

DIAGNOSIS

LABORATORY
- Cardiac enzymes
- Complete blood count (CBC)

PATHOLOGY FINDINGS
- Abnormal ECG findings

DIAGNOSTIC PROCEDURES/TESTS
- Cardiac catheterization
- Electrophysiologic tests
- Exercise ECG
- Coronary angiography
- Echocardiogram
- Chest radiograph
- Pulmonary function test
- Arterial blood gases

MEDICAL MANAGEMENT & TREATMENT

IMMEDIATE TREATMENT
- Initiate CPR.
- Set up automated external defibrillator (AED).
- Confirm rhythm.
- Defibrillate up to three times.

IF VENTRICULAR FIBRILLATION (VF) OR PULSELESS VENTRICULAR TACHYCARDIA (VT)
- Defibrillate again at 360 joules.
- Consider:
  - Amiodarone, 300 mg IV push; repeat with 150 mg IV in 3 to 5 minutes.
  - Lidocaine, 1 to 1.5 mg/kg IV push; repeat every 3 to 5 minutes to maximum of 3 mg/kg.

IF PULSELESS ELECTRICAL ACTIVITY (PEA)/ASYSTOLE
- Epinephrine, 1 mg IV push; repeat every 3 to 5 minutes.
- Atropine, 1 mg IV push every 3 to 5 minutes to total dose of 0.04 mg/kg if rhythm on monitor is slow.
- Transport to medical facility.

FOLLOW-UP
- Medical follow-up and long-term care should be guided by the primary health care physician.

MONITORING
- ECG
- AED

- Blood pressure
- Pulse
- Level of consciousness
- Signs/feeling of impending doom

PREVENTION/AVOIDANCE
- Identify patients at possible risk:
  - Ischemic heart disease
  - Dysrhythmias
    - Tachydysrhythmia
    - Bradydysrhythmia
  - Primary myocardial disease
    - Cardiomyopathies
    - Myocarditis: viral/rheumatic
  - Mitral valve prolapse
  - Muscular dystrophy
  - Marfan's syndrome
  - Patient on liquid protein diets for weight loss
  - Cocaine abuse
  - Kawasaki disease
  - Pulmonary hypertension
  - Asthma: status asthmaticus

COMPLICATIONS

- Ventricular fibrillation
- Pulseless ventricular fibrillation
- Pulseless electrical activity
- Asystole

PROGNOSIS

Prognosis is variable depending on the cause, timing on intervention, success of treatment, and post-MI management. A better prognosis is associated with early reperfusion, inferior wall infarct, and treatment with β-blockers, aspirin, and ACE inhibitors. Poor prognosis is associated with delay in reperfusion or unsuccessful reperfusion.

DENTAL SIGNIFICANCE

Brain death and permanent death can start to occur in just 4 to 6 minutes after the initial symptoms occur. Knowing those patients who are potential risks for sudden cardiac death and responding to the situation in a timely manner are of utmost importance. If treated within the first few minutes of the episode, long-term prognosis is greatly improved.

SUGGESTED REFERENCES
American Heart Association: http://www.americanheart.org
Lewis DP, et al. *Advanced Protocols for Medical Emergencies: An Action Plan for Office Response.*
Schwartz GR, et al. *Principles and Practice of Emergency Medicine.* Baltimore, Lippincott Williams & Wilkins, 1999.
The Washington Manual of Medical Therapeutics, ed 30. Philadelphia, Lippincott Williams & Wilkins, 2001.

AUTHOR: **DONALD P. LEWIS, JR., DDS, CFE**

SYNONYM(S)

Stroke
Cerebral vascular accident (CVA)
Cerebral accident

ICD-9CM/CPT CODE(S)

V17.1 Acute, but ill-defined, cerebro-
vascular disease
Apoplexy, Apoplectic:
NOS   Cerebral seizure
Attack
CVA NOS
Cerebral Stroke
Seizure
Stroke with family history

OVERVIEW

Stroke or cerebral vascular accident (CVA) is the onset of a
focal neurologic deficit of abnormality
that is caused by a decrease in blood
flow to that specific area of the brain.
This results in damage of brain tissue
when the flow of blood supplying the
brain is interrupted. Most strokes are
due to blood clots that block blood
flow.

ETIOLOGY & PATHOGENESIS

- A common cause of stroke is atherosclerosis. Plaques collecting on the walls
  of the arteries slowly begin to block the
  flow of the blood and may block the
  artery enough to cause a stroke.
- Strokes can also be caused by embolism
  caused by heart disorders. An embolism
  can originate in a major blood vessel as
  it branches off the heart. This clot then
  can travel to the brain to cause the
  block of blood flow. Dysrhythmias of
  the heart, such as atrial fibrillation, can
  also be associated with a stroke.

COMMON CONTRIBUTING RISK FACTORS

- Previous history of stroke
- Hypertension
- Atherosclerosis
- Coronary artery disease
- Diabetes mellitus
- Hypercholesterolemia
- Obesity
- Blood clotting disorders
- Embolus
- Aneurysm
- Cardiac dysrhythmias
- Tobacco use
- Drug/alcohol abuse
- Trauma
- Valvular heart disease

CLINICAL PRESENTATION / PHYSICAL FINDINGS

SIGNS & SYMPTOMS

- Weakness/paralysis of an arm, leg, side
  of face, or body
- Numbness
- Tingling
- Decreased sensation
- Visual changes/sudden blindness to one
  eye
- Slurred speech
- Inability to speak or understand com-
  mands
- Difficulty in reading
- Loss of memory
- Vertigo
- Severe headache
- Loss of balance
- Drowsiness/lethargy
- Loss of consciousness
- Uncontrollable eye movement
- Eyelid drooping
- Carotid bruit
- Syncope

DIAGNOSIS

DIFFERENTIAL DIAGNOSIS

- Carotid dissection
- Carotid stenosis
- Cocaine use
- Secondary to syphilis
- Arteriovenous malformation

LABORATORY TESTS

- Cerebral angiography

IMAGING STUDIES

- Head CT/head MRI
- ECG
- Heart monitor

MEDICAL MANAGEMENT & TREATMENT

- 100% oxygen.
- Elevate patient's head.
- Place monitors,
- Check and record vital signs.
- If hypotension is present, administer
  250 mL bolus of normal saline (NS).
- ACLS if indicated.
- Activate EMS.
- Transport to medical facility.

FOLLOW-UP

- Updated medical history.
- Use of anticoagulants.
- Use of aspirin.

MONITORING

- Blood pressure
- Cholesterol
- Weight
- Diet

PREVENTION/AVOIDANCE

- Medical history
- High blood pressure screening
- Cholesterol screening
- Low-fat diet
- Cessation of smoking
- Increased exercise
- Weight loss
- Avoidance of excess alcohol use/abuse

COMPLICATIONS

- Loss of mobility
- Permanent paralysis
- Decrease sensation loss
- Muscle spasticity
- Loss of brain function
- Reduced communication ability
- Aspiration
- Malnutrition

PROGNOSIS

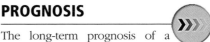

The long-term prognosis of a
patient suffering from a stroke
depends directly on the extent of the damage to the brain. It is also related to the
presence of associated medical problems.

DENTAL SIGNIFICANCE

Significant morbidity and mortality can arise from a cerebral
vascular accident (stroke). Recognition
of the early signs and initiating early
treatment is essential. By early diagnosis
and treatment, devastating effects of
brain infarction can be minimized or
even avoided. Care must be taken in the
postevent period to communicate with
the patient's primary healthcare provider
regarding the type of medication being
taken and the timing of continuance of
treatment.

DENTAL MANAGEMENT

In case of signs/symptoms of cerebral vascular accident during a dental procedure,
terminate the procedure immediately and
follow medical management guidelines.

SUGGESTED REFERENCES

Lewis DP, et al. *Advanced Protocols for
Medical Emergencies: An Action Plan for
Office Response.*
*The Washington Manual of Medical
Therapeutics,* ed 30. Philadelphia, Lippincott
Williams & Wilkins, 2001.

AUTHOR: **DONALD P. LEWIS, JR., DDS, CFE**

SYNONYM(S)

Alcohol withdrawal syndrome
DTs
Shakes
Jitters
Alcohol withdrawal seizures

ICD-9CM/CPT CODE(S)

291.0–291.81 Alcoholic psychoses
291.0   Alcohol withdrawal delirium
         Alcoholic delirium
         Delirium tremens
         Excludes: Alcohol withdrawal (291.81)
291.1   Alcohol amnesic syndrome
         Alcoholic polyneuritic psychosis
         Korsakoff's psychosis, alcoholic
493.2   Wernicke-Korsakoff syndrome (alcoholic)

OVERVIEW

Delirium tremens is a disorder most commonly associated with sudden and severe mental changes or neurologic changes resulting from the abrupt stopping of the use of alcohol. It can result in different clinical states depending on the severity of the abuse and the time interval since the last ingestion of alcohol.

ETIOLOGY & PATHOGENESIS

- Abruptly stopping consumption of alcohol, especially after heavy drinking.
- Minor symptoms commonly occur within 12 to 18 hours after last drink.
- Major symptoms commonly occur within 48 to 72 hours after last drink.
- Symptoms may occur up to 7 to 10 days after last drink.
- Excess alcohol consumption with lack of dietary intake.
- Head injury with history of alcohol abuse.
- Infection with history of alcohol abuse.
- Habitual alcohol abuse.
- Due to the toxic effects of the alcohol on the brain and nervous system.

CLINICAL PRESENTATION / PHYSICAL FINDINGS

SIGNS & SYMPTOMS

- Tremulous state
  - Early alcohol withdrawal
  - Impending DTs
  - Shakes
  - Jitters
  - Time to onset:
    - Six to 8 hours since last drink
    - Twelve to 48 hours after reduction of intake
    - Most pronounced at 4 to 36 hours

- Manifestations:
  - Tremors
  - Mild agitation
  - Insomnia
  - Tachycardia
  - Anorexia
  - Relieved by alcohol ingestion
- Hallucinogenic state
  - Usually auditory
  - Can be visual/tactile/olfactory
  - Can be clinically mistaken for acute schizophrenic episode
  - Most pronounced at 24 to 36 hours after cessation
- Alcohol withdrawal seizures
  - "Rum fits"
  - Brief, generalized convulsions with loss of consciousness
  - Occur 12 to 48 hours after cessation of alcohol intake
  - Exclude other types of seizure disorder
- Delirium tremens
  - Severe withdrawal
  - Tremors
  - Hallucination
  - Agitation
  - Confusion
  - Disorientation
  - Autonomic hyperactivity
    - Fever
    - Tachycardia
    - Diaphoresis
  - Occurs 72 to 96 hours after cessation
  - Symptoms generally resolve within 3 to 5 days
  - Chance of mortality

DIAGNOSIS

DIFFERENTIAL DIAGNOSIS

- Alcoholic liver disease
- Blood clotting disorders
- Alcoholic neuropathy
- Alcoholic cardiomyopathy
- Wernicke-Korsakoff syndrome
- Malnutrition
- Seizure disorder

LABORATORY

- CBC
- Platelets
- INR
- Toxicology screen
- Serum electrolytes
- Liver function tests
- Creatinine
- Fasting blood sugar
- Electrocardiogram
- Calcium
- Magnesium
- Albumin
- B_{12} and folic acid levels
- Stool guaiac
- Urinanalysis

MEDICAL MANAGEMENT & TREATMENT

- Admit to hospital for close observation.
- Monitor vital signs every 30 minutes.
- Neurologic evaluation.
- Treat immediate symptoms:
  - Tachycardia
  - Temperature
  - Blood pressure
- Fluid replacement: IV with glucose.
- Sedatives to depress the CNS to reduce symptoms (benzodiazepines).
- Thiamine, 100 mg IV q/day.
- Chlordiazepoxide (Librium®):
  - 100 mg IV or PO q 2 to 6 hours as needed.
  - Maximum dose 500 mg in first 24 hours.
  - One-half initial 24-hour dose over next 24 hours.
  - Reduce dose by 25 to 50 mg/day each day thereafter.
- Lorazepam (Ativan®), 2 mg IV every 4 hours; increase dose until patient is calm/not obtunded.
  - May be preferred over Librium in older patients

COMPLICATIONS

- Seizures
- Heart dysrhythmias
- Injury from seizures/decreased mental state
- Death

PROGNOSIS

Social rehabilitation is necessary after the initial treatment of alcohol withdrawal. The diagnosis and treatment of alcohol abuse needs to consist of concomitant medical, surgical, and psychiatric modalities.

DENTAL SIGNIFICANCE

- Awareness of patient's propensity to alcohol abuse and therefore the potential effects of withdrawal is necessary. Patients with apparent alcohol abuse problems should be referred for evaluation.
- The liver changes that can occur with long-standing alcohol use or abuse can be a significant factor in the treatment of the dental patient, not only psychologically but also from a bleeding standpoint. Long-term alcohol users/abusers should be considered to have some degree of decreased liver function. This dysfunction can cause alteration in the coagulation factors and will lead to prolonged bleeding.
- Delayed wound healing, alteration of the effectiveness of medications, and

the increased incidence of oral cancer should all be considered in alcoholic patients.

SUGGESTED REFERENCES

Amos JJ, Crowe R, Doebbeling CC, Lievsveld J. *Treatment of Alcohol Withdrawal.* Iowa City, IA, The University of Iowa, 2001.

Ferri FF (ed): *Practical Guide to the Care of the Medical Patient.* St Louis, Mosby, 2004.

The Washington Manual of Medical Therapeutics, ed 30. Philadelphia, Lippincott Williams & Wilkins, 2001.

AUTHOR: **DONALD P. LEWIS, JR., DDS, CFE**

SYNONYM(S)

Hypoglycemia
Insulin shock
Low blood sugar

ICD-9CM/CPT CODE(S)

250.80 Diabetes with other specified
manifestations
    Diabetic hypoglycemia
    Hypoglycemic shock
    Use additional E codes to
    identify if drug-induced
Diabetes with other coma
    Diabetic coma (with keto-
    acidosis)
    Diabetic hypoglycemic coma
    Insulin coma NOS
    Excludes: Diabetes with hyper-
    osmolar coma

OVERVIEW

Hypoglycemia is an arbitrary
reduction in blood glucose levels (< 50 mg/dL), which results in the
deprivation of blood glucose to the
brain. Hypoglycemia (low blood sugar)
occurs when blood sugar levels drop to
low levels that cannot properly fuel the
body's metabolism. Insulin is produced
in the pancreas in response to increased
glucose levels in the blood.

ETIOLOGY & PATHOGENESIS

- Body uses glucose too rapidly
- Glucose release is slower than needed
- Excessive insulin therapy
- Excessive oral hypoglycemics
- Alcohol ingestion
- Excessive exercise
- Missed/delayed meals
- Illness
- Infection
- Gestational diabetes

CLINICAL PRESENTATION / PHYSICAL FINDINGS

- Mild hypoglycemia (blood glucose < 60 to 65 mg/dL):
  - Nausea
  - Extreme hunger
  - Pallor
  - Cold/clammy skin
  - Tachycardia/palpitations
  - Numbness/tingling of lips and finger-tips
  - Trembling
- Moderate (blood glucose < 50 mg/dL):
  - Irritability
  - Anxiety
  - Restlessness
  - Anger
  - Blurred vision
  - Dizziness
  - Headache
  - Weakness
  - Lethargy

- Poor coordination
- Impaired concentration
- Slurred speech
- Fatigue/lethargy
- Severe (blood glucose < 30 mg/dL):
  - Aphasia
  - Seizures
  - Convulsion
  - Cardiac ischemia
  - Dysrhythmias
  - Loss of consciousness
  - Coma
  - Hypothermia

DIAGNOSIS

DIFFERENTIAL DIAGNOSIS

- Drug-induced: hypoglycemic drugs
- Relative hypoglycemia: after rich meal
- Syncope
- Seizure disorder
- Malnourished state
- Sepsis
- Shock

LABORATORY

- Serum blood glucose
- Serum electrolytes
- Insulin level: increased
- Blood and urine toxicologic tests

TESTS

- Serum glucose
- Plasma insulin level and proinsulin level
- Glucose tolerance test
- CSF collection
- Blood glucose monitoring
- Urinalysis: urine sulfonylurea levels

RISK FACTORS

- Pregnancy
- Skipped meals
- Insufficient meals
- Unaccustomed to physical exercise
- Alcohol ingestion
- Medication overdose

MEDICAL MANAGEMENT & TREATMENT

EARLY TREATMENT

- Stop dental treatment.
- Place patient in supine position.
- Maintain airway.
- Monitor vital signs.
- Check blood glucose levels (glucometer).
- Treat blood glucose levels < 50 mg/dL, even with no symptoms.
- Oral glucose (responsive patient):
  - Glucose tablets
  - Soft drink/fruit juice
  - Quick, sugar-based foods

ADVANCED TREATMENT

- Unconscious patient: basic life support (BLS).
- Activate EMS.
- Establish IV access.
- 1 ampule IV glucose (50 mL of 50% glucose solution).

- Recheck blood glucose in 15 minutes.
- IV infusion of 5–20% dextrose solution.
  - Without IV access:
    - 1 mg of glucagon IM.
    - Recheck blood glucose in 15 minutes.
    - Repeat glucagon PRN based on blood glucose levels.
    - Recheck blood glucose levels.

FOLLOW-UP

- After initial treatment of the hypo-glycemic patient has been achieved, the patient should continue to be monitored for recurring hypoglycemia. The duration of this observation should be at least 2 to 4 hours.

MONITORING

- Blood glucose levels
- Responsiveness of patient
- Level of consciousness

PREVENTION/AVOIDANCE

- Thorough medical history and physical exam.
- Update health history at each dental appointment.
- Stringent control of diet, medication, and exercise.
- Maintain normal glycemic control.
- Avoid hypoglycemia.
- Avoid excessive hyperglycemia.
- Keep appointments short.
- Keep appointments at time of peak insulin coverage.
- Early identification and management.
- Preoperative with insulin-dependent diabetics (IDDM) for general anesthesia:
  - Consider one-half normal insulin dose.
  - Measure blood glucose.
  - Start IV with D5W.
  - Sliding scale postoperatively as indicated.

COMPLICATIONS

- Syncope
- Headache
- Visual disturbances
- Loss of consciousness
- Coma
- Permanent damage to the nervous system

PROGNOSIS

Severe hypoglycemia can most
often be prevented or avoided
by the recognition of the early warning
signs and followed with rapid and
appropriate treatment. If left untreated,
hypoglycemia can lead to unconsciousness and, if the brain is exposed to
reduced glucose for an extended period
of time, there may be permanent brain
damage. After initial treatment of the
hypoglycemic patient has been achieved,
the patient should continue to be monitored for recurring hypoglycemia. The
duration of this observation should be at
least 2 to 4 hours.

DENTAL SIGNIFICANCE

Isolated, mild episodes of hypoglycemia may not require specific treatment. Readily absorbable nondiabetic carbohydrates (fruit juice or other sugar-containing beverages) should be available in the office. Recurrent episodes of hypoglycemia need to be medically evaluated. The type and consequential therapy of the hypoglycemia should be discussed with the medical consult. This information should be used to modify the treatment of these susceptible individuals.

SUGGESTED REFERENCES

Branch Jr WT. *Office Practice of Medicine,* ed 4. Philadelphia, WB Saunders, 2003.

Ferri FF (ed): *Practical Guide to the Care of the Medical Patient.* St Louis, Mosby, 2004.

Lewis DP, et al. *Advanced Protocols for Medical Emergencies: An Action Plan for Office Response.*

The Washington Manual of Medical Therapeutics, ed 30. Philadelphia, Lippincott Williams & Wilkins, 2001.

AUTHOR: **DONALD P. LEWIS, JR., DDS, CFE**

SYNONYM(S)

DKA

ICD-9CM/CPT CODE(S)
ICD-9CM
250.1 Diabetic ketoacidosis
790.6 Hyperglycemia
CPT
80048 Basic metabolic panel
81002 Urinalysis
82803 Arterial blood gas

OVERVIEW

- Diabetic ketoacidosis (DKA) is an acute, serious complication of diabetes. It typically occurs in patients with type I diabetes but rarely occurs in patients with type II diabetes.
- DKA is defined as acute and severe uncontrolled diabetes requiring emergency treatment with insulin and intravenous fluids.
- DKA may be the first presentation of type I diabetes mellitus or may result from the increased insulin requirements of surgery, trauma, infection, or other physiologically stressful situations.
- DKA is characterized by hyperglycemia, acidosis, and ketonuria. This type of hormonal imbalance enhances hepatic gluconeogenesis, glycogenolysis, and lipolysis.

EPIDEMIOLOGY & DEMOGRAPHICS

INCIDENCE/PREVALENCE IN USA:
The annual incidence is from 5 to 8 per 1000 diabetic subjects.

ETIOLOGY & PATHOGENESIS

- Hyperglycemia is a result of increased hepatic glucose production and poor peripheral glucose uptake. Coma may occur at serum osmolality of 320 to 330 mg/dL. Ketoacidemia results from low insulin as well as elevated levels of catecholamines, glucagon, and growth hormone. This contributes to increased lipolysis and ketogenesis in the liver. Hepatic metabolism of free fatty acids as an alternative energy source results in the buildup of keto-acid intermediates and endproducts. The keto-acids include acetone, beta-hydroxybutyric acid, and acetoacetic acid.
- Ketones (beta-hydroxybutyric acid) induce nausea and vomiting and magnify fluid and electrolyte disturbances already existing in DKA. Moreover, acetone accumulation results in the characteristic fruity breath odor of ketotic patients.
- The increased concentration of these organic acids initially results in ketonemia. The body buffers these ketones in the early stages of ketonemia. When the ketones surpass the body's metabolic capacity, they spill into the urine (ketonuria). When not treated promptly, further accumulation of organic acids leads to metabolic acidosis (ketoacidosis), with a decrease in serum pH and bicarbonate levels. Respiratory compensation then occurs, which manifests as rapid, deep breathing (Kussmaul respirations).
- Hyperglycemia often exceeds the renal threshold of glucose absorption and results in glycosuria. There is a resultant osmotic diuresis induced by the glycosuria. This moderate to severe diuresis results in profound dehydration, thirst, hypoperfusion, and lactic acidosis.

CLINICAL PRESENTATION / PHYSICAL FINDINGS

SIGNS & SYMPTOMS
- One or more days of polyuria and polydipsia
- Nausea and vomiting
- Fatigue
- Stupor

ON EXAMINATION
- Fruity odor of acetone on breath
- Hypotension
- Tachycardia
- Rapid, deep breathing (Kussmaul respirations)

DIAGNOSIS

- Hyperglycemia > 250 mg/dL
- Acidosis with a blood pH < 7.3
- Serum bicarbonate < 15 mEq/L
- Serum positive for ketones
- Glycosuria and ketonuria

MEDICAL MANAGEMENT & TREATMENT

- Intravenous insulin.
- Isotonic intravenous fluids (fluid deficit of 3 to 5 liters).
- Five percent glucose solutions to be added later.
- Potassium replacement (potassium levels fall rapidly after initiating therapy).
- Bicarbonate may be indicated with severe acidosis.

COMPLICATIONS

- Vascular thrombosis
- Acute respiratory distress syndrome
- Pneumonia
- Myocardial infarction
- Cerebral edema

PROGNOSIS

Mortality rate is 10%, though most mortality is from late complications of DKA (sepsis, myocardial infarction).

DENTAL SIGNIFICANCE

Elective care should be discontinued, and the patient should be transported to a hospital setting where DKA can be appropriately managed. Blood glucose should be checked with a glucometer. If available, isotonic IV fluids should be administered, and the patient should be placed on a monitor until emergency medical transport can be accomplished.

SUGGESTED REFERENCES

Masharani U. Diabetes mellitus and hypoglycemia, in Tierney LM, et al. (eds): *Current Medical Diagnosis and Treatment*, ed 44. New York, McGraw-Hill, 2005, pp 1190–1194.
Powers AC. Diabetes mellitus, in Fauci AS, et al. (eds): *Harrison's Principles of Internal Medicine*, ed 14. New York, McGraw-Hill, 2005, pp 2158–2161.

AUTHOR: **JOHN F. CACCAMESE, JR., DMD, MD**

SYNONYM(S)

Alveolar osteitis
Osteitis sicca
Fibrinolytic osteitis

ICD-9CM/CPT CODE(S)
ICD-9CM
526.5 Dry socket
CPT
70355 Panorex

OVERVIEW

- Dry socket is the most common complication following the extraction of permanent teeth.
- It occurs due to the premature dissolution, loss, or necrosis of the alveolar blood clot resulting in exposed bone.
- Moderate to severe pain follows (often exceeding that which accompanied the initial surgery) and may be refractory to the usual analgesics.
- The onset is usually within a few days of surgery and may last well over a week, requiring multiple appointments before symptoms are controlled.

EPIDEMIOLOGY & DEMOGRAPHICS

INCIDENCE/PREVALENCE IN USA:
The frequency for all extractions is 3–4%, with impacted mandibular third molars accounting for the majority of cases at a rate of 1–30%.
PREDOMINANT SEX: Females are five times more likely than males to be affected.

ETIOLOGY & PATHOGENESIS

- The cause of dry socket is as yet unestablished. Bacterial fibrinolysis of the alveolar clot has been strongly implicated as a causal factor. Multiple bacterial species have been isolated from affected alveoli, and systemic antibiotics have had little success in preventing this problem.
- The cause is most likely multifactorial, involving both local and systemic factors such as tobacco use, oral contraceptives use, local bacterial count, presence of pericoronitis, age, gender, and practitioner experience.

CLINICAL PRESENTATION / PHYSICAL FINDINGS

- Moderate to severe pain that radiates to the ipsilateral ear
- Onset 2 to 5 days following extraction; may last for weeks
- Pain often refractory to systemic analgesics, both narcotic and nonnarcotic
- Visible alveolar bone or the presence of a necrotic clot
- Foul smell

DIAGNOSIS

- There are no laboratory abnormalities.
- There are no radiologic abnormalities; however, radiographs to rule out the presence of sequestra or root tips may be obtained.

MEDICAL MANAGEMENT & TREATMENT

- Prevention may be improved by preoperative chlorhexidine rinses or tetracycline in lower sockets, patient counseling, and the careful handling of hard and soft tissues.
- Treatment for dry socket is largely symptom management. Pain continues to be managed with oral analgesics in addition to the application of local sedative dressings (e.g., Dentalone, zinc oxide eugenol). The wound is irrigated, and the dressing is changed every second or third day until symptoms resolve.
- Long-acting local anesthetic blocks (bupivacaine) can be administered to alleviate more urgent pain.
- Consultation: oral-maxillofacial surgeon.

PROGNOSIS

Excellent long-term; there are no permanent sequelae.

DENTAL SIGNIFICANCE

Further elective treatment may be postponed until symptoms resolve.

DENTAL MANAGEMENT

- Must differentiate from postoperative infection
- Topical sedative dressings
- Narcotic analgesics
- Oral hygiene

SUGGESTED REFERENCES

Bergdahl M, Hedstrom L. Metronidazole for the prevention of dry socket after removal of a partially impacted mandibular third molar: a randomised controlled trial. *Br J Oral Maxillofac Surg* 2004;42:555–558.

Hermesch CD, Hilton TJ, Biesbrock AR, Baker RA, Cain-Hamlin J, McClanahan SF, Gerlach RW. Perioperative use of 0.12% chlorhexidine gluconate for the prevention of alveolar osteitis. *Oral Surg Oral Med Oral Pathol Oral Radiol Endod* 1998;85:381–387.

Larsen PE. Alveolar osteitis after surgical removal of impacted mandibular third molars. *Oral Surg Oral Med Oral Path* 1992;73:393–397.

Torres-Lagares D, Serrera-Figallo MA, Romero-Ruiz MM, Infante-Cossio P, Garcia Calderon M, Guitierrez-Perez JL. Update on dry socket: a review of the literature. *Med Oral Patol Oral Cir Bucal* 2005;10:77–85.

AUTHOR: JOHN F. CACCAMESE, JR., DMD, MD

SYNONYM(S)

Nose bleed

ICD-9CM/CPT CODE(S)

ICD-9CM
784.7   Epistaxis
448.0   Hereditary epistaxis
CPT
30901   Cauterization and/or packing anterior nose, simple
30903   Cauterization and/or packing anterior nose, complex
30905   Cauterization and/or packing posterior nose
30915   Ligation of arteries ethmoidal
30920   Ligation of arteries internal maxillary transantral
37600   Ligation of external carotid artery

OVERVIEW

- Epistaxis is more commonly due to trauma in the younger population and secondary to pathology in the older population.
- Epistaxis is divided into two categories: anterior bleeds and posterior bleeds.
- Bleeding typically occurs when the mucosa is eroded and vessels become exposed.
- More than 90% of bleeds occur anteriorly and arise from Kiesselbach plexus on the nasal septum.
- Posterior bleeds arise farther in the roof of the nasal cavity; are more profuse; often are of arterial origin; are a greater risk of airway compromise and aspiration; and are more difficult to control.

EPIDEMIOLOGY & DEMOGRAPHICS

Although epistaxis is common in occurrence, the true incidence of epistaxis is not known because most cases are self-limiting and thus are not reported.

ETIOLOGY & PATHOGENESIS

- Trauma
- Foreign bodies (pediatrics)
- Hypertensive crisis
- Bleeding disorders
- Infection
- Inflammation
- Neoplasm
- Idiopathic
- Drugs (warfarin, aspirin)
- Chemical

CLINICAL PRESENTATION / PHYSICAL FINDINGS

- Bleeding from bilateral nares or posterior pharynx

DIAGNOSIS

- Obtain a thorough medical history.
- Perform a thorough head and neck examination.
- Anterior rhinoscopy with topical administration of vasoconstrictor before and after exam.
- Fiberoptic endoscopy to inspect the nasopharynx.
- Laboratory tests such as a complete blood count, prothrombin time, activated partial thromboplastin time, and comprehensive chemistry panel that includes liver function tests.
- CT scanning or MRI to evaluate the presence of foreign bodies, neoplasms, and inflammation.
- Angiography in severe cases.

MEDICAL MANAGEMENT & TREATMENT

- Head elevation and nasal pressure.
- Topical anesthetics and vasoconstrictors with 4% lidocaine and 0.05% oxymetazoline are applied via aerosolizing spray or cotton pledgets.
- Electrocautery or silver nitrate cauterization.
- Anterior packing with petroleum impregnated gauze or Merocel packs.
- Posterior packs with rolled gauze or tonsil sponges, 12 or 14 FR Foley catheter, or specially designed epistaxis packs with inflatable balloons.
- Patients with posterior packs should be placed in a monitored setting (ICU), observing oxygenation, pain control, and fluid status.
- Surgical ligation of the internal maxillary artery or ethmoid arteries via a formal surgical approach, or endoscopy.
- Embolization of the internal maxillary artery or ethmoid arteries.
- Managing medical etiologies (e.g., coagulopathies).

COMPLICATIONS

- Hemorrhagic shock
- Sepsis from leaving nasal packing in place longer than 3 to 4 days

PROGNOSIS

Generally good if not due to severe coagulopathy.

DENTAL MANAGEMENT

See Medical Management & Treatment, preceding.

SUGGESTED REFERENCES

Kucik CJ, Clenney T. Management of epistaxis. *Am Fam Phys* 2005;71(2):305–311.
Randall DA, Freeman SB. Management of anterior and posterior epistaxis. *Am Fam Phys* 1991;43(6):2007–2014.

AUTHOR: **DOMENICK COLETTI, DDS, MD**

SYNONYM(S)

Overbreathing
Fast, deep breathing
Hyperventilation
Hyperventilation syndrome

ICD-9CM/CPT CODE(S)

786.01–306.01 Hyperventilation
Excludes: Hyperventilation, psychogenic

OVERVIEW

Hyperventilation is the condition where the patient is breathing at a faster rate than their normal breathing pattern and/or breathing more deeply than the body requires to maintain the normal oxygen/carbon dioxide balance. Hyperventilation is usually triggered by an imbalance in the body's natural levels of O_2 and CO_2.

ETIOLOGY & PATHOGENESIS

- Anxiety
- Nervousness
- Stress
- Pain
- Panic attacks
- Low oxygen levels in blood (hypoxia):
  ○ Asthma
  ○ Pneumonia
  ○ Pulmonary edema
  ○ Pulmonary embolus
  ○ Anemia
  ○ Pulmonary fibrosis
- Ingestion of medications/drugs:
  ○ Amphetamine
  ○ Aspirin
  ○ β-2 agonists (asthma mediations)
  ○ Cocaine
  ○ Iron
  ○ LSD
  ○ Methamphetamine
  ○ Methanol
- Increased metabolism:
  ○ Exercise
  ○ Fever
  ○ Infection
  ○ Hyperthyroidism, thyroid storm

CLINICAL PRESENTATION / PHYSICAL FINDINGS

- Symptoms usually last 20 to 30 minutes.
- Feeling of anxiety, nervousness.
- Yawning.
- Feeling of air hunger/shortness of breath.
- Pounding/racing heartbeat/palpitations.
- Pericordial discomfort.
- Lightheadedness.
- Vertigo.
- Numbness/tingling of hands, feet, perioral region.
- Epigastric pain.
- Headache.
- Diaphoresis.
- Blurred vision.
- Loss of consciousness.
- Muscle cramping/pain.
- Tetany/carpal-pedal spasm.
- Nausea.
- Vomiting.

DIAGNOSIS

DIFFERENTIAL DIAGNOSIS

- Diabetic ketoacidosis
- Panic disorder
- Drug abuse
- Thyroid storm
- Drug ingestion: salicylate
- Asthma
- Malignant hyperthermia
- Pulmonary embolus
- Congestive heart failure

MEDICAL MANAGEMENT & TREATMENT

EARLY TREATMENT

- Terminate procedure.
- Place patient in upright position.
- Maintain airway.
- Attempt to verbally calm patient.
- Monitor blood pressure/pulse.
- Oxygen not indicated.
- Reduce CO_2 elimination: rebreathing into paper bag:
  ○ Instruct patient to hold paper bag.
  ○ Patient takes 6 to 12 easy/normal breaths, then repeats without bag.
  ○ Alternate until return to normal breathing and symptoms disappear.

ADVANCED TREATMENT

- Midazolam (Versed®), 1 to 2 mg IV slowly; or
- Diazepam (Valium®), 1 to 2 mg IV slowly.
- Continue to monitor vital signs.
- Discontinue breathing bag when breathing returns to normal.
- Activate EMS if patient does not respond.

MONITORING

- Blood pressure
- Pulse
- Pulse oximeter

PREVENTION/AVOIDANCE

- Check if preoperative history of hyperventilation.
- Screen patient for anxiety disorders.
- Observe the initial signs of impending hyperventilation:
  ○ Increased anxiety
  ○ Perspiration
  ○ Mild tachycardia
  ○ Elevation in blood pressure
- Consider antianxiety protocol.
- Reschedule patient.

COMPLICATIONS

- Loss of consciousness.
- Vital signs are unstable.

PROGNOSIS

- Patient's breathing should return to normal.
- Symptoms will disappear.
- Patient should have medical consultation if etiology of the episode is not clear.

DENTAL SIGNIFICANCE

While hyperventilation is a dental office emergency that is most commonly caused by anxiety, it is important to rule out other potential etiologies. Previous history of hyperventilation or psychiatric disorders (e.g., panic attacks) should be documented. Medications for psychiatric disorders should all be reviewed.

SUGGESTED REFERENCES

Bennet JD, Rosenberg MB. *Medical Emergencies in Dentistry*. Philadelphia, WB Saunders, 2002.
Lewis DP, et al. *Advanced Protocols for Medical Emergencies: An Action Plan for Office Response*.

AUTHOR: **DONALD P. LEWIS, JR., DDS, CFE**

SECTION III

SYNONYM(S)

Low blood sugar

ICD-9CM/CPT CODE(S)

ICD-9CM
251.1 or 251.2	Hypoglycemia

CPT
80048	Basic metabolic panel
82947	Fasting glucose
82951 or 82952	Oral glucose tolerance
83525	Insulin
80432	C-peptide
74160	CT scan, abdomen
74185	MRI, abdomen

OVERVIEW

- Characterized by decreased plasma glucose concentration to a level (< 50 mg/dL) that may induce symptoms of low blood sugar.
- More acutely dangerous than hyperglycemia since glucose is the primary source of energy for the brain.
- Symptoms occur as a result of neuroglycopenia and stimulation of the sympathetic nervous system. The sympathetic-mediated symptoms often herald the onset of more ominous neuroglycopenic symptoms, alerting the patient to an imminent medical crisis.

EPIDEMIOLOGY & DEMOGRAPHICS

INCIDENCE/PREVALENCE IN USA: The true incidence of hypoglycemia in a population is difficult to establish. It is frequently attributed to anxiety and irritability associated with hunger without subjective documentation of low blood glucose. The prevalence of true hypoglycemia (with blood glucose levels below 50 mg/dL) occurs in only 5–10% of people presenting with symptoms consistent with hypoglycemia.

Hypoglycemia is a consequence of many medications and therapies; hence, the incidence of hypoglycemia in a population of patients with diabetes is different from that in a population of patients without diabetes. Insulinomas (insulin-producing tumors) are rare, with an annual incidence of 1 to 2 cases per million persons per year.

PREDOMINANT SEX: Postprandial (reactive) hypoglycemia is reported most frequently by women ages 25 to 35 years. Other causes of hypoglycemia are not associated with a sex predilection.

GENETICS: No known racial predilection exists.

ETIOLOGY & PATHOGENESIS

- Postprandial (reactive): rapid discharge of carbohydrates into the small bowel, followed by rapid glucose absorption and hypersecretion of insulin.
  - Idiopathic
  - Alimentary
  - Congenital enzyme deficiencies: hereditary fructose intolerance and galactosemia
- Fasting hypoglycemia
  - Drugs: ethanol, haloperidol, pentamidine, quinine, salicylates, and sulfonamides
  - B-cell disorders: insulinoma and islet-cell hyperplasia
  - Non-B-cell tumors
  - Autoimmune hypoglycemia
  - Exogenous insulin
  - Occult oral hypoglycemic use/abuse
  - Hormonal deficiencies: cortisol, growth hormone (in children), glucagon, and epinephrine
  - Critical illness: cardiac, hepatic, and renal diseases; sepsis
  - Congenital

CLINICAL PRESENTATION / PHYSICAL FINDINGS

- Sweating.
- Dizziness.
- Tremor.
- Headache.
- Tachycardia.
- Decreased mentation.
- Hunger.
- Loss of fine motor skill.
- Anxiety.
- Unconsciousness.
- Abnormal behavior.
- Clouded vision.
- Seizures.
- The Whipple triad is commonly present. This includes documented low blood glucose, presence of symptoms (detailed previously), and recovery when the blood glucose level is restored to normal.

DIAGNOSIS

- Oral glucose tolerance test
- Home testing during hypoglycemic episodes
- Simultaneous glucose and insulin levels
- A supervised fast (the most reliable diagnostic test for the evaluation of fasting hypoglycemia)
- C-peptide levels (to rule out surreptitious exogenous insulin injection)
- CT scan or MRI of the abdomen
- Octreotide scanning

MEDICAL MANAGEMENT & TREATMENT

ACUTE

- Obtain subjective serum glucose measurement.
- Oral administration of glucose (juice, sugar) when patient is conscious.
- Administer d50 IV when patient is unconscious.
- Adjust insulin/oral hypoglycemics as needed.
- IV octreotide to suppress insulin secretion.

CHRONIC

- Fasting hypoglycemia: frequent meals/snacks, especially at night, with complex carbohydrates.
- Postprandial (reactive) hypoglycemia: carbohydrate restriction, avoid simple sugars, increase meal frequency, and reduce the size of meals.

SURGICAL

- The treatment for fasting hypoglycemia caused by a tumor is surgical resection.

COMPLICATIONS

- Seizures
- Coma
- Death

PROGNOSIS

- Postprandial (reactive) and fasting hypoglycemia are often treated successfully with diet modification and are associated with minimal morbidity.
- With the early recognition and treatment of most forms of hypoglycemia, morbidity is minimal and mortality is rare.
- The success rate for benign islet-cell adenomas is good, and the success rate for malignant islet-cell tumors is as high as 50%.
- Hypoglycemia occurring as a result of treatment for diabetes is common. Mild hypoglycemia occurs in 50% of patients with diabetes who are in therapy. Poorly regulated glycemic control in diabetics (labile diabetes) is one indication for pancreas or islet-cell transplantation.

DENTAL SIGNIFICANCE

- Fasting and postprandial hypoglycemia can be treated with the oral administration of glucose, and treatment can be completed.
- During the advanced states of hypoglycemia (i.e., seizure, coma), treatment should be stopped or postponed until the patient has received adequate medical care.

SUGGESTED REFERENCES

Cryer PE. Hypoglycemia, in Fauci AS, et al. (eds): *Harrison's Principles of Internal Medicine*, ed 14. New York, McGraw-Hill, 2005, pp 2180–2185.

Masharani U. Diabetes mellitus and hypoglycemia, in Tierney LM, et al. (eds): *Current Medical Diagnosis and Treatment*, ed 44. New York, McGraw-Hill, 2005, pp 1196–1201.

AUTHOR: **JOHN F. CACCAMESE, JR., DMD, MD**

SYNONYM(S)

Laryngospasm

ICD-9CM/CPT CODE(S)
478.75 Laryngeal spasm
Laryngismus (stridulus)

OVERVIEW

- Laryngospasm is the protective reflex of the vocal chords to prevent foreign matter from entering the larynx, trachea, or lungs. This is a result of a spasm in the adductor muscles which close the vocal chords. It is the normal response to prevent foreign matter from entering the trachea and lungs.
- The classic signs and symptoms of a laryngospasm are increased ventilatory effort accompanied by increasing difficulty in exchanging air.

ETIOLOGY & PATHOGENESIS

- Precipitated by foreign material in the region of the vocal chords
- Light general anesthesia

CLINICAL PRESENTATION / PHYSICAL FINDINGS

SIGNS & SYMPTOMS

- Increased respiratory effort
- Increased difficulty with exchanging of air
- "Crowing" sound: partial laryngospasm
- No air movement or sound: complete laryngospasm

DIAGNOSIS

DIFFERENTIAL DIAGNOSIS

- Laryngospasm
- Bronchospasm

MEDICAL MANAGEMENT & TREATMENT

EARLY TREATMENT

- Rapid diagnosis.
- Pack of operative site.
- Positive pressure with 100% oxygen.
- Immediate suction of oropharynx: tonsil suction.
- Establish head position: tongue/mandible forward.
- Position tongue anteriorly.
- Observe/listen for air exchange.

ADVANCED TREATMENT

- With complete spasm:
  ○ Attempt to break with positive pressure: 100% oxygen
- Continuing spasm:
  ○ Succinylcholine (Anectine®), 10 to 20 mg IV (partial spasm)
  ○ Succinylcholine (Anectine®), 20 to 40 mg IV (complete spasm)
  ○ Deepen anesthesia
- Assist ventilation

MONITORING

- ECG
- Blood pressure
- Pulse oximeter
- Pulse

PREVENTION/AVOIDANCE

- Proper throat packs
- Proper airway maintenance
- Adequate suctioning
- Prevention of foreign material into oropharynx
- Deepen anesthesia

COMPLICATIONS

- Developing cardiac dysrhythmias secondary to:
  ○ Hypoxia.
  ○ Hypercarbia.
  ○ Hyperkalemia: succinylcholine can raise the levels of potassium with the result being hyperkalemia (can result in dysrhythmias leading to severe bradycardia and cardiac arrest).
  ○ Bradycardia.

PROGNOSIS

- Return to spontaneous breathing

DENTAL MANAGEMENT

See Medical Management & Treatment, preceding.

SUGGESTED REFERENCE

Lewis DP, et al. *Advanced Protocols for Medical Emergencies: An Action Plan for Office Response.*

AUTHOR: **DONALD P. LEWIS, JR., DDS, CFE**

SECTION III

SYNONYM(S)

Natural latex allergy
Natural rubber latex (NRL) allergy
Latex allergy

ICD-9CM/CPT CODE(S)
V15.07 Allergy to latex

OVERVIEW

- An allergic reaction caused by the exposure to natural rubber latex (NRL); may be present as either an immediate or a delayed type of allergic reaction.
- The delayed hypersensitivity response is usually manifested primarily as an allergic contact dermatitis.
- Natural rubber latex is found in the form of gloves and other surgical, dental, and medical supplies.

ETIOLOGY & PATHOGENESIS

Exposure to natural rubber latex

CLINICAL PRESENTATION / PHYSICAL FINDINGS

DELAYED REACTION
- Onset: 4 to 6 hours
- Peak: within 48 hours
- Respiratory reaction from airborne antigens:
  ○ Rhinitis
  ○ Asthma (wheezing)
  ○ Cough

IMMEDIATE REACTION
- Onset: within 20 minutes

SIGNS & SYMPTOMS
- Delayed:
  ○ Allergic contact dermatitis (rash)
  ○ Contact urticaria (hives)
  ○ Vesicles (blisters)
  ○ Erythema (redness)
  ○ Induration (firmness)
- Immediate:
  ○ Mild:
    ▪ Localized urticaria (hives)
    ▪ Nonspecific pruritus (itching)

  ○ Severe:
    ▪ Anaphylaxis
    ▪ Respiratory distress
    ▪ Hypotension

MEDICAL MANAGEMENT & TREATMENT

DELAYED HYPERSENSITIVITY
- Early treatment:
  ○ Place patient in upright position.
  ○ Administer 100% oxygen.
  ○ Monitor pulse, blood pressure, and pulse oximeter (PaO_2).
- Advanced treatment:
  ○ Consider activating EMS.
  ○ Continue to monitor and record vital signs.
  ○ Diphenhydramine hydrochloride (Benadryl®), 25 to 50 mg PO every 4 to 6 hours. Maximum dose = 300 mg/day, or
  ○ Diphenhydramine hydrochloride (Benadryl®), 25 to 50 mg IM/IV every 2 to 4 hours. Maximum dose = 400 mg/day.

IMMEDIATE HYPERSENSITIVITY
- Advanced treatment:
  ○ Epinephrine, 0.3 to 0.5 mg (1:1000 solution) administered sublingual, subcutaneous, or intramuscular.
  ○ Monitor vital signs.
  ○ Communicate with EMS en route.
  ○ Start IV fluids (1000 mL or 500 mL of NS or Ringer's lactate).
  ○ Advanced cardiac life support (ACLS) when trained:
    ▪ Epinephrine, 3 to 5 mL (1:10,000 solution) IV; may repeat in 10 to 20 minutes if necessary.
- If patient is intubated:
  ○ Epinephrine:
    ▪ Adults: 5 to 10 mL of 1:10,000 concentration.
    ▪ Children: 0.01 mg/kg.
- Treatment of bronchospasm:
  ○ Albuterol, 2 to 4 puffs initially; may repeat after 10 to 20 minutes.

  ○ Dexamethasone (Decadron®), 4 mg IV or hydrocortisone, 100 mg IV push.
- Transfer patient to medical facility for further treatment.

FOLLOW-UP
- Allergy testing

MONITORING
- Continue to monitor and record all vital signs.

PREVENTION/AVOIDANCE
- Avoidance of all products with natural rubber latex

COMPLICATIONS

- Symptoms worsen
- Signs of anaphylaxis

PROGNOSIS

Symptoms subside

DENTAL SIGNIFICANCE

The most common place in the dental office to have natural latex rubber is the gloves that are used. The NRL protein allergen can become airborne and is capable of causing an allergic response if inhaled. Patients with natural latex rubber allergy should have appointments and treatment scheduled early in the day before the contaminants are released in the air. Also, supplies and equipment containing latex need to be identified and avoided in the treatment of these patients.

SUGGESTED REFERENCES

Bennet JD, Rosenberg MB. *Medical Emergencies in Dentistry*. Philadelphia, WB Saunders, 2002.

Lewis DP, et al. *Advanced Protocols for Medical Emergencies: An Action Plan for Office Response.*

AUTHOR: DONALD P. LEWIS, JR., DDS, CFE

SYNONYM(S)

Deep neck infection

ICD-9CM/CPT CODE(S)

ICD-9CM
528.3 Ludwig's angina
CPT
21501 I & D, soft tissue
31500 Emergency endotracheal intubation
31600 Tracheostomy, planned
31603 Tracheostomy, emergency procedure
41015 Extraoral I & D, sublingual
41016 Extraoral I & D, submental
41017 Extraoral I & D, submandibular
41018 Extraoral I & D, masseteric space
41800 Drainage of abscess from dentoalveolar structure
70350 Cephalogram
70355 Panorex
70360 Radiograph exam, soft tissue neck
87040 Culture, blood
87070 Culture, any source other than nose, throat, blood
87205 Smear, primary source
99000 Transport specimen to outside laboratory

OVERVIEW

Deep neck infection from an odontogenic source involving bilateral submandibular, sublingual, and submental spaces. If untreated, has a mortality rate approaching 100%.

ETIOLOGY & PATHOGENESIS

- Odontogenic infection most commonly from first, second, or third molars
- Oral surgical procedures
- Secondarily infected malignancies
- Local trauma to oral cavity or neck
- Salivary gland infections
- IV drug abuse
- Infected branchial cleft or thyroglossal duct cysts

CLINICAL PRESENTATION / PHYSICAL FINDINGS

- Bilateral swelling of the submandibular, submental, and sublingual spaces
- Odynophagia (painful swallowing)
- Dysphagia (difficulty swallowing)
- Dyspnea (shortness of breath)
- Difficulty speaking
- Trismus
- Inability to handle oral secretions (drooling)
- Fevers
- Malaise

DIAGNOSIS

- Thorough head and neck evaluation.
- CT scan or MRI; however, if patient's airway is involved he/she may not be able to lie supine for the study.
- Leukocytosis (elevated white blood cell count).

MEDICAL MANAGEMENT & TREATMENT

- All medical management is adjuvant to aggressive surgical treatment.
- Admission to intensive care unit for sepsis and ventilatory support.
- Broad-spectrum antibiotics (ampicillin/sulbactam), 3.0 grams IV every 6 hours. If penicillin-allergic, then clindamycin, 600 to 900 mg every 8 hours.

COMPLICATIONS

- Airway compromise
- Sepsis
- Mediastinitis
- Death

PROGNOSIS

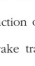

With the advent of aggressive surgical management and antibiotics, prognosis is favorable.

DENTAL SIGNIFICANCE

Deep neck infections of odontogenic etiology should be managed surgically and promptly. Antibiotic therapy is only adjuvant therapy and should rarely be used as the only treatment.

DENTAL MANAGEMENT

- Immediate and aggressive incision and drainage of all involved spaces.
- Send cultures and STAT gram stain from wound.
- Remove the source (i.e., extraction of all necessary teeth).
- May need to consider an awake tracheostomy.
- If decision is to intubate, then this should be done as an awake fiberoptic intubation.

SUGGESTED REFERENCES

Baqain ZH, Newman L, Hyde N. How serious are oral infections? *J Laryngol Otol* 2004;118(7):561–565.

Huang TT, Liu TC, Chen PR, Tseng FY, Yeh TH, Chen YS. Deep neck infection: analysis of 185 cases. *Head Neck* 2004;26(10):854–860.

AUTHOR: **DOMENICK COLETTI, DDS, MD**

SECTION III

Malignant Hypertension

SYNONYM(S)

Hypertensive crisis
Hypertensive emergencies
Hypertensive urgency
Malignant hypertension

ICD-9CM/CPT CODE(S)

995.86
401   Essential hypertension
        Includes: HPB
          Hyperpiesia
          Hypertension (arterial, essential, primary, systemic)
          Hypertensive vascular: degeneration, disease
        Excludes: Elevated BP without diagnosis of hypertension
          Pulmonary hypertension
          Involving vessels of brain and eye
401.0   Malignant hypertension

OVERVIEW

- Hypertension is an elevation in blood pressure that increases the risk of end-target organ damage including the central nervous system, cardiovascular system, and kidneys. It can be arbitrarily defined as a systolic blood pressure > 140 mmHg and/or a diastolic blood pressure of > 90 mmHg.
- Malignant hypertension is a potentially life-threatening situation that is secondary to the elevation of the blood pressure. The rate of the rise in the blood pressure is the critical measurement.
- Hypertensive emergencies are situations that require rapid (within 1 hour) lowering of the blood pressure to reduce end-organ damage and impairment. Hypertensive emergencies have been defined as a systolic blood pressure exceeding 210 mmHg and the diastolic > 130 mmHg along with blurred vision, headaches, and focal neurologic symptoms.

EPIDEMIOLOGY & DEMOGRAPHICS

Patients with the following conditions are at higher risk for developing malignant hypertension:
- Pulmonary edema
- Stroke
- Hypoperfusion
- Hypovolemia
- Hypertensive encephalopathy
- Intracranial hemorrhage
- Unstable angina
- Acute myocardial infarction

ETIOLOGY & PATHOGENESIS

- Abrupt increase in blood pressure in patients with chronic hypertension.
- Hypoxia can stimulate tachycardia and hypertension.
- Inadequate local/general anesthesia: pain.
- Excessive or intravascular injection of vasoconstrictor.
- Exacerbation of essential hypertension.
- Noncompliance with medications/self-withdrawal.
- Renal failure.
- Stroke.
- Acute anxiety.
- Drug overdose/withdrawal.
- Cocaine/amphetamine ingestion.
- Renovascular hypertension.
- Pheochromocytoma.

CLINICAL PRESENTATION / PHYSICAL FINDINGS

- Systolic blood pressure exceeding 210 mmHg
- Diastolic > 130 mmHg
- Focal neurologic symptoms

SIGNS & SYMPTOMS

- Sometimes there are no symptoms.
- Headache.
- Dizziness.
- Tinnitus.
- Retinal/visual changes.
- Chest pain.
- Shortness of breath.
- Symptoms of stroke.

DIAGNOSIS

DIFFERENTIAL DIAGNOSIS

- Stroke
- Hypovolemia
- Hypertensive encephalopathy
- Intracranial hemorrhage
- Unstable angina
- Acute myocardial infarction

LABORATORY

- Complete blood count (CBC)
- Electrolytes
- Urinalysis

TESTS

- ECG

IMAGING

- Chest radiograph
- CT scan

MEDICAL MANAGEMENT & TREATMENT

EARLY TREATMENT

- Cessation of current treatment.
- Confirm patient airway and adequate ventilation.
- Review medication and drugs.
- Reassess patient.
- 100% oxygen.
- Record vital signs every 5 minutes.

ADVANCED TREATMENT

- Activate EMS.
- Oral therapy:
  - Additional dose of patient's regular blood pressure medication.
  - Clonidine (Catapres®), 0.2 mg orally; may give additional doses every 1 hour to maximum of 0.6 mg.
- IV therapy:
  - β Blockers:
    - Labetalol (Trandate®, Normodyne®), 20 mg IV over 2 minutes followed by 40- to 80-mg dose every 10 minutes to maximum dose of 300 mg
    - Esmolol (Brevibloc®), 500 μg/kg bolus over 1 minute followed by 50 to 200 μg/kg/minute infusion to desired blood pressure
  - Vasodilators:
    - Nitroglycerin, 5 μg/minute IV and titrate to blood pressure (maximum 200 μg/minute)
    - Nitroprusside (Nipride®), 0.3 μg/ky/minute IV and titrate to blood pressure (maximum 10 μg/minute)
- Narcotic pain relief.

FOLLOW-UP

- A plan for long-term follow-up, treatment, and care should be instituted. Communications with the patient's primary care physician need to be documented.

MONITORING

- Blood pressure
- Pulse

PREVENTION/AVOIDANCE

- Consultation with medical physician.
- Continuation of antihypertensive drug therapy.
- Determine amount and type of antihypertensive being taken.
- Check adequacy of blood pressure control.
- Consider oral antianxiety control.

COMPLICATIONS

- Stroke
- Hypoperfusion
- Hypovolemia
- Hypertensive encephalopathy
- Intracranial hemorrhage
- Unstable angina
- Acute myocardial infarction
- Pulmonary edema

PROGNOSIS

The initial goal in the treatment of the hypertensive crisis is gradual reduction of the blood pressure.

DENTAL SIGNIFICANCE

With updated medical histories and recent vital signs, the impending hypertensive crisis may be avoided. The use of profound local anesthetics and the judicious use of vasoconstrictors also need to be taken into account in the treatment of patients with a history of malignant hypertension.

SUGGESTED REFERENCES

Ferri FF (ed): *Practical Guide to the Care of the Medical Patient*. St Louis, Mosby, 2004.

Lewis DP, et al. *Advanced Protocols for Medical Emergencies: An Action Plan for Office Response.*

The Washington Manual of Medical Therapeutics, ed 30. Philadelphia, Lippincott Williams & Wilkins, 2001.

AUTHOR: **DONALD P. LEWIS, JR., DDS, CFE**

SECTION III

SYNONYM(S)

Malignant hyperpyrexia

ICD-9CM/CPT CODE(S)
995.86 Malignant hyperthermia
Malignant hyperpyrexia due to
anesthesia

OVERVIEW

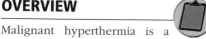

Malignant hyperthermia is a genetically transmitted myopathy manifested by an increase in body metabolism, muscle rigidity, and high fever. Serum creatine kinase is markedly elevated and cardiac dysrhythmias caused by electrolyte imbalance can be life-threatening.

ETIOLOGY & PATHOGENESIS

Malignant hyperthermia is characterized by muscle breakdown after certain stimuli including certain forms of anesthetic agents, extremes in physical exercise, or fever. It is inherited as an autosomal dominant trait and may be associated with other muscular diseases (i.e. muscular dystrophy).

- Anesthetic triggers:
  - Succinylcholine (Anectine®)
  - Inhalation anesthetics: Desflurane, Sevoflurane
- Other trigger agents:
  - Cocaine
  - Amphetamine (Speed)
  - Ecstasy
- Safe drugs:
  - Nitrous oxide
  - Methohexital (Brevital®)
  - Sublimaze (Fentanyl®)
  - Meperidine (Demerol®)
  - Benzodiazepine (Valium®)
  - Ester/amide local anesthetics
  - Ketamine
  - Propofol
  - Etomidate
  - Vecuronium
  - Pancuronium
  - Atracurium
  - Catecholamines

CLINICAL PRESENTATION / PHYSICAL FINDINGS

- Often noted for the first time during the administration of general anesthesia
- Develops rapidly a high fever and muscle rigidity

SIGNS & SYMPTOMS

- Tachycardia
- Tachypnea
- Masseter muscle spasms
- Onset may be delayed 10 to 30 minutes
- Unanticipated increase in end tidal CO_2 (10 to 20 minutes)
- Hyperkalemia
- Cardiac arrest
- Total body rigidity
- Unstable blood pressure
- Ventricular dysrhythmias
- ECG changes
  - Elevated T waves
  - Widened QRS complex leading to ventricular fibrillation
- Respiratory/metabolic acidosis
- Temperature elevation—late sign

DIAGNOSIS

LABORATORY

- Increased levels of CPK, potassium, uric acid, and phosphate
- Urine myoglobin—elevated

TESTS

- Genetic testing—ryanodine receptor (RYR1) shows gene abnormalities

DIAGNOSTIC PROCEDURES

- Muscle biopsy—increased levels of CPK

MEDICAL MANAGEMENT & TREATMENT

- Discontinuation of volatile inhalation anesthesia
- Discontinuation of succinylcholine (Anectine®)
- Hyperventilate with 100% oxygen
- Dantrolene sodium 2 to 3 mg/kg rapid initial bolus
  - Continue until symptoms subside
- IV cold saline (not LR) 15 mL/kg every 15 minutes × 3
- Hypothermic blanket
- Treat hyperkalemia with hyperventilation
- ACLS
- Transport to medical facility

MONITORING

- Blood pressure
- Temperature
- Pulse
- Muscle rigidity
- CO_2

PREVENTION/AVOIDANCE

- Family history
- Careful history taking
- Dantrolene preoperatively 2.5 mg/kg IV over 30 minutes preop
- Hypothermic blankets available

COMPLICATIONS

- Myopathy
- Muscular dystrophy
- Rhabdomyolysis/muscle breakdown
- Kidney damage due to excess myoglobin
- Acute kidney failure—repeated or untreated episodes
- Death

PROGNOSIS

- Malignant hyperthermia can often be prevented. The use of Dantrolene has greatly reduced the morbidity and mortality of this potentially fatal condition.

DENTAL SIGNIFICANCE

Malignant hyperthermia is commonly associated with abnormal elevation in intracellular calcium following triggering factors such as halothane anesthesia or succinylcholine. Patients with certain muscle disorders (i.e., muscular dystrophy) are at risk. Successful management of malignant hyperthermia requires prompt recognition and initiation of treatment including discontinuation of the offending agent, aggressive supportive care, and medication to reduce muscular rigidity.

SUGGESTED REFERENCES

Lewis DP, et al. *Advanced Protocols for Medical Emergencies: An Action Plan for Office Response.*

The Washington Manual of Medical Therapeutics, ed 30. Philadelphia, Lippincott, Williams, Wilkins 2001.

AUTHOR: **DONALD P. LEWIS, JR., DDS, CFE**

SYNONYM(S)

Epinephrine overdose
Epinephrine toxicity

ICD-9CM/CPT CODE(S)

E855   Accidental poisoning by drugs acting on central and autonomic nervous system
E855.5 Sympathomimetics
Epinephrine (adrenalin)
Levarterenol (nonadrenaline)

OVERVIEW

Adverse reactions to epinephrine are often erroneously described as a sensitivity or idiosyncrasy to the local anesthetic used. It can usually be explained on the basis of the amounts used; even though they may have been in exceedingly small amounts, they can still cause an adverse reaction. This reaction results from the local anesthetic being absorbed in the bloodstream and causing reactions in the central nervous system, respiratory system, and cardiovascular system. Epinephrine should be used judiciously in patients with myocardial disease or coronary arteriosclerosis because it can cause an increase workload of the heart due to its positive chronotropic and inotropic actions.

CLINICAL PRESENTATION / PHYSICAL FINDINGS

SIGNS & SYMPTOMS

- Rapid elevation in blood pressure
- Increase in pulse rate
- Anxiety/apprehension
- Tremor
- Pallor
- Sweating

MEDICAL MANAGEMENT & TREATMENT

- Place patient upright, in comfortable position.
- Provide 100% oxygen.
- Reassure patient.
- Monitor vital signs.
- Activate EMS if other signs/symptoms develop (e.g., blood pressure does not return to normal range).

MONITORING

- Vital signs
- Respiration
- Level of consciousness
- Appropriate responsiveness

PREVENTION/AVOIDANCE

- Monitor amount of epinephrine administered.
- Consider local anesthetic without vasoconstrictor.

COMPLICATIONS

- Increased blood pressure with hypertensive condition
- Development of dysrhythmias

PROGNOSIS

- Blood pressure should return to normal range within 20 minutes.
- Body redistributes/metabolizes the epinephrine.
- Heart rate should return to normal.

DENTAL SIGNIFICANCE

See "Medication Overdose: Local Anesthetic" in Section III, p 368 for Dental Significance.

SUGGESTED REFERENCES

Bennet JD, Rosenberg MB. *Medical Emergencies in Dentistry.* Philadelphia, WB Saunders, 2002.
Lewis DP, et al. *Advanced Protocols for Medical Emergencies: An Action Plan for Office Response.*
Longnecker DE, Murphy FL (eds): *Dripps, Eckenhoff, Vandam: Introduction to Anesthesia,* ed 9. Philadelphia, WB Saunders, 1997.
The Washington Manual of Medical Therapeutics, ed 30. Philadelphia, Lippincott Williams & Wilkins, 2001.

AUTHOR: **DONALD P. LEWIS, JR., DDS, CFE**

SECTION III

SYNONYM(S)

Local anesthetic overdose
Local anesthetic toxicity

ICD-9CM/CPT CODE(S)

E850	Accidental poisoning by analgesics, antipyretics, antirheumatics
E850.2	Other opiates and related narcotics
	Codeine
	Morphine
	Meperidine
	Opium
E850.3	Salicylates
	Acetylsalicylic acid (ASA)
	Amino derivatives of salicylic acid
	Salicylic acid salts
E851	Accidental poisoning by barbiturates
	Amobarbital
	Pentobarbital
	Barbital
	Phenobarbital
	Butabarbital
	Secobarbital
E853.2	Benzodiazepine-based tranquilizers
	Chlordiazepoxide
	Lorazepam
	Diazepam
	Medazepam
	Flurazepam
	Nitrazepam
E854	Accidental poisoning by other psychotropic agents
E854.3	Central nervous system stimulants
	Analeptics
	Opiate antagonists
E855	Accidental poisoning by drugs acting on central and autonomic nervous system
E855.1	Other central nervous system depressants
	Ether
	Gaseous anesthetics
	Intravenous anesthetics
E855.2	Local anesthetics
	Cocaine
	Lidocaine
	Procaine
	Tetracaine
E855.4	Parasympatholytics and spasmolytics
	Atropine
E855.5	Sympathomimetics
	Epinephrine (adrenalin)
	Levarterenol (nonadrenaline)

OVERVIEW

Adverse reactions to local anesthetics are often erroneously described as a sensitivity or idiosyncrasy to the local anesthetic used. It can usually be explained on the basis of the amounts used; even though they may have been in exceedingly small amounts, they can still cause an adverse reaction. This reaction results from the local anesthetic being absorbed in the bloodstream and causing reactions in the central nervous system, respiratory system, and cardiovascular system.

ETIOLOGY & PATHOGENESIS

- Injection of local anesthetic
- Intraarterial injection

CLINICAL PRESENTATION / PHYSICAL FINDINGS

SIGNS & SYMPTOMS

- Central nervous system
  - Drowsiness
  - Seizures/convulsions
  - Unconsciousness
  - Excitement
- Apprehension
- Tremors
- Restlessness
- Rapid pulse
- Anxiety
- Confusion
- Rapid breathing

MEDICAL MANAGEMENT & TREATMENT

- Administer 100% oxygen.
- Monitor vital signs.
- Activate EMS if continued symptoms.
- Place in supine position.
- Maintain airway.
- Observe for and manage resultant seizures.
  - Diazepam (Valium®), 5 to 10 mg IV (5 mg/minute).
- Provide basic life support (BLS).

FOLLOW-UP

- Monitor postictal state of seizures.
- Reappoint patient.

MONITORING

- Vital signs
- Respiration
- Airway
- Level of consciousness

PREVENTION/AVOIDANCE

- Careful injection of local anesthetic with aspiration on injection.
  - Least possible amount should be used
  - Minimum effective concentration
- Monitor amount of local anesthetic given.
- Use of epinephrine to decrease the rate of absorption of the anesthetic.
- Slow/repeated aspiration on injection.

COMPLICATIONS

- Depression of central nervous system
- Seizures

PROGNOSIS

Usually self-limiting and with reassurance the patient will be discharged from the office. The patient needs to be informed about possible adverse reactions. If there is any doubt whether or not it was an allergic reaction vs an adverse reaction, then the patient should be referred for allergy testing.

DENTAL SIGNIFICANCE

The entire dental staff should be aware of the types and amounts of local anesthetics being used. Monitoring the patient's vital signs and determining the amount of local anesthetic used is important. Any adverse reaction needs to be noted on the patient's records; this will allow a different approach at the next appointment.

SUGGESTED REFERENCES

Bennet JD, Rosenberg MB. *Medical Emergencies in Dentistry.* Philadelphia, WB Saunders, 2002.

Lewis DP, et al. *Advanced Protocols for Medical Emergencies: An Action Plan for Office Response.*

Longnecker DE, Murphy FL (eds): *Dripps, Eckenhoff, Vandam: Introduction to Anesthesia,* ed 9. Philadelphia, WB Saunders, 1997.

The Washington Manual of Medical Therapeutics, ed 30. Philadelphia, Lippincott Williams & Wilkins, 2001

AUTHOR: **DONALD P. LEWIS, JR., DDS, CFE**

SYNONYM(S)

Narcotic overdose
Narcotic toxicity

ICD-9CM/CPT CODE(S)

E850 Accidental poisoning by analgesics, antipyretics, antirheumatics
E850.2 Other opiates and related narcotics
    Codeine
      Morphine
    Meperidine
      Opium

OVERVIEW

The use of narcotics in the control of pain has a usual and predictable outcome. Adverse reactions and side effects are usually secondary to an inappropriate amount of drug given; an overdose may occur.

CLINICAL PRESENTATION / PHYSICAL FINDINGS

SIGNS & SYMPTOMS

- Respiratory depression
- CNS depression
- Miosis
- Hypotension
- Cheyne-Stokes breathing
- Recurrent ventilatory depression
- Constricted pupils
- Obtundation
- Cyanosis
- Comatose

MEDICAL MANAGEMENT & TREATMENT

- Activate EMS.
- Place in supine position.
- Maintain airway; supportive care is critical.
- Provide 100% oxygen.
- Assist ventilation if respiration is depressed or arrested.
- Administer Naloxone (Narcan®), 0.4 to 2 mg IV:
  - Repeat at 2- to 3-minute intervals.
  - Not to exceed 10 mg.
  - IM or SC may be used if IV not available.
- IV fluids: hypotension.
- Inducing emesis is contraindicated.

FOLLOW-UP

- Continue to monitor until normal responsiveness.
- Do not allow patient to drive home.

MONITORING

- Blood pressure
- Pulse
- Pulse oximeter
- Level of consciousness

PREVENTION/AVOIDANCE

- Knowledge of patient's physical status
- Knowledge of drug doses/interactions
- Risk factors:
  - Underlying hepatic disease
  - Chronic pulmonary dysfunction
  - Age-related: elderly
  - Synergistic effects with other medications/drugs

COMPLICATIONS

- Respiratory depression
- Coma
- Death

PROGNOSIS

Reversal of respiratory depression and disorientation after metabolism of drug

DENTAL SIGNIFICANCE

Narcotics are used to provide pain control and management during conscious sedation for dental procedures. Care should be taken to know the correct dose and the different possible responses to medications used. The healthcare practitioner should also be aware of possible overdose in patients who recreationally use/abuse narcotics.

SUGGESTED REFERENCES

Bennet JD, Rosenberg MB. *Medical Emergencies in Dentistry.* Philadelphia, WB Saunders, 2002.

Lewis DP, et al. *Advanced Protocols for Medical Emergencies: An Action Plan for Office Response.*

Longnecker DE, Murphy FL (eds): *Dripps, Eckenhoff, Vandam: Introduction to Anesthesia,* ed 9. Philadelphia, WB Saunders, 1997.

The Washington Manual of Medical Therapeutics, ed 30. Philadelphia, Lippincott Williams & Wilkins, 2001.

AUTHOR: **DONALD P. LEWIS, JR., DDS, CFE**

SYNONYM(S)

Sedative overdose
Sedative/hypnotic toxicity

ICD-9CM/CPT CODE(S)

E850   Accidental poisoning by analgesics, antipyretics, antirheumatics

E853.2   Benzodiazepine-based tranquilizers

      Chlordiazepoxide
       Lorazepam
      Diazepam
       Medazepam
      Flurazepam
       Nitrazepam

OVERVIEW

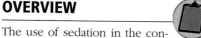

The use of sedation in the control of anxiety has a usual and predictable outcome. Adverse reactions and side effects are usually secondary to an inappropriate amount of drug given.

ETIOLOGY & PATHOGENESIS

- Drug overdose
- Inappropriate dose of medication
- Inappropriate response to normal dose

CLINICAL PRESENTATION / PHYSICAL FINDINGS

SIGNS & SYMPTOMS

- Respiratory depression
- Hypoxemia
- Hypercapnia
- Bradycardia
- Hypotension
- Hypersomnolence
- Behavior modification
- Confusion
- Auditory/visual hallucinations
- Drowsiness
- Ataxia
- Slurred speech
- Agitation
- Disorientation
- Nystagmus
- Tremor
- Cyanosis

MEDICAL MANAGEMENT & TREATMENT

- Place in supine position.
- Maintain airway.
- Positive pressure: 100% oxygen.
- Monitor vital signs.
- EMS if necessary.
- Consider Flumazenil (Romazicon®), 0.2 mg:
  - May repeat every 1 minute to maximum of 1 mg.
- Do not induce emesis with oral overdose ingestion.
- Support/treat bradycardia.

FOLLOW-UP

- Continue to monitor until normal responsiveness.
- Do not allow patient to drive home.

MONITORING

- Blood pressure
- Pulse
- Pulse oximeter
- Level of consciousness

PREVENTION/AVOIDANCE

- Knowledge of patient's physical status
- Knowledge of drug doses/interactions
- Risk factors:
  - Underlying hepatic disease
  - Chronic pulmonary dysfunction
  - Age-related: elderly
  - Synergistic effects with other medications/drugs

COMPLICATIONS

- Respiratory depression
- Coma
- Death

PROGNOSIS

Reversal of respiratory depression and disorientation after metabolism of drug

DENTAL SIGNIFICANCE

Sedatives are used to provide anxiolysis, sedation, amnesia, and muscle relaxation during conscious sedation for dental procedures. Care should be taken to know the correct dose and the different possible responses of medications used. The healthcare practitioner should also be aware of possible overdose in patients who recreationally use/abuse sedatives.

SUGGESTED REFERENCES

Bennet JD, Rosenberg MB. *Medical Emergencies in Dentistry.* Philadelphia, WB Saunders, 2002.

Lewis DP, et al. *Advanced Protocols for Medical Emergencies: An Action Plan for Office Response.*

Longnecker DE, Murphy FL (eds): *Dripps, Eckenhoff, Vandam: Introduction to Anesthesia,* ed 9. Philadelphia, WB Saunders, 1997.

The Washington Manual of Medical Therapeutics, ed 30. Philadelphia, Lippincott Williams & Wilkins, 2001.

AUTHOR: DONALD P. LEWIS, JR., DDS, CFE

SYNONYM(S)

Myocardial infarction (MI)
Acute myocardial infarction (AMI)
Heart attack

ICD-9CM/CPT CODE(S)

411.81 Acute myocardial infarction (410)

Includes: Cardiac infarction
Coronary
Embolism
Occlusion
Rupture
Thrombosis
Infarction of heart, myocardium, or ventricle
Rupture of heart, myocardium, or ventricle

OVERVIEW

Myocardial infarction is caused by inadequate blood flow and oxygen to the heart resulting in an irreversible injury to the myocardium. This is a result of the narrowing of the cardiac blood vessels with either partial or complete occlusion. This lack of cardiac perfusion to the myocardium can result in irreversible myocardial necrosis.

EPIDEMIOLOGY & DEMOGRAPHICS

Usually seen in:
- Diabetics
- Elderly
  Those with the following conditions/traits are typically more at risk:
- Older age
- Smoking
- Hypercholesterolemia/hypertriglyceridemia
- Diabetes mellitus
- Poorly controlled hypertension
- Type A personality
- Family history
- Lack of exercise

ETIOLOGY & PATHOGENESIS

- Decreased oxygen flow to the myocardium.
- Coronary atherosclerosis:
  ○ Complete or partial blockage of coronary arteries.
- Predominant cause is a rupture of atherosclerotic plaque with spasm and clot formation.
- Hypoxia.
- Coronary emboli.
- Induced coronary spasm:
  ○ Cocaine
  ○ Amphetamines
  ○ Ephedrine
- Aneurysm: dissection of coronary arteries.
- Congenital abnormalities.
- Polycythemia vera: increased blood viscosity.
- Trauma.

CLINICAL PRESENTATION / PHYSICAL FINDINGS

SIGNS & SYMPTOMS

- Chest pain: resembles angina pectoris but differentiates:
  ○ More severe
  ○ Vise-like
  ○ Choking
  ○ Oppressive
  ○ Longer than 20 minutes
  ○ Crushing
  ○ Squeezing
- Pain continues at rest
- Shortness of breath
- Elevated or reduced blood pressure
- Pain not immediately relieved by nitroglycerin
- May originate under sternum
- May radiate to arm, neck, and mandible, either left or right side
- Nausea
- Vomiting
- Skin:
  ○ Diaphoretic
  ○ Cool
  ○ Pallor
- Anxiety
- Sense of impending doom
- Dyspnea
- Evidence of ischemia on ECG
- Syncope
- Apical systolic murmur caused by mitral regurgitation
- Increased levels of cardiac enzymes
- Congestive heart failure (CHF) may occur:
  ○ Neck vein distension
  ○ Rales on pulmonary examination
- Fatigue
- Dizziness/lightheadedness
- May occur without chest pain (20% of patients)

DIAGNOSIS

DIFFERENTIAL DIAGNOSIS

- Angina pectoris
- Anxiety
- Asthma
- Congestive heart failure
- Pneumothorax
- Acute cholecystitis
- Acute aortic dissection
- Myocarditis
- Pericarditis
- Gastroenteritis
- Pulmonary embolism
- Shock

LABORATORY

- Complete blood count
- Creatine kinase: increased
- Myoglobin: rapidly released
- Troponin I
- Cardiac enzymes: elevated

TESTS

- Electrocardiogram (ECG)
  ○ Consistent with ischemia/necrosis
  ○ ST–T wave changes: inverted T waves
  ○ Elevated ST segments
  ○ New Q waves
- Angiography

IMAGING

- Chest radiograph
- Echocardiography

MEDICAL MANAGEMENT & TREATMENT

EARLY TREATMENT

- Place in upright/semireclined position.
- Active EMS.
- Establish airway.
- Monitor vital signs.

ADVANCED TREATMENT

- Activate automatic external defibrillator (AED).
- Begin ACLS.
- Aspirin (ASA), 160 to 325 mg (if not allergic).
- Nitroglycerin, 400 μg SL tablet or spray every 5 minutes up to three doses.
- Establish IV access.
- Provide 100% oxygen (face mask or nasal canula).
- Pain management:
  ○ Nitroglycerin, 0.2 to 0.6 mg sublingually; repeat every 5 minutes up to three doses over 15 minutes.
  ○ Morphine, 2 to 4 mg IV every 5 to 10 minutes as needed; or Meperidine (Demerol®), 12.5 0 25 mg IV every 20 to 30 minutes PRN; or Sublimaze (Fentanyl®), 25 μg IV every 10 to 20 minutes PRN.
- Reassess pain management after each dose.
- Monitor vital signs.
- Continue ACLS with unconscious patient.
- Transport to medical facility.

MONITORING

- ECG rhythms
- Vital signs
- Patient responsiveness
- Patient consciousness
- Pain control

PREVENTION/AVOIDANCE

- Identification of risk/history (medical and family).
- Physician consultation.
- Consider stress reduction protocol.
  ○ Administer 5 to 10 mg Diazepam (Valium®) prior to appointment.
- Continue antihypertensives.
- Consider preoperative nitroglycerin.
- Avoid hypoxia (low $PaCO_2$).

COMPLICATIONS

- Tachydysrhythmia: sinus tachycardia
- Bradydysrhythmia: type I, type II second-degree heart block
- Cardiogenic shock
- Valvular insufficiency

SECTION III

- Recurrent chest pain
- Recurrent ischemia
- Acute pericarditis
- Right ventricular infarct
- Ventricular septal defect (VSD)
- Myocardial rupture
- Systemic embolism
- Left ventricular aneurysm
- Pulmonary embolism

PROGNOSIS

- Prognosis is variable depending on the cause, timing of intervention, success of treatment, and post-MI management.
- A better prognosis is associated with early reperfusion, inferior wall infarct, and treatment with β-blockers, aspirin, and ACE inhibitors.
- Poor prognosis is associated with delay in reperfusion or unsuccessful reperfusion.

- Approximately 33% of patients with ST elevation myocardial infarction die, one-half of them within the first hour after onset of symptoms.

DENTAL SIGNIFICANCE

The signs and symptoms of acute myocardial infarction are similar to angina. The diagnostic difference between the two is determined by the duration of the pain. In angina, the pain is transient and is relieved by nitroglycerin, whereas the pain associated with an acute myocardial infarctions is unrelenting. Unless proven otherwise, all chest pain not relieved by nitroglycerin and rest should be considered and treated as an acute myocardial infarction.

SUGGESTED REFERENCES

Ferri FF (ed): *Practical Guide to the Care of the Medical Patient.* St Louis, Mosby, 2004.

Lewis DP, et al. *Advanced Protocols for Medical Emergencies: An Action Plan for Office Response.*

Schwartz GR, et al. *Principles and Practice of Emergency Medicine.* Baltimore, Lippincott Williams & Wilkins, 1999.

Stahmer S. *Myocardial Infarction.* Department of Emergency Medicine, University of Medicine and Dentistry or New Jersey, Robert Wood Johnson Medical School.

The Washington Manual of Medical Therapeutics, ed 30. Philadelphia, Lippincott Williams & Wilkins, 2001.

AUTHOR: **DONALD P. LEWIS, JR., DDS, CFE**

SYNONYM(S)

Aspiration
Emesis
Vomiting

ICD-9CM/CPT CODE(S)

7876.0–787.01
787.0	Nausea and vomiting
787.03.1	Vomiting alone
787.01	Nausea with vomiting

OVERVIEW

- Nausea and vomiting are common complications of multiple conditions.
- Emesis and aspiration of the stomach contents can result in the infiltration of the lungs, which can cause potentially serious or fatal pulmonary complications. In the acute phase of emesis, the body reacts to a noxious stimulus. The chronic form of emesis usually signifies an underlying gastrointestinal disorder that may affect the gastric motility. In either the acute or chronic forms of emesis, the body needs to have the protective mechanism to prevent the aspiration of the contents into the lungs.
- Therapy for nausea and vomiting should be directed at specific mechanisms that have been shown to cause the nausea.

EPIDEMIOLOGY & DEMOGRAPHICS

The following are more likely to cause nausea/emesis/aspiration in patients:
- Codeine preparations
- NSAIDs
- Erythromycin
- Swallowing of blood: gastric irritation
- Long-term effects of general anesthesia
- Pregnancy

ETIOLOGY & PATHOGENESIS

NAUSEA/EMESIS
- Stress
- Fear
- Pain

EMESIS/ASPIRATION
- Aspiration of liquid/semiliquid
- Aspiration of solids
- Foreign body aspiration
- Gastric contents
- Unprotected airway
- Loss of vocal cord protective reflex

CLINICAL PRESENTATION / PHYSICAL FINDINGS

SIGNS & SYMPTOMS
Aspiration
- Vary according to the type/amount aspirated
- Liquid aspiration (most common):
  ○ Rales
  ○ Dyspnea

○ Tachycardia
○ Bronchospasm
○ Partial airway obstruction
○ Cyanosis
○ Occurs in matter of seconds
○ Followed by rapid/progressively developing hypotension
○ pH of gastric contents (less than 2.5) and volume more than 25 mL have increased morbidity

Solid Aspiration
- Acute respiratory obstruction
- Asphyxia

Large Foreign Body
- Coughing, choking sensation
- Stridorous breathing
- Crowing sound
- Severe dyspnea
- Inability to breathe
- Cyanosis
- Loss of consciousness

Gastric Contents Are Acid in Nature
- Coughing
- Strider breathing
- Wheezing/rales
- Tachycardia
- Hypotension
- Dyspnea
- Cyanosis

MEDICAL MANAGEMENT & TREATMENT

TREATMENT: NAUSEA
- Tigan (Trimethobenzamide)
- Phenergan (Promethazine)
- Compazine (Prochlorperazine)

EARLY TREATMENT: EMESIS
- Assess level of anesthesia/assess patient responsiveness.
- Coughing patient: allow to clear contents.
- Position: sit upright and allow patient to clear contents.
- Provide 100% oxygen.

ADVANCED TREATMENT: ASPIRATION
- Head down and to the right side.
- Clear vomitus from oropharynx (suction).
- Provide 100% oxygen.
- Use large-volume suction.
- Do not use positive pressure ventilation.
- Consider intubation.
- Monitor vital signs.
- Tracheobronchial lavage.
- Intravenous steroids.
- Activate EMS.
- CPR if indicated.
- Manage hypotension/cardiac dysrhythmias.
- Manage bronchospasm:
  ○ Inhaled β-agonist drugs
    ▪ Bronchodilating medications:
      - Albuterol (Ventolin®), 2 puffs STAT, repeat every 10 to 20 minutes, *or*

0.5 mL nebulized solution mixed in 3 to 6 mL NS; repeat every 20 minutes.
- Ipratropium bromide (Atrovert®), 2 puffs STAT; repeat every 20 minutes, *or* 0.5 mL of 0.02% solution nebulized solution; repeat every 20 minutes.
- Epinephrine, 0.3 to 0.5 mg (1:1000) subcutaneous (SC); repeat every 20 minutes to maximum of 1 mg total.
- Prednisone, 40 to 60 mg orally (PO) (one-time dose).
- Aminophylline, 50 mg per minute (alternative).

Note: To administer medication, the patient must be awake (PO) or endotracheal intubation must be placed for delivery.

OBTUNDED PATIENTS
- Epinephrine (SC), 5 mL of 1:10,000 solution.
- Epinephrine (sublingual), 0.5 mL of 1:1000 solution if anaphylaxis is suspected and/or hypotension is present.

FOLLOW-UP
- Refer for follow-up immediate medical evaluation.

PREVENTION/AVOIDANCE OF NAUSEA/EMESIS
- Sedation prior to appointment (e.g., Valium®).
- Nitrous oxide/oxygen.
- Use of long-acting local anesthetic to decrease postoperative pain.
- Careful screening of patients.
- Consider parenteral sedation or general anesthesia.
- Patients receiving sedation/general anesthetic: NPO 8 hours prior to appointment.
- Clear liquids for adults/children for no less than 2 hours prior to anesthetic.

COMPLICATIONS

- Hypoglycemia (i.e., diabetic patient)
- Dehydration
- Electrolyte imbalance
- Inability to absorb medication
- Severe complications include:
  ○ Esophageal rupture
  ○ Rib fracture
  ○ Gastric herniation

PROGNOSIS

The expected prognosis for the patient experiencing nausea and/or vomiting would be a return to normal. Those patients who have aspirated vomitus contents have a more guarded prognosis.

DENTAL SIGNIFICANCE

Due to multiple factors, the dental patient is always a candidate for experiencing nausea and/or vomiting. Care should be taken to be cognizant of the possibility and to treat the episode quickly and efficiently.

SUGGESTED REFERENCE

Lewis DP, et al. *Advanced Protocols for Medical Emergencies: An Action Plan for Office Response.*

AUTHOR: **DONALD P. LEWIS, JR., DDS, CFE**

SYNONYM(S)

Collapsed lung

ICD 9CM/CPT CODE(S)

IDC-9CM
512.1 Postoperative pneumothorax
512.8 Pneumothorax
860.0 Traumatic pneumothorax without open wound
860.1 Traumatic pneumothorax with open wound
CPT
32000 Thoracocentesis for aspiration
32002 Thoracocentesis with insertion of tube

OVERVIEW

Pneumothorax is the presence of air within the pleural space. Pneumothorax is one of the more common forms of thoracic disease and can be life-threatening, especially when there is significant lung collapse or tension, which can cause cardiac and great vessel compression. Air enters the pleural space either through puncture of the chest wall and/or lung parenchyma and is caused by penetrating or blunt trauma, spontaneously (either primary or secondary), or iatrogenically.

ETIOLOGY & PATHOGENESIS

- Trauma (blunt, penetrating, rib fracture, barotrauma)
- Therapeutic or diagnostic procedures: central venous cauterization, positive pressure ventilation, thoracocentesis, needle aspiration biopsy, hyperbaric oxygen therapy, and radiation and chemotherapy for malignancies
- Can develop spontaneously due to presence of lung blebs or can be seen in patients with a history of endometriosis
- Airway diseases: COPD, cystic fibrosis, and asthma
- Interstitial lung diseases: Langerhans cell histiocytosis, sarcoidosis, tuberous sclerosis, rheumatoid disease, pulmonary fibrosis, radiation fibrosis, Wegener's granulomatosis, and lymphangioleiomyomatosis
- Infectious diseases: polymicrobial pneumonias, AIDS with *P. carinii* pneumonia, and tuberculosis
- Connective tissue diseases: Marfan's syndrome
- Malignancies
- Pneumoconiosis: silicosis and berylliosis
- Drugs and toxins: aerosolized pentamidine therapy in AIDS patients

CLINICAL PRESENTATION / PHYSICAL FINDINGS

- Shortness of breath
- Diaphoresis
- Chest pain (splinting chest wall)
- Tachypnea
- Tachycardia
- Hypotension, mediastinal and tracheal deviation, jugular venous distention (tension pneumothorax)
- Diminished or absent breath sounds on affected side
- Hyperresonance to percussion of affected side
- Noted sucking chest wound

DIAGNOSIS

- Good clinical exam
- Chest radiograph
- CT scan

MEDICAL MANAGEMENT & TREATMENT

Provide 100% oxygen, and depending upon the severity of the pneumothorax, treatment can vary:
- Simple observation
- Fine-needle aspiration (thoracocentesis)
- Chest tube thoracotomy
- Immediate needle decompression and chest tube placement (tension pneumothorax)

COMPLICATIONS

- Persistent air leak (requiring pleurodesis)
- Acute respiratory failure
- Empyema (infection of the pleural space)
- Systemic infection
- Death

PROGNOSIS

Pneumothorax is a potentially life-threatening condition; however, prognosis is excellent if a prompt diagnosis is made and aggressive management is performed.

DENTAL SIGNIFICANCE

No specific dental implications

SUGGESTED REFERENCES

Iannettoni M. Management of non-penetrating chest trauma, in Fonseca RJ, Walker R (eds): *Oral and Maxillofacial Trauma*. Philadelphia, WB Saunders, 1997.
Weisberg D, et al. Pneumothorax. *Chest* 2000;117:1279.

AUTHOR: **DOMENICK COLETTI, DDS, MD**

SYNONYM(S)

None

ICD-9CM/CPT CODE(S)

ICD-9CM
528.9   Bleeding from mouth
998.1   Postoperative bleeding
523.8   Unspecified
CPT
35800   Exploration postoperative hemorrhage, neck
37204   Transcatheter embolization
37600   Ligation external carotid
37799   Unlisted procedure, vascular surgery
40800   Drainage of hematoma, vestibule of mouth, simple
40801   Drainage of hematoma, vestibule of mouth, complex
41000   Intraoral drainage of hematoma, floor of mouth
        41015 Extraoral
41800   Drainage of dentoalveolar hematoma
41899   Unlisted procedure, dentoalveolar structures
85002   Bleeding time

OVERVIEW

- Bleeding from the socket or the surrounding soft tissue following a surgical extraction.
- Bleeding is classified as primary (direct bleeding from an injured vessel) or secondary (poor clot formation or lysis of clot).

ETIOLOGY & PATHOGENESIS

- Direct injury to vessels (inferior alveolar neurovascular bundle) or nutrient vessels
- Traumatic injury to surrounding soft tissue
- Inadequately removing granulation tissue

- History of liver disease
- History of renal disease (hemodialysis, uremia)
- History of bleeding disorder (e.g., hemophilia, von Willebrand's disease)
- Medications (e.g., warfarin, aspirin, Plavix®, low-molecular-weight heparin)
- Extraction associated with vascular lesion
- Infected hematoma

CLINICAL PRESENTATION / PHYSICAL FINDINGS

- Bleeding that is profuse and bright red is most consistent with an arterial injury.
- Bleeding that is dark red and has a persistent ooze is most consistent with a venous etiology.
- Presence of "liver" clot and chronic ooze from surrounding tissue.
- Sudden facial swelling, tenderness and/or firmness.
- Ecchymosis surrounding skin, vestibule, or floor of mouth.
- In severe cases, patients may develop hypovolemic shock with initial signs of tachycardia and hypotension.

DIAGNOSIS

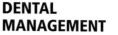

- Adequate physical examination
- Adequately obtained medical history
- Coagulation panel: PT, PTT, INR
- Complete blood count
- Basic metabolic panel
- Liver function tests

MEDICAL MANAGEMENT & TREATMENT

- Direct pressure with gauze pack for 15 minutes.
- Consider use of AMICAR mouth washes.
- Correct coagulopathies (i.e. platelets, frozen plasma, desmopressin, protamine, vitamin K).

- In cases of shock, patient will require aggressive fluid resuscitation and possible angiography.

COMPLICATIONS

- Airway compromise secondary to blood clots
- Hypovolemic shock

PROGNOSIS

Good

DENTAL MANAGEMENT

- First obtain adequate lighting, retraction, and suction.
- Irrigate socket with normal saline to attempt visualization of source.
- Remove any remaining granulation with curettage if noted as etiology.
- Consider application of bone wax if bleeding is noted from nutrient or neurovascular bundle.
- Consider application of gel foam, fibrin glue, Surgicel®, and thrombin with or without primary closure.
- Consider obtaining primary closure of tissue with watertight seal.

SUGGESTED REFERENCES

Carter G, Goss A, Lloyd J, Tocchetti R. Tranexamic acid mouthwash versus autologous fibrin glue in patients taking warfarin undergoing dental extractions: a randomized prospective clinical study. *J Oral Maxillofac Surg* 2003;61(12):1432–1435.

Piot B, Sigaud-Fiks M, Huet P, Fressinaud E, Trossaert M, Mercier J. Management of dental extractions in patients with bleeding disorders. *Oral Surg Oral Med Oral Pathol Oral Radiol Endod* 2002;93(3):247–250.

AUTHOR: **DOMENICK COLETTI, DDS, MD**

SYNONYM(S)

Seizure, petit mal
Absence seizure
Seizure, absence
Seizure, tonic-clonic
Seizure, grand mal
Grand mal seizure

ICD-9CM/CPT CODE(S)

345 Epilepsy
345.0 Generalized nonconvulsive epilepsy
Absences: atonic
Typical
Minor epilepsy
Petit mal
345.1 Generalized convulsive epilepsy
Epileptic seizures: clonic, myoclonic, tonic, tonic-clonic, grand mal, major epilepsy
345.2 Petit mal status
345.3 Grand mal status—status epilepticus
345.9 Epilepsy—unspecified
Epileptic convulsion, fits, seizures
Excludes: Convulsive seizure or fit

OVERVIEW

- Seizure disorders are caused by a sudden and abnormal electrical activity in the brain. This abnormal electrical activity causes a temporary cessation of brain function as a result of the excessive discharge of cortical neurons.
- Seizures can range from being unnoticed to (in severe cases) producing a change or loss of consciousness with involuntary muscles spasms called convulsions.
- Seizures can range from the grand mal seizure with clonic contractions to petit mal seizures with only a blank stare.
- See also "Seizure Disorders" in Section I, p 189.

EPIDEMIOLOGY & DEMOGRAPHICS

Patients with the following conditions are more at risk:
- Pregnancy
- Lack of sleep
- Missing doses of seizure medication
- Use/abuse of alcohol or recreational drug use

ETIOLOGY & PATHOGENESIS

- A seizure can be associated with or caused by an underlying condition.
- Epilepsy is a pathologic condition that is associated with recurrent and unprovoked seizures.
- Seizures can also result from a reaction to various anesthetic agents or can result from a combination of other factors.
- Seizures can be injury-induced or a result of alcohol abuse and/or withdrawal.

CLINICAL PRESENTATION / PHYSICAL FINDINGS

- Sustained unconsciousness
- Continuous or intermittent generalized convulsions

SIGNS & SYMPTOMS

Seizure symptoms can vary widely. These symptoms are related to the area of the brain affected and the amount of abnormal electrical activity being discharged.
- Petit mal seizure:
  - Muscle activity changes.
    - No movement
    - Hand fumbling
  - Blank stare/eye fluttering: 10 to 30 seconds.
    - Unintentional
  - Brief/sudden loss of awareness.
  - Resumes activity immediately after recovery.
  - Recurs multiple times.
  - Most often occurs in children.
- Grand mal seizure (generalized tonic-clonic seizures):
  - Sometimes preceded by an aura
  - Loss of consciousness
  - Muscle rigidity (stiffness)
  - Convulsions
  - Temporary cessation of breathing
  - "Sighing" after cessation of breathing
  - Possible loss of bladder control (incontinence)
  - Cheek/tongue biting
  - Regains consciousness with confusion and exhaustion
  - Weakness
- Simple partial (focal) seizures:
  - Muscle contraction of specific part(s) of the body
  - Abnormal sensations
  - Involuntary movements
  - Nausea/diaphoresis
  - Pupils dilated
  - No loss of consciousness
- Complex partial seizure:
  - Initial disorientation
  - Abnormal sensations
  - May have focal symptoms
  - Strange movement of extremities
  - Odd vocalization for 1 to 3 minutes
  - Possible loss of consciousness
  - Olfactory (smell) or gustatory (taste) hallucinations
- Jacksonian:
  - Muscle twitching
  - Begins in one area and progresses

CAUSES

- Hyperventilation
- Blinking lights
- Syncope
- Epilepsy (can be hereditary)
- Brain tumors
  - Any age: most after 30
  - Partial (focal) seizure: most common initially
  - May progress to tonic-clonic (grand mal) seizures
- Brain injury
  - Most common in young adults
  - Usually begin within 2 years of injury
- Previous head trauma/head injuries
- During administration of local/general anesthetic:
  - Ketamine (Ketalar®) and methohexital (Brevital®) can increase electrical activity.
  - Epinephrine: most likely precipitating factor.
    - Seizure is one sign of clinical overdose (see "Medication Overdose: Epinephrine" in Section III, p 367).
- Hypoxia
- Elevated body temperature (e.g., malignant hyperthermia)
- Hypoglycemia
- Hypocalcemia
- Hypernatremia
- Hyponatremia
- Hypomagnesemia
- Stroke
  - Most common after age 60
  - TIA (transient ischemic attack)
- Brain tumor/infection
  - May be reversible
  - Meningitis or encephalitis
  - Brain abscess
  - Neurosyphilis
  - Complication of AIDS
- Electrolyte imbalance
- Medications
  - Antipsychotics
  - Asthma medications
- Withdrawal
  - Medication
  - Alcohol
- Drug abuse
  - Cocaine
  - Heroin
- Cancer

DIAGNOSIS

DIFFERENTIAL DIAGNOSIS

- Syncope
  - Reflex syncope
  - Decreased cardiac output
  - Dysrhythmias
- Hypoglycemia: drug-induced (insulin/sulfonylureas)
- Recent head trauma
- Alcohol ingestion/withdrawal
- History of encephalitis
- History of meningitis
- Hyperventilation
- Stroke
- Transient ischemic attacks
- Positional vertigo
- Psychogenic seizures
- Extrapyramidal reactions
- Narcolepsy

LABORATORY TESTS

- Complete blood count (CBC)
  - Rule out sepsis/meningitis/encephalitis/thrombocytopenia.

- Blood chemistry/serum electrolytes
  - Glucose: rule out hypoglycemia.
  - Calcium: rule out hypocalcemia.
  - Magnesium: rule out hypomagnesemia.
- Liver function tests

DIAGNOSTIC PROCEDURES
- CT scan of head.
- MRI of head.
- Electroencephalogram (EEG).
- Lumbar puncture (spinal tap): rule out meningitis/encephalitis.
- Blood tests.

MEDICAL MANAGEMENT & TREATMENT

EARLY TREATMENT
- Place patient in supine position.
- Loosen clothing.
- Relocate instruments/supplies: safety of patient.
- Establish airway and monitor.
- Possible vomit: position head to right side.
- High-volume suction.
- Basic life support (BLS): with apnea > 30 seconds.
- Monitor vital signs.
- 100% oxygen via clear face mask.

ADVANCED TREATMENT
- Initiate BLS.
- Establish IV access.
- Consider IV medication for treatment of continued seizures:
  - Diazepam (Valium®), 5 mg/minute IV, up to 10 mg
    - Pediatric: 0.2 to 0.5 mg/kg IV
  - Midazolam (Versed®), 3 mg/minute IV or IM, up to 10 mg
- With suspected hypoglycemia:
  - Dextrose, 50 mL bolus of 50% glucose solution (adult) or 2 mL/kg of 25% solution (pediatric).
  - Observe:
    - Increased respiratory depression.
    - Discontinuance of seizure activity.

- Continued seizure activity: activate EMS.
- ECG monitoring: treat arrhythmias.
- Transfer to medical facility.
- Record details of seizure.

MONITORING
- Observe for 1 hour after seizure activity.
- Support respiration during recovery period.
- Place patient on right side.
- Continue to monitor vital signs.
- Continue 100% oxygen.
- Transfer to medical facility if concerned or patient is not responding to treatment.

PREVENTION/AVOIDANCE
- Limit amounts of precipitating drugs.
- Avoid rapid injection of local anesthetic.
- Aspiration of injection.
- Patient should wear a medical alert tag.
- Report seizure activity to patient's physician.
- Medication should be taken as prescribed.
- Monitor compliance of taking medication.
- Avoidance of recreational drugs.
- Avoid excessive alcohol.

COMPLICATIONS

- Loss of consciousness
- Aspiration of secretions/vomitus: aspiration pneumonia
- Loss of airway
- Bodily injury from equipment
- Biting of tongue
- Prolonged/numerous seizures without complete recovery (status epilepticus)
- Permanent brain damage

PROGNOSIS

- Most seizures are self-limiting.
- Early recognition and treatment results in better prognosis.

- Patient will usually regain consciousness and be in a confused state and/or exhausted.
- May be weak for 24 to 48 hours (Todd's paralysis).

DENTAL SIGNIFICANCE

Emergency treatment of the seizure patient should include complete recognition of the situation. Misdiagnosis and failure to recognize early signs and symptoms of the seizure will delay treatment. The delay in treatment may increase the morbidity of the seizure.

DENTAL MANAGEMENT

- Terminate procedure and follow preceding directions for medical management and treatment.
- Allow patient to recover without restraint.
- Do not place anything between patient's teeth.
- Do not move patient unless in hazardous position.
- Do not give patient anything by mouth until fully recovered.
- Do not allow patient to drive home.

SUGGESTED REFERENCES

Bennet JD, Rosenberg MB. *Medical Emergencies in Dentistry*. Philadelphia, WB Saunders, 2002.
Ferri FF (ed): *Practical Guide to the Care of the Medical Patient*. St Louis, Mosby, 2004.
Lewis DP, et al. *Advanced Protocols for Medical Emergencies: An Action Plan for Office Response*.
Schwartz GR, et al. *Principles and Practice of Emergency Medicine*. Baltimore, Lippincott Williams & Wilkins, 1999.
The Washington Manual of Medical Therapeutics, ed 30. Philadelphia, Lippincott Williams & Wilkins, 2001.

AUTHOR: **DONALD P. LEWIS, JR., DDS, CFE**

SYNONYM(S)

Nonconvulsive status epilepticus
Convulsive status epilepticus

ICD-9CM/CPT CODE(S)

345   Epilepsy
345.0   Generalized—nonconvulsive
        epilepsy
            Absences: atonic
            Typical
            Minor epilepsy
            Petit mal
345.1   Generalized—convulsive epi-
        lepsy
        Epileptic seizures: clonic, myo-
        clonic, tonic, tonic-clonic, grand
        mal, major epilepsy
345.2   Petit mal status
345.3   Grand mal status—status epi-
        lepticus
345.71 Epilepsia partialis continua,
        with intractable epilepsy, so
        stated
345.9   Epilepsy—unspecified
            Epileptic convulsion, fits,
            seizures
            Excludes: convulsive seizure or
            fit

OVERVIEW

- Status epilepticus is considered in the event of either a prolonged seizure that is not responding to conventional treatment or recurrent seizures without full recovery.
- Usually status epilepticus is considered the diagnosis when the seizure activity is longer than 30 minutes or there is absence of full recovery of consciousness between seizures. The increase in serious complications and an unfavorable prognosis are seen in this time period.
- Convulsive status epilepticus is a medical emergency that requires prompt and focused treatment. The treatment needs to be aimed at controlling the seizure activity and maintaining the patient's airway. The inability to control or stop the seizure activity can cause great morbidity or mortality.

ETIOLOGY & PATHOGENESIS

- Anticonvulsant withdrawal
- Alcohol withdrawal
- Hysteria
- Tumor
- Other
- Vascular (stroke, aneurysm, subdural hematoma)
- Infections (viral, bacterial)
- Toxic (poisons, drugs)
- Head trauma
- Idiopathic
- Immune (lupus, multiple sclerosis)
- Degenerative (Alzheimer's disease)
- Iatrogenic: change in anticonvulsant levels

CLINICAL PRESENTATION / PHYSICAL FINDINGS

SIGNS & SYMPTOMS

- Sustained unconsciousness
- Continuous or intermittent generalized, convulsive seizure activity
- Seizure activity lasting > 10 minutes without recovery of consciousness
- Warrants IV anticonvulsant therapy

DIAGNOSIS

DIFFERENTIAL DIAGNOSIS

- Syncope
  - Reflex syncope
  - Decreased cardiac output
  - Dysrhythmias
- Hypoglycemia: drug-induced (insulin/sulfonylureas)
- Recent head trauma
- Alcohol ingestion/withdrawal
- History of encephalitis
- History of meningitis
- Hyperventilation
- Stroke
- Transient ischemic attacks
- Positional vertigo
- Psychogenic seizures
- Extrapyramidal reactions
- Narcolepsy

LABORATORY TESTS

- Glucose levels
- Electrolytes
- Calcium
- Magnesium
- BUN
- Creatinine
- Antiepileptic drug levels
- CBC
- Urinanalysis

MEDICAL MANAGEMENT & TREATMENT

INITIAL TREATMENT (beginning of seizure to 5 minutes):

- Terminate procedure.
- Place patient in supine position.
- Loosen clothing.
- Relocate instruments/supplies: safety of patient.
- Establish airway and monitor.
- Possible vomit: position head to right side.
- High-volume suction.
- Provide basic life support (BLS): with apnea > 30 seconds.
- Monitor vital signs.
- Provide 100% oxygen via clear face mask.
- Activate EMS when seizure > 2 minutes.

ADVANCED TREATMENT (5 to 10 minutes):

- Initiate BLS.
- Establish IV access.
- Draw blood samples (include anticonvulsant levels).

- Consider IV medication for treatment of continued seizures:
  - Diazepam (Valium®), 5 mg/minute IV, up to 10 mg.
    - Pediatric: 0.2 to 0.5 mg/kg IV
  - Note: Observe side effects: hypotension, bradycardia, respiratory depression, depressed mental status, cardiac arrest.
- With suspected hypoglycemia:
  - Dextrose, 50 mL bolus of 50% glucose solution (adult) or 2 mL/kg of 25% solution (pediatric).
  - Phenytoin, 17 mg/kg (1 gm minimum) at 50 mg/minute with monitoring of vital signs and ECG. Administer either directly into the vein or close, never as drip.
- With continued seizure:
  - Phenobarbital, 400 mg/10 minutes (powerful depressant)
- Observe:
  - Increased respiratory depression
  - Discontinuance of seizure activity
- Continued seizure activity: activate EMS.
- ECG monitoring: treat dysrhythmias.
- Transfer to medical facility.
- Record details of seizure.

CONTINUED ADVANCED TREATMENT (10 to 30 minutes)

- Longer-acting anticonvulsant required.
- Consider intubation.
- Transport to medical facility should be complete.

MONITORING

- Vital signs
- Oximetry
- ECG

PREVENTION/AVOIDANCE

- Proper medical history
- Observance for early signs/symptoms

COMPLICATIONS

- Hypoxemia
- Pulmonary edema
- Hypotension
- Bradycardia
- Hypoglycemia
- Rhabdomyolysis with acute renal failure
- Brain damage

PROGNOSIS

- Most seizures are self-limiting.
- Status epilepticus needs prompt treatment.
- Transport to medical facility.

DENTAL SIGNIFICANCE

- Convulsive status epilepticus is a medical emergency that requires prompt and focused treatment. The treatment needs to be aimed at controlling the seizure activity and maintaining the patient's airway.

- The inability to control or stop the seizure activity can cause great morbidity or mortality.

SUGGESTED REFERENCES

Bennet JD, Rosenberg MB. *Medical Emergencies in Dentistry*. Philadelphia, WB Saunders, 2002.

Lewis DP, et al. *Advanced Protocols for Medical Emergencies: An Action Plan for Office Response*.

Ooommen, KJ. Status epilepticus in adults, at http//w3.ouhsc.edu/neuro/division/cope/status/htm

Schwartz GR, et al. *Principles and Practice of Emergency Medicine*. Baltimore, Lippincott Williams & Wilkins, 1999.

The Washington Manual of Medical Therapeutics, ed 30. Philadelphia, Lippincott Williams & Wilkins, 2001.

AUTHOR: **DONALD P. LEWIS, JR., DDS, CFE**

SYNONYM(S)

Vasovagal syncope
Fainting
Passed out

ICD-9CM/CPT CODE(S)

780 Syncope
780.2 Syncope and collapse
    Blackout
    Fainting
    Presyncope
    Vasovagal attack
  Excludes:
    Carotid sinus syncope (337.0)
    Heat syncope (992.1)
    Neurocirculatory asthenia (306.2)
    Orthostatic hypotension (478.0)
    Shock (785.5)

OVERVIEW

Syncope is the temporary loss of consciousness due to a decrease in blood flow to the brain. This is usually temporary in nature and is followed by a rapid and complete recovery.

EPIDEMIOLOGY & DEMOGRAPHICS

Patients with the following conditions are at greater risk:
- Seizure disorder
- Preexisting history of syncope
- History of coronary disease
- Congestive heart failure
- Dehydration

ETIOLOGY & PATHOGENESIS

- Panic or anxiety attacks
- Low blood sugar (hypoglycemia)
- Vasovagal reaction
- Orthostatic hypotension
  - Hypovolemia
  - Hypotensive drugs
  - Pheochromocytoma
- Hyperventilation
- Familial history of fainting
- Seizures
- Transient ischemic attack
- Conditions of the nervous system:
  - Diabetes
  - Alcoholism
  - Malnutrition
  - Hypertensive medications
  - Dehydration
- Conditions of the cardiovascular system:
  - Heart block
  - Sinus node conditions
  - Heart dysrhythmias/asystole
    - Extreme tachycardia (> 160 to 180 bpm)
    - Severe bradycardia (< 30 to 40 bpm)
    - Sick sinus syndrome
    - Ventricular tachycardia/fibrillation
  - Blood clot in lungs
  - Narrowed aortic valve
  - Cardiac tamponade
  - Mitral stenosis

- Other conditions:
  - Micturition syncope (fainting during/after urination)
  - Straining during bowel movement
  - Cough syncope
  - Stretch syncope (stretching of neck and arms)
  - Swallowing syncope

CLINICAL PRESENTATION / PHYSICAL FINDINGS

- Presyncope
  - Nausea
  - Sensation of warmth
  - Lightheadedness
  - Diaphoresis
  - Pallor (loss of color)
  - Tachycardia
- Syncope
  - Hypotension
  - Bradycardia
  - Dilation of pupils
  - Peripheral chill
  - Visual disturbance
  - Loss of consciousness

DIAGNOSIS

DIFFERENTIAL DIAGNOSIS

- Primary cardiac syncope
  - Cardiac myopathy
  - Valvular stenosis
  - Aortic dissection
  - Pulmonary embolism
  - Dysrhythmias
    - Bradyarrhythmias
      - Sinus node disease
      - AV node disease
      - Conduction system disease
      - Pacemaker malfunction
    - Tachydysrhythmias
      - Supraventricular tachycardia (SVT)
      - Ventricular tachycardia (VT)
  - Neurocardiogenic syncope
    - Micturition
    - Defecation
    - Coughing
    - Swallowing
  - Orthostatic hypotension
  - Drug toxicities
  - Hypoglycemia
  - Hypoxia
  - Seizures
  - Cerebrovascular events
  - Psychiatric disorders/anxiety
  - Hyperventilation
  - Vasovagal syncope

LABORATORY TESTS

- ECG
- Holter monitor
- Chest radiograph
- Echocardiogram
- EEG
- Toxicology screening
- Neurologic/psychiatric testing
- Arterial blood gases (ABGs): rule out pulmonary embolism/hyperventilation

MEDICAL MANAGEMENT & TREATMENT

EARLY TREATMENT

- Trendelenburg position in chair (head below legs).
  - Note: Pregnant patient: place in left lateral decubitus position.
- Assess level of consciousness.
- Assess airway, breathing, and circulation (ABCs).
- Head tilt for proper airway.
- Provide 100% oxygen.
- Monitor/record vital signs.
- Consider crushed ammonia under nose.
- Cold compress to neck.
- Reassure patient.
- Expect full recovery within less than 20 minutes.

ADVANCED TREATMENT

- Differential Diagnosis to be considered:
  - Medication-related hypotension
  - Hypoglycemia
  - CVA
  - Seizure disorder
  - Dysrhythmias
  - Anaphylaxis
  - Anxiety/panic attack
  - Hyperventilation syndrome
- Activate EMS if loss of consciousness is > than 5 minutes or recovery is > 20 minutes.
- Start ACLS.
- With bradycardia:
  - Atropine, 0.5 to 1 mg IV.
  - Repeat atropine every 5 minutes to maximum dose of 3 mg as needed, based on heart monitoring.

FOLLOW-UP

- Low risk: patients whose apparent cause of syncope is responsive to therapy can be discharged.
- High risk: patients thought to have cardiac cause of syncope need to be referred for physical exam and diagnostic testing.

MONITORING

- Blood pressure
- Pulse
- Pulse oximeter
- Respiration rate and depth
- Electrocardiogram

PREVENTION/AVOIDANCE

- Control predisposing factors.
- Implement stress reduction protocol.
- Consider preoperative sedation.
- Monitor patient.
- Start patient in supine position.
- Beware of early recognition.

COMPLICATIONS

- Cardiac myopathy
- Pulmonary embolism
- Dysrhythmias
  - Bradydysrhythmias

- ○ Tachydysrhythmias
- Neurocardiogenic syncope
- Orthostatic hypotension
- Seizures
- Cerebrovascular events
- Psychiatric disorders/anxiety
- Hyperventilation

PROGNOSIS

- Benign prognosis:
  - ○ Patient < 30 years of age and noncardiac syncope
  - ○ Patient < 70 years of age and having vasovagal/psychogenic syncope
- Poor prognosis: patient with cardiogenic syncope

DENTAL SIGNIFICANCE

Syncope is a transient loss of consciousness that is probably the most common type of emergency encountered in the dental office. It may also signal an undiagnosed, underlying, potentially lethal cardiac condition. Therefore, with any syncopal event careful evaluation is necessary.

DENTAL MANAGEMENT

Patients considered to be low-risk can be discharged after recovery. Patients considered as being high-risk (i.e., patients with suspected cardiac syncope) need to be referred to a healthcare facility.

SUGGESTED REFERENCES

Ferri FF (ed): *Practical Guide to the Care of the Medical Patient.* St Louis, Mosby, 2004.
Lewis DP, et al. *Advanced Protocols for Medical Emergencies: An Action Plan for Office Response.*
Schwartz GR, et al. *Principles and Practice of Emergency Medicine.* Baltimore, Lippincott Williams & Wilkins, 1999.
The Washington Manual of Medical Therapeutics, ed 30. Philadelphia, Lippincott Williams & Wilkins, 2001.

AUTHOR: **DONALD P. LEWIS, JR., DDS, CFE**

SYNONYM(S)

Thyroid crisis
Thyrotoxic crisis

ICD-9CM/CPT CODE(S)

242 Thyrotoxicosis
242.4 Thyrotoxicosis from ectopic thyroid nodule
242.8 Thyrotoxicosis of other specified origin
   Overproduction of TSH
242.9 Thyrotoxicosis without mention of goiter or other cause
   Hyperthyroidism

OVERVIEW

Thyroid storm is a life-threatening condition that is more likely to develop when a patient has a serious health problem (e.g., infection) in addition to having hyperthyroidism. Thyroid storm is an acute exacerbation of the hypermetabolic symptoms and can develop suddenly; medical treatment is necessary. It is a metabolic event that is characterized by hyperthermia, tachycardia, and altered mental status.

See also "Hyperthyroidism" in Section I, p 119.

ETIOLOGY & PATHOGENESIS

Thyroid storm develops when the thyroid gland releases large amounts of thyroid hormone in a short period of time. This hypermetabolic state results in a sudden shift from the protein-bound thyroid hormone to the relatively free and metabolically active hormone. This can be the result of:

- Infection
- Surgery
- Trauma
- Sepsis
- Pregnancy
- Physiologic/emotional stress
- Pulmonary embolism
- Autoimmune trigger
- Diabetic ketoacidosis
- Insulin-induced hypoglycemia
- Attempted surgical treatment of hyperthyroidism
- Withdrawal of antithyroid medication
- Radioactive iodine
- Thyroid hormone overdose
- Cardiovascular events
- Psychiatric disturbances

CLINICAL PRESENTATION / PHYSICAL FINDINGS

SIGNS & SYMPTOMS

- Predisposed signs:
  o Tremor
  o Tachycardia
  o Weight loss
  o Hypertension
  o Irritability
  o Intolerance to heat
  o Exophthalmus

- Elevation of temperature > 41°C/105°F
- Nervousness
- Agitation
- Hypotension < 90 mmHg
- Weakness
- Exhaustion
- Palpitations
- Fatigue
- Dyspnea
- Nausea
- Vomiting
- Abdominal pains
- Partial or complete loss of consciousness
- Bruit over thyroid
- Goiter
- Dermatologic:
  o Warm, moist, velvety skin
  o Palmar erythema
  o Fingernails: onycholysis
  o Hair: fine and silky
- Neuromuscular:
  o Fine tremor of fingers and tongue
  o Hyperkinesia
  o Rapid speech
  o Quadriceps weakness
- Ophthalmologic:
  o Staring/infrequent blinking
  o Widened palpebral fissures
  o Chemosis
  o Lid lad
  o Proptosis
  o Periorbital edema
- Cardiovascular:
  o Increased blood pressure/systolic hypertension
  o Dysrhythmia
  o Atrial fibrillation
  o Tachycardia > 140 bpm

DIAGNOSIS

DIFFERENTIAL DIAGNOSIS

- Adrenal tumors (i.e., pheochromocytoma)
- Cocaine/amphetamine overdose
- Cardiac tachydysrhythmias
- Extreme anxiety
- Aggressive psychiatric disorders
- Malignant hyperthermia

LABORATORY TESTS

- TSH Test
- CPK
- ABGs
- ECG
- Chest radiograph
- Urinanalysis

MEDICAL MANAGEMENT & TREATMENT

- Terminate procedure.
- Activate EMS.
- Provide 100% oxygen.
- Place in comfortable position.
- Acetaminophen for hyperthermia.
- Monitor vital signs.
- Initiate BLS as indicated.
- Establish IV line: D5LR or NS.

- Dexamethasone (Decadron®), 4 mg IV, slow.
- Crystalloid solution IV (150 mL/hour).
- Transport to medical facility.

PREVENTION/AVOIDANCE

- Awareness of medical history of:
  o Rapid heartbeat
  o Palpitations
  o Weight loss
  o Mental changes
  o "Nerve disorders"
- Avoidance of stressful situations
- Minimal use of vasoconstrictors
- Consultation with primary physician
- Determination of adequacy of excessive thyroid hormone production
- Determination of precipitating cause

COMPLICATIONS

- Severe hypotension
- Cardiac complication
- Pulmonary edema
- High-output cardiac failure
- Coma

PROGNOSIS

Metabolic disorders leading to emergencies caused by thyroid dysfunction should be avoided.

DENTAL SIGNIFICANCE

A patient suspected to be in thyroid storm needs to receive prompt and aggressive treatment. This is a life-threatening situation and failure to recognize and treat the condition is essential to prevent an adverse result.

DENTAL MANAGEMENT

- Terminate procedure.
- Activate EMS/transport to medical facility.
- Not treating the underlying cause, such as infection or pulmonary embolism, is the most common oversight in the management of thyroid storm.

SUGGESTED REFERENCES

Lewis DP, et al. *Advanced Protocols for Medical Emergencies: An Action Plan for Office Response.*

Schwartz GR, et al. *Principles and Practice of Emergency Medicine.* Baltimore, Lippincott Williams & Wilkins, 1999.

AUTHOR: **DONALD P. LEWIS, JR., DDS, CFE**

SYNONYM(S)

TIA
Transient cerebral ischemia

ICD-9CM/CPT CODE(S)

435 Transient cerebral ischemia
Includes: Cerebrovascular insufficiency (acute)
Insufficiency of basilar, carotid, and vertebral arteries
Spasm of cerebral arteries
435.9 Unspecified transient cerebral ischemia
Impending cerebrovascular accident
Intermittent cerebral ischemia
Transient ischemic attack (TIA)

OVERVIEW

- A transient ischemic attack (TIA) is defined as a brief episode of neurological dysfunction caused by focal brain or retinal ischemia with clinical symptoms typically lasting less than 1 hour and without evidence of acute infarction.
- TIA is a sudden and/or rapid onset of signs and symptoms. This definition shows the urgency of recognizing a TIA as an important warning sign of impending stroke and to rapidly start the evaluation and treatment to prevent permanent brain ischemia.

EPIDEMIOLOGY & DEMOGRAPHICS

Patients with the following conditions are at greater risk:
- Hypertension
- Diabetes
- Cardiac disease
- Elevated blood lipid levels
- Carotid artery stenosis
- Smoking
- Oral contraceptive use
- Postmenopausal estrogen use
- Sickle cell anemia
- Excessive alcohol abuse
- Obesity
- Inactivity

ETIOLOGY & PATHOGENESIS

- Result of large or small vessel disease
- Arteriosclerosis
- Cardiac emboli:
  - Atrial fibrillation
  - Sick sinus syndrome
  - Prosthetic heart valves
  - Bacterial endocarditis
  - Cardiomyopathies
  - Mitral valve disease:
    - Mitral stenosis
    - Mitral regurgitation
    - Mitral valve prolapse
- Hematologic disorders:
  - Red blood cell disorders:
    - Polycythemia vera

- Sickle cell anemia
- Erythrocytosis
  - Platelet disorders:
    - Thrombocytosis
    - Thrombocytopenia
    - Thrombocytopenic purpura
- Brain tumor/abscess
- Compression of neck vessels during rotation of head
- Cocaine abuse
- Hypoglycemia
- Fat emboli
- Air emboli

CLINICAL PRESENTATION / PHYSICAL FINDINGS

- Rapid onset
- Maximum intensity (usually within minutes)
- Fleeting episodes lasting 1 to 2 seconds
- Visual disturbance/graying
- Lightheadedness

SIGNS & SYMPTOMS

- Visual loss in one or both eyes
- Vertigo
- Dizziness
- Difficulty in swallowing
- Unilateral/bilateral weakness of the face, arm, or leg
- Decreased sensation, numbness
- Slurring of speech
- Incoordination of limbs
- Affected gait
- Apathy
- Inappropriate behavior
- Excessive somnolence
- Agitation

DIAGNOSIS

DIFFERENTIAL DIAGNOSIS

- Migraine headaches: headache, nausea, photophobia
- Focal seizure: postictal state
- Tumors
- Acute hemorrhage: subdural hematoma
- Hypoglycemia
- Hyperglycemia

LABORATORY TESTS

- CBC
- Platelet count
- INR (international normalized ratio)
- Partial thromboplastin time
- Glucose
- Electrolytes
- BUN
- Creatinine

DIAGNOSTIC TESTS

- MR with venography/cerebral angiography
- Blood cultures
- CT scan of brain
- Electrocardiogram (ECG): rule out atrial fibrillation
- Holter monitor

DIAGNOSTIC PROCEDURES/IMAGING

- Cerebrovascular arterial imaging: non-invasive ultrasound evaluation
- Cardiac imaging
- Echocardiogram
- Chest radiograph

MEDICAL MANAGEMENT & TREATMENT

- MRI/CT of head.
- Hematologic screen.
- Cardiac evaluation.
- Assess risk factors.
- Assess blood pressure.
- Anticoagulation:
  - Initially heparin
  - Followed by Coumadin (warfarin)

SURGICAL THERAPY

- Carotid endarterectomy
- Failure of medical protocol

FOLLOW-UP

- Medical consultation

MONITORING

- Vital signs
- ECG
- Level of alertness

PREVENTION/AVOIDANCE

- Aspirin therapy
- Anticoagulants: Coumadin
- Modification of smoking/alcohol
- Diet
- Exercise

COMPLICATIONS

TIA patients are at high risk for stroke.

PROGNOSIS

Patients who have TIAs have a much higher risk of stroke and therefore poorer prognosis than the general population.

DENTAL SIGNIFICANCE

When treating patients with a history of TIAs, it is important to understand the treatment and medications being prescribed. It is also important to consider other conditions that may mimic TIAs.

DENTAL MANAGEMENT

- Discontinue dental treatment.
- Refer to nearest healthcare facility.
- Notify healthcare provider.
- Do not allow patient to drive.
- Hypertension to be treated.

SUGGESTED REFERENCES

Branch Jr WT. *Office Practice of Medicine*, ed 4. Philadelphia, WB Saunders, 2003.

Ferri FF (ed): *Practical Guide to the Care of the Medical Patient*. St Louis, Mosby, 2004.

Lewis DP, et al. *Advanced Protocols for Medical Emergencies: An Action Plan for Office Response*.

Schwartz GR, et al. *Principles and Practice of Emergency Medicine*. Baltimore, Lippincott Williams & Wilkins, 1999.

The Washington Manual of Medical Therapeutics, ed 30. Philadelphia, Lippincott Williams & Wilkins, 2001.

AUTHOR: **DONALD P. LEWIS, JR., DDS, CFE**

Venous Thrombosis

SYNONYM(S)

Thrombophlebitis
Deep venous thrombosis (DVT)
Superficial venous thrombosis (SVT)

ICD-9CM/CPT CODE(S)

ICD-9CM

451.9	Thrombophlebitis
451.82	Superficial arm
451.0	Superficial leg
453.8	Deep venous thrombosis, upper extremity
453.40	Deep venous thrombosis, lower extremity
415.19	Pulmonary artery

CPT

85610–85611	Prothrombin time
85730–85732	Partial thromboplastin time
82803	Arterial blood gas
93970-93971	Venous duplex, extremity
71250	Spiral CT scan, chest
75825	Venography, inferior vena cava
75827	Venography, superior vena cava
73219	MRI, upper extremity
73719	MRI, lower extremity
73719	MRI, pelvis

OVERVIEW

- The presence of thrombus in either a superficial or deep vein and the accompanying inflammatory response in the vessel wall is referred to as venous thrombosis or thrombophlebitis (DVT).
- The most important consequence of DVT is pulmonary embolism. This most commonly occurs as a result of thrombosis in the iliac, femoral, or popliteal venous systems. DVT occurs less frequently in the lower extremity than in the upper extremity; in the upper extremity, it is most often associated with indwelling venous catheters.
- The bedside diagnosis of venous thrombosis is insensitive and inaccurate. Many conditions produce signs and symptoms suggestive of DVT. Multiple studies have documented the difficulty of the clinical diagnosis of lower extremity DVT.
- Superficial venous thrombosis (SVT) is associated with intravenous catheters, varicose veins, and sometimes with DVT. When found in the absence of DVT, it does not result in pulmonary embolism. SVT is usually of little consequence, but it can be recurrent and persistent.

EPIDEMIOLOGY & DEMOGRAPHICS

- The exact incidence of DVT is unknown since most studies are limited by the inherent imprecision of clinical diagnosis. Most DVTs are occult and resolve without treatment or complication.

- Estimated at 80 cases per 100,000 persons occur annually. As many as 800,000 hospitalizations for DVT occur annually in the U.S.
- Treatment costs approach $1 to $2.5 billion annually.
- In hospitalized patients, the incidence of venous thrombosis is significantly higher and has been reported from 20–70%.
- Eighty percent begin in the deep veins of the calf.
- DVT usually affects individuals > 40 years of age.
- Patients with superficial thrombophlebitis and no obvious cause (IV catheters, IV drug abuse, varicose veins) are at high risk because DVT is found in as many as 40% of these patients.

ETIOLOGY & PATHOGENESIS

- The etiology varies depending on other associated medical conditions. However, in the 1820s Rudolf Virchow defined three factors that predispose to thrombus formation: stasis, intimal (endothelial) injury, and hypercoagulability.
- Thrombogenesis:
  - Although the etiology is often multifactorial, the events that predispose a vein to thrombophlebitis are illustrated by Virchow's triad.
  - Thrombus is composed primarily of fibrin and platelets.
  - Red blood cells are entrapped within the thrombus, which tends to propagate in the direction of blood flow.
  - Vessel inflammation is variable, dependent on the extent of vessel damage and granulocyte infiltration.
  - Eventual recanalization occurs, and flow through the vein is reestablished.
  - Permanent valve damage can result in chronic venous insufficiency.
- Numerous clinical conditions are associated with an increased risk of venous thrombosis, including:
  - Trauma (particularly spine and lower extremity)
  - Cancer (pancreas, lung, breast, and stomach)
  - Pregnancy
  - Myelodysplastic disorders
  - Certain autoimmune disorders
  - Vasculitides
  - Hypercoagulability disorders
  - Type A blood group
  - Oral contraceptive use
  - Obesity
  - Previous thrombus

CLINICAL PRESENTATION/PHYSICAL FINDINGS

- Unilateral extremity edema.
- Leg pain occurs commonly. Pain on dorsiflexion of the foot (Homan's sign) is nonspecific and only occurs in 50% of cases.

- Tenderness occurs in 75% of patients but is also found in 50% of patients without objectively confirmed DVT.
- Clinical signs and symptoms of pulmonary embolism as the primary manifestation of DVT occur in 10% of patients with confirmed DVT.
  - Dyspnea, chest pain, tachycardia
- Warmth and erythema of the skin may be present in the affected extremity.
- Venous distension and prominence of the subcutaneous veins.
- Patients may have a fever, usually low-grade.
- Superficial thrombophlebitis is characterized by the finding of a palpable, indurated, cordlike, tender, subcutaneous venous segment.
- Phlegmasia cerulean dolens: resultant cyanosis and pain of the involved extremity associated with proximal DVT.
- Phlegmasia alba dolens: resultant pallor and pain of the involved extremity associated with proximal DVT and arterial spasm.

DIAGNOSIS

IMAGING

- Duplex venous ultrasonography (two-dimensional imaging and pulse wave Doppler interrogation)
  - Sensitivity/specificity > 95%
- Magnetic resonance imaging
  - Proximal DVTs (iliac system)
- Venography
  - Gold standard
    - Sensitivity/specificity: 100% and 96%, respectively
  - Rarely utilized
- Impedance plethysmography
  - Detects outflow obstruction
- Spiral CT scan, ventilation/perfusion scan, pulmonary arteriogram (pulmonary embolism)

LABS

- Prothrombin time (PT), international normalized ratio (INR)
- Adjusted partial thromboplastin time (aPTT)
- Hypercoagulable state: protein(s) C & S, antithrombin III, Factor V Leiden, antiphospholipid antibodies, antithrombin III, homocysteine
- D-dimer
- Arterial blood gas (pulmonary embolism)

MEDICAL MANAGEMENT & TREATMENT

DVT

- Anticoagulation for 3 to 6 months (goal: INR 2.0 to 3.0)
  - IV heparin
  - Low-molecular-weight heparin (LMWH)
  - Warfarin
- Elevation of affected extremity
- Placement of a vena cava filter

SVT

- Elevation of affected extremity.
- Warm compresses.
- Nonsteroidal antiinflammatory drugs.
- Septic or suppurative thrombophlebitis requires treatment with antibiotics.

PREVENTION

- Subcutaneous heparin (unfractionated heparin or LMWH).
- Sequential compression boot/devices (SCDs).
- Graduated compression stockings.
- Early ambulation.
- High-risk patients should be double-covered (e.g., subcutaneous heparin and SCDs).

COMPLICATIONS

- Suppurative thrombophlebitis
- Pulmonary embolism
- Venous ulceration
- Chronic venous insufficiency

PROGNOSIS

- Death from superficial thrombophlebitis without complication is rare. If the thrombus extends into the deep venous system, it can be the source of pulmonary emboli.
- Death from DVT is attributed to massive pulmonary embolism, which causes 200,000 deaths annually in the U.S. Pulmonary embolism is the leading cause of preventable in-hospital mortality.

DENTAL SIGNIFICANCE

Therapeutic anticoagulation may affect dental treatment plan (e.g., tooth extractions, periodontal surgery).

DENTAL MANAGEMENT

Consult primary care physician regarding anticoagulation parameters.

See "Deep Venous Thrombosis (Thrombophlebitis)" in Section I, p 68 for more information.

SUGGESTED REFERENCES

Creager MA, Dzau VJ. Vascular diseases of the extremities, in Fauci AS, et al. (eds): *Harrison's Principles of Internal Medicine*, ed 14. New York, McGraw-Hill, 2005, pp 1491–1493.

Messina LM, Tierney LM. Blood vessels and lymphatics, in Tierney LM, et al. (eds): *Current Medical Diagnosis and Treatment*, ed 44. New York, McGraw-Hill, 2005, pp 453–456.

AUTHOR: **JOHN F. CACCAMESE, JR., DMD, MD**

SECTION III

SYNONYM(S)

V. tach
Wide complex tachycardia

ICD-9CM/CPT CODE(S)

427   Cardiac dysrhythmias
       Paroxysmal ventricular tachycardia
427.1 Ventricular tachycardia
427.9 Cardiac dysrhythmias
785.0 Tachycardia, unspecified—rapid heart beat

OVERVIEW

Ventricular tachycardia (VT) is a rapid heartbeat that originates in the ventricle of the heart. It is characterized by three or more consecutive premature ventricular beats. This is a potentially fatal complication due to the disruption of the normal heartbeat. This disruption will cause the heart to be unable to pump adequate blood to the body. Ventricular fibrillation can have a rate between 160 and 240 bpm. It can also occur in the absence of apparent heart disease. There are different types of ventricular tachycardia, including torsade de pointes, long QT syndrome, and bidirectional ventricular tachycardia.

See "Cardiac Dysrhythmias" in Section I, p 35 for more information.

EPIDEMIOLOGY & DEMOGRAPHICS

Patients with the following significant histories/conditions are more at risk:
- Previous myocardial infarction
- Antidysrhythmic medications
- Altered blood chemistry
- Altered pH changes
- Insufficient oxygenation
- Cardiomyopathies
- Drugs/toxins
- Mitral valve prolapse
- Myocarditis

ETIOLOGY & PATHOGENESIS

- Previous myocardial infarction
- Antidysrhythmic medications: undesired effects
- Altered blood chemistry
  - Hypokalemia (low potassium)
  - Hypomagnesemia (low magnesium)
- Altered pH changes
- Insufficient oxygenation

- Cardiomyopathies: difficulty in conduction
- Drugs/toxins
  - Quinidine
  - Tricyclic antidepressants
- Mitral valve prolapse
- Myocarditis

CLINICAL PRESENTATION / PHYSICAL FINDINGS

SIGNS & SYMPTOMS

- Palpitations
- Tachycardia
- Lightheadedness
- Syncope
- Shortness of breath
- Angina
- Abrupt starting/stopping
- Blood pressure: may by normal or low
- Loss of consciousness

DIAGNOSIS

DIFFERENTIAL DIAGNOSIS

- Supraventricular tachycardia
- Ventricular fibrillation
- Asystole
- ECG artifact

LABORATORY TESTS

- Electrocardiogram (ECG)
- Holter monitor
- Intracardiac electrophysiology
- Blood chemistries
- Echocardiogram

MEDICAL MANAGEMENT & TREATMENT

- Varies with symptoms/situation/underlying cardiac disorder.
- Provide basic life support (BLS).
- Alert EMS.
- Attach automatic external defibrillator (AED).
- Intravenous antiarrhythmic medications.
- Surgical ablation.
- Implantable cardioverter defibrillator.

FOLLOW-UP

- Medical consultation

MONITORING

- ECG
- AED

PREVENTION/AVOIDANCE

- In some cases, this disorder is not preventable.

- Treatment of underlying cardiac disorders.
- Correction of blood chemistries.

COMPLICATIONS

- Major cause of sudden cardiac death
- Hypotension
- Loss of consciousness
- Death

PROGNOSIS

The prognosis depends on underlying disease. If ventricular fibrillation (VF) develops within 6 weeks of an acute myocardial infarction, this has a poor prognosis (75% mortality at 1 year). Patients who experience nonsustained VT after an MI have a threefold greater risk of death than those who had not had an MI. However, patients without heart disease and monomorphic VT patterns have a good prognosis and low risk of death.

DENTAL SIGNIFICANCE

The heart beating too fast for the patient's cardiovascular condition can cause insufficient and inadequate blood flow through the heart. An unstable condition can arise that requires immediate diagnosis and treatment. When treating patients with a known history of an unstable tachydysrhythmia, care should be taken to prevent recurrence or prevent complications associated with the specific tachydysrhythmia.

SUGGESTED REFERENCES

Hupp JR, Williams TP, Vallerand WP. *The Clinical Consult for Dental Professionals.* Philadelphia, Lippincott Williams & Wilkins, 1995.

Lewis DP, et al. *Advanced Protocols for Medical Emergencies: An Action Plan for Office Response.*

The Washington Manual of Medical Therapeutics, ed 30. Philadelphia, Lippincott Williams & Wilkins, 2001.

AUTHOR: **DONALD P. LEWIS, JR., DDS, CFE**

Drugs

IMPORTANT READER INFORMATION

The Drugs section of this book is designed to be a supportive element to other sections of the book rather than a stand-alone source of complete information on medications. The author has made an attempt to focus almost exclusively on drugs unlikely to be prescribed by dentists but commonly used by physicians for patients coming to dental facilities. The drugs selected for coverage are those most commonly prescribed in 2004 in the United States, as ranked by the online magazine *Drug Topics*.

Each drug entry is listed according to its U.S. generic drug name followed by commonly used brand names available in the United States. The General Uses section of each entry typically lists those uses for which the drug is labeled for use by the manufacturer. The Side/Adverse Effects section is not an exhaustive list of potential problems. Instead, it tends to list those side/adverse effects with a reported incidence of greater than 1%. Some specific drug interactions are listed for many drugs, but in some entries, no effort is made to list the multitude of drugs that affect the availability or metabolism of the drug via stimulation or inhibition of particular enzymes. The interested reader should consult more comprehensive drug information sources for that information.

It is a contraindication of all drugs to give them to someone with a known hypersensitivity to that drug or drugs in the same chemical class; this is usually not mentioned in drug entries. Dosing parameters are provided to give readers a general idea of typical dosing regimens. With many drugs, however, the dose varies with the condition being managed, the patient's overall state of health, body weight, and other factors. Therefore, no effort was made to give extensive dosing information. Finally, the Dental Considerations section gives dental professionals an idea of what impact the drug may have on the safe delivery of dental care.

The reader seeking information in greater depth or coverage for drugs being prescribed by the dentist is urged to use the sources used for most of the information provided in this book's drug entries. These are:

1. Gage TW, Pickett FA (eds): *Mosby's Dental Drug Reference*, ed 7. St Louis, Mosby, 2005.
2. *2006 Mosby's Drug Consult,* ed 16. St Louis, Mosby, 2006.
3. Wynn RL, Meiller TF, Crossley HL (eds): *Drug Information Handbook for Dentistry*, ed 10. Hudson, OH, Lexi-Comp, 2005.

Every attempt has been made throughout this book to have the information provided be accurate and up-to-date. However, like all of science, changes occur in the understanding of disease and treatments. Therefore, the reader is strongly urged to stay current on all aspects of clinical care via other sources of clinical information, including peer-reviewed journals, well-researched online reference sources, and continuing education programs.

BRAND NAME(S)
Proventil, Ventolin

OVERVIEW

Bronchodilator available in oral and inhaler forms that relax bronchial smooth muscle

TYPE OF DRUG

β-2 adrenergic agonist

GENERAL USES

Used to manage reversible airway obstruction due to diseases such as asthma or COPD. Also useful to prevent exercise-induced bronchospasm.

CAUTIONS

Optimize antiinflammatory treatment since respiratory obstruction is usually due, in part, to airway inflammation. Use with caution in patients with tendency for cardiac dysrhythmias.

SIDE/ADVERSE EFFECTS

- Cardiac dysrhythmias
- Hypertension flushing
- Central nervous system stimulation
- Angioedema
- Erythema multiforme
- Gastrointestinal disturbances

IMPORTANT DRUG INTERACTIONS

Cardiac risks increase if used concurrently with MAO inhibitors, tricyclic antidepressants, or sympathomimetic amines.

CONTRAINDICATIONS

Hypersensitivity to adrenergic amines

USUAL DOSING PARAMETERS: ADULTS/CHILDREN

- Adults:
  - Oral: 2 to 4 mg 3 to 4 times/day.
  - Inhale 4 to 8 puffs every 20 minutes up to 4 hours, then q 1 to 4 hr PRN.
- Children:
  - Age 6 to 12: 2 mg 3 to 4 times/day.

DENTAL CONSIDERATIONS

Causes xerostomia. Possible altered taste and tooth discoloration.

AUTHOR: **JAMES R. HUPP, DMD, MD, JD, MBA**

FIGURE IV-1 Albuterol

SECTION IV

BRAND NAME(S)
Fosamax

OVERVIEW

Drug inhibits bone resorption by inhibiting osteoclasts.

TYPE OF DRUG

Bisphosphonate derivative

GENERAL USES

Generally used to decrease bone loss in conditions such as Paget's disease, in postmenopausal women, and in those chronically taking corticosteroids.

CAUTIONS

- Use with caution in patients with renal impairment.
- Ensure adequate vitamin D and calcium intake.
- Watch for esophageal problems.

SIDE/ADVERSE EFFECTS

- Abdominal pain
- Headache
- Dyspepsia
- Diarrhea
- Constipation
- Muscle pain

IMPORTANT DRUG INTERACTIONS

Use with aspirin-like drugs may increase gastrointestinal problems. Oral drugs containing calcium (such as antacids) may decrease absorption.

CONTRAINDICATIONS

- Hypocalcemia
- Functional esophageal disorders

USUAL DOSING PARAMETERS: ADULTS/CHILDREN

- Adults:
  - Usually 5 to 10 mg qd or 35 to 70 mg q per week

DENTAL CONSIDERATIONS

May produce osteonecrosis in the jaws, especially the mandible after bone exposure from surgery (extraction) and/or trauma. It is unclear how frequently this occurs.

AUTHOR: **JAMES R. HUPP, DMD, MD, JD, MBA**

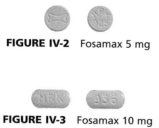

FIGURE IV-2   Fosamax 5 mg

FIGURE IV-4   Fosamax 35 mg

FIGURE IV-3   Fosamax 10 mg

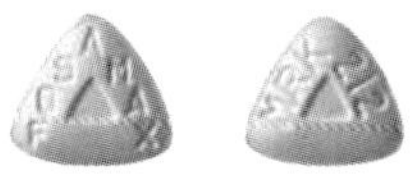

FIGURE IV-5   Fosamax 40 mg

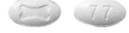

BRAND NAME(S)
Xanax
Xanax XR
Niravam

OVERVIEW

Intermediate-duration antianxiety drug that binds to GABA receptors in the limbic system and reticular formation for the CNS.

TYPE OF DRUG

Benzodiazepine

GENERAL USES

Used for managing chronic anxiety disorders as well as short-term treatment of acute anxiety. Useful for premedication prior to surgery.

CAUTIONS

- Avoid abrupt discontinuation if used chronically.
- Use with great caution in elderly and debilitated patients.
- Use with care in those with severe hepatic or renal insufficiency.
- Use with caution in depressed or suicidal patients.

SIDE/ADVERSE EFFECTS

- Sedation, respiratory depression.
- May cause prolonged memory impairment and psychomotor disturbance.
- Can cause sleep disturbance.

IMPORTANT DRUG INTERACTIONS

Additive sedating effects with other sedating drugs, including ethanol

CONTRAINDICATIONS

Avoid in patients with acute narrow-angle glaucoma, with severe respiratory problems, or during pregnancy or breastfeeding.

USUAL DOSING PARAMETERS: ADULTS/CHILDREN

- Adults:
  - 0.5 to 4 mg/day in divided doses. Usual dose 0.25 mg tid.
- Children:
  - 0.005 to 0.124 mg/kg/dose tid, titrated for effect.

DENTAL CONSIDERATIONS

May cause xerostomia. Can produce orthostatic hypotension, especially in older patients.

AUTHOR: **JAMES R. HUPP, DMD, MD, JD, MBA**

SECTION IV

BRAND NAME(S)
Norvasc

OVERVIEW

Vasodilating drug that inhibits calcium movement through slow membrane channels, relaxing vascular smooth muscle and myocardium.

TYPE OF DRUG

Calcium channel blocker (antagonist)

GENERAL USES

Generally used for treating essential hypertension alone or in combination with other drugs. Also used to manage angina, particularly when due to coronary vasospasm.

CAUTIONS

Use with caution with impaired hepatic or renal function and in patients with cardiac conduction abnormalities or impaired myocardial performance.

SIDE/ADVERSE EFFECTS

- Hypotension
- Constipation, especially in the elderly
- Peripheral edema
- Headaches
- Flushing
- Palpitations
- Fatigue
- Pulmonary edema

IMPORTANT DRUG INTERACTIONS

A large variety of drugs can increase or decrease effects of amlodipine.

CONTRAINDICATIONS

Allergy to drug

USUAL DOSING PARAMETERS: ADULTS/CHILDREN

- Adults:
  - 2.5 to 10 mg qd

DENTAL CONSIDERATIONS

May promote gingival hyperplasia. Severity can be reduced by reduction of dose and good oral hygiene.

AUTHOR: **JAMES R. HUPP, DMD, MD, JD, MBA**

FIGURE IV-6   Norvasc 2.5 mg

FIGURE IV-7   Norvasc 5 mg

FIGURE IV-8   Norvasc 10 mg

BRAND NAME(S)
Augmentin

OVERVIEW

Antibiotic that interferes with cell wall replication; useful against aerobic gram-positive and -negative bacteria when compounded with clavulanic acid, which inhibits β-lactamase.

TYPE OF DRUG

Aminopenicillin with β-lactamase inhibitor

GENERAL USES

Generally used for treatment of otitis media, sinusitis, and other respiratory infections or urinary tract infections due to susceptible organisms. Used for infectious endocarditis prophylaxis prior to dental or other surgical procedures.

CAUTIONS

Use with caution in renally impaired patients or those with bone marrow depression.

SIDE/ADVERSE EFFECTS

- Rash
- Nausea/vomiting
- Elevated liver enzymes

IMPORTANT DRUG INTERACTIONS

May increase action of warfarin

CONTRAINDICATIONS

Penicillin allergy

USUAL DOSING PARAMETERS: ADULTS/CHILDREN

- Adults:
  - All solid forms contain 125 mg clavulanic acid. Tablets and capsules come with 250, 500, or 875 mg amoxicillin.
- Children:
  - Powder for suspension and chewable tablets available.

DENTAL CONSIDERATIONS

May promote oral candidiasis outbreak. Can also cause tongue discoloration, glossitis.

AUTHOR: **JAMES R. HUPP, DMD, MD, JD, MBA**

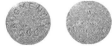

FIGURE IV-9   Augmentin 200 mg chew

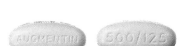

FIGURE IV-12   Augmentin 250 mg

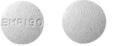

FIGURE IV-10   Augmentin 250 mg chew

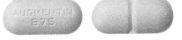

FIGURE IV-13   Augmentin 500 mg

FIGURE IV-11   Augmentin 400 mg chew

FIGURE IV-14   Augmentin 875 mg

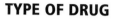
BRAND NAME(S)
Tenormin

OVERVIEW

Antihypertensive agent that does not cause the problematic side effects of nonselective agents such as a pressor response to epinephrine.

TYPE OF DRUG

β-1-selective β-blocker

GENERAL USES

Used primarily to control hypertension but also useful to control heart rate in patients prone to angina pectoris or those having suffered a myocardial infarction.

CAUTIONS

- May be useful for migraine headaches.
- Avoid withdrawing drug abruptly.
- May mask symptoms of hypoglycemia in diabetics.
- Use with caution in renally impaired patients.

SIDE/ADVERSE EFFECTS

- Bradycardia
- Hypotension
- Heart conduction blocks
- Impotence
- Cold extremities
- GI disturbances

IMPORTANT DRUG INTERACTIONS

Prolonged use of NSAIDs can reduce hypotensive effects of atenolol.

CONTRAINDICATIONS

- Preexisting heart blocks
- Cardiac failure
- Pregnancy

USUAL DOSING PARAMETERS: ADULTS/CHILDREN

- Adults:
  - 50 mg/day, increased to maximum of 200 mg/day
- Children:
  - 0.8 to 1 mg/kg/day with maximum of 2 mg/kg/day

DENTAL CONSIDERATIONS

May produce xerostomia. Monitor vital signs carefully. Watch for orthostatic hypotension. Use vasoconstrictors with some caution.

AUTHOR: **JAMES R. HUPP, DMD, MD, JD, MBA**

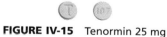

FIGURE IV-15   Tenormin 25 mg

BRAND NAME(S)
Lipitor

OVERVIEW

Drug used to reduce harmful forms of cholesterol by inhibiting enzyme of the rate-limiting step in cholesterol synthesis (HMG-CoA reductase).

TYPE OF DRUG

Antilipidemic agent

GENERAL USES

Used to reduce total and low-density cholesterol and triglycerides in patients with primary hypercholesterolemia.

CAUTIONS

- Monitor liver function regularly.
- Watch for signs of rhabdomyolysis or renal failure.

SIDE/ADVERSE EFFECTS

- Headache
- Diarrhea

IMPORTANT DRUG INTERACTIONS

A large number of drugs increase the effects of atorvastatin.

CONTRAINDICATIONS

- Active liver disease
- Pregnancy
- Breastfeeding

USUAL DOSING PARAMETERS: ADULTS/CHILDREN

- Adults:
  - 10 to 20 mg/day

DENTAL CONSIDERATIONS

No specific dental considerations

AUTHOR: JAMES R. HUPP, DMD, MD, JD, MBA

FIGURE IV-16 Lipitor 10 mg

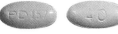

FIGURE IV-18 Lipitor 40 mg

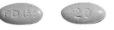

FIGURE IV-17 Lipitor 20 mg

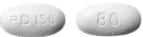

FIGURE IV-19 Lipitor 80 mg

BRAND NAME(S)
Wellbutrin
Zyban

OVERVIEW

Antidepressant with poorly understood mechanism of action but thought to interfere with function of dopamine in CNS.

TYPE OF DRUG

Dopamine reuptake inhibitor, aminoketone antidepressant

GENERAL USES

Used to treat depression and as part of nicotine addiction therapy. Sometimes used for patients with attention deficit/hyperactivity syndrome.

CAUTIONS

- Use with caution with other drugs known to lower the seizure threshold.
- Use with care with other antidepressant or sedating drugs.

SIDE/ADVERSE EFFECTS

- Headache
- Dizziness
- Insomnia
- Nausea
- Pharyngitis

IMPORTANT DRUG INTERACTIONS

- Hypertension can occur if used in conjunction with nicotine supplements.
- Cimetidine inhibits bupropion metabolism.

CONTRAINDICATIONS

- Recent use of MAO inhibitors
- Seizure disorder
- Anorexia (bulimia)
- Recent abstinence from excessive EtOH use

USUAL DOSING PARAMETERS: ADULTS/CHILDREN

- Adults:
  - 100 mg bid up to maximum of 450 mg/day
- Children:
  - 1.4 to 6 mg/kg/day

DENTAL CONSIDERATIONS

Xerostomia is common; alters taste sensation.

AUTHOR: **JAMES R. HUPP, DMD, MD, JD, MBA**

FIGURE IV-20 Zyban 150 mg

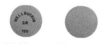

FIGURE IV-23 Wellbutrin-sr 100 mg

FIGURE IV-25 Wellbutrin-sr 200 mg

FIGURE IV-21 Wellbutrin 75 mg

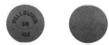

FIGURE IV-24 Wellbutrin-sr 150 mg

FIGURE IV-26 Wellbutrin-xl 150 mg

FIGURE IV-22 Wellbutrin 100 mg

BRAND NAME(S)
BuSpar

OVERVIEW

Antianxiety drug with unknown mechanism of action

TYPE OF DRUG

Antianxiety agent

GENERAL USES

Used for treatment of various anxiety disorders. Sometimes used to reduce aggression in mentally handicapped patients and as an adjunct to antidepressants.

CAUTIONS

Pregnancy risk: B

SIDE/ADVERSE EFFECTS

- Dizziness
- Headache
- Depression

IMPORTANT DRUG INTERACTIONS

- Avoid concurrent use with serotonin reuptake inhibitors, trazodone, nefazodone, or MAO inhibitors.
- Some antimicrobials and anticonvulsants lessen effects of buspirone.

CONTRAINDICATIONS

- Allergy to drug
- Hepatic or renal insufficiency
- Pregnancy or lactation

USUAL DOSING PARAMETERS: ADULTS/CHILDREN

- Adults:
  - 15 mg/day, increased to maximum of 60 mg/day as needed
- Children:
  - 5 mg/day, increased to maximum of 60 mg/day in divided doses

DENTAL CONSIDERATIONS

Xerostomia potential

AUTHOR: **JAMES R. HUPP, DMD, MD, JD, MBA**

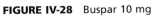

FIGURE IV-27 Buspar 5 mg

FIGURE IV-28 Buspar 10 mg

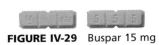

FIGURE IV-29 Buspar 15 mg

BRAND NAME(S)
Soma
Vanadom

OVERVIEW

Causes skeletal muscle relaxation, probably due to effects on central nervous system.

TYPE OF DRUG

Muscle relaxant

GENERAL USES

Typically used as an adjunct to analgesics for treatment of musculoskeletal pain.

CAUTIONS

Watch for general central nervous system depression.

SIDE/ADVERSE EFFECTS

- Drowsiness
- Dizziness
- Weakness

IMPORTANT DRUG INTERACTIONS

Additive sedating effects to other sedation-producing drugs, including ethanol

CONTRAINDICATIONS

- Porphyria
- Allergy to drug or meprobamate

USUAL DOSING PARAMETERS: ADULTS/CHILDREN

- Adults:
  - 350 mg, 3 to 4 times/day, with final dose hs

DENTAL CONSIDERATIONS

Watch for glossitis or lip swelling.

AUTHOR: **JAMES R. HUPP, DMD, MD, JD, MBA**

BRAND NAME(S)
Biocef
Keflex
Keftab
Zartan

OVERVIEW

Antibacterial drug with spectrum that includes gram-positive and -negative aerobes including staphylococci and many oral anaerobes.

TYPE OF DRUG

First-generation cephalosporin, β-lactam

GENERAL USES

Used to prevent and treat infections of the orofacial region, respiratory tract, ear, and skin. Also may be used for genitourinary tract infections due to susceptible bacteria. Can serve as a drug for infectious endocarditis prophylaxis.

CAUTIONS

- Modify dosage in patients with renal insufficiency.
- Monitor for antibiotic associated colitis in debilitated patients.
- Pregnancy risk: B.

SIDE/ADVERSE EFFECTS

- Rare except for allergy, but rarely causes dermatologic problems.
- Can cause candidal or other superinfections to occur.

IMPORTANT DRUG INTERACTIONS

Concurrent use of aminoglycosides increases nephrogenic potential.

CONTRAINDICATIONS

Hypersensitivity to any cephalosporin

USUAL DOSING PARAMETERS: ADULTS/CHILDREN

- Adults:
  - 500 to 1000 mg q 6 h
- Children:
  - 50 to 100 mg/kg/day in 4 equal doses

DENTAL CONSIDERATIONS

May promote candidal infection.

AUTHOR: **JAMES R. HUPP, DMD, MD, JD, MBA**

Cetirizine

BRAND NAME(S)
Virlix
Zyrtec

OVERVIEW

Active metabolite of terfenadine that competes with histamine for H1-receptors reducing histamine response of GI and respiratory tracts.

TYPE OF DRUG

Antihistamine

GENERAL USES

Used to manage symptoms of seasonal allergies and for chronic idiopathic urticaria

CAUTIONS

Use with caution in patients with renal or hepatic insufficiency.

SIDE/ADVERSE EFFECTS

- Headache
- Somnolence
- Fatigue
- Abdominal pain
- Diarrhea
- Pharyngitis
- Bronchospasm

IMPORTANT DRUG INTERACTIONS

Increased toxicity may occur with concurrent use with CNS depressants or anticholinergics.

CONTRAINDICATIONS

Allergy to cetirizine or hydroxyzine

USUAL DOSING PARAMETERS: ADULTS/CHILDREN

- Adults:
  - 5 to 10 mg qd
- Children:
  - Age 6 to 12 months: 2.5 mg qd
  - 1 to 2 years: 2.5 to 5 mg qd
  - 2 to 5 years: 5 mg qd

DENTAL CONSIDERATIONS

Xerostomia in some patients; increased salivation in others.

AUTHOR: **JAMES R. HUPP, DMD, MD, JD, MBA**

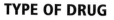

FIGURE IV-30 Zyrtec 5 mg

FIGURE IV-31 Zyrtec 10 mg

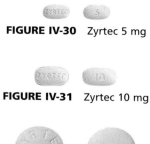

FIGURE IV-32 Zyrtec D

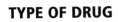

BRAND NAME(S)
Cipro

OVERVIEW

Broad-spectrum, bactericidal agent that interferes with bacterial DNA replication.

TYPE OF DRUG

Quinolone antibiotic

GENERAL USES

Used primarily to prevent and treat infections due to gram-negative aerobic bacteria, including those commonly responsible for urinary tract infections, pneumonia, sinus infections, and wound infections. Can be used for anthrax prophylaxis or treatment.

CAUTIONS

- Can cause photosensitivity.
- May exacerbate myasthenia gravis.
- Use with caution in patients with renal insufficiency.

SIDE/ADVERSE EFFECTS

Low incidence; sometimes see GI upset in children.

IMPORTANT DRUG INTERACTIONS

- May increase risk of tendon rupture when used with corticosteroids.
- Enhances action of warfarin.

CONTRAINDICATIONS

Hypersensitivity to drug

USUAL DOSING PARAMETERS: ADULTS/CHILDREN

- Adults:
  - Depends upon condition. Generally oral 250 to 500 mg/bid
- Children:
  - 20 to 30 mg/kg/day in 2 divided doses

DENTAL CONSIDERATIONS

- May promote candidal overgrowth. Can cause unpleasant taste.
- Some practitioners use in combination with metronidazole for managing periodontitis.

AUTHOR: **JAMES R. HUPP, DMD, MD, JD, MBA**

FIGURE IV-33 Cipro 250 mg

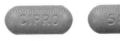

FIGURE IV-34 Cipro 500 mg

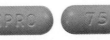

FIGURE IV-35 Cipro 750 mg

BRAND NAME(S)
Celexa

OVERVIEW

Antidepressant drug used for a large variety of anxiety disorders

TYPE OF DRUG

Selective serotonin reuptake inhibitor (SSRI) antidepressant

GENERAL USES

Used for treatment of major depressive disorders.

CAUTIONS

Use with caution in patients with hepatic or renal insufficiency, or prone to seizures. Use with caution in suicidal patients.

SIDE/ADVERSE EFFECTS

- Somnolence
- Insomnia
- Nausea
- Diaphoresis

IMPORTANT DRUG INTERACTIONS

Many drugs increase or decrease the effects of citalopram.

CONTRAINDICATIONS

Avoid use in patients taking MAO inhibitors or antipsychotic agents thioridazine or mesoridazine.

USUAL DOSING PARAMETERS: ADULTS/CHILDREN

- Adults:
  - 20 to 40 mg qd
- Children:
  - 10 to 40 mg qd

DENTAL CONSIDERATIONS

May cause xerostomia, taste abnormalities

AUTHOR: **JAMES R. HUPP, DMD, MD, JD, MBA**

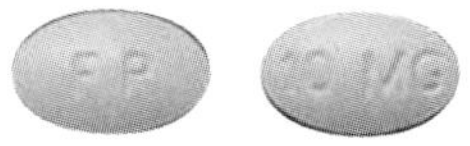

FIGURE IV-36 Celexa 10 mg

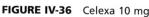

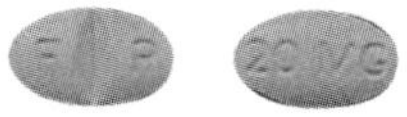

FIGURE IV-37 Celexa 20 mg

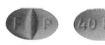

FIGURE IV-38 Celexa 40 mg

BRAND NAME(S)
Cleocin

OVERVIEW

Antimicrobial that inhibits bacteria protein synthesis by reversibly binding to ribosomes. Can be either bacteriostatic or bactericidal.

TYPE OF DRUG

Lincomycin group antibiotic

GENERAL USES

- Useful to treat or prevent infections due to aerobic or anaerobic gram-positive bacteria except enterococci, as well as bacteroides and actinomyces.
- Alternate drug to amoxicillin for infectious endocarditis prophylaxis.

CAUTIONS

- Like many antibiotics, can provoke pseudomembranous colitis in debilitated patients.
- Alter dose in those with severe hepatic insufficiency.
- Pregnancy risk: B.

SIDE/ADVERSE EFFECTS

- Diarrhea
- Abdominal pain
- Bone marrow depression

IMPORTANT DRUG INTERACTIONS

Can increase duration of certain neuromuscular blockers.

CONTRAINDICATIONS

- Neonates
- Previous episode of pseudomembranous colitis

USUAL DOSING PARAMETERS: ADULTS/CHILDREN

- Adults:
  - 300 to 450 mg q 6 to 8 h
- Children:
  - 8 to 25 mg/kg/day in divided doses

DENTAL CONSIDERATIONS

May cause candidal overgrowth

AUTHOR: **JAMES R. HUPP, DMD, MD, JD, MBA**

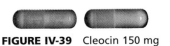

FIGURE IV-39 Cleocin 150 mg

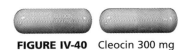

FIGURE IV-40 Cleocin 300 mg

Clonazepam

BRAND NAME(S)
Klonopin

OVERVIEW

Intermediate-duration antianxiety drug that binds to GABA receptors in limbic system and reticular formation.

TYPE OF DRUG

Benzodiazepine

GENERAL USES

Primarily used for management of certain types of seizure disorders alone or in combination with other antiseizure drugs. Also useful for panic disorder.

CAUTIONS

- Use with extra care in elderly and debilitated patients.
- Abrupt discontinuation can cause depression.
- Dependence on drug can occur.
- Pregnancy risk: D.

SIDE/ADVERSE EFFECTS

- Ataxia
- Drowsiness
- Somnolence
- Behavioral problems
- Confusion
- Respiratory depression
- Bone marrow suppression

IMPORTANT DRUG INTERACTIONS

- Additive sedating and respiratory depressing effects with other drugs known to produce these problems.
- Affects metabolism of large number of other drugs.

CONTRAINDICATIONS

- Acute narrow-angle glaucoma, serious hepatic disease
- Pregnancy

USUAL DOSING PARAMETERS: ADULTS/CHILDREN

- Adults:
  ○ 0.05 to 0.2 mg/kg up to maximum dose of 20 mg/day
- Children:
  ○ 0.01 to 0.03 mg/kg/day in 2 to 3 divided doses

DENTAL CONSIDERATIONS

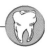

Xerostomia may be severe.

AUTHOR: **JAMES R. HUPP, DMD, MD, JD, MBA**

FIGURE IV-41 Klonopin 0.5 mg

FIGURE IV-42 Klonopin 1 mg

BRAND NAME(S)
Plavix

OVERVIEW

Drug works to interfere with platelet adhesion and aggregation by blocking ADP receptors, which prevents fibrinogen binding.

TYPE OF DRUG

Platelet aggregation inhibitor

GENERAL USES

Used to prevent thrombosis in coronary arteries and other sites affected by atherosclerosis and after coronary artery stenting.

CAUTIONS

- Can produce acute thrombotic thrombocytopenic purpura.
- Use with care in patients with hepatic insufficiency.

SIDE/ADVERSE EFFECTS

- GI side effects but may be due, in part, to concurrent use of aspirin
- Chest pain
- Edema
- Hypertension
- Dizziness
- Headache
- Rash
- Pruritus
- Dyspnea
- Arthralgia
- Back pain
- Flu-like symptoms

IMPORTANT DRUG INTERACTIONS

- Additive effects with other drugs that interfere with coagulation.
- Many drugs can increase or decrease the effects of clopidogrel.

CONTRAINDICATIONS

Active bleeding and coagulation disorders

USUAL DOSING PARAMETERS: ADULTS/CHILDREN

- Adults:
  - 75 mg qd

DENTAL CONSIDERATIONS

This drug acts as an anticoagulant and therefore may promote prolonged bleeding after moderately invasive procedures.

AUTHOR: **JAMES R. HUPP, DMD, MD, JD, MBA**

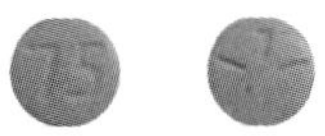

FIGURE IV-43   Plavix 75 mg

BRAND NAME(S)
Flexeril

OVERVIEW

Centrally acting skeletal muscle relaxant that reduces tonic somatic motor activity of alpha and gamma motor neurons.

TYPE OF DRUG

Muscle relaxant

GENERAL USES

Used to manage muscle spasms due to musculoskeletal disorders or trauma.

CAUTIONS

Use with caution with patients with urinary hesitancy, glaucoma, and hepatic insufficiency, and with the elderly.

SIDE/ADVERSE EFFECTS

- Drowsiness
- Dizziness
- Fatigue

IMPORTANT DRUG INTERACTIONS

- Additive effects with other CNS depressants.
- Quinoline antibiotics increase drug levels.

CONTRAINDICATIONS

- Do not use within 2 weeks of use of MAO inhibitors.
- Hyperthyroidism.
- Dysrhythmia.
- Recent MI.
- Congestive heart failure.

USUAL DOSING PARAMETERS: ADULTS/CHILDREN

- Adults:
  - 5 mg tid, up to 10 mg tid as needed

DENTAL CONSIDERATIONS

Xerostomia potential

AUTHOR: **JAMES R. HUPP, DMD, MD, JD, MBA**

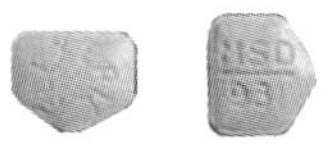

FIGURE IV-44 Flexeril 10 mg

BRAND NAME(S)
Cardizem
Cartia
Dilacor
Taztia
Tiazac

OVERVIEW

First-generation calcium channel blocker that inhibits calcium from entering "slow channels," thereby relaxing vascular smooth muscle and myocardial tissues.

TYPE OF DRUG

Calcium channel blocker (antagonist)

GENERAL USES

Used to manage hypertension as well as stable angina secondary to coronary artery spasm. Also useful for atrial and supraventricular tachydysrhythmias.

CAUTIONS

Use cautiously in patients with compromised cardiac status, hypotension, renal insufficiency, or hepatic insufficiency.

SIDE/ADVERSE EFFECTS

- Edema
- Headache
- Heart blocks
- Hypotension
- Dizziness
- Dyspepsia
- Constipation
- Rhinitis
- Pharyngitis

IMPORTANT DRUG INTERACTIONS

- Additive effects causing conduction problems with other antidysrhythmias.
- Increases or decreases potency of a large number of other drugs.

CONTRAINDICATIONS

- Preexisting heart blocks
- Low blood pressure
- Acute myocardial infarction

USUAL DOSING PARAMETERS: ADULTS/CHILDREN

- Adults:
  - 30 mg qid, increased gradually to 180 to 360 mg/day in divided doses

DENTAL CONSIDERATIONS

- Causes gingival hyperplasia that regresses if dose is reduced or drug is discontinued.
- Xerostomia.
- May cause altered taste or mucosal ulceration.

AUTHOR: **JAMES R. HUPP, DMD, MD, JD, MBA**

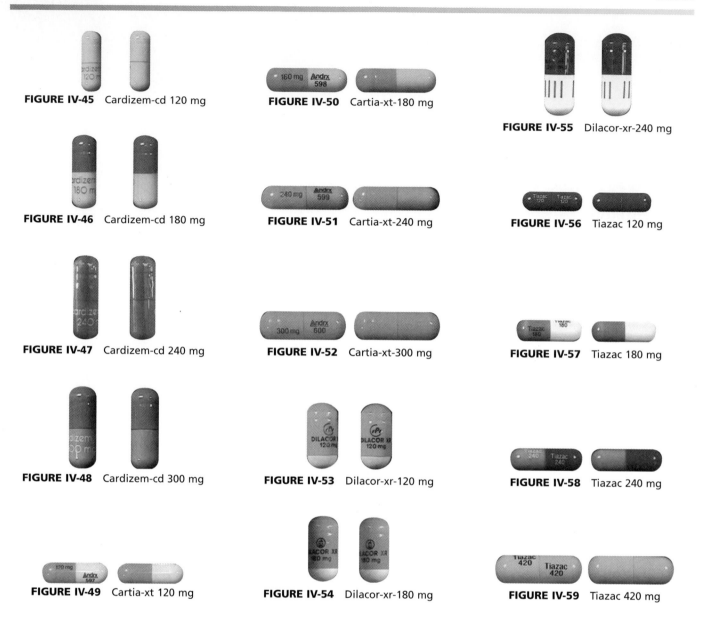

FIGURE IV-45 Cardizem-cd 120 mg

FIGURE IV-46 Cardizem-cd 180 mg

FIGURE IV-47 Cardizem-cd 240 mg

FIGURE IV-48 Cardizem-cd 300 mg

FIGURE IV-49 Cartia-xt 120 mg

FIGURE IV-50 Cartia-xt-180 mg

FIGURE IV-51 Cartia-xt-240 mg

FIGURE IV-52 Cartia-xt-300 mg

FIGURE IV-53 Dilacor-xr-120 mg

FIGURE IV-54 Dilacor-xr-180 mg

FIGURE IV-55 Dilacor-xr-240 mg

FIGURE IV-56 Tiazac 120 mg

FIGURE IV-57 Tiazac 180 mg

FIGURE IV-58 Tiazac 240 mg

FIGURE IV-59 Tiazac 420 mg

BRAND NAME(S)
Vasotec

OVERVIEW

This drug is a competitive inhibitor of the enzyme that converts angiotensin I into the potent vaso constrictor angiotensin II. This causes an increase in plasma renin levels and lowers serum aldosterone.

TYPE OF DRUG

Angiotensin-converting enzyme (ACE) inhibitor

GENERAL USES

Primarily used to treat moderate to severe hypertension. Also useful for myocardial dysfunction causing congestive heart failure.

CAUTIONS

- Monitor for angioedema even during first dose.
- Monitor renal function carefully.

SIDE/ADVERSE EFFECTS

- Hypotension
- Headache
- Dizziness
- Compromised renal function
- Cough
- Angioedema

IMPORTANT DRUG INTERACTIONS

- Concurrent use with diuretics may cause electrolyte disturbances.
- Hypotensive effects additive with other antihypertensive drugs.

CONTRAINDICATIONS

- Severe renal disease, adverse reaction to any ACE inhibitor drug
- Pregnancy

USUAL DOSING PARAMETERS: ADULTS/CHILDREN

- Adults:
  - 2.5 to 5 mg/day, increased to 40 mg/day in 2 divided doses as needed
- Children:
  - 0.08 mg/kg/day, up to maximum of 5 mg

DENTAL CONSIDERATIONS

- Loss or alteration of taste, mucosal ulceration, angioedema possible.
- Watch for orthostatic hypotension.

AUTHOR: **JAMES R. HUPP, DMD, MD, JD, MBA**

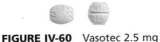

FIGURE IV-60 Vasotec 2.5 mg

FIGURE IV-62 Vasotec 10 mg

FIGURE IV-61 Vasotec 5 mg

FIGURE IV-63 Vasotec 20 mg

BRAND NAME(S)
Lexapro

OVERVIEW

This drug interferes with uptake of serotonin at receptor sites with little effect on dopamine or norepinephrine.

TYPE OF DRUG

Selective serotonin reuptake inhibitor antidepressant

GENERAL USES

Used to manage major depressive disorders and general anxiety disorders

CAUTIONS

Avoid use as single agent for bipolar disorders

SIDE/ADVERSE EFFECTS

- Headache
- Somnolence
- Insomnia
- Nausea
- Fatigue
- Dizziness
- Decreased libido
- Diarrhea
- Constipation
- GI upset
- Rhinitis
- Diaphoresis
- Flu-like symptoms

IMPORTANT DRUG INTERACTIONS

A large number of drugs can increase or decrease effects of this drug.

CONTRAINDICATIONS

- Concurrent or recent use of MAO inhibitors
- Allergy to escitalopram or citalopram

USUAL DOSING PARAMETERS: ADULTS/CHILDREN

- Adults:
  - 10 to 20 mg/day

DENTAL CONSIDERATIONS

Xerostomia is common.

AUTHOR: **JAMES R. HUPP, DMD, MD, JD, MBA**

BRAND NAME(S)
Nexium

OVERVIEW

This drug reduces gastric parietal cell acid secretion by inhibiting H+/K+-ATPase.

TYPE OF DRUG

Substituted benzimidazole proton pump inhibitor

GENERAL USES

Used for short-term therapy of esophagitis and gastroesophageal reflux syndrome. Also can be part of a multidrug *H. pylori* eradication program.

CAUTIONS

Rule out other causes of GI tract symptoms before assuming relief from esomeprazole proves an inflammatory origin to the patient's problems.

SIDE/ADVERSE EFFECTS

- Headache
- Diarrhea
- Nausea/vomiting
- Abdominal pain

IMPORTANT DRUG INTERACTIONS

May increase levels of benzodiazepines and carbamazepine. A number of drugs decrease effects of esomeprazole or are decreased by this drug.

CONTRAINDICATIONS

Allergy to this drug or lansoprazole, omeprazole, or other substituted benzimidazoles

USUAL DOSING PARAMETERS: ADULTS/CHILDREN

- Adults:
  - 20 to 40 mg qd
- Children:
  - Safety not established

DENTAL CONSIDERATIONS

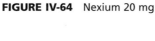

Xerostomia

AUTHOR: **JAMES R. HUPP, DMD, MD, JD, MBA**

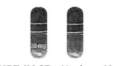

FIGURE IV-64 Nexium 20 mg

FIGURE IV-65 Nexium 40 mg

SECTION IV

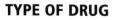

BRAND NAME(S)
Allegra

OVERVIEW

Active metabolite of terfenadine that competes with histamine for H1-receptors reducing histamine response of GI and respiratory tracts.

TYPE OF DRUG

Nonsedating antihistamine

GENERAL USES

Used to manage symptoms of seasonal allergies and for chronic idiopathic urticaria.

CAUTIONS

- Safety in children under age 6 is not clear.
- Pregnancy risk: C.

SIDE/ADVERSE EFFECTS

- Headache
- Back pain
- Cough

IMPORTANT DRUG INTERACTIONS

Effects increased by erythromycin and ketoconazole

CONTRAINDICATIONS

Allergy to this class of antihistamines

USUAL DOSING PARAMETERS: ADULTS/CHILDREN

- Adults:
  - 60 mg bid or 120 mg qd
- Children:
  - Age 6 to 12: 30 mg bid

DENTAL CONSIDERATIONS

No specific dental considerations

AUTHOR: **JAMES R. HUPP, DMD, MD, JD, MBA**

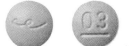

FIGURE IV-66 Allegra 30 mg tab

FIGURE IV-69 Allegra 60 mg capsule

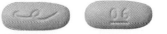

FIGURE IV-67 Allegra 60 mg tab

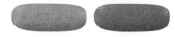

FIGURE IV-70 Allegra D

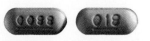

FIGURE IV-68 Allegra 180 mg tab

BRAND NAME(S)
Prozac
Sarafem

OVERVIEW

Antidepressant drug used for large variety of anxiety disorders

TYPE OF DRUG

Selective serotonin reuptake inhibitor

GENERAL USES

Used for treatment of major depressive disorders as well as obsessive-compulsive disorder, panic attacks, and bulimia.

CAUTIONS

- Use with caution in patients with hepatic or renal insufficiency, or prone to seizures.
- Use with caution in suicidal patients.

SIDE/ADVERSE EFFECTS

- Headache
- Insomnia
- Nervousness
- Somnolence
- Anorexia
- Nausea
- Diarrhea
- Pharyngitis
- Weakness
- Tremor
- May interfere with platelets

IMPORTANT DRUG INTERACTIONS

May increase serum levels of diazepam, lidocaine, phenytoin, β-blockers, and lithium

CONTRAINDICATIONS

Avoid use in patients taking MAO inhibitors or antipsychotic agents thioridazine or mesoridazine.

USUAL DOSING PARAMETERS: ADULTS/CHILDREN

- Adults:
  - 20 mg/day, titrated to maximum of 80 mg/day
- Children:
  - Age 8 to 18: 10 to 20 mg/day

DENTAL CONSIDERATIONS

- Causes xerostomia
- May affect taste
- Occasional problems with bruxism

AUTHOR: **JAMES R. HUPP, DMD, MD, JD, MBA**

FIGURE IV-71 Prozac 10 mg tab

FIGURE IV-72 Prozac 10 mg

FIGURE IV-73 Prozac 20 mg

SECTION IV

BRAND NAME(S)
Flonase

OVERVIEW

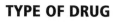

Extremely potent corticosteroid with strong antiinflammatory effects and ability to cause vaso-constriction due to unique ester linkage.

TYPE OF DRUG

Inhalent corticosteroid

GENERAL USES

Regularly used to prevent acute asthma in susceptible people and for managing seasonal allergic rhinitis. Not for use for acute asthmatic bronchospasm or status asthmaticus.

CAUTIONS

- Prolonged use can suppress hypothalamic-pituitary-adrenal axis, especially in children.
- Extended use can also affect growth in children.
- Immune suppression may occur.

SIDE/ADVERSE EFFECTS

- Headache
- Superinfection
- Respiratory tract irritation
- Diarrhea
- GI upset
- Fever

IMPORTANT DRUG INTERACTIONS

A large number of drugs can increase or decrease effects of fluticasone.

CONTRAINDICATIONS

Allergy to drug

USUAL DOSING PARAMETERS: ADULTS/CHILDREN

- Adults:
  - 50 µg/spray: 100 µg per nostril once or twice daily for rhinitis. Higher doses may be needed for asthma prevention.
- Children:
  - 4 yrs of age to adult: 50 µg per nostril once or twice daily.

DENTAL CONSIDERATIONS

Infections by yeast or fungi can occur in oral cavity or upper respiratory tract. May require antimicrobial treatment.

AUTHOR: **JAMES R. HUPP, DMD, MD, JD, MBA**

BRAND NAME(S)
Lasix

OVERVIEW

Potent diuretic that limits reabsorption of sodium and chloride in the renal loop of Henle and the distal tubule, causing excretion of water and other ions.

TYPE OF DRUG

Loop diuretic

GENERAL USES

Used primarily for treating edema associated with congestive heart failure or other systemic diseases causing serious fluid retention. Also used for hypertension management.

CAUTIONS

- Use cautiously in diabetics and patients on digoxin.
- Pregnancy risk: C.

SIDE/ADVERSE EFFECTS

- Hypotension
- Hypokalemia
- Rashes
- Electrolyte deficiencies
- Hyperglycemia
- Renal insufficiency
- Thrombocytopenia

IMPORTANT DRUG INTERACTIONS

- May increase risk of lithium or salicylate toxicity.
- Additive hypotensive effects with other drugs used to manage hypertension.

CONTRAINDICATIONS

- Renal or hepatic failure
- Uncorrected electrolyte problems

USUAL DOSING PARAMETERS: ADULTS/CHILDREN

- Adults:
  - 20 to 80 mg, repeated as needed to produce desired diuresis
- Children:
  - 2 mg/kg, increased up to 6 mg/kg as needed

DENTAL CONSIDERATIONS

- Watch for orthostatic hypotension.
- Monitor vital signs carefully.
- Xerostomia common.

AUTHOR: **JAMES R. HUPP, DMD, MD, JD, MBA**

BRAND NAME(S)
Neurontin

OVERVIEW

Antiseizure medication with chemical structure similar to GABA but does not appear to affect GABA receptors.

TYPE OF DRUG

Anticonvulsant

GENERAL USES

Primarily used to manage partial seizures in patients with epilepsy. Also useful for treating the pain of post-herpetic neuralgia.

CAUTIONS

- Abrupt withdrawal can provoke seizures.
- Use with caution in patients with renal insufficiency.

SIDE/ADVERSE EFFECTS

- Somnolence
- Dizziness
- Ataxia
- Fatigue
- Tremor
- Nystagmus
- Rhinitis
- In children may also see fever, hostility, nausea/vomiting

IMPORTANT DRUG INTERACTIONS

- Drugs lowering gastric acidity decrease absorption.
- Additive sedative effects with other sedation-producing drugs.

CONTRAINDICATIONS

Allergy to drug

USUAL DOSING PARAMETERS: ADULTS/CHILDREN

- Adults:
  - Slowly increase dosing up to 600 to 900 mg tid
- Children:
  - Age 3 to 13: 10 to 15 mg/kg/day in 3 divided doses

DENTAL CONSIDERATIONS

Xerostomia

AUTHOR: **JAMES R. HUPP, DMD, MD, JD, MBA**

FIGURE IV-74 Neurontin 100 mg

FIGURE IV-76 Neurontin 400 mg

FIGURE IV-75 Neurontin 300 mg

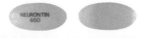

FIGURE IV-77 Neurontin 600 mg

BRAND NAME(S)
Glucotrol

OVERVIEW

This drug lowers serum glucose by stimulating release of insulin from pancreatic beta cells, reduces hepatic glucose output, and sensitizes peripheral insulin receptors.

TYPE OF DRUG

Second-generation oral sulfonylurea hypoglycemic agent

GENERAL USES

Drug used to help control serum glucose in noninsulin-dependent (type II) diabetes mellitus.

CAUTIONS

- Use with great caution in patients with compromised hepatic function.
- Can cause serious cardiac problems in higher doses.
- Pregnancy risk: C.

SIDE/ADVERSE EFFECTS

- Headache
- Hypoglycemia
- Bone marrow depression
- Hepatic toxicity

IMPORTANT DRUG INTERACTIONS

Affects drug levels (in both positive and negative directions) of a large number of other drugs.

CONTRAINDICATIONS

Sensitivity to any sulfonylurea drug or patients with sulfa drug allergies

USUAL DOSING PARAMETERS: ADULTS/CHILDREN

- Adults:
  - 5 mg/day, increased to 15 mg/day as needed.
  - Use reduced dose in elderly patients.

DENTAL CONSIDERATIONS

- Monitor for signs and symptoms of hypoglycemia.
- Treat infections aggressively in diabetics.

AUTHOR: **JAMES R. HUPP, DMD, MD, JD, MBA**

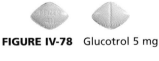

FIGURE IV-78 Glucotrol 5 mg

FIGURE IV-81 Glucotrol-xl 5 mg

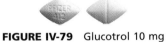

FIGURE IV-79 Glucotrol 10 mg

FIGURE IV-82 Glucotrol-xl 10 mg

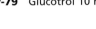

FIGURE IV-80 Glucotrol-xl 2.5 mg

Glyburide

BRAND NAME(S)
DiaBeta
Glynase
Micronase

OVERVIEW

This drug lowers serum glucose by stimulating release of insulin from pancreatic beta cells, reduces hepatic glucose output, and sensitizes peripheral insulin receptors.

TYPE OF DRUG

Second-generation sulfonylurea oral hypoglycemic agent

GENERAL USES

Drug used to help control serum glucose in noninsulin-dependent (type II) diabetes mellitus.

CAUTIONS

- Use with great caution in patients with compromised hepatic function.
- Can cause serious cardiac problems in higher doses.
- Pregnancy risk: C.

SIDE/ADVERSE EFFECTS

- Headache
- Hypoglycemia
- Bone marrow depression
- Hepatic toxicity

IMPORTANT DRUG INTERACTIONS

Affects drug levels (in both positive and negative directions) of a large number of other drugs.

CONTRAINDICATIONS

Sensitivity to any sulfonylurea drug or patients with sulfa drug allergies

USUAL DOSING PARAMETERS: ADULTS/CHILDREN

- Adults:
  - 2.5 to 5 mg/day, increased to maximum of 20 mg/day.
  - Reduce dosage in the elderly.

DENTAL CONSIDERATIONS

- Use all standard precautions for managing diabetic patients.
- Manage infections aggressively.

AUTHOR: **JAMES R. HUPP, DMD, MD, JD, MBA**

FIGURE IV-83 Glynase 3 mg

FIGURE IV-84 Glynase 6 mg

BRAND NAME(S)
Aquazide
Microzide
Oretic

OVERVIEW

Diuretic drug that inhibits sodium reabsorption in distal tubules of kidney, causing loss of sodium, potassium, hydrogen, and water

TYPE OF DRUG

Diuretic

GENERAL USES

Used to promote diuresis in the management of hypertension. Also helps control edema in cases of congestive heart failure and nephrotic syndrome.

CAUTIONS

- Monitor for electrolyte disturbances.
- Use with caution in patients with systemic lupus and in patients with significantly elevated cholesterol levels.

SIDE/ADVERSE EFFECTS

- Can precipitate gout
- Hypokalemia, hypotension, and disturbed glucose control in diabetics

CONTRAINDICATIONS

- Severe renal insufficiency
- Untreated hypokalemia
- Pregnancy

USUAL DOSING PARAMETERS: ADULTS/CHILDREN

- Adults:
  - 12.5 to 100 mg/day, titrated for effect
- Children:
  - Age > 6 months: 2 mg/kg/day in 2 divided doses

DENTAL CONSIDERATIONS

Xerostomia, orthostatic hypotension, and low blood pressure are possible.

AUTHOR: **JAMES R. HUPP, DMD, MD, JD, MBA**

FIGURE IV-85. Microzide 12.5 mg

BRAND NAME(S)
Compounded with acetaminophen:
Lortab, Lorcet, Vicodin, others
Compounded with ibuprofen:
Vicoprofen

OVERVIEW

Useful narcotic pain reliever for use for moderate pain. Typically compounded with other pain-relieving drugs or drugs used for symptomatic relief of respiratory tract infections.

TYPE OF DRUG

Semisynthetic, centrally-acting, opioid analgesic

GENERAL USES

Used for reduction of moderate pain for short time periods (10 days or less)

CAUTIONS

- Avoid use in those hypersensitive to hydrocodone or associated drugs.
- Avoid ethanol and herbals, including valerian and St. John's wort.
- Pregnancy risk: C.

SIDE/ADVERSE EFFECTS

- Respiratory depression in high doses
- Nausea, constipation
- Suppresses cough reflex
- Can produce drug dependence

IMPORTANT DRUG INTERACTIONS

Additive with other drugs causing sedation or respiratory depression

CONTRAINDICATIONS

Head-injured patients

USUAL DOSING PARAMETERS: ADULTS/CHILDREN

- Adults:
  - 2.5 to 10 mg every 4 to 6 hours (maximum 60 mg/day)
- Children:
  - 0.135 mg/kg/dose

DENTAL CONSIDERATIONS

Usual precautions for narcotic drugs

AUTHOR: **JAMES R. HUPP, DMD, MD, JD, MBA**

BRAND NAME(S)
Imdur
Ismo
Monoket

OVERVIEW

Long-acting metabolite of isosorbide dinitrate used for its systemic vasodilatory capabilities. Helpful to lower preload and afterload on the heart.

TYPE OF DRUG

Long-acting vasodilator

GENERAL USES

Used most commonly to prevent angina pectoris in susceptible patients. Also beneficial for patients in congestive heart failure.

CAUTIONS

Transient hypotension, dizziness, and weakness can occur.

SIDE/ADVERSE EFFECTS

- Headache
- Dizziness
- Nausea/vomiting
- Postural hypotension

IMPORTANT DRUG INTERACTIONS

- A large number of antimicrobial drugs and calcium channel blockers increase the effects of isosorbide.
- Ethanol potentiates effects.

CONTRAINDICATIONS

- Hypersensitivity to nitrates in any form.
- Narrow-angle glaucoma, patients with elevated CNS pressure, severely anemic patients.
- Avoid concurrent use with erectile dysfunction drugs.

USUAL DOSING PARAMETERS: ADULTS/CHILDREN

- Adults:
  ○ 5 to 10 mg bid

DENTAL CONSIDERATIONS

Closely monitor vital signs. Xerostomia if excessive dose used.

AUTHOR: **JAMES R. HUPP, DMD, MD, JD, MBA**

SECTION IV

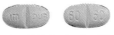

FIGURE IV-86   Imdur 60 mg

BRAND NAME(S)
Prevacid

OVERVIEW

Gastric acid-reducing drug that decreases parietal cell acid production by interfering with proton pump

TYPE OF DRUG

Proton pump inhibitor

GENERAL USES

Used for short-term treatment of active gastric ulcers, as an adjunct to *H. pylori* eradication, and also useful for GERD and reflux esophagitis management.

CAUTIONS

- Reduce dose in presence of severe liver disease
- Pregnancy risk: B

SIDE/ADVERSE EFFECTS

- Headache
- Abdominal pain
- Diarrhea

IMPORTANT DRUG INTERACTIONS

Drug effects can be increased or decreased when used with certain other drugs.

CONTRAINDICATIONS

Allergy to substituted benzimidazoles

USUAL DOSING PARAMETERS: ADULTS/CHILDREN

- Adults:
  - Varies based on problem being managed. Generally 15 to 30 mg/day.
- Children:
  - Varies. Weight < 30 kg: 15 mg qd; > 30 kg: 30 mg/day.

DENTAL CONSIDERATIONS

No specific dental considerations

AUTHOR: **JAMES R. HUPP, DMD, MD, JD, MBA**

FIGURE IV-87 Prevacid 15 mg

FIGURE IV-88 Prevacid 30 mg

BRAND NAME(S)
Prinivil
Zestril

OVERVIEW

ACE inhibitor used to lower angiotensin II levels, thereby reducing aldosterone secretion

TYPE OF DRUG

Angiotensin-converting enzyme (ACE) inhibitor

GENERAL USES

Primarily used for the drug's antihypertensive effects and control of intravascular volume to treat congestive heart failure and myocardial infarction patients with compromised cardiac performance.

CAUTIONS

- Use with caution with diuretics.
- Pregnancy risk: C/D.

SIDE/ADVERSE EFFECTS

- Hypotension
- Headaches
- Dizziness
- Cough
- Hyperkalemia
- Diarrhea
- Angioedema

IMPORTANT DRUG INTERACTIONS

- Aspirin, antacids, rifampin, NSAIDs
- Additive with diuretics

CONTRAINDICATIONS

- Pregnancy in second and third trimesters
- Allergy to ACE inhibitors

USUAL DOSING PARAMETERS: ADULTS/CHILDREN

- Adults:
  - 10 mg/day, increased up to 40 mg/day as needed
- Children:
  - 0.07 mg/kg/day

DENTAL CONSIDERATIONS

Xerostomia

AUTHOR: **JAMES R. HUPP, DMD, MD, JD, MBA**

FIGURE IV-89 Prinivil 5 mg

FIGURE IV-92 Prinivil 40 mg

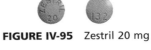

FIGURE IV-95 Zestril 20 mg

FIGURE IV-90 Prinivil 10 mg

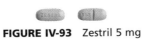

FIGURE IV-93 Zestril 5 mg

FIGURE IV-96 Zestril 30 mg

FIGURE IV-91 Prinivil 20 mg

FIGURE IV-94 Zestril 10 mg

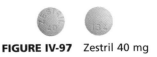

FIGURE IV-97 Zestril 40 mg

SECTION IV

BRAND NAME(S)
Ativan

OVERVIEW

Relatively long-duration antianxiety drug that binds to GABA receptor in limbic system and reticular formation

TYPE OF DRUG

Benzodiazepine

GENERAL USES

- Used for managing chronic anxiety disorders as well as short-term treatment of acute anxiety
- Useful as premedication prior to surgery

CAUTIONS

- Use with great caution in elderly and debilitated patients.
- Use with care in those with severe hepatic or renal insufficiency.
- Use with caution in depressed or suicidal patients.

SIDE/ADVERSE EFFECTS

- Sedation, respiratory depression
- May cause prolonged memory impairment and psychomotor disturbance
- Can cause sleep disturbance

IMPORTANT DRUG INTERACTIONS

Additive sedating effects with other sedating drugs, including ethanol

CONTRAINDICATIONS

Avoid in patients with acute narrow-angle glaucoma, with severe respiratory problems, or during pregnancy or breastfeeding.

USUAL DOSING PARAMETERS: ADULTS/CHILDREN

- Adults:
  - 1 to 10 mg/day in 2 to 3 divided doses. Usual dose is 2 to 6 mg/day individual doses.
- Children:
  - 0.01 to 0.03 mg/kg, titrated for effect. Usual dose is 0.05 mg/kg/dose.

DENTAL CONSIDERATIONS

May cause xerostomia. Can produce orthostatic hypotension, especially in older patients.

AUTHOR: **JAMES R. HUPP, DMD, MD, JD, MBA**

FIGURE IV-98 Ativan 1 mg

FIGURE IV-99 Ativan 2 mg

BRAND NAME(S)
Altocor
Mevacor

OVERVIEW

Cholesterol-lowering drug that acts by competitively inhibiting the enzyme that catalyzes the rate-limiting step in cholesterol synthesis

TYPE OF DRUG

Lipid-lowering, HMG-CoR reductive inhibitor

GENERAL USES

- Used in combination with dietary program to reduce levels of total and low-density lipoprotein cholesterols.
- Helps slow or prevent progression of atherosclerosis.

CAUTIONS

Monitor aminotransferase levels periodically and warn patient to report myalgias.

SIDE/ADVERSE EFFECTS

- Elevated CPK
- GI disturbances
- Flatulence
- Myalgia

IMPORTANT DRUG INTERACTIONS

Many drugs (including antifungal and antibacterial agents) increase the effects of lovastatin.

CONTRAINDICATIONS

- Elevated hepatic transaminases
- Pregnancy, breastfeeding

USUAL DOSING PARAMETERS: ADULTS/CHILDREN

- Adults:
  - 10 to 80 mg/day with evening meal
- Children:
  - Age 10 to 17: 10 to 40 mg/day with evening meal

DENTAL CONSIDERATIONS

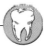

No specific dental considerations

AUTHOR: **JAMES R. HUPP, DMD, MD, JD, MBA**

BRAND NAME(S)
Fortamet
Glucophage
Riomet

OVERVIEW

Oral hypoglycemic agent often used with a sulfonylurea or insulin for glycemic control

TYPE OF DRUG

Biguanide

GENERAL USES

Used primarily to treat hyperglycemia due to type II (NIDDM) diabetes that does not respond to dietary therapy.

CAUTIONS

- Stop drug prior to use of contrast agents used for imaging.
- Pregnancy risk: B.

SIDE/ADVERSE EFFECTS

- Nausea/vomiting
- Diarrhea
- Flatulence
- Weakness
- Headache

IMPORTANT DRUG INTERACTIONS

- Furosemide and cimetidine increase drug levels.
- Drugs eliminated by kidneys may decrease metformin rate of elimination.

CONTRAINDICATIONS

- Allergy, renal insufficiency
- Avoid in patients with significant hepatic dysfunction

USUAL DOSING PARAMETERS: ADULTS/CHILDREN

- Adults:
  - 500 mg bid or 850 mg qd. Can be increased to 2000 mg as needed.
- Children:
  - Age 10 to 16 years: 500 mg bid up to 2000 mg/day.

DENTAL CONSIDERATIONS

May predispose to hypoglycemia if insufficient caloric intake

AUTHOR: **JAMES R. HUPP, DMD, MD, JD, MBA**

FIGURE IV-100 Glucophage 500 mg

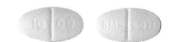

FIGURE IV-102 Glucophage 1000 mg

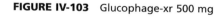

FIGURE IV-101 Glucophage 850 mg

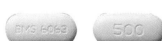

FIGURE IV-103 Glucophage-xr 500 mg

BRAND NAME(S)
Lopressor

OVERVIEW

Selective inhibitor of β-1-receptor in sympathetic nervous system; thus inhibits ability of epinephrine to raise heart rate and blood pressure.

TYPE OF DRUG

β-1-selective β-adrenergic blocker

GENERAL USES

Drug used primarily to treat essential hypertension and prevent angina. Also used in myocardial infarction patients, management of atrial dysrhythmias, and in patients with congestive heart failure.

CAUTIONS

- Avoid abrupt withdrawal of this drug.
- Use with caution in patients with bronchospastic tendency.
- Can mask signs and symptoms of hypoglycemia in diabetics.

SIDE/ADVERSE EFFECTS

- Drowsiness
- Insomnia
- Impotence
- Bradycardia
- Bronchospasm

IMPORTANT DRUG INTERACTIONS

Metoprolol has increased and decreased effects in the presence of a large number of other drugs.

CONTRAINDICATIONS

- Bradycardia
- Second- and third-degree heart block
- Cardiogenic shock
- Second and third trimesters of pregnancy

USUAL DOSING PARAMETERS: ADULTS/CHILDREN

- Adults:
  - 100 to 450 mg/day in 2 to 3 divided doses
- Children:
  - 1 to 5 mg/kg/day in 2 divided doses

DENTAL CONSIDERATIONS

None, but carefully record vital signs.

AUTHOR: **JAMES R. HUPP, DMD, MD, JD, MBA**

Minocycline

BRAND NAME(S)
Dynacin
Minocin

OVERVIEW

Antibiotic that inhibits bacterial protein synthesis by binding to ribosome of susceptible bacteria; bacteriostatic.

TYPE OF DRUG

Tetracycline derivative antibiotic

GENERAL USES

Used for treatment of gram-positive and -negative bacterial infections. Often used for treating acne and the meningococcal carrier state. Some practitioners use this drug for certain forms of periodontal infection.

CAUTIONS

- May trigger photosensitivity
- Pregnancy risk: D

SIDE/ADVERSE EFFECTS

Low incidence of headache, pharyngitis

IMPORTANT DRUG INTERACTIONS

- Antacids can limit absorption.
- Can get increased drug levels of warfarin or digoxin with concurrent use.

CONTRAINDICATIONS

Pregnancy

USUAL DOSING PARAMETERS: ADULTS/CHILDREN

- Adults:
  - Oral: 50 mg 1 to 3 times/day after 200 mg loading dose
- Children:
  - Age 7 to 8 years: 2 mg/kg every 12 hours after 4 mg/kg loading dose

DENTAL CONSIDERATIONS

Staining of developing teeth is likely; avoid in pregnant, lactating, or young patients. Candidal superinfections can occur, especially with prolonged use.

AUTHOR: **JAMES R. HUPP, DMD, MD, JD, MBA**

FIGURE IV-104 Dynacin 75 mg

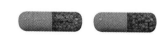

FIGURE IV-106 Minocin 100 mg pellets

FIGURE IV-105 Dynacin 100 mg

BRAND NAME(S)
Remeron

OVERVIEW

Tetracyclic antidepressant that antagonizes central, presynaptic α-2 receptors; increases release of serotonin and norepinephrine but does not inhibit their reuptake.

TYPE OF DRUG

α-2 antagonist antidepressant

GENERAL USES

Used to treat depression

CAUTIONS

Use with care in those with hepatic insufficiency or renal impairment.

SIDE/ADVERSE EFFECTS

- Somnolence very common
- Constipation
- Increased appetite
- Dizziness
- Abnormal thoughts

IMPORTANT DRUG INTERACTIONS

Causes increased or decreased effects of a large number of other drugs

CONTRAINDICATIONS

MAO inhibitor use

USUAL DOSING PARAMETERS: ADULTS/CHILDREN

- Adults:
  - 15 to 45 mg/day, slowly titrated for effect

DENTAL CONSIDERATIONS

Xerostomia is common.

AUTHOR: **JAMES R. HUPP, DMD, MD, JD, MBA**

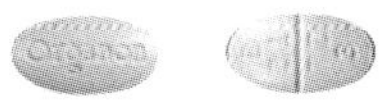

FIGURE IV-107   Remeron 15 mg

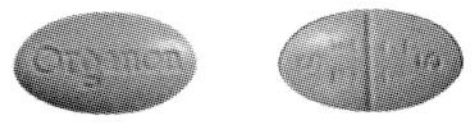

FIGURE IV-108   Remeron 30 mg

SECTION IV

Montelukast

BRAND NAME(S)
Singulair

OVERVIEW

This drug reduces airway edema, smooth muscle contraction, and abnormal airway cellular activity by inhibiting the cysteinyl leukotriene receptors.

TYPE OF DRUG

Leukotriene-receptor antagonist

GENERAL USES

Used to prevent and manage asthma and for the reduction of symptoms seen in seasonal allergic rhinitis.

CAUTIONS

Do not use to treat bronchospasm in acute asthma attacks or use alone for exercise-induced asthma.

SIDE/ADVERSE EFFECTS

- Headache
- Flu-like symptoms
- Abdominal pain
- Cough

IMPORTANT DRUG INTERACTIONS

A number of drugs have their effects decreased by montelukast, or this drug's effects are reduced by others.

CONTRAINDICATIONS

- Allergy to drug
- Avoid in phenylketonuric children

USUAL DOSING PARAMETERS: ADULTS/CHILDREN

- Adults:
  - 10 mg/day hs
- Children:
  - Age 1 to 5 years: 4 mg/day hs; 6 to 14 years: 5 mg qd hs

DENTAL CONSIDERATIONS

No special dental considerations

AUTHOR: **JAMES R. HUPP, DMD, MD, JD, MBA**

OVERVIEW

NSAID whose major active metabolite increases production of endoperoxide and prostaglandins E_2 and I_2, inhibiting inflammation-producing prostaglandins.

TYPE OF DRUG

Nonsteroidal antiinflammatory drug (NSAID)

GENERAL USES

Primarily used to control inflammation and resulting pain in patients with rheumatoid arthritis and osteoarthritis.

CAUTIONS

- Has GI upset and platelet aggregation inhibitory effects similar to other NSAIDs.
- Can cause renal problems with long-term use.
- May provoke bronchospasm in aspirin-sensitive asthmatics.
- Pregnancy risk: C.

SIDE/ADVERSE EFFECTS

- Dizziness
- Rash
- Abdominal pain
- Diarrhea
- Heartburn

IMPORTANT DRUG INTERACTIONS

- Increased GI problems if given with corticosteroids
- May decrease effect of antihypertensives
- Increases renal toxicity effect of ACE inhibitors

CONTRAINDICATIONS

Sensitivity to aspirin or other NSAIDs

USUAL DOSING PARAMETERS: ADULTS/CHILDREN

- Adults:
  - 1 g qd, increased to 1.5 to 2 g if needed in single or divided daily dose

DENTAL CONSIDERATIONS

Xerostomia potential. Interferes with platelet function; monitor bleeding closely.

AUTHOR: **JAMES R. HUPP, DMD, MD, JD, MBA**

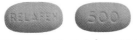

FIGURE IV-109 Relafen 500 mg

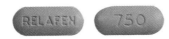

FIGURE IV-110 Relafen 750 mg

BRAND NAME(S)
Adalat
Nifedical
Procardia

OVERVIEW

First-generation calcium channel blocker that inhibits calcium from entering "slow channels," thereby relaxing vascular smooth muscle and myocardial tissues.

TYPE OF DRUG

Calcium channel blocker (antagonist)

GENERAL USES

Due to extremely potent hypotensive effect, used primarily to manage acute angina due to coronary vasospasm and serious hypertension. Also useful for treating pulmonary edema.

CAUTIONS

- Angina may occur when starting drug or increasing dose.
- Use with caution in patients prone to congestive heart failure.

SIDE/ADVERSE EFFECTS

- Flushing
- Peripheral edema
- Lightheadedness
- Headache
- Nausea
- Weakness
- Palpitations
- Hypotension
- Nervousness

IMPORTANT DRUG INTERACTIONS

This drug causes increases or decreases in serum levels of a large number of other drugs.

CONTRAINDICATIONS

- Do not use immediate-release form for severe hypertensive episodes.
- Avoid during acute myocardial infarction.

USUAL DOSING PARAMETERS: ADULTS/CHILDREN

- Adults:
  - 10 to 30 mg tid, up to maximum dose of 120 to 180 mg/day
- Children:
  - 0.6 to 0.9 mg/kg/day in 3 to 4 divided doses

DENTAL CONSIDERATIONS

Gingival hyperplasia is common but improves as dose is reduced. Hyperplasia is less severe when good hygiene is maintained.

AUTHOR: **JAMES R. HUPP, DMD, MD, JD, MBA**

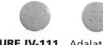

FIGURE IV-111 Adalat-cc 30 mg

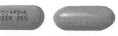

FIGURE IV-114 Procardia 10 mg

FIGURE IV-117 Procardia-xl 90 mg

FIGURE IV-112 Adalat-cc 60 mg

FIGURE IV-115 Procardia-xl 30 mg

FIGURE IV-113 Adalat-cc 90 mg

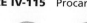

FIGURE IV-116 Procardia-xl 60 mg

BRAND NAME(S)
Prilosec
Zegerid

OVERVIEW

This drug lowers gastric acid by inhibiting the parietal cell H^+/K^+ ATP pump.

TYPE OF DRUG

Proton pump inhibitor

GENERAL USES

Used short-term for treatment of duodenal or gastric ulcers, heartburn, gastroesophageal reflux, and erosive esophagitis. Available over-the-counter for heartburn.

CAUTIONS

- Long-term use may increase risk of developing GI tumors.
- Pregnancy risk: C.

SIDE/ADVERSE EFFECTS

- Headache
- GI complaints
- Dizziness
- Rash
- Back pain

IMPORTANT DRUG INTERACTIONS

- Increases levels of benzodiazepines
- Slows elimination of phenytoin and warfarin
- Interferes with certain antiviral and antifungal drugs

CONTRAINDICATIONS

Allergy to this or other proton pump inhibitors

USUAL DOSING PARAMETERS: ADULTS/CHILDREN

- Adults:
  - 20 to 40 mg/day for 2 to 8 weeks, taken before eating
- Children:
  - 10 to 20 mg/day

DENTAL CONSIDERATIONS

Commonly causes xerostomia. Also may alter taste, cause atrophy of glossal mucosa, and promote appearance of esophageal candidiasis.

AUTHOR: **JAMES R. HUPP, DMD, MD, JD, MBA**

FIGURE IV-118 Prilosec 10 mg

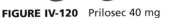

FIGURE IV-120 Prilosec 40 mg

FIGURE IV-119 Prilosec 20 mg

SECTION IV

BRAND NAME(S)
OxyContin
Roxicodone

OVERVIEW

Analgesic drug that acts by binding to opioid receptors in the CNS, inhibiting ascending pain pathways. Also produces euphoria.

TYPE OF DRUG

Narcotic analgesic

GENERAL USES

• Used for the management of moderate to severe pain
• Typically given in combination or compounded with other nonnarcotic analgesics

CAUTIONS

• Highly addictive.
• Use with caution in patients with GI motility disorders, biliary disease, or pancreatitis.
• Take care when using in patients with hepatic or renal insufficiency, or in the elderly.
• Pregnancy risk: B.

SIDE/ADVERSE EFFECTS

• Sedation
• Dizziness
• Respiratory depression
• GI upset
• Constipation
• Euphoria

IMPORTANT DRUG INTERACTIONS

Additive respiratory and sedating effects with other drugs known to cause these problems

CONTRAINDICATIONS

Preexisting respiratory insufficiency or paralytic ileus

USUAL DOSING PARAMETERS: ADULTS/CHILDREN

• Adults:
  ○ 10 to 30 mg q 4 h PRN pain

DENTAL CONSIDERATIONS

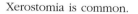

Xerostomia is common.

AUTHOR: **JAMES R. HUPP, DMD, MD, JD, MBA**

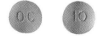

FIGURE IV-121 OxyContin 10 mg

FIGURE IV-124 OxyContin 80 mg

FIGURE IV-122 OxyContin 20 mg

FIGURE IV-125 Roxicodone 5 mg

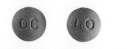

FIGURE IV-123 OxyContin 40 mg

BRAND NAME(S)
Protonix

OVERVIEW

This drug suppresses parietal cell gastric acid secretion by interfering with the H^+/K^+ ATP pump.

TYPE OF DRUG

Substituted benzimidazole proton pump inhibitor

GENERAL USES

Generally used for preventing and treating erosive esophagitis seen in patients with GERD and other hypersecretory disorders.

CAUTIONS

- Relief of gastric tract pain does not rule out malignancy.
- Not advised for use for more than 4 months.

SIDE/ADVERSE EFFECTS

- Chest pain
- Diarrhea
- Flu-like symptoms

IMPORTANT DRUG INTERACTIONS

A large number of drugs can increase or decrease effects.

CONTRAINDICATIONS

Allergy to substituted benzimidazole drugs

USUAL DOSING PARAMETERS: ADULTS/CHILDREN

- Adults:
  - 40 mg qd

DENTAL CONSIDERATIONS

No specific dental considerations

AUTHOR: **JAMES R. HUPP, DMD, MD, JD, MBA**

  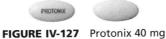

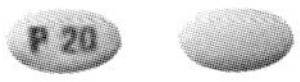

FIGURE IV-126 Protonix 20 mg

FIGURE IV-127 Protonix 40 mg

BRAND NAME(S)
Paxil

OVERVIEW

Selective serotonin reuptake inhibitor used to treat various anxiety disorders.

TYPE OF DRUG

Antidepressant

GENERAL USES

- Used primarily to manage depression, panic disorder, obsessive-compulsive disorder, and general anxiety disorders.
- Also considered for eating disorders and premenstrual disorders.

CAUTIONS

- Rapid discontinuation without tapering can cause dizziness, dysphasia, irritability, confusion, and paresthesia.
- Pregnancy risk: C.

SIDE/ADVERSE EFFECTS

- Headaches
- Sedation
- Nausea
- Diarrhea
- Ejaculatory problems
- Weakness
- Diaphoresis

IMPORTANT DRUG INTERACTIONS

- MAO inhibitors
- Ethanol
- Can potentiate effects of drugs with anticoagulant properties
- Additive with other drugs causing sedation
- Increases half-life of diazepam

CONTRAINDICATIONS

Recent use of MAO inhibitors

USUAL DOSING PARAMETERS: ADULTS/CHILDREN

- Adults:
  - 20 mg daily; can increase 10 mg per day up to 50 mg/day if needed.
- Children:
  - Not recommended for children.

DENTAL CONSIDERATIONS

- Causes xerostomia, postural hypotension, and taste disorder
- Can trigger bruxism in susceptible patients

AUTHOR: **JAMES R. HUPP, DMD, MD, JD, MBA**

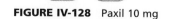

FIGURE IV-128 Paxil 10 mg

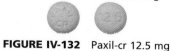

FIGURE IV-131   Paxil 40 mg

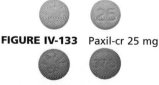

FIGURE IV-133 Paxil-cr 25 mg

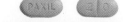

FIGURE IV-129 Paxil 20 mg

FIGURE IV-132 Paxil-cr 12.5 mg

FIGURE IV-134 Paxil-cr 37.5 mg

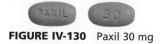

FIGURE IV-130 Paxil 30 mg

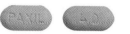

BRAND NAME(S)
Pravachol

OVERVIEW

Drug used to reduce harmful forms of cholesterol by inhibiting enzyme of the rate-limiting step in cholesterol synthesis (HMG-CoA reductase).

TYPE OF DRUG

Antilipidemic agent

GENERAL USES

Used to reduce total and low-density cholesterol and triglycerides in patients with primary hypercholesterolemia.

CAUTIONS

- Monitor liver function regularly.
- Have patient report unexplained myalgias.
- Pregnancy risk: X.

SIDE/ADVERSE EFFECTS

- Headache
- Fatigue
- Nausea
- Vomiting
- Diarrhea
- Rash
- Cough

IMPORTANT DRUG INTERACTIONS

Large number of drugs (including some antimicrobials) can increase risk of renal toxicity.

CONTRAINDICATIONS

- Acute liver disease, elevated transaminases
- Pregnancy
- Breastfeeding

USUAL DOSING PARAMETERS: ADULTS/CHILDREN

- Adults:
  - 40 to 80 mg qd
- Children:
  - Age 8 to 13 years: 20 mg qd; 14 to 18 years: 40 mg qd

DENTAL CONSIDERATIONS

No specific dental considerations

AUTHOR: **JAMES R. HUPP, DMD, MD, JD, MBA**

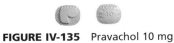

FIGURE IV-135 Pravachol 10 mg

FIGURE IV-137 Pravachol 40 mg

FIGURE IV-136 Pravachol 20 mg

FIGURE IV-138 Pravachol 80 mg

BRAND NAME(S)
Deltasone
Sterapred

OVERVIEW

Corticosteroid that suppresses inflammation-like endogenous cortisol, reducing white blood cell migration, capillary permeability, and other immune functions.

TYPE OF DRUG

Systemic corticosteroid antiinflammatory agent

GENERAL USES

Generally used for wide variety of autoimmune disorders, following organ transplantation, in the treatment of malignancies, for adrenocortical insufficiency, and when suppression of inflammatory response is desired.

CAUTIONS

- Taper drug when planning to stop medication.
- Use with caution in patients with hypothyroidism, hepatic insufficiency, tendency to GI ulceration, diabetics, cataracts, and osteoporosis.

SIDE/ADVERSE EFFECTS

- Nervousness
- Increased appetite
- Glucose intolerance
- Indigestion

IMPORTANT DRUG INTERACTIONS

Increases GI toxic tendency of NSAIDs

CONTRAINDICATIONS

- Presence of serious infection
- GI ulceration

USUAL DOSING PARAMETERS: ADULTS/CHILDREN

Complex dosing regimen that varies with condition being managed

DENTAL CONSIDERATIONS

Consider possibility of adrenal suppression and need for supplementation if major surgery is planned.

AUTHOR: **JAMES R. HUPP, DMD, MD, JD, MBA**

FIGURE IV-139 Deltasone 5 mg

FIGURE IV-140 Deltasone 10 mg

BRAND NAME(S)
Darvocet

OVERVIEW

Opioid that depresses pain perception in the CNS by binding to opioid receptors combined with drug that interferes with prostaglandin synthesis.

TYPE OF DRUG

Synthetic opioid analgesic in combination with acetaminophen (nonnarcotic analgesic)

GENERAL USES

Used to manage mild to moderate pain.

CAUTIONS

- Can be addictive.
- Use with caution in patients with renal or hepatic insufficiency and in elderly or debilitated patients.
- Pregnancy risk: C.

SIDE/ADVERSE EFFECTS

- Respiratory problems
- Depression
- Sedation
- Confusion
- Weakness

IMPORTANT DRUG INTERACTIONS

Additive effect with other CNS and respiratory depressants

CONTRAINDICATIONS

- CNS pressure elevation, acute myocardial infarction, severe heart or respiratory disease
- Concurrent use of MAO inhibitors

USUAL DOSING PARAMETERS: ADULTS/CHILDREN

- Adults:
  - 100 mg propoxyphene of 4 h PRN, up to maximum of 600 mg/day

DENTAL CONSIDERATIONS

Xerostomia potential. Avoid concurrently giving other CNS or respiratory depressants.

AUTHOR: **JAMES R. HUPP, DMD, MD, JD, MBA**

FIGURE IV-141   Darvocet-n 50 mg

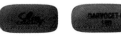

FIGURE IV-142   Darvocet-n 100 mg

OVERVIEW

ACE inhibitor used to lower angiotensin II levels, thereby reducing aldosterone secretion.

TYPE OF DRUG

Angiotensin-converting enzyme (ACE) inhibitor

GENERAL USES

Primarily used for this drug's antihypertensive effects and control of intravascular volume to treat congestive heart failure and myocardial infarction patients with compromised cardiac performance.

CAUTIONS

- Use with caution with diuretics.
- Pregnancy risk: C/D.

SIDE/ADVERSE EFFECTS

- Hypotension
- Headaches
- Dizziness
- Cough
- Hyperkalemia
- Diarrhea
- Angioedema

IMPORTANT DRUG INTERACTIONS

- Aspirin, antacids, rifampin, NSAIDs
- Additive with diuretics

CONTRAINDICATIONS

- Pregnancy in second and third trimesters
- Allergy to ACE inhibitors

USUAL DOSING PARAMETERS: ADULTS/CHILDREN

- Adults:
  - 2.5 to 20 mg qd for hypertension; 2.5 to 5 mg bid for post-MI heart failure

DENTAL CONSIDERATIONS

Angioedema can occur but is relatively rare.

AUTHOR: **JAMES R. HUPP, DMD, MD, JD, MBA**

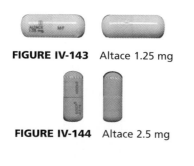

FIGURE IV-143 Altace 1.25 mg

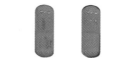

FIGURE IV-145 Altace 5 mg

FIGURE IV-144 Altace 2.5 mg

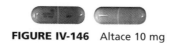

FIGURE IV-146 Altace 10 mg

BRAND NAME(S)
Zantac

OVERVIEW

Gastric acid controller that competitively inhibits histamine at H2 receptors of gastric parietal cells, lessening acid secretion

TYPE OF DRUG

H2 histamine antagonist

GENERAL USES

- Helps treat gastric peptic ulcers, gastric reflux, and erosive esophagitis
- Also used in multidrug regimens to eradicate *H. pylori* and associated duodenal ulcers

CAUTIONS

- Use with caution in patients with hepatic or renal insufficiency.
- Can cause vitamin B_{12} deficiency with chronic use.
- Pregnancy risk: B.

SIDE/ADVERSE EFFECTS

Hepatotoxicity

IMPORTANT DRUG INTERACTIONS

- Increases effects of cyclosporine, gentamicin, midazolam, β-blockers, and oral hypoglycemics
- Lowers absorption of drugs dependent upon gastric acidity for uptake

CONTRAINDICATIONS

Acute porphyria

USUAL DOSING PARAMETERS: ADULTS/CHILDREN

- Adults:
  - 300 mg/day in single or divided doses

DENTAL CONSIDERATIONS

Avoid NSAID use in patients prone to serious gastric disease.

AUTHOR: **JAMES R. HUPP, DMD, MD, JD, MBA**

BRAND NAME(S)
Zoloft

OVERVIEW

Antidepressant that inhibits presynaptic serotonin reuptake with only weak effects on norepinephrine and dopamine reuptake.

TYPE OF DRUG

Selective serotonin reuptake inhibitor (SSRI) antidepressant

GENERAL USES

Used primarily to treat major depression as well as obsessive-compulsive and panic disorders, posttraumatic stress syndrome, premenstrual dysphoric state, and social anxiety disorder.

CAUTIONS

- Lower dose in presence of hepatic disease
- Pregnancy risk: C

SIDE/ADVERSE EFFECTS

- Insomnia
- Somnolence
- Dizziness
- Headache
- Fatigue
- Diarrhea
- Nausea
- Ejaculatory disturbance

IMPORTANT DRUG INTERACTIONS

A large number of other drugs can increase or decrease effects of sertraline.

CONTRAINDICATIONS

Use of MAO inhibitors

USUAL DOSING PARAMETERS: ADULTS/CHILDREN

- Adults:
  - 25 to 100 mg/day
- Children:
  - Age 6 to 12 years: 25 mg/day; 13 to 17 years: 50 mg qd

DENTAL CONSIDERATIONS

Xerostomia potential

AUTHOR: **JAMES R. HUPP, DMD, MD, JD, MBA**

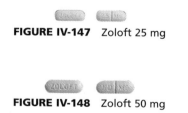

FIGURE IV-147 Zoloft 25 mg

FIGURE IV-148 Zoloft 50 mg

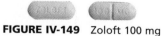

FIGURE IV-149 Zoloft 100 mg

BRAND NAME(S)
Zocor

OVERVIEW

This drug reduces harmful forms of cholesterol by inhibiting the enzyme of the rate-limiting step in cholesterol synthesis (HMG-CoA reductase).

TYPE OF DRUG

Antilipidemic agent

GENERAL USES

Used to reduce total and low-density cholesterol and triglycerides in patients with primary hypercholesterolemia.

CAUTIONS

- Monitor liver function regularly.
- Have patient report unexplained myalgias.

SIDE/ADVERSE EFFECTS

- Constipation
- Flatulence
- CPK elevation
- Renal failure

IMPORTANT DRUG INTERACTIONS

A large number of drugs (including some antimicrobials) can increase risk of renal toxicity.

CONTRAINDICATIONS

- Acute liver disease, elevated transaminases
- Pregnancy
- Breastfeeding

USUAL DOSING PARAMETERS: ADULTS/CHILDREN

- Adults:
  - 20 to 80 mg qd hs
- Children:
  - Age 10 to 17 years: 10 to 40 mg qd hs

DENTAL CONSIDERATIONS

No special dental considerations

AUTHOR: **JAMES R. HUPP, DMD, MD, JD, MBA**

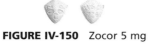

FIGURE IV-150   Zocor 5 mg

FIGURE IV-153   Zocor 40 mg

FIGURE IV-151   Zocor 10 mg

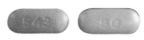

FIGURE IV-154   Zocor 80 mg

FIGURE IV-152   Zocor 20 mg

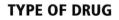

BRAND NAME(S)
Zanaflex

OVERVIEW

This drug decreases excitatory input to α motor neurons at the level of the spinal cord.

TYPE OF DRUG

α-2-adrenergic agonist

GENERAL USES

Skeletal muscle relaxant

CAUTIONS

Reduce dose in patients with hepatic or renal insufficiency and in the elderly.

SIDE/ADVERSE EFFECTS

- Hypotension
- Sedation
- Somnolence

IMPORTANT DRUG INTERACTIONS

- May increase in potency if patient is on oral contraceptives.
- Additive hypotensive effects when given with antihypertensive agents.

CONTRAINDICATIONS

None, other than hypersensitivity to drug

USUAL DOSING PARAMETERS: ADULTS/CHILDREN

- Adults:
  - 2 to 4 mg tid, increased to maximum of 36 mg/day as needed

DENTAL CONSIDERATIONS

Xerostomia potential

AUTHOR: **JAMES R. HUPP, DMD, MD, JD, MBA**

FIGURE IV-155 Zanaflex 4 mg

BRAND NAME(S)
Ultram

OVERVIEW

This narcotic analgesic is able to block pain by binding to the opiate receptors in the CNS, inhibiting ascending pain pathways.

TYPE OF DRUG

Synthetic opioid analgesic

GENERAL USES

Used for relief of moderate to moderately severe pain

CAUTIONS

• Use with caution in patients on MAO inhibitors.
• May cause seizures if given to patients on serotonin reuptake inhibitors, tricyclic antidepressants, or neuroleptic drugs.

SIDE/ADVERSE EFFECTS

• Dizziness
• Headache
• Sedation
• Vertigo
• Constipation
• Nausea

IMPORTANT DRUG INTERACTIONS

• Carbamazepine (Tegretol) decreases half-life.
• Additive with other CNS and respiratory depressants.

CONTRAINDICATIONS

• Opioid dependency
• Respiratory insufficiency
• Increased intracranial pressure

USUAL DOSING PARAMETERS: ADULTS/CHILDREN

• Adults:
  ○ 50 to 100 mg q 4h, up to maximum of 400 mg/day.
  ○ Reduce dosage in elderly patients.

DENTAL CONSIDERATIONS

Xerostomia may occur. Stomatitis is possible.

AUTHOR: **JAMES R. HUPP, DMD, MD, JD, MBA**

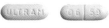

FIGURE IV-156   Ultram

BRAND NAME(S)
Desyrel

OVERVIEW

Antidepressant drug that inhibits the reuptake of serotonin changing sensitivity of adrenoreceptors. Also blocks histamine (H-1) and α-adrenergic receptors.

TYPE OF DRUG

Serotonin reuptake inhibitor

GENERAL USES

Used for the management of depression, alone or in combination with other drugs

CAUTIONS

- Use with caution in patients with cardiac disease.
- Can be extremely sedating.

SIDE/ADVERSE EFFECTS

- Sedation
- Dizziness
- Headache
- Nausea
- Blurred vision

IMPORTANT DRUG INTERACTIONS

A large number of drugs increase or decrease the effects of trazodone.

CONTRAINDICATIONS

Children under the age of 18

USUAL DOSING PARAMETERS: ADULTS/CHILDREN

- Adults:
  - 50 mg tid, increased to 200 mg tid as indicated.
  - May take weeks to see desired effects.

DENTAL CONSIDERATIONS

Xerostomia, but less than in other antidepressants

AUTHOR: **JAMES R. HUPP, DMD, MD, JD, MBA**

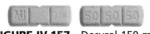
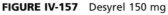

FIGURE IV-157 Desyrel 150 mg

BRAND NAME(S)
Dyrenium

OVERVIEW

Diuretic that interferes with sodium/potassium exchange in the renal distal tubule and other sites. In contrast to other diuretics, tends to preserve potassium.

TYPE OF DRUG

Potassium-sparing diuretic

GENERAL USES

- Drug used alone or in combination with potassium-wasting diuretics to manage hypertension.
- Also used to manage peripheral edema seen with congestive heart failure.

CAUTIONS

- Be careful to monitor serum potassium levels, particularly if potassium supplements are planned.
- Pregnancy risk: B.

SIDE/ADVERSE EFFECTS

- Hypotension
- Dizziness
- Fatigue
- Thrombocytopenia
- Azotemia

IMPORTANT DRUG INTERACTIONS

Avoid concurrent use with ACE inhibitors or spironolactone, especially in patients with renal impairment.

CONTRAINDICATIONS

- Patients already taking other potassium-sparing diuretics
- Severe renal insufficiency

USUAL DOSING PARAMETERS: ADULTS/CHILDREN

- Adults:
  - 100 mg bid

DENTAL CONSIDERATIONS

Xerostomia; carefully monitor vital signs.

AUTHOR: **JAMES R. HUPP, DMD, MD, JD, MBA**

BRAND NAME(S)
Diovan

OVERVIEW

This drug directly antagonizes angiotensin II receptors, lowering blood pressure, limiting aldosterone release, and limiting angiotensin I vasoconstrictive effects.

TYPE OF DRUG

Angiotensin II receptor blocker

GENERAL USES

Valsartan is used alone or with other antihypertensive drugs to manage essential hypertension or congestive heart failure, particularly in patients unable to take ACE inhibitors.

CAUTIONS

Potassium abnormalities can lead to major complications; careful monitoring of serum K^+ is critical.

SIDE/ADVERSE EFFECTS

- Dizziness.
- Fatigue.
- Abdominal pain.
- Coughs.
- If being used to manage heart fatigue, add hypotension, diarrhea, and musculoskeletal pain.

IMPORTANT DRUG INTERACTIONS

- Several drugs can increase or decrease effects of this drug.
- Take care when using potassium-sparing diuretics or giving K^+ supplements.

CONTRAINDICATIONS

- Renal artery stenosis
- Second and third trimesters of pregnancy

USUAL DOSING PARAMETERS: ADULTS/CHILDREN

- Adults:
  - Hypertension therapy: 80 to 160 mg qd
  - Heart failure: 40 to 160 mg bid as tolerated

DENTAL CONSIDERATIONS

None, other than possible postural hypotension

AUTHOR: **JAMES R. HUPP, DMD, MD, JD, MBA**

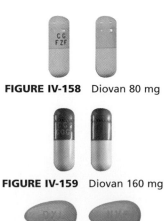

FIGURE IV-158 Diovan 80 mg

FIGURE IV-159 Diovan 160 mg

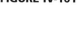

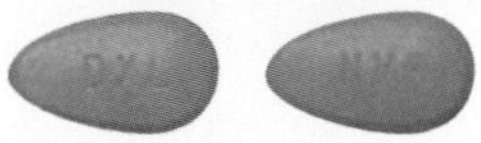

FIGURE IV-160 Diovan 320 mg

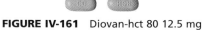

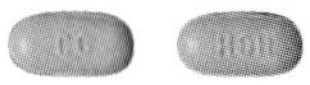

FIGURE IV-161 Diovan-hct 80 12.5 mg

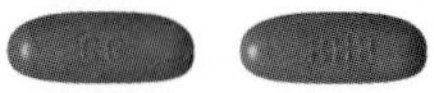

FIGURE IV-162 Diovan-hct 160 12.5 mg

BRAND NAME(S)
Calan
Isoptin
Verelan

OVERVIEW

First-generation calcium channel blocker that inhibits calcium from entering "slow channels," thereby relaxing vascular smooth muscle and myocardial tissues.

TYPE OF DRUG

Calcium channel blocker (antagonist)

GENERAL USES

- Used to manage hypertension as well as stable angina secondary to coronary artery spasm.
- Also useful for atrial and supraventricular tachydysrhythmia.

CAUTIONS

- Use with caution in patients prone to cardiac conduction problems.
- Grapefruit juice may increase potency.
- Avoid abrupt discontinuation.

SIDE/ADVERSE EFFECTS

- Hypotension
- Heart blocks
- Dizziness
- Constipation

IMPORTANT DRUG INTERACTIONS

- Concurrent use with aspirin may increase bleeding time.
- A large number of drugs have serum concentrations affected by verapamil.

CONTRAINDICATIONS

- Serious cardiac dysfunction
- Hypotension
- Preexisting heart blocks

USUAL DOSING PARAMETERS: ADULTS/CHILDREN

Complex dosing regimens that depend upon condition being managed

DENTAL CONSIDERATIONS

Gingival hyperplasia is very frequent and responds to decreasing the dose or stopping the drug. Good hygiene decreases severity.

AUTHOR: **JAMES R. HUPP, DMD, MD, JD, MBA**

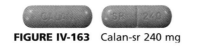

FIGURE IV-163   Calan-sr 240 mg

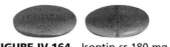
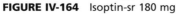

FIGURE IV-164   Isoptin-sr 180 mg

BRAND NAME(S)
Coumadin

OVERVIEW

Slow-onset, long-duration oral anticoagulant that interferes with synthesis of vitamin K-dependent clotting factors (II, VII, IX, X) by the liver.

TYPE OF DRUG

Anticoagulant

GENERAL USES

- This drug is used for the prevention and treatment of undesired intravascular clotting such as in venous thrombosis, pulmonary embolism, atrial fibrillation, and thromboembolic disorders.
- Also regularly used during care for myocardial infarction.

CAUTIONS

Use with great caution in patients with preexisting bleeding disorders or recent major surgery.

SIDE/ADVERSE EFFECTS

- Unwanted bleeding
- Osteoporosis
- Elevated liver enzymes

IMPORTANT DRUG INTERACTIONS

- Antifungal agents and NSAIDs may increase warfarin potency.
- A large number of other possible interactions.

CONTRAINDICATIONS

- Recent major surgery or trauma
- Preexisting major disorders of coagulation

USUAL DOSING PARAMETERS: ADULTS/CHILDREN

- Adults:
  - 1 to 10 mg qd, titrated to desired INR value
- Children:
  - 0.05 to 0.34 mg/kg/day, titrated to desired INR value

DENTAL CONSIDERATIONS

Prolonged bleeding after procedures, especially if INR > 2.5–3.0; local anesthetic blocks may cause hematomas.

AUTHOR: **JAMES R. HUPP, DMD, MD, JD, MBA**

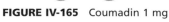
FIGURE IV-165 Coumadin 1 mg

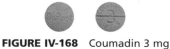
FIGURE IV-168 Coumadin 3 mg

FIGURE IV-171 Coumadin 6 mg

FIGURE IV-166 Coumadin 2 mg

FIGURE IV-169 Coumadin 4 mg

FIGURE IV-172 Coumadin 7.5 mg

FIGURE IV-167 Coumadin 2.5 mg

FIGURE IV-170 Coumadin 5 mg

FIGURE IV-173 Coumadin 10 mg

BRAND NAME(S)
Ambien

OVERVIEW

Has a chemical structure similar to benzodiazepines but does not act in the same way in the central nervous system. Does have hypnotic and anxiolytic properties.

TYPE OF DRUG

Hypnotic agent

GENERAL USES

Used for short-term treatment of insomnia

CAUTIONS

- Eliminate other causes of sleep disturbance that depend upon other therapeutic approaches.
- Has additive effects with other sedating drugs and EtOH.
- Pregnancy risk: B.

SIDE/ADVERSE EFFECTS

- Headache
- Drowsiness
- Dizziness
- Lethargy

IMPORTANT DRUG INTERACTIONS

A large variety of drugs either increase or decrease effects of this drug.

CONTRAINDICATIONS

Allergy to drug

USUAL DOSING PARAMETERS: ADULTS/CHILDREN

- Adults:
  - 5 or 10 mg qd hs as needed

DENTAL CONSIDERATIONS

No specific dental considerations

AUTHOR: **JAMES R. HUPP, DMD, MD, JD, MBA**

FIGURE IV-174 Ambien 5 mg

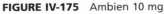

FIGURE IV-175 Ambien 10 mg

Anesthesia

BRAND NAME(S)
Septocaine

OVERVIEW

A newer local anesthetic in the United States but has been used since 1970 in Europe and Canada. The formulation available in the U.S. is a 4% solution with 1:100,000 epinephrine.

TYPE OF DRUG

Local anesthetic, amide type with an ester side chain.

GENERAL USES

Infiltration and nerve block (see Side/Adverse Effects below) for dental procedures.

CAUTIONS

Although the rapid hydrolysis via the ester side chain reduces the risk of toxic overdosage from local resorption, the 4% formulation does increase the risk of toxicity following an intravascular injection.

SIDE/ADVERSE EFFECTS

- Toxicity due to the higher concentration.
- Articaine is associated with an increased nerve toxicity with block injections. May be due to the higher concentration or inherent local neurotoxicity of the drug.

IMPORTANT DRUG INTERACTIONS

Local anesthetic agents containing epinephrine should be used sparingly in patients taking tricyclic antidepressants (severe, prolonged hypertension may develop).

CONTRAINDICATIONS

- Allergy or hypersensitivity to the components (articaine and epinephrine)
- Allergy or hypersensitivity to sulfites

USUAL DOSING PARAMETERS: ADULTS/CHILDREN

7 mg/kg for adults and children

DENTAL CONSIDERATIONS

Although some dentists report anecdotally that articaine diffuses through tissue more rapidly than lidocaine and can achieve profound local anesthesia in areas of inflammation, this has not been scientifically proven. The risks of permanent paresthesia should be taken into account if a nerve block injection is given.

SUGGESTED REFERENCES

Haas DA, Lennon D. A 21-year retrospective study of the reports of paresthesia following local anesthetic administration. *J Can Dent Assoc* 1995;61:319–330.
Malamed SF, Gagnon S, Leblanc D. Efficacy of articaine: a new amide local anesthetic. *J Am Dent Assoc* 2000;131:635–642.

AUTHOR: **STUART E. LIEBLICH, DMD**

BRAND NAME(S)
Sal-Tropine

OVERVIEW

By blocking the action of acetylcholine at receptor sites, it causes drying of the mouth, antagonizes histamine, and increases cardiac output.

TYPE OF DRUG

Anticholinergic

GENERAL USES

- Intravenous form: to treat acute bradycardia
- Orally: to create reversible xerostomia

CAUTIONS

Patients should be cardiovascularly stable enough to tolerate the expected increase in heart rate. Atropine crosses the blood–brain barrier, which can present as an acute psychosis.

SIDE/ADVERSE EFFECTS

- Flushing
- Blurry vision
- Increased heart rate
- Delirium (atropine psychosis)

IMPORTANT DRUG INTERACTIONS

In combination with the epinephrine in local anesthetics, severe tachycardias may develop.

CONTRAINDICATIONS

- Glaucoma
- Thyrotoxicosis

USUAL DOSING PARAMETERS: ADULTS/CHILDREN

- For acute treatment of bradycardia (IV): 0.5 mg children; 1.0 mg in adolescents and adults to a maximum of 3 mg. If the IV route is not available, it can be administered intratracheally at 2 to 2.5 times the IV dose.
- For dental procedures to reduce salivation (orally): 0.1 mg per 10 lb to a maximum of 0.4 mg.

DENTAL CONSIDERATIONS

The significant xerostomia may be beneficial in certain situations where a dry field is needed. Also, atropine is occasionally mixed with ketamine to reduce the increased secretions associated with that agent.

SUGGESTED REFERENCE

Dowd F. Antimuscarinic drugs, in Yagiela JA, Dowd FJ, Neidle EA (eds): *Pharmacology and Therapeutics for Dentistry*. St Louis, Elsevier (Mosby), 2004, pp 139–146.

AUTHOR: **STUART E. LIEBLICH, DMD**

Bupivacaine with Epinephrine

BRAND NAME(S)
Marcaine with epinephrine (1:200,000)

OVERVIEW

Bupivacaine is related to mepivacaine but with a substitution to increase its lipid solubility. It has a significantly higher protein binding (96% vs 64% for lidocaine), accounting for its longer duration of action. The increased protein binding and high lipid solubility reduce the efficacy and duration of action when used for infiltration-type injections; this gives it even a shorter duration of action of pulpal anesthesia with maxillary infiltration injections in comparison to lidocaine with epinephrine. Bupivacaine has a higher pKa (8.1 vs 7.8 for lidocaine), thereby increasing the time of onset.

TYPE OF DRUG

Local anesthetic, amide type

GENERAL USES

Local anesthesia for dental procedures

CAUTIONS

Maximum doses must be observed to avoid overdosage, especially in children. Toxic effects are increased with hypoxia.

SIDE/ADVERSE EFFECTS

Toxicity is often manifested as initial restlessness and agitation. However, may also present as drowsiness, slurred speech, and unconsciousness, particularly with bupivacaine. Higher CNS levels lead to seizures. Bupivacaine has an increased tendency (tropism) to binding in the cardiac conduction system, leading to bradycardia that can progress to heart block (even with subtoxic doses). The cardiac manifestations often present prior to the CNS signs with bupivacaine. Epinephrine causes heart palpitations, tachycardia, and premature ventricular contractions (PVCs).

IMPORTANT DRUG INTERACTIONS

Epinephrine and nonselective β-blockers (e.g., propranolol) may cause initial hypertension followed by bradycardia. It is less likely with the selective β-1 blockers.

CONTRAINDICATIONS

- Known allergy or hypersensitivity to the agents
- Recent myocardial infarction (wait at least 6 months for elective treatment)
- Pregnancy

USUAL DOSING PARAMETERS: ADULTS/CHILDREN

- Adults: 1.5 mg/kg to a maximum total dose of 90 mg for the bupivacaine (if using with a vasoconstrictor). Epinephrine should be limited to 0.2 mg in an adult.
- Children: pediatric doses are not established (current data is not available for using it in children under 12 years of age). There is a concern that prolonged anesthesia of the lip may lead to self-inflicted injuries in the child and mentally handicapped individual.

DENTAL CONSIDERATIONS

The long duration of action of bupivacaine is beneficial if prolonged anesthesia is indicated following surgical procedures. The duration of analgesia averages 5 hours in the maxilla and 8 hours in the mandible. This may reduce the need for postoperative narcotics.

Slow injection (1 mL/minute) may avoid toxic reactions if an inadvertent intravascular injection is given. Toxic effects are increased if respiratory acidosis is present. Toxicity is treated by hyperventilation, monitoring, and cardiovascular support as needed. If asystole develops, prolonged resuscitation should be attempted due to the duration of action of bupivacaine.

SUGGESTED REFERENCE

Yagiela JA. Local anesthetics, in Yagiela JA, Dowd FJ, Neidle EA (eds): *Pharmacology and Therapeutics for Dentistry.* St Louis, Elsevier (Mosby), 2004, pp 251–270.

AUTHOR: **STUART E. LIEBLICH, DMD**

BRAND NAME(S)
Suprane

OVERVIEW

An inhalational general anesthetic agent with a blood/gas solubility close to nitrous oxide. This causes a rapid onset of the agent and a rapid recovery. Its increased potency creates true general anesthesia. It has a low toxicity since very little is actively metabolized. Due to its high pungency and respiratory irritation it is associated with coughing, breath-holding, and the potential for laryngospasm during induction. This makes it a less than ideal agent to induce anesthesia in children, but it is very good for the maintenance of anesthesia.

TYPE OF DRUG

Halogenated volatile general anesthetic

GENERAL USES

For maintenance of general anesthesia

CAUTIONS

If used for induction, must be titrated slowly due to respiratory irritant properties.

SIDE/ADVERSE EFFECTS

- Coughing, breath-holding, laryngospasm
- Tachycardia, hypotension
- Respiratory depression

IMPORTANT DRUG INTERACTIONS

Additive effects with other anesthetic and CNS depressants

CONTRAINDICATIONS

If history or suspected risk of malignant hyperthermia

USUAL DOSING PARAMETERS: ADULTS/CHILDREN

- Adults: 2.5–8%, (MAC = 6% in oxygen, 2.8% with 60% nitrous oxide). Induction dose (adults only, limited by respiratory irritation): start at 3%, increase 0.5% every 2 to 5 breaths as tolerated.
- Children: 5.2–10%.

DENTAL CONSIDERATIONS

Used primarily in the operating room setting since sedation cannot be reliably achieved with this agent. Its low blood solubility permits rapid recovery from the anesthetic and faster discharge in comparison to some of the other volatile anesthetic agents. In comparison to halothane, it does not sensitize the heart to exogenous catecholamines.

SUGGESTED REFERENCE

Eger EI. New inhaled anesthetics. *Anesthesiology* 1993;80:906–922.

AUTHOR: **STUART E. LIEBLICH, DMD**

Diazepam

BRAND NAME(S)
Diazemuls
Valium

OVERVIEW

A benzodiazepine agent that has a long duration due to the presence of active metabolites. Diazepam has been used as an oral as well as intravenous agent for anxiolysis and sedation for dental procedures. Diazepam acts in the central nervous system (CNS) with very few cardiovascular effects.

TYPE OF DRUG

Anxiolytic and sedative agent with muscle relaxant properties

GENERAL USES

- Orally for preoperative sedation, intravenously as a sole agent or in combination with other drugs for deep sedation/general anesthesia.
- Its skeletal muscle relaxant properties may improve patients with temporomandibular dysfunction due to muscle spasms.
- Diazepam is effective at raising the seizure threshold and may be used emergently for the treatment of status epilepticus as well as seizures due to an overdose of local anesthesia.

CAUTIONS

- Drowsiness and sedation.
- Active metabolites are stored in the gallbladder, and a second peak level may occur following a meal during which the gallbladder empties and reabsorption occurs.
- Prolonged and more profound effect in elderly patients, with a risk of falls.
- The intravenous formulation typically contains propylene glycol and is associated with an increased incidence of phlebitis. Consider using an alternative water-soluble benzodiazepine (such as midazolam), or an oil emulsion formulation should be given.
- Intramuscular absorption is poor and erratic whereas oral administration is more predictable.

SIDE/ADVERSE EFFECTS

- Drowsiness, ataxia, amnesia (can persist for extended periods of time, sometimes over 24 hours due to the long half-life and active metabolites)
- Xerostomia
- Apnea (especially with rapid administration in the elderly)

IMPORTANT DRUG INTERACTIONS

- Additive effects with other CNS depressants and narcotics
- Increased serum level and potential toxicity: cimetidine, ciprofloxacin, ritonavir, grapefruit juice
- Increased metabolism rate (decreased effectiveness): phenobarbital, phenytoin, rifampin
- Direct antagonism: theophylline

CONTRAINDICATIONS

- Hypersensitivity to the agent, drug class, or vehicle agents
- Acute narrow angle glaucoma
- Pregnancy

USUAL DOSING PARAMETERS: ADULTS/CHILDREN

Note: intramuscular route gives erratic and unpredictable absorption.
- Adults:
  - Oral: 2 to 10 mg
  - IV: 2 to 10 mg titrated to effect. Avoid doses over 5 mg in elderly patients and administer each 1-mg increment at least 5 minutes apart.
- Children:
  - Oral: 0.2 to 0.3 mg/kg to 10 mg maximum.
  - IV: 0.1 to 0.3 mg/kg titrated to effect.
- Status epilepticus (IV):
  - Adults: 5 to 10 mg every 10 to 20 minutes to a total dose of up to 30 mg.
  - Children: 0.2 mg/kg over 2 to 3 minutes, repeated every 15 minutes until effective.

DENTAL CONSIDERATIONS

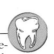

The benzodiazepines are excellent agents for reducing the anxiety associated with dental procedures. Diazepam is well absorbed orally and is effective in 45 to 60 minutes. Its prolonged length of action may be a limiting factor, and other agents such as midazolam or triazolam should be considered. Similarly, the intravenous form with its associated risks of phlebitis has led most practitioners to substitute midazolam for sedation and anesthesia in dentistry. Elderly patients are more sensitive to the prolonged action and have had an increase in the rate of falls following its use.

SUGGESTED REFERENCE

Finder RA, Moore P. Benzodiazepines for intravenous conscious sedation: agonists and antagonists. *Compendium* 1993;14:972–980.

AUTHOR: **STUART E. LIEBLICH, DMD**

Diphenhydramine

BRAND NAME(S)
Benadryl

OVERVIEW

Diphenhydramine is an antihistamine drug with many useful properties. It is effective at reducing the rash and hives following a mild allergic reaction, such as the dermatologic responses after taking an antibiotic. Diphenhydramine is also a mild sedative and often used to aid sleep in over-the-counter preparations (e.g., Sominex, Nytol). Additionally, its antinausea properties may act as an antiemetic, especially with nausea induced by ambulation following anesthesia or preventively in patients susceptible to motion sickness. Diphenhydramine has mild antitussive properties as well.

TYPE OF DRUG

Antihistamine

GENERAL USES

- Treatment of mild allergic reactions
- To induce sleep
- Motion sickness prophylaxis
- Topical anesthetic
- Treatment of extrapyramidal reactions following phenothiazine drugs

CAUTIONS

- Sedative effects may cause ataxia and risk of falls, especially in the elderly.
- Prolonged elimination in the elderly (13 hours vs 6 hours in adults).
- Anticholinergic effects may cause blurred vision.

SIDE/ADVERSE EFFECTS

- Dizziness, blurred vision, ataxia
- Sleepiness
- Xerostomia
- Urinary retention

IMPORTANT DRUG INTERACTIONS

Additive effects with other CNS depressants (e.g., ethanol, benzodiazepines, narcotics, barbiturates)

CONTRAINDICATIONS

As an injectable for nerve block (may cause necrosis of the nerve with permanent neurosensory effects)

USUAL DOSING PARAMETERS: ADULTS/CHILDREN

- Adults:
  - Oral:
    - 25 to 50 mg
  - IV:
    - 25 to 50 mg
- Children:
  - Oral:
    - 2 to 6 years: 6.25 mg
    - 6 to 12 years: 12.5 to 25 mg
    - > 12 years: 25 to 50 mg
  - IV:
    - 0.5 to 1.0 mg/kg to a maximum of 50 mg

DENTAL CONSIDERATIONS

Doses of 25 to 50 mg 4 times per day can be used to treat mild allergic reactions. It may assist patients to achieve sleep the night before an appointment if they have mild anxiety about an upcoming dental procedure. The mild, local anesthetic effect and its antihistamine properties make it useful in a topical solution for reducing the discomfort of recurrent aphthous ulcerations and mucositis following chemotherapy. An effective combination is to compound 1 part diphenhydramine elixir, 1 part viscous lidocaine, and 1 part Maalox. Patients are instructed to use 15 mL "swish and spit" every 2 to 4 hours for control of pain.

SUGGESTED REFERENCE

Simons FER, Simons KJ. The pharmacology and use of H-1 receptor antagonist drugs. *N Engl J Med* 1994;330: 1663–1670.

AUTHOR: STUART E. LIEBLICH, DMD

BRAND NAME(S)
Duragesic
Sublimaze

OVERVIEW

A narcotic analgesic that is used as an adjunctive agent in patients undergoing sedation and general anesthesia. It has a rapid peak effect when given intravenously and a short duration of only 30 minutes. Fentanyl is more lipid soluble than morphine; thus, it acts sooner and also has a shorter duration of action.

TYPE OF DRUG

Narcotic analgesic

GENERAL USES

- In conjunction with intravenous sedation/general anesthesia in dentistry
- For control of severe chronic pain and breakthrough cancer pain with the use of a transdermal patch

CAUTIONS

- Risks of respiratory depression.
- Administer over 3 to 5 minutes to avoid development of stiff chest syndrome (see Side/Adverse Effects following).

SIDE/ADVERSE EFFECTS

- Respiratory depression.
- Nausea/vomiting.
- Constipation.
- Rapid administration may cause chest wall rigidity and difficulty in ventilation that may require treatment with a nondepolarizing muscle relaxant.

IMPORTANT DRUG INTERACTIONS

Although the risks of meperidine and MAO inhibitors are well known, there are isolated reports that risks may occur with fentanyl as well. The U.S. manufacturer's recommendations are that if the patient has received an MAO inhibitor within 14 days, vasodilators and β-blockers must be available to treat hypertension.

CONTRAINDICATIONS

Hypersensitivity to the agent

USUAL DOSING PARAMETERS: ADULTS/CHILDREN

As an adjunct to sedative administrations:
- Adults:
  - 50 to 100 µg, repeated every 30 to 60 minutes
- Children:
  - 1 to 2 µg/kg, repeated every 30 to 60 minutes

DENTAL CONSIDERATIONS

Useful in combination with other intravenous drugs such as midazolam for a balanced intravenous sedation.

Death has been reported with the use of the transdermal patch for control of postoperative dental pain. Therefore, this formulation is contraindicated for this use in dentistry.

SUGGESTED REFERENCES

Dionne RA, Yagiela JA, Moore PA. Comparing efficacy and safety of four intravenous sedation regimens in dental outpatients. *J Am Dent Assoc* 2001;132:740–751.
Sublimaze (fentanyl citrate) U.S. prescribing information. Decatur, IL, Taylor Pharmaceuticals, 2005.

AUTHOR: **STUART E. LIEBLICH, DMD**

BRAND NAME(S)
Robinul

OVERVIEW

An anticholinergic agent similar to atropine. It is a quaternary amine; it does not cross the blood–brain barrier, resulting in a lower incidence of central nervous system side effects.

TYPE OF DRUG

Anticholinergic

GENERAL USES

- Inhibits excessive salivation and upper respiratory secretions
- Adjunctive treatment for peptic ulcers

CAUTIONS

- Spastic paralysis
- Glaucoma
- Benign prostatic hypertrophy
- Myasthenia gravis

SIDE/ADVERSE EFFECTS

- Dry skin
- Constipation
- Xerostomia

IMPORTANT DRUG INTERACTIONS

- Pramlintide (Symlin) combination is clearly contraindicated due to additive effects of decreased gastric emptying.
- Phenothiazines—additive and adverse reactions with the combination of agents.

CONTRAINDICATIONS

Paralytic ileus

USUAL DOSING PARAMETERS: ADULTS/CHILDREN

- Orally to control secretions:
  - Adults: 1 to 2 mg
  - Children: 40 to 100 µg/kg
- IV:
  - Adults: 0.1 to 0.2 mg
  - Children: 4 to 10 µg/kg

DENTAL CONSIDERATIONS

Useful for the temporary control of salivation for dental procedures. Its poor oral absorption requires approximately 1 hour to achieve peak effect. Due to the slow onset with intravenous administration, it is not indicated for the emergency treatment of bradycardia.

AUTHOR: **STUART E. LIEBLICH, DMD**

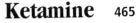

BRAND NAME(S)
Ketalar

OVERVIEW

Ketamine produces dissociative anesthesia different from other general anesthetic agents. It is characterized by profound analgesia, amnesia, and catalepsy while maintaining spontaneous respirations. Most protective reflexes are maintained, including coughing and the corneal responses. Ketamine has sympathomimetic properties that support circulation and blood pressure. It also has bronchodilating effects that may be beneficial in the asthmatic patient.

TYPE OF DRUG

A phencyclidine derivative

GENERAL USES

For the induction and maintenance of deep sedation/general anesthesia. Ketamine can be used in conjunction with other agents to provide a balanced anesthetic.

CAUTIONS

Increased secretions may cause laryngospasm. Consider administering with an anticholinergic agent (see "Atropine" or "Glycopyrrolate" in Section V, pp 457 and 464). Emergence delirium has been reported. This often is abated by concomitant administration with a benzodiazepine and allowing recovery in a darkened room with little stimulation.

SIDE/ADVERSE EFFECTS

- Hypertension, tachycardia.
- Hypersecretions, coughing, laryngospasm.
- Increased intracranial pressure.
- Tonic clonic movements, tremors.
- Nystagmus may blur vision.

IMPORTANT DRUG INTERACTIONS

- Other sympathomimetic drugs (epinephrine, cocaine) have additive cardiovascular responses.
- Halothane may increase dysrhythmias.

CONTRAINDICATIONS

Closed head injury

USUAL DOSING PARAMETERS: ADULTS/CHILDREN

Ketamine is predictably absorbed via the oral, IM, and IV routes of administration.
- Adults:
  - IM: 3 to 8 mg/kg
  - IV: 1 to 2 mg/kg
- Children:
  - Oral: 6 to 10 mg/kg
  - IM: 3 to 7 mg/kg
  - IV: 0.5 to 2 mg/kg

DENTAL CONSIDERATIONS

Ketamine is an effective agent to induce dissociative anesthesia. Because it can be administered intramuscularly, it is useful in the uncooperative child or adult patient. It can be mixed in the same syringe with other agents such as atropine (to reduce secretions), meperidine (for additive effects), and midazolam (to improve the sedation and reduce the tendency for emergence delirium) to allow one effective intramuscular injection. General anesthesia will commence in 1 to 2 minutes following intravenous, 3 to 10 minutes following intramuscular, and 15 to 30 minutes after oral administration.

SUGGESTED REFERENCE
White PF, Way WL, Trevor AJ. Ketamine: its pharmacology and therapeutic uses. *Anesthesiology* 1982;56:119–136.

AUTHOR: STUART E. LIEBLICH, DMD

BRAND NAME(S)
Xylocaine with epinephrine

OVERVIEW

Lidocaine with epinephrine is the most commonly used local anesthetic for infiltration and nerve blocks. The usual concentration is 2% lidocaine with 1:100,000 epinephrine. For surgical hemostasis, the limited use of 1:50,000 concentration may be used but is associated with local tissue necrosis. Lidocaine without a vasoconstrictor is not effective for achieving pulpal anesthesia, and the rapid absorption may lead to toxic reactions.

TYPE OF DRUG

Local anesthetic, amide type

GENERAL USES

- Local anesthesia for dental procedures
- Antidysrhythmia therapy (lidocaine without epinephrine)

CAUTIONS

Maximum doses must be observed to avoid overdosage, especially in children. Toxic effects are increased with hypoxia.

SIDE/ADVERSE EFFECTS

- Toxicity often is manifested as initial restlessness and agitation. However, it may also present as drowsiness, slurred speech, and unconsciousness, particularly with lidocaine. Higher central nervous system levels lead to seizures.
- Epinephrine causes heart palpitations, tachycardia, and premature ventricular contractions (PVCs).

IMPORTANT DRUG INTERACTIONS

Epinephrine and nonselective β-blockers (e.g., propranolol) may cause initial hypertension followed by bradycardia. It is less likely with the selective β-1 blockers.

CONTRAINDICATIONS

- Known allergy or hypersensitivity to the agents
- Recent myocardial infarction (wait at least 6 months for elective treatment)

USUAL DOSING PARAMETERS: ADULTS/CHILDREN

7 mg/kg to a maximum total dose of 500 mg for the lidocaine (if using with a vasoconstrictor). Epinephrine should be limited to 0.2 mg in an adult.

DENTAL CONSIDERATIONS

The safety of lidocaine with epinephrine is well-documented in dentistry. Slow injection (1 mL/minute) will avoid toxic reactions if an inadvertent intravascular injection is given. Toxic effects are increased if respiratory acidosis is present. Toxicity is treated by hyperventilation, monitoring, and cardiovascular support as needed.

SUGGESTED REFERENCE

Yagiela JA. Local anesthetics, in Yagiela JA, Dowd FJ, Neidle EA (eds): *Pharmacology and Therapeutics for Dentistry.* St Louis, Elsevier (Mosby), 2004, pp 251–270.

AUTHOR: **STUART E. LIEBLICH, DMD**

TABLE V-1 **Comparison of Local Anesthetics Used in Dentistry**

Preparation contents	Proprietary (trade) name	Maximum dose* (mg/kg)	Maximum dose* (mg)	Duration of anesthesia (soft tissue) Maxillary infiltration (min)	Duration of anesthesia (soft tissue) Inferior alveolar block (min)
2% Lidocaine hydrochloride; 1:100,000 epinephrine	Xylocaine with epinephrine	7	500	170	190
2% Lidocaine	Xylocaine	4.5	300	40†	100†
2% Mepivacaine hydrochloride; 1:20,000 levonordefrin	Scandonest 2%	6.6	400	130	185
3% Mepivacaine hydrochloride	Carbocaine	6.6	400	90	165
4% Prilocaine hydrochloride; 1:200,000 epinephrine	Citanest Forte	8	600	140	220
4% Prilocaine hydrochloride	Citanest	8	600	105	190
0.5% Bupivacaine hydrochloride; 1:200,000 epinephrine	Marcaine with epinephrine	—	90	340	440
4% Articaine hydrochloride; 1:100,000 epinephrine	Septocaine	7	—	190	230

* The maximum dose is the smaller of the two values (e.g., 7 mg/kg lidocaine up to a maximum dose of 500 mg).
† Lidocaine without epinephrine produces unreliable pulpal anesthesia.
From: Yagiela JA. Local anesthetics, in Yagiela JA, Dowd FJ, Neidle EA (eds): *Pharmacology and Therapeutics for Dentistry*. St Louis, Elsevier (Mosby), 2004.

SECTION V

Meperidine

BRAND NAME(S)
Demerol

OVERVIEW

A narcotic analgesic used for the treatment of moderate to severe pain. Meperidine is usually administered intravenously or intramuscularly due to erratic oral absorption. There are some patients deficient in the enzymes (CP450, 2D6) necessary to metabolize the more commonly used oral analgesics such as codeine and oxycodone who may respond positively to meperidine. This enzyme deficiency may affect 5–10% of Caucasians. Although not an ideal oral analgesic due to the potential for the accumulation of toxic metabolites, it is a useful alternative in this class of patients.

TYPE OF DRUG

Centrally acting narcotic agonist

GENERAL USES

- Treatment of moderate to severe pain
- As an adjunct agent for deep sedation/general anesthesia

CAUTIONS

Associated with respiratory depression. Risks are greater in the elderly. When used for longer than a 14-day period, normeperidine can accumulate, causing seizures and increased intracranial pressure.

SIDE/ADVERSE EFFECTS

- Respiratory depression
- Nausea/vomiting
- Xerostomia
- Rash, urticaria due to histamine release
- Constipation

IMPORTANT DRUG INTERACTIONS

- MAO inhibitors can precipitate acute serotonin crisis.
- Phenytoin decreases the analgesic effects.

CONTRAINDICATIONS

Use of MAO inhibitors within the past 14 days

USUAL DOSING PARAMETERS: ADULTS/CHILDREN

- Children:
  - 25 to 50mg every 4 to 6 hours
- Adults:
  - 50 to 100 mg orally every 4 to 6 hours as needed for management of acute pain
  - 50 to 100 mg IV as an adjunct for deep sedation/general anesthesia

DENTAL CONSIDERATIONS

Due to the acute risks of abuse, the use of oral meperidine should be reserved for those allergic or nonresponsive to codeine or its congeners (i.e., oxycodone, hydrocodone). Limited use to no more than 5 to 7 days is indicated.

SUGGESTED REFERENCE

Fletcher MC, Spera JF. Pre-emptive and postoperative analgesia for dentoalveolar surgery. *Oral Maxillofacial Clin No Am* 2002;14:137–151.

AUTHOR: **STUART E. LIEBLICH, DMD**

BRAND NAME(S)
Carbocaine
Carbocaine with neocobefrin
Polocaine

OVERVIEW

Mepivacaine with and without levonordefrin is an effective agent for maxillary infiltration and inferior alveolar nerve block. Because mepivacaine is less potent than lidocaine, the plain solution is provided as a 3% solution. The addition of the levonordefrin will significantly increase the duration of an infiltration pulpal anesthesia (from 90 to 130 minutes) but has little effect on the duration of an inferior alveolar nerve block (165 vs 185 minutes). The systemic absorption of the drug is not reduced with the addition of the vasoconstrictor; the maximal recommended dosages do not differ.

TYPE OF DRUG

Local anesthetic, amide type

GENERAL USES

Local anesthesia for dental procedures

CAUTIONS

Maximum doses must be observed to avoid overdosage, especially in children. Toxic effects are increased with hypoxia.

SIDE/ADVERSE EFFECTS

Toxicity is often manifested as initial restlessness and agitation. However, may also present as drowsiness, slurred speech, and unconsciousness, particularly with mepivacaine. Higher central nervous system levels lead to seizures. See Table V-1, p XXX.

IMPORTANT DRUG INTERACTIONS

Levonordefrin and nonselective β-blockers (e.g., propranolol) may cause initial hypertension followed by bradycardia. This is less likely with the selective β-1 blockers. Interactions of levonordefrin with tricyclic antidepressants may also cause an increase in pressor response to the alpha adrenergic properties.

CONTRAINDICATIONS

- Known allergy or hypersensitivity to the agents
- Recent myocardial infarction (wait at least 6 months for elective treatment)

USUAL DOSING PARAMETERS: ADULTS/CHILDREN

- Adults:
  - 6.6 mg/kg to a maximum total dose of 400 mg for the mepivacaine
- Children:
  - Under age 10: 6.6 mg/kg to a maximum of 180 mg

DENTAL CONSIDERATIONS

The safety of mepivacaine is well-documented in dentistry. Slow injection (1 mL/minute) will avoid toxic reactions if an inadvertent intravascular injection is given. Toxic effects are increased if respiratory acidosis is present. Toxicity is treated by hyperventilation, monitoring, and cardiovascular support as needed. Use of the 3% solution in children should be accompanied by appropriate maximum dosage considerations. See Table V-1, p 467.

SUGGESTED REFERENCES

Chin KL, Yagiela JA, Quinn CL, et al. Serum mepivacaine concentrations after intraoral injection in young children. *J Calif Dent Assoc* 2003;31(10):757–764.
Yagiela JA. Local anesthetics, in Yagiela JA, Dowd FJ, Neidle EA (eds): *Pharmacology and Therapeutics for Dentistry.* St Louis, Elsevier (Mosby), 2004, pp 251–270.

AUTHOR: **STUART E. LIEBLICH, DMD**

BRAND NAME(S)
Brevital

OVERVIEW

An ultrashort-acting barbiturate, methohexital previously was the most common intravenous agent for inducing general anesthesia used by oral maxillofacial surgeons. Due to a lack of supply and the substitution for it with propofol, it is less commonly used. Propofol causes less tachycardia, nausea, and risks of laryngospasm as compared with methohexital, leading to its continued use even after methohexital became available. Nonetheless, methohexital has a long history for deep sedation/general anesthesia in dentistry and is compatible with many anesthetic regimens.

TYPE OF DRUG

Ultrashort-acting barbiturate

GENERAL USES

For inducing and maintaining deep sedation/general anesthesia. Due to the short duration of action, incremental bolus administration can be given during more noxious portions of oral surgical procedures (e.g., local anesthetic administration, luxation of an infected tooth). The rapid redistribution of the drug permits fast awakening at the conclusion of the procedure.

CAUTIONS

Use with caution in patients with cardiovascular disease or asthma.

SIDE/ADVERSE EFFECTS

- Coughing, hiccups, laryngospasm
- Tachycardia, hypotension
- Nausea, vomiting
- Seizures (may trigger temporal lobe seizure in susceptible patients)
- Decreased respirations, apnea, dyspnea

IMPORTANT DRUG INTERACTIONS

- Sodium oxybate (Xyrem) combination is contraindicated due to increased sleep duration and CNS depression.
- Toxic effects of acetaminophen may be induced. Reduce daily acetaminophen to < 2g/day.

CONTRAINDICATIONS

- Hypersensitivity to the agent or other barbiturates
- Porphyria

USUAL DOSING PARAMETERS: ADULTS/CHILDREN

- Intravenous:
  - Children (> 3 years): 1 to 2 mg/kg initial induction dose, then 0.5 to 1.0 mg/kg as needed every 5 to 10 minutes
  - Adults: 50 to 120 mg initial bolus, then 20 to 50 mg every 5 to 10 minutes as needed
- Rectal: 25 mg/kg as a 10% solution

DENTAL CONSIDERATIONS

Intravenous methohexital has proven to be an effective agent for the induction and maintenance of planes of deep sedation/general anesthesia in dentistry. A trained anesthesia team of at least two staff plus the doctor along with appropriate monitoring (e.g., ECG, pulse oximetry, and automated blood pressures) are necessary for the safe administration of this agent. Rectal administration has been described for extremely uncooperative children in whom intravenous access cannot be achieved. Methohexital is reconstituted as a 1% solution and is stable for over 6 weeks at room temperature. The high pH does not support bacterial growth.

SUGGESTED REFERENCE

Lieblich SE. Methohexital versus propofol for outpatient anesthesia. Part I. *J Oral Maxillofac Surg* 1995;53:811–815.

AUTHOR: **STUART E. LIEBLICH, DMD**

BRAND NAME(S)
Versed

OVERVIEW

Sedative/anxiolytic agent with anterograde amnesic properties. Midazolam is water-soluble in pH of 4.0 or less but becomes highly lipid-soluble once absorbed or infused into the central circulation with a higher pH. It binds to GABA receptors in the central nervous system, facilitating the inhibitory effects of this naturally occurring neurotransmitter.

TYPE OF DRUG

Benzodiazepine

GENERAL USES

- For sedation as a sole agent or in conjunction with other agents.
- Can be administered intravenously, intramuscularly, or orally. Intravenous administration permits titration to desired levels of anxiolysis or sedation.

CAUTIONS

Patients must be monitored for potential respiratory depression. Administration by trained dentists with appropriately trained staff and monitoring is mandatory. Increased risks of respiratory depression in the elderly should be expected, and lower doses with longer intervals between repeated doses should be used. With concomitant drugs such as narcotics and other sedative agents, the doses should be reduced by 30% (by at least 50% in patients over the age of 65).

SIDE/ADVERSE EFFECTS

Overdosage can lead to respiratory depression. Patients should be observed and monitored based on level of sedation. Training in respiratory support and reversal agents (flumazenil) is indicated.

IMPORTANT DRUG INTERACTIONS

- Additive effects with other respiratory depressants, especially narcotics. The metabolism may be increased, causing a decreased effect with the use of phenytoin, carbamazine, rifampin, and phenobarbital. CYP3A inhibitors can increase the effect and cause toxic reactions. These drugs include cimetidine, clarithromycin, fluoxetine, ketoconazole, and the protease inhibitors (saquinavir, ritonavir, amprenavir).
- Grapefruit juice is a potent inhibitor of the CYP3A enzymes and should not be used to take the oral formulation.

CONTRAINDICATIONS

- Known allergy to the benzodiazepines and benzyl alcohol (present in the parenteral formulation) Concomitant use of certain protease inhibitors (amprenavir, ritonavir)

USUAL DOSING PARAMETERS: ADULTS/CHILDREN

Oral: 0.25 to 0.5 mg/kg administered 30 to 45 minutes preoperatively for adults and children over 6 years of age; onset of action is 20 to 30 minutes.
Intranasal: 0.2 to 0.4 mg/kg; onset of sedation is 10 to 15 minutes.
IM: 0.1 to 0.15 mg/kg 30 to 60 minutes preoperatively; onset is 5 to 15 minutes.
IV (over the age of 6): 0.025 to 0.05 mg/kg titrated to effect; onset is 1 to 5 minutes.

DENTAL CONSIDERATIONS

No interaction with local anesthetics and epinephrine; can be used to treat status epilepticus and seizures due to local anesthetic toxicity.

SUGGESTED REFERENCE

Smith TC. Hypnotics and intravenous anaesthetic agents, in Pinnock C, Lin T, Smith T (eds): *Fundamentals of Anaesthesia*. London, Greenwich Medical Media, 2003, pp 611–613.

AUTHOR: **STUART E. LIEBLICH, DMD**

Nitrous Oxide

BRAND NAME(S)
None

OVERVIEW

A sedative/analgesic vapor that rapidly equilibrates from the inhaled concentration to the brain. Nitrous oxide has been used in dentistry for over 175 years, initially as a sole agent but now as a sedative adjunct in conjunction with local anesthesia.

TYPE OF DRUG

An inorganic vapor

GENERAL USES

In concentrations of under 100% (higher concentrations can be achieved with hyperbaric chambers), nitrous oxide does not create true general anesthesia. It does produce central nervous system depression with the patient typically feeling relaxed and calm. It has some mild analgesic properties as well.

CAUTIONS

- Although nonflammable, it will support combustion since at high temperatures it will dissociate into oxygen and nitrogen.
- Since it is stored as a liquid, the gas pressure gauge maintains a constant pressure until the liquid is consumed; then the pressure will drop rapidly.
- Although diffusion hypoxia (the rapid drop in arterial oxygen levels upon abrupt cessation of the agent) is not likely to have clinical significance in dentistry, patients should be given 100% oxygen for at least 5 minutes at the completion of the administration and assisted to standing position. Elderly patients are at risk for falls following nitrous oxide administration if they are moved abruptly.
- Because nitrous oxide cannot support respiration, supplemental oxygen of at least 30% must be given. New installations should be professionally verified so that the oxygen and nitrous oxide pipelines are not crossed. Fail-safe and pin indexing of the gas canisters must be checked regularly. Leak testing of all connections and tubing should be done at least yearly.

SIDE/ADVERSE EFFECTS

- Dizziness, nausea, and vomiting
- Orthostatic hypotension
- Prolonged use/abuse interferes with vitamin B_{12}, causing neurologic symptoms similar to multiple sclerosis that may be irreversible
- Hypoxia if administered at levels greater than 70% or if fail-safe mechanisms malfunction
- May decrease fertility in female dental staff exposed to unscavenged nitrous oxide greater than 5 hours per week

IMPORTANT DRUG INTERACTIONS

- Additive effects with other sedative and anesthetic agents.
- Patients with previous bleomycin chemotherapy can develop pulmonary fibrosis due to the higher oxygen concentrations given with nitrous oxide.

CONTRAINDICATIONS

- Closed head injuries
- Previous middle ear surgery
- Pregnancy
- Administration directly after a large meal

USUAL DOSING PARAMETERS: ADULTS/CHILDREN

Titrated to levels usually up to 50% in adults and children. Patients should be allowed to breathe 100% oxygen at the completion of the procedure for 5 to 10 minutes.

DENTAL CONSIDERATIONS

A rapidly acting, well-tolerated agent safely used in adults and children. Although not a substitute for local anesthesia, the relaxing effects may improve patient acceptance of the local injection. The additional oxygen administered concurrently with the nitrous oxide may be of benefit for patients with a history of cardiovascular disease, along with the sedative properties of the agent itself. The anxiolytic effects of nitrous oxide may also lower the blood pressure in patients exhibiting mild to moderate hypertension in response of the anticipated stress of the dental procedure.

SUGGESTED REFERENCES

Rowland AS, Baird DD, Weinberg CR. Reduced fertility among women employed as female dental assistants exposed to high levels of nitrous oxide. *N Engl J Med* 1992;327:993–997.

Smith TC. Anaesthetic gases and vapours, in Pinnock C, Lin T, Smith T (eds): *Fundamentals of Anaesthesia*. London, Greenwich Medical Media, 2003, pp 598–600.

AUTHOR: **STUART E. LIEBLICH, DMD**

Prilocaine

BRAND NAME(S)
Citanest
Citanest Forte

OVERVIEW

Prilocaine and prilocaine with epinephrine are rapidly acting, local anesthetics. The toxicity of prilocaine is approximately half that of lidocaine, but the agent is less potent. Therefore, it is used in a 4% solution, making it about as toxic as lidocaine on an equal volume basis. The duration of mandibular nerve block is about the same whether epinephrine is included or not (190 minutes without epinephrine and 220 minutes with epinephrine). Thus the plain agent may be useful in cases when the use of epinephrine is limited or contraindicated.

TYPE OF DRUG

Local anesthetic, amide type

GENERAL USES

Local anesthesia for dental procedures

CAUTIONS

Maximum doses must be observed to avoid overdosage, especially in children. Toxic effects are increased with hypoxia.

SIDE/ADVERSE EFFECTS

Toxicity is often manifested as initial restlessness and agitation. Higher CNS levels lead to seizures. Epinephrine causes heart palpitations, tachycardia, and premature ventricular contractions (PVCs).

Prilocaine and benzocaine are unique among the local anesthetic agents in potentially causing methemoglobemia. This is due to the hepatic metabolism of the drug to *o*-toluidine. Since it typically occurs 2 to 3 hours following administration of the agent, the relationship of the drug to the development of respiratory symptoms (dyspnea, cyanosis) may not immediately be recognized. Children and those receiving doses greater than 400 mg are more susceptible, as well as patients taking other oxidative agents (acetaminophen, nitrates, phenytoin, and sulfonamides). The diagnosis is confirmed by the presence of methemoglobin on an arterial blood gas sample and is treated with intravenous administration of methylene blue.

IMPORTANT DRUG INTERACTIONS

Epinephrine and nonselective β-blockers (e.g., propranolol) may cause initial hypertension followed by bradycardia. It is less likely with the selective β-1 blockers. Use caution with patients taking tricyclic antidepressants and MAO inhibitors since an increased pressor response can occur (not with typical epinephrine doses used in dental procedures). Methemoglobemia risks are increased with concomitant use of other oxidative drugs (e.g., acetaminophen, nitrates, phenytoin, and sulfonamides).

CONTRAINDICATIONS

- Known allergy or hypersensitivity to the agents
- Recent myocardial infarction (wait at least 6 months for elective treatment)

USUAL DOSING PARAMETERS: ADULTS/CHILDREN

8 mg/kg to a maximum total dose of 600 mg for the prilocaine. Epinephrine should be limited to 0.2 mg in an adult.

DENTAL CONSIDERATIONS

The safety of prilocaine and prilocaine with epinephrine is well-documented in dentistry. Slow injection (1 mL/minute) will avoid toxic reactions if an inadvertent intravascular injection is given. Toxic effects are increased if respiratory acidosis is present. Toxicity is treated by hyperventilation, monitoring, and cardiovascular support as needed. See Table V-1, p 467.

SUGGESTED REFERENCE

Yagiela JA. Local anesthetics, in Yagiela JA, Dowd FJ, Neidle EA (eds): *Pharmacology and Therapeutics for Dentistry.* St Louis, Elsevier (Mosby), 2004, pp 251–270.

AUTHOR: **STUART E. LIEBLICH, DMD**

BRAND NAME(S)
EMLA
Oraqix

OVERVIEW

These agents combine prilocaine and lidocaine for use as a topical application. EMLA cream is applied under an occlusive dressing and provides skin anesthesia for venipuncture. Due to the poor distribution through the skin surface, it takes approximately 1 hour to be effective. Oraqix is a similar compound but formulated to change to an elastic gel after application to the gingival sulcus. Absorption through the mucosa is much faster and provides anesthesia for scaling and root planing procedures.

TYPE OF DRUG

Topically applied local anesthetics

GENERAL USES

- EMLA: topical anesthesia on skin for venipuncture
- Oraqix: topical anesthesia for scaling and root planing

CAUTIONS

- Sensitivity to the agents or the additives.
- Prilocaine can cause methemoglobemia.

SIDE/ADVERSE EFFECTS

Toxicits can be manifested by restlessness and agitation or even CNS depression.

IMPORTANT DRUG INTERACTIONS

Methemoglobemia risks are increased with concomitant use of other oxidative drugs (e.g., acetaminophen, nitrates, phenytoin, and sulfonamides).

CONTRAINDICATIONS

Sensitivity to prilocaine, lidocaine, or other associated agents

USUAL DOSING PARAMETERS: ADULTS/CHILDREN

Doses under 400 mg of prilocaine should be maintained to reduce the chance of methemoglobemia. Additive amounts with supplemental injected local anesthetics (if used) need to be accounted for to prevent toxicity due to absolute overdose.

DENTAL CONSIDERATIONS

Oral formulation is useful for alleviating the pain associated with scaling and root planing.

SUGGESTED REFERENCE

Donaldson D, Meechan JG. A comparison of the effects of EMLA cream and topical 5% lidocaine on discomfort during gingival probing. *Anesth Prog* 1995;42:7–10.

AUTHOR: **STUART E. LIEBLICH, DMD**

Propofol

BRAND NAME(S)
Diprivan

OVERVIEW

An agent for the induction and maintenance of deep sedation/general anesthesia. It has a very rapid onset of action (within 30 seconds) and a short duration of action (only 3 to 10 minutes, depending on dose).

TYPE OF DRUG

General anesthetic agent unrelated to benzodiazepines, barbiturates, or opioids

GENERAL USES

For the induction and maintenance of deep sedation/general anesthesia

CAUTIONS

The lipid emulsion solution supports rapid bacterial growth. Unused, opened vials must be discarded within 6 to 8 hours, and strict aseptic technique must be utilized when drawing up the solution.

SIDE/ADVERSE EFFECTS

- Pain on injection
- Hypotension
- Respiratory depression, apnea

IMPORTANT DRUG INTERACTIONS

The combination with fentanyl in pediatric ICU patients had led to an increased frequency of cardiovascular collapse.

CONTRAINDICATIONS

Sensitivity to the agent or the additives. In order to put the drug into an emulsion, it is mixed with glycerol, egg, and soybean oils.

USUAL DOSING PARAMETERS: ADULTS/CHILDREN

- Adults:
  - 2 to 2.5 mg/kg every 10 seconds until induction
  - Reduced amounts for ASA III/IV and elderly
  - Maintenance for adults: bolus 20 to 50 mg as needed
- Children:
  - 3 to 16 years: 2.5 to 3.5 mg/kg for induction of anesthesia

DENTAL CONSIDERATIONS

For ambulatory deep sedation/general anesthesia, propofol has begun to replace methohexital as the agent of choice. Its antiemetic properties are also of benefit.

SUGGESTED REFERENCE

Lieblich SE. Methohexital versus propofol for outpatient anesthesia. Part I. *J Oral Maxillofac Surg* 1995;53:811–815.

AUTHOR: STUART E. LIEBLICH, DMD

BRAND NAME(S)
Ultane

OVERVIEW

Sevoflurane is a volatile anesthetic agent that is well-tolerated. It is suitable for mask induction since it has low pungency and respiratory irritation properties. It is quite potent with a MAC of 2.1% in adults, which is decreased to 1.1% if used in combination with 65% nitrous oxide. Sevoflurane is relatively highly metabolized with a biotransformation rate of 2–3%. Although the metabolism yields inorganic fluorine (which has been implicated in nephrotoxicity with other volatile agents), the plasma levels decline rapidly, and this complication has not been reported.

TYPE OF DRUG

Volatile anesthetic agent

GENERAL USES

For inducing and maintaining general anesthesia

CAUTIONS

- Respiratory depression
- Cardiac depression

SIDE/ADVERSE EFFECTS

- Decreased cardiac output
- Hypotension

IMPORTANT DRUG INTERACTIONS

Additive effects with other sedative and anesthetic agents

CONTRAINDICATIONS

History or suspicion of malignant hyperthermia

USUAL DOSING PARAMETERS: ADULTS/CHILDREN

- Adults:
  - Induction: 0.5–3%, titrate to effect.
  - Maintenance: 2–3%, reduce in combination with nitrous oxide.
- Children:
  - Induction: 0.5–3%, titrate to effect.
  - Maintenance: 2–3%, reduce if using in combination with nitrous oxide.

DENTAL CONSIDERATIONS

Sevoflurane is well-tolerated for mask induction and can be used in dentistry for induction of general anesthesia. It does not sensitize the heart to catecholamines, and therefore local anesthetic agents with epinephrine can be used more safely than with halothane.

AUTHOR: **STUART E. LIEBLICH, DMD**

BRAND NAME(S)
Halcion

OVERVIEW

An oral premedication to reduce anxiety associated with dental procedures. It is rapidly cleared with a mean half-life of approximately 3 hours (vs diazepam with a half-life of 30 to 60 hours). Triazolam is well-absorbed when taken orally and is effective within 60 minutes of oral administration.

TYPE OF DRUG

Sedative/hypnotic benzodiazepine; short to intermediate time of onset of action; has a shorter duration of action than even midazolam

GENERAL USES

- Used for the short-term treatment of insomnia in medicine
- Preoperative anxiolytic agent

CAUTIONS

Causes sedation, drowsiness, and anterograde amnesia

SIDE/ADVERSE EFFECTS

- Dizziness
- Confusion
- Nervousness
- Ataxia
- Paradoxical excitement, especially in the elderly and the very young

IMPORTANT DRUG INTERACTIONS

- Additive sedative and respiratory depression with the other central nervous system depressants, especially narcotics.
- Other CYP3A3 enzyme inhibitor drugs will cause an increase in blood levels and increased time of elimination, which may lead to toxic effects (i.e., cimetidine, clarithromycin, erythromycin, fluoxetine, ketoconazole).
- Contraindicated with the use of protease inhibitors such as ritonavir and saquinavir.
- Grapefruit juice should not be used to take the medication due to increased serum concentration.

CONTRAINDICATIONS

- Hypersensitivity or allergy to triazolam or other benzodiazepines (e.g., diazepam, lorazepam).
- Pregnancy.

USUAL DOSING PARAMETERS: ADULTS/CHILDREN

- For adults, 0.25 to 0.5 mg the night before the procedure and 1 to 2 hours prior to the dental appointment.
- For patients over the age of 65, use 0.125 mg.
- Dosage in children under the age of 18 has not been established.

DENTAL CONSIDERATIONS

- Patients have greater acceptance of local anesthetic injections and less anxiety about the procedure, which may prevent syncopal episodes. Better acceptance for the starting of an intravenous line has also been reported.
- Patients should not drive for 6 to 8 hours following the taking of the medication (geriatric patients may take longer to have ataxia resolved).
- The addition of nitrous oxide may produce deeper levels of sedation, and the patient should be monitored for adequate respiratory exchange.

SUGGESTED REFERENCES

Kurzrock M. Triazolam and dental anxiety. *J Am Dent Assoc* 1994;125(4):358–360.
Lieblich SE, Horswell B. Attenuation of anxiety in ambulatory oral surgery patients with oral triazolam. *J Oral Maxillofac Surg* 1991;49(8):792–797.

AUTHOR: **STUART E. LIEBLICH, DMD**

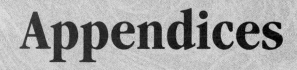

Appendices

Appendix A: Common Helpful Information for Medical Diseases and Conditions
Appendix B: Clinical Algorithms

Common Helpful Information for Medical Diseases and Conditions

---

BOX A-1 Antibiotic Prophylaxis Recommendations by the American Heart Association for the Prevention of Bacterial Endocarditis (June 11, 1997)

Antibiotic Prophylaxis IS Recommended for:
- Dental extractions
- Periodontal procedures, including surgery, scaling and root planing, probing, and recall maintenance
- Dental implant placement and reimplantation of avulsed teeth
- Endodontic (root canal) instrumentation or surgery only beyond the apex
- Subgingival placement of antibiotic fibers or strips
- Initial placement of orthodontic bands but not brackets
- Intraligamentary local anesthetic injections
- Prophylactic cleaning of teeth or implants where bleeding is anticipated

Antibiotic Prophylaxis Is NOT Recommended for:
- Restorative dentistry* (operative and prosthodontic) with or without retraction cord‡
- Local anesthetic injections (nonintraligamentary)
- Intracanal endodontic treatment; post placement and buildup
- Placement of removable prosthodontic or orthodontic appliances
- Postoperative suture removal
- Shedding of primary teeth
- Taking of oral impressions
- Taking of oral radiographs
- Fluoride treatments
- Orthodontic appliance adjustment

* This includes restoration of decayed teeth and replacement of missing teeth.
‡ Clinical judgment may indicate antibiotic use in selected circumstances that may create significant bleeding.
Adapted from Dajani AS, Taubert KA, Wilson W, Bolger AF, Bayer A, Ferrieri P, et al. Prevention of bacterial endocarditis. Recommendations by the American Heart Association. *JAMA* 1997;277(22):1794–1801.

TABLE A-1   **Prophylactic Regimens for Dental, Oral, Respiratory Tract, or Esophageal Procedures**

Situation	Agent	Regimen*
Standard general prophylaxis	Amoxicillin	Adults: 2.0 g; children: 50 mg/kg orally 1 hour before procedure
Unable to take oral medications	Ampicillin	Adults: 2.0 g intramuscularly (IM) or intravenously (IV); children: 50 mg/kg IM or IV within 30 minutes before procedure
Allergic to penicillin	Clindamycin *or*	Adults: 600 mg; children: 20 mg/kg orally 1 hour before procedure
	Cephalexin † or Cefadroxil † *or*	Adults: 2.0 g; children: 50 mg/kg orally 1 hour before procedure
	Azithromycin or Clarithromycin	Adults: 500 mg; children 15 mg/kg orally 1 hour before procedure
Allergic to penicillin and unable to take oral medications	Clindamycin *or*	Adults: 600 mg; children: 20 mg/kg IV within 30 minutes before procedure
	Cefazolin †	Adults: 1.0 g; children: 25mg/kg IM or IV within 30 minutes before procedure

* Total children's dose should not exceed adult dose.

† Cephalosporins should not be used in individuals with immediate-type hypersensitivity reaction (i.e., urticaria, angioedema, or anaphylaxis) to penicillins.

Adapted from Dajani AS, Taubert KA, Wilson W, Bolger AF, Bayer A, Ferrieri P, et al. Prevention of bacterial endocarditis. Recommendations by the American Heart Association. *JAMA* 1997;277(22):1794–1801.

BOX A-2   **Presurgical and Postsurgical Antibiotic Prophylaxis for Patients at Increased Risk for Postoperative Infections**

Suggested regimens for adult patients not allergic to penicillin:
- Penicillin V potassium, 1 to 2 grams, 1 hour before the procedure, then 500 mg, q6h for 7 days postop or longer until sufficient wound healing has occurred to minimize the risk of infection.

For adult, penicillin allergic patients, choices include:
- Erythromycin ethylsuccinate, 800 mg, 1 hour before the procedure, then 400 mg, q6h for 7 days postop or longer until sufficient wound healing has occurred to minimize the risk of infection.

OR
- Azithromycin 500 mg, 1 hour before the procedure, then 250 mg, qd for 5 days postop or longer until sufficient wound healing has occurred to minimize the risk of infection.

OR
- Clindamycin 300 to 600 mg, 1 hour before the procedure, then 150 to 300 mg, q6h for 7 days postop or longer until sufficient wound healing has occurred to minimize the risk of infection.

BOX A-3   **Local Anesthetic with Vasoconstrictor Dose Restriction Guidelines[1]**

- **Limit total vasoconstrictor dose per appointment:**
  - 0.036 mg epinephrine (e.g., 2 cartridges* of 2% lidocaine with 1:100,000 epinephrine).
  - 0.18 mg of levonordefrin (e.g., 2 cartridges* of 2% mepivacaine with 1:20,000 levonordefrin).

- ***Do not* use epinephrine impregnated gingival retraction cord.**
  - Aluminum potassium sulfate impregnated gingival retraction cord is a safe alternative.

- ***Do not* use local anesthetics containing vasoconstrictors for:**
  - Direct hemostasis to control bleeding
  - Intraligamentary or intrabony infiltrations

* 1 cartridge (Carpule®) = 1.8 mL

1. Adapted from Little JW, Falace DA, Miller CS, Rhodus NL. *Dental Management of the Medically Compromised Patient,* ed 6. St Louis, Mosby, 2002, pp 75,90.

Box A-4   Dental Management of Patients at Risk for Acute Adrenal Insufficiency[1]

General Guidelines
1. Schedule dental treatment or surgery in the morning, when cortisol levels usually are highest.
2. Minor surgeries require minimal steroid coverage. The patient's usual daily dose typically is sufficient. Major surgeries and those lasting more than 1 hour or involving general anesthesia should be performed in a hospital with (intravenous) steroid supplementation (see "Corticosteroid Supplementation Guidelines" following).
   - Avoid general anesthesia for outpatient procedures, since it increases glucocorticoid demand.
3. Discontinue drug therapy that decreases cortisol levels (e.g., ketoconazole) at least 24 hours before surgery, with the consent of the patient's physician. Avoid the use of barbiturates, since these drugs increase the metabolism of cortisol and reduce blood levels of cortisol.
4. Provide adequate pain control during the operative and postoperative phases of care.
   - Clinicians should ensure good postoperative pain control by administering long-acting local anesthetics (e.g., bupivacaine) at the end of the procedure, as well as regular analgesic dosing.
5. Provide proper stress reduction, since anxiety can increase cortisol demand.
   - Use of nitrous oxide-oxygen, intravenous, or oral benzodiazepine conscious sedation is helpful, since plasma cortisol levels are not reduced by these agents.
6. For surgical or other procedures that present a risk for postoperative infection, consider the use of presurgical and postsurgical antibiotic prophylaxis to minimize the risk of infection if significant soft tissue manipulation is anticipated.
7. Blood and other fluid volume loss, as well as the use of anticoagulants, can exacerbate hypotension and increase the risk of adrenal insufficiency-like symptoms. Thus, methods to reduce blood loss should be used.
8. Monitor blood pressure throughout the procedure and before the patient leaves the dental office. Patients whose blood pressure is at or below 100/60 mmHg should receive intravenous fluid replacement (5% dextrose), vasopressors or, if needed, corticosteroids.
9. Recognize the signs of hypotension, hypoglycemia, and hypovolemia and take corrective action quickly.

Corticosteroid Supplementation Guidelines
1. Patients Currently Taking Corticosteroids:
   - Nonsurgical Dental Procedures (Negligible Risk)
     - This includes any routine nonsurgical (e.g., restorative, periodontic) dental treatment using local anesthesia.
     - **Regimen:** No corticosteroid supplementation required (patients currently taking corticosteroids may maintain their usual dose regimen).
   - Minor Oral Surgery (Mild Risk)
     - This includes a few simple extractions, soft tissue biopsy or surgery, performed under local anesthesia.
     - **Regimen:** The glucocorticoid target is the equivalent of ~25 mg of cortisol (~5 mg of prednisone) the day of surgery, 2 hours prior to the procedure.
     - The clinician should confirm that the patient has taken the recommended dose of steroid within 2 hours prior to the surgical procedure and should schedule the surgery in the morning when normal cortisol levels are highest. Stress reduction measures should be implemented. Benefits can be gained from use of:
       - oral, inhalation, or intravenous sedation that provides stress reduction
       - long-acting local anesthetics and adequate postoperative analgesics
       - intravenous fluids (e.g., 5% dextrose) that can prevent hypovolemia and hypoglycemia
   - Major Oral Surgery (Moderate to High Risk)
     - This includes:
       - multiple extractions, quadrant periodontal surgery, extraction of bony impactions, osseous surgery, osteotomy, bone resections, implant placement, or oral cancer surgery using local anesthesia
       - any surgical procedures involving general anesthesia
       - surgical procedures lasting more than 1 hour
       - procedures associated with significant blood loss
     - **Regimen:** The glucocorticoid target is the equivalent of ~50 to 100 mg of cortisol (~12.5 to 25 mg of prednisone) within 2 hours prior to surgery and for at least 1 to 2 postoperative days (or longer until postoperative pain has abated).
     - Higher steroid doses may be needed if excessive bleeding or complications are encountered. Patients should take their usual steroid dose before the procedure, and supplemental intravenous hydrocortisone should be administered during surgery to achieve a total glucocorticoid level the equivalent of 100 mg of cortisol. Clinicians should consider hospitalizing these patients since blood pressure can be more closely monitored after surgery in this setting. Hydrocortisone (25 mg) usually is prescribed every 8 hours after surgery for 24 to 48 hours (or longer), depending on the procedure and the level and duration of postoperative pain.
2. Patients Previously Taking Corticosteroids:
   - In patents where therapeutic corticosteroid administration has been discontinued, it may take weeks or months to regain normal adrenal function, and theoretically during this period patients are susceptible to adrenal crisis from the decreased adrenocortical response. However, a review of the literature disclosed that most patients regain an adequate clinical response to stress within 2 weeks after cessation of corticosteroid administration, in spite of persistent subnormal plasma cortisol levels.
   - If dental treatment is needed for patients who have received the equivalent of ~30 mg of cortisol (~7.5 mg of prednisone) per day for at least 7 days in the past 2 weeks, the guidelines listed previously for patients currently taking corticosteroids should provide the necessary corticosteroid supplementation.

1. Adapted from Miller CS, Little JW, Falace DA. Supplemental corticosteroids for dental patients with adrenal insufficiency: Reconsideration of the problem. *JADA* 2001;132:1570–1579. Copyright (c) 2001, American Dental Association. All rights reserved. Adapted 2006 with permission.

BOX A-5 Dental Management of Patients Taking Coumarin Anticoagulants [1,2,3]

Low Risk Dental Procedures:
Dental procedures that do not create gingival insult to any great extent are considered low risk procedures. They include:
- supragingival prophylaxis
- routine restorations without subgingival margins
- local anesthetic injections that are confined to areas over bone (as opposed to those to loose connective tissue areas including regional infiltrations and blocks)

Moderate Risk Dental Procedures:
Moderate risk procedures in dentistry can include:
- subgingival scaling and root planing
- subgingival restorations
- uncomplicated forceps extraction of 1 to 3 teeth that are amenable to primary closure
- endodontic procedures
- injections of local anesthetics that are not confined to well-defined areas over bone, including regional infiltrations and blocks

Treatment Modifications:
1. Regardless of a patient's medical risk status, if a low risk dental procedure is planned, no change in the anticoagulation medication is indicated. Provided that the dental treatment is not invasive, with the exception of an atraumatic injection, the continued anticoagulant medication is the protocol of choice.
2. If bleeding does occur because of the local anesthetic injection, local measures can usually be used with successful results.
3. With this protocol, the patient is not placed at risk for thrombolytic complications and is placed at only minimal risk for uncontrolled bleeding episodes.

Treatment Modifications:
If any of these procedures are planned for the anticoagulated patient, the practitioner should use a reduction- or withdrawal-of-medication protocol for proper treatment:

Preoperative:
1. Consultation with patient's physician:
   a. Determine the current status of underlying medical problem(s) that require anticoagulation therapy.
   b. Determine the level of anticoagulation expressed in PT or INR:
      - If PT is < 2.5 times control or INR is < 3.5, Coumarin dosage usually does not need to be altered.
      - If PT is > 2.5 times control or INR is > 3.5 then Coumarin dosage should be altered prior to moderate-risk dental procedures.
2. To achieve an acceptable PT/INR level, it may be necessary to withdraw the anticoagulation medication (with physician's approval) 2 to 3 days before treatment in order to achieve the desired effect on the patient's hemostasis. This should be sufficient to place the patient's PT/INR levels within the acceptable range.
3. The patient's physician is informed of the planned procedures, and the patient's dental appointment is (ideally) scheduled on a day when their PT/INR level is to be routinely monitored. (Combining multiple procedures into longer scheduled appointments helps to minimize the overall number of alterations in the anticoagulation medication).

Operative:
1. The patient's PT/INR values should be verified within an acceptable level for treatment (PT < 2.5 times control or INR < 3.5) on the day of dental treatment.
2. Control bleeding by local means. Suturing, pressure packs, and absorbable hemostatic agents are helpful, especially after routine extractions, for controlling postoperative bleeding.

Postoperative:
1. Analgesics: Avoid aspirin, aspirin-containing compounds, and other NSAIDs (COX-2 inhibitors can be used but may require a reduction in anticoagulant medication dose). Acetaminophen and narcotic analgesics can be used unless contraindicated for some other reason. Limit acetaminophen use to the minimal amount needed for pain relief.
2. Instruct the patient to call if bleeding occurs during the first 24 to 48 hours.
3. Coumarin therapy is usually resumed on the day of or the day following the procedure (as agreed upon in consultation with patient's physician) because warfarin takes 4 to 5 days to reach therapeutic levels and has no effect on formed blood clots. With this method, the risk of a thrombolytic event is minimized, and bleeding from the dental procedures is no longer an immediate threat.
4. In all situations in which dental treatment is rendered to anticoagulated patients, the risk of hemorrhage immediately after the procedure and up to 5 to 7 days after treatment calls for providing the patient with a strict recall protocol and instructions for recognizing signs and symptoms of abnormal bleeding.

a. See the patient 48 to 72 hours after treatment and observe for: healing, infection (treat if present), or bleeding (control by local means if present), with additional postoperative visits as needed.

High Risk Dental Procedures:

High risk procedures in dentistry can include:

- periodontal surgical procedures
- insertion of dental implants
- extensive (i.e., more than 3 teeth) or complex oral surgery procedures including those involving removal of bone (e.g., extraction of impacted or unerupted third molars, preprosthetic alveoloplasty, or tuberosity reduction)

Treatment Modifications:

- Any extensive surgical procedure in dentistry can place the anticoagulated patient at risk for uncontrolled bleeding, regardless of the patient's medical risk. To properly treat these patients, it is recommended that a low-dose subcutaneous heparin protocol or a hospitalization protocol with intravenous (IV) heparin administration be used, depending on the physician's assessment and recommendations.
- The hospitalization protocol for high-risk dental surgery includes:
  1. Withdrawal of Coumarin therapy 24 hours before the patient is admitted to the hospital.
  2. On admission, the patient's PT/INR levels should be checked and IV heparin administration should be started. As soon as the PT levels are within normal limits, the patient can be prepared for surgery, and the IV heparin is halted 6 to 8 hours before surgery is begun. Immediately before surgery, the patient's PT/INR and PTT levels are again verified to be within normal limits.
  3. During the procedure, local hemostatic measures are used.
  4. After surgery, heparin is resumed 12 to 24 hours postoperatively, and the Coumarin therapy is resumed on the same evening of the surgery. As soon as the patient's PT/INR level has reached therapeutic range, the IV heparin is stopped. This leaves the patient at risk for thromboembolic episodes resulting from lack of anticoagulation for less than 1 day.
- An alternative to the preceding hospitalization protocol using heparin involves the use of low-molecular-weight heparin (LMWH) such as enoxaparin (Lovenox). Enoxaparin has a half-life of about 3 to 5 hours, and any clinically significant effect on hemostasis in relation dental surgery usually resolves within 12 hours.

The protocol for use of LMWH for high-risk dental surgery includes:

Preoperative:
1. Consultation with patient's physician to determine the status of underlying medical problem(s) that require anticoagulation therapy and approval of the use of LMWH.
2. Withdrawal of coumarin therapy 4 days prior to the day of surgery and the start of subcutaneous injections of 30 mg of enoxaparin every 12 hours (usually at 9 a.m. and 9 p.m.) administered by the patient (or a household member) on an outpatient basis.
3. Instruct the patient to discontinue the enoxaparin injections 12 hours prior to surgery (e.g., the evening before a 9 a.m. surgery on the following day).

Operative:
1. Immediately before surgery, the patient's PT/INR and PTT levels are verified to be within acceptable limits.
2. During the procedure, local hemostatic measures are used.

Postoperative:
1. Coumarin therapy can be restarted the evening after surgery, and subcutaneous injections of 30 mg of enoxaparin every 12 hours are continued for 3 days to allow the patient's PT/INR to return to a therapeutic level.
2. Analgesic precautions and postoperative patient follow-up are the same as previously described for patients undergoing moderate risk dental procedures.

1. Ball JH, Land ES. Management of the anticoagulated dental patient. *Compend Contin Educ Dent* 1996;17(11):1100–1111.
2. Johnson-Leong C, Rada RE. The use of low-molecular-weight heparins in outpatient oral surgery for patients receiving anticoagulation therapy. *JADA* 2002;133:1083–1087.
3. Jeske AH, Suchko GD. Lack of scientific basis for routine discontinuation of oral anticoagulation therapy before dental treatment. *JADA* 2003;134:1492–1497.

BOX A-6   Drug Use in Hepatic Dysfunction[1]

- Patients with liver disease may have an unpredictable hepatic metabolism of drugs that can lead to atypical effects of prescribed dental medications. However, the hepatic reserve appears to be large, and liver disease has to be severe before important changes in drug metabolism take place. The ability to eliminate a specific drug may or may not correlate with liver's synthetic capacity for substances such as albumin or clotting factors, which tends to decrease as hepatic function declines. Unlike renal disease, where estimates of renal function based on creatinine clearance correlate with parameters of drug elimination such as clearance and half-life, routine liver function tests do not reflect actual liver function but are rather markers of liver cellular damage. However, as a general guideline, a dosage reduction of drugs metabolized by the liver should be considered if one (or more) of the following are present:
  - aminotransferase (AST, ALT) levels elevated greater than 4 times normal
  - serum bilirubin elevated above 2.0 mg/dL
  - serum albumin less than 3.5 g/dL
  - signs of ascites or encephalopathy attributable to hepatic failure
- Patients with mild to moderate alcoholic liver disease may demonstrate increased tolerance to drugs like local anesthetics and sedative-hypnotic drugs due to significant enzyme induction and may possibly require increased dosage to obtain the desired effect (e.g., increased doses of local anesthetics may be needed to control pain).
- Patients with more advanced liver disease or cirrhosis may demonstrate a significant decrease in hepatic drug metabolism resulting in an increased or unpredictable effect at normal doses. Therefore, the clinician should be careful to avoid the use of *or* limit (reduce) the dose of hepatically metabolized drugs used or prescribed in dental treatment including:
  - amide local anesthetics (e.g., lidocaine, mepivacaine)
  - benzodiazepines and other sedative-hypnotics (e.g., diazepam, alprazolam)
  - barbiturates
  - antibiotics (e.g., ampicillin, tetracycline, erythromycin, metronidazole)
  - analgesics (e.g., aspirin and NSAIDs[*]; acetaminophen[†]; opioid analgesics)
- Some imidazole antifungal drugs (e.g., ketoconazole) have been implicated in drug-induced hypotoxicity and must therefore be used with caution in patients with known liver disease.
- In patients with severe liver disease, increased sensitivity to the effects of some drugs can further impair cerebral function and may precipitate hepatic encephalopathy (e.g., morphine and other opioid analgesics).
- Edema and ascites in chronic liver disease may be exacerbated by drugs that cause fluid retention (e.g., aspirin, ibuprofen, prednisolone, dexamethasone).

[*] Aspirin and non-COX-selective nonsteroidal antiinflammatory drugs (e.g., ibuprofen) should be used cautiously in patients with significant liver disease because they contribute to an increased antiplatelet effect and exacerbate impaired hemostasis.

[†] Acetaminophen should not be used in patients with significant liver disease because therapeutic doses have induced severe hepatic failure.

1. Douglas LR, Douglass JB, Sieck JO, Smith PJ. Oral management of the patient with end-stage liver disease and the liver transplant patient. *Oral Surg Oral Med Oral Pathol Oral Radiol Endod* 1998;86(1):55–64.

TABLE A-2   Drug Therapy in Chronic Renal Disease[1]

| Drug | Route of metabolism (M) and excretion (E) | Normal dosage okay? | Dose Adjustment in Renal Failure | | | | Removed by dialysis?* | Dosage supplementation required after hemodialysis? |
| | | | Method | GFR (mL/min) | | | | |
				> 50	10–50	< 10		
ANALGESICS								
Acetaminophen	M = liver E = kidneys	No	Increase dose interval	q4h	q6h	q8h	Yes. HD (minimally)	No
Aspirin	M = liver E = kidneys	No	Increase dose interval	q4h	q6h	Avoid	Yes: HD, PD	Yes
Codeine Hydrocodone Oxycodone	M = liver E = kidneys	No	Dosage reduction	100%	75%	50%	No (?)	No
Ibuprofen	M = liver E = kidneys	Yes [2]	None	-	-	-	No (?)	No
ANTIMICROBIALS								
Acyclovir	M= liver 85-95% excreted unchanged by kidneys	No	Increase dose interval	q8h	q12-24h	q24-48h and reduce dose by 50%	Yes: HD	Yes
Amoxicillin	M = liver E = kidney	No	Increase dose interval	q8h	q8-12h	q24h	Yes: HD	Yes
Azithromycin	M = liver E = bile (feces)	Yes	None	-	-	-	No	No
Cephalexin	90-100% excreted unchanged by kidneys	No	Increase dose interval	q8h	q12h	q12h	Yes: HD, PD	Yes: 50% of previous dose
Clindamycin	M = liver E = kidney and bile (feces)	Yes	None	-	-	-	No	No
Doxycycline	M = none [3] E = kidneys and bile (feces)	Yes	None	-	-	-	No	No
Erythromycin	M = liver E = bile (feces) and kidneys	No	Dose reduction	100%	100%	50-75%	Yes: HD (minimally)	No
Fluconazole	60-80% excreted unchanged by kidneys	No	Dose reduction [4]	See note 4	See note 4	See note 4	Yes: HD, PD	Yes
Metronidazole	M = liver E = kidney and bile (feces)	No	Dose reduction	100%	100%	75%	Yes: HD	Yes
Penicillin V	90-100% excreted unchanged by kidneys	Yes	None	-	-	-	Yes: HD, PD	Yes
LOCAL ANESTHETIC								
Lidocaine	M = liver E = kidneys	Yes	None	-	-	-	No	No
SEDATIVE/HYPNOTICS								
Benzodiazepines: - **Diazepam** - **Triazolam**	M = liver E = kidneys	Yes[5]	None	-	-	-	No	No

* HD = Hemodialysis; PD = Peritoneal Dialysis

1. Adapted in part from:
  a. Brenner BM, Rector FC. *The Kidney*, ed 7. St Louis, Elsevier, 2004, pp 2856–2868;
  b. Little JW, Falace DA, Miller CS, Rhodus NL. *Dental Management of the Medically Compromised Patient*, ed 6. St Louis, Mosby, 2002, p 156;
  c. Livomese LL et al. Use of antibacterial agents in renal failure. *Infect Dis Clin N Am* 2004:18;551–579.

Footnote continued on following page

2. Ibuprofen and other NSAIDs should be used cautiously in patients with decreased renal function. NSAIDs may cause a sudden decrease in renal function related to the hemodynamic effects of decreased renal prostaglandin production. Patients at greatest risk are those in whom renal vasoconstrictors are upregulated and the renal vasodilatory properties of prostaglandins are the most important. Patients with congestive heart failure, volume contraction, and ascites or edema from liver failure are at greatest risk. Hyperkalemia and sodium retention may also occur in patients with impaired renal function treated with NSAIDs. These drugs should not be used in patients with renal impairment without a specific indication, and when they are required, renal function and other signs of toxicity should be monitored.

3. Although it was previously suggested that doxycycline is partially metabolized in the liver, recent studies indicate that the drug is not metabolized but is partially deactivated in the intestine by chelate formation.

4. Prescribing information from the manufacturer[‡] recommends that adults with impaired renal function receive an initial loading dose of 50–400 mg of fluconazole (based on the type of infection being treated), then patients with creatinine clearances exceeding 50 mL/min should receive 100% of the usual daily dose and those with creatinine clearances of 50 mL/min or less should receive 50% of the usual daily dose.

[‡] Pfizer. Diflucan® (fluconazole) tablets, for oral suspension, and injection prescribing information. New York, NY; 1998 Jun.

5. Active polar metabolites of benzodiazepines, including diazepam and flurazepam, are normally excreted by the kidneys and are likely to accumulate in patients with renal impairment and produce enhanced, prolonged sedation. Because of the potential for drug or metabolite accumulation, the chronic use of these agents and others in this drug class should be discouraged in patients with decreased renal function.

Appendix A compiled by F. John Firriolo, DDS, PhD

Clinical Algorithms

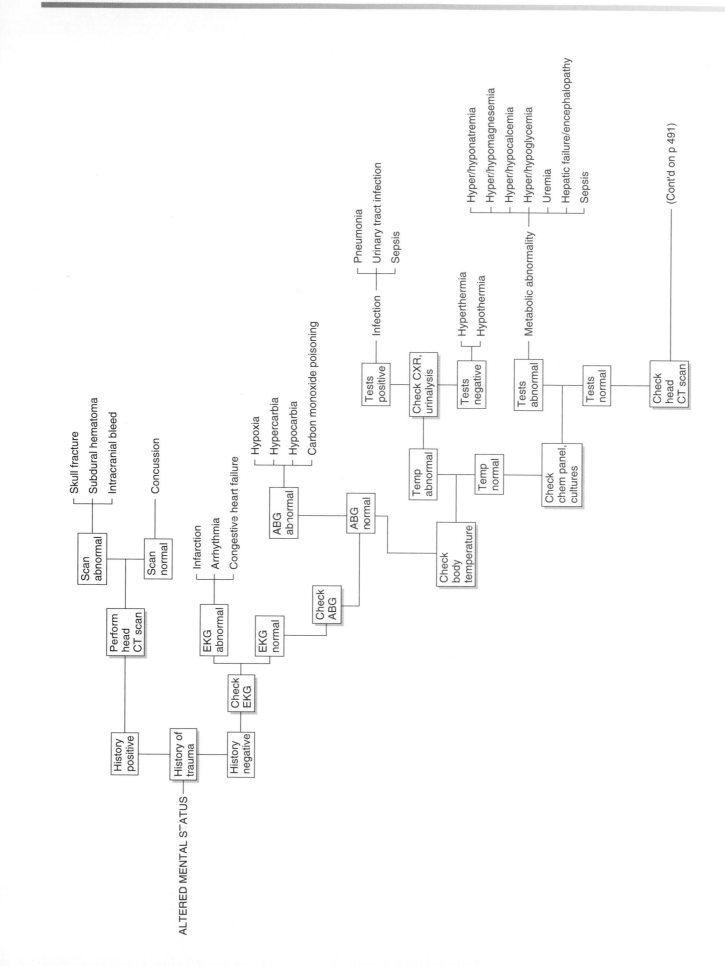

ALTERED MENTAL STATUS

History positive ── Perform head CT scan

Scan abnormal
├─ Skull fracture
├─ Subdural hematoma
└─ Intracranial bleed

Scan normal ── Concussion

History of trauma

History negative ── Check EKG

EKG abnormal
├─ Infarction
├─ Arrhythmia
└─ Congestive heart failure

EKG normal ── Check ABG

ABG abnormal
├─ Hypoxia
├─ Hypercarbia
├─ Hypocarbia
└─ Carbon monoxide poisoning

ABG normal ── Check body temperature

Temp abnormal ── Check CXR, urinalysis

Tests positive ── Infection
├─ Pneumonia
├─ Urinary tract infection
└─ Sepsis

Tests negative
├─ Hyperthermia
└─ Hypothermia

Temp normal ── Check chem panel, cultures

Tests abnormal ── Metabolic abnormality
├─ Hyper/hyponatremia
├─ Hyper/hypomagnesemia
├─ Hyper/hypocalcemia
├─ Hyper/hypoglycemia
├─ Uremia
├─ Hepatic failure/encephalopathy
└─ Sepsis

Tests normal ── Check head CT scan

(Cont'd on p 491)

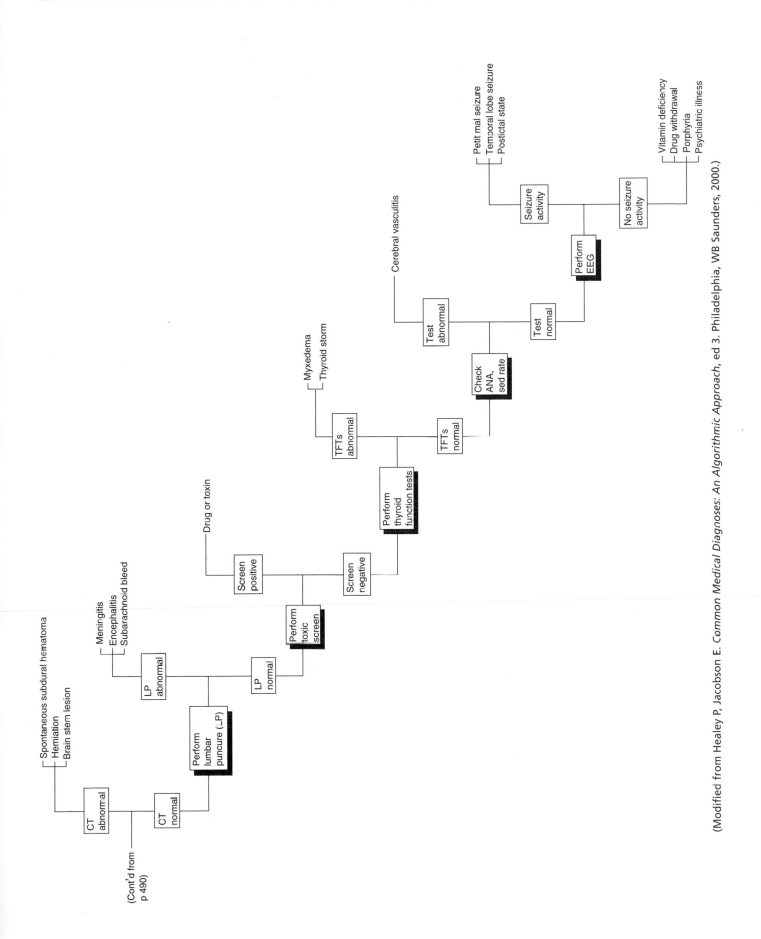

(Modified from Healey P, Jacobson E. *Common Medical Diagnoses: An Algorithmic Approach*, ed 3. Philadelphia, WB Saunders, 2000.)

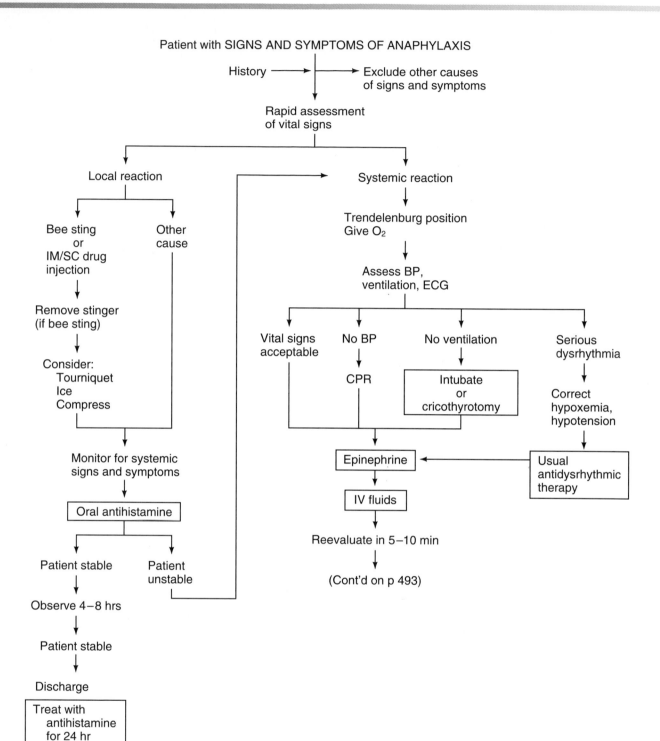

Patient with SIGNS AND SYMPTOMS OF ANAPHYLAXIS

History ⟶ Exclude other causes of signs and symptoms

Rapid assessment of vital signs

Local reaction

- Bee sting or IM/SC drug injection
  - Remove stinger (if bee sting)
  - Consider: Tourniquet / Ice / Compress
- Other cause

Monitor for systemic signs and symptoms

Oral antihistamine

- Patient stable
  - Observe 4–8 hrs
  - Patient stable
  - Discharge
  - Treat with antihistamine for 24 hr
- Patient unstable

Systemic reaction

Trendelenburg position / Give O₂

Assess BP, ventilation, ECG

- Vital signs acceptable
- No BP → CPR
- No ventilation → Intubate or cricothyrotomy
- Serious dysrhythmia → Correct hypoxemia, hypotension → Usual antidysrhythmic therapy

Epinephrine

IV fluids

Reevaluate in 5–10 min

(Cont'd on p 493)

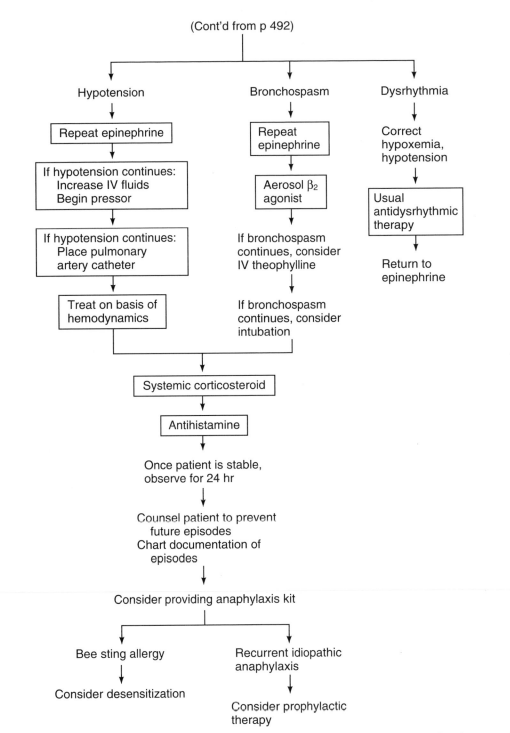

(Cont'd from p 492)

Hypotension	Bronchospasm	Dysrhythmia
Repeat epinephrine	Repeat epinephrine	Correct hypoxemia, hypotension
If hypotension continues: Increase IV fluids Begin pressor	Aerosol β₂ agonist	Usual antidysrhythmic therapy
If hypotension continues: Place pulmonary artery catheter	If bronchospasm continues, consider IV theophylline	Return to epinephrine
Treat on basis of hemodynamics	If bronchospasm continues, consider intubation	

Systemic corticosteroid

Antihistamine

Once patient is stable, observe for 24 hr

Counsel patient to prevent future episodes
Chart documentation of episodes

Consider providing anaphylaxis kit

Bee sting allergy

Consider desensitization

Recurrent idiopathic anaphylaxis

Consider prophylactic therapy

(Modified from Greene H, Johnson W, Lemcke D. *Decision Making in Medicine: An Algorithmic Approach*, ed 2. St Louis, Mosby, 1999.)

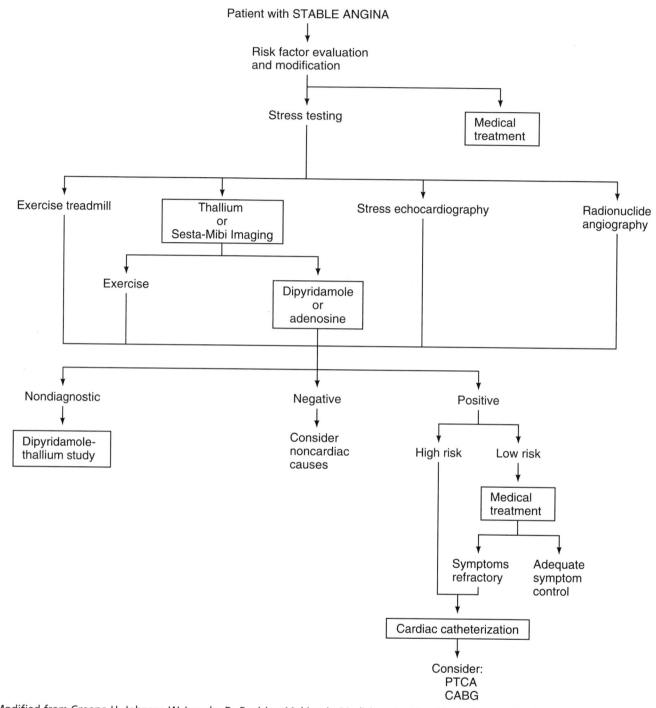

Patient with STABLE ANGINA

Risk factor evaluation
and modification

Stress testing

Medical
treatment

Exercise treadmill

Thallium
or
Sesta-Mibi Imaging

Stress echocardiography

Radionuclide
angiography

Exercise

Dipyridamole
or
adenosine

Nondiagnostic

Dipyridamole-
thallium study

Negative

Consider
noncardiac
causes

Positive

High risk   Low risk

Medical
treatment

Symptoms   Adequate
refractory   symptom
                  control

Cardiac catheterization

Consider:
PTCA
CABG

(Modified from Greene H, Johnson W, Lemcke D. *Decision Making in Medicine: An Algorithmic Approach*, ed 2. St Louis, Mosby, 1999.)

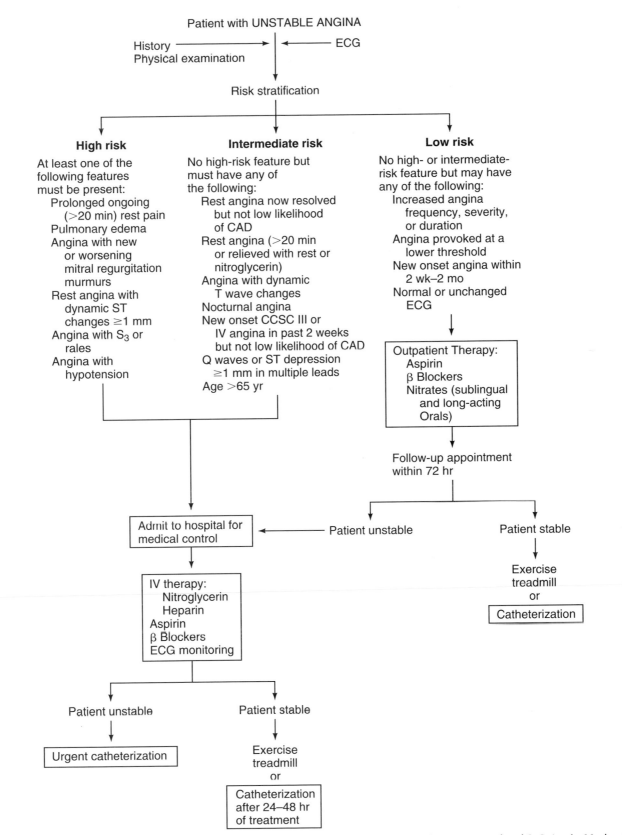

Patient with UNSTABLE ANGINA

History ——→ ←—— ECG
Physical examination

Risk stratification

High risk

At least one of the
following features
must be present:
  Prolonged ongoing
    (>20 min) rest pain
  Pulmonary edema
  Angina with new
    or worsening
    mitral regurgitation
    murmurs
  Rest angina with
    dynamic ST
    changes ≥1 mm
  Angina with S₃ or
    rales
  Angina with
    hypotension

Intermediate risk

No high-risk feature but
must have any of
the following:
  Rest angina now resolved
    but not low likelihood
    of CAD
  Rest angina (>20 min
    or relieved with rest or
    nitroglycerin)
  Angina with dynamic
    T wave changes
  Nocturnal angina
  New onset CCSC III or
    IV angina in past 2 weeks
    but not low likelihood of CAD
  Q waves or ST depression
    ≥1 mm in multiple leads
  Age >65 yr

Low risk

No high- or intermediate-
risk feature but may have
any of the following:
  Increased angina
    frequency, severity,
    or duration
  Angina provoked at a
    lower threshold
  New onset angina within
    2 wk–2 mo
  Normal or unchanged
    ECG

Outpatient Therapy:
  Aspirin
  β Blockers
  Nitrates (sublingual
    and long-acting
    Orals)

Follow-up appointment
within 72 hr

Admit to hospital for
medical control   ←——— Patient unstable   Patient stable

IV therapy: Exercise
  Nitroglycerin   treadmill
  Heparin   or
  Aspirin   Catheterization
  β Blockers
  ECG monitoring

Patient unstable   Patient stable

Urgent catheterization   Exercise
                                 treadmill
                                   or
                                 Catheterization
                                 after 24–48 hr
                                 of treatment

(Modified from Greene H, Johnson W, Lemcke D. *Decision Making in Medicine: An Algorithmic Approach*, ed 2. St Louis, Mosby, 1999.)

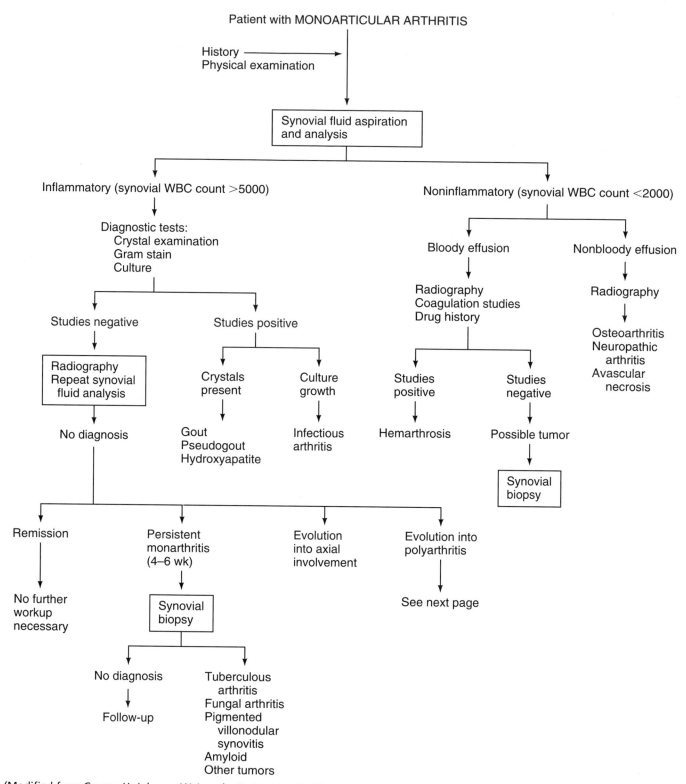

(Modified from Greene H, Johnson W, Lemcke D. *Decision Making in Medicine: An Algorithmic Approach,* ed 2. St Louis, Mosby, 1999.)

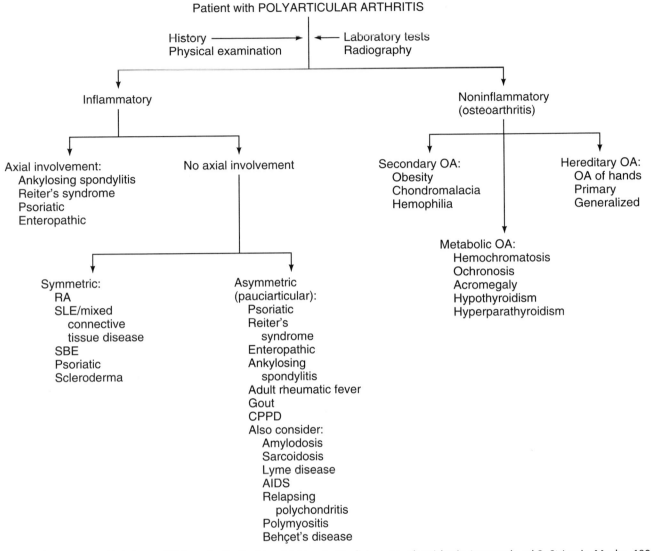

Patient with POLYARTICULAR ARTHRITIS

History ⟶ ← Laboratory tests
Physical examination   Radiography

Inflammatory

Axial involvement:
Ankylosing spondylitis
Reiter's syndrome
Psoriatic
Enteropathic

No axial involvement

Symmetric:
RA
SLE/mixed
connective
tissue disease
SBE
Psoriatic
Scleroderma

Asymmetric
(pauciarticular):
Psoriatic
Reiter's
syndrome
Enteropathic
Ankylosing
spondylitis
Adult rheumatic fever
Gout
CPPD
Also consider:
Amylodosis
Sarcoidosis
Lyme disease
AIDS
Relapsing
polychondritis
Polymyositis
Behçet's disease

Noninflammatory
(osteoarthritis)

Secondary OA:
Obesity
Chondromalacia
Hemophilia

Hereditary OA:
OA of hands
Primary
Generalized

Metabolic OA:
Hemochromatosis
Ochronosis
Acromegaly
Hypothyroidism
Hyperparathyroidism

(Modified from Greene H, Johnson W, Lemcke D. *Decision Making in Medicine: An Algorithmic Approach,* ed 2. St Louis, Mosby, 1999.)

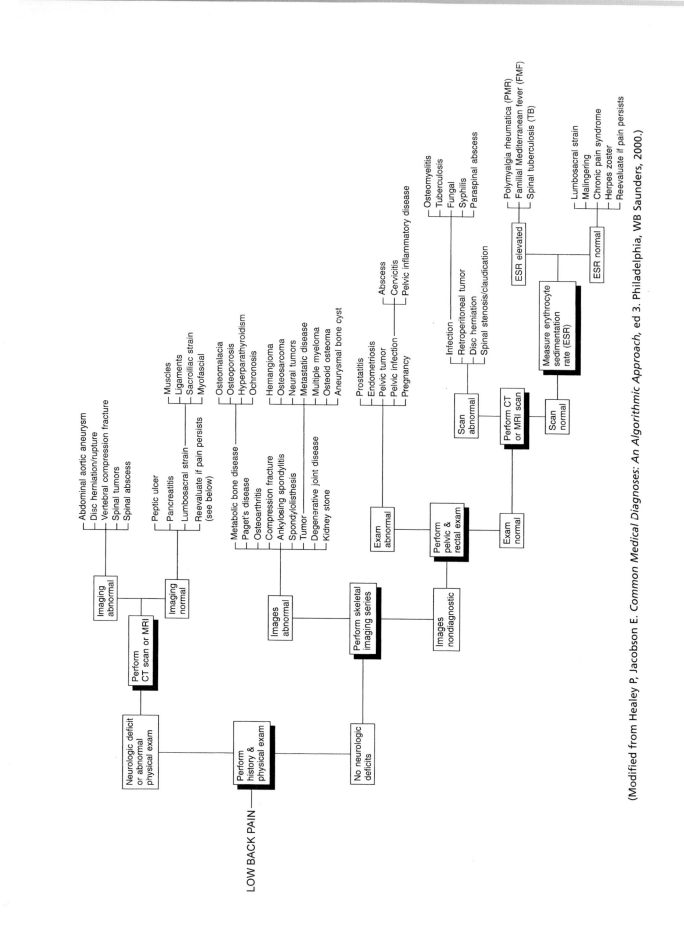

(Modified from Healey P, Jacobson E. *Common Medical Diagnoses: An Algorithmic Approach*, ed 3. Philadelphia, WB Saunders, 2000.)

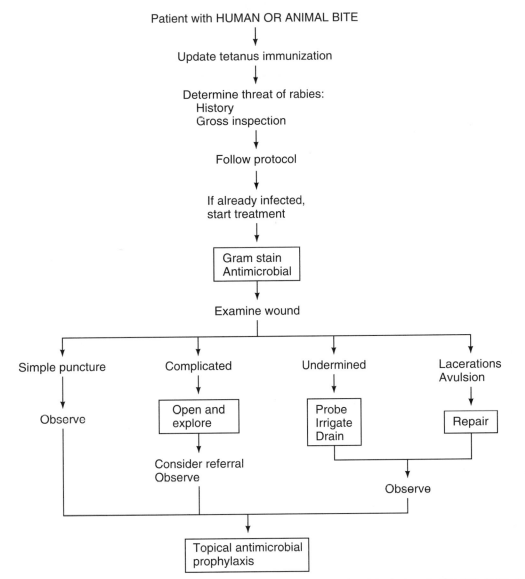

Patient with HUMAN OR ANIMAL BITE

Update tetanus immunization

Determine threat of rabies:
History
Gross inspection

Follow protocol

If already infected,
start treatment

Gram stain
Antimicrobial

Examine wound

| Simple puncture | Complicated | Undermined | Lacerations Avulsion |

Observe

Open and explore

Probe Irrigate Drain

Repair

Consider referral
Observe

Observe

Topical antimicrobial prophylaxis

(Modified from Greene H, Johnson W, Lemcke D. *Decision Making in Medicine: An Algorithmic Approach,* ed 2. St Louis, Mosby, 1999.)

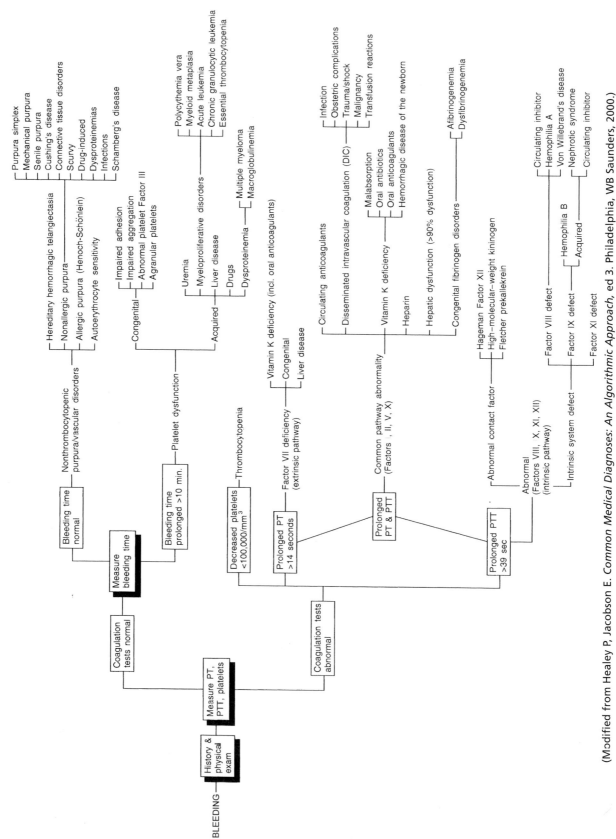

(Modified from Healey P, Jacobson E. *Common Medical Diagnoses: An Algorithmic Approach*, ed 3. Philadelphia, WB Saunders, 2000.)

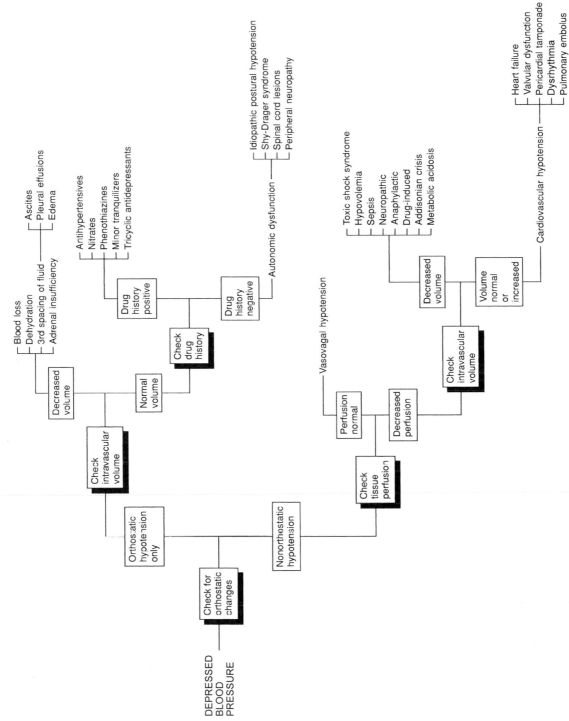

Orthostatic hypotension only

Check intravascular volume

Decreased volume
- Blood loss
- Dehydration
- 3rd spacing of fluid
  - Ascites
  - Pleural effusions
  - Edema
- Adrenal insufficiency

Normal volume

Check drug history

Drug history positive
- Antihypertensives
- Nitrates
- Phenothiazines
- Minor tranquilizers
- Tricyclic antidepressants

Drug history negative
- Autonomic dysfunction
  - Idiopathic postural hypotension
  - Shy-Drager syndrome
  - Spinal cord lesions
  - Peripheral neuropathy

DEPRESSED BLOOD PRESSURE

Check for orthostatic changes

Nonorthostatic hypotension

Check tissue perfusion

Perfusion normal
- Vasovagal hypotension

Decreased perfusion

Check intravascular volume

Decreased volume
- Toxic shock syndrome
- Hypovolemia
- Sepsis
- Neuropathic
- Anaphylactic
- Drug-induced
- Addisonian crisis
- Metabolic acidosis

Volume normal or increased
- Cardiovascular hypotension
  - Heart failure
  - Valvular dysfunction
  - Pericardial tamponade
  - Dysrhythmia
  - Pulmonary embolus

(Modified from Healey P, Jacobson E. *Common Medical Diagnoses: An Algorithmic Approach*, ed 3. Philadelphia, WB Saunders, 2000.)

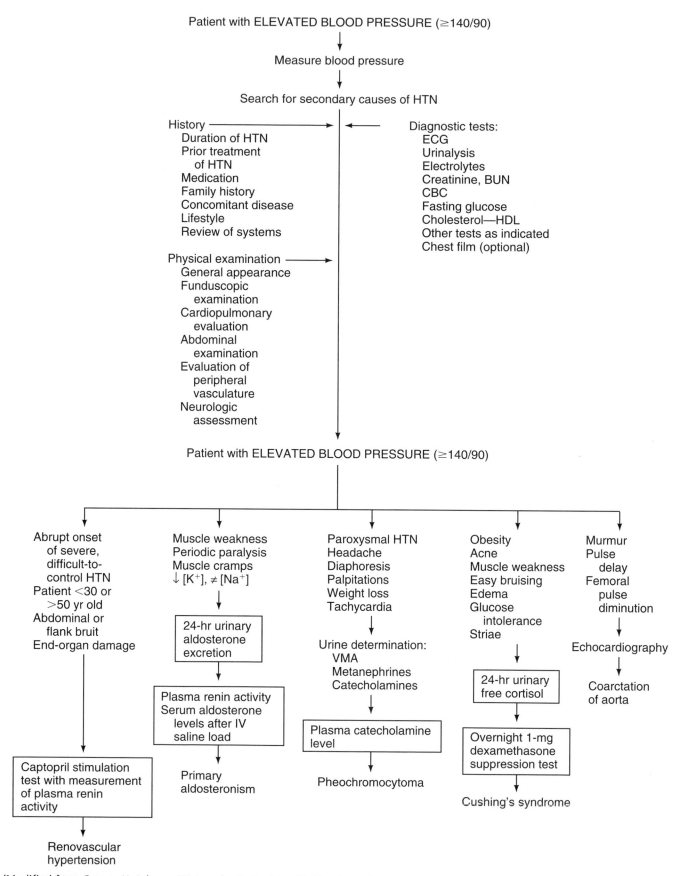

Patient with ELEVATED BLOOD PRESSURE (≥140/90)

Measure blood pressure

Search for secondary causes of HTN

History
  Duration of HTN
  Prior treatment
    of HTN
  Medication
  Family history
  Concomitant disease
  Lifestyle
  Review of systems

Diagnostic tests:
  ECG
  Urinalysis
  Electrolytes
  Creatinine, BUN
  CBC
  Fasting glucose
  Cholesterol—HDL
  Other tests as indicated
  Chest film (optional)

Physical examination
  General appearance
  Funduscopic
    examination
  Cardiopulmonary
    evaluation
  Abdominal
    examination
  Evaluation of
    peripheral
    vasculature
  Neurologic
    assessment

Patient with ELEVATED BLOOD PRESSURE (≥140/90)

Abrupt onset
  of severe,
  difficult-to-
  control HTN
Patient <30 or
  >50 yr old
Abdominal or
  flank bruit
End-organ damage

Muscle weakness
Periodic paralysis
Muscle cramps
↓ [K$^+$], ≠ [Na$^+$]

24-hr urinary
aldosterone
excretion

Plasma renin activity
Serum aldosterone
  levels after IV
  saline load

Primary
aldosteronism

Paroxysmal HTN
Headache
Diaphoresis
Palpitations
Weight loss
Tachycardia

Urine determination:
  VMA
  Metanephrines
  Catecholamines

Plasma catecholamine
level

Pheochromocytoma

Obesity
Acne
Muscle weakness
Easy bruising
Edema
Glucose
  intolerance
Striae

24-hr urinary
free cortisol

Overnight 1-mg
dexamethasone
suppression test

Cushing's syndrome

Murmur
Pulse
  delay
Femoral
  pulse
  diminution

Echocardiography

Coarctation
of aorta

Captopril stimulation
test with measurement
of plasma renin
activity

Renovascular
hypertension

(Modified from Greene H, Johnson W, Lemcke D. *Decision Making in Medicine: An Algorithmic Approach,* ed 2. St Louis, Mosby, 1999.)

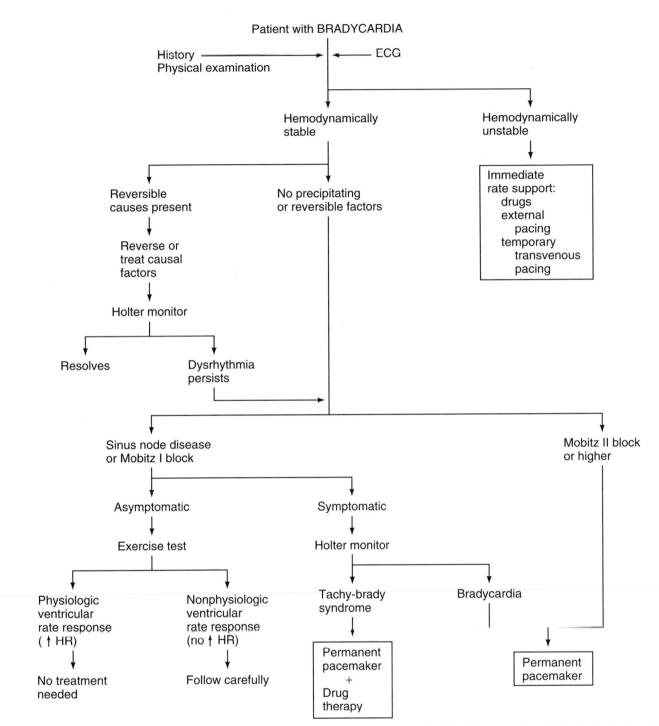

Patient with BRADYCARDIA

History ⟶ ← ECG
Physical examination

Hemodynamically stable

Hemodynamically unstable

Immediate
rate support:
  drugs
  external
    pacing
  temporary
    transvenous
    pacing

Reversible causes present

No precipitating or reversible factors

Reverse or treat causal factors

Holter monitor

Resolves

Dysrhythmia persists

Sinus node disease or Mobitz I block

Mobitz II block or higher

Asymptomatic

Symptomatic

Exercise test

Holter monitor

Physiologic ventricular rate response (↑ HR)

Nonphysiologic ventricular rate response (no ↑ HR)

Tachy-brady syndrome

Bradycardia

No treatment needed

Follow carefully

Permanent pacemaker + Drug therapy

Permanent pacemaker

(Modified from Greene H, Johnson W, Lemcke D. *Decision Making in Medicine: An Algorithmic Approach,* ed 2. St Louis, Mosby, 1999.)

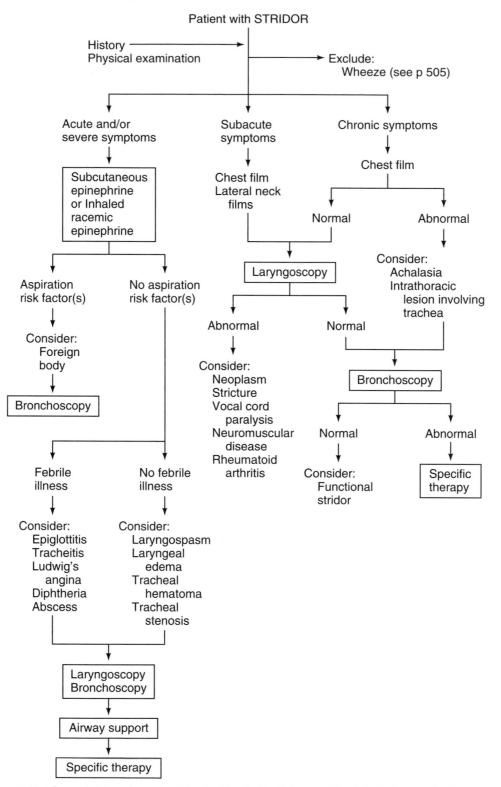

(Modified from Greene H, Johnson W, Lemcke D. *Decision Making in Medicine: An Algorithmic Approach,* ed 2. St Louis, Mosby, 1999.)

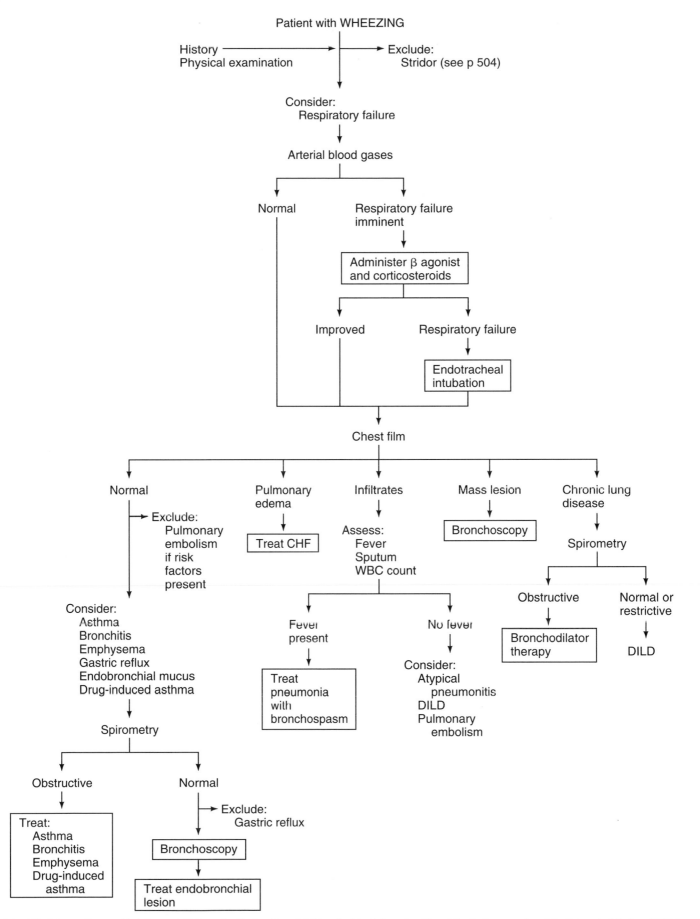

(Modified from Greene H, Johnson W, Lemcke D. *Decision Making in Medicine: An Algorithmic Approach,* ed 2. St Louis, Mosby, 1999.)

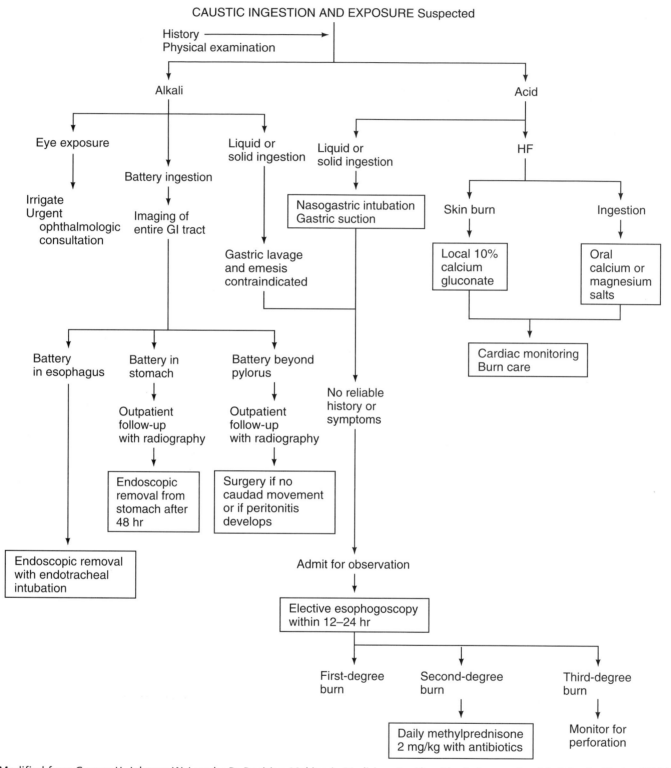

CAUSTIC INGESTION AND EXPOSURE Suspected

(Modified from Greene H, Johnson W, Lemcke D. *Decision Making in Medicine: An Algorithmic Approach,* ed 2. St Louis, Mosby, 1999.)

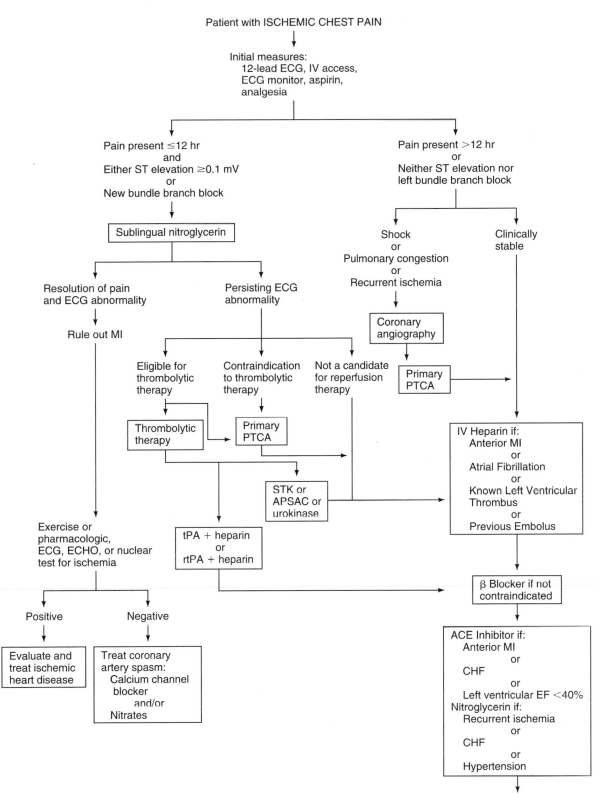

(Cont'd on p 508)

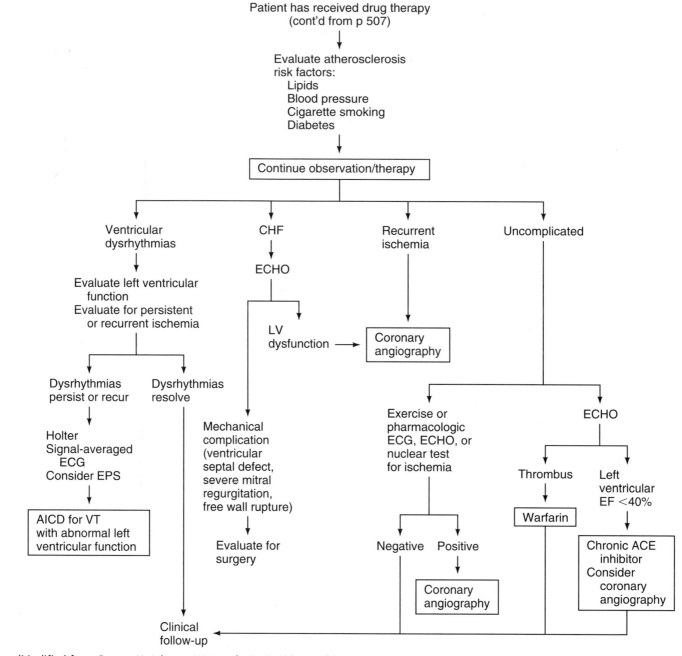

(Modified from Greene H, Johnson W, Lemcke D. *Decision Making in Medicine: An Algorithmic Approach,* ed 2. St Louis, Mosby, 1999.)

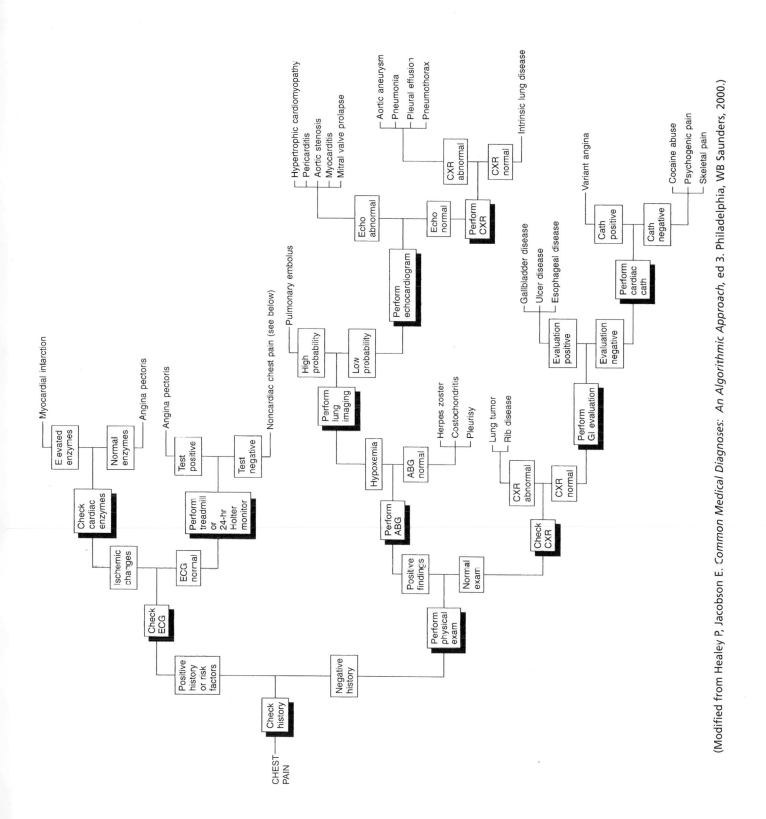

(Modified from Healey P, Jacobson E. *Common Medical Diagnoses: An Algorithmic Approach*, ed 3. Philadelphia, WB Saunders, 2000.)

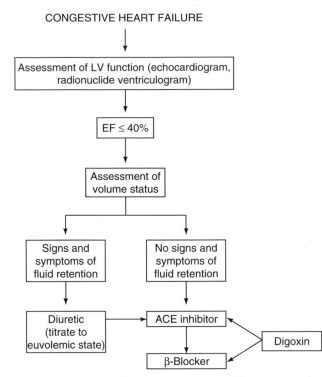

CONGESTIVE HEART FAILURE

↓

Assessment of LV function (echocardiogram, radionuclide ventriculogram)

↓

EF ≤ 40%

↓

Assessment of volume status

Signs and symptoms of fluid retention → No signs and symptoms of fluid retention

Diuretic (titrate to euvolemic state) → ACE inhibitor

β-Blocker

Digoxin

(Modified from Packer M, Cohn JN. *Am J Cardiol* 1999;83:1A–38A with permission from Excerpta Medica, Inc.)

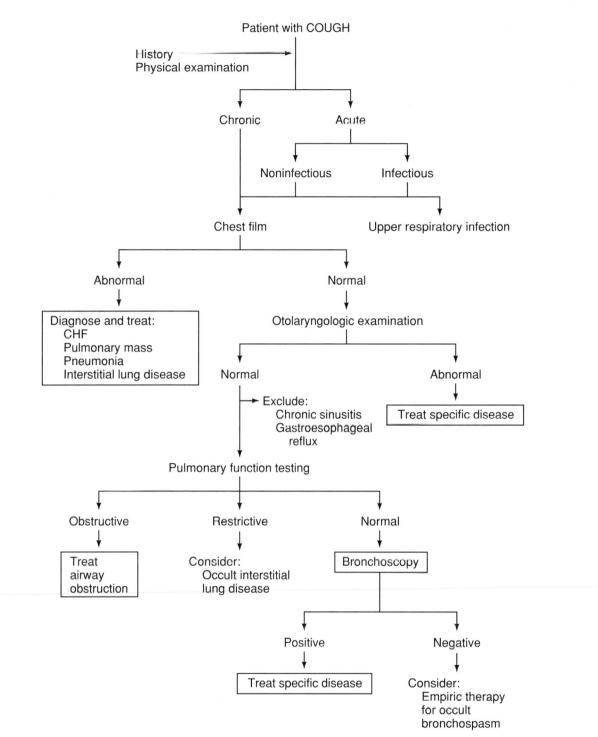

(Modified from Greene H, Johnson W, Lemcke D. *Decision Making in Medicine: An Algorithmic Approach,* ed 2. St Louis, Mosby, 1999.)

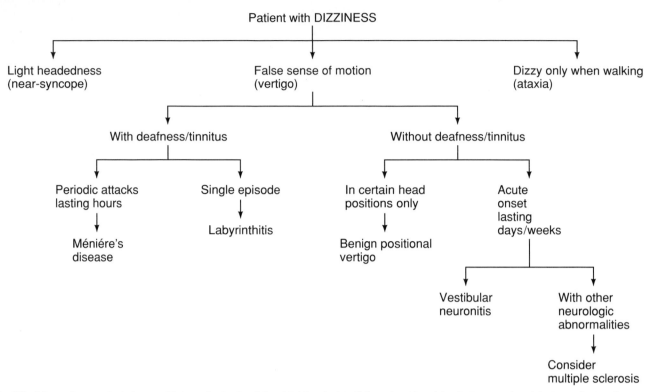

(Modified from Greene H, Johnson W, Lemcke D. *Decision Making in Medicine: An Algorithmic Approach,* ed 2. St Louis, Mosby, 1999.)

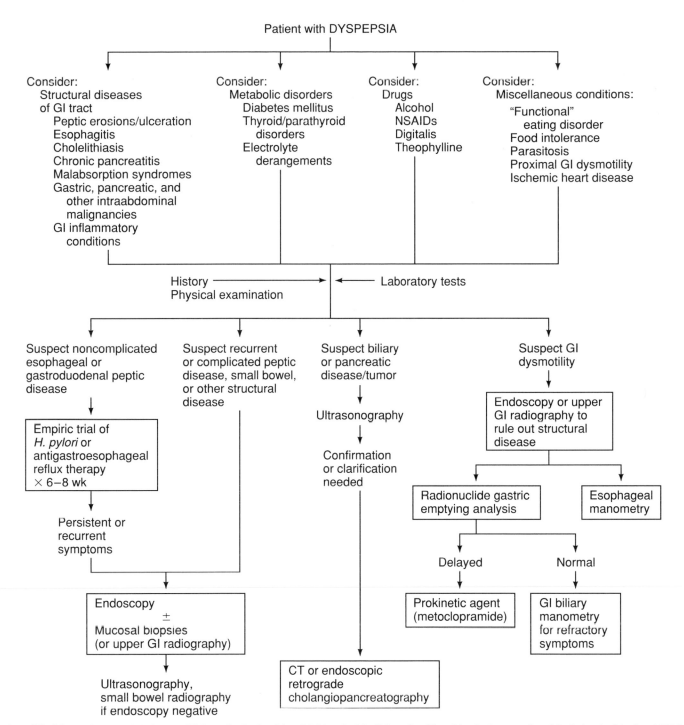

Patient with DYSPEPSIA

Consider:
Structural diseases
of GI tract
Peptic erosions/ulceration
Esophagitis
Cholelithiasis
Chronic pancreatitis
Malabsorption syndromes
Gastric, pancreatic, and
other intraabdominal
malignancies
GI inflammatory
conditions

Consider:
Metabolic disorders
Diabetes mellitus
Thyroid/parathyroid
disorders
Electrolyte
derangements

Consider:
Drugs
Alcohol
NSAIDs
Digitalis
Theophylline

Consider:
Miscellaneous conditions:
"Functional"
eating disorder
Food intolerance
Parasitosis
Proximal GI dysmotility
Ischemic heart disease

History ——→ ←—— Laboratory tests
Physical examination

Suspect noncomplicated
esophageal or
gastroduodenal peptic
disease

Suspect recurrent
or complicated peptic
disease, small bowel,
or other structural
disease

Suspect biliary
or pancreatic
disease/tumor

Suspect GI
dysmotility

Empiric trial of
H. pylori or
antigastroesophageal
reflux therapy
× 6–8 wk

Ultrasonography

Endoscopy or upper
GI radiography to
rule out structural
disease

Confirmation
or clarification
needed

Radionuclide gastric
emptying analysis

Esophageal
manometry

Persistent or
recurrent
symptoms

Delayed

Normal

Endoscopy
±
Mucosal biopsies
(or upper GI radiography)

Prokinetic agent
(metoclopramide)

GI biliary
manometry
for refractory
symptoms

CT or endoscopic
retrograde
cholangiopancreatography

Ultrasonography,
small bowel radiography
if endoscopy negative

(Modified from Greene H, Johnson W, Lemcke D. *Decision Making in Medicine: An Algorithmic Approach,* ed 2. St Louis, Mosby, 1999.)

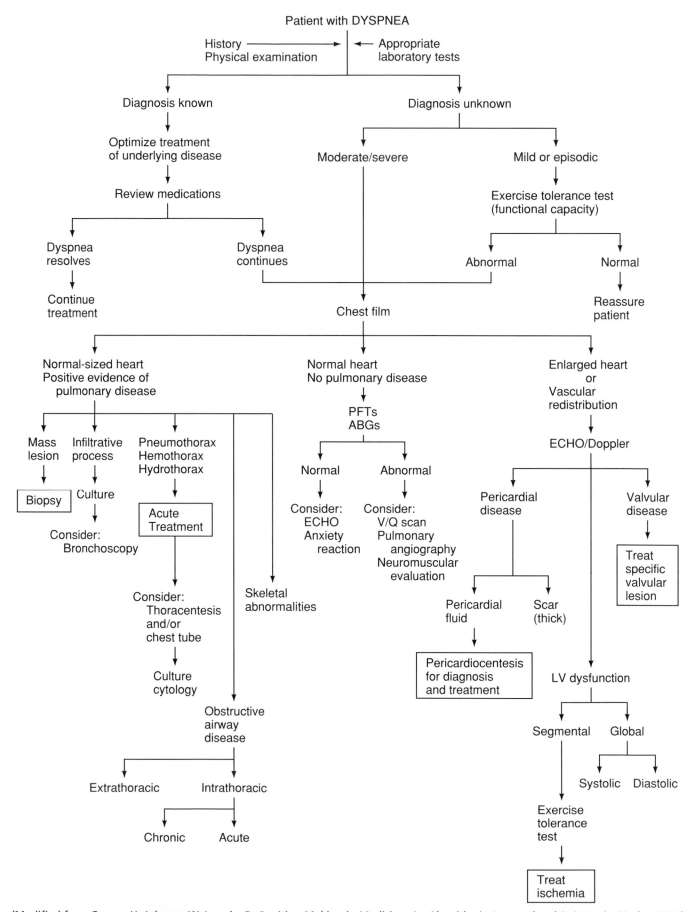

(Modified from Greene H, Johnson W, Lemcke D. *Decision Making in Medicine: An Algorithmic Approach,* ed 2. St Louis, Mosby, 1999.)

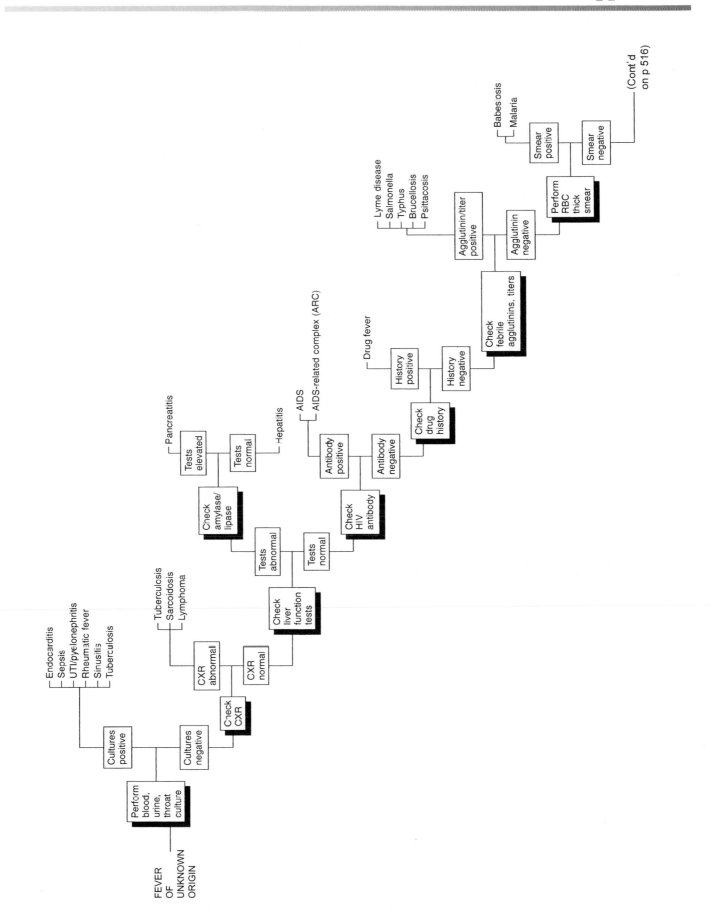

(Cont'd on p 516)

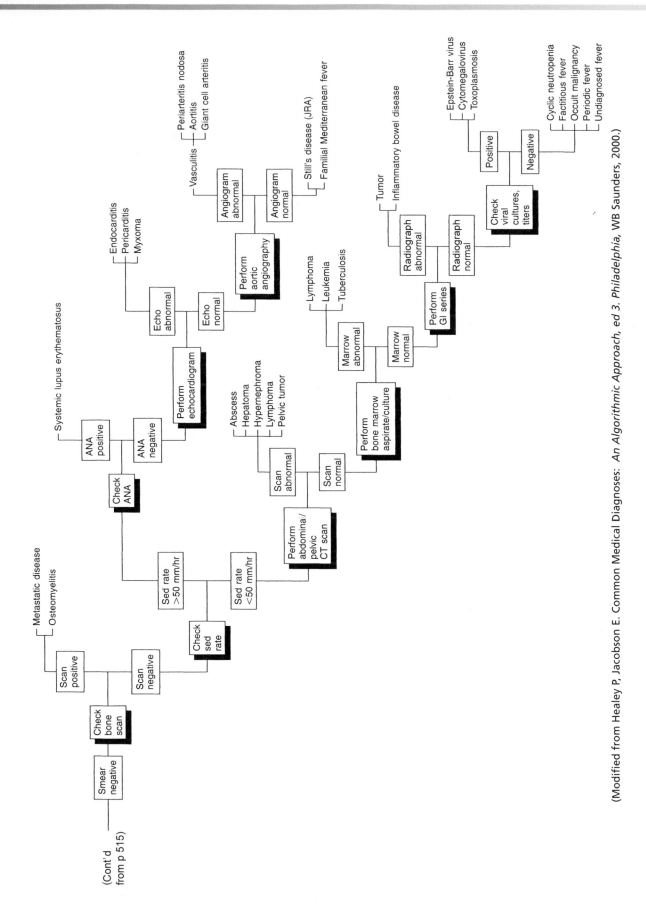

(Modified from Healey P, Jacobson E. Common Medical Diagnoses: *An Algorithmic Approach, ed 3. Philadelphia*, WB Saunders, 2000.)

Patient with INGESTED FOREIGN BODY

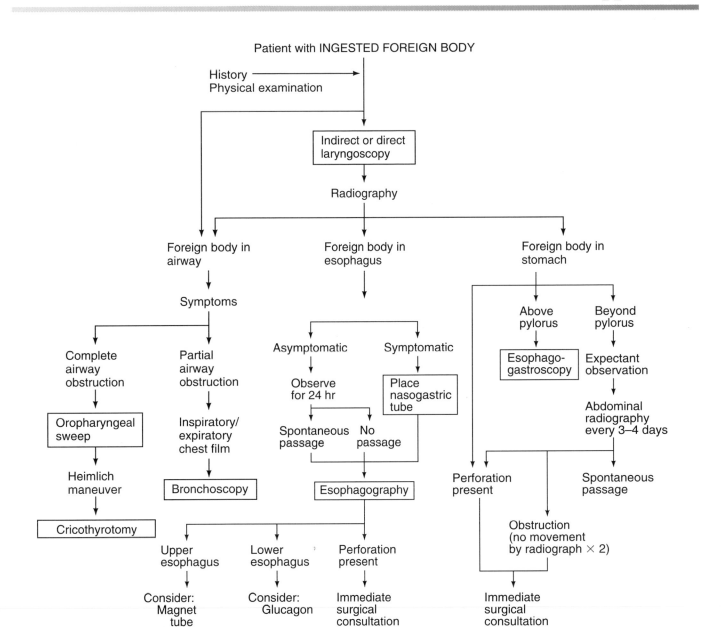

(Modified from Greene H, Johnson W, Lemcke D. *Decision Making in Medicine: An Algorithmic Approach,* ed 2. St Louis, Mosby, 1999.)

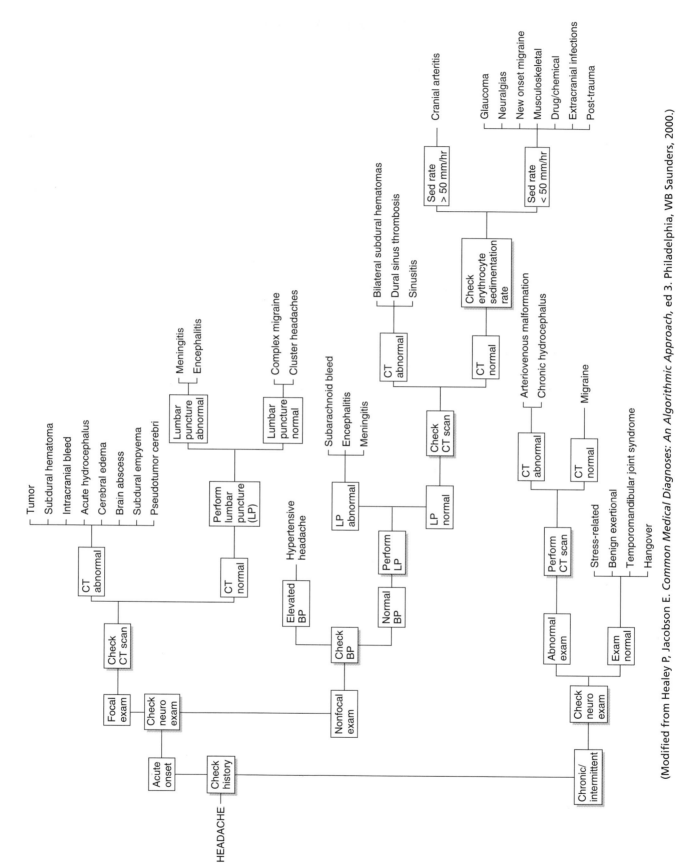

(Modified from Healey P, Jacobson E. *Common Medical Diagnoses: An Algorithmic Approach*, ed 3. Philadelphia, WB Saunders, 2000.)

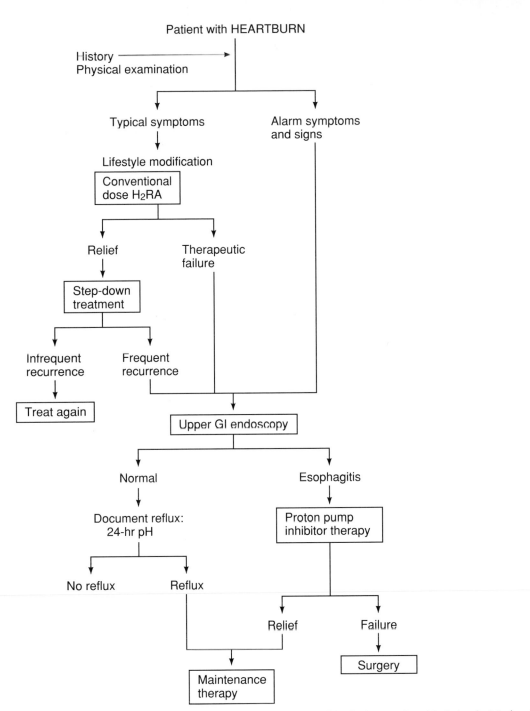

Patient with HEARTBURN

History
Physical examination

Typical symptoms

Alarm symptoms
and signs

Lifestyle modification

Conventional
dose H₂RA

Relief

Therapeutic
failure

Step-down
treatment

Infrequent
recurrence

Frequent
recurrence

Treat again

Upper GI endoscopy

Normal

Esophagitis

Document reflux:
24-hr pH

Proton pump
inhibitor therapy

No reflux

Reflux

Relief

Failure

Surgery

Maintenance
therapy

(Modified from Greene H, Johnson W, Lemcke D. *Decision Making in Medicine: An Algorithmic Approach,* ed 2. St Louis, Mosby, 1999.)

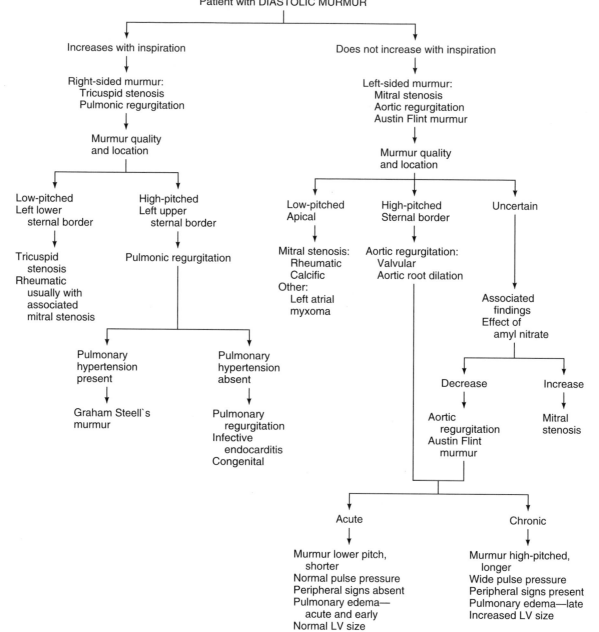

(Modified from Greene H, Johnson W, Lemcke D. *Decision Making in Medicine: An Algorithmic Approach,* ed 2. St Louis, Mosby, 1999.)

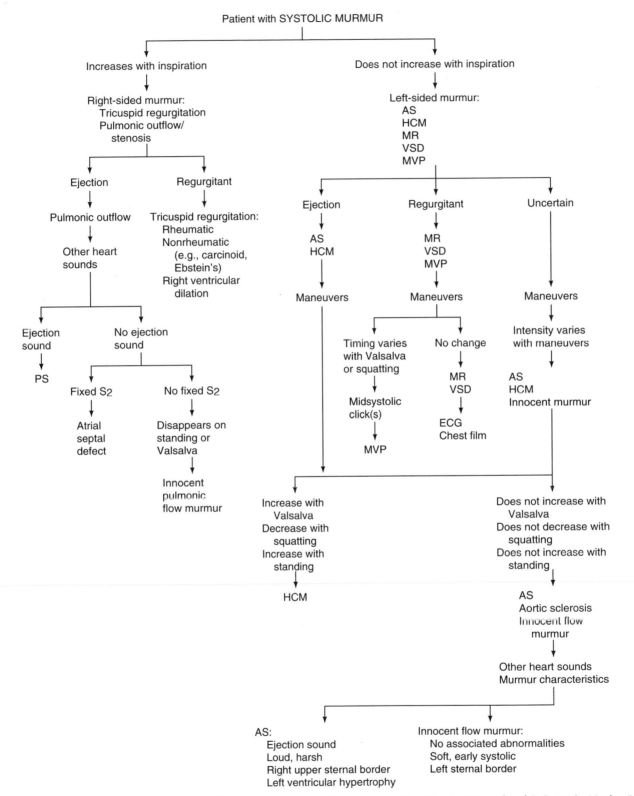

(Modified from Greene H, Johnson W, Lemcke D. *Decision Making in Medicine: An Algorithmic Approach,* ed 2. St Louis, Mosby, 1999.)

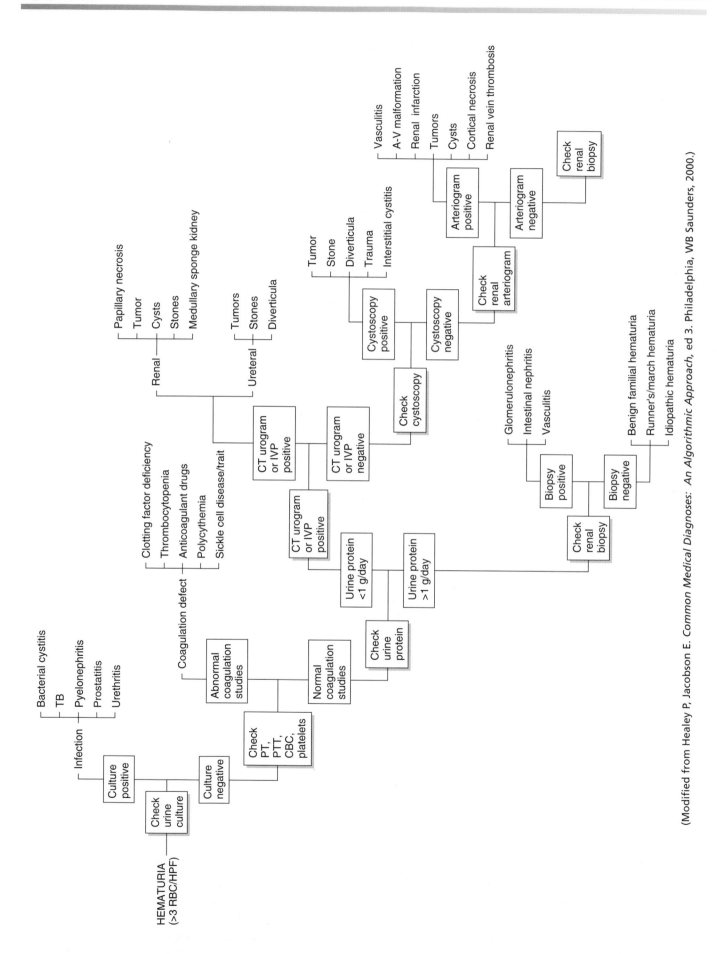

HEMATURIA (>3 RBC/HPF)

Check urine culture

Culture positive → Infection
- Bacterial cystitis
- TB
- Pyelonephritis
- Prostatitis
- Urethritis

Culture negative → Check PT, PTT, CBC, platelets

Abnormal coagulation studies → Coagulation defect
- Clotting factor deficiency
- Thrombocytopenia
- Anticoagulant drugs
- Polycythemia
- Sickle cell disease/trait

Normal coagulation studies → CT urogram or IVP positive

CT urogram or IVP positive
- Renal
  - Papillary necrosis
  - Tumor
  - Cysts
  - Stones
  - Medullary sponge kidney
- Ureteral
  - Tumors
  - Stones
  - Diverticula

CT urogram or IVP negative → Check cystoscopy

Cystoscopy positive
- Tumor
- Stone
- Diverticula
- Trauma
- Interstitial cystitis

Cystoscopy negative → Check renal arteriogram

Arteriogram positive
- Vasculitis
- A-V malformation
- Renal infarction
- Tumors

Arteriogram negative → Check renal biopsy
- Cysts
- Cortical necrosis
- Renal vein thrombosis

Check urine protein

Urine protein <1 g/day → CT urogram or IVP positive

Urine protein >1 g/day → Check renal biopsy

Biopsy positive
- Glomerulonephritis
- Intestinal nephritis
- Vasculitis

Biopsy negative
- Benign familial hematuria
- Runner's/march hematuria
- Idiopathic hematuria

(Modified from Healey P, Jacobson E. *Common Medical Diagnoses: An Algorithmic Approach*, ed 3. Philadelphia, WB Saunders, 2000.)

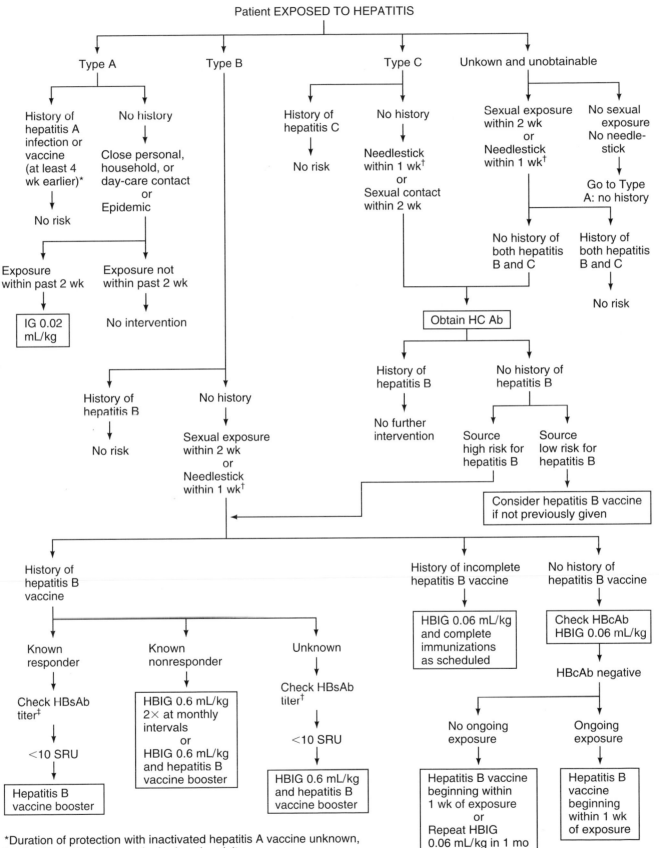

Patient EXPOSED TO HEPATITIS

Type A — Type B — Type C — Unkown and unobtainable

Type A

History of hepatitis A infection or vaccine (at least 4 wk earlier)* → No risk

No history → Close personal, household, or day-care contact or Epidemic

Exposure within past 2 wk → IG 0.02 mL/kg

Exposure not within past 2 wk → No intervention

Type B

History of hepatitis B → No risk

No history → Sexual exposure within 2 wk or Needlestick within 1 wk†

History of hepatitis B vaccine:
- Known responder → Check HBsAb titer‡ → <10 SRU → Hepatitis B vaccine booster
- Known nonresponder → HBIG 0.6 mL/kg 2× at monthly intervals or HBIG 0.6 mL/kg and hepatitis B vaccine booster
- Unknown → Check HBsAb titer† → <10 SRU → HBIG 0.6 mL/kg and hepatitis B vaccine booster

History of incomplete hepatitis B vaccine → HBIG 0.06 mL/kg and complete immunizations as scheduled

No history of hepatitis B vaccine → Check HBcAb HBIG 0.06 mL/kg → HBcAb negative
- No ongoing exposure → Hepatitis B vaccine beginning within 1 wk of exposure or Repeat HBIG 0.06 mL/kg in 1 mo
- Ongoing exposure → Hepatitis B vaccine beginning within 1 wk of exposure

Type C

History of hepatitis C → No risk

No history → Needlestick within 1 wk† or Sexual contact within 2 wk → Obtain HC Ab
- History of hepatitis B → No further intervention
- No history of hepatitis B:
  - Source high risk for hepatitis B
  - Source low risk for hepatitis B → Consider hepatitis B vaccine if not previously given

Unkown and unobtainable

Sexual exposure within 2 wk or Needlestick within 1 wk†
- No history of both hepatitis B and C → Obtain HC Ab
- History of both hepatitis B and C → No risk

No sexual exposure No needle-stick → Go to Type A: no history

*Duration of protection with inactivated hepatitis A vaccine unknown, but is at least 1 yr after a single dose in adults.

†Treat permucosal exposure to blood similarly to a needlestick.

‡If not known to be >10 SRU in the last 24 mo.

(Modified from Greene H, Johnson W, Lemcke D. *Decision Making in Medicine: An Algorithmic Approach,* ed 2. St Louis, Mosby, 1999.)

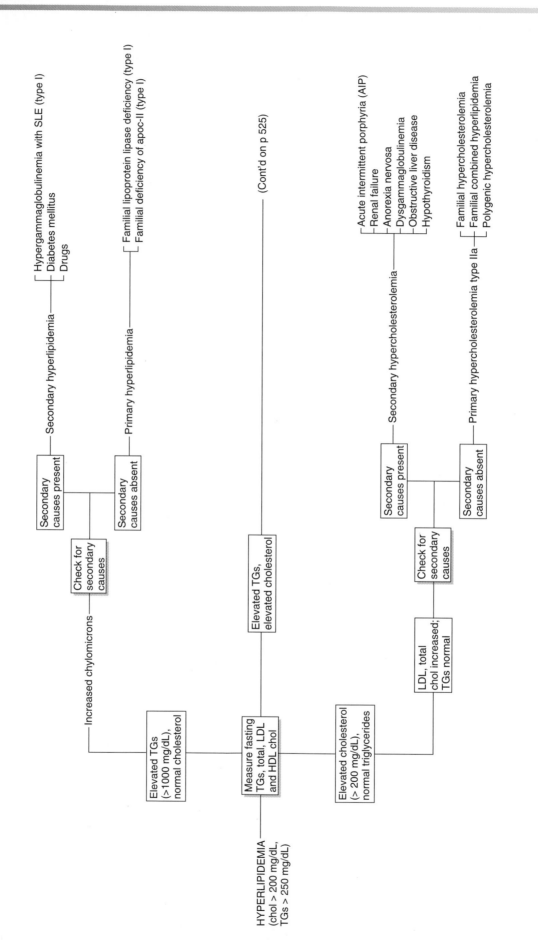

HYPERLIPIDEMIA
(chol > 200 mg/dL,
TGs > 250 mg/dL)

Measure fasting
TGs, total, LDL
and HDL chol

Elevated TGs
(>1000 mg/dL),
normal cholesterol

Increased chylomicrons

Check for
secondary
causes

Secondary
causes present

Secondary hyperlipidemia

Hypergammaglobulinemia with SLE (type I)
Diabetes mellitus
Drugs

Secondary
causes absent

Primary hyperlipidemia

Familial lipoprotein lipase deficiency (type I)
Familial deficiency of apoc-II (type I)

Elevated TGs,
elevated cholesterol

(Cont'd on p 525)

Elevated cholesterol
(> 200 mg/dL),
normal triglycerides

LDL, total
chol increased;
TGs normal

Check for
secondary
causes

Secondary
causes present

Secondary hypercholesterolemia

Acute intermittent porphyria (AIP)
Renal failure
Anorexia nervosa
Dysgammaglobulinemia
Obstructive liver disease
Hypothyroidism

Secondary
causes absent

Primary hypercholesterolemia type IIa

Familial hypercholesterolemia
Familial combined hyperlipidemia
Polygenic hypercholesterolemia

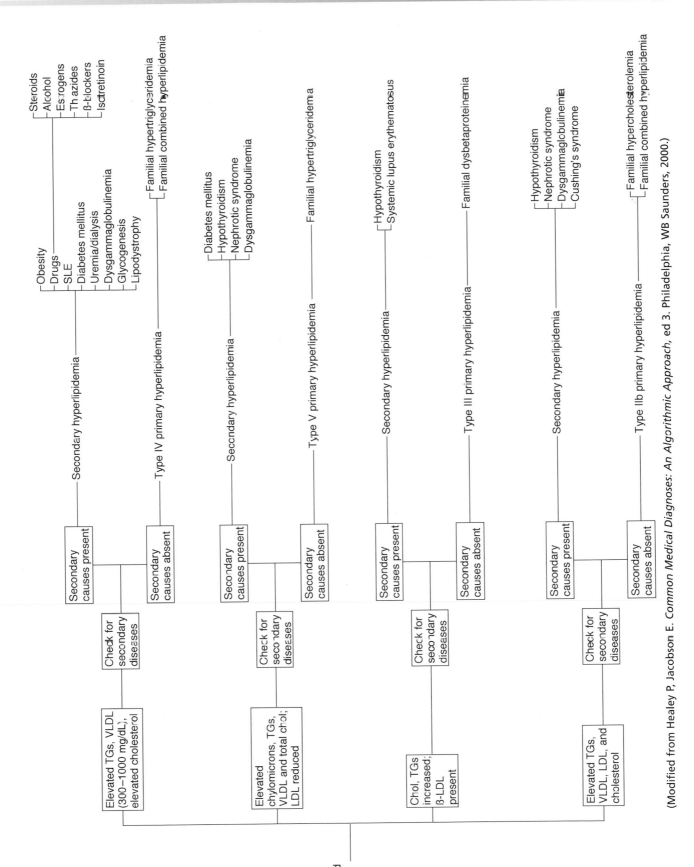

(Modified from Healey P, Jacobson E. *Common Medical Diagnoses: An Algorithmic Approach*, ed 3. Philadelphia, WB Saunders, 2000.)

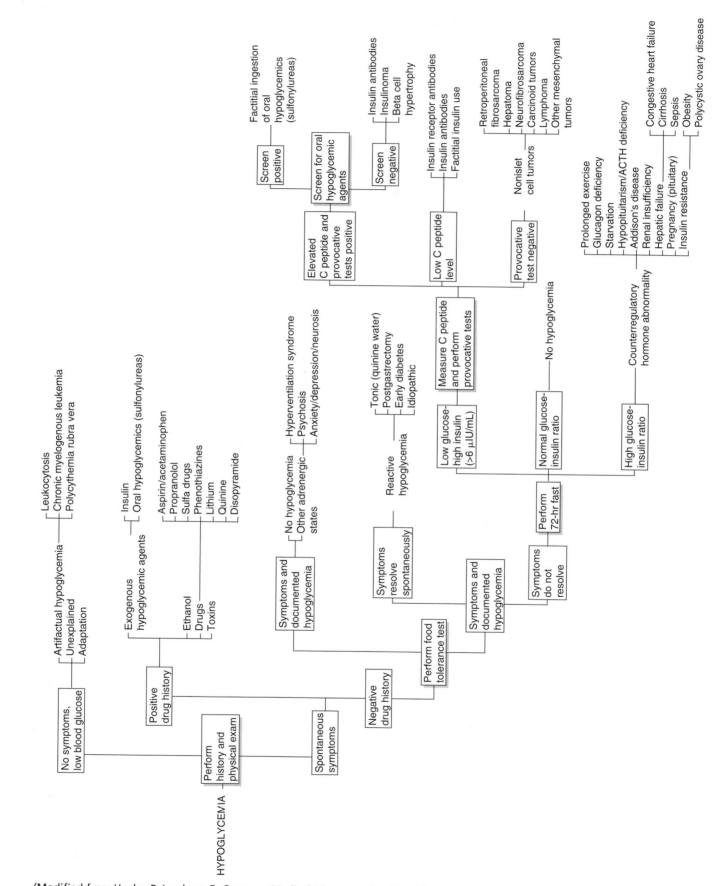

(Modified from Healey P, Jacobson E. *Common Medical Diagnoses: An Algorithmic Approach,* ed 3. Philadelphia, WB Saunders, 2000.)

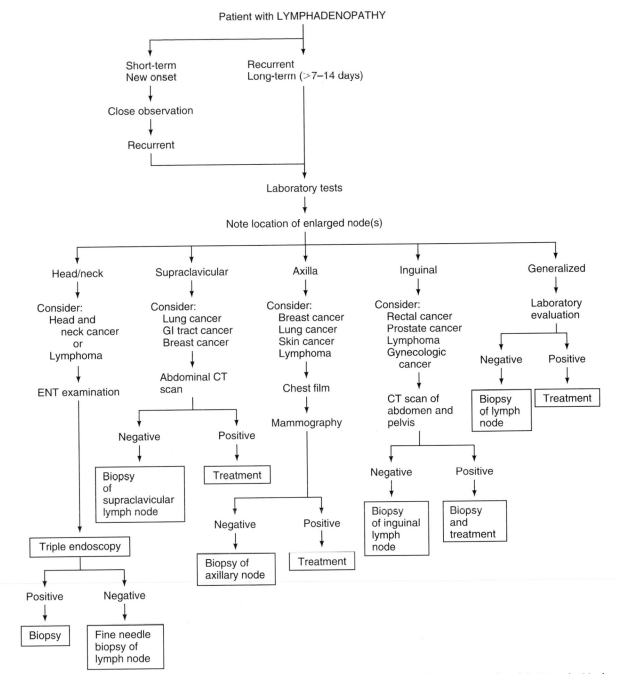

(Modified from Greene H, Johnson W, Lemcke D. *Decision Making in Medicine: An Algorithmic Approach,* ed 2. St Louis, Mosby, 1999.)

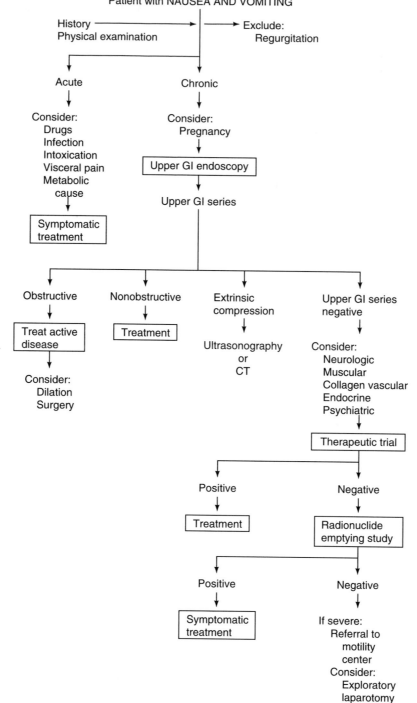

(Modified from Greene H, Johnson W, Lemcke D. *Decision Making in Medicine: An Algorithmic Approach,* ed 2. St Louis, Mosby, 1999.)

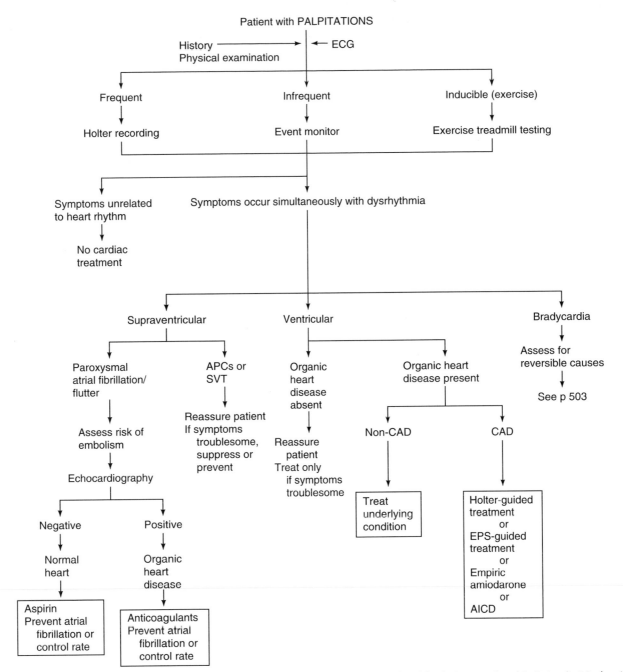

Patient with PALPITATIONS

History ——→ ←— ECG
Physical examination

Frequent   Infrequent   Inducible (exercise)

Holter recording   Event monitor   Exercise treadmill testing

Symptoms unrelated to heart rhythm   Symptoms occur simultaneously with dysrhythmia

No cardiac treatment

Supraventricular   Ventricular   Bradycardia

Paroxysmal atrial fibrillation/flutter   APCs or SVT   Organic heart disease absent   Organic heart disease present   Assess for reversible causes

See p 503

Assess risk of embolism

Reassure patient
If symptoms troublesome, suppress or prevent

Reassure patient
Treat only if symptoms troublesome

Non-CAD   CAD

Echocardiography

Negative   Positive

Normal heart   Organic heart disease

Treat underlying condition

Holter-guided treatment
or
EPS-guided treatment
or
Empiric amiodarone
or
AICD

Aspirin
Prevent atrial fibrillation or control rate

Anticoagulants
Prevent atrial fibrillation or control rate

(Modified from Greene H, Johnson W, Lemcke D. *Decision Making in Medicine: An Algorithmic Approach,* ed 2. St Louis, Mosby, 1999.)

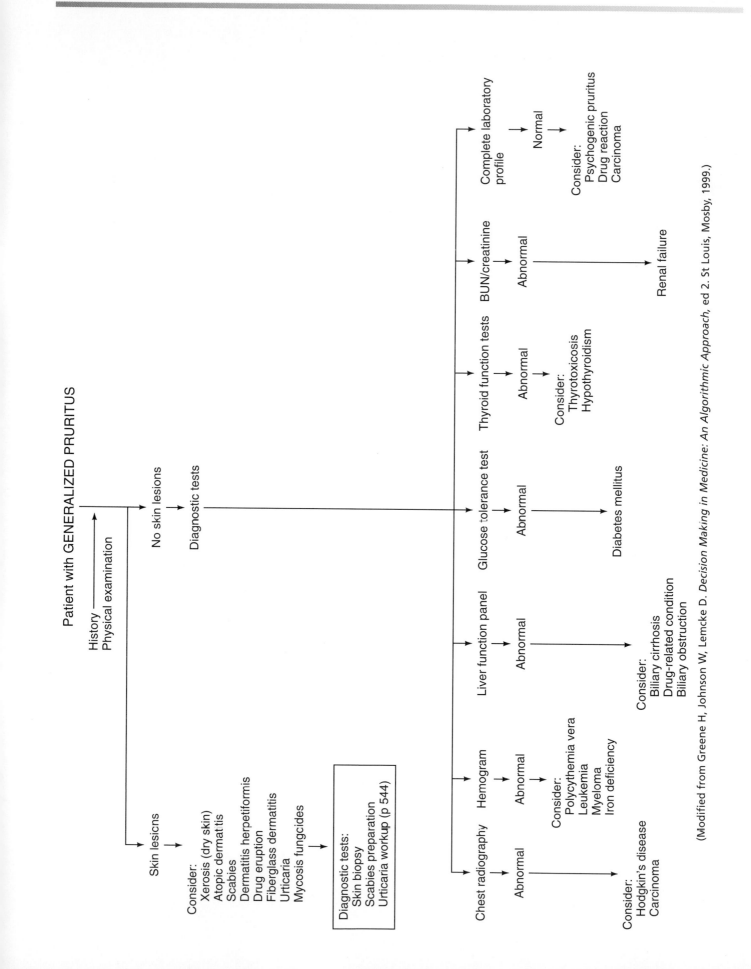

Patient with GENERALIZED PRURITUS

History
Physical examination

Skin lesions

Consider:
Xerosis (dry skin)
Atopic dermatitis
Scabies
Dermatitis herpetiformis
Drug eruption
Fiberglass dermatitis
Urticaria
Mycosis fungoides

Diagnostic tests:
Skin biopsy
Scabies preparation
Urticaria workup (p 544)

No skin lesions

Diagnostic tests

Chest radiography   Hemogram   Liver function panel   Glucose tolerance test   Thyroid function tests   BUN/creatinine   Complete laboratory profile

Abnormal   Abnormal   Abnormal   Abnormal   Abnormal   Abnormal   Normal

Consider:
Hodgkin's disease
Carcinoma

Consider:
Polycythemia vera
Leukemia
Myeloma
Iron deficiency

Consider:
Biliary cirrhosis
Drug-related condition
Biliary obstruction

Diabetes mellitus

Consider:
Thyrotoxicosis
Hypothyroidism

Renal failure

Consider:
Psychogenic pruritus
Drug reaction
Carcinoma

(Modified from Greene H, Johnson W, Lemcke D. *Decision Making in Medicine: An Algorithmic Approach*, ed 2. St Louis, Mosby, 1999.)

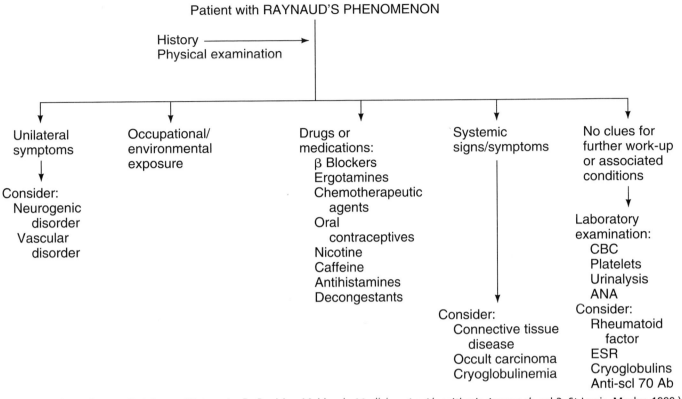

Patient with RAYNAUD'S PHENOMENON

History ⟶
Physical examination

Unilateral symptoms

Consider:
Neurogenic
disorder
Vascular
disorder

Occupational/ environmental exposure

Drugs or medications:
β Blockers
Ergotamines
Chemotherapeutic
agents
Oral
contraceptives
Nicotine
Caffeine
Antihistamines
Decongestants

Systemic signs/symptoms

Consider:
Connective tissue
disease
Occult carcinoma
Cryoglobulinemia

No clues for further work-up or associated conditions

Laboratory
examination:
CBC
Platelets
Urinalysis
ANA
Consider:
Rheumatoid
factor
ESR
Cryoglobulins
Anti-scl 70 Ab

(Modified from Greene H, Johnson W, Lemcke D. *Decision Making in Medicine: An Algorithmic Approach,* ed 2. St Louis, Mosby, 1999.)

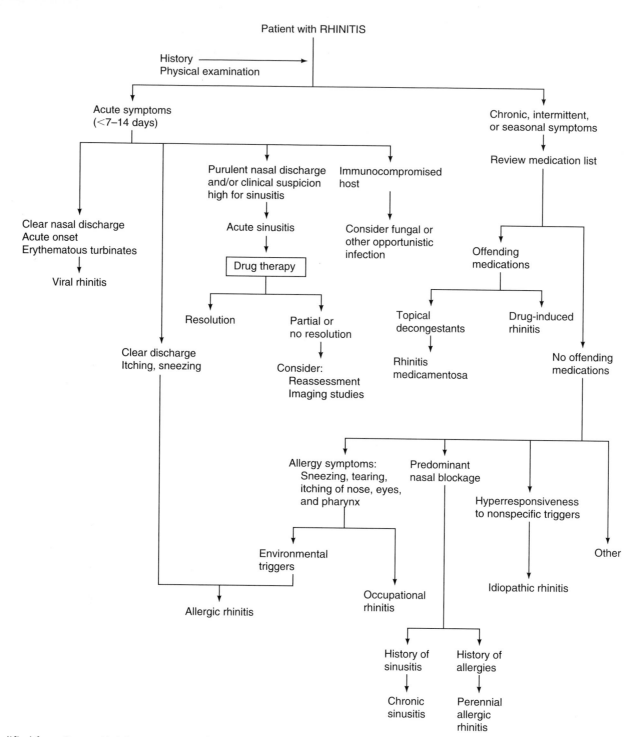

(Modified from Greene H, Johnson W, Lemcke D. *Decision Making in Medicine: An Algorithmic Approach,* ed 2. St Louis, Mosby, 1999.)

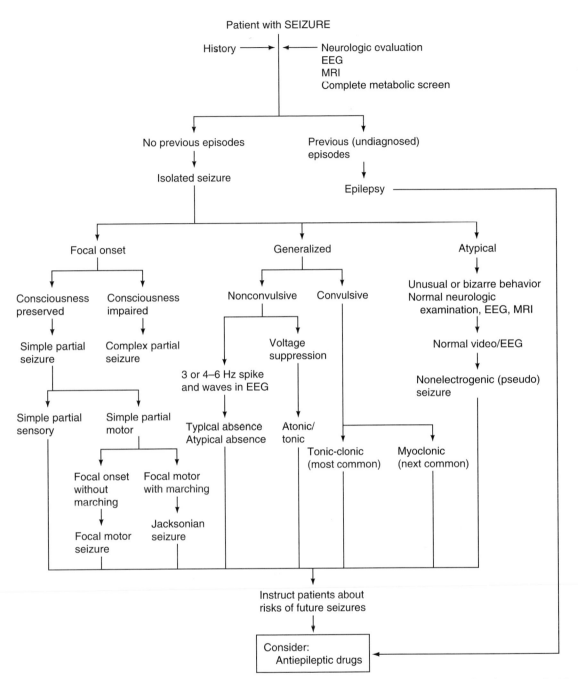

Patient with SEIZURE

History → ← Neurologic evaluation
EEG
MRI
Complete metabolic screen

No previous episodes

Previous (undiagnosed) episodes

Isolated seizure

Epilepsy

Focal onset

Generalized

Atypical

Consciousness preserved

Consciousness impaired

Nonconvulsive

Convulsive

Unusual or bizarre behavior
Normal neurologic examination, EEG, MRI

Simple partial seizure

Complex partial seizure

Voltage suppression

Normal video/EEG

3 or 4–6 Hz spike and waves in EEG

Nonelectrogenic (pseudo) seizure

Simple partial sensory

Simple partial motor

Typical absence
Atypical absence

Atonic/ tonic

Focal onset without marching

Focal motor with marching

Tonic-clonic (most common)

Myoclonic (next common)

Focal motor seizure

Jacksonian seizure

Instruct patients about risks of future seizures

Consider:
Antiepileptic drugs

(Modified from Greene H, Johnson W, Lemcke D. *Decision Making in Medicine: An Algorithmic Approach,* ed 2. St Louis, Mosby, 1999.)

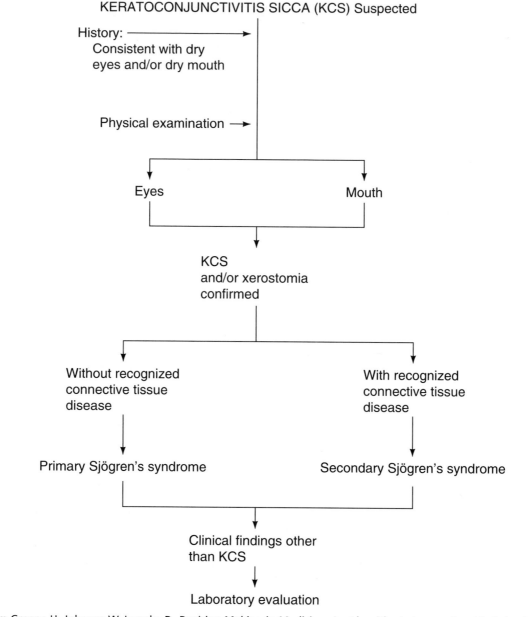

KERATOCONJUNCTIVITIS SICCA (KCS) Suspected

History: ⟶
Consistent with dry
eyes and/or dry mouth

Physical examination ⟶

Eyes   Mouth

KCS
and/or xerostomia
confirmed

Without recognized
connective tissue
disease

With recognized
connective tissue
disease

Primary Sjögren's syndrome   Secondary Sjögren's syndrome

Clinical findings other
than KCS

Laboratory evaluation

(Modified from Greene H, Johnson W, Lemcke D. *Decision Making in Medicine: An Algorithmic Approach,* ed 2. St Louis, Mosby, 1999.)

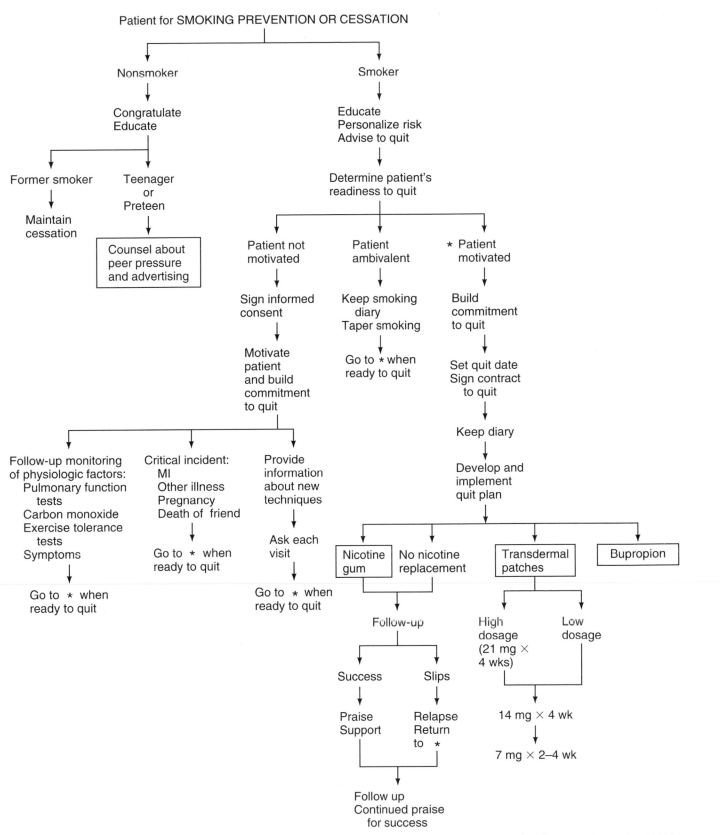

Patient for SMOKING PREVENTION OR CESSATION

Nonsmoker

Congratulate
Educate

Former smoker

Maintain
cessation

Teenager
or
Preteen

Counsel about
peer pressure
and advertising

Smoker

Educate
Personalize risk
Advise to quit

Determine patient's
readiness to quit

Patient not
motivated

Sign informed
consent

Motivate
patient
and build
commitment
to quit

Patient
ambivalent

Keep smoking
diary
Taper smoking

Go to * when
ready to quit

* Patient
motivated

Build
commitment
to quit

Set quit date
Sign contract
to quit

Keep diary

Develop and
implement
quit plan

Follow-up monitoring
of physiologic factors:
  Pulmonary function
    tests
  Carbon monoxide
  Exercise tolerance
    tests
  Symptoms

Go to * when
ready to quit

Critical incident:
  MI
  Other illness
  Pregnancy
  Death of friend

Go to * when
ready to quit

Provide
information
about new
techniques

Ask each
visit

Go to * when
ready to quit

Nicotine
gum

No nicotine
replacement

Transdermal
patches

Bupropion

Follow-up

Success

Praise
Support

Slips

Relapse
Return
to *

High
dosage
(21 mg ×
4 wks)

Low
dosage

14 mg × 4 wk

7 mg × 2–4 wk

Follow up
Continued praise
for success

(Modified from Greene H, Johnson W, Lemcke D. *Decision Making in Medicine: An Algorithmic Approach,* ed 2. St Louis, Mosby, 1999.)

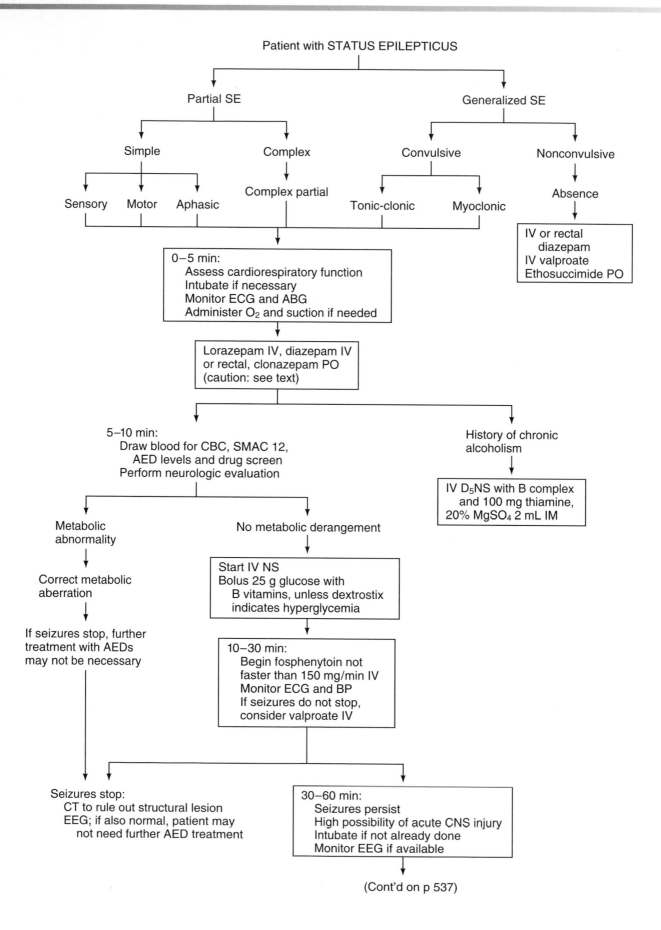

Patient with STATUS EPILEPTICUS

Partial SE

Generalized SE

Simple

Complex

Convulsive

Nonconvulsive

Sensory   Motor   Aphasic

Complex partial

Tonic-clonic   Myoclonic

Absence

IV or rectal
    diazepam
IV valproate
Ethosuccimide PO

0–5 min:
    Assess cardiorespiratory function
    Intubate if necessary
    Monitor ECG and ABG
    Administer O₂ and suction if needed

Lorazepam IV, diazepam IV
or rectal, clonazepam PO
(caution: see text)

5–10 min:
Draw blood for CBC, SMAC 12,
    AED levels and drug screen
Perform neurologic evaluation

History of chronic
alcoholism

IV D₅NS with B complex
    and 100 mg thiamine,
20% MgSO₄ 2 mL IM

Metabolic
abnormality

No metabolic derangement

Correct metabolic
aberration

Start IV NS
Bolus 25 g glucose with
    B vitamins, unless dextrostix
    indicates hyperglycemia

If seizures stop, further
treatment with AEDs
may not be necessary

10–30 min:
    Begin fosphenytoin not
    faster than 150 mg/min IV
    Monitor ECG and BP
    If seizures do not stop,
    consider valproate IV

Seizures stop:
    CT to rule out structural lesion
    EEG; if also normal, patient may
        not need further AED treatment

30–60 min:
    Seizures persist
    High possibility of acute CNS injury
    Intubate if not already done
    Monitor EEG if available

(Cont'd on p 537)

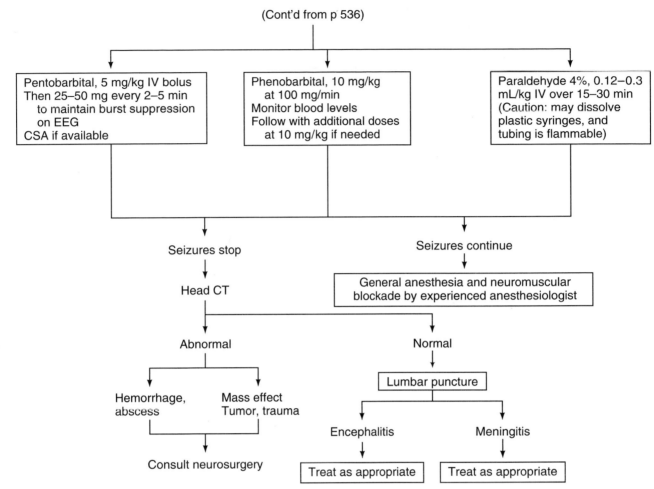

(Cont'd from p 536)

| Pentobarbital, 5 mg/kg IV bolus
Then 25–50 mg every 2–5 min
to maintain burst suppression
on EEG
CSA if available | Phenobarbital, 10 mg/kg
at 100 mg/min
Monitor blood levels
Follow with additional doses
at 10 mg/kg if needed | Paraldehyde 4%, 0.12–0.3
mL/kg IV over 15–30 min
(Caution: may dissolve
plastic syringes, and
tubing is flammable) |

Seizures stop → Head CT

Seizures continue → General anesthesia and neuromuscular blockade by experienced anesthesiologist

Head CT → Abnormal / Normal

Abnormal → Hemorrhage, abscess / Mass effect Tumor, trauma → Consult neurosurgery

Normal → Lumbar puncture → Encephalitis / Meningitis

Encephalitis → Treat as appropriate

Meningitis → Treat as appropriate

(Modified from Greene H, Johnson W, Lemcke D. *Decision Making in Medicine: An Algorithmic Approach,* ed 2. St Louis, Mosby, 1999.)

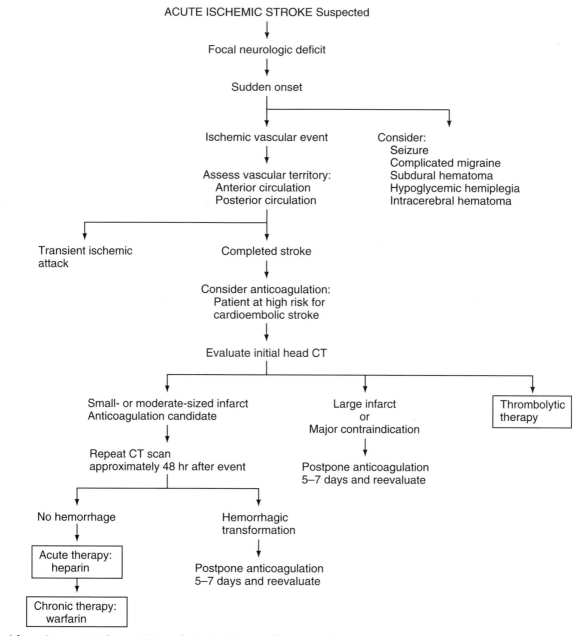

ACUTE ISCHEMIC STROKE Suspected

↓

Focal neurologic deficit

↓

Sudden onset

↓

Ischemic vascular event   Consider:
                            Seizure
                            Complicated migraine

Assess vascular territory: Subdural hematoma
   Anterior circulation   Hypoglycemic hemiplegia
   Posterior circulation   Intracerebral hematoma

Transient ischemic   Completed stroke
attack

Consider anticoagulation:
Patient at high risk for
cardioembolic stroke

↓

Evaluate initial head CT

Small- or moderate-sized infarct   Large infarct   Thrombolytic
Anticoagulation candidate   or   therapy
                       Major contraindication

Repeat CT scan
approximately 48 hr after event   Postpone anticoagulation
                             5–7 days and reevaluate

No hemorrhage   Hemorrhagic
                   transformation

Acute therapy:
heparin   Postpone anticoagulation
               5–7 days and reevaluate

Chronic therapy:
warfarin

(Modified from Greene H, Johnson W, Lemcke D. *Decision Making in Medicine: An Algorithmic Approach,* ed 2. St Louis, Mosby, 1999.)

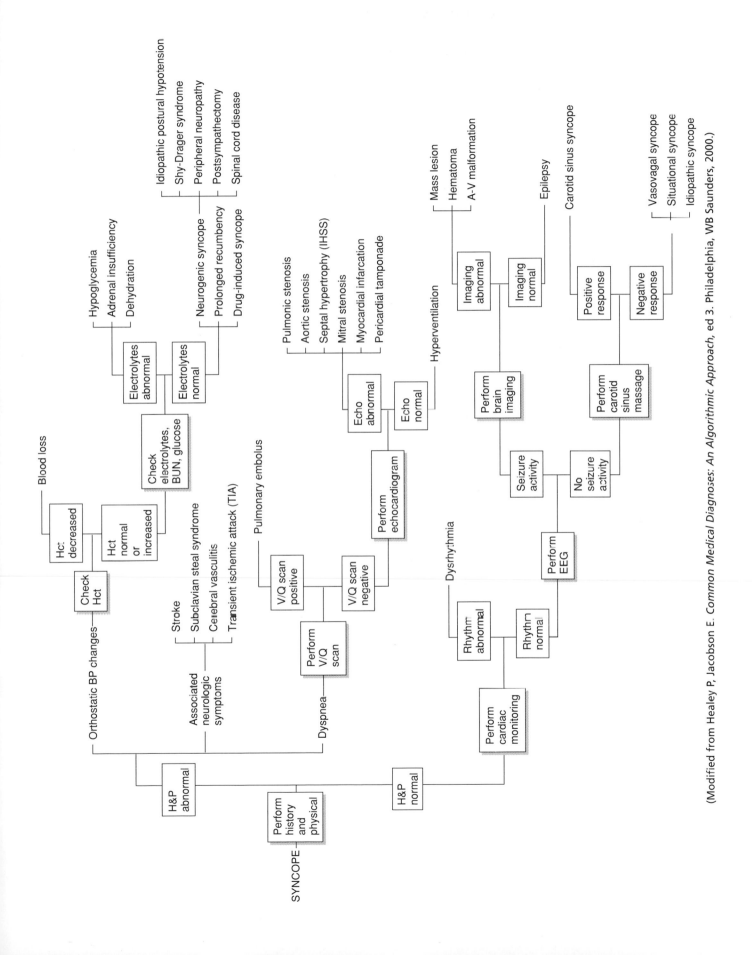

(Modified from Healey P, Jacobson E. *Common Medical Diagnoses: An Algorithmic Approach*, ed 3. Philadelphia, WB Saunders, 2000.)

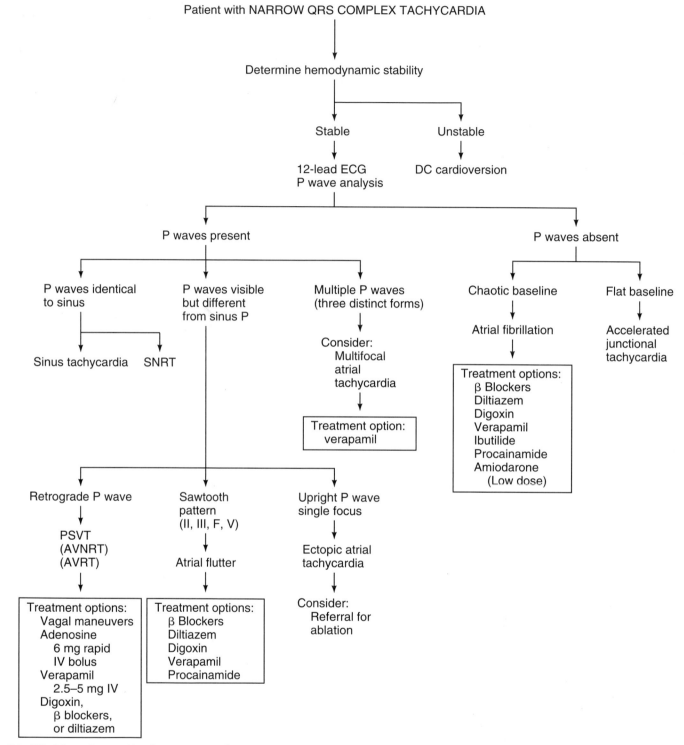

Patient with NARROW QRS COMPLEX TACHYCARDIA

Determine hemodynamic stability

Stable — Unstable

12-lead ECG
P wave analysis — DC cardioversion

P waves present — P waves absent

P waves identical to sinus — P waves visible but different from sinus P — Multiple P waves (three distinct forms) — Chaotic baseline — Flat baseline

Sinus tachycardia — SNRT

Consider:
Multifocal
atrial
tachycardia

Atrial fibrillation

Accelerated
junctional
tachycardia

Treatment option:
verapamil

Treatment options:
β Blockers
Diltiazem
Digoxin
Verapamil
Ibutilide
Procainamide
Amiodarone
(Low dose)

Retrograde P wave — Sawtooth pattern (II, III, F, V) — Upright P wave single focus

PSVT
(AVNRT)
(AVRT)

Atrial flutter

Ectopic atrial
tachycardia

Treatment options:
Vagal maneuvers
Adenosine
6 mg rapid
IV bolus
Verapamil
2.5–5 mg IV
Digoxin,
β blockers,
or diltiazem

Treatment options:
β Blockers
Diltiazem
Digoxin
Verapamil
Procainamide

Consider:
Referral for
ablation

(Modified from Greene H, Johnson W, Lemcke D. *Decision Making in Medicine: An Algorithmic Approach,* ed 2. St Louis, Mosby, 1999.)

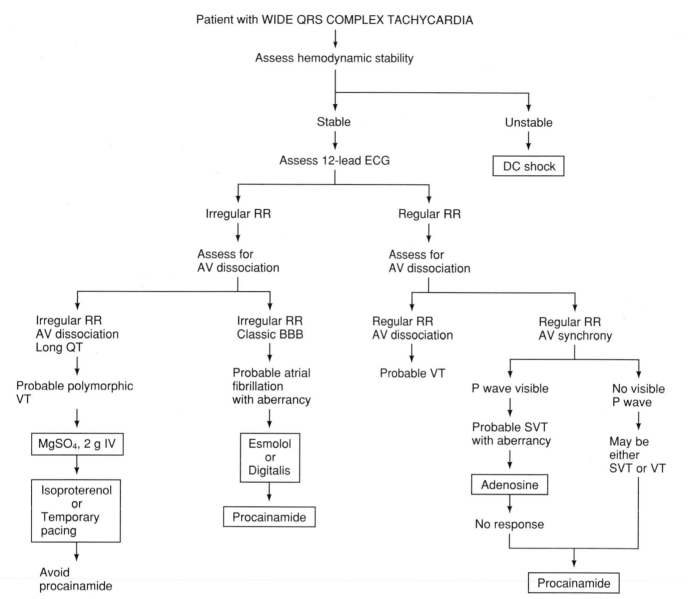

(Modified from Greene H, Johnson W, Lemcke D. *Decision Making in Medicine: An Algorithmic Approach,* ed 2. St Louis, Mosby, 1999.)

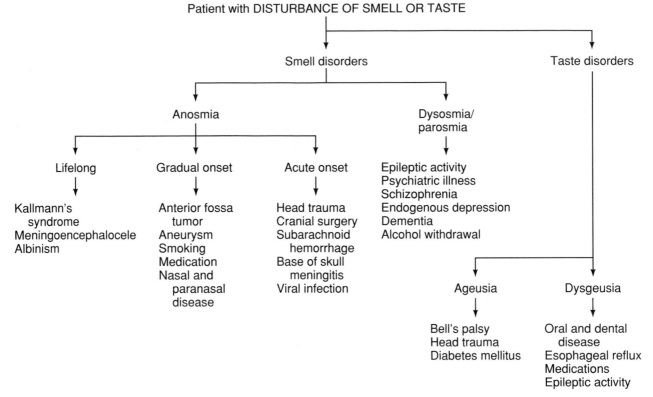

(Modified from Greene H, Johnson W, Lemcke D. *Decision Making in Medicine: An Algorithmic Approach,* ed 2. St Louis, Mosby, 1999.)

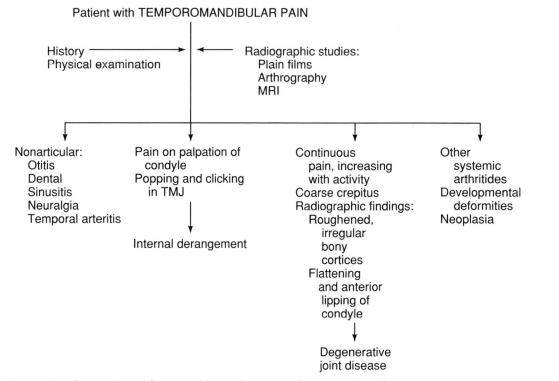

Patient with TEMPOROMANDIBULAR PAIN

History ⟶ ⟵ Radiographic studies:
Physical examination   Plain films
                          Arthrography
                          MRI

Nonarticular:
 Otitis
 Dental
 Sinusitis
 Neuralgia
 Temporal arteritis

Pain on palpation of
 condyle
Popping and clicking
 in TMJ

 ↓

Internal derangement

Continuous
 pain, increasing
 with activity
Coarse crepitus
Radiographic findings:
 Roughened,
  irregular
  bony
  cortices
Flattening
 and anterior
 lipping of
 condyle

 ↓

Degenerative
joint disease

Other
 systemic
 arthritides
Developmental
 deformities
Neoplasia

(Modified from Greene H, Johnson W, Lemcke D. *Decision Making in Medicine: An Algorithmic Approach,* ed 2. St Louis, Mosby, 1999.)

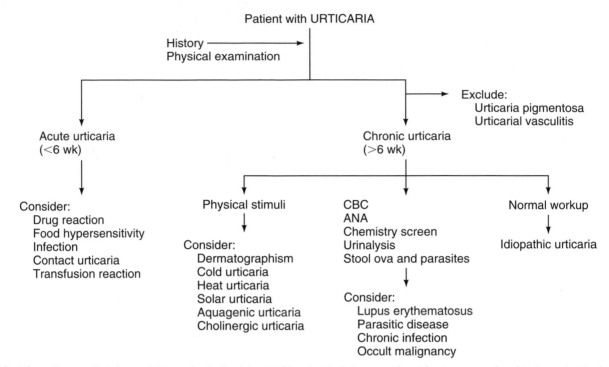

Patient with URTICARIA

History ———————→
Physical examination

Acute urticaria
(<6 wk)

Chronic urticaria
(>6 wk)

Exclude:
  Urticaria pigmentosa
  Urticarial vasculitis

Consider:
  Drug reaction
  Food hypersensitivity
  Infection
  Contact urticaria
  Transfusion reaction

Physical stimuli

Consider:
  Dermatographism
  Cold urticaria
  Heat urticaria
  Solar urticaria
  Aquagenic urticaria
  Cholinergic urticaria

CBC
ANA
Chemistry screen
Urinalysis
Stool ova and parasites

Consider:
  Lupus erythematosus
  Parasitic disease
  Chronic infection
  Occult malignancy

Normal workup

Idiopathic urticaria

(Modified from Greene H, Johnson W, Lemcke D. *Decision Making in Medicine: An Algorithmic Approach,* ed 2. St Louis, Mosby, 1999.)

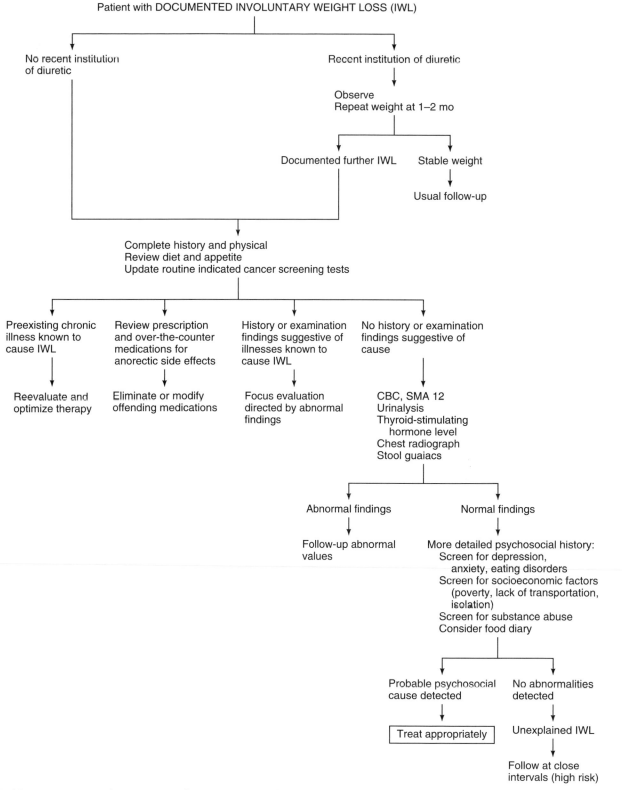

(Modified from Greene H, Johnson W, Lemcke D. *Decision Making in Medicine: An Algorithmic Approach,* ed 2. St Louis, Mosby, 1999.)

Index

A

AA amyloidosis. *See* Amyloidosis
Abnormal platelet function. *See* Thrombocytopathies (congenital and acquired)
Absence seizures. *See* Seizures
Acetaminophen, compounds with, 422
Acquired fibrinolytic hemorrhage. *See* Disseminated intravascular coagulation
Acquired immune deficiency syndrome (AIDS)
　dental management of, 111
　dental significance of, 111
　diagnosis of, 110
　medical management and treatment of, 110
　prognosis of, 110–111
Acquired thrombocytopathia. *See* Thrombocytopathies (congenital and acquired)
Acquired toxoplasmosis. *See* Toxoplasmosis
Acrodermatitis chronica atrophicans. *See* Lyme disease
Actinomycetes. *See* Actinomycosis
Actinomycosis, 226
　dental management of, 226
　dental significance of, 226
　diagnosis of, 226
　medical management and treatment of, 226
　prognosis of, 226
Active tuberculosis disease, 212
Acute adrenal insufficiency, 340
　complications of, 340
　dental management of, 340, 483
　diagnosis of, 340
　etiology of, 340
　medical management of, 340
　pathogenesis of, 340
　prognosis of, 340
Acute atrial tachycardia. *See* Atrial tachycardia
Acute atrophic candidosis. *See* Candidosis
Acute bradycardia. *See* Bradycardia
Acute bronchospasm. *See* Bronchospasm
Acute coarctation. *See* Coarctation of aorta
Acute coronary syndrome. *See* Angina pectoris
Acute gingivostomatitis. *See* Herpes simplex virus
Acute GVHD. *See* Graft-*versus*-host disease
Acute infectious mononucleosis. *See* Epstein-Barr virus diseases: infectious mononucleosis
Acute lymphoblastic leukemia. *See* Leukemias

Acute myelogenous leukemia. *See* Leukemias
Acute myocardial infarction (AMI). *See* Myocardial infarction
Acute osteomyelitis. *See* Osteomyelitis
Adalat, 434f. *See also* Nifedipine
Addisonian crisis. *See* Acute adrenal insufficiency
Addison's disease, 2–3
　complications of, 3
　dental management of, 3
　dental significance of, 2–3
　diagnosis of, 2
　medical management of, 2
　prognosis of, 2
Adenomatoid odontogenic tumor, 227
　complications of, 227
　dental management of, 227
　dental significance of, 227
　diagnosis of, 227
　medical management and treatment of, 227
　prognosis of, 227
Adrenal crisis. *See* Acute adrenal insufficiency
Adult-onset diabetes mellitus. *See* Diabetes mellitus
Afibrinogenemia. *See* Disseminated intravascular coagulation
African Burkitt's lymphoma. *See* Burkitt's lymphoma
Agnogenic myeloid metaplasia. *See* Myeloproliferative disorders
Agonal rhythm, 37
AIDS. *See* Acquired immune deficiency syndrome
Airway obstruction, 341
　dental significance of, 341
　etiology of, 341
　medical management of, 341
　pathogenesis of, 341
　prognosis of, 341
AL amyloidosis. *See* Amyloidosis
Albuterol, 391, 391f
　contraindications of, 391
　dental considerations of, 391
　dosing of, 391
　drug interactions of, 391
　side effects of, 391
　uses of, 391
Alcohol withdrawal seizures. *See* Delirium tremens
Alcohol withdrawal syndrome. *See* Delirium tremens
Alcoholic liver disease. *See* Hepatitis: alcoholic
Alcoholism
　complications of, 4
　dental management of, 5
　dental significance of, 5
　diagnosis of, 4
　medical management of, 4
　prognosis of, 4
Alendronate, 392
　contraindications of, 392
　dental considerations of, 392

Alendronate—cont'd
　dosing of, 392
　interactions of, 392
　side effects of, 392
　uses of, 392
Aleukia hemorrhagica. *See* Aplastic anemia
ALL. *See* Leukemias
Allegra, 414f. *See also* Fexofenadine
Allergic asthma. *See* Asthma
Allergic reactions, 6–7. *See also* Bronchitis
　complications of, 6–7
　dental management of, 7
　dental significance of, 7
　diagnosis of, 6
　medical management and treatment of, 6
　prognosis of, 7
　types of, 6t
Alprazolam, 393
　contraindications of, 393
　dental considerations of, 393
　dosing of, 393
　interactions of, 393
　side effects of, 393
　uses of, 393
Altace, 442f. *See also* Ramipril
Altered mental status, algorithm for, 470–471
Altocor. *See* Lovastatin
Alveolar osteitis. *See* Dry socket
Alzheimer's disease, 8–9
　complications of, 8–9
　dental management of, 9
　dental significance of, 9
　diagnosis of, 8
　medical management and treatment of, 8
　prognosis of, 9
Amalgam tattoo, 229
　complications of, 229
　dental management of, 229
　dental significance of, 229
　diagnosis of, 229
　medical management and treatment of, 229
　prognosis of, 229
Ambien, 453f. *See also* Zolpidem
Ameloblastic fibroma, 230
　complications of, 230
　dental management of, 230
　dental significance of, 230
　diagnosis of, 230
　medical management and treatment of, 230
　prognosis of, 230
Ameloblastoma, 231–232
　complications of, 232
　dental management of, 232
　dental significance of, 232
　diagnosis of, 231–232
　medical management and treatment of, 232
　prognosis of, 232
AMI. *See* Myocardial infarction

AML. *See* Leukemias
Amlodipine, 394
  contraindications of, 394
  dental considerations of, 394
  dosing of, 394
  interactions of, 394
  sides effects of, 394
  uses of, 394
Amoxicillin acid, 395
  contraindications of, 395
  dental considerations of, 395
  dosing of, 395
  interactions of, 395
  side effects of, 395
  uses of, 395
Amyloidosis, 10
  dental management of, 10
  dental significance of, 10
  diagnosis of, 10
  medical management and treatment
    of, 10
  prognosis of, 10
Anaphylactic reaction. *See*
  Anaphylaxis
Anaphylactic shock. *See* Anaphylaxis
Anaphylaxis, 342–343
  algorithm for, 492–493
  complications of, 342
  dental significance of, 343
  diagnosis of, 342
  etiology of, 342
  medical management of, 342
  pathogenesis of, 342
  prognosis of, 342
ANE. *See* Angioneurotic edema
Anemia: hemolytic (congenital and
    acquired), 12–14
  complications of, 12
  dental management of, 12
  dental significance of, 12
  diagnosis of, 12
  medical management and treatment,
    12
Anemia: iron deficiency, 13
  complications of, 13
  dental management of, 14
  dental significance of, 13
  diagnosis of, 13
  medical management of, 13
  prognosis of, 13
Anemia: pernicious, 15
  complications of, 15
  dental management of, 15
  dental significance of, 15
  diagnosis of, 15
  medical management and treatment
    of, 15
  prognosis of, 15
Anemia: sickle cell, 17–18
  complications of, 18
  dental management of, 18
  dental significance of, 18
  diagnosis of, 17
  medical management and treatment
    of, 17–18
  prognosis of, 18

Aneurysmal bone cyst, 233
  complications of, 233
  dental management of, 233
  dental significance of, 233
  diagnosis of, 233
  medical management and treatment
    of, 233
  prognosis of, 233
Angina. *See also* Angina pectoris
  algorithm for, 494–495
Angina pectoris, 19–21, 344
  complications of, 19, 344
  dental management of, 19, 344
  dental significance of, 19
  diagnosis of, 19, 344
  etiology of, 344
  functional classification of, 19t
  medical management and treatment
    of, 19–20
  medical management of, 344
  pathogenesis of, 344
  prognosis of, 19, 344
Angioedema, 22–23
  complications of, 22
  dental management of, 22–23
  dental significance of, 22
  diagnosis of, 22
  medical management and treatment
    of, 22
  prognosis of, 22
Angiohemophilia. *See* Von Willebrand's
  disease
Angioneurotic edema, 345. *See also*
    Angioedema
  complications of, 345
  dental significance of, 345
  diagnosis of, 345
  etiology of, 345
  medical management of, 345
  pathogenesis of, 345
  prognosis of, 345
Angioneurotic edema. *See*
    Angioedema
Angular cheilitis, 234
  complications of, 234
  dental management of, 234
  dental significance of, 234
  diagnosis of, 234
  medical management and treatment
    of, 234
  prognosis of, 234
Angular cheilosis. *See* Angular
  cheilitis
Anorexia nervosa, 24–27
  complications of, 25
  dental management of, 26
  dental significance of, 25–26
  diagnosis of, 24–25
  medical management and treatment
    of, 24–25
Anterior triangle masses, 294
Antibiotic prophylaxis, 481, 482
Anticoagulant therapy. *See*
    Coagulopathies (clotting factor
    defects, acquired)
Anticonvulsant drugs, 190f

Antidiuretic hormone secretion. *See*
  Inappropriate secretion of
  antidiuretic hormone
Antidysrhythmic drugs, 37–39
  classifications of, 38t
Antihemophilic globulin deficiency. *See*
  Hemophilia (Types A, B, C)
Aortic coarctation. *See* Coarctation of
  aorta
Aortic insufficiency. *See* Cardiac valvular
  disease
Aortic regurgitation, 44
Aortic stenosis. *See* Cardiac valvular
  disease
Aphthous pharyngitis. *See* Herpangina
Aphthous stomatitis, 235–236
  complications of, 235
  dental management of, 236
  dental significance of, 236
  diagnosis of, 235
  medical management and treatment
    of, 235
  prognosis of, 236
Aplastic anemia, 27–28
  complications of, 27
  dental management of, 28
  dental significance of, 27
  diagnosis of, 27
  medical management and treatment
    of, 27
  prognosis of, 27
Apneic sleep. *See* Sleep apnea
Aquazide. *See* Hydrochlorothiazide
Aregeneratory anemia. *See* Aplastic
  anemia
Arterial venous malformation. *See*
  Hemangioma
Arthritis, algorithm for, 496–497
Articaine with epinephrine, 456
  contraindications of, 456
  dental considerations of, 456
  dosing of, 456
  interactions of, 456
  side effects of, 456
  uses of, 456
Aspiration. *See* Nausea
Asthma, 29–31
  classification of, 30t
  complications of, 29
  dental management of, 29–30
  dental significance of, 29
  diagnosis of, 29
  medical management and treatment
    of, 29
  medications, 31t
  prognosis of, 29
Asystole, 37
Atenolol, 396
  contraindications of, 396
  dental considerations of, 396
  dosing of, 396
  interactions of, 396
  side effects of, 396
  uses of, 396
Ativan, 426f. *See also* Lorazepam
Atorvastatin, 397

Atorvastatin—cont'd
    contraindications of, 397
    dental considerations of, 397
    dosing of, 397
    interactions of, 397
    side effects of, 397
    uses of, 397
Atrial fibrillation, 36
Atrial flutter, 36
Atrial septal defects. *See* Cardiac septal
    defects: atrial and ventricular
Atrial tachycardia, 36, 346
    complications of, 346
    dental significance of, 346
    diagnosis of, 346
    etiology of, 346
    medical management of, 346
    pathogenesis of, 346
    prognosis of, 346
Atrioventricular septal defects. *See*
    Cardiac septal defects: atrial and
    ventricular
Atrophic glossitis. *See* Glossitis
Atropine, 457
    contraindications of, 457
    dental considerations of, 457
    dosing of, 457
    interactions of, 457
    side effects of, 457
    uses of, 457
Augmentin, 395f. *See also* Amoxicillin
    acid
Autoimmune hemolytic anemia. *See*
    Anemia: hemolytic (congenital and
    acquired)
Autoimmune thrombocytopenic
    purpura. *See* Idiopathic
    thrombocytopenic purpura (ITP)
AV heart block, 36

B
Back pain, algorithm for, 498
Bacterial endocarditis, 481. *See also*
    Endocarditis (infective)
Bald tongue of pernicious anemia. *See*
    Glossitis
Bannwarth's syndrome. *See* Lyme
    disease
Basal cell carcinoma, 237
    complications of, 237
    dental significance of, 237
    medical management and treatment
        of, 237
    prognosis of, 237
Basal cell epithelioma. *See* Basal cell
    carcinoma
B-cell lymphoma. *See* Burkitt's
    lymphoma
Behcet's syndrome, 32
    dental management of, 32
    dental significance of, 32
    diagnosis of, 32
    medical management and treatment
        of, 32
    prognosis of, 32
Benadryl. *See* Diphenhydramine

Benign fibroosseous lesions. *See* Fibrous
    dysplasia
Benign inoculation lymphoreticulosis.
    See Cat-scratch disease
Benign lymphoepithelial cysts, 238
    complications of, 238
    dental management of, 238
    dental significance of, 238
    diagnosis of, 238
    medical management and treatment
        of, 238
    prognosis of, 238
Benign mixed tumor. *See* Pleomorphic
    adenoma
Beriberi, 335
Bernard-Soulier syndrome. *See*
    Thrombocytopathies (congenital
    and acquired)
Biocef. *See* Cephalexin
Bites, algorithm for, 499
Bleeding
    algorithm for, 500
    platelet count effects on, 208t
Blood pressure
    algorithm for, 501–502
    classification, 116t
Boeck's sarcoid. *See* Sarcoidosis
Bone marrow failure syndrome. *See*
    Aplastic anemia
Bony exostoses. *See* Exostosis
Brachial cleft cysts. *See* Benign
    lymphoepithelial cysts; Neck
    masses (differential diagnosis)
Brachycardias, 36
Bradycardia, 347
    algorithm for, 503
    complications of, 347
    dental significance of, 347
    diagnosis of, 347
    etiology of, 347
    medical management of, 347
    pathogenesis of, 347
    prognosis of, 347
Brain attack. *See* Stroke
Branchial cleft cysts. *See* Benign
    lymphoepithelial cysts
Breathing difficulty, algorithm for,
    504–505
Brevital. *See* Methohexital
Brittle bone disease. *See*
    Osteoporosis
Bronchial asthma. *See* Asthma
Bronchitis (acute), 33–34
    complications of, 34
    dental management of, 34
    dental significance of, 34
    diagnosis of, 33
    medical management and treatment
        of, 33–34
    prognosis of, 34
Bronchitis (chronic). *See* Chronic
    obstructive pulmonary disease
Bronchoalveolar carcinoma. *See* Lung:
    primary malignancy
Bronchoalveolar carcinoma. *See* Lung:
    primary malignancy

Bronchospasm, 29, 348–349
    complications of, 349
    dental significance of, 349
    diagnosis of, 348
    etiology of, 348
    medical management of, 348
    pathogenesis of, 348
    prognosis of, 349
Bulimia nervosa, 24–27
    complications of, 25
    dental management of, 26
    dental significance of, 25–26
    diagnosis of, 24–25
Bupivacaine with epinephrine, 458
    contraindications of, 458
    dental considerations of, 458
    dosing of, 458
    interactions of, 458
    side effects of, 458
    uses of, 458
Bupropion
    contraindications of, 398
    dental considerations of, 398
    dosing of, 398
    interactions of, 398
    side effects of, 398
    uses of, 398
Burkitt's lymphoma, 239–240. *See also*
    Non-Hodgkin's lymphoma
    complications of, 239
    dental management of, 239–240
    dental significance of, 239
    diagnosis of, 239
    medical management and treatment
        of, 239
    prognosis of, 239
Burning mouth syndrome, 241–242
Burning tongue. *See* Burning mouth
    syndrome
BuSpar, 399f. *See also* Buspirone
Buspirone
    contraindications of, 399
    dental considerations of, 399
    dosing of, 399
    interactions of, 399
    side effects of, 399
    uses of, 399

C
Cachexia. *See* Bulimia nervosa; Anorexia
    nervosa
Calan, 451f. *See also* Verapamil
Calcific degeneration, 44
Calcifying epithelial odontogenic tumor,
    242
    complications of, 242
    dental management of, 242
    dental significance of, 242
    diagnosis of, 242
    medical management and treatment
        of, 242
    prognosis of, 242
Calcifying fibrous epulis. *See* Peripheral
    odontogenic fibroma
Calcifying odontogenic tumor. *See* Calci-
    fying epithelial odontogenic tumor

Calculi. *See* Sialolithiasis
Candidiasis. *See* Candidosis
Candidosis, 243–244
    complications of, 243
    dental management of, 244
    dental significance of, 243
    diagnosis of, 243
    management of, 243t
    medical management and treatment
      of, 243
    prognosis of, 243
Canker sores. *See* Aphthous stomatitis
Capillary hemangioma. *See*
    Hemangioma
Carbocaine, 467t. *See also* Mepivacaine
Carbocaine with neocobefrin. *See*
    Mepivacaine
Cardiac arrest, 37, 350
    complications of, 350
    dental significance of, 350
    diagnosis of, 350
    etiology of, 350
    medical management of, 350
    pathogenesis of, 350
    prognosis of, 350
Cardiac arrhythmias. *See* Cardiac
    dysrhythmias
Cardiac dysrhythmias, 35–40
    anesthesia considerations, 40
    complications of, 39
    dental management of, 39–40
    dental significance of, 39
    diagnosis of, 37
    prognosis of, 39
Cardiac septal defects: atrial and
    ventricular, 41–43
    complications of, 42
    dental management of, 43
    dental significance of, 42–43
    diagnosis of, 42
    genetic syndromes associated with,
      41t
    medical management and treatment
      of, 42
    prognosis of, 42
Cardiac valvular disease, 44–46
    complications of, 45
    dental management of, 45–46
    dental significance of, 45
    diagnosis of, 45
    medical management and treatment
      of, 45
    prognosis of, 45
    rheumatic fever, 44
Cardiomyopathy, 47–49
    characteristics of, 48t
    complications of, 48
    dental management of, 49
    diagnosis of, 48
    medical management and treatment
      of, 48
    prognosis of, 49
Cardioversion, 38
Cardizem, 410f. *See also* Diltiazem
Carisoprodol
    contraindications of, 400

Carisoprodol—cont'd
    dental considerations of, 400
    dosing of, 400
    interactions of, 400
    side effects of, 400
    uses of, 400
Carotid body tumor. *See* Neck masses
    (differential diagnosis)
Cartia, 410f. *See also* Diltiazem
Cat-scratch disease, 50. *See also*
    Neck masses (differential
    diagnosis)
    complications of, 50
    dental management of, 50
    dental significance of, 50
    diagnosis of, 50
    medical management and treatment
      of, 50
    prognosis of, 50
Caustic ingestion and exposure,
    algorithm for, 506
Cavernous hemangioma. *See*
    Hemangioma
Celexa, 404f. *See also* Citalopram
Cementifying fibromas
    complications of, 299
    dental management of, 300
    dental significance of, 299
    diagnosis of, 299
    medical management and treatment
      of, 299
    prognosis of, 299
Cementoblastoma. *See* Osteoblastoma
Central diabetes insipidus. *See* Diabetes
    insipidus
Central giant cell granuloma, 245
    complications of, 245
    dental management of, 245
    dental significance of, 245
    diagnosis of, 245
    medical management and treatment
      of, 245
    prognosis of, 245
Central papillary atrophy of the
    tongue. *See* Median rhomboid
    glossitis
Central sleep apnea. *See* Sleep apnea
Cephalexin, 401
    contraindications of, 401
    dental considerations of, 401
    dosing of, 401
    interactions of, 401
    side effects of, 401
    uses of, 401
Cerebral accident. *See* Cerebral vascular
    accident
Cerebral vascular accident, 351
    complications of, 351
    dental management of, 351
    dental significance of, 351
    diagnosis of, 351
    etiology of, 351
    medical management of, 351
    pathogenesis of, 351
    prognosis of, 351
Cerebrovascular accident. *See* Stroke

Cervical adenitis. *See* Cervical
    lymphadenitis
Cervical lymphadenitis
    complications of, 246
    dental management of, 246
    dental significance of, 246
    diagnosis of, 246
    medical management and treatment
      of, 246
    prognosis of, 246
Cervical lymphadenopathy. *See* Cervical
    lymphadenitis
Cervicofacial actinomycosis. *See*
    Actinomycosis
Cetirizine, 402
    contraindications of, 402
    dental considerations of, 402
    dosing of, 402
    interactions of, 402
    side effects of, 402
    uses of, 402
Cherubism, 247
    dental management of, 247
    dental significance of, 247
    diagnosis of, 247
    medical management and treatment
      of, 247
    prognosis of, 247
Chest cold. *See* Bronchitis (acute)
Chest pain
    ischemic, algorithm for, 507–508
    nonspecific, algorithm for, 509
Chicken pox. *See* Varicella-Zoster virus
    diseases
Child abuse and neglect, 51–53
    complications of, 52
    dental management of, 52–53
    dental significance of, 52
    diagnosis of, 51–52
    medical management and treatment
      of, 52
    prognosis of, 52
Child sexual abuse. *See* Child abuse and
    neglect
Chondroma, 248
    complications of, 248
    dental management of, 248
    dental significance of, 248
    diagnosis of, 248
    medical management and treatment
      of, 248
    prognosis of, 248
Chondrosarcoma, 285
Christmas disease. *See* Hemophilia
    (Types A, B, C)
Chronic atrophic candidosis. *See*
    Candidosis
Chronic cutaneous lupus
    erythematosus. *See* Discoid lupus
    erythematosus
Chronic GVHD. *See* Graft-*versus*-host
    disease
Chronic headaches. *See* Headaches:
    tension
Chronic hypertrophic candidosis. *See*
    Candidosis

Chronic lymphocytic leukemia. *See* Leukemias
Chronic myelocytic leukemia. *See* Leukemias; Myeloproliferative disorders
Chronic obstructive lung disease. *See* Chronic obstructive pulmonary disease
Chronic obstructive pulmonary disease, 54–57
  clinical characteristics of, 55t
  clinical classification of, 55
  complications of, 56
  dental management of, 56
  dental significance of, 56–57
  diagnosis of, 55
  medical management and treatment of, 55–56
  prognosis of, 56
  risk assessment of treatment of, 56t
Chronic osteomyelitis. *See* Osteomyelitis
Chronic renal disease, 487t. *See also* Renal disease, dialysis, and transplant
Cipro, 403f. *See also* Ciprofloxacin
Ciprofloxacin, 403
  contraindications of, 403
  dental considerations of, 403
  dosing of, 403
  interactions of, 403
  side effects of, 403
  uses of, 403
Citalopram, 404
  contraindications of, 404
  dental considerations of, 404
  dosing of, 404
  interactions of, 404
  side effects of, 404
  uses of, 404
Citanest, 467t. *See also* Prilocaine
Citanest Forte, 467t. *See also* Prilocaine
Clavulanic acid. *See* Amoxicillin acid
Cleidocranial dysplasia, 249
  complications of, 249
  dental management of, 249
  dental significance of, 249
  diagnosis of, 249
  medical management and treatment of, 249
  prognosis of, 249
Cleocin, 405f. *See also* Clindamycin
Clindamycin, 405
  contraindications of, 405
  dental considerations of, 405
  dosing of, 405
  interactions of, 405
  side effects of, 405
  uses of, 405
CLL. *See* Leukemias
Clonazepam, 406
  contraindications of, 406
  dental considerations of, 406
  dosing of, 406
  interactions of, 406
  side effects of, 406

Clonazepam—cont'd
  uses of, 406
Clopidogrel, 407
  contraindications of, 406
  dental considerations of, 406
  dosing of, 406
  interactions of, 406
  side effects of, 406
  uses of, 406
Clotting factor defects. *See* Coagulopathies (clotting factor defects, acquired)
Clotting factor deficiency. *See* Coagulopathies (clotting factor defects, acquired)
Cluster headaches. *See* Headaches: cluster
CML. *See* Leukemias
Coagulopathies (clotting factor defects, acquired), 58–59. *See also* Disseminated intravascular coagulopation
  complications of, 58
  dental management of, 59
  dental significance of, 58
  diagnosis of, 58
  prognosis of, 58
Coarctation of aorta, 60–61
  complications of, 60
  dental management of, 61
  dental significance of, 61
  diagnosis of, 60
  medical management and treatment of, 60
  prognosis of, 60
Cold sore. *See* Herpes simplex virus
Colitis. *See* Ulcerative colitis
Collapsed lung. *See* Pneumothorax
Common angina. *See* Angina pectoris
Conduction disorders. *See* Cardiac dysrhythmias
Condyloma acuminatum, 250. *See also* Human papilloma virus diseases
  complications of, 250
  dental significance of, 250
  diagnosis of, 250
  medical management and treatment of, 250
  prognosis of, 250
Congenital syphilis, 326
Congenital thrombocytopathia. *See* Thrombocytopathies (congenital and acquired)
Congenital toxoplasmosis. *See* Toxoplasmosis
Congestive cardiomyopathy. *See* Cardiomyopathy
Congestive heart failure, 62–64
  algorithm for, 510
  classification of, 62t
  complications of, 63
  dental management of, 63
  dental significance of, 63
  diagnosis of, 62–63

Congestive heart failure—cont'd
  medical management and treatment of, 63
  prognosis of, 63
Constitutional thrombopathy. *See* Von Willebrand's disease
Consumption coagulopathy. *See* Disseminated intravascular coagulation
Consumption. *See* Tuberculosis
Convulsive status epilepticus. *See* Status eplilepticus
Coronary artery atherosclerosis, 150
Coronary artery spasm. *See* Angina pectoris
Coronary failure. *See* Congestive heart failure
Coronary occlusion. *See* Myocardial infarction
Coronary thrombosis. *See* Myocardial infarction
Coronavirus, 33
Corticoadrenal insufficiency. *See* Addison's disease
Cough, algorithm for, 511
Coumadin, 452f. *See also* Warfarin
Coumarin anticoagulants, 484–485
Cranial arteritis, 251
  complications of, 251
  dental management of, 251
  dental significance of, 251
  diagnosis of, 251
  medical management and treatment of, 251
Craniofacial fibrous dysplasia. *See* Fibrous dysplasia
Craniopharyngioma, 252
  complications of, 252
  dental management of, 252
  dental significance of, 252
  diagnosis of, 252
  medical management and treatment of, 252
  prognosis of, 252
Crohn's disease, 65–66, 66
  complications of, 65
  dental management of, 66
  dental significance of, 66
  diagnosis of, 65
  medical management and treatment of, 65
  prognosis of, 65–66
Crown variation, 78
CVA. *See* Cerebral vascular accident
Cyclobenzaprine, 408
  contraindications of, 408
  dental considerations of, 408
  dosing of, 408
  interactions of, 408
  side effects of, 408
  uses of, 408
Cystic fibrosis, 67
  complications of, 67
  dental management of, 67
  dental significance of, 67
  diagnosis of, 67

Cystic fibrosis—cont'd
  medical management of, 67
  prognosis of, 67
Cystic hygroma. *See* Neck masses
  (differential diagnosis)

D

Darling's disease. *See* Histoplasmosis
Darvocet, 441f. *See also*
  Propoxyphene
Decreased platelet count. *See*
  Thrombocytopenia
Deep neck infection. *See* Ludwig's
  angina
Deep venous thrombosis (DVT), 68–69.
  See also Venous thrombosis
  complications of, 68
  dental management of, 68–69
  dental significance of, 68
  diagnosis of, 68
  medical management and treatment
    of, 68
  prognosis of, 68
Defibrillation, 38
Defibrination syndrome. *See*
  Disseminated intravascular
  coagulation
Degenerative joint disease. *See*
  Osteoarthritis
Delirium tremens, 352–353
  complications of, 352
  dental significance of, 352–353
  diagnosis of, 352
  etiology of, 352
  medical management of, 352
  pathogenesis of, 352
  prognosis of, 352
Deltasone, 440f. *See also* Prednisone
Demerol. *See* Meperidine
Dental caries, 78
Dentigerous cyst, 274
Dermatomyositis, 70
  complications of, 70
  dental management of, 70
  dental significance of, 70
  diagnosis of, 70
  medical management and treatment
    of, 70
  prognosis of, 70
Dermoid cyst
  complications of, 253
  dental management of, 253
  dental significance of, 253
  diagnosis of, 253
  medical management and treatment
    of, 253
  prognosis of, 253
Desflurane, 459
  contraindications of, 459
  dental considerations of, 459
  dosing of, 459
  interactions of, 459
  side effects of, 459
  uses of, 459
Desyrel, 448f. *See also* Trazodone

DiaBeta. *See* Glyburide
Diabetes insipidus, 71
  complications of, 71
  dental management of, 71
  dental significance of, 71
  diagnosis of, 71
  medical management and treatment
    of, 71
  prognosis of, 71
Diabetes mellitus, 72–74
  complications of, 73
  dental management of, 74–75
  dental significance of, 74
  diagnosis of, 73
  medical management and treatment
    of, 73
  prognosis of, 74
Diabetic hypoglycemia, 354–355
  complications of, 354
  dental significance of, 355
  diagnosis of, 354
  etiology of, 354
  medical management of, 354
  pathogenesis of, 354
  prognosis of, 354
Diabetic ketoacidosis (DKA), 73, 356
  complications of, 356
  dental significance of, 356
  diagnosis of, 356
  etiology of, 356
  medical management of, 356
  pathogenesis of, 356
  prognosis of, 356
Diazemuls. *See* Diazepam
Diazepam, 460–461
  contraindications of, 460
  dental considerations of, 461
  dosing of, 460
  interactions of, 460
  side effects of, 460
  uses of, 460
Diffuse intravascular coagulation. *See*
  Disseminated intravascular
  coagulation
Diffuse large B-cell lymphoma. *See*
  Non-Hodgkin's lymphoma
Digitalis, 40
Dilacor, 410f. *See also* Diltiazem
Dilated cardiomyopathy. *See*
  Cardiomyopathy
Diltiazem, 409–410
  contraindications of, 409
  dental considerations of, 409
  dosing of, 409
  interactions of, 409
  side effects of, 409
  uses of, 409
Diovan, 450f. *See also* Valsartan
Diphenhydramine, 462
  contraindications of, 462
  dental considerations of, 462
  dosing of, 462
  interactions of, 462
  side effects of, 462
  uses of, 462

Diprivan. *See* Propofol
Discoid lupus erythematosus, 254
  complications of, 254
  dental management of, 254
  dental significance of, 254
  diagnosis of, 254
  medical management and treatment
    of, 254
  prognosis of, 254
Disseminated intravascular coagulation,
  76. *See also* Coagulopathies
  (clotting factor defects, acquired)
  complications of, 76
  dental management of, 76
  dental significance of, 76
  diagnosis of, 76
  medical management and treatment
    of, 76
  prognosis of, 76
Disseminated lupus erythematosous. *See*
  Systemic lupus erythematosus
Disseminated sclerosis. *See* Multiple
  sclerosis
Dizziness, algorithm for, 512
DKA. *See* Diabetic ketoacidosis
Down syndrome, 77–79
  dental management of, 79
  dental significance of, 78–79
  diagnosis of, 78
  medical management and treatment
    of, 78
  prognosis of, 78
Dry eye syndrome. *See* Sjögren's
  syndrome
Dry mouth syndrome. *See* Sjögren's
  syndrome
Dry socket, 357
  complications of, 357
  dental management of, 357
  dental significance of, 357
  diagnosis of, 357
  etiology of, 357
  medical management of, 357
  pathogenesis of, 357
  prognosis of, 357
DTs. *See* Delirium tremens
Duragesic. *See* Fentanyl
DVT. *See* Venous thrombosis
Dynacin, 430f. *See also* Minocycline
Dyrenium. *See* Triamterene
Dyspepsia, algorithm for, 513
Dyspnea, algorithm for, 514

E

Eating disorder. *See* Bulimia nervosa;
  Anorexia nervosa
EBV. *See* Epstein-Barr virus diseases:
  infectious mononucleosis
Eclampsia. *See* Pregnancy
Eczema herpeticum. *See* Herpes simplex
  virus
EM. *See* Erythema multiforme (Stevens-
  Johnson syndrome)
Emesis. *See* Nausea
EMLA. *See* Prilocaine-Lidocaine

Emotional abuse. *See* Child abuse and neglect
Emphysema. *See* Chronic obstructive pulmonary disease
Enalapril, 411
  contraindications of, 411
  dental considerations of, 411
  dosing of, 411
  interactions of, 411
  side effects of, 411
  uses of, 411
Enchondroma. *See* Chondroma
Endemic Burkitt's lymphoma. *See* Burkitt's lymphoma
Endemic parotitis. *See* Mumps
Endocarditis (infective), 44, 80–81
  complications of, 81
  dental management of, 81
  dental significance of, 81
  diagnosis of, 80–81
  medical management and treatment of, 81
  prognosis of, 81
Endolymphatic hydrops. *See* Ménière's disease
Endothelial cell sarcoma. *See* Kaposi's sarcoma
End-stage liver disease. *See* Hepatic cirrhosis
End-stage renal disease (ESRD). *See* Renal disease, dialysis, and transplant
Enterobacter, 33
Enterovirus, 33
Eosinophilic granuloma. *See* Langerhans cell histiocytosis
Epidemic parotitis. *See* Mumps
Epidermoid carcinoma of floor of mouth. *See* Squamous cell carcinoma of floor of mouth
Epidermoid carcinoma of lip. *See* Squamous cell carcinoma of lip
Epidermoid carcinoma of tongue. *See* Squamous cell carcinoma of tongue
Epidermoid cyst. *See* Dermoid cyst
Epilepsy. *See* Seizure disorders
Epinephrine. *See* Articaine with epinephrine; Bupivacaine with epinephrine; Lidocaine; Medication overdose: epinephrine
Epistaxis, 358
  complications of, 358
  dental management of, 358
  diagnosis of, 358
  etiology of, 358
  medical management of, 358
  pathogenesis of, 358
  prognosis of, 358
Epstein-Barr virus diseases: Hairy leukoplakia, 82
  dental management of, 82
  dental significance of, 82
  diagnosis of, 82

Epstein-Barr virus diseases: Hairy leukoplakia—cont'd
  medical management and treatment of, 82
  prognosis of, 82
Epstein-Barr virus diseases: infectious mononucleosis, 83–84
  complications of, 83–84
  dental management of, 84
  dental significance of, 84
  diagnosis of, 83
  medical management and treatment of, 83
  prognosis of, 84
Erythema multiforme, 85–86. *See also* Stevens-Johnson syndrome
  complications of, 85
  dental management of, 85
  dental significance of, 85
  diagnosis of, 85
  medical management and treatment of, 85
  prognosis of, 85
Erythroblastphthisis. *See* Aplastic anemia
Erythroleukoplakia. *See* Leukoplakia
Escitalopram, 412
  contraindications of, 412
  dental considerations of, 412
  dosing of, 412
  interactions of, 412
  side effects of, 412
  uses of, 412
Esomeprazole, 413
  contraindications of, 413
  dental considerations of, 413
  dosing of, 413
  interactions of, 413
  side effects of, 413
  uses of, 413
Essential hypertension. *See* Hypertension
Essential thrombocytosis. *See* Myeloproliferative disorders
Ethanol abuse. *See* Alcoholism
Ewing's sarcoma, 285
Exercise-induced asthma. *See* Asthma
Exostosis
  complications of, 328
  dental management of, 328–329
  diagnosis of, 328
  medical management and treatment of, 328
  prognosis of, 328
Exposure, algorithm for, 506
Extrinsic asthma. *See* Asthma

F
Factor IX deficiency. *See* Hemophilia (Types A, B, C)
Factor VIII deficiency. *See* Hemophilia (Types A, B, C)
Factor VIII deficiency with vascular defect. *See* Von Willebrand's disease
Factor XI deficiency. *See* Hemophilia (Types A, B, C)

Fainting. *See* Syncope
Familial fibrous dysplasia. *See* Cherubism
Fast, deep breathing. *See* Hyperventilation
FBO. *See* Airway obstruction
Fentanyl, 463
  contraindications of, 463
  dental considerations of, 463
  dosing of, 463
  interactions of, 463
  side effects of, 463
  uses of, 463
Fetation. *See* Pregnancy
Fever, algorithm for, 515–516
Fever blister. *See* Herpes simplex virus
Fexofenadine, 414
  contraindications of, 414
  dental considerations of, 414
  dosing of, 414
  interactions of, 414
  side effects of, 414
  uses of, 414
Fibrinolytic osteitis. *See* Dry socket
Fibrinolytic purpura. *See* Disseminated intravascular coagulation
Fibrocystic disease of pancreas. *See* Cystic fibrosis
Fibroma. *See* Traumatic fibroma
Fibrooseous lesions. *See* Fibrous dysplasia
Fibrous dysplasia, 255
  complications of, 256
  dental management of, 256
  dental significance of, 256
  diagnosis of, 255
  medical management and treatment of, 255–256
  prognosis of, 256
Fibrous nodule. *See* Traumatic fibroma
Filiform papilloma. *See* Human papilloma virus diseases
Flexeril, 408f. *See also* Cyclobenzaprine
Flonase. *See* Fluticasone
Fluoxetine, 415
  contraindications of, 415
  dental considerations of, 415
  dosing of, 415
  interactions of, 415
  side effects of, 415
  uses of, 415
Fluticasone, 416
  contraindications of, 416
  dental considerations of, 416
  dosing of, 416
  interactions of, 416
  side effects of, 416
  uses of, 416
Focal epithelial hyperplasia. *See* Human papilloma virus diseases
Focal fibrous hyperplasia. *See* Traumatic fibroma
Follicular ameloblastoma. *See* Ameloblastoma

Follicular lymphoma. *See* Non-Hodgkin's lymphoma
Foreign body ingestion, algorithm for, 517
Foreign body obstruction (FBO). *See* Airway obstruction
Fortamet. *See* Metformin
Fosamax, 392f. *See also* Alendronate
Fothergill's disease. *See* Trigeminal neuralgia
Furosemide, 417
  contraindications of, 417
  dental considerations of, 417
  dosing of, 417
  interactions of, 417
  side effects of, 417
  uses of, 417

G
Gabapentin, 418
  contraindications of, 418
  dental considerations of, 418
  dosing of, 418
  interactions of, 418
  side effects of, 418
  uses of, 418
Gastroesophageal reflux disease, 87–88
  complications of, 87
  dental management of, 87–88
  dental significance of, 87
  diagnosis of, 87
  medical management and treatment of, 87
  prognosis of, 87
Genital herpes. *See* Herpes simplex virus
GERD. *See* Gastroesophageal reflux disease
Gestation. *See* Pregnancy
Gestational diabetes. *See* Pregnancy
Giant cell arteritis. *See* Cranial arteritis; Polymyalgia rheumatica
Giant cell tumor. *See* Central giant cell granuloma
Glandular fever. *See* Epstein-Barr virus diseases: Infectious mononucleosis
Glanzmann's thrombasthenia. *See* Thrombocytopathies (congenital and acquired)
Glipizide, 419
  contraindications of, 419
  dental considerations of, 419
  dosing of, 419
  interactions of, 419
  side effects of, 419
  uses of, 419
Glossitis, 257
  complications of, 257
  dental management of, 257
  dental significance of, 257
  diagnosis of, 257
  medical management and treatment of, 257
  prognosis of, 257

Glossodynia exfoliativa. *See* Glossitis
Glossodynia. *See* Burning mouth syndrome
Glossopharyngeal neuralgia, 258
  complications of, 258
  dental management of, 258
  diagnosis of, 258
  medical management and treatment of, 258
Glottic carcinoma. *See* Laryngeal carcinoma
Glucophage, 428f. *See also* Metformin
Glucotrol, 419f. *See also* Glipizide
Glyburide, 420
  contraindications of, 420
  dental considerations of, 420
  dosing of, 420
  interactions of, 420
  side effects of, 420
  uses of, 420
Glycopyrrolate, 464
  contraindications of, 464
  dental considerations of, 464
  dosing of, 464
  interactions of, 464
  side effects of, 464
  uses of, 464
Glynase, 420f. *See also* Glyburide
Goitrous hypothyroidism. *See* Hypothyroidism
Gougerot-Sjögren disease. *See* Sjögren's syndrome
Gout, 89, 259
  complications of, 89, 259
  dental management of, 89, 259
  dental significance of, 89, 259
  diagnosis of, 89, 259
  medical management and treatment of, 89, 259
  prognosis of, 89, 259
Graft-*versus*-host disease, 90–91
  complications of, 90
  dental management of, 91
  dental significance of, 90–91
  diagnosis of, 90
  medical management and treatment of, 90
  prognosis of, 90
Grand mal seizures. *See* Seizures
Granuloma pyogenicum. *See* Pyogenic granuloma
Graves' disease. *See* Hyperthyroidism
Gravidism. *See* Pregnancy
"Great imitator." *See* Syphilis
GVHD. *See* Graft-*versus*-host disease

H
Hairy cell leukemia. *See* Leukemias
Hairy tongue, 260
  complications of, 260
  dental management of, 260
  diagnosis of, 260
  medical management and treatment of, 260
  prognosis of, 260

Halcion. *See* Triazolam
Hand-Schüller-Christian syndrome. *See* Langerhans cell histiocytosis
Hashimoto's thyroiditis. *See* Hyperthyroidism
Headache, algorithm for, 518
Headaches: cluster, 92
  complications of, 92, 261
  dental management of, 92, 261
  dental significance of, 92
  diagnosis of, 92, 261
  medical management of, 92, 261
  prognosis of, 92, 261
Headaches: migraine, 93
  complications of, 93, 262
  dental management of, 93, 262
  dental significance of, 93
  diagnosis of, 93, 262
  medical management and treatment of, 93, 262
  prognosis of, 93, 262
Headaches: tension
  complications of, 94
  dental management of, 94
  dental significance of, 94
  diagnosis of, 94
  medical management and treatment of, 94
  prognosis of, 94
Heart attack. *See* Myocardial infarction
Heart failure. *See* Congestive heart failure
Heart murmur, algorithm for, 520–521
Heartburn, algorithm for, 519
Hemangioma, 263
  complications of, 263
  dental management of, 263
  dental significance of, 263
  diagnosis of, 263
  medical management and treatment of, 263
  prognosis of, 263
Hemangioma (soft tissue), 264
  complications of, 264
  dental management of, 264
  diagnosis of, 264
  medical management and treatment of, 264
  prognosis of, 264
Hematuria, algorithm for, 522
Hemicrania. *See* Headaches: migraine
Hemifacial spasm. *See* Trigeminal neuralgia
Hemoglobin S disease. *See* Anemia: sickle cell
Hemophilia (Types A, B, C), 95
  complications of, 95
  dental management of, 95
  dental significance of, 95
  diagnosis of, 95
  medical management and treatment of, 95
Hemorrhagic fibrinogenolysis. *See* Disseminated intravascular coagulation

Hepatic cirrhosis, 96–97
  complications of, 97
  dental management of, 97
  dental significance of, 97
  diagnosis of, 96–97
  medical management and treatment
    of, 97
  prognosis of, 97
Hepatic dysfunction, 486
Hepatic failure. *See* Thrombocytopathies
  (congenital and acquired)
Hepatitis A virus. *See* Hepatitis: Viral
Hepatitis: alcoholic, 100–101
  complications of, 100
  dental management of, 100
  dental significance of, 100
  diagnosis of, 100
  medical management and treatment
    of, 100–101
  prognosis of, 100
Hepatitis B virus. *See* Hepatitis: viral
Hepatitis C virus. *See* Hepatitis: viral
Hepatitis D virus. *See* Hepatitis: viral
Hepatitis E virus. *See* Hepatitis: viral
Hepatitis, exposure to, algorithm for,
  523
Hepatitis: general concepts, 98–99
  complications of, 99
  dental management of, 99
  dental significance of, 99
  diagnosis of, 99
  etiologies and clinical signs associated
    with, 98t
  medical management and treatment
    of, 99
  prognosis of, 99
Hepatitis: viral, 102–104
  complications of, 103
  dental management of, 104
  dental significance of, 104
  diagnosis of, 103
  medical management and treatment
    of, 103
  prognosis of, 103–104
Hereditary angioedema, 22
Hereditary angioneurotic edema (HAE).
  See Angioneurotic edema
Hereditary hemorrhagic telangiectasia,
  105
  complications of, 105
  dental management of, 105
  dental significance of, 105
  diagnosis of, 105
  medical management and treatment
    of, 105
  prognosis of, 105
Hereditary intestinal polyposis
  syndrome. *See* Peutz-Jeghers
  syndrome
Herpangina, 265
  dental management of, 265
  diagnosis of, 265
  medical management and treatment
    of, 265
  prognosis of, 265

Herpes digitalis. *See* Herpes simplex
  virus
Herpes gladiatorum. *See* Herpes simplex
  virus
Herpes simplex virus, 106–107, 266
  complications of, 107, 266
  dental management of, 107, 266
  dental significance of, 107, 266
  diagnosis of, 107, 266
  medical management and treatment
    of, 107, 266
  prognosis of, 107, 266
Herpes zoster, 267. *See also*
  Varicella-Zoster virus diseases
  complications of, 267
  dental management of, 267
  dental significance of, 267
  diagnosis of, 267
  medical management and treatment
    of, 267
  prognosis of, 267
HHT. *See* Hereditary hemorrhagic
  telangiectasia
High blood pressure. *See* Hypertension
Histamine cephalgia. *See* Headaches:
  cluster
Histamine headache. *See* Headaches:
  cluster
Histiocytosis X. *See* Langerhans cell
  histiocytosis
Histoplasmosis, 268
  dental management of, 268
  diagnosis of, 268
  medical management and treatment
    of, 268
  prognosis of, 268
HIV. *See* Human immunodeficiency
  virus
Hodgkin's disease, 108–109, 269
  complications of, 108–109, 269
  dental management of, 109
  dental significance of, 109
  diagnosis of, 108, 269
  medical management and treatment
    of, 108, 269
  prognosis of, 109, 269
Homozygous HbS condition. *See*
  Anemia: sickle cell
Horton headache. *See* Headaches:
  cluster
HSV. *See* Herpes simplex virus
Human herpes virus 4 (HHV-4). *See*
  Epstein-Barr virus diseases:
  infectious mononucleosis
Human immunodeficiency virus (HIV),
  110–111
  complications of, 110
  dental management of, 111
  dental significance of, 111
  diagnosis of, 110
  medical management and treatment
    of, 110
  prognosis of, 110–111
Human papilloma virus diseases,
  112–113

Human papilloma virus diseases
  —cont'd
  complications of, 112
  dental management of, 113
  dental significance of, 113
  diagnosis of, 112
  medical management and treatment
    of, 112
  prognosis of, 112
Hunter's glossitis. *See* Glossitis
Hydrochlorothiazide, 421
  contraindications of, 421
  dental considerations of, 421
  dosing of, 421
  interactions of, 421
  side effects of, 421
  uses of, 421
Hydrocodone, 422
  with acetaminophen, 422
  contraindications of, 422
  dental considerations of, 422
  dosing of, 422
  with ibuprofen, 422
  interactions of, 422
  side effects of, 422
  uses of, 422
Hyperkeratosis. *See* Leukoplakia
Hyperlipidemia, algorithm for, 524–525
Hyperosmolar hyperglycemic nonketotic
  coma (HHNC), 73
Hyperparathyroidism, 114–115, 271
  complications of, 114, 271
  dental management of, 115, 271
  dental significance of, 115, 271
  diagnosis of, 114, 271
  medical management and treatment
    of, 114, 271
  prognosis of, 114, 271
Hyperplastic scar. *See* Traumatic fibroma
Hyperreactive airway disease. *See*
  Asthma
Hypersensitivity reactions (types I-IV).
  See Allergic reactions
Hypertension, 116–118. *See also*
  Pregnancy
  complications of, 117
  dental management of, 117–118
  dental significance of, 117
  diagnosis of, 117
  medical management and treatment
    of, 117
  prognosis of, 117
Hypertensive crisis. *See* Malignant
  hypertension
Hypertensive emergencies. *See*
  Malignant hypertension
Hypertensive urgency. *See* Malignant
  hypertension
Hyperthyroidism, 119–121. *See also*
  Neck masses (differential
  diagnosis)
  complications of, 120
  dental management of, 120–121
  dental significance of, 120
  diagnosis of, 119–120

Hyperthyroidism—cont'd
  medical management and treatment
    of, 120
  prognosis of, 120
Hypertrophic cardiomyopathy. *See*
  Cardiomyopathy
Hypertrophic obstructive
  cardiomyopathy. *See*
  Cardiomyopathy
Hyperventilation, 359
  complications of, 359
  dental significance of, 359
  diagnosis of, 359
  etiology of, 359
  medical management of, 359
  pathogenesis of, 359
  prognosis of, 359
Hyperventilation syndrome. *See*
  Hyperventilation
Hypocalcification, 78
Hypodontia, 78
Hypoglycemia, 360. *See also* Diabetic
  hypoglycemia
  algorithm for, 526
  complications of, 360
  dental significance of, 360
  diagnosis of, 360
  etiology of, 360
  medical management of, 360
  pathogenesis of, 360
  prognosis of, 360
Hypokinetic syndrome. *See* Parkinson's
  disease
Hypoplasia, 78
Hypoplasia of hematopoietic stem cells,
  208
Hypoplastic anemia. *See* Aplastic
  anemia
Hypoprothrombinemia. *See*
  Coagulopathies (clotting factor
  defects, acquired)
Hypothyroidism, 122–124
  complications of, 123
  dental management of, 123–124
  dental significance of, 123
  diagnosis of, 123
  medical management and treatment
    of, 123

I

Ibuprofen, compounds with, 422
Idiopathic histiocytosis. *See* Langerhans
  cell histiocytosis
Idiopathic hypertension. *See*
  Hypertension
Idiopathic hypertrophic subaortic
  stenosis. *See* Cardiomyopathy
Idiopathic inflammatory myopathy. *See*
  Dermatomyositis
Idiopathic thrombocytopenic purpura
  (ITP), 125
  complications of, 125
  dental management of, 125
  dental significance of, 125
  diagnosis of, 125

Idiopathic thrombocytopenic purpura
  (ITP)—cont'd
  medical management and treatment
    of, 125
Idiosyncratic asthma. *See* Asthma
IgE-mediated angioedema, 22
Imdur, 423f. *See also* Isosorbide
  mononitrate
Immune thrombocytopenic purpura. *See*
  Idiopathic thrombocytopenic
  purpura
Implantable cardioverter-defibrillator,
  38
Inappropriate secretion of antidiuretic
  hormone, 126–128
  complications of, 127
  conditions associated with, 127t
  dental management of, 127–128
  dental significance of, 127
  diagnosis of, 126
  medical management and treatment
    of, 126–127
  prognosis of, 127
Ineffective endocarditis, 44
Ineffective thrombocytopoiesis, 208
Infectious mononucleosis. *See also*
  Epstein-Barr virus diseases
  complications of, 272–273
  dental significance of, 273
  diagnosis of, 272
  medical management and treatment
    of, 272
  prognosis of, 273
Infective endocarditis, 44. *See also*
  Endocarditis (infective)
Inflammatory bowel disease. *See*
  Crohn's disease; Ulcerative colitis
Insulin shock. *See* Diabetic
  hypoglycemia
Insulin-dependent diabetes mellitus. *See*
  Diabetes mellitus
Intrinsic asthma. *See* Asthma
Iron deficiency anemia. *See* Anemia:
  iron deficiency
Irritation fibroma. *See* Traumatic
  fibroma
Ismo. *See* Isosorbide mononitrate
Isolated ectopic beats, 35–36
Isoptin, 451f. *See also* Verapamil
Isosorbide mononitrate, 423
  contraindications of, 423
  dental considerations of, 423
  dosing of, 423
  interactions of, 423
  side effects of, 423
  uses of, 423
ITP. *See* Idiopathic thrombocytopenic
  purpura

J

Jaw cancer. *See* Malignant jaw tumors
Jaw cysts, 274
  dental management of, 274
  dental significance of, 274
  diagnosis of, 274

Jaw cysts—cont'd
  medical management and treatment
    of, 274
  prognosis of, 274
Jitters. *See* Delirium tremens
Juvenile onset diabetes mellitus. *See*
  Diabetes mellitus

K

Kahler's disease. *See* Multiple
  myeloma
Kaposi's sarcoma, 275–276
  diagnosis of, 275
  medical management and treatment
    of, 275
  prognosis of, 275
Keflex. *See* Cephalexin
Keftab. *See* Cephalexin
Keratoacanthoma, 277
  diagnosis of, 277
  medical management and treatment
    of, 277
  prognosis of, 277
Keratoconjunctivitis sicca. *See* Sjögren's
  syndrome
Keratosis: actinic, 278
  complications of, 278
  diagnosis of, 278
  medical management and treatment
    of, 278
  prognosis of, 278
Ketalar. *See* Ketamine
Ketamine, 465
  contraindications of, 465
  dental considerations of, 465
  dosing of, 465
  interactions of, 465
  side effects of, 465
  uses of, 465
Kidney disease. *See* Renal disease,
  dialysis, and transplant
Kidney transplant. *See* Renal disease,
  dialysis, and transplant
Kissing disease. *See* Epstein-Barr virus
  diseases: infectious mononucleosis
Klonopin, 406f. *See also* Clonazepam

L

Labial herpes. *See* Herpes simplex
  virus
Langerhans cell histiocytosis, 129–131
  complications of, 130
  dental management of, 131
  dental significance of, 131
  diagnosis of, 129–130
  medical management and treatment
    of, 130
  prognosis of, 130
Lansoprazole, 424
  contraindications of, 424
  dental considerations of, 424
  dosing of, 424
  interactions of, 424
  side effects of, 424
  uses of, 424

Laryngeal carcinoma, 279
  dental management of, 279
  diagnosis of, 279
  medical management of, 279
  prognosis of, 279
Laryngospasm, 361
  complications of, 361
  dental management of, 361
  diagnosis of, 361
  etiology of, 361
  medical management of, 361
  pathogenesis of, 361
  prognosis of, 361
Lasix. *See* Furosemide
Latent tuberculosis infection, 212
Latex allergy, 362
  complications of, 362
  delayed hypersensitivity of, 362
  dental significance of, 362
  diagnosis of, 362
  etiology of, 362
  immediate hypersensitivity of, 362
  medical management of, 362
  pathogenesis of, 362
  prognosis of, 362
Lermoyez's syndrome. *See* Ménière's
    disease
Letterer-Siwe disease. *See* Langerhans
    cell histiocytosis
Leukemias, 132–135
  categories of, 132f
  complications of, 134
  dental management of, 135
  dental significance of, 134
  diagnosis of, 133
  medical management and treatment
    of, 133–134
  prognosis of, 134
  survival rates for, 134t
Leukokeratosis. *See* Leukoplakia
Leukoplakia, 280
  complications of, 280
  diagnosis of, 280
  medical management and treatment
    of, 280
  prognosis of, 280
Lexapro. *See* Escitalopram
Lichen planus, 281
  diagnosis of, 281
  medical management and treatment
    of, 281
  prognosis of, 281
Lidocaine, 466
  contraindications of, 466
  dental considerations of, 466
  dosing of, 466
  interactions of, 466
  side effects of, 466
  uses of, 466
Lipitor, 397f. *See also* Atorvastatin
Lisinopril, 425
  contraindications of, 425
  dental considerations of, 425
  dosing of, 425
  interactions of, 425

Lisinopril—cont'd
  side effects of, 425
  uses of, 425
Liver cirrhosis. *See* Hepatic cirrhosis
Local anesthetic, 482. *See also*
    Medication overdose: local
    anesthetic
Lockjaw. *See* Tetanus
Lopressor. *See* Metoprolol
Lorazepam, 426
  contraindications of, 426
  dental considerations of, 426
  dosing of, 426
  interactions of, 426
  side effects of, 426
  uses of, 426
Lorcet. *See* Hydrocodone
Lortab. *See* Hydrocodone
Lovastatin, 427
  contraindications of, 427
  dental considerations of, 427
  dosing of, 427
  interactions of, 427
  side effects of, 427
  uses of, 427
Low blood sugar. *See* Diabetic
    hypoglycemia; Hypoglycemia
Low platelet count. *See*
    Thrombocytopenia
Ludwig's angina, 282, 363
  complications of, 282, 363
  dental management of, 282, 363
  diagnosis of, 282, 363
  etiology of, 363
  medical management and treatment
    of, 282
  medical management of, 363
  pathogenesis of, 363
  prognosis of, 282, 363
Lues. *See* Syphilis
Lumpy jaw. *See* Actinomycosis
Lung: primary malignancy, 283
  dental management of, 283
  diagnosis of, 283
  medical management and treatment
    of, 283
  prognosis of, 283
Lyme borreliosis. *See* Lyme disease
Lyme disease, 284
  complications of, 284
  diagnosis of, 284
  medical management and treatment
    of, 284
  prognosis of, 284
Lymph node cancer. *See* Hodgkin's
    disease
Lymph node masses, 294
Lymphadenitis. *See* Cervical
    lymphadenitis
Lymphadenopathy, algorithm for,
    527

M
Major erythema multiforme. *See*
    Erythema multiforme

Malignant hyperpyrexia. *See* Malignant
    hyperthermia
Malignant hypertension, 364–365
  complications of, 364
  dental significance of, 364
  diagnosis of, 364
  etiology of, 364
  medical management of, 364
  pathogenesis of, 364
  prognosis of, 364
Malignant hyperthermia, 366
  complications of, 366
  dental significance of, 366
  diagnosis of, 366
  etiology of, 366
  medical management of, 366
  pathogenesis of, 366
  prognosis of, 366
Malignant jaw tumors, 285
  diagnosis of, 285
  medical management and treatment
    of, 285
  prognosis of, 285
Malignant lymphoma. *See* Hodgkin's
    disease
Malignant melanoma. *See* Melanoma
Malocclusion, 79
Mandibular tori. *See* Tori
Marcaine with epinephrine. *See*
    Bupivacaine with epinephrine
Marfan-Achard syndrome. *See* Marfan's
    syndrome
Marfan's syndrome, 136–137
  complications of, 136
  dental management of, 137
  dental significance of, 136–137
  diagnosis of, 136
  medical management and treatment
    of, 136
  prognosis of, 136
Marie-Sainton syndrome. *See*
    Cleidocranial dysplasia
MAT. *See* Atrial tachycardia
Median rhomboid glossitis, 286
  diagnosis of, 286
  medical management and treatment
    of, 286
  prognosis of, 286
Medication overdose
  epinephrine, 367
    complications of, 367
    dental significance of, 367
    medical management of, 367
    prognosis of, 367
  local anesthetic, 368
    complications of, 368
    dental management of, 368
    etiology of, 368
    medical management of, 368
    pathogenesis of, 368
    prognosis of, 368
  narcotic/analgesic, 369
    complications of, 369
    dental significance of, 369
    medical management of, 369

Medication overdose—cont'd
    prognosis of, 369
    sedative, 370
      complications of, 370
      dental significance of, 370
      etiology of, 370
      medical management of, 370
      pathogenesis of, 370
      prognosis of, 370
Megaloblastic anemia. *See* Anemia:
    pernicious
Melanocarcinoma. *See* Melanoma
Melanoma, 287
    diagnosis of, 287
    medical management and treatment
      of, 287
    prognosis of, 287
Ménière's disease, 138
    complications of, 138
    dental management of, 138
    dental significance of, 138
    diagnosis of, 138
    medical management and treatment
      of, 138
    prognosis of, 138
Meperidine, 468
    contraindications of, 468
    dental considerations of, 468
    dosing of, 468
    interactions of, 468
    side effects of, 468
    uses of, 468
Mepivacaine, 469
    contraindications of, 469
    dental considerations of, 469
    dosing of, 469
    interactions of, 469
    side effects of, 469
    uses of, 469
Mesothelioma. *See* Lung: primary
    malignancy
Metastatic tumor, 285
Metformin, 428
    contraindications of, 428
    dental considerations of, 428
    dosing of, 428
    interactions of, 428
    side effects of, 428
    uses of, 428
Methohexital, 470
    contraindications of, 470
    dental considerations of, 470
    dosing of, 470
    interactions of, 470
    side effects of, 470
    uses of, 470
Metoprolol, 429
    contraindications of, 429
    dental considerations of, 429
    dosing of, 429
    interactions of, 429
    side effects of, 429
    uses of, 429
Mevacor. *See* Lovastatin
MI. *See* Myocardial infarction

Microdontia, 78
Micronase. *See* Glyburide
Microzide, 421f. *See also*
    Hydrochlorothiazide
Midazolam, 471
    contraindications of, 471
    dental considerations of, 471
    dosing of, 471
    interactions of, 471
    side effects of, 471
    uses of, 471
Migraine headaches. *See* Headaches:
    migraine
Migrainous neuralgia. *See* Headaches:
    cluster
Minocin, 430f. *See also* Minocycline
Minocycline, 430
    contraindications of, 430
    dental considerations of, 430
    dosing of, 430
    interactions of, 430
    side effects of, 430
    uses of, 430
Mirtazapine, 431
    contraindications of, 431
    dental considerations of, 431
    dosing of, 431
    interactions of, 431
    side effects of, 431
    uses of, 431
Mitral insufficiency. *See* Cardiac valvular
    disease
Mitral stenosis. *See* Cardiac valvular
    disease
Mitral valve prolapse, 44
Moeller's glossitis. *See* Glossitis
Mongoloidism. *See* Down syndrome
Mono. *See* Epstein-Barr virus diseases:
    infectious mononucleosis
Monocytic angina. *See* Infectious
    mononucleosis
Monoket. *See* Isosorbide mononitrate
Monostotic fibrous dysplasia. *See*
    Fibrous dysplasia
Montelukast, 432
    contraindications of, 432
    dental considerations of, 432
    dosing of, 432
    interactions of, 432
    side effects of, 432
    uses of, 432
MS. *See* Multiple sclerosis
Mucocele (mucus retention
    phenomenon), 289
    diagnosis of, 289
    medical management and treatment
      of, 289
    prognosis of, 289
Mucocutaneous ocular syndrome. *See*
    Behçet's syndrome
Mucoepidermoid carcinoma, 290
    complications of, 290
    diagnosis of, 290
    medical management and treatment
      of, 290

Mucoepidermoid carcinoma—cont'd
    prognosis of, 290
Mucosa-associated lymphoid tissue
    lymphoma. *See* Non-Hodgkin's
    lymphoma
Mucoviscidosis. *See* Cystic fibrosis
Mucus escape reaction. *See* Mucocele
    (mucus retention phenomenon)
Mucus extravasation phenomena. *See*
    Mucocele (mucus retention
    phenomenon)
Mucus retention cyst. *See* Mucocele
    (mucus retention phenomenon)
Multifocal atrial tachycardia (MAT). *See*
    Atrial tachycardia
Multiple drug-resistant tuberculosis, 213
Multiple endocrine neoplasia
    syndromes, 291
    complications of, 291
    dental management of, 291
    dental significance of, 291
    diagnosis of, 291
    medical management and treatment
      of, 291
    prognosis of, 291
Multiple myeloma, 139–140
    complications of, 139–140
    dental management of, 140
    dental significance of, 140
    diagnosis of, 139
    medical management and treatment
      of, 139
    prognosis of, 140
Multiple sclerosis, 141–142
    complications of, 141
    dental management of, 141
    dental significance of, 141
    diagnosis of, 141
    medical management and treatment
      of, 141
    prognosis of, 141
Mumps, 143
    complications of, 143
    dental management of, 143
    dental significance of, 143
    diagnosis of, 143
    medical management and treatment
      of, 143
    prognosis of, 143
Muscle contraction headaches. *See*
    Headaches: tension
Muscular dystrophy, 144–146
    clinical features of, 145t
    complications of, 144
    dental management of, 146
    dental significance of, 146
    diagnosis of, 144
    major types of, 144t
    medical management and treatment
      of, 144
    prognosis of, 144–146
Myasthenia gravis
    complications of, 148
    dental management of, 148–149
    dental significance of, 148

Myasthenia gravis—cont'd
diagnosis of, 147–148
medical management and treatment of, 148
prognosis of, 148
Myelofibrosis. *See* Myeloproliferative disorders
Myeloma. *See* Multiple myeloma
Myeloproliferative disorders, 292–293. *See also* Thrombocytopathies (congenital and acquired)
complications of, 293
dental significance of, 293
diagnosis of, 292
medical management and treatment of, 292–293
prognosis of, 293
Myocardial infarction, 150–152, 371–372
complications, 151–152
complications of, 151–152, 371–372
dental significance of, 372
diagnosis of, 151, 371
etiology of, 371
medical management and treatment of, 151, 371
pathogenesis of, 371
prognosis of, 372
Myocardial ischemia. *See* Angina pectoris
Myocardial necrosis, 150
Myxedema. *See* Hypothyroidism
Myxomatous degeneration, 44

N

Nabumetone, 433
contraindications of, 433
dental considerations of, 433
dosing of, 433
interactions of, 433
side effects of, 433
uses of, 433
Narcotic overdose. *See* Medication overdose: narcotic/analgesic
Natural latex allergy. *See* Latex allergy
Natural rubber latex (NRL) allergy. *See* Latex allergy
Nausea, 373–374
algorithm for, 528
complications of, 373
dental significance of, 374
etiology of, 373
medical management of, 373
pathogenesis of, 373
prognosis of, 373
Neck masses (differential diagnosis), 294–295
complications of, 295
dental management of, 295
diagnosis of, 294
medical management and treatment of, 294
prognosis of, 295
Neglect. *See* Child abuse and neglect

Nephrosis. *See* Nephrotic syndrome
Nephrotic syndrome, 153–154
complications of, 154
dental management of, 154
dental significance of, 154
diagnosis of, 153–154
medical management and treatment of, 154
prognosis of, 154
Neurogenic diabetes insipidus. *See* Diabetes insipidus
Neurontin, 418f. *See also* Gabapentin
Nexium, 413f. *See* Esomeprazole
NHL. *See* Non-Hodgkin's lymphoma (NHL)
Nicotine palatinus. *See* Nicotine stomatitis
Nicotine stomatitis, 296
complications of, 296
dental management of, 296
dental significance of, 296
diagnosis of, 296
medical management and treatment of, 296
prognosis of, 296
Nifedical. *See* Nifedipine
Nifedipine, 434
contraindications of, 434
dental considerations of, 434
dosing of, 434
interactions of, 434
side effects of, 434
uses of, 434
Niravam. *See* Alprazolam
Nitrous oxide, 472–473
contraindications of, 472
dental considerations of, 472
dosing of, 472
interactions of, 472
side effects of, 472
uses of, 472
Nonautoimmune hypothyroidism. *See* Hypothyroidism
Nonbacterial regional lymphadenitis. *See* Cat-scratch disease
Nonconvulsive status epilepticus. *See* Status eplilepticus
Non-Hodgkin's lymphoma (NHL), 155–156
complications of, 155
dental management of, 156
dental significance of, 156
diagnosis of, 155
medical management and treatment of, 155
prognosis of, 155–156
staging of, 156t
Noninsulin-dependent diabetes mellitus. *See* Diabetes mellitus
Nonodontogenic cysts. *See* Jaw cysts
Norvasc, 394f. *See also* Amlodipine
Nose bleed. *See* Epistaxis
NRL allergy. *See* Natural rubber latex

O

Obliterative cardiomyopathy. *See* Cardiomyopathy
Obstructive sleep apnea. *See* Sleep apnea
Odontogenic cysts. *See* Jaw cysts
Odontogenic infection. *See* Ludwig's angina
Odontogenic myxoma, 297
complications of, 297
dental management of, 297
dental significance of, 297
diagnosis of, 297
medical management and treatment of, 297
prognosis of, 297
Odontoma, 298
complications of, 298
dental management of, 298
dental significance of, 298
diagnosis of, 298
medical management and treatment of, 298
prognosis of, 298
Omeprazole, 435
contraindications of, 435
dental considerations of, 435
dosing of, 435
interactions of, 435
side effects of, 435
uses of, 435
Oral hairy leukoplakia. *See* Epstein-Barr virus diseases
Oral leukoplakia. *See* Leukoplakia
Oral lymphoepithelial cysts. Benign lymphoepithelial cysts
Oraqix. *See* Prilocaine-Lidocaine
Oretic. *See* Hydrochlorothiazide
Osler-Weber-Rendu disease. *See* Hereditary hemorrhagic telangiectasia
Ossifying fibromas
complications of, 299
dental management of, 300
dental significance of, 299
diagnosis of, 299
medical management and treatment of, 299
prognosis of, 299
Osteitis sicca. *See* Dry socket
Osteoarthritis (Degenerative joint disease), 157–158
complications of, 157
dental management of, 157
dental significance of, 157
diagnosis of, 157
medical management and treatment of, 157
prevention of, 158t
prognosis of, 157
Osteoblastoma, 301
complications of, 301
dental management of, 301
dental significance of, 301
diagnosis of, 301

Osteoblastoma—cont'd
  medical management and treatment
    of, 301
  prognosis of, 301
Osteodental dysplasia. *See* Cleidocranial
    dysplasia
Osteoid osteoma. *See* Osteoblastoma
Osteomalacia, 335
Osteomyelitis, 159
  complications, 159
  dental management of, 159
  dental significance of, 159
  diagnosis of, 159
  medical management and treatment
    of, 159
Osteopenia. *See* Osteoporosis
Osteoporosis, 160–161
  complications of, 161
  dental management of, 161
  dental significance of, 161
  diagnosis of, 160–161
  medical management and treatment
    of, 161
  prognosis of, 161
Osteosarcoma, 285
Overbreathing. *See* Hyperventilation
Oxycodone, 436
  contraindications of, 436
  dental considerations of, 436
  dosing of, 436
  interactions of, 436
  side effects of, 436
  uses of, 436
OxyContin, 436f. *See also* Oxycodone

P
Pacemakers, 37–38, 40
Palatal tori. *See* Tori
Palpitations, algorithm for, 529
Panmyelopathy. *See* Aplastic anemia
Panmyelophthisis. *See* Aplastic anemia
Pantoprazole, 437
  contraindications of, 437
  dental considerations of, 437
  dosing of, 437
  interactions of, 437
  side effects of, 437
  uses of, 437
Parainfluenza, 33
Paralysis agitans. *See* Parkinson's disease
Paramyxosvirus. *See* Mumps
Parkinson's disease, 162–164
  complications of, 163
  dental management of, 164
  dental significance of, 163
  diagnosis of, 162–163
  medical management and treatment
    of, 163
  prognosis of, 163
Parotid swellings. *See* Neck masses
    (differential diagnosis)
Paroxetine, 438
  contraindications of, 438
  dental considerations of, 438
  dosing of, 438

Paroxetine—cont'd
  interactions of, 438
  side effects of, 438
  uses of, 438
Passing out. *See* Syncope
Paterson-Brown-Kelly syndrome. *See*
    Plummer-Vinson syndrome
Paterson-Kelly syndrome. *See* Plummer-
    Vinson syndrome
Pathological fibrinolysis. *See*
    Disseminated intravascular
    coagulation
Paxil, 438f. *See also* Paroxetine
Pellagra, 335
Peptic ulcer disease, 165–166
  complications of, 165–166
  dental management of, 166
  dental significance of, 166
  diagnosis of, 165
  medical management and treatment
    of, 165
  prognosis of, 166
Periapical cyst, 274
Periodontal breakdown, 79
Perioral dermatitis, 302
  complications of, 302
  dental management of, 302
  dental significance of, 302
  diagnosis of, 302
  medical management and treatment
    of, 302
  prognosis of, 302
Peripheral giant cell granuloma, 303
  complications of, 303
  dental management of, 303
  dental significance of, 303
  diagnosis of, 303
  medical management and treatment
    of, 303
  prognosis of, 303
Peripheral odontogenic fibroma, 304
  complications of, 304
  dental significance of, 304
  diagnosis of, 304
  medical management and treatment
    of, 304
  prognosis of, 304
Peripheral pancytopenia. *See* Aplastic
    anemia
Perlèche. *See* Angular cheilitis
Petit mal seizures. *See* Seizures
Peutz-Jeghers syndrome, 167
  dental management of, 167
  dental significance of, 167
  diagnosis of, 167
  medical management and treatment
    of, 167
  prognosis of, 167
Pfieffer's disease. *See* Infectious
    mononucleosis
Pharyngitis. *See* Ludwig's angina
Physical abuse. *See* Child abuse and
    neglect
Pindborg tumor. *See* Calcifying epithelial
    odontogenic tumor

Pipe smoker's palate. *See* Nicotine
    stomatitis
Pituitary adamantinoma. *See*
    Craniopharyngioma
Plasma cell myeloma. *See* Multiple
    myeloma
Plasma thromboplastin component
    deficiency. *See* Hemophilia (Types
    A, B, C)
Plastocytopenia. *See* Thrombocytopenia
Platelet counts, bleeding and, 208t
Platybasia, 79
Plavix, 407f. *See also* Clopidogrel
Pleomorphic adenoma, 305
  complications of, 305
  dental significance of, 305
  diagnosis of, 305
  medical management and treatment
    of, 305
  prognosis of, 305
Plummer-Vinson syndrome, 306
  complications of, 306
  dental management of, 306
  dental significance of, 306
  diagnosis of, 306
  medical management and treatment
    of, 306
  prognosis of, 306
Pneumothorax, 375
  complications of, 375
  diagnosis of, 375
  medical management of, 375
  prognosis of, 375
Polocaine. *See* Mepivacaine
Polyarteritis nodosa, 307
  dental management of, 307
  diagnosis of, 307
  medical management and treatment
    of, 307
  prognosis of, 307
Polycythemia vera, 308. *See also*
    Myeloproliferative disorders
  dental management of, 308
  dental significance of, 308
  diagnosis of, 308
  medical management and treatment
    of, 308
  prognosis of, 308
Polymorphous low-grade
    adenocarcinoma, 309
  dental significance of, 309
  diagnosis of, 309
  medical management and treatment
    of, 309
  prognosis of, 309
Polymyalgia rheumatica, 168–169
  complications of, 168
  dental significance of, 168–169
  diagnosis of, 168
  medical management and treatment
    of, 168
  prognosis of, 168
Polymyositis, 170–171
  complications of, 170
  dental management of, 171

Polymyositis—cont'd
dental significance of, 170–171
diagnosis of, 170
medical management and treatment
of, 170
prognosis of, 170
Polyostotic fibrous dysplasia. *See*
Fibrous dysplasia
Port wine stain. *See* Hemangioma (soft
tissue)
Postablative hypothyroidism. *See*
Hypothyroidism
Posterior triangle masses, 294
Postextraction Hemorrhage, 376
complications of, 376
dental management of, 376
diagnosis of, 376
medical treatment of, 376
prognosis of, 376
Postherpetic neuralgia, 310
diagnosis of, 310
medical management and treatment
of, 310
prognosis of, 310
Postherpetic trigeminal neuralgia. *See*
Postherpetic neuralgia
Pravachol, 439f. *See also* Pravastatin
Pravastatin, 439
contraindications of, 439
dental considerations of, 439
dosing of, 439
interactions of, 439
side effects of, 439
uses of, 439
Prednisone, 440
contraindications of, 440
dental considerations of, 440
dosing of, 440
interactions of, 440
side effects of, 440
uses of, 440
Pregnancy, 172–175
breastfeeding during, 174t
complications of, 172–173
dental management of, 173
dental significance of, 173
diagnosis of, 172
medical management and treatment
of, 172
prognosis of, 173
risk category descriptions, 173t
Pregnancy epulis. *See* Pyogenic
granuloma
Pregnancy tumor. *See* Pyogenic
granuloma
Preinfarction angina. *See* Prinzmetal's
angina; Unstable angina;
Vasospastic angina
Premature AV beats, 36
Premature ventricular beats, 36
Prevacid, 424f. *See also* Lansoprazole
Prilocaine, 474
contraindications of, 474
dental considerations of, 474
dosing of, 474

Prilocaine—cont'd
interactions of, 474
side effects of, 474
uses of, 474
Prilocaine-Lidocaine, 475
contraindications of, 475
dental considerations of, 475
dosing of, 475
interactions of, 475
side effects of, 475
uses of, 475
Prilosec, 435f. *See also* Omeprazole
Primary adrenocortical insufficiency. *See*
Addison's disease
Primary HSV-1. *See* Herpes simplex
Primary hyperparathyroidism. *See*
Hyperparathyroidism
Primary hypertension. *See* Hypertension
Primary hypothyroidism. *See*
Hypothyroidism
Primary idiopathic polymyositis. *See*
Polymyositis
Primary PD. *See* Parkinson's disease
Primary Raynaud's phenomenon. *See*
Raynaud's phenomenon
Primary syphilis, 326
Primary tooth eruption, 78
Primary tuberculosis, 212
Prinivil, 425f. *See also* Lisinopril
Procardia, 434f. *See also* Nifedipine
Progressive hypocythemia. *See* Aplastic
anemia
Propofol, 476
contraindications of, 476
dental considerations of, 476
dosing of, 476
interactions of, 476
side effects of, 476
uses of, 476
Propoxyphene, 441
contraindications of, 441
dental considerations of, 441
dosing of, 441
interactions of, 441
side effects of, 441
uses of, 441
Prosthetic valve endocarditis, 80
Protonix, 437f. *See also* Pantoprazole
Proventil. *See* Albuterol
Prozac, 415f. *See also* Fluoxetine
Pruritus, algorithm for, 530
Pseudohemophilia type B. *See* Von
Willebrand's disease
Pseudomembranous candidosis. *See*
Candidosis
Psoriasis, 311
complications of, 311
dental management of, 311
dental significance of, 311
diagnosis of, 311
medical management and treatment
of, 311
prognosis of, 311
Psychomyogenic headaches. *See*
Headaches: tension

PUD. *See* Peptic ulcer disease
Purpura fulminans. *See* Disseminated
intravascular coagulation
Pyogenic granuloma, 312
dental management of, 312
diagnosis of, 312
medical management and treatment
of, 312
prognosis of, 312

Q
Qualitative platelet disorder. *See*
Thrombocytopathies (congenital
and acquired)

R
Radicular cyst, 274
Radiofrequency catheter ablation,
38–39
Ramipril, 442
contraindications of, 442
dental considerations of, 442
dosing of, 442
interactions of, 442
side effects of, 442
uses of, 442
Ranitidine, 443
contraindications of, 443
dental considerations of, 443
dosing of, 443
interactions of, 443
side effects of, 443
uses of, 443
Ranula, 313. *See also* Neck masses
(differential diagnosis)
dental significance of, 313
diagnosis of, 313
medical management and treatment
of, 313
prognosis of, 313
Rathke's pouch tumor. *See*
Craniopharyngioma
Raynaud's phenomenon, 176–177
algorithm for, 531
complications of, 176
dental management of, 176
dental significance of, 176
diagnosis of, 176
medical management and treatment
of, 176
prognosis of, 176
Reactivation tuberculosis infection, 212
Reactive arthritis. *See* Reiter's syndrome
Refractory anemia. *See* Aplastic anemia
Regional enteritis. *See* Crohn's disease
Reiter's syndrome, 178–179, 314
complications of, 178
dental management of, 178
dental significance of, 178, 314
diagnosis of, 178, 314
medical management and treatment
of, 178, 314
prognosis of, 178, 314
Relafen, 433f. *See also* Nabumetone
Relapsing syphilis. *See* Syphilis

Relative AI. *See* Acute adrenal insufficiency

Remeron, 431f. *See also* Mirtazapine

Renal disease, dialysis, and transplant, 180–182
  complications of, 181
  dental management of, 181–182
  dental significance of, 181
  diagnosis of, 180–181
  medical management and treatment of, 181
  prognosis of, 181

Renal failure. *See* Thrombocytopathies (congenital and acquired)

Respiratory syncytial virus, 33

Restrictive cardiomyopathy. *See* Cardiomyopathy

Rheumatic fever, 44

Rheumatoid arthritis, 183–186
  complications of, 184
  dental management of, 186
  dental significance of, 186
  diagnosis of, 183–184
  disease-modifying drugs for, 185t
  medical management and treatment of, 184
  prognosis of, 184–185

Rhinitis, algorithm for, 532

Rickets, 335

Riomet. *See* Metformin

Robinul. *See* Glycopyrrolate

Rodent ulcer. *See* Basal cell carcinoma

Rosenthal's disease. *See* Hemophilia (Types A, B, C)

Roxicodone, 436f. *See also* Oxycodone

S

SA heart block, 36

Salivary gland tumor. *See* Neck masses (differential diagnosis)

Salivary stones. *See* Sialolithiasis

Sal-Tropine. *See* Atropine

Sarafem. *See* Fluoxetine

Sarcoidosis, 187–188, 315
  complications of, 187
  dental management of, 187
  dental significance of, 187, 315
  diagnosis of, 187, 315
  medical management and treatment of, 187, 315
  prognosis of, 187, 315

Scandonest 296, 467t

Scurvy, 335

Secondary HSV-1. *See* Herpes simplex

Secondary hyperparathyroidism. *See* Hyperparathyroidism

Secondary hypothyroidism. *See* Hypothyroidism

Secondary PD. *See* Parkinson's disease

Secondary Raynaud's phenomenon. *See* Raynaud's phenomenon

Secondary syphilis, 326

Secondary tooth eruption, 78–79

Sedative overdose. *See* Medication overdose: sedative

Sedative/hypnotic toxicity. *See* Medication overdose: sedative

Seizure disorders, 189–192
  complications of, 190
  dental management of, 192
  dental significance of, 191
  diagnosis of, 190
  drugs used in treatment of, 191t
  medical management and treatment of, 190
  prognosis of, 191

Seizures, 377
  algorithm for, 533
  causes of, 377
  complications of, 378
  dental management of, 378
  diagnosis of, 377–378
  medical management of, 378
  prognosis of, 378
  symptoms of, 377

Senile dementia. *See* Alzheimer's disease

Septal defects. *See* Cardiac septal defects: atrial and ventricular

Septocaine, 467t. *See also* Articaine with epinephrine

Seronegative myasthenia gravis. *See* Myasthenia gravis

Seronegative spondyloarthropathy. *See* Reiter's syndrome

Sertraline, 444
  contraindications of, 444
  dental considerations of, 444
  dosing of, 444
  interactions of, 444
  side effects of, 444
  uses of, 444

Sevoflurane, 477
  contraindications of, 477
  dental considerations of, 477
  dosing of, 477
  interactions of, 477
  side effects of, 477
  uses of, 477

Shakes. *See* Delirium tremens

Shaking palsy. *See* Parkinson's disease

Shingles. *See* Postherpetic neuralgia; Varicella-Zoster virus diseases

SIADH. *See* Inappropriate secretion of antidiuretic hormone

Sialadenitis, 316
  complications of, 316
  dental significance of, 316
  diagnosis of, 316
  medical management and treatment of, 316
  prognosis of, 316

Sialolithiasis, 317
  dental significance of, 317
  diagnosis of, 317
  medical management and treatment of, 317
  prognosis of, 317

Sicca syndrome. *See* Sjögren's syndrome

Sickle cell disease. *See* Anemia: sickle cell

Sideropenia dysphagia. *See* Plummer-Vinson syndrome

Simvastatin, 445
  contraindications of, 445
  dental considerations of, 445
  dosing of, 445
  interactions of, 445
  side effects of, 445
  uses of, 445

Singulair. *See* Montelukast

Sinus brachycardia, 36

Sinus bradycardia. *See* Bradycardia

Sinus infection. *See* Sinusitis

Sinus tachycardia, 36

Sinusitis, 318
  complications of, 318
  dental significance of, 318
  diagnosis of, 318
  medical management and treatment of, 318
  prognosis of, 318

Sipple syndrome. *See* Multiple endocrine neoplasia syndromes

Sjögren's syndrome, 319–320
  algorithm for, 534
  complications of, 320
  dental management of, 320
  dental significance of, 320
  diagnosis of, 319–320
  medical management and treatment of, 320
  prognosis of, 320

SJS. *See* Erythema multiforme (Stevens-Johnson syndrome)

SLE. *See* Systemic lupus erythematosus

Sleep apnea, 193–194
  complications of, 194
  dental management of, 194
  dental significance of, 194
  diagnosis of, 193
  medical management and treatment of, 194
  prognosis of, 194

Sleep-disordered breathing. *See* Sleep apnea

Small cell lymphoma. *See* Burkitt's lymphoma

Smell disturbance, algorithm for, 542

Smoking, algorithm for, 535

Solar cheilitis. *See* Keratosis: actinic

Solar keratosis. *See* Keratoacanthoma; Keratosis: actinic

Soma. *See* Carisoprodol

Soprane. *See* Desflurane

Sphenopalatine neuralgia. *See* Headaches: cluster

Squamous cell carcinoma of floor of mouth. *See also* Neck masses (differential diagnosis)
  dental management of, 321
  diagnosis of, 321
  medical management and treatment of, 321
  prognosis of, 321

Squamous cell carcinoma of lip, 322

Squamous cell carcinoma of lip
—cont'd
diagnosis of, 322
medical management and treatment
of, 322
prognosis of, 322
Squamous cell carcinoma of tongue. *See
also* Neck masses (differential
diagnosis)
dental management of, 323
diagnosis of, 323
medical management and treatment
of, 323
prognosis of, 323
Squamous cell carcinoma. *See*
Keratoacanthoma
Squamous odontogenic tumor, 324
complications of, 324
dental significance of, 324
diagnosis of, 324
medical management and treatment
of, 324
prognosis of, 324
Squamous papilloma. *See* Human
papilloma virus diseases
Stable angina, 19. *See* Angina pectoris
Status asthmaticus. *See* Bronchospasm
Status eplilepticus, 379
algorithm for, 536–537
complications of, 379
dental significance of, 379–380
diagnosis of, 379
prognosis of, 379
Steatosis. *See* Hepatitis: Alcoholic
Sterapred. *See* Prednisone
Stevens-Johnson syndrome, 325. *See
also* Erythema multiforme
complications of, 325
dental significance of, 325
diagnosis of, 325
medical management and treatment
of, 325
prognosis of, 325
Stomatitis nicotina. *See* Nicotine
stomatitis
Stomatodynia. *See* Burning mouth
syndrome
Storage pool disease. *See*
Thrombocytopathies (congenital
and acquired)
Strawberry nevus. *See* Hemangioma
(soft tissue)
Stress headaches. *See* Headaches: tension
Stridor, algorithm for, 504
Stroke, 195–197. *See also* Cerebral
vascular accident
algorithm for, 538
complications of, 196
dental management of, 196–197
dental significance of, 196
diagnosis of, 195
medical management and treatment
of, 196
prognosis of, 196
Struma ovarii. *See* Hyperthyroidism

Subacute thyroiditis. *See*
Hyperthyroidism
Sublimaze. *See* Fentanyl
Submandibular triangle masses, 294
Sudden cardiac arrest. *See* Cardiac arrest
Sudden cardiac death. *See* Cardiac arrest
Sudden death. *See* Cardiac arrest
Superficial venous thrombosis (SVT).
See Venous thrombosis
Supine hypotensive syndrome. *See*
Pregnancy
Suprane. *See* Desflurane
SVT. *See* Venous thrombosis
Symptomatic hyperviscosity. *See*
Multiple myeloma
Syncope, 381–382
algorithm for, 539
complications of, 381–382
demographics of, 381
dental management of, 381–382
diagnosis of, 381
epidemiology of, 381
medical management of, 381
prognosis of, 381–382
Syphilis, 198–199, 326
complications of, 198–199, 326
dental management of, 199
dental significance of, 199, 326
diagnosis of, 198, 326
medical management and treatment
of, 198, 326
prognosis of, 199, 326
Systemic lupus erythematosus, 200–201
complications of, 200
dental management of, 201
dental significance of, 200–201
diagnosis of, 200
medical management and treatment
of, 200
prognosis of, 200

T
Tachycardias, 36
algorithm for, 540–541
Taste disturbance, algorithm for,
542
Taurodontism, 78
Taztia, 410f. *See also* Diltiazem
TB. *See* Tuberculosis
Temporal arteritis. *See* Cranial arteritis;
Polymyalgia rheumatica
Temporomandibular pain, algorithm for,
543
Tenormin, 396f. *See also* Atenolol
Tension headaches. *See* Headaches:
tension
Teratoid cyst. *See* Dermoid cyst
Tertiary hyperparathyroidism. *See*
Hyperparathyroidism
Tertiary hypothyroidism. *See*
Hypothyroidism
Tertiary syphilis, 326
Tetanus, 202–204
complications of, 203
dental management of, 203

Tetanus—cont'd
dental significance of, 203
diagnosis of, 202
medical management and treatment
of, 202–203
prognosis of, 203
prophylaxis, 204t
vaccination schedules for,
203t
Thrombocytopathies (congenital and
acquired), 205–207
complications of, 206
dental management of, 206–207
dental significance of, 206
diagnosis of, 206
laboratory tests for, 207t
medical management and treatment
of, 206
prognosis of, 206
Thrombocytopenia, 208–209
complications of, 208–209
dental management of, 209
dental significance of, 209
diagnosis of, 208
medical management and treatment
of, 208
prognosis of, 209
Thrombophlebitis. *See* Deep venous
thrombosis; Venous thrombosis
Thrush. *See* Candidosis
Thyroglossal cyst. *See* Neck masses
(differential diagnosis)
Thyroglossal duct cyst, 327
dental management of, 327
diagnosis of, 327
medical management and treatment
of, 327
prognosis of, 327
Thyroglossal tract cyst. *See* Thyroglossal
duct cyst
Thyrotoxicosis. *See* Hyperthyroidism
Tiazac, 410f. *See also* Diltiazem
Tic douloureux. *See* Trigeminal
neuralgia
Tizanidine, 446
contraindications of, 446
dental considerations of, 446
dosing of, 446
interactions of, 446
side effects of, 446
uses of, 446
TN. *See* Trigeminal neuralgia
Tonic-clonic seizures. *See* Seizures
Tori, 328–329
complications of, 328
dental management of, 328–329
diagnosis of, 328
medical management and treatment
of, 328
prognosis of, 328
Torus mandibularis. *See* Tori
Toxic multinodular goiter. *See*
Hyperthyroidism
Toxic paralytic anemia. *See* Aplastic
anemia

Toxic uninodular goiter. *See* Hyperthyroidism

Toxoplasma gondii. See Toxoplasmosis

Toxoplasmosis, 210–211
  complications of, 211
  dental management of, 211
  dental significance of, 211
  diagnosis of, 210
  medical management and treatment of, 210–211
  prognosis of, 211

Tracheobronchitis. *See* Bronchitis (acute)

Tramadol, 447
  contraindications of, 447
  dental considerations of, 447
  dosing of, 447
  interactions of, 447
  side effects of, 447
  uses of, 447

Traumatic fibroma, 330
  dental management of, 330
  dental significance of, 330
  diagnosis of, 330
  medical management and treatment of, 330
  prognosis of, 330

Trazodone, 448
  contraindications of, 448
  dental considerations of, 448
  dosing of, 448
  interactions of, 448
  side effects of, 448
  uses of, 448

Triamterene, 449
  contraindications of, 449
  dental considerations of, 449
  dosing of, 449
  interactions of, 449
  side effects of, 449
  uses of, 449

Triazolam, 478
  contraindications of, 478
  dental considerations of, 478
  dosing of, 478
  interactions of, 478
  side effects of, 478
  uses of, 478

Trifacial neuralgia. *See* Trigeminal neuralgia

Trigeminal neuralgia, 331–332
  complications of, 331
  dental significance of, 332
  diagnosis of, 331
  medical management and treatment of, 331
  prognosis of, 331–332

Trisomy 21. *See* Down syndrome

True/false vocal cord carcinoma. *See* Laryngeal carcinoma

Tubercles. *See* Tori

Tuberculosis, 212–215, 333–334. *See also* Neck masses (differential diagnosis)
  complications of, 214
  dental management of, 214–215, 334
  dental significance of, 214, 334

Tuberculosis—cont'd
  diagnosis of, 213, 333
  medical management and treatment of, 214, 333
  prognosis of, 214, 334

Type 1 diabetes. *See* Diabetes mellitus

Type 2 diabetes. *See* Diabetes mellitus

Type 3B euvolemic hyponatremia. *See* Inappropriate secretion of antidiuretic hormone

Type A hemophilia. *See* Hemophilia (Types A, B, C)

Type B hemophilia. *See* Hemophilia (Types A, B, C)

Type C hemophilia. *See* Hemophilia (Types A, B, C)

Type I hypersensitivity reactions. *See* Allergic reactions

Type II hypersensitivity reactions. *See* Allergic reactions

Type III hypersensitivity reactions. *See* Allergic reactions

Type IV hypersensitivity reactions. *See* Allergic reactions

U

Ulcerative colitis, 216–217
  complications of, 216
  dental management of, 216–217
  dental significance of, 216
  diagnosis of, 216
  medical management and treatment of, 216
  prognosis of, 216

Ulcerative enteritis. *See* Ulcerative colitis

Ultane. *See* Sevoflurane

Ultram, 447f. *See also* Tramadol

Unstable angina, 19. *See* Angina pectoris

Urticaria, algorithm for, 544

V

V. tach. *See* Ventricular tachycardia

Vagal tone. *See* Bradycardia

Valium. *See* Diazepam

Valsartan, 450
  contraindications of, 450
  dental considerations of, 450
  dosing of, 450
  interactions of, 450
  side effects of, 450
  uses of, 450

Vanadom. *See* Carisoprodol

Variant angina, 19. *See* Angina pectoris

Varicella-Zoster virus diseases, 218–219
  complications of, 219
  dental management of, 219
  dental significance of, 219
  diagnosis of, 218
  medical management and treatment of, 218
  prognosis of, 219

Vascular hemophilia. *See* Von Willebrand's disease

Vascular nevus. *See* Hemangioma (soft tissue)

Vasoconstrictors, 482

Vasotec, 411f. *See also* Enalapril

Vasovagal syncope. *See* Syncope

Venereal wart. *See* Condyloma acuminatum

Venous thrombosis, 386–387
  complications of, 387
  dental management of, 387
  dental significance of, 387
  diagnosis of, 386
  etiology of, 386
  medical management of, 386–387
  pathogenesis of, 386

Ventolin. *See* Albuterol

Ventricular failure. *See* Congestive heart failure

Ventricular fibrillation, 37

Ventricular septal defects. *See* Cardiac septal defects: atrial and ventricular

Ventricular tachycardia, 36, 388
  complications of, 388
  demographics of, 388
  dental significance of, 388
  diagnosis of, 388
  epidemiology of, 388
  prognosis of, 388

Verapamil, 451
  contraindications of, 451
  dental considerations of, 451
  dosing of, 451
  interactions of, 451
  side effects of, 451
  uses of, 451

Verelan. *See* Verapamil

Verruca vulgaris. *See* Human papilloma virus diseases; Keratoacanthoma

Versed. *See* Midazolam

Vesicular pharyngitis. *See* Herpangina

Vicodin. *See* Hydrocodone

Vicoprofen. *See* Hydrocodone

Virlix. *See* Cetirizine

Vitamin deficiencies, 335–336
  dental significance of, 336
  diagnosis of, 335
  medical management and treatment of, 335–336
  prognosis of, 336

Vomiting. *See* Nausea

Von Willebrand's disease, 220–222. *See also* Thrombocytopathies (congenital and acquired)
  complications of, 220
  dental management of, 220
  dental significance of, 220
  diagnosis of, 220
  medical management and treatment of, 220
  prognosis of, 220

W

Waldenström's disease. *See* Plummer-Vinson syndrome

Warfarin, 452
  contraindications of, 452
  dental considerations of, 452

Warfarin—cont'd
    dosing of, 452
    interactions of, 452
    side effects of, 452
    uses of, 452
Wasting. *See* Bulimia nervosa; Anorexia
    nervosa
Wear and tear arthritis. *See* Osteoarthritis
    (Degenerative joint disease)
Wegener's granulomatosis, 222–223, 337
    complications of, 222–223, 337
    dental management of, 223, 337
    dental significance, 223
    diagnosis of, 222, 337
    medical management and treatment
        of, 222, 337
    prognosis of, 223, 337
Weight loss, algorithm for, 545
Wellbutrin, 398f. *See also* Bupropion

Wermer's syndrome. *See* Multiple
    endocrine neoplasia syndromes
Wernicke-Korsakoff syndrome, 335
Wheezing, algorithm for, 505
Wide complex tachycardia. *See*
    Ventricular tachycardia
Wolff-Parkinson-White syndrome,
    36–37

X
Xanax. *See* Alprazolam
Xanax XR. *See* Alprazolam
Xylocaine, 467t
Xylocaine with epinephrine, 467t. *See
    also* Lidocaine

Z
Zanaflex, 446f. *See also* Tizanidine
Zantac. *See* Ranitidine

Zartan. *See* Cephalexin
Zegerid. *See* Omeprazole
Zestril, 425f. *See also* Lisinopril
Zocor, 445f. *See also* Simvastatin
Zoloft, 444f. *See also* Sertraline
Zolpidem, 453
    contraindications of, 453
    dental considerations of, 453
    dosing of, 453
    interactions of, 453
    side effects of, 453
    uses of, 453
Zona. *See* Postherpetic neuralgia
Zyban, 398f. *See also* Bupropion
Zyrtec, 402f. *See also* Cetirizine